The Pharmacologic Approach
to the
Critically Ill Patient

SECOND EDITION

The Pharmacologic Approach to the

Critically Ill Patient

SECOND EDITION

EDITOR

Bart Chernow, M.D., F.A.C.P., F.C.C.P.

Associate Professor of Anesthesia (Critical Care)
Harvard Medical School
Associate Director, Respiratory-Surgical Intensive Care Unit
Co-Director, Henry K. Beecher Anesthesia Research Laboratories
Massachusetts General Hospital
Boston, Massachusetts

Associate Editors:

John W. Holaday, Ph. D., Washington, D.C.
Gary P. Zaloga, M.D., Winston-Salem, North Carolina
Arno L. Zaritsky, M.D., Chapel Hill, North Carolina

Editorial Assistants:

Robert M. Burke
Donia M. Goss
Anne L. Macaulay

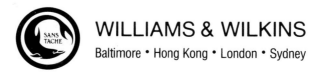

WILLIAMS & WILKINS
Baltimore • Hong Kong • London • Sydney

Editor: Timothy R. Grayson
Associate Editor: Carol Eckhart
Copy Editors: Elia A. Flanegin, Linda Hansford
Design: Alice Johnson
Illustration Planning: Annie Och
Production: Anne G. Seitz

Copyright © 1988
William & Wilkins
428 East Preston Street
Baltimore, MD 21202, USA

The authors, editor, and publisher have made every effort to provide
accurate indications, adverse reactions, and dosage schedules for drugs
discussed in this book, but it is possible that they may change.
**The reader is urged to review the package information data of the
manufacturers of the medications mentioned.**

Printed in the United States of America

First Edition 1983
Library of Congress Cataloging-in-Publication Data

The Pharmacologic approach to the critically ill
  patient.

  Includes bibliographies and index.
  1. Chemotherapy. 2. Pharmacology. 3. Critical
care medicine. I. Chernow, Bart. [DNLM: 1. Critical
Care. 2. Drug Therapy. 3. Pharmacology, Clinical.
QV 38 P5355]
RM147.P48 1988   615.5′8   87-28040
ISBN 0-683-01521-4

To Shandee and Peggy Chernow
for their never ending love and support.

To Dr. Richard J. Kitz for his leadership,
suggestions, help, and friendship.

Preface

The responses of readers and reviewers of the first edition of this book were gratifying. This second edition is an attempt to extend and update knowledge available on the pharmacologic approach to critically ill patients. In order to achieve this goal, I have enlisted the help of three associate editors—Drs. John W. Holaday, Gary P. Zaloga, and Arno L. Zaritsky. Their expertise in experimental therapeutics, metabolism, and pediatric pharmacology, respectively, has been invaluable in organizing this text. I am greatly indebted to each of them and I am confident that readers will appreciate the improvements in this second edition.

In the five years since publication of the first edition of this book, many pharmacologic advances have been made. For this reason, every previously published chapter has been completely revised and updated. More importantly, new chapters on adjustment of medications in heart failure, adrenergic receptors, red cell substitutes, thrombolytic therapy, digitalis, glucocorticoids in sepsis, fibronectin, management of patients requiring bone marrow transplantation, special problems in pediatric pharmacotherapy, and calcium in shock states have been added.

All chapters have extensive bibliographies that permit the reader to investigate the basis for statements made in the text. Some "overlap" of topics exists so that the reader is provided with information about a medication from different viewpoints. For example, thrombolytic therapy is discussed as a therapeutic agent in one place, and then again in the chapter on anticoagulants. Similarly, catecholamines are reviewed under resuscitation pharmacology and in the chapter dedicated to the pharmacology of these agents. I have included an extensive index, so that clinicians at the bedside can find information rapidly.

In one of the journal reviews of the first edition, this book was called, "a scholarly work." If this adjective holds true for the second edition, it will be because the contributors whom my associates and I have enlisted as chapter authors are scholars. I am honored and grateful that so many experts were willing to give their time and energy to this book. I hope that the multidisciplinary nature of the contributors (anesthesiologists, internists, neurologists, pediatricians, pharmacists, pharmacologists, physiologists, and surgeons) helps to provide a balance in the suggestions for various pharmacologic approaches to critically ill patients.

Critical care medicine has evolved into a large and important subspecialty of anesthesiology, medicine, pediatrics, and surgery. With its growth, and the complexity of patient problems now seen in critical care units, reference sources have become essential. This book is written for all those who contribute to the care of critically ill patients. I sincerely hope that physicians, nurses, therapists, pharmacists, students, nutritionists, and physician assistants will find the book to be a valuable resource providing both clinically useful prescribing information, as well as basic science data and advanced pharmacokinetic principles, to enhance our care of critically ill patients.

Bart Chernow, M.D., F.A.C.P.

Acknowledgment

The editor wishes to thank Donia Goss, Robert Burke,
Stephan Bamberger, Dr. Lena Napolitano, and Dr. Gregory G. Stanford
for all of their help.

Contributors

Patricia A. Arns, M.D.
Research Fellow
Division of Clinical Pharmacology
Vanderbilt University School of Medicine
Nashville, Tennessee

Frank J. Balestrieri, D.D.S., M.D.
Assistant Professor of Anesthesia
Georgetown University School of Medicine
Staff Anesthetist
Fairfax Hospital
Falls Church, Virginia

Timothy P. Blair, M.D.
Assistant Professor of Medicine
Uniformed Services University of the Health
  Sciences
F. Edward Hebert School of Medicine
Director, Coronary Care Unit
Bethesda Naval Hospital
Bethesda, Maryland

William F. Boyer, M.D.
Clinical Fellow in Psychopharmacology
Feighner Research Institute
Instructor in Psychiatry
University of California, San Diego
San Diego, California
Instructor in Psychiatry
Uniformed Services University of the Health
  Sciences
Bethesda, Maryland

Robert A. Branch, M.D.
Professor of Medicine and Pharmacology
Vanderbilt University School of Medicine
Nashville, Tennessee

D. Craig Brater, M.D.
Professor of Medicine
Indiana University School of Medicine
Director of Clinical Pharmacology
Wishard Memorial Hospital
Indianapolis, Indiana

Kenneth D. Burman, M.D., Col., M.C.
Professor of Medicine
Uniformed Services University of the Health
  Sciences
F. Edward Hebert School of Medicine
Bethesda, Maryland
Assistant Chief, Endocrine-Metabolic Unit
Departments of Medicine and Clinical
  Investigation
Walter Reed Army Medical Center
Washington, D.C.

Hugh J. Carroll, M.D.
Professor of Medicine
State University of New York
Health Science Center at Brooklyn
Director, Hypertension Division
Down State Medical Center
Brooklyn, New York

Edwin H. Cassem, M.D.
Associate Professor of Psychiatry
Harvard Medical School
Chief, Psychiatric Consultation Service
Massachusetts General Hospital
Boston, Massachusetts

Edward L. Cattau, Jr., M.D.
Associate Professor of Medicine
Georgetown University School of Medicine
Chief, Clinical Endoscopy
Georgetown University Medical Center
Washington, D.C.

Bart Chernow, M.D.
Associate Professor of Anesthesia (Critical Care)
Harvard Medical School
Associate Director, Respiratory-Surgical
  Intensive Care Unit
Co-Director Henry K. Beecher Anesthesia
  Research Laboratories
Massachusetts General Hospital
Boston, Massachusetts

Robert Chin, Jr., MD.
Staff Physician
Goddard Medical Associates, P.C.
Pulmonologist
Goddard Memorial Hospital
Stoughton, Massachusetts

Larry F. Cohler, M.D.
Postdoctoral Fellow, Physiology
Surgical Resident
Albany Medical College of Union University
Albany, New York

James A. Cook, Ph.D.
Professor of Physiology
Medical University of South Carolina
Charleston, South Carolina

Joseph P. Coyle, M.D.
Assistant Professor of Anesthesia
  and Medicine
Uniformed Services University of the Health
  Sciences
F. Edward Hebert School of Medicine
Director, Recovery Room
National Naval Medical Center
Bethesda, Maryland

David J. Cullen, M.D.
Professor of Anesthesia
Harvard Medical School
Director, Recovery Room
Massachusetts General Hospital
Boston, Massachusetts

Imbesat Daudi, M.D.
Postdoctoral Fellow
Albany Medical College of Union University
Department of Physiology
Albany Hospital
Albany, New York

H. Joachim Deeg, M.D.
Professor of Medicine
Georgetown University School of Medicine
Director, Marrow Transplant Unit
Lombardi Cancer Research Center
Washington, D.C.

Harold J. DeMonaco, M.S.
Director of Pharmacy
Massachusetts General Hospital
Boston, Massachusetts

Douglas S. DeWitt, Ph.D.
Assistant Professor of Anesthesia
Bowman Gray School of Medicine
Director, Basic Cerebrovascular Research
  Laboratory
Wake Forest University Medical Center
Winston-Salem, North Carolina

John P. DiMarco, M.D., Ph.D.
Associate Professor
University of Virginia School of Medicine
Director, Clinical Electrophysiology
  Laboratory
Department of Internal Medicine
Division of Cardiology
University of Virginia Medical Center
Charlottesville, Virginia

Paul R. Eisenberg, M.D., M.P.H.
Assistant Professor of Medicine
Cardiovascular Division
Washington University School of Medicine
Assistant Director, Cardiac Care Unit
Barnes Hospital
St. Louis, Missouri

James F. English, M.D.
Departments of Anesthesia and Critical Care
Bethesda Naval Hospital
Bethesda, Maryland

Glenn C. Freas, M.D.
Clinical Assistant Professor
Department of Military and Emergency
  Medicine
Uniformed Services University of the Health
  Sciences
F. Edward Hebert School of Medicine
Head, Emergency Medicine Department
Bethesda Naval Hospital
Bethesda, Maryland

Steven A. Gould, M.D.
Associate Professor of Surgery
University of Chicago Pritzker School
  of Medicine
Director, Blood Flow Laboratory
Michael Reese Hospital and Medical Center
Chicago, Illinois

John P. Grant, M.D.
Associate Professor of Surgery
Duke University School of Medicine
Director, Nutritional Support
Duke University Medical Center
Durham, North Carolina

John M. Hallenbeck, M.D.
Acting Vice Chairman and Professor of
  Neurology and Physiology
Uniformed Services University of the Health
  Sciences
F. Edward Hebert School of Medicine
Chairman, Department of Neurology
Bethesda Naval Hospital
Bethesda, Maryland

Paul M. Heerdt, M.D., Ph.D.
Clinical Fellow in Anesthesia
Harvard Medical School
Boston, Massachusetts

John W. Holaday, Ph.D.
Associate Professor of Pharmacology
Uniformed Services University of the Health
  Sciences
F. Edward Herbert School of Medicine
Bethesda, Maryland
Chief, Neuropharmacology Branch
Department of Medical Neuroscience
Division of Neuropsychiatry
Walter Reed Army Institute of Research
Walter Reed Army Medical Center
Washington, D.C.

John W. Hoyt, M.D.
Associate Clinical Professor of
  Anesthesiology and Critical Care Medicine
University of Pittsburgh School of Medicine
Medical Director,
Medical/Surgical Intensive Care Unit
St. Francis Medical Center
Pittsburgh, Pennsylvania

Karl F. Hubner, M.D.
Professor of Radiology
The University of Tennessee Medical Center
  at Knoxville
Director, Nuclear Medicine and Radiologic
  Research
University of Tennessee Hospital
Knoxville, Tennessee

Allan S. Jaffe, M.D.
Associate Professor of Medicine
Cardiovascular Division
Washington University School of Medicine
Director, Cardiac Care Unit
Barnes Hospital
St. Louis, Missouri

Thomas C. Jannett, Ph.D.
Assistant Professor of Electrical Engineering
The University of Alabama at Birmingham
Birmingham, Alabama

David A. Johnson, M.D.
Assistant Professor of Medicine
Uniformed Services University of the Health
  Sciences
F. Edward Hebert School of Medicine
Staff Gastroenterologist
Bethesda Naval Hospital
Bethesda, Maryland

Carl H. June, M.D.
Assistant Professor of Medicine
Uniformed Services University of the Health
  Sciences
F. Edward Hebert School of Medicine
Head, Tissue Bank
Naval Medical Research Institute
Bethesda, Maryland

C. Raymond Lake, M.D., Ph.D.
Professor of Psychiatry and Pharmacology
Uniformed Services University of the Health
  Sciences
F. Edward Hebert School of Medicine
Bethesda, Maryland

John F. Maher, M.D.
Professor of Medicine
Uniformed Services University of the Health
  Sciences
F. Edward Hebert School of Medicine
Director, Nephrology Division
Bethesda Naval Hospital
Bethesda, Maryland

Diana S. Malcolm, Ph.D.
Assistant Professor of Surgery
Uniformed Services University of the Health
  Sciences
F. Edward Hebert School of Medicine
Bethesda, Maryland

Eric S. Marks, M.D.
Associate Professor of Medicine
Uniformed Services University of the Health
  Sciences
F. Edward Hebert School of Medicine
Staff Physician
Bethesda Naval Hospital
Staff Physician
Walter Reed Army Medical Center
Adjunct Scientist
National Heart, Lung and Blood Institute
National Institutes of Health
Bethesda, Maryland

Henry Masur, M.D.
Professor of Medicine
George Washington University
Chief, Critical Care Medicine Department
Clinical Center
National Institutes of Health
Bethesda, Maryland

Joseph A. Miller, M.D.
Associate Professor of Neurology
Uniformed Services University of the Health
  Sciences
F. Edward Hebert School of Medicine

Director, EEG Laboratory
Staff Neurologist
Bethesda Naval Hospital
Bethesda, Maryland

Gerald S. Moss, M.D.
Professor of Surgery
University of Chicago, Pritzker School
of Medicine
Chairman, Department of Surgery
Michael Reese Hospital and Medical Center
Chicago, Illinois

Charles Myers, M.D.
Chief, Clinical Pharmacology
National Cancer Institute
National Institutes of Health
Bethesda, Maryland

John J. Nanfro, M.D.
Hematology/Oncology Section
Harbin Clinic
Rome, Georgia

Daniel A. Notterman, M.D.
Assistant Professor of Pediatrics and
Pediatrics in Surgery
Cornell Medical School
Director, Division of Critical Care Pediatrics
Department of Pediatrics
The New York Hospital-Cornell Medical
Center
New York, New York

Man S. Oh, M.D.
Associate Professor of Medicine
State University of New York
Health Science Center at Brooklyn
Brooklyn, New York

Joseph E. Parrillo, M.D.
Chief, Critical Care Medicine
National Institutes of Health
Bethesda, Maryland

H.D. Peterson, D.D.S., M.D.
Oliver R. Rowe Distinguished Professor
of Surgery
University of North Carolina School
of Medicine
Director, North Carolina Jaycee Burn Center
University of North Carolina Hospital
Chapel Hill, North Carolina

Patricia T. Pisciotto, M.D.
Associate Professor of Laboratory Medicine
and Pediatrics
University of Connecticut Medical School
Assistant Blood Bank Director
University of Connecticut Health Center
Farmington, Connecticut

Donald S. Prough, M.D.
Associate Professor of Anesthesia (Critical Care)
and Neurology
Bowman Gray School of Medicine
Head, Section on Critical Care
Medical Director, Regional Cerebral Blood Flow
Laboratory
Wake Forest University Medical Center
Winston-Salem, North Carolina

Albert W. Pruitt, M.D.
Ellington Charles Hawes Professor and
Chairman of Pediatrics
Medical College of Georgia
Chief, Pediatrics
Medical Center of Georgia Hospital and
Clinics
Augusta, Georgia

Thomas G. Rainey, M.D.
Associate Professor of Medicine
Uniformed Services University of the Health
Sciences
F. Edward Hebert School of Medicine
Head, Critical Care Medicine
Bethesda Naval Hospital
Bethesda, Maryland

H. David Reines, M.D.
Associate Professor of
Anesthesiology/Surgery
Division of Respiratory/Critical Care
Medical University of South Carolina
Charleston, South Carolina

Arthur L. Rosen, Ph.D.
Research Associate and Assistant Professor
University of Chicago, Pritzker School
of Medicine
Department of Surgery
Michael Reese Hospital and Medical Center
Chicago, Illinois

Laurence H. Ross, M.D.
Staff Physician
Department of Surgery
Duke University School of Medicine
Durham, North Carolina

Robert R. Ruffolo, Jr., Ph.D.
Chief, Cardiovascular and Renal
Pharmacology
Smith Kline & French Laboratories
King of Prussia, Pennsylvania

Thomas M. Saba, Ph.D.
Harold C. Wiggers Professor and Chairman
of Physiology
Albany Medical College of Union University
Albany, New York

Rodney W. Savage, M.D.
Attending Physician
White House
Washington, D.C.

Hansa L. Sehgal, B.S.
Laboratory Manager
Department of Surgical Research
Michael Reese Hospital and Medical Center
Chicago, Illinois

Lakshman R. Sehgal, Ph.D.
Assistant Professor of Surgery
University of Chicago, Pritzker School
  of Medicine
Director, Surgery Research
Michael Reese Hospital and Medical Center
Chicago, Illinois

Marissa Seligman, Pharm.D.
Pharmacy Coordinator
Drug Information/Staff Development
Pharmacist, Respiratory/Surgical Intensive
  Care Unit
Massachusetts General Hospital
Boston, Massachusetts

John N. Sheagren, M.D.
Professor of Internal Medicine
University of Michigan Medical School
Chief of Staff
Veterans Administration Medical Center
Ann Arbor, Michigan

Louis C. Sheppard, Ph.D.
Professor and Chairman
Biomedical Engineering
Associate Professor of Surgery
The University of Alabama at Birmingham
  Medical School
Birmingham, Alabama

Edward L. Snyder, M.D.
Associate Professor of Laboratory Medicine
Yale University School of Medicine
Associate Director, Blood Transfusion Service
Yale-New Haven Hospital
New Haven, Connecticut

Curt M. Steinhart, M.D.
Assistant Professor of Pediatrics and Surgery
Medical College of Georgia
Chief, Section of Pediatric Critical Care
Director, Pediatric Intensive Care Unit
Medical College of Georgia
Augusta, Georgia

Antonella Surbone, M.D.
Visiting Scientist
National Cancer Institute

National Institutes of Health
Bethesda, Maryland

Craig B. Thompson, M.D., Ph.D.
Assistant Professor of Medicine
University of Michigan Medical Center
Assistant Investigator, Howard Hughes
  Medical Institute
Ann Arbor, Michigan

Michael R. Vasko, Ph.D.
Assistant Professor of Pharmacology
The University of Texas Health Science
  Center at Dallas
Chief, Pharmacology Section
Veterans Administration Medical Center
Dallas, Texas

Charles B. Watson, M.D.
Associate Clinical Professor of Anesthesia
University of Connecticut Medical School
Assistant Chairman of Anesthesiology and
  Critical Care Medicine
Bridgeport Hospital
Bridgeport, Connecticut

Peter J. Wedlund, Ph.D.
Assistant Professor
College of Pharmacy
University of Kentucky
Lexington, Kentucky

Gary P. Zaloga, M.D.
Associate Professor of Anesthesia and
  Medicine
Section on Critical Care
Bowman Gray School of Medicine
Wake Forest University
Staff Physician
North Carolina Baptist Hospital
Winston-Salem, North Carolina

Arno L. Zaritsky, M.D.
Assistant Professor of Pediatrics
University of North Carolina School
  of Medicine
Director, Pediatric Intensive Care Unit
North Carolina Memorial Hospital
Chapel Hill, North Carolina

Michael G. Ziegler, M.D.
Associate Professor of Medicine
University of California, San Diego, School
  of Medicine
Director, Hypertension Program
University of California, San Diego, Medical
  Center
San Diego, California

Contents

Section 3   MEDICATION GROUPS 302

Clinical Pharmacology in the ICU

1

Pharmacokinetics

D. Craig Brater, M.D.
Michael R. Vasko, Ph.D.

When administering drugs to patients, one is concerned with the relationship between the dose of drug given and the response elicited. The obvious goal is to attain a therapeutic effect while minimizing toxicity. To attain this goal, clinicians need a working knowledge of the principles of drug absorption, distribution, and elimination and of how these processes are related to intensity and duration of drug action (pharmacokinetics). Using pharmacokinetic principles, therefore, can assist the clinician in determining the relationship between the dose administered and the concentration of drug achieved in the blood. There are several advantages to utilizing pharmacokinetic parameters, especially in the critically ill patient: *(a)* The proper use of kinetics can improve the overall care of the patient by more accurately attaining desired drug concentrations and response as compared with "hit or miss" therapy. *(b)* It can decrease the incidence of toxicity from drugs with a narrow margin of safety. *(c)* It can eliminate as causative factors alterations in absorption, distribution, and elimination in problem patients and thus allow the clinician to focus on pharmacodynamic efficacy (see below). *(d)* Finally, it can help reduce the incidence of drug inter-

actions that can complicate therapy (see Chapter 2).

When used properly, kinetic principles can be extremely helpful in the critical care setting; however, clinicians must also be aware of the limitations of applying pharmacokinetic principles. Clearly, the endpoint of drug therapy is clinical efficacy, not simply attaining a certain blood concentration of drug. Thus, to utilize blood concentrations without proper history, diagnosis, and clinical judgment would be a grave error. Indeed, the concentration of drug in the blood is only one tool to be used in assessing outcome. The relationship between the concentration of drug in blood and the clinical response (pharmacodynamics) is most critical (25). This relationship is a function of each patient's dose (concentration)-response curve and must be judged on an individual basis. In clinical practice we evaluate this parameter by clinical measures of response which can then be related to drug concentration and to dose in the individual patient. For example, in the use of quinidine to suppress ventricular ectopic beats, one can evaluate the decrease in ectopy as a measure of efficacy. Since widening of the QRS complex and prolongation of the Q-T interval are

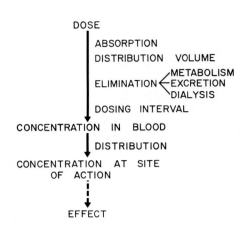

Figure 1.1. Schematic representation of the determinants of the relationship between the dose of a drug and the response it elicits. (From Brater DC: The pharmacological role of the kidney. *Drugs* 19:31–48, 1980.)

associated with quinidine toxicity, one can measure these as toxic endpoints in individual patients. Obviously, a dose of quinidine is sought that results in diminished ectopy (efficacy) without ECG changes of toxicity. This ratio of efficacy to toxicity (the therapeutic index) and the dose of drug that optimizes the ratio is highly individual. We know "average" doses of drugs that achieve "average" blood concentrations and "average" response in "average" patients. However, variability among patients is quite large, and disease states impact upon both handling of and responses to drugs in patients. Therefore, to practice good therapeutics, we must attempt in each individual patient to define the optimal dose-response relationship.

The relationship between dose and response can be influenced by a variety of pharmacokinetic and pharmacodynamic parameters (Fig. 1.1). Using these parameters in concert with knowledge of how disease states influence absorption, distribution, and elimination of drugs and knowledge of the pharmacology of drugs, we can attempt to optimize drug therapy to the individual patient and measure clinical indices of response. In this chapter, principles of pharmacokinetics and pharmacodynamics are discussed in a general fashion using specific, illustrative examples. The principles can then be applied in succeeding chapters. Rather than citing a voluminous literature, references are focused on timely reviews from which the interested reader can pursue more specific and detailed listings.

PHARMACOKINETIC PRINCIPLES (10, 17, 18, 20, 32, 45, 55, 61)

In using and reading about drugs one encounters a variety of symbols and terminology (Table 1.1).

Derivation of Pharmacokinetic Parameters

It is important to understand the symbols and terminology (Table 1.1) used in discussing pharmacokinetics and the derivation of some simple pharmacokinetic parameters. These pharmacokinetic calculations can be useful in determining drug dosing and therefore in the optimal care of the patient.

The majority of drugs used clinically obey first order or linear kinetics as opposed to saturable kinetics, which may also be termed zero order, nonlinear, or Michaelis-Menten kinetics. With first order kinetics, a constant percentage of drug is removed per unit time;

Table 1.1
Glossary of Pharmacokinetic Terms

$t_{1/2}$—Half-life: the amount of time required for the concentration of drug to decrease by one-half.

K_e or K_d—Elimination rate constant; determined by the slope of the terminal phase of a plot of the logarithm of the concentration of drug versus time.

K_a—Absorption rate constant.

K_r—Elimination rate constant for the renal component of drug elimination.

K_{nr}—Elimination rate constant for the nonrenal component of drug elimination.

V_d—Volume of distribution, which relates the concentration of drug achieved to a given dose.

Cl—Clearance: the amount of blood, plasma, or serum from which all drug is removed per unit time.

Cl_r—The component of clearance accounted for by renal elimination.

Cl_{nr}—The component of clearance accounted for by nonrenal elimination.

f_e—Fraction of dose excreted unchanged in the urine.

F—Fraction of dose absorbed after oral administration (bioavailability).

τ—Dosing interval: the time between doses.

Cp_{ave}—Average concentration of drug at steady state.

Cp_{max}—The maximum or peak concentration of drug at steady state.

Cp_{min}—The minimum or trough concentration of drug at steady state.

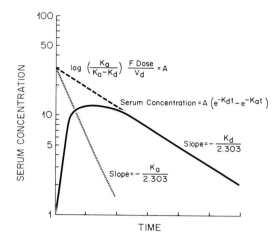

Figure 1.2. Pharmacokinetic parameters after oral administration of a drug. See text for explanation.

that is, as drug concentration increases, proportionally more drug is removed. The elimination half-life remains constant. With saturable kinetics, the percentage eliminated is different at different drug concentrations, usually resulting in long elimination half-lives with higher concentrations. The relevance of drugs obeying this latter type of elimination is discussed subsequently. Figure 1.2 shows an example of an orally administered drug obeying first order kinetics. A plot of the logarithm of the serum concentration versus time allows derivation of a number of parameters. The straight, terminal segment of the curve, called the log-linear phase, can be extrapolated back to the Y axis. This component of the curve represents elimination, and from the slope of this line one can calculate K_d, the elimination rate constant (Fig. 1.2). For example,

$$\text{Slope} = \frac{\Delta Y}{\Delta X}$$

$$= \frac{\Delta \text{concentration}}{\Delta \text{time}}$$

$$= \frac{\log 7.5 - \log 4.8}{3 - 4}$$

$$= \frac{0.875 - 0.681}{-1}$$

$$= -0.194 \text{ (in units of reciprocal time)}$$

Therefore, $-0.194 = \dfrac{-K_d}{2.303}$

(2.303 is for conversion from logarithm to the base 10 to natural logarithms).

or $K_d = 0.447$ (in units of reciprocal time)

The elimination half-life can then be calculated as $t_{1/2}$ elimination $= 0.693/K_d$. Therefore, in Figure 1.2, $t_{1/2}$ elimination $= 0.693/0.447 = 1.55$ (the units of time would be those used in the graph). The value in the numerator is the natural logarithm of 2. Alternatively, and probably more simply, any elimination half-life can be determined graphically by measuring the time interval for the serum concentration to decrease by one-half (for example from 10 to 5)—in the case shown in Figure 1.2, approximately 1.5, i.e., the same as that calculated above.

Parameters for absorption can be calculated by the method of residuals. By subtracting data points on the curve from the extrapolated log-linear phase (heavy dashed line), another straight line can be defined (small dashed line), the slope of which is a function of the absorption rate constant, K_a (Fig. 1.2). The half-life of absorption is then equal to $0.693/K_a$. The volume of distribution can also be calculated using the intercept (A) of these straight lines with the Y axis, if one knows F, the fraction absorbed (bioavailability). This calculation is done using the equation:

$$\log \left(\frac{K_a}{K_a - K_d} \right) \cdot \frac{F \text{ dose}}{V_d} = A \text{ or}$$

$$V_d = \log \left(\frac{K_a}{K_a - K_d} \right) \cdot \frac{F \text{ dose}}{A}$$

A similar graph can be made for an intravenously administered drug. In this instance, the plasma decay curve has two components, the α phase (rapid or early phase), which usually represents a distribution phase; i.e., the drug is distributing into tissues; and the β phase, which represents elimination (Fig. 1.3). The terms α and β are both rate constants from which respective half-lives can be calculated; A and B are intercepts with the Y axis. The extrapolation of the β phase (heavy dashed line) defines B. Generation of another line (small dashed line) by subtracting the extrapolated β phase from the curve defines α and A. From A, B, α, and β, clearance and volume of distribution can be calculated (Table 1.2).

At clinically used doses, some drugs, particularly ethanol, phenytoin, salicylates, and mezlocillin, obey saturable or Michaelis-Menten kinetics. At usual therapeutic blood concentrations these drugs can saturate elimination pathways. Their handling, then, is best characterized by parameters for V_{max} and K_m rather

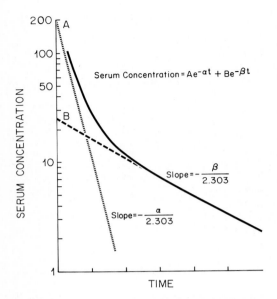

Figure 1.3. Pharmacokinetic parameters after intravenous administration of a drug. See text for explanation.

than by volume of distribution and clearance. For drugs such as these, clearance decreases and half-life increases with increasing doses of drug. Clinically, this characteristic means that at higher dosages a small increase in dose can result in a large increase in serum concentration of these drugs with a longer half-life. For example, increasing a patient's phenytoin dose from 200 to 300 mg/day may result in a proportional increase in steady state blood concentration from 10 to 15 μg/ml. However, as metabolizing enzymes become saturated, a

Table 1.2
Calculation of Pharmacokinetic Parameters after Intravenous Administration of a Drug[a]

$Cp = Ae^{-\alpha t} + Be^{-\beta t}$ (see Fig. 1.3)

V_d area or $V_{d\beta} = \dfrac{dose}{\beta AUC} = \dfrac{dose}{\beta\left(\dfrac{A}{\alpha}+\dfrac{B}{\beta}\right)}$

$Cl = \dfrac{dose}{AUC} = \dfrac{dose}{\dfrac{A}{\alpha}+\dfrac{B}{\beta}}$

$t_{1/2\,\alpha} = \dfrac{0.693}{\alpha}$ or measure directly

$t_{1/2\,\beta} = \dfrac{0.693}{\beta}$ or measure directly

[a] AUC refers to the *area under the curve* relating serum concentration to time.

further increase in dose from 300 to 400 mg/day may cause the blood concentration to rise from 15 to 30 μg/ml or more. The clinical lesson from this example is that dosage increments above the "usual normal dose" should be small with these drugs.

Disease states or drug interactions can adversely affect the elimination of drugs, and this is of greatest concern for drugs that are cleared by saturable kinetics. A patient with hepatic disease, for example, may have a significantly lower V_{max} for a drug than a healthy individual. Consequently, lower concentrations could result in saturation of metabolizing enzymes. Thus, as discussed in the phenytoin example above, saturation may occur between 200- and 300-mg doses in the critically ill patient and cause unpredictably high drug concentrations at much lower dosages.

Clinical Application of Pharmacokinetic Parameters

In the clinical setting, the most important pharmacokinetic parameters are bioavailability *(F)*, half-life $(t_{1/2})$, clearance *(Cl)*, and volume of distribution (V_d). Proper knowledge of what these parameters represent and how they are used can assist in delivering proper dosing, in correctly utilizing therapeutic drug monitoring, and in optimizing drug therapy.

BIOAVAILABILITY (F)

Bioavailability is defined as the percentage of an administered dose of drug that reaches the systemic circulation. If a drug is administered intravenously, for example, the bioavailability is obviously 100% and F equals 1.0. When drugs are administered by other routes, however, the bioavailability in most instances is less than 100%. The degree of bioavailability is determined by the extent of drug absorption and degree of metabolism prior to entering the systemic circulation. This subject is discussed in detail below under "Extent of Absorption." The clinician should have some quantitative estimate of bioavailability to correctly decide the dose of a drug the patient should receive. For example, morphine has an oral bioavailability of 20–30% due to rapid metabolism by the liver prior to entering the systemic circulation (first pass effect). Consequently, the dose given orally is usually three to five times larger than the dose administered by parenteral routes.

HALF-LIFE ($t_{1/2}$)

The most commonly used pharmacokinetic parameter is half-life, which is defined as the time it takes for the blood concentration of a drug to diminish by 50%. This term is often used inappropriately by clinicians as a term to define drug elimination. In contrast, half-life is a hybrid term, being a function of both clearance and volume of distribution. A change in half-life caused by a change in clearance has different therapeutic implications than does a change occurring because of an altered volume of distribution.

The most important use of half-life is to predict how long it takes for a dosing regimen to achieve steady state concentrations of drug in blood. With initiation of therapy, if a loading dose is not administered—i.e., the patient is not "instantly" affixed at a desired serum drug concentration that is to be maintained throughout therapy—four to five half-lives will elapse before the patient reaches steady state drug concentrations. For a drug such as digoxin then, which has an average half-life of approximately 36 hours in patients with normal renal function, approximately 1 week must elapse before steady state is achieved. If one evaluates such a patient clinically by obtaining a serum concentration of digoxin after only 2 days, and erroneously assumes that a steady state has been reached, the drug concentration will be misinterpreted and the clinician may have little, if any, insight into the patient's current status as well as the patient's therapeutic or toxic state in the future.

Similarly, if the dose of a drug is either increased or decreased, four to five times the half-life must elapse to reattain steady state. Also, if drug half-life changes, such as may occur with a change in the patient's disease state, a new steady state occurs after four to five times the new half-life (Fig. 1.4).

One must always try to maintain the perspective of whether or not the patient is at steady state. Interpreting blood drug concentration data is very difficult, if not impossible, unless one has some idea of this factor. Changing doses of a drug before the patient has reached steady state with one dose often be-

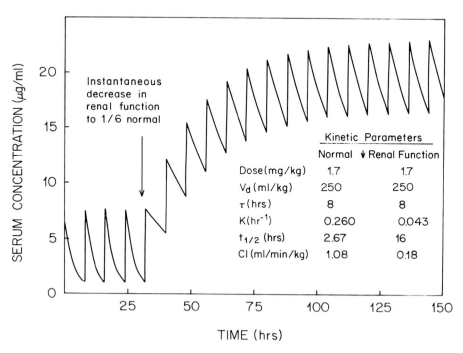

Figure 1.4. Schematic representing the effect of a 6-fold increase in half-life on the reattainment of steady state blood concentrations of a drug. This schematic applies specifically to gentamicin or tobramycin if an instantaneous decrease of renal function to one-sixth of normal occurred. See text for explanation of kinetic parameters. (From Chennavasin P, Brater DC: Nomograms for drug use in renal disease. *Clin Pharmacokinet* 6:193–214, 1981.)

comes a ludicrous, confusing, and potentially hazardous exercise. In the critically ill patient, this concept is exceedingly important, because the status of the patient's disease and other coadministered drugs can change rapidly and dramatically with concomitant effects on drug handling and half-life.

VOLUME OF DISTRIBUTION (V_d)

The volume of distribution defines the size of the compartment into which drug distributes. It is useful to define the concentration of drug attained in serum by a given dose of drug; namely, concentration achieved = dose/V_d. Therefore, if one achieves an initial concentration of 10 μg/ml by administering a 1-g dose of a drug:

$$V_d = \frac{dose}{concentration\ achieved}$$
$$= \frac{1\ g}{10\ \mu g/ml} = \frac{1,000,000\ \mu g}{10\ \mu g/ml}$$
$$= 100,000\ ml = 100\ liters$$

This volume should not be ascribed physiologic meaning. It is a derived parameter. One might best think of the body as a bathtub; the volume of distribution simply describes the size of the bathtub for a given drug. Clinically, one may use the volume of distribution to calculate the loading dose of a drug required to reach an initial, target concentration of drug in blood. For example, if one wishes to achieve a drug concentration of 10 μg/ml and the volume of distribution is 100 liters, the loading dose would be 1000 mg:

$$Concentration\ achieved = \frac{dose}{V_d}$$
$$10\ \mu g/ml = \frac{dose}{100,000\ ml}$$
$$Dose = 1,000,000\ \mu g = 1000\ mg$$

This calculation is independent of a drug's clearance or its half-life. Importantly, diseases can change a drug's volume of distribution, and the clinician who is not aware of this possibility can cause a serious disservice to the patients. In the example just discussed, if the patient's disease caused the volume of distribution of the drug to decrease from 100 to 50 liters and this effect was not realized, resulting in the patient's being administered the same 1000-mg loading dose, the patient's serum concentration would predictably be 1000/50 = 20 μg/ml as opposed to the desired concentration of 10 μg/ml. This type of mistake could result in toxicity.

CLEARANCE (Cl)

Clearance is usually referred to as blood, plasma, or serum clearance depending on whether concentrations of drug are measured in whole blood, plasma, or serum, respectively. With each use, clearance quantifies the amount of blood, or whatever, from which all drug is removed per unit time. Therefore, a serum clearance of 100 ml/minute means that all drug can be removed from 100 ml of serum in 1 minute. This removal can occur through distribution to tissues, metabolism, or excretion (see below).

Clinically, clearance is important for determining the amount of drug needed to maintain the concentration of drug at steady state. By definition, at steady state:

$$Rate\ of\ drug\ in = rate\ of\ drug\ out$$

The rate of drug entering is, in turn, a function of the dose administered, the fraction, F, of that dose absorbed if administered orally or intramuscularly, and the time interval over which it is administered (τ):

$$Rate\ in = F \times dose/\tau$$

The rate of drug leaving the body is a function of its steady state concentration (Cp_{ave}) and its clearance:

$$Rate\ out = Cp_{ave} \times Cl$$

Therefore, at steady state

$$F \times dose/\tau = Cp_{ave} \times Cl$$

or, rearranging the equation:

$$Cp_{ave} = \frac{F \times dose}{\tau \times Cl}$$

It is obvious from this relationship that changes or individual differences in bioavailability, in dosing regimen (dose and dosing interval), and in clearance can influence the steady state concentration of a drug (Fig. 1.4). Changes in clearance of a drug caused by disease must be compensated for by changes in dosing regimen.

CLINICAL USE OF PHARMACOKINETIC PARAMETERS

Table 1.3 summarizes the clinical importance of the various pharmacokinetic parameters discussed above. Briefly, *the volume of*

Table 1.3
Pharmacokinetic Principles

Initial concentration achieved	$= \dfrac{\text{loading dose}}{\text{volume of distribution}}$
Steady state concentration maintained	$= \dfrac{\text{fraction absorbed} \times \text{maintenance dose}}{\text{dosing interval} \times \text{clearance}}$
Half-life	$= \dfrac{0.693 \times \text{volume of distribution}}{\text{clearance}}$

distribution is important for determining the loading dose, clearance for maintenance dose, and half-life for determining the time needed to reach steady state. A change in half-life can occur by changes in volume of distribution and/or by changes in clearance. Therefore, for example, knowing only that the half-life of a drug is altered in a particular disease state does not allow one to decide appropriate adjustment of therapy. One must dissect this parameter into its component terms of volume of distribution and clearance and alter therapy accordingly.

These points can be illustrated with the drugs digoxin and lidocaine, showing how effects on volume of distribution and/or clearance affect therapeutic decisions (Table 1.4). As can be readily appreciated, the actual quantitative change in half-life is a function of the relative magnitude of change of each of its determinants. For example, assessing the effect of congestive heart failure only on the half-life of lidocaine would result in no dose adjustment while, clearly, V_d and Cl are both different, requiring changes in both loading and maintenance doses of this drug.

ABSORPTION (2, 4, 19, 21, 30, 36, 52)

Drug absorption is influenced by a variety of factors including site of absorption, ratio of ionized to nonionized drug, amount of drug metabolized before entry into the systemic circulation, and drug interactions. These factors can be highly variable among individuals and in different disease states. In fact, in many critical care situations, to circumvent these potential vagaries, one administers drugs intravenously if at all possible.

General Principles of Absorption

Absorption can occur from many sites. Some drugs, such as dermatologics or nitroglycerin ointment, are absorbed through the skin. Others are injected intradermally, subcutaneously, or intramuscularly. Inherent variability in blood flow to these sites, disease-induced changes in perfusion, scarring from multiple injections, or injury can influence absorption characteristics from such sites. The nature of the drug and its formulation may also be important. For example, the injectable formulation of phenytoin is only soluble at a highly alkaline pH. When injected into muscle, the drug precipitates so that incomplete, erratic and prolonged absorption occurs (49, 58). A similar phenomenon occurs with some of the benzodiazepines, emphasizing the inappropriateness of intramuscular administration of some of these tranquilizers (22, 28, 38). They are better and

Table 1.4
Clinical Illustration of Pharmacokinetic Principles

Clinical Setting	Kinetic Parameter			Dose		Time to Reach Steady State
	V_d	Cl	$t_{1/2}$	Loading	Maintenance	
Digoxin in mild to moderate renal failure	—	↓	↑	—	↓	↑
Digoxin in end-stage renal failure	↓	↓↓	↑	↓	↓↓	↑
Lidocaine in liver disease	—	↓	↑	—	↓	↑
Lidocaine in congestive heart failure	↓	↓	—	↓	↓	—

more predictably absorbed through the gastrointestinal tract.

Drugs can be absorbed throughout the length of the intestinal tract. Although most drug absorption occurs in the small intestine, in some instances drug absorption occurs through the oral mucosa. There are two important pharmacologic principles illustrated by absorption within the oropharynx. The general principle of passive, nonionic diffusion is well illustrated here. Drugs that are nonionized more readily cross a lipid membrane than do ionized species. Therefore, an ambient pH favoring nonionized drug favors drug diffusion across membranes. In the gastrointestinal tract this characteristic favors absorption, whereas in the kidney it could favor elimination (see below). The degree to which absorption is modified is influenced by the pK_a of the drug as well as non–pH-dependent factors such as molecular size and lipid solubility. This principle and its application to absorption of drugs through the oral mucosa have been known by various cultures for centuries. Cocaine and betel nut are both weak bases with pK_a values above 9. Local formulations of these drugs mix them with limestone to make the saliva more alkaline, thereby increasing the amount of nonionized drug and increasing absorption.

Another principle illustrated by absorption through the oral mucosa is the importance of the *first pass effect* or *presystemic elimination.* Drugs absorbed distal to the oropharynx enter the portal system and are delivered to the liver before reaching the systemic circulation. If the drug is rapidly metabolized in the liver, a substantial portion of the dose, although absorbed across the intestinal epithelium, may never reach circulating levels in the body. A clue that the first pass effect is quantitatively important is that the dose of a drug given intravenously is considerably less than that administered by mouth. With propranolol, for example, a standard intravenous dose is 1–5 mg, whereas an oral dose needed to achieve similar serum concentrations is 40–80 mg. The difference is accounted for by the amount removed during the first pass through the liver after oral administration.

Drugs absorbed through the oral mucosa do not enter the portal circulation and the first pass effect is avoided. For example, nitroglycerin has sufficient first pass metabolism that very large doses must be given if it is swallowed. Consequently, patients place tablets under the tongue to achieve a rapid therapeutic effect. A direct analogy can be used to account for the similar efficacy of nitrates administered through the skin.

Gastric absorption is highly dependent on passive nonionic diffusion. Because of the acidic environment, appreciable absorption only occurs with weak acids such as salicylate and phenobarbital. Quantitatively, most absorption, even of weak acids, occurs in the proximal small intestine, which has a large surface area. Many drugs are also readily absorbed through the rectal mucosa, although the time course of absorption may differ compared with administration by mouth. Data assessing quantitative rectal absorption and its time course are scanty at best. The formulation administered rectally markedly influences absorption characteristics but not in a fashion that allows a priori predictions. This area is in need of further study (13).

In the gastrointestinal tract, a number of factors can influence drug absorption, and these are best considered in terms of three aspects: (a) the lag time for absorption to occur, (b) the extent of absorption, and (c) the rate of absorption.

Lag Time for Absorption

Lag time is defined as the time it takes for orally administered drug to enter the systemic circulation. It can vary from zero to many hours. For gastrointestinal absorption, the most important determinants of lag time are product formulation and gastric emptying time. For example, if a tablet is highly compressed, some time may be needed before dissolution occurs and drug becomes available for absorption. Since quantitatively most absorption occurs in the small bowel, the stomach must empty the drug to that site for the drug to enter the circulation. Disease states such as duodenal ulcer with gastric outlet obstruction, and drugs such as anticholinergics and narcotic analgesics, may delay gastric emptying, importantly affecting lag time. Similarly, a drug such as metoclopramide, which hastens gastric emptying, may diminish lag time (46, 47, 50).

EXTENT OF ABSORPTION (BIOAVAILABILITY)

The extent of absorption (bioavailability) is obviously important, because it influences the total amount of drug entering the body, which in turn is directly related to the concentration of drug achieved in plasma at steady state as shown in the equation:

$$\text{Concentration at steady state} = \frac{F \times \text{dose}}{\tau \times \text{clearance}}$$

A representation of potential effects of changed bioavailability is shown in Figure 1.5. If one first considers the *upper dashed horizontal line* as representing the concentration of drug needed for efficacy, a decrease in bioavailability could result in lack of efficacy. If one then considers the *lower horizontal line* to be the effective blood concentration, a decrease in bioavailability results in still maintaining effective concentrations but for a shorter time.

One must also consider the impact of changes in bioavailability in the opposite direction—namely, increases. If in Figure 1.5 the *lower horizontal line* represents an effective drug concentration and the *upper horizontal line* a toxic concentration, an increase in bioavailability could provide a longer time above the therapeutic concentration but at the expense of toxicity.

Product formulation and intestinal transit time may be important determinants of drug bioavailability. If a formulation dissolves very slowly and the patient has a shortened bowel or rapid intestinal transit because of disease or other drugs, the medication may not spend sufficient time in the intestinal tract for "normal" absorption to occur. Physical complexing of drugs within the gastrointestinal tract may also occur, such as milk products with tetra-cycline antibiotics, or cholestyramine or antacids with a number of drugs (see Chapter 2).

Finally, the magnitude of the first pass effect is an important determinant of overall bioavailability. If the liver's capacity to metabolize a drug changes, the total amount of drug reaching the systemic circulation can change. Changes in the liver's metabolic capacity can occur by several means:

1. Changed blood flow. For example, in cirrhosis or in treatment of patients with cimetidine or β-blockers, liver blood flow decreases.
2. Changed capacity of metabolizing enzymes, either (a) induced, such as with administration of rifampin (see Chapter 2), or (b) inhibited, such as occurs in cirrhosis or by enzyme-inhibiting drugs such as cimetidine (see below) (see Chapter 2).

A decrease in the liver's ability to metabolize drugs or a decrease in hepatic blood flow can increase bioavailability of drugs, having a substantial first pass effect. This characteristic has been clearly demonstrated with propranolol, labetalol, and a few other drugs (26, 62). This effect can have a considerable impact on the circulating concentration of drugs.

Recall that concentration at steady state = $(F \times \text{dose})/(\tau \times \text{clearance})$. If bioavailability (F) is increased, and in addition the ability to metabolize the drug is also decreased (clearance has decreased), then the overall effect on the serum concentration at steady state has undergone a "multiplier" effect and is dispro-

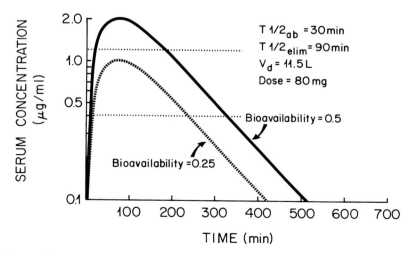

Figure 1.5. Schematic representation of the effect on serum concentration versus time curves of changes in bioavailability. Pharmacokinetic parameters are those of furosemide. See text for discussion.

portionate to the effect that would have occurred by changing bioavailability or clearance alone. Thus, critically ill patients may require substantial dosing modifications in order to avoid toxicity from some orally administered drugs.

Rate of Absorption

Changes in rate of drug absorption are also important. Figure 1.6 depicts serum concentration curves with different absorption half-lives, but all having the same bioavailability.

If one first considers the *lower horizontal line* as the effective blood concentration, the curve with the slowest absorption half-life provides effective concentrations for the longest period of time. This phenomenon is the rationale for development of sustained-release preparations. However, such a phenomenon should not be expected necessarily to occur in all circumstances. For example, if the effective concentration were the *upper horizontal line*, the change to a slower absorption would result in lack of efficacy (fig. 1.6). Assuming the *lower horizontal line* to represent efficacy and the *upper horizontal line* toxicity (Fig. 1.6), changes in rate of absorption also influence whether toxicity occurs and its duration.

One cannot predict a priori which phenomenon will occur in individual patients or in the presence of significant disease. Consequently, it is a clinician's responsibility to obtain serum drug concentrations and to assess clinical endpoints in individual patients to discern the overall effect of a change in time course of absorption on response.

Rate of absorption is influenced by product formulation (as discussed with bioavailability), by drug interactions (see Chapter 2), and probably by gastrointestinal physiology-pathology, which has been little studied but likely occurs.

Any permutation and combination of all of the effects discussed can and will occur in individual patients.

DISTRIBUTION (5, 11, 16, 27, 29, 53)

The determinants of distribution of drugs throughout the body are incompletely understood. Some drugs reach tissues by active transport, and their degree of distribution to a particular tissue may depend on their affinity for transport pumps, access to the pump(s), pump activity, distribution away from the tissue after reaching it, etc.

Lipid solubility and, in turn, ambient pH related to the drug's pK_a can influence distribution to certain tissues. For example, salicylate and phenobarbital have restricted access through the blood-brain barrier to the central nervous system (CNS). If the blood pH becomes more acidic, favoring the nonionized form of these weak acids, lipid permeability increases and more drug distributes into the CNS (24). This phenomenon explains the importance of reversing systemic acidemia in

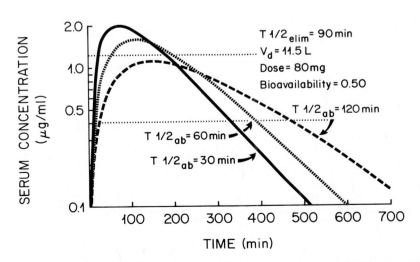

Figure 1.6. Schematic representation of the effect on serum concentration versus time curves of changes in the rate of absorption with bioavailability remaining constant. See text for discussion.

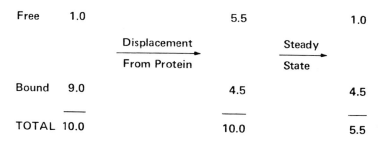

Free	1.0		5.5		1.0
		Displacement → From Protein		Steady → State	
Bound	9.0		4.5		4.5
TOTAL	10.0		10.0		5.5

Figure 1.7. Schematic representation of the effect of decreased protein binding on phenytoin concentrations in serum. (From Brater DC: The pharmacological role of the kidney. *Drugs* 19:31–48, 1980.)

treating toxicity to facilitate exit of these agents from the CNS.

Binding of drugs to circulating proteins is an important determinant of distribution. Only unbound drug in blood can diffuse or be transported into tissues. Thus, the influence of protein binding is a limiting factor in drug distribution, especially with those drugs that are highly protein bound—in excess of 90--95%. Such drugs include penicillins, cephalosporins, sulfonamides, anticoagulants, nonsteroidal antiinflammatory drugs, propranolol, and others. The protein binding of these drugs can be affected by their relative concentrations in the blood (drug interactions), by changes in circulating protein concentration, and by diseases such as uremia that can result in accumulation of endogenous competitors for binding and/or alter the binding characteristics of protein (23).

In general, one needs to be concerned about changes in distribution with drugs that are highly protein bound and/or drugs that have a small volume of distribution. Quantitatively important distribution-related effects have been described with phenytoin (41, 42), thiopental (9), valproic acid (8), warfarin (3), salicylates (24), and diazoxide (37).

In both hypoalbuminemia and uremia, phenytoin, valproic acid, and warfarin are displaced from albumin, increasing the amount of free drug in plasma. This displacement from binding in itself should cause an increased effect inasmuch as the amount of drug accessible to its site of action is related to the amount of free drug in plasma. However, this free drug is also available for elimination and for distribution into tissues in which the drug is not active. The overall result is that a new steady state is reached in which the concentration of free drug in plasma is virtually the same as in the unperturbed condition; the pharmacologic effect is the same, but the total concentration

of drug in blood (free plus bound) is less than that before displacement. This consequence is illustrated schematically for phenytoin in Figure 1.7.

The clinical importance of this phenomenon is that the amount of drug administered to the patient remains the same—i.e., for phenytoin approximately 300 mg/day. The "therapeutic" blood concentration of phenytoin in patients with the nephrotic syndrome or uremia, however, is one-half to one-third that in normal subjects. Consequently, the importance of this effect is in interpretation of measurements of phenytoin blood concentrations. "Low" total concentrations of phenytoin, thiopental, or valproic acid in a uremic or nephrotic patient should not be misinterpreted as subtherapeutic. This interpretive problem does not occur with warfarin, for one monitors the response to the anticoagulant rather than its blood concentration.

Digoxin, although not highly protein bound, can have clinically relevant changes in drug distribution. In end-stage renal failure, the volume of distribution of digoxin is decreased and a smaller loading dose is needed to achieve a given blood concentration (Table 1.4) (1). The reduced maintenance dose of digoxin required in end-stage renal disease relates to decreased ability of the kidney to eliminate digoxin; additionally, the drug distributes into a smaller volume so that a diminished loading dose is also necessary.

Other influences on drug distribution might include factors such as overall tissue perfusion. For example, a diabetic who develops peripheral osteomyelitis often must undergo amputation because the disease has affected perfusion so severely that antibiotics never distribute to the site of infection. Patients with severe cirrhosis and portosystemic shunts do not distribute drug to the liver, where metabolism can occur.

It is important to reemphasize the difference between distribution to tissues and volume of distribution. They are undoubtedly related but not rigidly so. The latter should be thought of in the context discussed previously—namely, its therapeutic implications regarding loading dose and as one determinant of half-life. No physiologic implications should be attached to the magnitude of the volume of distribution, and disease-induced changes in volume of distribution do not warrant speculation as to actual effects on drug access to various tissues.

ELIMINATION

Metabolism (15, 59, 60)

Most metabolism occurs in the liver, where drugs are converted to polar compounds that are then excreted by the kidney. Importantly, their metabolism does not necessarily imply that the metabolite is inactive. In fact, for some drugs such as chloral hydrate, encainide, and sulindac the parent drug is inactive and metabolism to the active component must occur. For many other drugs, metabolites are also active and may cause pharmacologic effects, particularly in the setting of decreased renal function if their excretion is impaired and they accumulate (6, 14, 32, 54). For example, procainamide is acetylated to N-acetylprocainamide (NAPA), which is itself an antiarrhythmic, eliminated by the kidney. Consequently, in renal failure NAPA accumulates in preference to procainamide and may do so in amounts that become toxic. Interpretation of serum concentrations of procainamide in a patient with azotemia becomes difficult, because both procainamide and NAPA contribute to the pharmacologic effect but only the former is measured in many assays and "therapeutic" concentrations for the latter have not been well defined. Clinical assessment of pharmacologic effect is essential rather than reliance on and possible misinterpretation of serum concentration measurements.

Some of the oral sulfonylureas are converted to active metabolites that accumulate in uremia, potentially causing prolonged and long-lasting hypoglycemia. Meperidine (pethidine) and propoxyphene are metabolized to normeperidine and norpropoxyphene, which depend on the kidney for elimination. Excess accumulation of these metabolites can result in seizures or cardiovascular collapse, respectively. These few examples illustrate the need

for clinicians to understand the pharmacology of the drugs they use, including the pharmacology of metabolites.

The liver has a variety of pathways by which it can metabolize drugs, the microsomal enzyme system with cytochrome P-450 playing a pivotal role. This system is important for oxidative reactions such as dealkylation, hydroxylation, oxidation, sulfoxide formation, deamination, and desulfuration. Glucuronide synthesis and conjugation also occur in the microsomal system. Other metabolizing pathways also occur mainly in the liver but not via the microsomal enzyme system. These include reactions such as acetylation, methylation and conjugation with glycine and sulfate, hydrolysis, and reduction reactions.

The microsomal enzyme system can be induced to greater activity or can be inhibited (see Chapter 2). The "classic" inducers of this system are the barbiturates; however, many agents can act as inducers. Inhibitors of the system include cimetidine and a variety of antituberculous drugs. These actions can affect the blood concentrations of drugs by impacting on bioavailability (for drugs with a substantial first pass effect) and on clearance. Such changes, via effects on hepatic metabolism, whether caused by disease or other drugs, must be anticipated to select proper dosing regimens for individual patients.

Excretion (6, 7)

By far the most important excretory route for both parent drug and metabolites is the kidney. It is easiest to consider renal modes of elimination in terms of the kidney's physiologic functions of filtration, active transport, and passive transport. In addition, the kidney metabolizes some drugs and conjugates others. These processes have been little explored, but there have been no reports of disease-induced changes or of drug interactions.

FILTRATION

The clinically relevant determinants of a drug's capacity to be filtered are molecular size and charge and the number of filtering nephrons.

Effective molecular size is a limiting factor for excretion of mixed and high molecular weight dextrans. The dextran 40 used clinically is actually a mixture of different molecular weight species; the high molecular weight component (approximately 70,000) is selectively retained because it cannot be filtered (12, 56). Consequently, these preparations remain in patients for extended periods of time. Other drugs have sufficiently small molecular weights that there are essentially no size limitations to filtration.

Most studies and clinical attention are directed to influences of decreased numbers of functioning nephrons on the renal elimination of drugs. The effect of decreased creatinine clearance on the elimination of digoxin and aminoglycoside antibiotics is particularly well known. In general, if 40% or more of the administered drug (or its active metabolites) is eliminated unchanged in the urine, decreased renal function will change handling of the drug and require dose adjustment (see Chapter 3).

ACTIVE TRANSPORT

The renal tubule can both actively secrete and actively reabsorb a variety of substrates. Active reabsorption appears to be inconsequential except for iodipamide (a cholecystographic agent), which can induce marked uricosuria, presumably by decreasing the active reabsorption of uric acid in the proximal tubule (34). The uricosuria could cause the acute renal failure occasionally reported with this contrast agent. The same mechanism accounts for the uricosuria caused by probenecid. The uptake by pinocytosis from the proximal tubular lumen of gentamicin and other aminoglycoside antibiotics might be considered another example of active reabsorption (40). Sequestration of these drugs within tubular cells most likely contributes to nephrotoxicity, the mechanisms of which are being actively investigated.

The pars recta (straight segment) of the proximal tubule actively secretes into the tubular lumen a variety of organic acids (43, 57) and bases (39, 44). The pathways for acids and for bases appear to be separate, but within a group there is lack of specificity such that a variety of organic acids can compete with each other for transport, as can a variety of organic bases (see Chapter 2). If competing agents are coadministered, changes in clearance may occur, requiring a compensatory alteration of the dosing regimen.

A clinically important drug transport that is not of acids or bases is a secretory component of digoxin elimination, which can be competed for by spironolactone, quinidine, and verapamil (see Chapter 2). Patients to whom these drugs are coadministered develop higher serum concentrations of cardiac glycoside. The site of digitalis transport appears to be the distal nephron.

PASSIVE TRANSPORT

Passive transport of drugs is an important mechanism for both excretion and reabsorption of drugs in the kidney. Both weak acids and weak bases can be passively reabsorbed in the collecting duct (33, 35, 48), accounting for retention of many drugs. For this reabsorption to occur, these drugs must have gained entry into the tubular lumen at more proximal portions of the nephron by either glomerular filtration or active secretion. Even drugs with high rates of entry into the kidney can be almost completely reabsorbed in the collecting duct. This reabsorption is dependent mainly on two factors: urinary pH and flow rate through the lumen.

As discussed earlier, drugs in the nonionized state more readily pass through membranes, a fact that is important for drug absorption. The same principle applies for passive reabsorption in the collecting duct. Thus, if a large percentage of the drug is in the nonionized state, more drug is passively reabsorbed. For weak acids, as the pH decreases, the concentration of nonionized drug increases; for weak bases, an increase in pH results in more nonionized drug. Consequently, altering urinary pH can be a clinically important determinant of elimination for some drugs (Table 1.5).

Alkalinization of the urine, by favoring excretion of the ionized congener of phenobarbital or salicylate, is a mainstay of therapy for toxicity due to these agents. The small changes

Table 1.5
Drugs with Clinically Important Urine pH-Dependent Elimination

Weak acids (alkaline urine increases excretion)
Phenobarbital
Salicylates
Sulfonamide derivatives
Trimethoprim
Weak bases (acid urine increases excretion)
Amphetamine
Ephedrine
Mexiletine
Pseudoephedrine
Quinine
Tocainide

in urinary pH caused by modest doses of antacids can enhance the elimination of salicylate sufficiently to prevent attaining concentrations in blood necessary for an antiinflammatory effect.

The effect of urinary pH on the elimination of amphetamine may be better known to abusers of this drug than to clinicians. Since amphetamine is a weak base, alkalinizing the urine increases the amount of nonionized drug, favoring reabsorption. Amphetamine abusers regularly ingest baking soda to prolong the "high." Therapeutically, it would be important to acidify the urine of a patient with an overdose of amphetamine. The supposedly nontoxic pseudoephedrine accumulates to toxic levels in children with renal tubular acidosis in whom a persistently alkaline urine favors passive reabsorption of the drug. A similar phenomenon occurs with tocainide, an orally available lidocaine-like agent, for which the administration of bicarbonate decreases the elimination rate.

Not all weak acids and bases demonstrate urine pH-dependent elimination, however, and one cannot assume that these principles will apply to all weak acids and bases. Part of the lack of effect with some drugs probably relates to the drug's pK_a and the lipid solubility of the congeners. For example, if even the nonionized species is poorly soluble in lipid, its ability to cross the tubular plasma membrane would not be enhanced. In this setting, changes in urinary pH would not cause changes in renal elimination.

Another modulator of the ability of the nonionized congener to pass across the lipid membrane may be antidiuretic hormone, which can increase by 50–100% the ability of lipophilic compounds to pass across the toad urinary bladder, a structure functionally analogous to the mammalian collecting duct (31). These findings have not been extrapolated to studies in humans. In many critical care settings, nonosmotic stimuli promote antidiuretic hormone release, which could conceivably affect renal drug handling. Other modulators of the effects of urinary pH on drug reabsorption are less well defined.

Urinary flow rate can affect excretion of some drugs by decreasing the concentration gradient for reabsorption, because the urine is dilute, and by decreasing the time available for a drug to diffuse out of the urine. Urinary flow rate is an important determinant of elimination for chloramphenicol, ephedrine, phenobarbital,

pseudoephedrine, and theophylline. This fact is probably clinically important only in patients with high urinary flow rates for prolonged periods of time.

Clinicians seem to pay little attention to the importance of urinary pH and flow rate except in the case of salicylate or barbiturate overdose. As discussed above, more thought should be given to the importance of the urine pH for excretion of a broader gamut of drugs (Table 1.5).

Dialysis (6)

Elimination of drugs by dialysis is not discussed in great detail here and, in particular, dialysis techniques are not addressed. It is important, however, to review pharmacokinetic and pharmacologic aspects of some of the more pertinent determinants of a drug's dialyzability.

DETERMINANTS OF DIALYZABILITY

Molecular size influences a drug's dialyzability. In general, compounds of molecular weight less than 500 have flow-dependent dialyzability, while elimination of higher molecular weight drugs depends on dialyzer surface area. Vancomycin, with a molecular weight of 1800, has such a large molecular size that it is not dialyzable. Other drugs for which molecular size is clinically important are amphotericin B, erythromycin, morphine, and digoxin, all of which have poor dialyzability that is limited by membrane surface area. All other drugs have a sufficiently small molecular size for their dialysance to be determined by flow rate of blood and dialysate and by other factors to be discussed subsequently.

For a drug to be dialyzable, it must be water soluble (this rule does not apply to resin hemoperfusion). Many of the sedative-hypnotics (such as glutethimide, methaqualone, meprobamate, ethchlorvynol, etc.) and the tricyclic antidepressants, although of small molecular weight, are relatively insoluble in water and are poorly dialyzable by conventional hemodialysis. Resin or charcoal hemoperfusion is not dependent on water solubility and therefore can remove these drugs effectively. In addition, drugs highly bound to serum proteins are, in general, poorly dialyzable. Protein binding is not a limiting factor with sorbent hemoperfusion.

QUANTITATIVE ASPECTS OF DIALYZABILITY

Whether dialysis can contribute to a drug's removal from the body relates to a drug's intrinsic plasma clearance—namely, how fast the body can eliminate the drug exclusive of dialysis. For dialysis to add a clinically important increment to overall drug elimination, clearance by dialysis should increase overall clearance by at least 30%. Some general principles can be appreciated by reconsidering the determinants of the clearance of a drug. Clearance is equal to the product of the elimination rate constant and the volume of distribution:

$$Cl = K_e \times V_d$$

but, as noted previously, $K_e = 0.693/t_{1/2}$; consequently,

$$Cl = 0.693 \ V_d/t_{1/2}$$

From this relationship, it is clear that if the volume in which a drug distributes is large, clearance is large; for dialysis to add to clearance, dialyzability would have to be great. This observation seems to make sense intuitively in that a large volume of distribution means much of the body burden of the drug is in the peripheral tissues; dialysis can only remove the amount in the blood. Consequently, drug in the tissues is not accessible to the dialyzer, and the body burden of the drug is not significantly decreased by dialysis. The converse is true for a drug with a small volume of distribution unless it is highly protein bound and therefore does not cross the dialysis membrane.

Similarly, if the half-life is short (i.e., elimination is fast) the intrinsic clearance is great and dialysis would be less likely to have an effect. The converse is also true. The effect of dialysis on the clearance of aminoglycosides illustrates the validity of this concept. In a patient with normal renal function, the half-life of an aminoglycoside antibiotic is relatively short (2–3 hours). Therefore, clearance is large and dialysis in such a patient would not remove large amounts of the drug. However, aminoglycosides have long half-lives in patients with end-stage renal failure. Therefore, clearance is low and dialysis can eliminate enough of the antibiotic to require dosing after each dialysis.

In overdose settings, saturation of elimination pathways may occur (6, 7). If so, intrinsic clearance may be low at high blood concentra-

Table 1.6
Guidelines for Dialysis Treatment of the Poisoned Patient

1. Severe clinical intoxication with life-threatening cardiovascular instability despite adequate volume replacement.
2. Ingestion and probable absorption of a potentially lethal dose.
3. A blood level of the drug that is in the range resulting in considerable mortality.
4. Impaired ability to eliminate the drug by endogenous routes by either disease, toxicity of the drug, or saturation of pathways of elimination.
5. Prolonged coma in a setting where expertise in hemodialysis exceeds expertise in respiratory care.
6. Methanol or ethylene glycol ingestion.

tions of the drug and increase as concentrations decrease. In this situation, dialysis may contribute an important increment to elimination when drug concentrations are highest. This situation occurs with chloral hydrate and ethchlorvynol.

HEMODIALYSIS

When to use hemodialysis or hemoperfusion (see below) for patients with drug overdoses is often debated and must be highly individualized to both patient status and the capacities of the hospital. For example, an identical patient might be treated differently depending on whether the local expertise is pulmonary care or technical skill in performing dialysis. A modification (6) of guidelines proposed by Schreiner is predicated on the ability of dialysis to contribute to elimination of the drug (Table 1.6).

Methanol and ethylene glycol ingestion warrant more detailed comments. Poisoning with either of these two agents is a clear indication for hemodialysis. Toxicity of massive doses can be completely prevented by appropriate treatment. Both methanol and ethylene glycol are benign and their toxicity is mediated by metabolic by-products. The first step in the metabolism of both of these compounds involves alcohol dehydrogenase for which ethanol is a preferred substrate. Consequently, adequate therapy entails not only hemodialysis to remove the parent methanol and ethylene glycol and any metabolites that may have formed, but also administration of sufficient ethanol to block formation of the toxic metabolites. The latter can be complicated, because ethanol itself is dialyzable and its infusion rate must be

Table 1.7
Dose of Ethanol for Achieving a Target Concentration of 100 mg/100 ml in the Treatment of Methanol or Ethylene Glycol Ingestions

Loading dose[a]:	0.6 g/kg
Maintenance dose:	
Nondrinkers	66 mg/kg/hr
Chronic drinkers	154 mg/kg/hr
During hemodialysis	170 mg/kg/hr or 95% ethanol to achieve a dialysate concentration of 100 mg/100 ml

[a] Four and one-half 1-ounce shots of 80-proof whiskey in a 70-kg patient.

Table 1.8
Drugs for Which Resin Hemoperfusion Has Been Demonstrated to Remove Clinically Important Amounts

Barbiturates
Chloral hydrate (trichloroethanol)[a]
Chloroquine
Digitalis glycosides
Disopyramide
Ethchlorvynol
Glutethimide
Meprobamate
Methaqualone
N-Dexmethylmethsuximide
Phenylbutazone
Salicylate
Theophylline
Tricyclic antidepressants

[a] Trichloroethanol is the active metabolite; the parent, chloral hydrate, is rapidly converted to the metabolite.

adjusted to maintain enzyme-blocking serum concentrations of ethanol (target concentration = 100–200 mg/100ml). In addition, chronic (alcohol) drinkers have a higher capacity to metabolize ethanol and require higher maintenance infusion rates, unless, of course, they have liver disease. Clearly, the ethanol dose must be tailored to the individual patient and followed by determinations of serum concentrations if possible. Table 1.7 offers recommendations as a first approximation of the required ethanol dose. Hemodialysis for 4–6 hours appears sufficient for treatment of even massive overdoses. Ethanol infusion should probably be continued for up to 24 hours.

Many hospitals do not have the ability to measure serum concentrations of methanol or ethylene glycol. A reasonably accurate estimation of their concentrations can be obtained by measuring serum osmolality. The total number of osmoles in the sample includes the contribution of the agent in question, electrolytes, urea, and glucose. The last three can be calculated from their chemical measurement. The number of osmoles contributed by methanol or ethylene glycol can then be estimated by subtracting the osmolal contribution of normal blood constituents from total osmolality. Concentration of methanol or ethylene glycol can then be calculated based on its molecular weight (32 and 62, respectively). However, if ethanol is being administered, both ethanol and either methanol or ethylene glycol will contribute to the serum osmolality, with no means other than specific assay to ascertain the contribution of each.

HEMOPERFUSION

Recently, attempts have been made to increase the dialyzability of water-insoluble drugs that are severely toxic in overdose settings.

Resins or activated charcoal have been used to bind these drugs and irreversibly extract them from the patient's blood. It is clear that these drugs can be removed efficiently by resin hemoperfusion. In fact, dialysis clearance for many of them is equal to blood flow through the dialyzer. Unfortunately, however, many of these drugs have large volumes of distribution so that the maximal reduction in blood concentrations is only short-lived, and the drug stores in peripheral tissues serve as a reservoir to refill the blood with drug as soon as hemoperfusion is stopped. In addition, the procedure itself can cause decrements in circulating formed elements in the blood. Clearer indications for use of resin hemoperfusion are likely to evolve. At present, the general indications for dialysis for poisoning (Table 1.6) would also apply for hemoperfusion, since hemoperfusion removes important amounts of a number of drugs in overdose settings (Table 1.8).

DOSING REGIMENS (10, 17, 18, 20, 32, 45, 55, 61)

The aforementioned determinants of the relationship between the dose of drug administered to a patient and the concentration of that drug achieved in blood are a function of the individual characteristics of the patient, that patient's disease, and effects of coadministered drugs (see Chapter 2). On the other hand, dosing regimens are solely in the physician's control. Used wisely, they can mean the difference between success and failure; failure may result from allowing the disease to go untreated (lack of efficacy) or from drug-induced toxicity. A clinical example of this is the case of aminoglycoside antibiotics. Efficacy in Gram-negative bacteremia or pneumonia requires attainment of peak concentrations of tobramycin or gentamicin of more than 5 μg/ml (>20 μg/ml for amikacin). On the other hand, minimizing ototoxicity and/or nephrotoxicity from these drugs requires trough concentrations of less than 2 μg/ml (<5 μg/ml for amikacin). To achieve these goals the clinician must have a knowledge of dosing regimens, which in turn is a logical extrapolation of the pharmacokinetic principles discussed above.

The multiplicity of influences on the relationship between dose of a drug and its serum concentration (Fig. 1.1) emphasizes the importance of dosing regimens and use of assays of drug concentrations. Because so many factors affect this relationship, there is tremendous variability from patient to patient in handling of drugs and therefore in the concentration achieved by a dosing regimen. Tailoring the dosage regimen to the individual patient is the clinician's only tool to compensate for this variability and truly individualize therapy. To do so, the clinician must understand pharmacokinetic principles, know the medical literature on the handling of specific drugs in patients relative to their demographic characteristics and disease state, and use clinical endpoints of pharmacologic effect and measured drug concentrations to adjust therapy to the individual patient. These principles are illustrated schematically in Figure 1.8. For example, by knowing that a patient has congestive heart failure and that published data indicate that, on average, such patients have a decreased volume of distribution and clearance of lidocaine, an appropriate starting dosing regimen can be devised. Clearly, however, a patient may not be "average," which would be reflected by a measured lidocaine concentration that differed from the desired or predicted concentration. Presuming that clinical assessment corroborates conclusions based on the measured lidocaine concentration, an estimate of the individual patient's handling of lidocaine can be made with revision of the dosing regimen appropriate for the individual patient.

Loading Dose

A loading dose is administered to achieve therapeutic drug concentrations rapidly. Otherwise, one must wait four to five times the elimination half-life for steady state to occur. As discussed previously, the loading dose is determined by the volume of distribution of the drug; to reiterate:

$$\text{Loading dose} = \text{desired concentration} \times \text{volume of distribution}$$

In emergent situations, loading doses are usually administered by vein. So doing ensures 100% bioavailability and a rapid attainment of desired serum drug concentrations. In less emergent situations, loading doses can be administered by other routes. When administered intravenously very high serum concentrations may be achieved for transient periods of time. The height of concentrations achieved and their duration depends on the rate of administration and the rate at which drug distributes from blood into tissues. A loading dose given intravenously should be given over 3–5 minutes; to administer the drug faster is unnecessary and risky.

Studies with lidocaine demonstrate the types of problems that may occur when giving a loading dose (51). Considerable effort has been expended to develop a reasonable method for loading patients with lidocaine, minimizing excursions into the toxic range while achieving desired concentrations quickly. To date, the best method in patients with a normal volume of distribution is to administer 75 mg

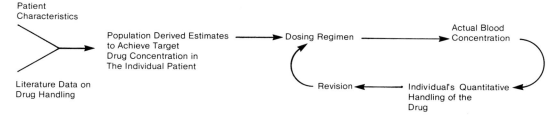

Figure 1.8. Steps for tailoring drug therapy to the individual patient.

over 2 minutes followed by 150 mg by continuous intravenous infusion over 18 minutes (8.33 mg/min). This infusion is then followed by the maintenance infusion rate. A study comparing this rapid infusion method with three bolus injections of 50 mg over the same period found that all of six patients with bolus injections developed toxicity, compared with one of 12 after the infusion method (51).

No similar data exist for other drugs commonly used in emergent situations. Even with drugs in which bolus administration may pose no dangers, however, it seems logical to be conservative and administer the drug slowly. One may always increase the rate of infusion if deemed necessary; on the other hand, if too much drug has been administered too quickly, no recourse exists.

As was discussed in previous sections and as will be addressed in subsequent chapters for specific drugs and specific clinical conditions, a patient's disease state can influence the volume of distribution of a drug. The impact of such effects on dosing regimens is on loading rather than maintenance doses (Tables 1.3 and 1.4). The impact of disease on the volume of distribution of many drugs has not been explored. Consequently, it behooves the clinician to realize that changes from "normal" may exist in the individual patient. Consequently, one should err on the cautious side in estimating the needed loading dose. If an underestimate is made, it is easy to give more drug, in contrast to the potential consequences of having overestimated and administered too much.

Maintenance Dose

The maintenance dose determines the average concentration of drug at steady state. To reiterate:

$$Cp_{ave} = \frac{F \times dose}{dosing\ interval \times clearance}$$

Disease can influence both bioavailability of drugs (*F*) and their clearance. Such effects can be compensated for by changing the dose, the frequency with which it is administered, or both. The method selected for adjusting the dosing regimen influences the magnitude of difference between peak and trough concentrations of drug, i.e., the fluctuation above and below the average drug concentration. The more frequently a drug is administered, the less fluctuation, and the converse. One can estimate

peak (Cp_{max}) and trough (Cp_{min}) concentrations of drug knowing pharmacokinetic parameters:

$$Cp_{max} = \frac{dose/V_d}{1 - e^{-K_d t}} \text{ and } Cp_{min} = Cp_{max} \times e^{-K_d t}$$

Such calculations might become important when using a drug with a narrow therapeutic range, when one is concerned about fluctuating from toxic to subtherapeutic concentrations of drug. For example, this phenomenon occurs in some patients when procainamide is administered in 750-mg doses every 6 hours as opposed to administering 375 mg every 3 hours. Because of variability among individuals, calculating estimated values for Cp_{max} and Cp_{min} is probably less informative than clinical evaluation of the patient at times of predicted peak and trough concentration of drug and obtaining measurements of actual drug concentration at these times.

No "best" method can be promulgated for adjusting the maintenance dose of a drug (10). Knowing the general relationship between dosing frequency and fluctuation of drug concentrations must be coupled with knowledge of the influence of specific disease states on the pharmacokinetics and dynamics of specific drugs. So doing allows approximation of a starting point for adjustment of dosing regimens, which must then be "fine tuned" to the individual patient by assessing clinical endpoints of response and measuring serum drug concentrations (Fig. 1.8).

DETERMINANTS OF THE RELATIONSHIP BETWEEN RESPONSE AND CONCENTRATIONS OF DRUG IN BLOOD

Understanding pharmacokinetics can help to clarify and compensate for the multitude of factors that influence the concentration of drug achieved in blood, relative to an administered dose. Many additional factors affect response. Their impact on the individual patient requires clinical assessment and cannot be quantified in pharmacokinetic terms. Optimal compensation for vagaries in response, however, then requires reapplication of pharmacokinetic principles to the modified goals derived from clinical assessment of pharmacodynamics.

Many clinical examples exist of changes in response to drugs; the increased toxicity of digitalis glycosides with hypokalemia, the decreased response to catecholamines in the acidemic patient, and the resistance to diuretics in severe congestive heart failure are all well known. Other examples must certainly exist. This entire area represents the "art" of therapeutics. Pharmacokinetics has evolved from a qualitative art to a quantitative science. Optimal therapeutics requires wedding the art of pharmacodynamic assessment to the science of pharmacokinetics.

Clearly, the use of therapeutic drug monitoring (TDM) has assisted clinicians' use of drugs. We now speak of therapeutic ranges, those serum concentrations at which the probability is high that the patient will receive optimal therapy and minimal toxicity. In critically ill patients especially, TDM has improved pharmacologic management.

It is important, however, for clinicians to utilize TDM correctly to optimize therapy and not overinterpret the serum drug concentration. Several confounding factors are important in interpreting serum drug concentrations, and many have been discussed in this chapter. For example, *if serum concentrations are measured during the distribution phase of drug dosing or prior to steady state, the use of the concentrations may lead to erroneous conclusions and inappropriate changes in therapy.* In addition, many drugs have active metabolites and these are rarely measured. Lastly, the implications of free compared to protein-bound drug have been discussed.

Measurement of serum drug concentrations is useful if the clinician knows what information can be derived from the test and if the pharmacodynamic effect correlates with the serum concentration, Clearly, concentration can be critical in individualizing dosing, assuming that the true relationship between dose and sample collection is known. The concentration may not be useful if it does not correlate with therapeutic endpoints or if pharmacokinetic principles are ignored.

References

1. Aronson JK: Clinical pharmacokinetics of digoxin 1980. *Clin Pharmacokinet* 5:137–149, 1980.
2. Azarnoff DL, Huffmann DH: Therapeutic implications of bioavailability. *Annu Rev Pharmacol Toxicol* 16:53–66, 1976.
3. Bachmann K, Shapiro R, Mackiewicz J: Influence of renal dysfunction on warfarin plasma protein binding. *J Clin Pharmacol* 16:468–472, 1976.
4. Benet LZ: Biopharmaceutics as a basis for the design of drug products. Ariens EJ (ed): *Drug Design.* New York, Academic Press, 1973, chapter I, pp 1–35.
5. Blaschke TF: Protein binding and kinetics of drugs in liver diseases. *Clin Pharmacokinet* 2:32–44, 1977.
6. Brater DC: Drug use in renal disease. Sydney, ADIS, 1983.
7. Brater DC: The pharmacological role of the kidney. *Drugs* 19:31–48, 1980.
8. Brewster D, Muir NC: Valproate plasma protein binding in the uremic condition. *Clin Pharmacol Ther* 27:76–82, 1980.
9. Burch PG, Stanski DR: Decreased protein binding and thiopental kinetics. *Clin Pharmacol Ther* 32:212–217, 1982.
10. Chennavasin P, Brater DC: Nomograms for drug use in renal disease. *Clin Pharmacokinet* 6:193–214, 1981.
11. Craig WA, Kunin CM: Significance of serum protein and tissue binding of antimicrobial agents. *Annu Rev Med* 27:287–300, 1976.
12. Data JL, Nies AS: Dextran 40. *Ann Intern Med* 81:500–504, 1974.
13. deBoer AG, Moolenaar F, deLeede LGJ, Breimer DD: Rectal drug administration: clinical pharmacokinetic considerations. *Clin Pharmacokinet* 7:285–311, 1982.
14. Drayer DE: Pharmacologically active drug metabolites: therapeutic and toxic-activities, plasma and urine data in man, accumulation in renal failure. *Clin Pharmacokinet* 1:426–443, 1976.
15. George CF: Drug metabolism by the gastrointestinal mucosa. *Clin Pharmacokinet* 6:259–274, 1981.
16. Gibaldi M, Koup JR: Pharmacokinetic concepts—drug binding, apparent volume of distribution and clearance. *Eur J Clin Pharmacol* 20: 299–305, 1981.
17. Gibaldi M, Levy G: Pharmacokinetics in clinical practice. *JAMA* 235:1864–1867, 1987–1992, 1976.
18. Gibaldi M, Perrier D: *Pharmacokinetics.* New York, Marcel Dekker, 1975.
19. Goldman P: Rate-controlled drug delivery. *N Engl J Med* 307:286–290, 1982.
20. Greenblatt DJ, Koch-Weser J: Clinical pharmacokinetics. *N Engl J Med* 293:702–705, 964–969, 1975.
21. Greenblatt DJ, Koch-Weser J: Intramuscular injection of drugs. *N Engl J Med* 295:542–546, 1976.
22. Greenblatt DJ, Shader RI, MacLeod SM, Sellers EM, Franke K, Giles HG: Absorption of oral and intramuscular chlordiazepoxide. *Eur J Clin Pharmacol* 13:267–274, 1978.
23. Gugler R, Shoeman DW, Huffman DH, Cohlmia JB, Azarnoff DL: Pharmacokinetics of drugs in patients with the nephrotic syndrome. *J Clin Invest* 55:1182–1189, 1975.
24. Hill JB: Salicylate intoxication. *N Engl J Med* 288:110–113, 1973.
25. Holford NHG, Sheiner LB: Understanding the dose-effect relationship: clinical application of pharmacokinetic-pharmacodynamic models. *Clin Pharmacokinet* 6:429–453, 1981.
26. Homeida M, Jackson L, Roberts CJC: Decreased first-pass metabolism of labetalol in chronic liver disease. *Br Med J* 2:1048–1050, 1978.
27. Jusko WJ, Gretch M: Plasma and tissue protein binding of drugs in pharmacokinetics. *Drug Metab Rev* 5:43–140, 1976.
28. Kanto J: Plasma concentrations of diazepam and its metabolites after peroral, intramuscular, and rectal administration: correlation between plasma concentration and sedatory effect of diazepam. *Int J Clin Pharmacol* 12:427–432, 1975.
29. Klotz U: Pathophysiological and disease-induced changes in drug distribution volume: pharmacokinetic implications. *Clin Pharmacokinet* 1:204–218, 1976.
30. Koch-Weser J: Bioavailability of drugs. *N Engl J Med* 291:233–236, 503–506, 1974.
31. Levine SD, Franki N, Einhorn R, Hays RM: Vasopressin-stimulated movement of drugs and uric acid across the toad urinary bladder. *Kidney Int* 9:30–35, 1976.
32. Melmon KL, Morrelli HF: *Clinical Pharmacology—Basic Principles in Therapeutics.* New York, Macmillan, 1972.

33. Milne MD, Scribner BH, Crawford MA: Non-ionic diffusion and the excretion of weak acids and bases. *Am J Med* 24:709–729, 1958.

34. Mudge GH: Uricosuric action of cholecystographic agents. *N Engl J Med* 284:929–933, 1971.

35. Mudge GH, Silva P, Stibitz GR: Renal excretion by nonionic diffusion. *Med Clin North Am* 59:681–698, 1975.

36. Parsons RL: Drug absorption in gastrointestinal disease with particular reference to malabsorption syndromes. *Clin Pharmacokinet* 2:45–60, 1977.

37. Pearson RM: Pharmacokinetics and response to diazoxide in renal failure. *Clin Pharmacokinet* 2:198–204, 1977.

38. Perry PJ, Wilding DC, Fowler RC, Hepler CD, Caputo JF: Absorption of oral and intramuscular chlordiazepoxide by alcoholics. *Clin Pharmacol Ther* 23:535–541, 1978.

39. Peters L: Renal tubular excretion of organic bases. *Pharmacol Rev* 12:1–35, 1960.

40. Porter GA, Bennett WM: Nephrotoxic acute renal failure due to common drugs. *Am J Physiol* 241:F1–F8, 1981.

41. Reidenberg MM: The binding of drugs to plasma proteins and the interpretation of measurements of plasma concentrations of drugs in patients with poor renal function. *Am J Med* 62:466–470, 1977.

42. Reidenberg MM, Affrime M: Influence of disease on binding of drugs to plasma proteins. *Ann NY Acad Sci* 226:115–126, 1973.

43. Rennick BR: Renal excretion of drugs: tubular transport and metabolism. *Annu Rev Pharmacol* 12:141–156, 1972.

44. Rennick BR: Renal tubule transport of organic cations. *Am J Physiol* 240:F83–F89, 1981.

45. Rowland M, Tozer TN: *Clinical Pharmacokinetics—Concepts and Applications.* Philadelphia, Lea & Febiger, 1980.

46. Schulze-Delrieu K: Metoclopramide. *Gastroenterology* 77:768–779, 1979.

47. Schulze-Delrieu K: Metoclopramide. *N Engl J Med* 305:28–33, 1981.

48. Scribner BH, Crawford MA, Dempster WJ: Urinary excretion by nonionic diffusion. *Am J Physiol* 5:1135–1140, 1959.

49. Serrano EE, Roye DB, Hammer RH, Wilder BJ: Plasma diphenylhydantoin values after oral and intramuscular administration of diphenylhydantoin. *Neurology* 23:311–317, 1973.

50. Snape WJ, Battle WM, Schwartz SS, Braunstein SN, Goldstein HA, Alavi A: Metoclopramide to treat gastroparesis due to diabetes mellitus—double-blind, controlled trial. *Ann Intern Med* 96:444–446, 1982.

51. Stargel WW, Shand DG, Routledge PA, Barchowsky A, Wagner GS: Clinical comparison of rapid infusion and multiple injection methods for lidocaine loading. *Am Heart J* 102:872–876, 1981.

52. Ueda CT: Essentials of bioavailability and bioequivalence. In *Concepts in Clinical Pharmacology.* Kalamazoo, MI, Upjohn Company, 1971, pp 1–12.

53. Vallner JJ: Binding of drugs by albumin and plasma protein. *J Pharm Sci* 66:447–465, 1977.

54. Verbeck RK, Branch RA, Wilkinson GR: Drug metabolites in renal failure: pharmacokinetic and clinical implications. *Clin Pharmacokinet* 6:329–345, 1981.

55. Wagner JG: *Biopharmaceutics and Relevant Pharmacokinetics.* Drug Intelligence Publications, IL 1971.

56. Walkley JW, Tillman J, Bonnar J: The persistence of dextran 70 in blood plasma following its infusion, during surgery, for prophylaxis against thromboembolism. *J Pharm Pharmacol* 28:29–31, 1976.

57. Weiner IM, Mudge GH: Renal tubular mechanisms for excretion of organic acids and bases. *Am J Med* 36:743–762, 1964.

58. Wilensky AJ, Lowden JA: Inadequate serum levels after intramuscular administration of diphenylhydantoin. *Neurology* 23:318–324, 1973.

59. Williams RL, Benet LZ: Drug pharmacokinetics in cardiac and hepatic disease. *Annu Rev Pharmacol Toxicol* 20:389–413, 1980.

60. Williams RL, Mamelok RD: Hepatic disease and drug pharmacokinetics. *Clin Pharmacokinet* 5:528–547, 1980.

61. Winter ME, Katcher BS, Koda-Kimble MA: *Basic Clinical Pharmacokinetics.* San Francisco, Applied Therapeutics, 1980.

62. Wood AJJ, Kornhauser DM, Wilkinson GR, Shand DG, Branch RA: The influence of cirrhosis on steady-state blood concentrations of unbound propranolol after oral administration. *Clin Pharmacokinet* 3:478–487, 1978.

2

Drug Interactions

Michael R. Vasko, Ph.D.
D. Craig Brater, M.D.

In recent years, increasing emphasis has been placed on both the study and the clinical importance of drug interactions. Several books and reviews provide extensive listings of drug interactions, both observed and theoretical (128, 221, 272, 312, 328). These listings, although contributing valuable information, are often voluminous and include anecdotal case reports, extrapolations from animal data, and interactions of questionable clinical relevance. Literal use of these listings could, therefore, overcomplicate therapeutic decisions and hinder rather than assist the clinician. Since some drug interactions are critical for optimal patient care and since new interactions are routinely discovered, it is important for clinicians to be aware of various types of drug interactions and their mechanisms. This caveat is particularly true in critical care medicine in which multiple drugs with narrow therapeutic indices are frequently coadministered to severely ill patients. In such settings, the margin for error is small and a drug interaction can dictate the success or failure of therapy.

The purpose of this chapter is to illustrate pharmacologic principles that may be important in clinically relevant drug interactions. It is not the intent of this chapter to present comprehensive listings of drug interactions, but to use examples to illustrate the types of interactions that can occur. The reader should then be able to extrapolate these principles to individual patient situations (210).

GENERAL PRINCIPLES FOR DRUG INTERACTIONS

Pharmacokinetic Interactions

For the purpose of this chapter, pharmacokinetic drug interactions result from altered

Table 2.1
Types of Drug Interactions

Pharmacokinetic
  Absorption
    Physicochemical complexing
    Changes in pH
    Changes in gastrointestinal motility
  Distribution
    Protein binding
  Metabolism
    Induction
    Inhibition
    Excretion
Pharmacodynamic
  Receptor (pharmacologic)
  Physiologic
  Modification of conditions at the site of action
  Physicochemical complexing

absorption, distribution, metabolism, or excretion of a drug (Table 2.1). Some of these interactions are beneficial to the patient, whereas most result in untoward effects.

Drug interactions at sites of absorption alter either the rate or extent of drug absorption. In general, the latter are more important clinically, since they can result in considerable reductions in steady state plasma drug concentrations. Absorption of a drug has multiple determinants, including physicochemical properties of the drug, gastric pH, site of absorption in the gastrointestinal tract, rate of gastric emptying, intestinal motility, surface area for absorption, mucosal function, and blood flow to the absorption site. When two or more drugs are coadministered, interactions involving any of these factors may occur, particularly in critically ill patients whose condition may independently affect these same parameters.

Drug interactions can also occur by alterations in the tissue distribution of drugs. Many drugs bind reversibly to plasma proteins and this binding limits the free drug concentration

21

that is available to tissue sites of action. For example, a decrease from the normal 99% binding of coumarin to 96% may seem like a small decrement, but the concentration of free drug that is available to the site of action has quadrupled from 1 to 4%. In most instances, however, an increase in free drug concentration is transient and is rapidly compensated for by an increase in distribution of drug to nonpharmacologically active sites or an increase in metabolism and/or excretion of the free drug (207). If, however, the patient's disease or another drug interaction compromises drug elimination, the increased free concentration may be sustained and serious consequences may result.

The majority of pharmacokinetic drug interactions involve elimination of drug by either metabolism or excretion. Metabolic drug interactions can result in an increase or decrease in the clearance of drugs and can occur by multiple mechanisms including alterations in hepatic blood flow (affecting drugs for which the limiting step in metabolism is delivery to metabolic enzymes), competitive inhibition at sites of metabolism, or induction of liver microsomal enzymes. Because there are limited pathways for drug metabolism, many drugs are metabolized by similar pathways. Consequently, interactions involving competitive inhibition or induction of metabolic enzymes are common. It is important, therefore, for clinicians to be familiar with the metabolism of each drug administered to a patient to predict the possibility of an interaction.

Most drugs are metabolized by first order kinetics, i.e., the rate of metabolism is dependent on the drug concentration. Consequently, enzymatic sites of drug metabolism are not saturated and an increase in drug concentration does not alter the rate of metabolism. In some instances, however, drugs are metabolized by zero order kinetics, i.e., only a specific amount of drug is metabolized per unit time. In addition, drugs metabolized by first order kinetics are capable of saturating their metabolic sites and shifting to zero order kinetics. This phenomenon usually occurs only at high plasma concentrations. When two drugs are administered simultaneously, however, they may compete for the same metabolic sites, and lesser concentrations of each are needed to saturate the metabolic enzymes. Therefore, a drug interaction may result in a disproportional increase in the half-life and decreased clearance of drug if the interaction not only competes for metabolism but also causes a

change from a nonsaturated to a saturated state. One could speculate that this phenomenon is more likely to occur in critically ill patients in whom diminished hepatic perfusion or metabolic function would readily occur because of their primary disease.

Finally, pharmacokinetic drug interactions can occur at sites of drug excretion, mainly the kidney, by affecting blood flow to the kidneys, glomerular filtration rate, urine pH, and secretion or reabsorption of the drug. Drug interactions can occur via any of these possible mechanisms or their combination.

Pharmacodynamic Drug Interactions

Pharmacodynamic drug interactions result in an alteration in the biochemical or physiologic effects of a drug (Table 2.1). In general, interactions of this type can be divided into four classes: (a) interactions at the drug receptor (pharmacologic); (b) interactions due to different cellular mechanisms acting in concert or in opposition (physiologic); (c) interactions by one drug changing the cellular environment and thereby altering the actions of a second drug; and (d) chemical neutralization of drugs.

A majority of pharmacodynamic drug interactions involve drugs binding to the same receptor. To exert the desired effect, most drugs bind to specific receptor sites (affinity), which activates a biochemical event or series of events that result in the pharmacologic action (intrinsic activity). *Drugs that have both high affinity for the receptor site and intrinsic activity are called agonists; drugs that have high affinity for binding sites but little or no intrinsic activity are called antagonists; drugs with varying degrees of affinity and intrinsic activity are termed mixed agonist-antagonists.* The overall outcome of drug interactions at receptor sites is dependent on the varying affinities and intrinsic activities of the different agents involved.

In many instances, drug interactions between agonists and antagonists are clinically useful. For example, the specific narcotic antagonist, naloxone, attenuates the undesirable actions of opioids. β-adrenergic antagonists are used extensively to block the effects of both endogenous and exogenous catecholamines. In some instances, however, receptor interactions are deleterious to the patient. For example, congestive heart failure or chronic obstructive pulmonary disease may worsen with β-adrenergic receptor antagonists by their attenuating the beneficial effects of catecholamines.

Pharmacodynamic drug interactions of the physiologic type can also produce either an enhanced or attenuated response. The use of combinations of agents with different mechanisms of action to lower blood pressure is clearly beneficial to the patient. Conversely, indomethacin reduces the antihypertensive effects of captopril (221), β-adrenergic antagonists (86, 87, 88, 194), and hydralazine (65) and decreases the response to loop diuretics (42, 255), presumably by inhibiting prostaglandin synthesis.

The third type of pharmacodynamic interaction occurs when the action of one drug results in a change in the intracellular or extracellular environment that modifies the action of another drug. The best such example is the increased toxicity of cardiac glycosides when administered with drugs that cause potassium depletion (31, 48). Another example is the interaction between reserpine and indirectly acting sympathomimetic agents (37, 50). Since reserpine depletes norepinephrine in nerve terminals (50), there is less response to drugs that act primarily by releasing the neurotransmitter.

The final type of interaction involves chemical neutralization of one drug by another. Several interactions of this type occur in the gastrointestinal tract and are discussed in detail below ("Interactions Affecting Drug Absorption"). This type of interaction also occurs within the circulation and may be desirable, as is the case with the use of protamine to neutralize heparin, or deleterious, as is illustrated by the inactivation of gentamicin by ureidopenicillins in patients with end-stage renal disease (266, 332, 355).

SPECIFIC TYPES OF DRUG INTERACTIONS

Interactions Affecting Drug Absorption

In this chapter, we focus on drug interactions affecting oral absorption since a large majority of documented drug interactions occur in the gastrointestinal (GI) tract. The principles applied here are also applicable, however, to other sites of drug absorption. In addition, the discussion does not include drug-food interactions. For these interactions and for a more extensive discussion of interactions of specific drugs affecting absorption, the reader is referred to reviews on the subject (129, 227, 356).

Drug interactions at sites of absorption can alter the rate and/or extent of drug absorption. The rate determines how rapidly the drug enters the blood and when the peak plasma concentration is achieved. The extent of absorption affects the total amount of the drug systemically available. In general, drug interactions altering the extent of absorption are of greater clinical importance than those affecting rate. If the patient requires a known concentration of drug in a short time, as often occurs in critical care settings, then intravenous administration can be employed, thus obviating uncertainties about rate as well as extent of absorption. If one drug interferes with the total amount of another drug absorbed, then the relationship between dose and plasma concentrations achieved (and subsequently clinical effect) is altered and dosing adjustments are required. For the most part, drug interactions of this type result in a decrease in circulating drug concentrations, and if this decrease is substantial, the interaction can compromise therapy. Less frequently, the interaction can result in increased absorption and could subject the patient to drug toxicity.

Since oral absorption of drugs is dependent on many factors involving both the properties of the drug and the characteristics of the GI tract, it is not surprising that interactions involve a number of mechanisms. In general, a majority of drug interactions affecting absorption involve (a) formation of drug complexes due to absorption, chelation, or binding; (b) alterations in gastric pH that change the ionization of drugs; and (c) changes in GI motility that affect the transit time of drugs. Other interactions, such as alterations in the GI mucosa (function, area, blood flow, or metabolism) also occur, but their clinical importance is yet to be determined. Some of these drug interactions involve only one mechanism while others are multifactorial. Table 2.2 summarizes some of the major drug interactions occurring at sites of drug absorption.

Several drugs can alter absorption by forming complexes with other agents. These drugs include antacids, activated charcoal, kaolin-pectin, and the hypocholesterolemic agents, cholestyramine and colestipol (Table 2.2). In most instances, the complex formed between the drug and the ion is less soluble and thereby less absorbable, resulting in a decrease in the amount of drug absorbed. Compounds with reduced absorption include digoxin (46, 158),

Table 2.2
Drug Interactions at Sites of Absorption

Proposed Mechanism	Drug Affected	Drug Causing Effect	Results of Interaction	References
Formation of complexes, chelation, adsorption	Bishydroxycoumarin	Antacids	Increased absorption	8, 13
	Carbamazepine	Activated charcoal	Decreased absorption, increased elimination	229
	Cephalexin	Cholestyramine	Decreased absorption	254
	Chlorothiazide	Cholestyramine	Decreased absorption	154
	Chlorpromazine	Antacids	Decreased absorption	91, 267
	Diflunisal	Antacids	Decreased absorption	344
	Digitoxin	Cholestyramine	Decreased absorption, increased elimination	53, 56
	Digoxin	Activated charcoal	Decreased absorption	228
		Antacids	Decreased absorption	46, 158
		Cholestyramine	Decreased absorption	47
		Kaolin-pectin	Decreased absorption	9, 46
	Isoniazid	Antacids	Decreased absorption	141
	Penicillamine	Antacids	Decreased absorption	251
	Phenobarbital	Activated charcoal	Decreased absorption, increased elimination	27, 187, 229
	Phenytoin	Activated charcoal	Decreased absorption	228
	Propranolol	Antacids	Decreased absorption	83
		Cholestyramine	Decreased absorption	136
	Ranitidine	Antacids	Decreased absorption	211
	Tetracyclines	Antacids	Decreased absorption	20, 105
	Theophylline	Activated charcoal	Decreased absorption, increased elimination	29
	Tolbutamide	Activated charcoal	Decreased absorption	230
	Valproate	Activated charcoal	Decreased absorption	230
	Warfarin	Cholestyramine	Decreased absorption, increased elimination	144, 284
Alterations in gastric pH	Cimetidine	Antacids	Decreased absorption	122, 324
	Ketoconazole	Cimetidine	Decreased absorption	186
	Tetracyclines	Cimetidine	Decreased absorption	105
		Sodium bicarbonate	Decreased absorption	20
Alterations in gastric motility				
Increase in motility	Acetaminophen	Metoclopramide	Increased rate of absorption	237
	Chlorothiazide	Metoclopramide	Increased rate of absorption	252
	Cimetidine	Metoclopramide	Decreased absorption	122, 152
	Digoxin	Metoclopramide	Decreased absorption	202
	Ethanol	Metoclopramide	Increased rate of absorption	108
	Lithium	Metoclopramide	Increased rate of absorption	69
Decrease in motility	Acetaminophen	Narcotic analgesics	Decreased rate of absorption	238
		Propantheline	Decreased rate of absorption	237
	Benzodiazepines	Antacids	Decreased rate of absorption	116, 118
	Bishydroxycoumarin	Amitriptyline	Increased absorption	269
	Chlorothiazide	Propantheline	Decreased rate of absorption	252
	Digoxin	Propantheline	Increased absorption	202
	Ethanol	Propantheline	Decreased rate of absorption	108
	Isoniazid	Antacids	Decreased rate of absorption	141
	Lithium	Propantheline	Decreased rate of absorption	69
	Phenytoin	Antacids	Decreased rate of absorption	103, 171
	Propranolol	Antacids	Decreased rate of absorption	83
Effects on gastrointestinal mucosa	Aminoglycoside antibiotics	Ethanol	Increased absorption due to mucosal damage	161
	Digoxin	Neomycin	Decreased absorption	191
		Sulfasalazine	Decreased absorption	149
		Erythromycin	Increased absorption	192
	Furosemide	Phenytoin	Decreased absorption	96

chlorpromazine (91), quinine (140), penicillamine (251), tetracyclines (20, 105), isoniazid (141), propranolol (83), ranitidine (211), and diflunisal (344). The resultant decrease in absorption can be 10–80%, depending on the drug involved; consequently, the interaction may be clinically important. Rarely, the drug complexes formed by interaction with antacids are more soluble, and thus increased absorption of drug occurs. For example, bishydroxycoumarin chelates with magnesium to form a more absorbable complex (8, 13). Thus, patients taking this anticoagulant with magnesium hydroxide antacids may develop higher serum drug concentrations and a greater anticoagulant effect. Interestingly, warfarin absorption does not appear to be affected by antacids (8, 284).

Both activated charcoal (227–229) and kaolin-pectin (9, 10, 46) adsorb many drugs in the GI tract. This adsorption can cause significant reductions in the amount of drug absorbed. For example, activated charcoal can reduce the bioavailability of tolbutamide and valproate by 90% and 65%, respectively (230). In addition, this adsorption can result in a significant increase in clearance of drug from the body. Many drugs are secreted into the gut, and then reabsorbed (so-called enterohepatic circulation). In the presence of charcoal, however, the secreted drugs are adsorbed, preventing their reabsorption into the body; thus, they are cleared more rapidly. This increased clearance of drugs has been observed for phenobarbital, carbamazepine, and theophylline (29, 229). This type of interaction could be of benefit in the acutely intoxicated patient, but it could prove harmful in therapeutic settings by reducing the steady state plasma concentration of drugs below the therapeutic range. In a similar manner, cholestyramine and colestipol bind bile acids, cholesterol, and many other drugs in the GI tract (47, 53, 144, 186, 284). This binding results in the decreased absorption of many drugs, including chlorothiazide (154), propranolol (136), cephalexin (254), cardiac glycosides (47, 53), and anticoagulants (144, 284). To avoid the interaction rather than compensate for it, patients requiring these drug combinations should be administered drug (digoxin, digitoxin, or warfarin) 1 hour before or 4 hours after ingesting cholestyramine or colestipol.

The interaction between digitoxin or warfarin and cholestyramine is used to clinical advantage in patients who are toxic or poisoned with either of these agents. Both agents undergo enterohepatic circulation. Administration of cholestyramine sequesters drug in the gut, resulting in less reabsorption and decreasing serum concentrations (53, 56, 144, 284).

As mentioned above, some drugs affect the absorption of others by multiple mechanisms. For example, antacids not only form complexes with other drugs, but also affect absorption by altering gastric pH. Drug absorption is dependent on both dissolution of drug and extent of ionization. In the acidic environment of the stomach, drugs that are weak acids are less ionized and more rapidly absorbed. The opposite is true for weak bases. Thus, alteration in gastric pH by antacids and/or histamine H_2-antagonists can affect drug absorption (186) (Table 2.2). Fortunately, this interaction is rarely of clinical importance since most drugs, whether weak acids or weak bases, are predominantly absorbed in the small intestine via pathways that are not pH sensitive.

Since most drugs are absorbed in the small intestine, changes in gastric emptying can alter delivery to absorption sites and, thereby, alter the rate of drug absorption. Thus, antacids (356), narcotic analgesics (238), and drugs with anticholinergic properties that slow emptying decrease the rate of absorption of benzodiazepines (118), isoniazid (141), phenytoin (103, 171), and propranolol (83). In addition, the anticholinergic, propantheline, reduces gastric emptying and delays the absorption of acetaminophen (237), ethanol (108), and lithium (69).

Drugs that alter intestinal transit time can also affect the extent of drug absorption. Propantheline not only reduces gastric emptying but decreases GI motility. This slowed transit time increases the absorption of poorly soluble drugs such as chlorothiazide (252) and older preparations of digoxin (202). Presumably, amitriptyline increases the absorption of bishydroxycoumarin by the same mechanism (269). Many other drugs, including phenothiazines, other tricyclic antidepressants, antihistamines, and narcotic analgesics, may also reduce GI transit time, thereby altering either rate or extent of drug absorption.

In general, drugs that increase GI motility have the opposite effect on rate and extent of absorption (129). Thus, metoclopramide increases the rate of absorption of many drugs (69, 108, 237), and decreases quantitative absorption of cimetidine and of older preparations of digoxin (148, 152, 202).

Drug interactions affecting absorption also

occur as a result of one drug affecting the intestinal metabolism and/or transport of another. Although there are only limited reports of these interactions, they are worth discussing since they involve drugs that may be used in critical care medicine. The antibiotics, neomycin and sulfasalazine, decrease the absorption and plasma concentrations of digoxin, presumably by affecting the integrity of the GI mucosa (149, 191). In contrast, erythromycin can increase digoxin absorption, the proposed mechanism being a decrease in flora that metabolize digoxin in the small intestine of approximately 10% of patients (192). The latter interaction can result in sufficient increases in serum digoxin concentrations to cause toxicity.

Interactions Affecting Drug Distribution

Once a drug is absorbed into the systemic circulation, it is distributed to various tissues, including the site of action. Many drugs bind extensively to plasma proteins whereas only unbound drug is free to enter tissue storage sites or sites of action, or to be metabolized or excreted. The concentration of unbound drug in the circulation can be affected by competition of other drugs for binding sites. Consequently, displacement of one bound drug by another constitutes a major source of drug interaction. Recently, however, the relative clinical importance of displacement interactions has been questioned (207, 302), and it appears that these types of interactions are often misinterpreted.

The importance and occurrence of displacement interactions are dependent on three factors: the concentration of drug in the plasma, the relative binding affinity of the drug, and the volume of distribution (V_d). A high concentration of one drug relative to another will shift the binding equilibrium. Thus, assuming equal affinities, addition of large concentrations of one drug to the blood will rapidly decrease plasma protein binding of a second. Relative binding affinity is the second important factor. In general, only drugs with high binding affinity displace other drugs. These include digitoxin, bishydroxycoumarin, warfarin, diazoxide, phenytoin, clofibrate, valproic acid, hydralazine, quinidine, sulfonamides, tolbutamide, and most nonsteroidal antiinflammatory drugs including salicylates. Finally, if a drug has a small V_d, more of the displaced drug can remain in the plasma and

be delivered to sites of action with a concomitant increase in the pharmacologic effect.

The clinical relevance of displacement interactions is dependent on the therapeutic index of the drugs involved, the availability of other distribution sites, and the rate of elimination of the displaced drug. If a drug has a wide therapeutic index, then displacement from binding that results in higher free concentrations is of little concern. In addition, increasing the free drug concentration is less important clinically when the free drug can be distributed to other tissue storage sites. This is the reason that clinically important interactions are less likely with drugs that have a large V_d. Finally, for most drugs, elimination occurs by first order kinetics. Thus, increasing the free concentration of drug is rapidly compensated for by an increase in metabolism or excretion (207, 302). With increased elimination, a new steady state is achieved with a free drug concentration similar to that before the interaction. However, if elimination is compromised by disease or other drug interactions, a higher concentration of free drug may be maintained, creating a greater risk of toxicity. This rule especially applies to drugs with a low V_d, since the increase in free drug does not redistribute to other tissue storage sites. Thus, in patients with compromised hepatic or renal function there is a greater potential that the displacement interaction will result in increased free drug concentration and increased pharmacologic effect.

Even though the effect of displacement interactions is usually transient, during the period of increased free drug concentration an increased pharmacologic response may occur. Consequently, clinicians should exercise caution in treating patients during this transitional period. For example, the most important drug interactions involving displacement from plasma protein binding sites occur with coumarin anticoagulants (6, 33, 197). The transient period of increased unbound anticoagulant can result in bleeding. It is therefore important to determine successive prothrombin times when a potential interaction is suspected. The patient may remain relatively stable during the critical time of the interaction and return to the same baseline level of anticoagulation in a few days, but then again, he or she may not.

In drug displacement interactions, after a new steady state has been attained, the resulting *total* plasma concentration of drug may be below the "normal" therapeutic range. One

Table 2.3
Drug Interactions Due to Displacement from Protein Binding Sites

Drug Displaced	Causative Agent	References
Coumarin anticoagulants	Chloral hydrate	305, 340
	Clofibrate	33
	Diazoxide	304
	Ethacrynic acid	304
	Mefenamic acid	304
	Nalidixic acid	304
	Phenylbutazone	6
	Phenytoin	126, 197
	Salicylates	197
Diazepam	Heparin	290
	Valproic acid	82
Phenytoin	Phenylbutazone	231
	Salicylates	98
	Tolbutamide	357
	Valproic acid	204, 262
Tolbutamide	Phenylbutazone	167, 268
	Salicylates	167, 362
Valproic acid	Salicylates	250

should not misinterpret such "subtherapeutic" values, for they do not adequately reflect the concentration of free drug. The clinician must be aware of the potentially altered "therapeutic range" of that patient and also rely on clinical assessment of the drug effect.

In some instances, drug toxicity originally attributed to a displacement interaction is the result of multiple interactions, e.g., displacement plus impairment of metabolism. Phenylbutazone displaces warfarin from binding sites on serum proteins but also inhibits metabolism (6). Thus, the increased concentration of free anticoagulant is not compensated for by increased metabolism, increasing the likelihood of bleeding. A similar mechanism accounts for the increased incidence of phenytoin toxicity when tolbutamide is coadministered with the anticonvulsant (357). In contrast, lessening of potential toxicity can also occur with multiple drug interactions. Phenytoin displaces dicumarol from serum protein (126), but this has little importance in patients to whom phenytoin is chronically administered, because of induction of metabolism that increases elimination of the free dicumarol.

As mentioned above, displacement interactions with anticoagulants appear to be the most important clinically (Table 2.3). Several drugs can displace coumarin anticoagulants from plasma protein binding sites, including the active metabolite of chloral hydrate (305, 399), clofibrate (33), phenylbutazone (6), salicylates (197), and phenytoin (126, 197). Displacement

interactions with other drugs may also have clinical importance (Table 2.3). For example, patients taking tolbutamide may experience a hypoglycemic episode when started on high doses of salicylates (167, 362) or when administered phenylbutazone (268). In addition, the therapeutic range for total phenytoin in the plasma may be reduced in patients taking valproic acid, salicylates, or tolbutamide since these drugs increase the free fraction of phenytoin (98, 204, 262, 357). In a similar manner, salicylates can transiently displace valproic acid from binding sites (250).

The clinical importance of many displacement interactions is currently being reassessed. Clinicians should, however, closely monitor patients given multiple drugs that have high plasma protein binding. This monitoring is especially important during the initial period after adding another drug to the patient's regimen or when the patient has compromised drug elimination, as may occur in critical care settings because of the influence of other drugs or the patient's primary disease.

Interactions Due to Altered Drug Metabolism

Drug interactions of metabolism are numerous and of varying clinical relevance. The vast majority of metabolic interactions occur with induction or inhibition of the hepatic microsomal P-450 system (51, 68, 107). Indeed, drugs as well as environmental chemicals that are metabolized by these mixed function oxidases can induce their own metabolism (autoinduction) and also affect the metabolism of other agents. In like manner, drugs that are metabolized by the same enzyme system can act as competitive inhibitors and decrease the biotransformation of other agents.

There is a great deal of individual variability in the metabolic capacity of the hepatic enzyme systems and the degree to which it may be induced or inhibited by drugs (51, 107). In addition, the time course of drug interaction varies with different drugs and with the patient's ability to metabolize them (i.e., disease, genetics, age, etc.). Thus it is difficult to predict a priori the extent of an interaction in an individual patient. Each patient must be followed closely with clinical evaluation of therapeutic and toxic endpoints and drug toxicity, and if possible, with measurement of serum drug concentrations to assess the clinical importance of a drug interaction.

DRUG INTERACTIONS RESULTING IN ENHANCED METABOLISM

Although a number of agents induce the metabolism of other drugs (Table 2.4), emphasis is placed on a few drugs that induce the metabolism of many others, including the barbiturates (especially phenobarbital), ethanol, rifampin, and the anticonvulsants, phenytoin and carbamazepine. All of these agents induce the metabolism of oral anticoagulants, thereby increasing the dosage required to achieve therapeutic prolongation of the prothrombin time (70, 126, 127, 153, 168, 197, 309). For example, coadministration of rifampin with warfarin for 5–7 days doubles warfarin clearance, requiring an approximate 2-fold increase in dosing to maintain therapeutic plasma concentrations of the anticoagulant (16, 245, 247, 287). This type of interaction is important not only during the time of induced metabolism, but also after the inducing agent is withdrawn (168). When the inducing stimulus is no longer present, the hepatic enzyme activity slowly decreases, increasing serum concentrations and resulting in increased anticoagulation with the possible consequence of disastrous bleeding. Consequently, after removal of an inducing agent, the dose of anticoagulant needs to be readjusted.

Phenobarbital is a potent inducer of hepatic microsomal enzymes, resulting in reduced plasma concentrations and increased elimi-

nation of many drugs (Table 2.4), including chloramphenicol (360), cimetidine (320), phenytoin (49, 70, 173), dicumarol (70, 168, 197), nortriptyline (39), theophylline (177), and warfarin (168, 197). In a similar manner, phenytoin induces the metabolism of a large number of drugs (Table 2.4). Phenobarbital combined with phenytoin doubles the clearance of quinidine in humans, with a concomitant decrease in the elimination half-life of approximately 50% (73), presumably due to enzyme induction. Similarly, this anticonvulsant combination results in a significant increase in steroid clearance in transplant patients (102, 264). Since many epileptic patients receive long-term therapy with either phenytoin or phenobarbital or both, caution must be exercised when the patients receive additional medication.

Rifampin is one of the most potent inducers of metabolizing enzymes, increasing the clearance of warfarin (245, 247), glucocorticoids (28), digitoxin (31, 316), chloramphenicol (274), hexobarbital (366), metoprolol (25) and dapsone (367). Rifampin therapy also decreases the half-life of tolbutamide (51, 366), oral contraceptives (17), and theophylline (38, 285). Rifampin has a 2-fold effect on quinidine handling, decreasing quinidine's elimination half-life with no change in the volume of distribution (338). From the data, one would predict an approximate 3-fold increase in clearance with an identical decrement in the steady state plasma concentration or area under the curve (AUC) of plasma concentration versus time. The observed change in AUC of quinidine in these subjects, however, was a 6-fold decrease (338). The probable explanation for this discrepancy is a concomitant decrease in the bioavailability of quinidine due to an enhanced first pass effect through an induced hepatic enzyme system. The net result is a "multiplier" effect on drug concentrations achieved in plasma.

Nonprescription drugs, ethanol, and cigarette smoking also induce the microsomal enzyme system. Indeed, the clinician is not always aware of the chronic use of ethanol or cigarettes, and may initiate therapy with "normal doses" of drugs, which may not achieve therapeutic plasma concentrations. Consequently, it is important to be aware of possible drug interactions with "recreational" drugs. As is evident in Table 2.4, chronic ethanol use can result in increased metabolism of several drugs. However, the acute use of ethanol often has opposite effects on drug metabolism, as

Table 2.4
Examples of Drugs That Induce the Metabolism of Other Drugs

Drug Induced	Inducing Agent	References
Acetaminophen	Oral contraceptives	219
Carbamazepine	Phenytoin	62, 261, 262
Chloramphenicol	Phenobarbital	360
	Rifampin	274
Chlorpromazine	Phenobarbital	51
Cimetidine	Phenobarbital	320
Clonazepam	Phenytoin	261, 262
Cyclosporin	Phenytoin	99
Dapsone	Rifampin	367
Diazepam	Phenytoin	261, 262
Digoxin	Rifampin	106
Digitoxin	Phenobarbital	31, 316
	Phenytoin	31, 316
	Rifampin	31, 316
Doxycycline	Phenytoin	259
Fludrocortisone	Phenytoin	156
Glucocorticoids	Phenytoin	102, 264
	Rifampin	28
Griseofulvin	Phenobarbital	51
Meprobamate	Chronic ethanol (prior to hepatic impairment)	193, 216, 301, 303
Methadone	Phenytoin	261, 262
Metoprolol	Rifampin	25
Mexiletine	Rifampin	258
Oral anticoagulants	Carbamazepine	127, 168, 197
	Chronic ethanol	153, 309
	Gluthethimide	168, 197
	Griseofulvin	168, 197
	Phenobarbital	168, 197, 309
	Phenytoin	126, 168, 197
	Rifampin	245, 247, 287
Pentobarbital	Chronic ethanol	193, 216, 301, 303
Phenylbutazone	Phenobarbital	51
Phenytoin	Carbamazepine	127, 261, 262
	Chronic ethanol	193, 296, 301
	Phenobarbital	49, 70, 173
	Rifampin	155
Quinidine	Phenytoin	73
	Rifampin	338
Theophylline	Cigarette smoking	120
	Phenobarbital	177
	Phenytoin	212
	Rifampin	38, 285
Tolbutamide	Chronic ethanol	153, 193, 301, 303
	Rifampin	51, 358
Valproic acid	Phenytoin	261, 262, 293

discussed in the next section. Thus acute ethanol use appears to inhibit metabolism, while chronic use (prior to onset of liver disease) can result in enhanced metabolism due to enzyme induction (178). Finally, induction of the hepatic microsomal enzyme system by cigarette smoking may explain the increase in theophylline clearance in chronic smokers (120).

Several points regarding enzyme induction are important (Table 2.5). First, drug interactions involving induction are slow in onset and offset. It takes days or weeks before the enzymes are induced; consequently, patients need to be monitored for extended periods when clinically important interactions are predicted. For example, Romankiewicz and Ehrman (287) showed that the onset and offset of the increase in warfarin clearance produced by rifampin was maximal 5–7 days after starting and stopping rifampin therapy. Conse-

Table 2.5
Important Considerations Concerning Enzyme Induction

---

1. Slow in onset and offset
2. Dosage adjustment and clinical monitoring are as important during offset as during onset
3. Induction may be specific or nonspecific
4. Clinical relevance is a function of the therapeutic index of the interacting drugs

---

quently, the critical period of this interaction occurs approximately 1 week after initiation of therapy and 1 week after discontinuing the inducing agent. Second, offset of the drug interaction is as clinically important as onset. If, for example, a dosage adjustment is made when a patient has been receiving rifampin and warfarin to compensate for the increased metabolism, then another adjustment is needed some days after the rifampin is discontinued to readjust for the decreased clearance and to prevent excessive bleeding. Third, the induction of the microsomal enzyme system may be specific for one isoenzyme (i.e., one pathway) or nonspecific. For example, rifampin administration appears to selectively induce certain pathways of antipyrine metabolism (337) but does not appear selective in theophylline metabolism (285). Another example of selective induction is seen with acetaminophen and oral contraceptives (219). Oral contraceptives appear to increase the clearance of acetaminophen by selectively increasing glucuronidation. Whether this selectivity can be exploited for clinical use in acetaminophen poisoning is yet to be determined. Finally, the overall clinical relevance of drug interactions involving induction is clearly dependent on the therapeutic index of the drug involved. Affected drugs with a narrow therapeutic range are more clinically important than those with a wide range.

DRUG INTERACTIONS DUE TO INHIBITION OF METABOLISM

In general, drugs discussed above that are susceptible to induction of metabolism are also subject to inhibition (Table 2.6). Inhibitors are capable of decreasing the metabolism of any drug that is metabolized by the same enzyme system. As with induction, the clinical importance of these interactions is largely a function of the therapeutic index of the drugs involved. Unlike induction interactions, however, the onset and offset of these interactions are fairly rapid.

Most drug interactions involving inhibition of metabolism occur in the liver, and are due to competitive inhibition of enzymes involved in drug biotransformation. For example, cimetidine inhibits the metabolism of many drugs (Table 2.6), presumably by inhibiting the hepatic cytochrome P-450 mixed function oxidases (164, 276, 322). This inhibition results in a decrease in elimination of many drugs and often requires a change in the dosing regimen (Table 2.6). Of most clinical importance, however, are interactions between cimetidine and theophylline, lidocaine, and oral anticoagulants, since these latter drugs have a narrow margin of safety and thus critical toxicity can occur. Cimetidine decreases theophylline clearance by approximately 50% with a corresponding doubling of the elimination half-life (54, 66, 143, 270, 278, 347). Volume of distribution does not change. The result, if a patient's dosing regimen were not modified, would be a doubling of the serum theophylline concentration. In a similar manner, cimetidine reduces the clearance of oral anticoagulants, potentiating their actions and requiring a decrease in dosage (168, 197, 244, 309, 318). Cimetidine also decreases the clearance of lidocaine by 25–42%, presumably because of a decrease in metabolism of the antiarrhythmic

Table 2.6
Examples of Drugs that Inhibit the Metabolism of Other Drugs

Drug Causing Inhibition	Drugs Inhibited	References
Allopurinol	6-Mercaptopurine	19, 226
	Flecainide	311
Amiodarone	Phenytoin	114, 208
	Procainamide	292
	Quinidine	292
	Warfarin	350
Bishydroxycoumarin	Tolbutamide	168, 197
Chloramphenicol	Carbamazepine	32, 63, 261
	Chlorpropamide	32, 63

Drug Causing Inhibition	Drugs Inhibited	References
Chloramphenicol (*continued*)	Oral anticoagulants	32, 63, 168, 197
	Phenobarbital	32, 63, 169
	Phenytoin	32, 63, 169, 261, 262
	Tolbutamide	32, 63, 272
Chlorpromazine	Phenytoin	261, 348
	Propranolol	346
Cimetidine	Amitriptyline	71
	Benzodiazepines	78, 115, 162, 241, 291, 318
	Carbamazepine	200, 261
	5-Fluorouracil	19, 130
	Imipramine	4, 133
	Lidocaine	22, 92, 361
	Meperidine	121
	Metoprolol	25
	Phenytoin	11, 135, 232, 294
	Propranolol	93, 318
	Theophylline	54, 66, 143, 270, 278
	Tolbutamide	58
	Triamterene	222
	Warfarin	168, 244
Diltiazem	Antipyrine	23, 55
	Carbamazepine	45
Disulfiram	Benzodiazepines	198
	Phenytoin	159, 243
	Warfarin	168, 197, 246
Ethanol (acute)	Diazepam	196
	Meprobamate	193, 301, 303
	Pentobarbital	193, 301, 303
	Phenytoin	193, 261, 301, 303
	Tolbutamide	57, 193, 272
	Warfarin	168, 193, 197
Erythromycin	Carbamazepine	363, 365
	Cyclosporine	203
	Theophylline	41, 206, 282, 283
Isoniazid	Carbamazepine	341, 364
	Phenytoin	174, 225, 261
Ketoconazole	Methylprednisolone	112
Methylphenidate	Phenobarbital	104, 261
	Phenytoin	104, 261
	Primidone	104, 261
Oral contraceptives	Diazepam	2
	Imipramine	3
	Metoprolol	25
	Oral anticoagulants	80, 168, 197
	Prednisolone	184
	Theophylline	336
Propoxyphene	Carbamazepine	72
	Doxepin	5
	Phenytoin	5, 261
Propranolol	Diazepam	242
	Lidocaine	40, 240
Quinidine	Digitoxin	170
Sulfinpyrazone	Warfarin	335
Sulfonamides	Carbamazepine	32, 150
	Phenytoin	32, 150, 195, 261
	Tolbutamide	32, 195, 257, 272
	Warfarin	32, 168, 195, 197
Thymidine	5-Fluorouracil	19
Verapamil	Antipyrine	23
	Carbamazepine	199

(22, 92, 361); however, this interaction increases the lidocaine serum concentration by 50% indicating a concomitant decrease in volume of distribution (approximately 10–20%) (92, 361). Consequently, when coadministering lidocaine and cimetidine, one should decrease both the loading and maintenance lidocaine doses. Cimetidine may also decrease lidocaine clearance by reducing hepatic blood flow (92), thereby decreasing lidocaine access to the liver (327, 333), although the occurrence of this reduction in hepatic blood flow by cimetidine is controversial (134, 142, 361).

Other drugs clearly alter hepatic blood flow, resulting in a reduced elimination of drugs whose metabolism is limited by availability of drug to liver enzymes (drugs with a high extraction ratio). For example, the β-adrenergic blocking agents, propranolol, nadolol, and metoprolol, decrease lidocaine clearance by 20–50% (25, 297). In addition, hydralazine increases the peak concentration and AUC of metoprolol and propranolol after oral administration, by diminishing hepatic blood flow (25, 298). Aspirin and indomethacin decrease clearance of indocyanine green without altering antipyrine clearance (94), suggesting that inhibition of prostaglandin synthesis may alter hepatic blood flow. These results imply that inhibitors of prostaglandin synthesis may have important interactions with drugs such as lidocaine and propranolol.

Many other drug interactions inhibiting metabolism are clinically relevant (Table 2.6). For example, acute administration of ethanol inhibits the metabolism of many drugs (178, 193, 301, 303), including chloral hydrate (306), some benzodiazepines (79, 307, 308), propranolol (85), tolbutamide (57), phenytoin (193, 301, 303), and warfarin (193, 301, 303). As discussed earlier, chronic ethanol has an opposite effect on the clearance of many of these drugs because of induction of drug metabolism (Table 2.4). Tolbutamide metabolism is reduced by the coadministration of several drugs (63, 301), which can result in long-lasting and profound hypoglycemia. Drug inhibition of phenytoin and carbamazepine metabolism has resulted in many incidences of toxicity with these agents (63, 125, 174, 195, 225, 261, 263). This toxicity, although usually not life threatening, causes considerable trauma to the patient and often requires prolonged hospitalization. The potential consequences of drug interactions that inhibit metabolism of oral anticoagulants are obvious (80, 131, 166, 168, 195, 235, 246, 248, 249, 335), and to avoid

potential toxicity, compensatory changes in dosing are necessary when therapy with an interacting drug is commenced or discontinued.

Interactions affecting drug metabolism can also occur with extrahepatic enzymes. As a major example, a number of drugs used clinically act by inhibiting monoamine oxidase (313). The significance of interactions with these drugs is only lessened by the appropriate infrequent use of these agents. However, procarbazine (81), a drug used in treating Hodgkin's disease, and isoniazid (185, 315) have monoamine oxidase inhibitory activity. Concomitant use of sympathomimetic agents with these drugs requires awareness of this potential effect. Monoamine oxidase metabolizes sympathetic neurotransmitters that are retaken up into the sympathetic nerve ending from the synaptic cleft. During inhibition of this enzyme, administration of catecholamines or agents that release catecholamines, such as tyramine, ephedrine, pseudoephedrine, and amphetamines, can cause potentially fatal hypertensive crisis since metabolism of these drugs and of endogenous catecholamine is inhibited. In addition, some antihypertensive agents such as reserpine, guanethidine, methyldopa, and clonidine may (rarely) acutely release endogenous catecholamine stores, paradoxically raising blood pressure to dangerous levels.

Several important points regarding drug interactions due to metabolic inhibition should be stressed (Table 2.7). First, as mentioned above, the onset of these interactions may be quite rapid. An effect can be seen with the first dose; the maximum effect is dependent on attainment of a new steady state drug concentration, and therefore requires four to five times the *new* half-life of the drug. Second, the interaction between two drugs may be dependent on the amount of the drug administered and the total duration of administration. For

Table 2.7
Important Considerations Concerning Enzyme Inhibition

1. Onset can occur quickly
2. Time to maximum effect depends on the new half-life of the drug
3. Whether an interaction occurs may be dose-dependent
4. The patient's primary disease may increase susceptibility
5. The interaction may involve one but not other stereoisomers

example, allopurinol at a dosage of 300 mg/day for 7 days does not alter the metabolism of theophylline in normal individuals, yet if the dosage is increased to 300 mg every 12 hours for 14 days, the clearance of theophylline is reduced 21% while the half-life and AUC are significantly increased (201). Thus, physicians must be cautious not only when adding a new drug to the therapeutic regimen, but also when altering the dosage of a drug the patient is already taking. Third, other factors (i.e., liver function, genetics) affecting drug metabolism may influence the incidence of drug interactions. For example, Rollinghoff and Paumgartner (286) demonstrated that therapeutic doses of cimetidine reduced aminopyrine metabolism to a greater degree in patients with compromised liver function than in subjects with normal liver function. They concluded that patients with chronic liver disease may be at increased risk for drug interactions with drugs that compete for metabolism. Another factor involves the patient's inherited ability to metabolize drug. Genetic variability of drug metabolism is well documented (176, 345, 353). The acetylation of isoniazid, for example, is rapid in approximately half the population and slow in the other half (89). Slow acetylation appears to predispose patients to increased toxicity from drugs metabolized by microsomal enzymes. This fact may explain the increased incidence of phenytoin toxicity in slow acetylators of isoniazid as opposed to rapid acetylators (172). Phenytoin metabolism is also genetically controlled, certain individuals slowly metabolizing the drug (175, 343). This genetic variability may prove to be an additional, important determinant of susceptibility to drug interactions.

A fourth important point involves inhibition of drug metabolism that selectively affects one enantiomer of a racemic mixture of a drug. For example, warfarin used in therapy is a racemic mixture, the $S(-)$ enantiomer having the predominant anticoagulant effect. Several drugs, including metronidazole, (249), trimethoprim-sulfamethoxazole (248), and sulfinpyrazone (335), inhibit the metabolism of $S(-)$-warfarin. When the interaction between these drugs and racemic warfarin is assessed, significant changes are observed in prothrombin time, yet no consistent or significant changes are observed in the pharmacokinetics of warfarin. The lack of a pharmacokinetic interaction is probably due to a masking of the inhibition of $S(-)$-warfarin by $R(-)$-warfarin. Consequently, clinicians should be aware that observed, yet unex-plained, pharmacodynamic drug interactions may in fact have a pharmacokinetic component.

Finally, although this discussion has stressed drug interactions of metabolism that have deleterious consequences, some interactions of this type may be beneficial. For example, cimetidine selectively inhibits the oxidative metabolism of acetaminophen in the liver (1, 220). Since the oxidative metabolites of acetaminophen are more toxic than the conjugated metabolites, cimetidine-induced inhibition is potentially beneficial in treating acetaminophen overdose.

Ideally, the clinician should be aware of the metabolic pathways for various drugs, be able to predict potential drug interactions, and compensate for them. It is also possible, in some instances, for the clinician to substitute one drug for another if drug interactions are anticipated. For example, cimetidine inhibits the metabolism of several benzodiazepines, including diazepam and chlordiazepoxide, by inhibiting the mixed function oxidases in the liver (78, 115, 162, 241, 291, 318). It does not, however, usually inhibit glucuronidation or sulfation. Consequently, if a benzodiazepine is needed in a patient receiving cimetidine, one can select oxazepam or lorazepam since cimetidine does not block glucuronidation of these drugs (256). If a drug is needed to decrease gastric acid secretion and the patient is receiving other drugs metabolized by the hepatic P-450 enzyme system, the clinician could select antacids, sucralfate, or ranitidine instead of cimetidine for therapy. Cimetidine (as discussed above) inhibits liver metabolism of many drugs whereas ranitidine, a structurally different H_2-receptor blocker, does not appear to affect the metabolism of antipyrine, theophylline, warfarin, diazepam, tolbutamide, phenytoin, or β-adrenergic receptor blockers (43, 58, 132, 157, 163, 244, 270, 279, 310, 321, 351). Thus, ranitidine has the clinical advantage of limited potential for metabolic drug interactions.

Interactions Affecting Drug Excretion

As noted previously, most drug excretion occurs in the kidney; consequently, emphasis is placed on drug interactions involving renal excretion of both parent drug and metabolites. Drugs can be excreted by filtration or active secretion and can be reabsorbed into the systemic circulation. Logically, all three functions are potential sites for drug interaction. The other major route of drug excretion involves biliary secretion into the intestinal tract. For such drugs, interactions can occur in the GI tract with other drugs that bind or adsorb the secreted drugs (see "Interactions Affecting Drug Absorption"). This phenomenon is analogous to drug interactions decreasing the extent of absorption, as previously discussed.

Many drugs are eliminated by glomerular filtration; clinically important examples are the aminoglycoside antibiotics and digoxin. Theoretically, changes in glomerular filtration rate (GFR) affect handling of these and other drugs. Few studies, however, have addressed this potentially important area of drug interactions. Evidence suggests that furosemide causes a fall in GFR consequent to volume depletion (180). Presumably, by decreasing GFR, furosemide can reduce the clearance of digoxin and gentamicin (180, 334). Whether this interaction has clinical significance is yet to be determined. Furthermore, furosemide is a poor pharmacologic tool for assessing potential effects of GFR since the effect is most likely dependent on the degree of volume loss or replacement. Other pharmacologic agents can increase renal perfusion directly. For example, in dogs, dopamine increases GFR and the elimination of tobramycin (160). Such effects need further study in humans. However, many patients in critical care settings receive vasoactive drugs that can affect GFR. Similarly, many receive drugs dependent on glomerular filtration for excretion. It is important, therefore, for critical care physicians to consider the potential for these types of interactions, despite the paucity of available information.

A large number of drugs and metabolites are eliminated from the body by active secretion at the pars recta (straight segment) of the proximal tubule. This secretion occurs via two nonspecific transport systems, one for organic acids and one for bases. Since the transport is nonspecific, drugs can compete for transport with one another and the resultant interactions can be clinically important (271, 280, 354). There is also a secretory pathway for digoxin, located in the distal tubule, which is a site for drug interactions affecting digoxin (109, 325).

Several drugs that are organic acids have clinically important renal secretion (Table 2.8). These include many diuretics, nonsteroidal antiinflammatory drugs (15), penicillins (151), cephalosporins (119), methotrexate (7, 19, 234), and sulfa compounds (260). Clearly, the different acids compete with each other for se-

Table 2.8
Organic Acids Actively Secreted by the Kidney[a]

Acetazolamide
p-Aminohippurate
Captopril
Cephalosporins (most)
Dyphylline
Heparin
Loop-acting diuretics
Methotrexate
Nonsteroidal antiinflammatory agents
Penicillins
Probenecid
Salicylates
Sulfonamides
Sulfonylureas
Thiazide diuretics

[a]Data from references 7, 15, 19, 119, 151, 205, 234, 260, 288, 289, 295, 330, 357.

cretion; however, it is difficult to predict a priori the degree of competition.

The interaction between methotrexate and probenecid illustrates the interaction between organic acids. When probenecid is administered to patients taking methotrexate, most clinicians decrease the dosage of the anticancer drug (7). Few physicians are aware, however, of a similar need to decrease the dose if other drugs secreted by the organic acid transport system are coadministered with methotrexate (19, 234). Indeed, the increased sensitivity to methotrexate seen in some patients may be due to coadministration of drugs that inhibit its active secretion.

In addition to exogenous organic acids, endogenous organic acids can also compete for the transport system. This mechanism may account for the large doses of organic acid diuretics, such as furosemide, that are required to cause diuresis in uremic patients (288, 289). The endogenous acids produced in uremia may compete with the diuretics for transport into the renal tubular lumen, i.e., to their site of action.

The active transport system for organic bases and its clinical importance are less well understood. Like organic acids, many bases undergo potentially important active secretion (Table 2.9). Of these, the only interactions studied clinically are those between the H_2-receptor antagonists, cimetidine and ranitidine, and the antiarrhythmic, procainamide (64, 317, 319). Coadministration to healthy volunteers of cimetidine with procainamide results in a significant increase in AUC for procainamide and a significant decrease in the renal clearance of

Table 2.9
Organic Bases Actively Secreted by the Kidney[a]

Amantadine
Amiloride
Cimetidine
Ethambutol
Mecamylamine
Mepacrine (quinacrine)
N-Methylnicotinamide
Procainamide
Pseudoephedrine
Ranitidine
Tetraethylammonium

[a] Data from references 64, 265, 281, 317, 319.

both procainamide and its major metabolite, N-acetylprocainamide (64, 319). Ranitidine produces similar effects, which are dependent on the plasma concentrations of the H_2-receptor antagonist (317). Whether other clinically significant interactions occur between organic bases is yet to be determined.

The decrease in secretion of digoxin caused by several drugs is one of the most important drug interactions affecting secretion (24, 30, 60, 84, 123, 139, 181–183, 223, 299, 326, 358). This phenomenon is reviewed in detail elsewhere (30). The interaction occurs in at least 90% of patients with coadministration of quinidine and digoxin, with, on the average, a doubling of the serum digoxin concentration. The magnitude of the effect appears to be dependent on the serum quinidine concentration. The predominant mechanism of the interaction is decreased tubular secretion of digoxin (109), resulting in decreased overall clearance and a need to halve the dose (on average) to maintain the same serum concentration of digoxin. In addition, approximately two-thirds of patients also demonstrate a 10% or more decrease in digoxin's volume of distribution. The mechanism of this effect is presumably the displacement of digoxin from muscle binding sites by quinidine (147, 299).

If displacement of digoxin from muscle occurs, does displacement occur from sites of action on cardiac muscle? If so, the increase in serum concentrations of digoxin would not result in an increased pharmacological effect on the heart but may affect other systems. Data addressing this issue are inconsistent (24, 84, 138, 183, 299, 326, 358). Some studies report a decreased cardiac digoxin concentration with an increased concentration in the brain after quinidine administration (30). Although controversial, observations suggest enhanced elec-

trophysiologic action on the heart (24, 183, 223) with a decrease in inotropism (81, 138, 299, 326, 358). The electrophysiologic actions may be due to enhanced central nervous system effects on atrioventricular nodal conduction. If these effects occur as a result of the interaction, one clearly needs to decrease the dosage of digoxin to maintain the "therapeutic range." This decrease may thereby compromise the inotropic actions of the drug. In fact, in those patients who do not require digoxin for effects on conduction, alternative therapy may be more appropriate.

This interaction with digoxin is not unique to quinidine. Amiodarone, quinine, spironolactone, verapamil, and flecainide also increase serum digoxin concentrations (95, 182, 189, 349, 352). Like quinidine, spironolactone affects both the volume of distribution and the clearance of digoxin (95, 349). On average, clearance decreases 26%; however, there is great variability among patients, with a range of 0–74%. Similarly, the effect on volume of distribution is highly variable. Therefore, some patients may require dose adjustment while others will not. In general, loading and maintenance doses of digoxin are decreased by one-third in patients receiving spironolactone; some patients may need subsequent upward titration.

Some drugs are reabsorbed in the nephron after having gained access to the tubular lumen by filtration or secretion. Reabsorption of drugs in the distal tubule and collecting duct is related to urinary flow rate and pH (214). High rates of urine flow induced by diuretics or fluid loading increase excretion of phenobarbital and theophylline, but these increased flow rates would have to be maintained for long periods of time before they became clinically important. In animal studies, digoxin clearly has a reabsorptive component, presumably in the proximal tubule (110). Consequently, renal excretion of digoxin involves filtration, proximal reabsorption, and secretion at more distal tubular sites. The mechanism of digoxin's reabsorption is unclear but appears to follow general reabsorptive activity of the proximal tubule. Administration of saline or mannitol decreases proximal tubular reabsorption of sodium and of digoxin, whereas agents acting more distally to increase sodium excretion and urinary volume do not affect digoxin excretion (110). Whether drug interactions occur in humans via this pathway is unclear. These interactions may, however, be particularly important in critical care settings in which fluctuations in volume status may have major effects on proximal tubule reabsorption. In such cases, digoxin handling should be followed closely.

Lithium is reabsorbed in the nephron in parallel with sodium, and changes in sodium homeostasis (particularly in the proximal tubule) can therefore alter renal excretion of lithium. The mild volume depletion attending chronic administration of thiazide diuretics causes increased proximal tubular reabsorption of sodium and concomitantly decreases lithium excretion (77, 137). Furosemide, on the other hand, appears to have little effect (146). Administration of indomethacin or diclofenac increases steady state serum lithium concentrations by approximately 30%, presumably by facilitating the reabsorption of lithium in the proximal tubule (100, 277). Other agents affecting proximal reabsorption of sodium might also affect handling of lithium.

Finally, altering the pH of the urine could alter passive transport of weak acids and bases. For example, administration of therapeutic doses of antacids may raise urinary pH sufficient to change the excretion of some drugs in clinically important amounts (188).

Pharmacodynamic Drug Interactions

Many drug interactions do not involve changes in the absorption, distribution, or elimination of drugs, but involve modification of the biologic effect of the drugs. These interactions may involve drug receptor interactions, may involve different cellular mechanisms, may be due to alterations in cellular environment, or may result from chemical neutralization.

Drug interactions at receptor sites are widely known and often used to clinical advantage. Clearly, drug antagonists are synthesized specifically for their effects on receptors, as is illustrated by the substantial number of β-adrenergic receptor blockers that are available. There are numerous examples of agonist/antagonist drug interactions. Often, however, antagonists lack specificity with regard to their receptor blocking ability. For example, phenothiazines, tricyclic antidepressants, and butyrophenones have α-adrenergic antagonist properties, accounting for the enhanced activity of other α-adrenergic blockers used concomitantly. In addition, this antagonist activity accounts for the use of directly acting sympathomimetics to reverse toxic α-adrenergic blockade caused by these drugs.

In a similar manner, some tricyclic antidepressants have potent antimuscarinic effects (233, 239). Consequently, adverse drug interactions can occur when multiple drugs are administered that block similar receptor sites. The clinician, therefore, needs to be aware of possible multiple receptor effects of drugs, not just of the major classes of agonists or antagonists.

Unanticipated but predictable interactions may occur with use of agents that have multiple receptor effects. For example, epinephrine is both an α- and β-adrenergic agonist; the α effect predominates in most instances, causing arteriolar vasoconstriction. Concomitant use of an α-adrenergic antagonist not only attenuates the vasoconstriction, but also may unveil the vasodilation caused by the β effect. Similarly, the use of propranolol for the treatment of hypertension can, in rare instances, exacerbate the hypertension by blocking β-induced vasodilation and potentiate preexisting α-mediated vasoconstriction, especially in patients with a pheochromocytoma (209, 236, 273). By a similar mechanism, in patients treated with clonidine, withdrawal of the drug during continued administration of propranolol can cause accentuation of the α-adrenergic effect of endogenous catecholamines (18).

Pharmacodynamic drug interactions also occur when two drugs administered together have different cellular mechanisms that either enhance or diminish the physiologic response. For example, indomethacin administration decreases the antihypertensive effects of captopril (101, 221), hydralazine (65), and propranolol (21, 86, 87, 194). The effect of indomethacin, although not known, may be due to inhibition of synthesis of prostaglandins responsible for vasodilation. This hypothesis is controversial, since the attenuation of the antihypertensive effects does not seem to occur with other inhibitors of prostaglandin synthesis (88).

In a similar manner, indomethacin decreases the acute response to furosemide whereas aspirin has no effect in normal subjects (26, 42, 255, 340). The indomethacin effect is not a result of a change in the amount of furosemide reaching its intraluminal site of action (61). Whether this interaction is of clinical importance is unclear; patients chronically receiving both drugs show no effect on sodium excretion, although the antihypertensive effect of furosemide is blunted by indomethacin (255).

Tricyclic antidepressants and guanethidine block neuronal uptake of catecholamines at the synaptic cleft (36, 323). Because reuptake of catecholamines is the major mechanism of attenuation of their effect, the response to exogenously administered catecholamines may be increased if used with these agents (67). In studies of normal subjects given imipramine (25 mg three times daily) for 5 days, the pressor effect of phenylephrine was potentiated by two to three times, norepinephrine by four to eight times, and epinephrine by two to four times (35). In a similar study in subjects administered debrisoquine (a guanidinium antihypertensive agent that blocks the catecholamine reuptake system), the effects of phenylephrine were markedly potentiated and prolonged (12). Sympathomimetics that act indirectly would not be expected to have an enhanced effect with guanethidine-like drugs, and would more likely have a decreased effect, since guanethidine, debrisoquine, and bethanidine deplete endogenous catecholamines.

Another set of important drug interactions involving the catecholamine reuptake mechanism is that occurring between the guanidinium antihypertensives, guanethidine, bethanidine, and debrisoquine, and a number of psychoactive agents. The former guanethidine antihypertensives are taken into the nerve ending by the catecholamine reuptake system, where they cause release and depletion of endogenous catecholamine stores. Tricyclic antidepressants reverse the antihypertensive effects of these agents by inhibiting their uptake to this site of action (36, 113, 124, 217, 218, 314, 329). Doxepin has less tendency to produce this effect than other antidepressants (90). A similar reversal of effect that probably results from inhibition of uptake or displacement from the site of action also occurs with amphetamine, ephedrine, methylphenidate, phenothiazines, butyrophenones, thiothixene, and possibly reserpine (59, 75, 76, 145, 329). A similar interaction has been reported with use of a nasal decongestant containing chlorpheniramine, isopropamide, and phenylpropanolamine (215). This last interaction is probably not clinically important in most patients, but use of over-the-counter "cold" remedies should be avoided in patients receiving guanethidine-like drugs.

Reversal of the antihypertensive effect of clonidine by desipramine is well documented (44, 342), implying that caution should be used when other tricyclic antidepressants and psychoactive drugs are administered to patients receiving clonidine.

There are several other examples of pharmacodynamic drug interactions resulting from different drug mechanisms. Phenothiazines and tricyclic antidepressants can produce a quinidine-like decrease in cardiac conduction time, resulting in a prolonged QRS complex and arrhythmias (14, 74, 97, 359). Concomitant use of quinidine, procainamide, or similar agents with these drugs could therefore have additive effects. Treatment of arrhythmias caused by phenothiazines or tricyclic antidepressants therefore requires agents that will not further depress conduction; these include lidocaine, tocainide, mexiletine, phenytoin, and β-adrenergic receptor blockers.

Verapamil, the slow calcium channel antagonist, slows atrioventricular (A-V) nodal conduction by inhibition of calcium influx into the myocardial cells (190, 331). Both propranolol and digoxin can also slow A-V nodal conduction via other mechanisms. The concomitant administration of verapamil with either propranolol or digoxin could therefore result in additive suppression of A-V nodal conduction and cause bradycardia, A-V block, or ventricular asystole (253, 300). Thus although most patients can tolerate such combinations without difficulty, caution should be exercised when these drugs are given together.

The third type of pharmacodynamic drug interaction involves one drug changing the extracellular or cellular environment such that the action of a second drug is affected. Perhaps the best example of this is the changes in electrolyte status that affect the response to digitalis glycosides (31, 48). Many drugs, including diuretics (117, 165, 275), amphotericin B (213), ampicillin (111), carbenicillin (52), and lithium (224), can cause hypokalemia. Potassium depletion increases the risk of digoxin toxicity. This interaction is particularly easy to overlook because substantial decreases in intracellular potassium can occur with normokalemia. Hypercalcemia and hypomagnesemia similarly increase the sensitivity to digitalis.

Finally, drugs can neutralize each other by forming complexes either in solution or in situ. Perhaps the best example of this type of interaction in situ involves heparin and protamine. The administration of protamine to neutralize heparin is widely known and used to clinical advantage. Another important interaction of this type that can be critical to the patient's well-being is the neutralization of aminoglycoside antibiotics by certain penicillins in patients with renal disease (266, 332, 355). The penicillins, carbenicillin, ticarcillin, and piperacillin, complex with the aminoglycoside. The effect appears to be dependent on the patient's level of renal function (179) and is related to both concentration and time (34).

The preceding constitute but a few of the myriad pharmacodynamic drug interactions. It should be clear that anticipation of these interactions requires a collation of knowledge concerning the fundamental pharmacologic characteristics of the drugs administered to a patient and the pathophysiology of the patient's disease(s).

APPLICATIONS TO CRITICAL CARE PRACTITIONERS

Patients in critical care settings are particularly susceptible to drug interactions. They frequently receive multiple drugs that have narrow therapeutic indices and/or are frequently implicated in drug interactions. Antiarrhythmic agents, sympathomimetics, cardiac inotropes, and histamine H_2-receptor antagonists are but a few examples of drugs administered to many, if not most, patients in critical care medicine. To compound potential problems, the patient's primary disease can have great influence on drug disposition and response. For example, cardiovascular instability can affect hepatic and renal perfusion and thereby influence elimination of a number of drugs, especially those agents used in critical care settings. Examples include diminished hepatic elimination of lidocaine with congestive hepatopathy, diminished V_d of lidocaine in heart failure, and diminished renal excretion of digoxin or aminoglycoside antibiotics when renal perfusion is compromised. Not anticipating such effects can clearly lead to potentially disastrous drug-induced consequences. Unfortunately, critical care patients are often so sick that adverse drug effects can easily be misinterpreted as a manifestation of the patient's underlying condition. Because of this fact, and the great potential for drug interactions in this setting, the critical care practitioner must maintain a constant alert for drug interactions. So doing will allow one to avoid toxicity and maximize efficacy of the potent drugs at our disposal.

SUMMARY

In this chapter, drug interactions are discussed from a mechanistic point of view. We hope that the use of this approach provides a framework that assists clinicians in predicting potentially important drug interactions without memorizing extensive listings. Furthermore, as new drugs are introduced into clinical medicine, the principles discussed in this chapter can be applied to predict potential interactions prior to their documentation. For example, if aware that a new drug is metabolized by the liver microsomal enzyme system, the clinician is alerted to the potential for enzyme induction and/or inhibition by other agents handled in a similar manner. Conversely, knowing that a drug has a large V_d and is not extensively bound to plasma proteins, the clinician does not need to be concerned about displacement interactions.

With the increasing numbers of new drugs available to the clinician and with the use of multiple drugs in a given patient, it is essential to be aware of important drug interactions. By understanding basic pharmacokinetic principles and the characteristics of given drugs, the clinician can be alerted to potential drug interactions. The appropriate steps can then be taken: closely monitoring the patient, altering the dosing of one or both drugs, or changing one of the drugs to minimize the likelihood of an interaction.

References

1. Abernethy DR, Greenblatt DJ, Divoll M, Ameer B, Shader RI: Differential effect of cimetidine on drug oxidation (antipyrine and diazepam) vs. conjugation (acetaminophen and lorazepam): prevention of acetaminophen toxicity by cimetidine. *J Pharmacol Exp Ther* 224:508–515, 1982.
2. Abernethy DR, Greenblatt DJ, Divoll M, Arendt R, Ochs HR, Shader RI: Impairment of diazepam metabolism by low-dose estrogen-containing oral-contraceptive steroids. *N Engl J Med* 306:791-792, 1982.
3. Abernethy DR, Greenblatt DJ, Shader RI: Imipramine disposition in users of oral contraceptive steroids. *Clin Pharmacol Ther* 35:792–797, 1984.
4. Abernethy DR, Greenblatt DJ, Shader RI: Imipramine-cimetidine interaction: impairment of clearance and enhanced absolute bioavailability. *J Pharmacol Exp Ther* 229:702–705, 1984.
5. Abernethy DR, Greenblatt DJ, Steel K, Shader RI: Impairment of hepatic drug oxidation by propoxyphene. *Ann Intern Med* 97:223–224, 1982.
6. Aggeler PM, O'Reilly RA, Leong L: Potentiation of anticoagulant effect of warfarin by phenylbutazone. *N Engl J Med* 276:496–501, 1967.
7. Aherne GW, Piall E, Marks V, Mould G, White WF: Prolongation and enhancement of serum methotrexate concentrations by probenecid. *Br Med J* 1:1097–1099, 1978.
8. Akers MA, Lach JL, Fischer LJ: Alterations in the absorption of bishydroxycoumarin by various excipient materials. *J Pharm Sci* 62:391–395, 1973.

9. Albert KS, Ayres JW, DiSanto AR, Weidler DI, Sakmar E, Hallmark MR, Stoll RG, Desante KA, Wagner JG: Influence of kaolin-pectin suspension on digoxin bioavailability. *J Pharm Sci* 67:1582–1586, 1978.

10. Albert KS, DeSante KA, Welsh DD, DiSanto AR: Pharmacokinetic evaluation of a drug interaction between kaolin, pectin, and clindamycin. *J Pharm Sci* 67:1579–1582, 1978.

11. Algozzine GJ, Stewart RB, Springer PK: Decreased clearance of phenytoin with cimetidine (letter). *Ann Intern Med* 95:244–245, 1981.

12. Allum W, Aminu J, Bloomfield TH, Davies C, Scales AH, Vere DW: Interaction between debrisoquin and phenylephrine in man. *Br J Clin Pharmacol* 1:51–57, 1974.

13. Ambre JJ, Fisher LJ: Effect of coadministration of aluminum and magnesium hydroxides on absorption of anticoagulants in man. *Clin Pharmacol Ther* 14:231–238, 1973.

14. Arita M, Surawicz B: Electrophysiologic effects of phenothiazines on canine cardiac fibers. *J Pharmacol Exp Ther* 184:619–630, 1973.

15. Baber N, Halliday L, Sibeon R, Littler T, Orme ML'E: The interaction between indomethacin and probenecid. A clinical and pharmacokinetic study. *Clin Pharmacol Ther* 24:298–306, 1978.

16. Baciewicz AM, Self TH: Rifampin drug interactions. *Arch Intern Med* 144:1667–1671, 1984.

17. Back DJ, Breckenridge AM, Crawford FE: The effect of rifampin on the pharmacokinetics of ethynylestradiol in women. *Contraception* 21:135–143, 1980.

18. Bailey RR, Neale TJ: Rapid clonidine withdrawal with blood pressure overshoot exaggerated by beta blockade. *Br Med J* 1:942–943, 1976.

19. Balis FM: Pharmacokinetic drug interactions of commonly used anticancer drugs. *Clin Pharmacokinet* 11:223–235, 1986.

20. Barr WH, Adir J, Garrettson L: Decrease of tetracycline absorption in man by sodium bicarbonate. *Clin Pharmacol Ther* 12:779–784, 1971.

21. Barrientos A, Alcazar V, Ruilope L, Jarillo D, Rodio JL: Indomethacin and beta-blockers in hypertension. *Lancet* 1:227, 1978.

22. Bauer LA, Edwards AD, Randolph FP: Cimetidine-induced decrease in lidocaine metabolism. *Am Heart J* 108:413–414, 1984.

23. Bauer LA, Stenwall M, Horn JR, Davis R, Opheim K, Greene L: Changes in antipyrine and indocyanine green kinetics during nifedipine, verapamil, and diltiazem therapy. *Clin Pharmacol Ther* 40:239–242, 1986.

24. Belz GG, Doering W, Aust PE, Heinz M, Matthews J, Schneider B: Quinidine-digoxin interaction. Cardiac efficacy of elevated serum dogoxin concentration. *Clin Pharmacol Ther* 31:548–554, 1982.

25. Benfield P, Clissold SP, Brogden RN: Metoprolol: An updated review of its pharmacodynamic and pharmacokinetic properties, and therapeutic efficacy, in hypertension, ischaemic heart disease and related cardiovascular disorders. *Drugs* 31:376–429, 1986.

26. Berg KJ: Acute effects of acetylsalicylic acid on renal function in normal man. *Eur J Clin Pharmacol* 11:117–123, 1977.

27. Berg MJ, Berlinger WG, Goldberg MJ, Spector R, Johnson GF: Acceleration of the body clearance of phenobarbital by oral activated charcoal. *N Engl J Med* 307:642–644, 1982.

28. Bergrem H, Refvem OK: Altered prednisolone pharmacokinetics in patients treated with rifampicin. *Acta Med Scand* 213:339–343, 1983.

29. Berlinger WG, Spector R, Goldberg MJ, Johnson GF, Quee CK, Berg MJ: Enhancement of theophylline clearance by oral activated charcoal. *Clin Pharmacol Ther* 33:351–354, 1983.

30. Bigger JT, Leahey EB: Quinidine and digoxin. An important interaction. *Drugs* 24:229–239, 1982.

31. Binnion PF: Drug interaction with digitalis glycosides. *Drugs* 15:369–380, 1978.

32. Bint AJ, Burtt I: Adverse antibiotic drug interaction. *Drugs* 20:57–68, 1980.

33. Bjornsson TD, Meffin PJ, Swezey S, Blaschke TF: Clofibrate displaces warfarin from plasma proteins in man: an example of a pure displacement interaction. *J Pharmacol Exp Ther* 210:316–321, 1979.

34. Blair DC, Duggan DO, Schroeder ET: Inactivation of amikacin and gentamicin by carbenicillin in patients with end-stage renal failure. *Antimicrob Agents Chemother* 22:376–379, 1982.

35. Boakes AJ, Laurence DR, Teoh PC, Barar FSK, Benedikter LT, Prichard BNC: Interactions between sympathomimetic amines and antidepressant agents in man. *Br Med J* 1:311–315, 1973.

36. Boulline DJ: The action of antidepressants on the effects of other drugs. *Primary Care* 2:669–688. 1975.

37. Boura ALA, Green AF: Adrenergic neurone blockade and other acute effects caused by N-benzyl-N'-N''-dimethylguanidine and its orthochloro derivative. *Br J Pharmacol* 20:36–55, 1963.

38. Boyce EG, Dukes GE, Rollins DE, Sudds TW: The effect of rifampin on theophylline kinetics. *J Clin Pharmacol* 26:696–699, 1986.

39. Braitwaite RA, Flanagan RJ, Richens A: Steady state plasma nortriptyline concentrations in epileptic patients. *Br J Clin Pharmacol* 2:469–471, 1975.

40. Branch RA, Shand DG, Wilkinson GR, Nies AS: The reduction of lidocaine clearance by dl-propranolol: An example of hemodynamic drug interaction. *J Pharmacol Exp Ther* 184:515–519, 1973.

41. Branigan TA, Robbin RA, Cady WJ, Nickols JG, Ueda CT: The effects of erythromycin on the absorption and disposition kinetics of theophylline. *Eur J Clin Pharmacol* 21:115–120, 1981.

42. Brater DC: Analysis of the effect of indomethacin on the response to furosemide in man. Effect of dose of furosemide. *J Pharmacol Exp Ther* 210:386–390, 1979.

43. Breen KJ, Bury R, Desmond PV, Mashford ML, Morphett B, Westwood B, Shaw RG: Effects of cimetidine and ranitidine on hepatic drug metabolism. *Clin Pharmacol Ther* 31:297–300, 1982.

44. Briant RH, Reid JL, Dollery CT: Interaction between clonidine and desipramine in man. *Br Med J* 1:522–523, 1973.

45. Brodie MJ, MacPhee GJA: Carbamazepine neurotoxicity precipitated by diltiazem. *Br Med J.* 292:1170–1171, 1986.

46. Brown DD, Juhl RP: Decreased bioavailability of digoxin due to antacids and kaolin pectin. *N Engl J Med* 295:1034–1037, 1976.

47. Brown DD, Juhl RP, Warner SL: Decreased bioavailability of digoxin due to hypocholesterolemia interventions. *Circulation* 58:164–172, 1978.

48. Brown DD, Spector R, Juhl RP: Drug interactions with digoxin. *Drugs* 20:198–206, 1980.

49. Buchanan RA, Heffelfinger JC, Weiss CF: The effect of phenobarbital on diphenylhydantoin metabolism in children. *Pediatrics* 43:114–116, 1969.

50. Burn JH, Rand MJ: The action of sympathomimetic amines in animals treated with reserpine. *J Physiol* 144:314–336, 1958.

51. Burns JJ, Conney AH: Enzyme stimulation and inhibition in the metabolism of drugs. *Proc R Soc Med* 58:955–960, 1965.

52. Cabizuca SV, Desser KB: Carbenicillin associated hypokalemic alkalosis. *JAMA* 236:956–957, 1976.

53. Caldwell JH, Greenberger NJ: Interruption of the enterohepatic circulation of digitoxin by cholestyramine. I. Protection against lethal digitoxin intoxication. *J Clin Invest* 50:2626–2637, 1971.

54. Campbell MA, Plachetka JR, Jackson JE, Moon JF, Finley PR: Cimetidine decreases theophylline clearance. *Ann Intern Med* 95:68–69, 1981.

55. Carrum G, Egan JM, Abernethy DR: Diltiazem treatment impairs hepatic drug oxidation: studies of antipyrine. *Clin Pharmacol Ther* 40:140–143, 1986.

56. Carruthers SG, Dujovne CA: Cholestyramine and spironolactone and their combination in digitoxin elimination. *Clin Pharmacol Ther* 27:184–187, 1980.

57. Carulli N, Manenti F, Gallo M, Salvioli GF: Alcohol-drugs interaction in man: alcohol and tolbutamide. *Eur J Clin Invest* 1:421–424, 1971.

58. Cate EW, Rogers JF, Powell JR: Inhibition of tolbutamide elimination by cimetidine but not ranitidine. *J Clin Pharmacol* 26:372–377, 1986.

59. Chang CC, Costa E, Brodie BB: Reserpine-induced release of drugs from sympathetic nerve endings. *Life Sci* 3:839–844, 1964.

60. Chen T-S, Friedman HS: Alteration of digoxin pharmacokinetics by a single dose of quinidine. *JAMA* 244:669–672, 1980.

61. Chennavasin P, Seiwell R, Brater DC: Pharmacokinetic-dynamic analysis of the indomethacin-furosemide interaction in man. *J Pharmacol Exp Ther* 215:77–81, 1980.

62. Christiansen J, Dam M: Influence of phenobarbital and diphenylhydantoin on plasma carbamazepine levels in patients with epilepsy. *Acta Neurol Scand* 49:543–546, 1973.

63. Christensen LK, Skovested L: Inhibition of drug metabolism by chloramphenicol. *Lancet* 2:1397–1399, 1969.

64. Christian CD, Meridith CG, Speeg KV: Cimetidine inhibits renal procainamide clearance. *Clin Pharmacol Ther* 36:221–227, 1984.

65. Cinquegrani MP, Liang C-S: Indomethacin attenuates the hypotensive action of hydralazine. *Clin Pharmacol Ther* 39:564–570, 1986.

66. Cluxton RJ, Rivera JO, Ritschel WA, Pesce AJ, Hanenson IB: Cimetidine-theophylline interaction (letter). *Ann Intern Med* 96:684, 1982.

67. Cocco G, Ague C: Interactions between cardioactive drugs and antidepressants. *Eur J Clin Pharmacol* 11:389–393, 1977.

68. Conney AH: Pharmacological implications of microsomal enzyme induction. *Pharmacol Rev* 19:317–366, 1967.

69. Cramer JL, Rosser RM, Crane G: Blood levels and management of lithium treatment. *Br Med J* 3:650–654, 1974.

70. Cucinell SA, Conney AH, Sansur M, Burns JJ: Drug interaction in man. I. Lowering effect of phenobarbital on plasma levels of bishydroxycoumarin (Dicumarol) and diphenylhydantoin (Dilantin). *Clin Pharmacol Ther* 6:420–429, 1965.

71. Curry SH, DeVane CL, Wolfe MM: Cimetidine interaction with amitriptyline. *Eur J Clin Pharmacol* 29:429–433, 1985.

72. Dam M, Kristensen B, Hansen BS, Christiansen J: Interaction between carbamazepine and propoxyphene in man. *Acta Neurol Scand* 56:602–607, 1977.

73. Data JL, Wilkinson GR, Nies AS: Interaction of quinidine with anticonvulsant drugs. *N Engl J Med* 294:699–702, 1976.

74. Davis JM, Bartlett E, Termini BS: Overdosage of psychotropic drugs. A review. *Dis Nerv Syst* 29:157–164, 246–256, 1986.

75. Day MD: Effect of sympathomimetic amines on the blocking action of guanethidine, bretylium, xylocholine. *Br J Pharmacol* 18:421–439, 1962.

76. Day MD, Rand MJ: Antagonism of guanethidine by dexamphetamine and other related sympathomimetic amines. *J Pharm Sci* 14:541–549, 1962.

77. Depaulo JR Jr, Correa EI, Sapir DG: Renal toxicity of lithium and its implications. *Johns Hopkins Med J* 149:15–21, 1981.

78. Desmond PV, Patwardhan RV, Schenker S, Speeg KV: Cimetidine impairs elimination of chlordiazepoxide (Librium) in man. *Ann Intern Med* 93:266–268, 1980.

79. Desmond PV, Patwardhan RV, Schenker S, Speeg KV: Short term ethanol administration impairs the elimination of chlordiazepoxide in man. *Eur J Clin Pharmacol* 18:275–278, 1980.

80. DeTeresa E, Vera A, Ortigosa J, Pulpon LA, Arus AP, DeArtaza M: Interaction between anticoagulants and contraceptives: an unsuspected finding. *Br Med J* 2:1260–1261, 1979.

81. DeVita VT, Hahn MA, Oliverio VT: Monoamine oxidase inhibition by a new carcinostatic agent, N-isopropyl-α-(2-methyl-hydrazino)-p-toluamide (MIH). *Proc Soc Exp Biol Med* 120:561–565, 1965.

82. Dhillon S, Richens A: Serum protein binding of diazepam and its displacement by valproic acid *in vitro*. *Br J Clin Pharmacol* 12:591–592, 1981.

83. Dobbs JH, Skoutakis VA, Acchardio SR, Dobbs BR: Effects of aluminum hydroxide on the absorption of propranolol. *Curr Ther Res* 21:877–892, 1977.

84. Doering W: Quinidine-digoxin interaction. Pharmacokinetics, underlying mechanism and clinical implications. *N Engl J Med* 301:400–404, 1979.

85. Dorian P, Sellers EM, Carruthers G, Hamilton C, Fan T: Propranolol-ethanol pharmacokinetic interaction. *Clin Pharmacol Ther* 31:219, 1982.

86. Durao B, Rico JMGT: Modification by indomethacin of the blood pressure lowering effect of pindolol and propranolol in conscious rabbits. *Eur J Pharmacol* 43:377–381, 1977.

87. Durao V, Prata MM, Gonclaves LMP: Modifications of antihypertensive effect of β-adrenoceptor-blocking agents by inhibition of endogenous prostaglandin synthesis. *Lancet* 2:1005–1007, 1977.

88. Easton PA, Koval A: Hypertensive reaction with sulindac. *Can Med Assoc J* 122:1273–1274, 1980.

89. Evans DAA, Mantey KA, McKusick VA: Genetic control of isoniazid metabolism in man. *Br Med J* 2:485–491, 1960.

90. Fann WE, Cavanaugh JH, Kaufmann JS: Doxepin: effects of transport of biogenic amines in man. *Psychopharmacologia* 22:111–125, 1972.

91. Fann WE, Davis JM, Janowsky DS, Sekerke WJ, Schmidt DM: Chlorpromazine: effects of antacids on its gastrointestinal absorption. *J Clin Pharmacol* 13:388–390, 1973.

92. Feely J, Wilkinson GR, McAllister CB, Wood AJJ: Increased toxicity and reduced clearance of lidocaine by cimetidine. *Ann Intern Med* 96:592–594, 1982.

93. Feely J, Wilkinson GR, Wood AJJ: Reduction of liver blood flow and propranolol metabolism by cimetidine. *N Engl J Med* 304:692–695, 1981.

94. Feely J, Wood AJJ: Effect of inhibitors of prostaglandin synthesis on hepatic drug clearance. *Br J Clin Pharmacol* 15:109–111, 1983.

95. Fenster PE, Hager WD, Goodman MM: Digoxin-quinidine-spironolactone interaction. *Clin Pharmacol Ther* 36:70–73, 1984.

96. Fine A, Henderson IS, Morgan DR, Wilstone WJ: Malabsorption of furosemide caused by phenytoin. *Br Med J* 2:1061–1062, 1977.

97. Fowler NO, McCall D, Chou T, Holmes JC, Hanenson IB: Electrocardiographic changes and cardiac arrhythmias in patients receiving psychotropic drugs. *Am J Cardiol* 37:223–230, 1976.

98. Fraser DG, Ludden TM, Evans RP, Sutherland EW: Displacement of phenytoin from plasma binding sites by salicylate. *Clin Pharmacol Ther* 27:165–169, 1980.

99. Freeman DJ, Laupacis A, Keown PA, Stiller CR, Carruthers SC: Evaluation of cyclosporin-phenytoin interaction with observations on cyclosporin metabolites. *Br J Clin Pharmacol* 18:887–893, 1984.

100. Frolich JC, Leftwich R, Ragheb M, Oates JA, Reimann I, Buchanan D: Indomethacin increases plasma lithium. *Br Med J* 1:1115–1116, 1979.

101. Fujita T, Yamashita N, Yamashita K: Effect of indo-

methacin on antihypertensive action of captopril in hypertension patients. *Clin Exp Hypertension* 3:939–952, 1981.

102. Gambertoglio JH, Holford NHG, Kapusnik JE, Nishikawa R, Saltiel M, Stanik-Lizak P, Birnbaum JL, Hau T, Amend WJC Jr: Disposition of total and unbound prednisolone in renal transplant patients receiving anticonvulsants. *Kidney Int* 25:119–123, 1984.

103. Garnett WR, Carter BL, Bellock JM: Bioavailability of phenytoin administered with antacids. *Ther Drug Monitoring* 1:435–437, 1979.

104. Garrettson LK, Perel JM, Dayton PG: Methylphenidate interaction with both anticonvulsants and ethyl discoumacetate. *JAMA* 207:2053–2056, 1969.

105. Garty M, Hurwitz A: Effect of cimetidine and antacids on intestinal absorption of tetracycline. *Clin Pharmacol Ther* 28:203–207, 1980.

106. Gault H, Longerich L, Dawe M, Fine A: Digoxin-rifampin interaction. *Clin Pharmacol Ther* 35:750–754, 1984.

107. Geleherter TD: Enzyme induction. *N Engl J Med* 294:522–526, 589–595, 646–651, 1976.

108. Gibbons DO, Lant AF: Effects of intravenous and oral propantheline and metoclopramide on ethanol absorption. *Clin Pharmacol Ther* 17:578–584, 1975.

109. Gibson TP, Quintanilla AP: Effect of quinidine on the renal handling of digoxin. *J Lab Clin Med* 96:1062–1070, 1980.

110. Gibson TP, Quintanilla AP: Effect of volume expansion and furosemide diuresis on the renal clearance of digoxin. *J Pharmacol Exp Ther* 219:54–59, 1981.

111. Gill MA, DuBe JE, Young WW: Hypokalemic, metabolic alkalosis induced by high-dose ampicillin sodium. *Am J Hosp Pharm* 34:528–531, 1977.

112. Glynn AM, Slaughter RL, Brass C, D'Ambrosio R, Jusko WJ: Effects of ketoconazole on methylprednisolone pharmacokinetics and cortisol secretion. *Clin Pharmacol Ther* 39:654–659, 1986.

113. Gokhale SD, Gulati OD, Udwadia BP: Antagonism of the adrenergic neurone blocking action of guanethidine by certain antidepressant and antihistamine drugs. *Arch Int Pharmacodyn* 160:321–329, 1966.

114. Gore JM, Haffajee CI, Alpert JS: Interaction of amiodarone and diphenylhydantoin. *Am J Cardiol* 54:1145, 1984.

115. Greenblatt DJ, Abernethy DR, Morse DS, Harmatz JS, Shader RI: Clinical importance of the interaction of diazepam and cimetidine. *N Engl J Med* 310:1639–1643, 1984.

116. Greenblatt DH, Allen DA, Maclaughlin DS, Harmatz JS, Shader RJ: Diazepam absorption: effect of antacids and food. *Clin Pharmacol Ther* 24:600–609, 1978.

117. Greenblatt DJ, Duhme DW, Allen MD, Koch-Weser J: Clinical toxicity of furosemide in hospitalized patients. *Am Heart J* 94:6–13, 1977.

118. Greenblatt DJ, Shader RI, Harmatz JS, Franke K, Koch-Weser J: Influence of magnesium and aluminum hydroxide mixture on chlordiazepoxide absorption. *Clin Pharmacol Ther* 19:234–239, 1976.

119. Griffith RS, Black HR, Brier GL, Wolny JD: Effect of probenecid on the blood levels and urinary excretion of cefamandole. *Antimicrob Agents Chemother* 11:809–812, 1977.

120. Grygiel JJ, Brikett DJ: Cigarette smoking and theophylline clearance and metabolism. *Clin Pharmacol Ther* 30:491–496, 1981.

121. Guay DRP, Meatherall RC, Chalmers JL, Grahame GR: Cimetidine alters pethidine disposition in man. *Br J Clin Pharmacol* 18:907–914, 1984.

122. Gugler R, Brand M, Somogyi A: Impaired cimetidine absorption by antacids and metoclopramide. *Eur J Clin Pharmacol* 20:225–228, 1981.

123. Hager WD, Fenster P, Mayersohn M, Perrier D, Graves P, Marcus FI, Goldman S: Digoxin-quinidine interaction. Pharmacokinetic evaluation. *N Engl J Med* 300:1238–1241, 1979.

124. Hanahoe THP, Ireson JD, Large BJ: Interactions between guanethidine and inhibitors of noradrenaline uptake. *Arch Int Pharmacodyn* 182:349–353, 1969.

125. Hansen JM, Kristensen M, Skovsted L: Sulthiame (Opsollot^R) an inhibitor of diphenylhydantoin metabolism. *Epilepsia* 9:17–22, 1968.

126. Hansen JM, Siersbaek-Nielsen K, Kristensen M, Skovsted L, Christensen LK: Effects of diphenylhydantoin on the metabolism of dicoumarol in man. *Acta Med Scand* 189:15–19, 1971.

127. Hansen JM, Siersbaek-Nielsen K, Skovsted L: Carbamazepine-induced acceleration of diphenylhydantoin and warfarin metabolism in man. *Clin Pharmacol Ther* 12:539–543, 1971.

128. Hansen PD: *Drug Interactions*. Philadelphia, Lea & Febiger, 1985.

129. Harrington RA, Hamilton CW, Brogden RN, Linkewich JA, Romankiewicz JA, Heel RC: Metoclopramide: an updated review of its pharmacological properties and clinical use. *Drugs* 25:451–494, 1983.

130. Harvey VJ, Slevin ML, Dilloway MR, Clark PI, Johnston A, Lant AF: The influence of cimetidine on the pharmacokinetics of 5-fluorouracil. *Br J Clin Pharmacol* 18:421–430, 1984.

131. Haworth E, Burroughs AK: Disopyramide and warfarin interaction. *Br Med J* 2:866–867, 1977.

132. Heagerty AM, Castleden CM, Patel I: Failure of ranitidine to interact with propranolol. *Br Med J* 284:1304, 1982.

133. Henaver SA, Hollister LE: Cimetidine interaction with imipramine and nortriptyline. *Clin Pharmacol Ther* 35:183–187, 1984.

134. Henderson JM, Ibrahim SZ, Millikan WJ Jr, Santi M, Warren WD: Cimetidine does not reduce liver blood flow in cirrhosis. *Hepatology* 3:919–922, 1983.

135. Hetzel DJ, Bochner F, Hallpike F, Shearman DJC, Hann CS: Cimetidine interaction with phenytoin. *Br Med J* 282:1512, 1981.

136. Hibbard DM, Peters JR, Hunninghake DB: Effects of cholestyramine and colestipol on the plasma concentrations of propranolol. *Br J Clin Pharmacol* 18:337–342, 1984.

137. Himmelhoch JM, Poust RI, Mallinger AG: Adjustment of lithium dose during lithium-chlorothiazide therapy. *Clin Pharmacol Ther* 22:225–227, 1977.

138. Hirsh PD, Weiner HJ, North RL: Further insights into digoxin-quinidine interaction: lack of correlation between serum digoxin concentration and inotropic state of the heart. *Am J Cardiol* 46:863–867, 1980.

139. Holt DW, Hayler AM, Edmonds ME, Ashford RF: Clinically significant interaction between digoxin and quinidine. *Br Med J* 2:1401, 1979.

140. Hurwitz A: The effects of antacids on gastrointestinal drug absorption II. Effect on sulfadiazine and quinine. *J Pharmacol Exp Ther* 179:485–490, 1971.

141. Hurwitz A, Schlozman DL: Effects of antacids on gastrointestinal absorption of isoniazid in rat and man. *Am Rev Respir Dis* 109:41–47, 1974.

142. Jackson JE: Reduction of blood flow by cimetidine (letter). *N Engl J Med* 305:99–100, 1981.

143. Jackson JE, Powell JR, Wandell M, Bentley J, Dorr R: Cimetidine decreases theophylline clearance. *Am Rev Respir Dis* 123:615–617, 1981.

144. Jahnchen E, Meinertz T, Gilfrich H-J, Kersting F, Groth V: Enhanced elimination of warfarin during treatment with cholestyramine. *Br J Clin Pharmacol* 5:437–440, 1978.

145. Janowsky DS, El-Yousef MK, Davis JM, Fann WE: Antagonism of guanethidine by chlorpromazine. *Am J Psychiatry* 130:808–812, 1973.

146. Jefferson JW, Kalin NH: Serum lithium levels and long-term diuretic use. *JAMA* 241:1134–1136, 1979.

147. Jogestrand T, Schenck-Gustafsson K, Nordlander R, Dahlqvist R: Quinidine-induced changes in serum and skeletal muscle digoxin concentration; evidence of

saturable binding of digoxin to skeletal muscle. *Eur J Clin Pharmacol* 27:571–575, 1984.

148. Johnson BF, Bustrack JA, Urbach DR, Hull JH, Marwaha R: Effect of metoclopramide on digoxin absorption from tablets and capsules. *Clin Pharmacol Ther* 36:724–730, 1984.

149. Juhl RP, Summers RW, Guillory JK, Blang SM, Cheng RH, Brown DD: Effect of sulfasalazine on digoxin bioavailability. *Clin Pharmacol Ther* 20:387–394, 1976.

150. Kabins SA: Interactions among antibiotics and other drugs. *JAMA* 219:206–212, 1972.

151. Kampmann J, Hansen JM, Siersbaek-Nielsen K, Laursen H: Effect of some drugs on penicillin half-life in blood. *Clin Pharmacol Ther* 13:516–519, 1972.

152. Kanto J, Allonen HJ, Jalonen H, Mantyla R: The effect of metoclopramide and propantheline on the gastrointestinal absorption of cimetidine. *Br J Pharmacol* 11:527–530, 1981.

153. Kater RMH, Roggin G, Tobon F, Zieve P, Iber FL: Increased rate of clearance of drugs from the circulation of alcoholics. *Am J Med Sci* 258:35–39, 1969.

154. Kauffman RE, Azarnoff DL: Effect of colestipol on gastrointestinal absorption of chlorothiazide in man. *Clin Pharmacol Ther* 14:886–889, 1973.

155. Kay L, Kampmann JP, Svendsen TL, Vergman B, Hansen JE, Skovsted L, Kristensen M: Influence of rifampicin and isoniazid on the kinetics of phenytoin. *Br J Clin Pharmacol* 20:323–326, 1985.

156. Keilholz U, Guthrie GP Jr: Case Report: adverse effect of phenytoin on mineralocorticoid replacement with fludrocortisone in adrenal insufficiency. *Am J Med Sci* 291:280–283, 1986.

157. Kelly HW, Powell JR, Donohue JF: Ranitidine at very large doses does not inhibit theophylline elimination. *Clin Pharmacol Ther* 39:577–581, 1986.

158. Khalil SAH: Bioavailability of digoxin in presence of antacids. *J Pharm Sci* 63:1641–1642, 1974 (letter).

159. Kiorboe E: Phenytoin intoxication during treatment with Antabuse^R (disulfiram). *Epilepsia* 7:246–249, 1966.

160. Kirby MG, Dasta JF, Armstrong DK, Tallman R Jr: Effect of low-dose dopamine on the pharmacokinetics of tobramycin in dogs. *Antimicrob Agents Chemother* 29:168–170, 1986.

161. Kitto W: Antibiotics and the ingestion of alcohol. *JAMA* 193:411, 1965.

162. Klotz U, Reimann IW: Delayed clearance of diazepam due to cimetidine. *N Engl J Med* 304:1012–1014, 1980.

163. Klotz V, Reimann IW, Ohnhaus EE: Effect of ranitidine on the steady state pharmacokinetics of diazepam. *Eur J Clin Pharmacol* 24:357–360, 1983.

164. Knodell RG, Holtzman JL, Crankshaw DL, Steele NM, Stanley LN: Drug metabolism by rat and human hepatic microsomes in response to interaction with H_2-receptor antagonist. *Gastroenterology* 82:84–88, 1982.

165. Kochar MS, Itskovitz HD: Effects of hydrochlorothiazide in hypertensive patients and the need for potassium supplementation. *Curr Ther Res* 15:298–304, 1973.

166. Koch-Weser J: Drug interactions in cardiovascular therapy. *Am Heart J* 90:93–116, 1975.

167. Koch-Weser J, Sellers EM: Binding of drugs to serum albumin. *N Engl J Med* 294:311–316, 526–531, 1976.

168. Koch-Weser J, Sellers EM: Drug interactions with coumarin anticoagulants. *N Engl J Med* 285:487–498, 547–558, 1971.

169. Koup JR, Gilbaldi M, McNamara P, Hilligoss DM, Colburn WA, Bruck E: Interaction of chloramphenicol with phenytoin and phenobarbital. *Clin Pharmacol Ther* 24:571–575, 1978.

170. Kuhlmann J, Dohrmann M, Marcin S: Effects of quinidine on pharmacokinetics and pharmacodynamics of digitoxin achieving steady-state conditions. *Clin Pharmacol Ther* 39:288–294, 1986.

171. Kulshrestha VK, Thomas M, Wadsworth J, Richens A: Interaction of phenytoin and antacids. *Br J Clin Pharmacol* 6:177–179, 1978.

172. Kutt H, Brennan R, Dehejia H, Verebely K: Diphenylhydantoin intoxication. A complication of isoniazid therapy. *Am Rev Resp Dis* 101:377–384, 1970.

173. Kutt H, Haynes J, Verebely K, McDowell F: The effect of phenobarbital on plasma diphenylhydantoin level and metabolism in man and in rat liver microsomes. *Neurology* 19:611–616, 1969.

174. Kutt H, Verebely K, McDowell F: Inhibition of diphenylhydantoin metabolism in rats and in rat liver microsomes by antitubercular drugs. *Neurology* 18:706–710, 1968.

175. Kutt H, Wolk M, Scherman R, McDowell F: Insufficient para-hydroxylation as a cause of diphenylhydantoin toxicity. *Neurology* 14:542–548, 1964.

176. LaDu BN: Pharmacogenetics. *Med Clin North Am* 53:839–85, 1969.

177. Landay RA, Gonzalez MA, Taylor JC: Effect of phenobarbital on theophylline disposition. *J Allerg Clin Immunol* 62:27–29, 1978.

178. Lane EA, Guthrie S, Linnoila M: Effects of ethanol on drug and metabolite pharmacokinetics. *Clin Pharmacokinet* 10:228–247, 1985.

179. Lau A, Lee M, Flascha S, Prasad R, Sharifi R: Effect of piperacillin on tobramycin pharmacokinetics in patients with normal renal function. *Antimicrob Agents Chemother* 24:533–537, 1983.

180. Lawson DH, Tilstone WJ, Gray JMB, Srivastava PK: Effect of furosemide on the pharmacokinetics of gentamicin in patients. *J Clin Pharmacol* 22:254–258, 1982.

181. Leahey EB, Rieffel JA, Drusin RE, Heissenbuttel RH, Lovejoy WP, Bigger JT: Interaction between quinidine and digoxin. *JAMA* 240:533–534, 1978.

182. Leahey EB, Reiffel JA, Giardina E-GV, Bigger JT: The effect of quinidine and other oral antiarrhythmic drugs on serum digoxin. *Ann Intern Med* 92:605–608, 1980.

183. Leahey EB, Reiffel JA, Heissenbuttel RH, Drusin RE, Lovejoy WP, Bigger JT: Enhanced cardiac effect of digoxin during quinidine treatment. *Arch Intern Med* 139:519–521, 1979.

184. Legler UF, Benet LZ: Marked alterations in dose-dependent prednisolone kinetics in women taking oral contraceptives. *Clin Pharmacol Ther* 39:425–429, 1986.

185. Lejonc JL, Gusmini D, Brochard P: Isoniazid and reaction to cheese (letter). *Ann Intern Med* 91:793, 1979.

186. Levine RR: Factors affecting gastrointestinal absorption of drugs. *Am J Digest Dis* 15:171–188, 1970.

187. Levy G: Gastrointestinal clearance of drugs with activated treated charcoal (editorial). *N Engl J Med* 307:676–678, 1982.

188. Levy G, Lampman T, Kamath BL, Garrettson LK: Decreased serum salicylate concentration in children with rheumatic fever treated with antacid. *N Engl J Med* 293:323–325, 1975.

189. Lewis GP, Holtzman JL: Interaction of flecainide with digoxin and propranolol. *Am J Cardiol* 53:52B–57B, 1984.

190. Lewis JG: Adverse reactions to calcium antagonists. *Drugs* 25:196–222, 1983.

191. Lindenbaum J, Maulitz RM, Butler VP: Inhibition of digoxin absorption by neomycin. *Gastroenterology* 71:399–404, 1976.

192. Lindenbaum J, Rund DH, Butler VP, Tse-Eng D, Saha JR: Inactivation of digoxin by the gut flora: reversal by antibiotic therapy. *N Engl J Med* 305:789–794, 1981.

193. Linnoila M, Mattila MJ, Kitchell BS: Drug interactions with alcohol. *Drugs* 18:229–311, 1979.

194. Lopez-Ovejero JA, Weber MA, Drayer JIM, Sealey JE, Laragh JH: Effects of indomethacin alone and during diuretic or β-adrenoreceptor-blockade therapy on blood pressure and the renin system in essential hypertension. *Clin Sci Mol Med* 55:203–205, 1978.

195. Lumholtz B, Siersbaek-Nielsen K, Skovsted L, Kampmann J, Hensen JM: Sulfamethizole-induced inhibition of diphenylhydantoin, tolbutamide, and warfarin

metabolism. *Clin Pharmacol Ther* 17:731–734, 1975.

196. MacLeod SM, Giles HG, Patzalek G, Thiessen JJ, Sellers EM: Diazepam actions and plasma concentrations following ethanol ingestion. *Eur J Clin Pharmacol* 11:346–349, 1977.

197. MacLeod SM, Sellers EM: Pharmacodynamic and pharmacokinetic drug interactions with coumarin anticoagulants. *Drugs* 11:461–470, 1976.

198. MacLeod SM, Sellers EM, Giles HG, Billings BJ, Martin PR, Greenblatt DJ, Marshman JA: Interaction of disulfiram with benzodiazepines. *Clin Pharmacol Ther* 24:583–589, 1978.

199. Macphee GJA, Thompson GG, McInnes GT, Brodie MJ: Verapamil potentiates carbamazepine neurotoxicity: a clinically important inhibitory interaction. *Lancet* 1:700–703, 1986.

200. Macphee GJA, Thompson GG, Scobie G, Agnew E, Park BK, Murray T, McColl KEL, Brodie MJ: Effects of cimetidine on carbamazepine auto- and hetero-induction in man. *Br J Clin Pharmacol* 18:411–419, 1984.

201. Manfred RL, Vesell ES: Inhibition of theophylline metabolism by long-term allopurinol administration. *Clin Pharmacol Ther* 29:224–229, 1981.

202. Manninen V, Apajalahti A, Simonen H, Reissel P: Effect of propantheline and metoclopramide on absorption of digoxin. *Lancet* 1:398, 1973.

203. Martell R, Heinrichs D, Stiller CR, Jenner M, Keown PA, Dupre J: The effects of erythromycin in patients treated with cyclosporine. *Ann Intern Med* 104:660–661, 1986.

204. Mattson RH, Cramer JA, Williamson PC, Novelly RA: Valproic acid in epilepsy: clinical and pharmacological effects. *Ann Neurol* 3:20–25, 1978.

205. May CD, Jarboe CH: Inhibition of clearance of dyphylline by probenecid (letter). *N Engl J Med* 304:791, 1981.

206. May DC, Jarboe CH, Ellenburg DT, Roe EJ, Karibo J: The effects of erythromycin on theophylline elimination in normal males. *J Clin Pharmacol* 22:125–130, 1982.

207. McElnay JC, D'Arcy PF: Protein binding displacement interactions and their clinical importance. *Drugs* 25:495–513, 1983.

208. McGovern B, Geer VR, LaRaia PJ, Garan H, Ruskin JN: Possible interaction between amiodarone and phenytoin. *Ann Intern Med* 101:650–651, 1984.

209. McMurty RJ: Propranolol, hypoglycemia, and hypertensive crisis. *Ann Intern Med* 80:669–670, 1974.

210. Melmon KL, Nierenberg DW: Drug interactions and the prepared observer (editorial). *N Engl J Med* 304:723–724, 1981.

211. Mihaly GW, Marino AT, Webster LK, Jones DB, Louis WJ, Smallwood RA: High dose of antacid (Mylanta II) reduces bioavailability of ranitidine. *Br Med J* 285:998–999, 1982.

212. Miller M, Cosgriff J, Kwong T, Morken DA: Influence of phenytoin on theophylline clearance. *Clin Pharmacol Ther* 35:666–669, 1984.

213. Miller RP, Bates JH: Amphotericin B toxicity. A follow-up report of 53 patients. *Ann Intern Med* 71:1089–1095, 1969.

214. Milne MD, Scribner BH, Crawford MA: Non-ionic diffusion and the excretion of weak acids and bases. *Am J Med* 24:709–729, 1958.

215. Misage JR, McDonald RH: Antagonism of hypotensive action of bethanidine by "common cold" remedy. *Br Med J* 4:347, 1974.

216. Misra PS, Leferve A, Ishii H, Rubin E, Lieber CS: Increase of ethanol, mebrobamate and pentobarbital metabolism after chronic ethanol administration in man and rats. *Am J Med* 51:346–351, 1971.

217. Mitchell JR, Arias L, Oates JA: Antagonism of the antihypertensive action of guanethidine sulfate by desipramine hydrochloride. *JAMA* 202:973–976, 1967.

218. Mitchell JR, Cavanaugh JH, Arias L, Oates JA: Guaneth-

idine and related agents. III. Antagonism by drugs which inhibit the norepinephrine pump in man. *J Clin Invest* 49:1596–1604, 1970.

219. Mitchell MC, Hanew T, Meredith CG, Schenker S: Effects of oral contraceptive steroids on acetaminophen metabolism and elimination. *Clin Pharmacol Ther* 34:48–53, 1983.

220. Mitchell MC, Schnecker S, Speeg KV: Selective inhibition of acetaminophen oxidation and toxicity by cimetidine and other histamine H_2 receptor antagonists *in vivo* and *in vitro* in the rat and in man. *J Clin Invest* 73:383–391, 1984.

221. Moore TJ, Crantz TR, Hollenberg NK, Koletsky RJ, Leboff MS, Swartz SL, Levine L, Podolsky S, Dluhy RG, Williams GH: Contribution of prostaglandins to the antihypertensive action of captopril in essential hypertension. *Hypertension* 3:168–173, 1981.

222. Muirhead MR, Somogyi AA, Rolan PE, Bochner F: Effect of cimetidine on renal and hepatic drug elimination: studies with triamterene. *Clin Pharmacol Ther* 40:400–407, 1986.

223. Mungall DR, Robichaux RP, Perry W, Scott JW, Robinson A, Burelle T, Hurst D: Effects of quinidine on serum digoxin concentration. *Ann Intern Med* 93:689–693, 1980.

224. Murphy DL, Bunney WE, Jr: Total body potassium changes during lithium administration. *J Nerv Ment Dis* 152:381–389, 1971.

225. Murray FJ: Outbreak of unexpected reactions among epileptics taking isoniazid. *Am Rev Respir Dis* 86:729–732, 1962.

226. Murrell GAC, Rapeport WG: Clinical pharmacokinetics of allopurinol. *Clin Pharmacokinet* 11:343–353, 1986.

227. Neuvonen PJ: Clinical pharmacokinetics of oral activated charcoal in acute intoxication. *Clin Pharmacokinet* 7:465–489, 1982.

228. Neuvonen PJ, Elfring SM, Elonen E: Reduction of absorption of digoxin, phenytoin and aspirin by activated charcoal in man. *Eur J Clin Pharmacol* 13:213–218, 1978.

229. Neuvonen PJ, Elonen E: Effect of activated charcoal on absorption and elimination of phenobarbitone, carbamazepine, and phenylbutazone in man. *Eur J Clin Pharmacol* 17:51–57, 1980.

230. Neuvonen PJ, Kannisto H, Hirvisalo EL: Effect of activated charcoal on absorption of tolbutamide and valproate in man. *Eur J Clin Pharmacol* 24:243–246, 1983.

231. Neuvonen PJ, Lehtovaara R, Bardy A, Elonen E: Antipyrine analgesics in patients on antiepileptic drug therapy. *Eur J Clin Pharmacol* 15:263–268, 1979.

232. Neuvonen PJ, Tokola RA, Kaste M: Cimetidine-phenytoin interactions: effect on serum phenytoin concentration and antipyrine test in man. *Eur J Clin Pharmacol* 21:215–220, 1981.

233. Newton RW: Physostigmine salicylate in the treatment of tricyclic antidepressant overdosage. *JAMA* 231:941–944, 1974.

234. Nierenberg DW: Competitive inhibition of methotrexate in kidney slices by nonsteroidal anti-inflammatory drugs. *J Pharmacol Exp Ther* 226:1–6, 1983.

235. Nies AS: Adverse reactions and interactions limiting the use of antihypertensive drugs. *Am J Med* 58:495–503, 1975.

236. Nies AS, Shand DG: Hypertensive response to propranolol in a patient treated with methyl dopa—a proposed mechanism. *Clin Pharmacol Ther* 14:823–826, 1973.

237. Nimmo WS, Heading RC, Tothill P, Prescott LF: Pharmacological evaluation of gastric emptying: effect of propantheline and metoclopramide on paracetamol absorption. *Br Med J* 1:587–589, 1973.

238. Nimmo WS, Heading RC, Wilson J, Tothill P, Prescott LF: Inhibition of gastric emptying and drug absorption

by narcotic analgesics. *Br J Clin Pharmacol* 2:502–513, 1975.

239. Noble J, Matthew H: Acute poisoning by antidepressants: clinical features and management of 100 patients. *Clin Toxicol* 2:403–421, 1969.

240. Ochs HR, Carstens G, Greenblatt DJ: Reduction in lidocaine clearance during continuous infusion and by coadministration of propranolol. *N Engl J Med* 303:373–377, 1980.

241. Ochs HR, Greenblatt DJ, Gugler R: Cimetidine impairs nitrazepam clearance. *Clin Pharmacol Ther* 34:227–230, 1983.

242. Ochs HR, Greenblatt DJ, Verburg-Ochs B: Propranolol interactions with diazepam, lorazepam, and alprazolam. *Clin Pharmacol Ther* 36:451–455, 1984.

243. Olesen OV: Disulfiram (Antabuse^R) as inhibitor of phenytoin metabolism. *Acta Pharmacol Toxicol* 24:317–322, 1966.

244. O'Reilly RA: Comparative interaction of cimetidine and ranitidine with racemic warfarin in man. *Arch Intern Med* 144:989–991, 1984.

245. O'Reilly RA: Interaction of chronic daily warfarin therapy and rifampin. *Ann Intern Med* 83:506–508, 1975.

246. O'Reilly RA: Interaction of sodium warfarin and disulfiram (Antabuse^R) in man. *Ann Intern Med* 78:73–76, 1973.

247. O'Reilly RA: Interaction of sodium warfarin and rifampin. *Ann Intern Med* 81:337–340, 1974.

248. O'Reilly RA: Stereoselective interaction of trimethoprim-sulfamethoxazole with the separated enantiomers of racemic warfarin in man. *N Engl J Med* 302:33–35, 1980.

249. O'Reilly RA: The stereoselective interaction of warfarin and metronidazole in man. *N Engl J Med* 295:354–357, 1976.

250. Orr JM, Abott FS, Farrell K, Ferguson S, Sheppard L, Godolphin W: Interaction between valproic acid and aspirin in epileptic children: serum protein binding and metabolic effects. *Clin Pharmacol Ther* 31:642–649, 1982.

251. Osman MA, Patel RB, Schuna A, Sundstrom WR, Welling PG: Reduction in oral penicillamine absorption by food, antacid and ferrous sulfate. *Clin Pharmacol Ther* 33:465–470, 1983.

252. Osman MA, Welling PG: Influence of propantheline and metaclopramide on the bioavailability of chlorothiazide. *Curr Ther Res* 34:404–408, 1983.

253. Packer M, Meller J, Medina N, Yushak M, Smith H, Holt J, Guererro J, Todd GD, McAllister RG, Gorlin R: Hemodynamic consequences of combined beta-adrenergic and slow calcium channel blockade in man. *Circulation* 65:660–668, 1982.

254. Parsons, RL, Paddock GM: Absorption of two antibacterial drugs, cephalexin and co-trimoxazole in malabsorption syndromes. *J Antimicrob Chemother* 1(suppl):59–67, 1975.

255. Patak RV, Mookerjee BK, Bentzel CJ, Hysert PE, Babej M, Lee JB: Antagonism of the effects of furosemide by indomethacin in normal and hypertensive man. *Prostaglandins* 10:649–659, 1980.

256. Patwardhan RV, Yarborough GW, Desmond PV, Johnson RF, Schenker S, Speeg KV: Cimetidine spares the glucuronidation of lorazepam and oxazepam. *Gastroenterology* 79:912–916, 1980.

257. Pedersen AK, Jackobsen P, Kampmann JP, Hansen JM: Clinical pharmacokinetics and potentially important drug interactions of sulphinpyrazone. *Clin Pharmacokinet* 7:42–56, 1982.

258. Pentikainen PJ, Koivula IH, Hiltunen HA: Effect of rifampicin treatment on the kinetics of mexiletine. *Eur J Clin Pharmacol* 23:261–266, 1982.

259. Penttila O, Neuvonen PJ, Aho K, Lehtovarra R: Interaction between doxycycline and some antiepileptic drugs. *Br Med J* 2:470–472, 1974.

260. Perel JM, Dayton PG, Snell MM, Yu TF, Gutman AB: Studies of interactions among drugs in man at the renal level: probenecid and sulfinpyrazone. *Clin Pharmacol Ther* 10:834–840, 1969.

261. Perucca E: Pharmacokinetic interactions with antiepileptic drugs. *Clin Pharmacokinet* 7:57–84, 1982.

262. Perucca E, Hebdige S, Gatti G, Leccini S, Frigo BM, Crema A: Interaction between phenytoin and valproic acid: plasma protein binding and metabolic effects. *Clin Pharmacol Ther* 28:779–789, 1980.

263. Perucca E, Richens A: Drug interactions with phenytoin. *Drugs* 21:120–137, 1981.

264. Petereit LB, Meikle AW: Effectiveness of prednisolone during phenytoin therapy. *Clin Pharmacol Ther* 22:912–916, 1977.

265. Peters L: Renal tubular excretion of organic bases. *Pharmacol Rev* 12:1–35, 1960.

266. Pickering IK, Rutherford I: Effect of concentration and time upon inactivation of tobramycin, gentamicin, netilmicin and amikacin by azlocillin carbenicillin, mecillinam, mezlocillin and piperacillin. *J Pharmacol Exp Ther* 217:345–349, 1981.

267. Pinell OC, Fenimore DC, Davis GM, Fann WE: Drug-drug interactions of chlorpromazine and antacids (abstract). *Clin Pharmacol Ther* 23:125, 1978.

268. Pond SM, Birkett DJ, Wade DN: Mechanisms of inhibition of tolbutamide metabolism: phenylbutazone, oxyphenbutazone, sulfaphenazole. *Clin Pharmacol Ther* 22:573–579, 1978.

269. Pond SM, Graham GG, Birkett DJ, Wade DN: Effects of tricyclic antidepressants on drug metabolism. *Clin Pharmacol Ther* 18:191–199, 1975.

270. Powell JR, Rogers JF, Wargin WA, Cross RE, Eshelman FN: Inhibition of theophylline clearance by cimetidine but not ranitidine. *Arch Intern Med* 144:484–486, 1984.

271. Prescott LF: Mechanisms of renal excretion of drugs. *Br J Anaesth* 44:246–251, 1972.

272. Prescott LF: Pharmacokinetic drug interactions. *Lancet* 2:1239–1243, 1969.

273. Prichard BNC, Ross EJ: Use of propranolol in conjunction with alpha receptor blocking drugs in pheochromocytoma. *Am J Cardiol* 18:394–398, 1966.

274. Prober CG: Effect of rifampin on chloramphenicol levels. *N Engl J Med* 312:788–789, 1985.

275. Puschett JB, Rastegar A: Comparative study of the effects of metolazone and other diuretics on potassium excretion. *Clin Pharmacol Ther* 15:397–405, 1974.

276. Puurunen J, Solaniemi E, Pelkonen O: Effect of cimetidine on microsomal drug metabolism in man. *Eur J Clin Pharmacol* 18:185–187, 1980.

277. Reimann IW, Frolich JC: Effects of diclofenac on lithium kinetics. *Clin Pharmacol Ther* 30:348–352, 1981.

278. Reitberg DP, Bernhard H, Schentag JJ: Alteration of theophylline clearance and half-life by cimetidine in normal volunteers. *Ann Intern Med* 95:582–586, 1981.

279. Rendic S, Alebic-Kolbah T, Kajfez F: Interaction of ranitidine with liver microsomes. *Xenobiotica* 12:9–17, 1982.

280. Rennick BR: Renal excretion of drugs: tubular transport and metabolism. *Annu Rev Pharmacol* 12:141–156, 1972.

281. Rennick BR: Renal tubule transport of organic cations. *Am J Physiol* 240:F83–F89, 1981.

282. Renton KW, Gray JD, Hung OR: Depression of theophylline elimination by erythromycin. *Clin Pharmacol Ther* 30:422–426, 1981.

283. Richer C, Mathieu M, Bah H, Thuillex C, Duroux P, Giudicelli J-F: Theophylline kinetics and ventilatory flow in bronchial asthma and chronic airflow obstruction: influence of erythromycin. *Clin Pharmacol Ther* 31:579–586, 1982.

284. Robinson DS, Benjamin DM, McCormack JJ: Interaction of warfarin and nonsystemic gastrointestinal drugs. *Clin Pharmacol Ther* 12:491–495, 1971.

285. Robson RA, Miners JO, Wing LMH, Birkett DJ: Theophylline-rifampin interaction: non-selective induc-

tion of theophylline metabolic pathways. *Br J Clin Pharmacol* 18:445–448, 1984.

286. Rollinghoff W, Paumgartner G: Inhibition of drug metabolism by cimetidine in man: dependence on pretreatment microsomal liver function. *Eur J Clin Invest* 12:429–434, 1982.

287. Romankiewicz JA, Ehrman M: Rifampin and warfarin: a drug interaction. *Ann Intern Med* 82:224–225, 1975.

288. Rose HJ, Pruitt AW, Dayton PG, McNay JL: Relationship of urinary furosemide excretion rate to natriuretic effect in experimental azotemia. *J Pharmacol Exp Ther* 199:490–497, 1976.

289. Rose HJ, Pruitt AW, McNay J: Effect of experimental azotemia on renal clearance of furosemide in the dog. *J Pharmacol Exp Ther* 196:238–247, 1976.

290. Routledge PA, Kitchell BB, Bjornsson TD, Skinner T, Linnoila M, Shand DG: Diazepam and N-desmethyldiazepam redistribution after heparin. *Clin Pharmacol Ther* 27:528–532, 1980.

291. Ruffalo RL, Thompson JF, Segal JL: Diazepam-cimetidine drug interaction: a clinically significant effect. *South Med J* 74:1075–1078, 1981.

292. Saal AK, Werner JA, Greene HL, Sears GK, Graham EL: Effect of amiodarone on serum quinidine and procainamide levels. *Am J Cardiol* 53:1264–1267, 1984.

293. Sackellares JC, Sato S, Dreifuss FE, Penry JK: Reduction of steady state valproate levels by other antiepileptic drugs. *Epilepsia* 22:437–441, 1981.

294. Salem RB, Breland BD, Mishra SK, Jordan JE: Effect of cimetidine on phenytoin serum levels. *Epilepsia* 24:284–288, 1983.

295. Sanchez G: Enhancement of heparin effect by probenecid (letter). *N Engl J Med* 292:48, 1975.

296. Sandor P, Sellers EM, Dumbrell M, Klouw V: Effect of short and long term alcohol use on phenytoin kinetics in chronic alcoholics. *Clin Pharmacol Ther* 30:390–397, 1981.

297. Schneck DW, Luderer JR, Davis D, Vary JE: Effects of nadolol and propranolol on plasma lidocaine clearance. *Clin Pharmacol Ther* 36:584–587, 1984.

298. Schneck DW, Vary JE: Mechanism by which hydralazine increases propranolol bioavailability. *Clin Pharmacol Ther* 35:447–453, 1984.

299. Schenck-Gustafsson K, Jogestrand T, Nordlander R, Dahlqvist R: Effect of quinidine on digoxin concentration in skeletal muscle and serum in patients with atrial fibrillation. Evidence for reduced binding of digoxin in muscle. *N Engl J Med* 305:209–211, 1981.

300. Schwartz JB, Keefe D, Kates RE, Kirsten E, Harrison DC: Acute and chronic pharmacodynamic interaction of verapamil and digoxin in atrial fibrillation. *Circulation* 65:1163–1170, 1982.

301. Seixas FA: Alcohol and its drug interactions. *Ann Intern Med* 83:86–92, 1975.

302. Sellers EM: Plasma protein displacement interactions are rarely of clinical significance. *Pharmacology* 18:225–227, 1979.

303. Sellers EM, Holloway MR: Drug kinetics and alcohol ingestion. *Clin Pharmacokinet* 3:440–452, 1978.

304. Sellers EM, Koch-Weser J: Displacement of warfarin from human albumin by diazoxide and ethacrynic, mefenamic, and nalidixic acids. *Clin Pharmacol Ther* 11:524–529, 1970.

305. Sellers EM, Koch-Weser J: Potentiation of warfarin-induced hypoprothrombinemia by chloral hydrate. *N Engl J Med* 283:827–831, 1970.

306. Sellers EM, Lang M, Koch-Weser J, LeBlanc E, Kalant H: Interaction of chloral hydrate and ethanol in man. I. Metabolism. *Clin Pharmacol Ther* 13:37–49, 1972.

307. Sellers EM, Naranjo CA, Giles HG, Frecker RC, Beeching M: Intravenous diazepam and oral ethanol interaction. *Clin Pharmacol Ther* 28:638–645, 1980.

308. Sellman F, Kanto J, Raijola E, Pekkarinen A: Human and animal study on elimination from plasma and metabolism of diazepam after chronic alcohol intake. *Acta Pharmacol Toxicol* 36:33–38, 1975.

309. Serlin MJ, Breckenridge AM: Drug interactions with warfarin. *Drugs* 25:610–620, 1983.

310. Serlin MJ, Sibeon RG, Breckenridge AM: Lack of effect of ranitidine on warfarin action. *Br J Clin Pharmacol* 12:791–794, 1981.

311. Shea P, Lal R, Kim SS, Schechtman K, Ruffy R: Flecainide and amiodarone interaction. *J Am Coll Cardiol* 7:1127–1130, 1986.

312. Shinn AF, Shrewsbury RP: *Evaluation of Drug Interactions*. St. Louis, CV Mosby, 1985.

313. Sjoqvist F: Psychotropic drugs (2). Interaction between monoamine oxidase (MAO) inhibitors and other substances. *Proc R Soc Med* 58:967–977, 1965.

314. Skinner C, Coull DC, Johnston AW: Antagonism of the hypotensive action of bethanidine and debrisoquin by tricyclic antidepressants. *Lancet* 2:564–566, 1969.

315. Smith CK, Durack DT: Isoniazid and reaction to cheese. *Ann Intern Med* 88:520–521, 1978.

316. Solomon HM, Abrams WB: Interactions between digitoxin and other drugs in man. *Am Heart J* 83:277–280, 1972.

317. Somogyi A, Bochner F: Dose and concentration dependent effect of ranitidine on procainamide disposition and renal clearance in man. *Br J Clin Pharmacol* 18:175–181, 1984.

318. Somogyi A, Gugler R: Drug interactions with cimetidine. *Clin Pharmacokinet* 7:23–41, 1982.

319. Somogyi A, McLean A, Heinzow B: Cimetidine-procainamide pharmacokinetic interaction in man: evidence of competition for tubular secretion of basic drugs. *Eur J Clin Pharmacol* 25:339–345, 1983.

320. Somogyi A, Theilscher S, Gugler R: Influence of phenobarbital treatment on cimetidine kinetics. *Eur J Clin Pharmacol* 19:343–347, 1981.

321. Spahn H, Mutschler E, Kirch W, Ohnhaus EE, Janisch HD: Influence of ranitidine on plasma metoprolol and atenolol concentrations. *Br Med J* 286:1546–1547, 1983.

322. Speeg KV, Patwardham RV, Avant GR, Mitchell MC, Schenker S: Inhibition of microsomal drug metabolism by histamine H_2-receptor antagonist studied in vivo and in vitro in rodents. *Gastroenterology* 82:89–96, 1982.

323. Stafford JR, Fann WE: Drug interactions with guanidinium antihypertensives. *Drugs* 13:57–64, 1977.

324. Steinberg WM, Lewis JH, Katz DM: Antacids inhibit absorption of cimetidine. *N Engl J Med* 307:400–404, 1982.

325. Steiness E: Renal tubular secretion of digoxin. *Circulation* 50:103–107, 1974.

326. Steiness E, Waldorff S, Hansen PB, Kjaergard H, Buch J, Egeblad H: Reduction of digoxin-induced inotropism during quinidine administration. *Clin Pharmacol Ther* 27:791–795, 1980.

327. Stenson RE, Constantino RT, Harrison DC: Interrelationships of hepatic blood flow, cardiac output, and blood levels of lidocaine in man. *Circulation* 43:205–211, 1971.

328. Stockley I: *Drug Interactions*. Oxford, Blackwell Scientific Publications, 1981.

329. Stone CA, Porter CC, Stavorski JM, Ludden CT, Totaro JA: Antagonism of catecholamine-depleting agents by antidepressant and related drugs. *J Pharmacol* 144:196–204, 1964.

330. Sweeney KR, Chapron DJ, Brandt JL, Gomolin IH, Feig PU, Kramer PA: Toxic interaction between acetazolamide and salicylate: case reports and a pharmacokinetic explanation. *Clin Pharmacol Ther* 40:518–524, 1986.

331. Talbert RL, Bussey HI: Update on calcium-channel blocking agents. *Clin Pharm* 2:403–416, 1983.

332. Thompson MJB, Russo ME, Saxon BJ, Atkinthor E, Matsem JM: Gentamicin inactivation by piperacillin or carbenicillin in patients with end stage renal dis-

ease. *Antimicrob Agents Chemother* 21:268–273, 1982.

333. Thompson PD, Melmon KL, Richardson JA, Cohn K, Steinbrunn W, Cudihee R, Rowland M: Lidocaine pharmacokinetics in advanced heart failure, liver disease, and renal failure in humans. *Ann Intern Med* 78:499–508, 1973.

334. Tilstone WJ, Semple PF, Lawson DH, Boyle JA: Effects of furosemide on glomerular filtration rate and clearance of practolol, digoxin, cephaloridine, and gentamicin. *Clin Pharmacol Ther* 22:289–294, 1977.

335. Toon S, Low LK, Gibaldi M, Trager WF, O'Reilly RA, Motley CH, Goulart DA: The warfarin-sulfinpyrazone interaction: stereochemical considerations. *Clin Pharmacol Ther* 39:15–24, 1986.

336. Tornatore KM, Kanarkowski R, McCarthy TL, Gardner MJ, Yurchak AM, Jusko WJ: Effect of chronic oral contraceptive steroids on theophylline disposition. *Eur J Clin Pharmacol* 23:129–134, 1982.

337. Touerud EL, Boobis AR, Brodie MJ, Murray S, Bennett PN, Whitmarsh V, Davies DS: Differential induction of antipyrine metabolism by rifampicin. *Eur J Clin Pharmacol* 21:155–160, 1981.

338. Twun-Barima Y, Carruthers SG: Quinidine-rifampin interaction. *N Engl J Med* 304:1466–1469, 1981.

339. Udall JA: Warfarin-chloral hydrate interaction. Pharmacological activity and clinical significance. *Ann Intern Med* 81:341–344, 1974.

340. Valette H, Apoil E: Interaction between salicylate and two loop diuretics. *Br J Clin Pharmacol* 8:592–594, 1979.

341. Valsalan VC, Cooper GL: Carbamazepine intoxication caused by interaction with isoniazid. *Br Med J* 285:261–262, 1982.

342. VanZwieten PA: The reversal of clonidine-induced hypotension by protryptyline and desipramine. *Pharmacology* 14:227–231, 1976.

343. Vasko MR, Bell RD, Daly DD, Pippenger CE: Inheritance of phenytoin hypometabolism: a kinetic study of one family. *Clin Pharmacol Ther* 27:96–103, 1980.

344. Verbeeck R, Tjandramaga TB, Mullie A: Effect of aluminum hydroxide on diflunisal absorption. *Br J Clin Pharmacol* 13:519–522, 1979.

345. Vessell E: Introduction: genetic and environment factors affecting drug response in man. *Fed Proc* 31:1253–1269, 1972.

346. Vestal RE, Kornhauser DM, Hollifield JW, Shand DG: Inhibition of propranolol metabolism by chlorpromazine. *Clin Pharmacol Ther* 25:19–24, 1979.

347. Vestal RE, Thummel KE, Musser B, Mercer GD: Cimetidine inhibits theophylline clearance in patients with chronic obstructive pulmonary disease: a study using stable isotope methodology during multiple oral dose administration. *Br J Clin Pharmacol* 15:411–418, 1983.

348. Vincent FM: Phenothiazine-induced phenytoin intoxication (letter). *Ann Intern Med* 93:56–57, 1980.

349. Waldorff S, Andersen JD, Heeboll-Nielson N, Nielsen OG, Moltke E, Sorensen U, Steiness E: Spironolactone-induced changes in digoxin kinetics. *Clin Pharmacol Ther* 24:162–167, 1978.

350. Watt AH, Stephens MR, Buss DC, Routledge PA: Amiodarone reduces plasma warfarin clearance in man. *Br J Clin Pharmacol* 20:707–709, 1985.

351. Watts RW, Hetzel DJ, Bochner F, Hallpike JF, Hann CS, Shearman DJC: Lack of interaction between ranitidine and phenytoin. *Br J Clin Pharmacol* 15:499–500, 1983.

352. Weeks CE, Conard GJ, Kvam DC, Fox JM, Chang SF, Paone RP, Lewis GP: The effect of flecainide acetate, a new antiarrhythmic, on plasma digoxin levels. *J Clin Pharmacol* 26:27–31, 1986.

353. Weber WW: The relationship of genetic factors to drug reactions. In Heyler L, Peck NM (eds): *Drug-Induced Diseases*. Amsterdam, Excerpta Medica, vol 4, 1972.

354. Weiner IM, Mudge GJ: Renal tubular mechanisms for excretion of organic acids and bases. *Am J Med* 36:743–762, 1964.

355. Weibert R, Keane W, Shapiro F: Carbenicillin inactivation of aminoglycosides in patients with severe renal failure. *Trans Am Soc Artif Intern Organs* 22:439–443, 1976.

356. Welling PG: Interactions affecting drug absorption. *Clin Pharmacokinet* 9:404–434, 1984.

357. Wesseling H, Mols-Thurkow I: Interaction of diphenylhydantoin (DPH) and tolbutamide in man. *Eur J Clin Pharmacol* 8:75–78, 1975.

358. Williams JF, Mathew B: Effect of quinidine on positive inotropic action of digoxin. *Am J Cardiol* 47:1052–1055, 1981.

359. Williams RB, Sherter C: Cardiac complications of tricyclic antidepressant therapy. *Ann Intern Med* 74:395–398, 1971.

360. Windorfer A Jr, Pringshein W: Studies on the concentration of chloramphenicol in the serum and cerebrospinal fluid of neonates, infants and small children. Reciprocal reactions between chloramphenicol, penicillin and phenobarbitone. *Eur J Pediatr* 124:129–138, 1977.

361. Wing LMH, Miners JO, Birkett DJ, Fornander T, Lillywhite K, Wanwimolruk S: Lidocaine disposition—sex differences and effects of cimetidine. *Clin Pharmacol Ther* 35:695–701, 1984.

362. Wishinsky N, Glasser EJ, Peakal S: Protein interactions of sulfonylurea compounds. *Diabetes* 2(suppl):18–25, 1962.

363. Wong YY, Ludden TM, Bell RD: Effect of erythromycin on carbamazepine kinetics. *Clin Pharmacol Ther* 33:460–464, 1983.

364. Wright JM, Stokes EF, Sweeny VP: Isoniazid-induced carbamazepine toxicity and vice versa: a double drug interaction. *N Engl J Med* 307:1325–1327, 1982.

365. Wroblewski BA, Singer WD, Whyte J: Carbamazepine-erythromycin interaction. *JAMA* 255:1165–1167, 1986.

366. Zilly W, Breimer DD, Richter E: Induction of drug metabolism in man after rifampin treatment measured by increased hexobarbital and tolbutamide clearance. *Eur J Clin Pharmacol* 9:219–227, 1975.

367. Zuidema J, Hilbers-Modderman ESM, Merkus FWHM: Clinical pharmacokinetics of dapsone. *Clin Pharmacokinet* 11:299–315, 1986.

3

Pharmacokinetic Alterations with Renal Failure and Dialysis[a]

John F. Maher, M.D.

GENERAL CONSIDERATIONS

With few exceptions, patients with acute renal failure tolerate the usual dose of a drug, once. The major pharmacologic problem in such patients is how much to give as a maintenance dose and at what intervals. Although impaired drug elimination predominates, pharmacokinetics are more complex than simple dose adjustment based on the fractional reduction in glomerular filtration rate. Nevertheless, restricting the use of drugs in patients with renal failure to those unequivocally necessary, reducing doses according to established guidelines, limiting the duration of therapy, measuring blood levels where available, and careful clinical monitoring for signs of toxicity would eliminate most toxicologic problems encountered. Several reviews provide detailed information and abundant references about pharmacokinetic abnormalities in renal failure (1, 5, 9, 10, 44, 70, 90, 91, 92, 112, 140).

The effectiveness and safety of drugs in renal failure depend on bioavailability, the route of elimination, the activity of metabolites, the severity of the consequences of drug or metabolite retention, alterations in the substrate and target organs, metabolic loads presented by drugs, renal adaptive changes to nephron loss, the margin of safety of the drug, and the capability of removing excesses by dialysis or hemoperfusion.

[a]The opinions and assertions contained herein are those of the author and are not to be construed as official or as representing those of the Uniformed Services University of the Health Sciences or the Department of Defense.

Bioavailability

Clinicians knew several decades ago that mercurial diuretics injected into the edematous lower extremities were absorbed slowly and were not as effective as when given intramuscularly or subcutaneously in the arm. Renal failure can affect gastrointestinal absorption because of higher gastric pH due to ammonia buffering, impaired transport secondary to vitamin D deficiency, or binding, for example to antacids. First pass metabolism during absorptive transit through the liver can eliminate a high fraction of absorbed drug (5). Indeed, hepatic metabolism of cancer chemotherapeutics administered intraperitoneally can prevent toxic drugs from reaching the systemic circulation allowing localized treatment. The liver is generally not overtly impaired functionally in uremic patients, but hepatic drug metabolism is often submaximal. When acute renal failure follows ischemia, hepatic perfusion may also be subnormal, limiting metabolic disposition of drugs. Concurrent drug therapy may induce cytochrome P-450 or other enzymes augmenting biotransformation, so the amount of a given drug reaching the systemic circulation is poorly predictable. When in doubt, only a modest reduction of the loading dose (10–20%) is warranted and clinical assessment can be used before commencing maintenance therapy.

The peak plasma drug concentration relates directly to the absorbed dose and inversely to the distribution space. After a bolus injection, a high drug concentration decreases rapidly as the drug distributes. Distribution occurs predominantly by diffusion, and if the rate deviates in uremic patients, it may be faster be-

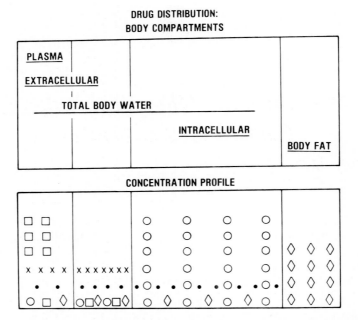

Figure 3.1. Illustration of potential distribution volumes of drugs and their impact on plasma concentrations. □, plasma protein bound; ×, extracellular fluid; •, total body water; ○, cellular protein bound; ◇, sequestered in fat.

cause of increased capillary permeability. Following the rapid decline there is a slower (β phase) decrease in concentration that correlates with the elimination rate. Using this exponential decay curve, a theoretical peak concentration at time zero can be calculated assuming instantaneous distribution. From this value the distribution space can be calculated as volume = dose/concentration.

Distribution Space

Each solute has a characteristic distribution space (Fig. 3.1). For some solutes this approximates total body water (e.g., antipyrine). Body water is ordinarily a higher fraction of body mass in uremic patients, so peak concentration at a given dose should be lower. Other drugs (e.g., bromide) distribute in extracellular fluid, which often is increased in uremic patients. Some drugs bind to plasma proteins (e.g., phenytoin), reducing the amount available for distribution into extravascular and plasma water, the concentration with which pharmacologic and toxic effects correlate best and from which elimination occurs directly. Uremia reduces fractional plasma protein binding of many drugs. Corollaries of such reduced binding are lower plasma concentrations, higher distribu-

tion volumes, and higher plasma water concentrations, and so potentially more pharmacologic activity and toxicity and more rapid hepatic elimination. Thus, the dosing interval may need to be shortened. For drugs eliminated by the kidney, the decreased elimination rate overrides the increased availability for elimination. Some drugs are bound by cellular proteins (e.g., digoxin). Such drugs have large apparent volumes of distribution, often exceeding body mass, and low plasma concentrations. Despite high clearances these drugs are eliminated slowly because the reservoir is so large. Uremia decreases intracellular binding of digoxin, raising plasma concentrations but lowering the fraction in muscle such as myocardium. Other drugs sequester preferentially in body fat (e.g., phenothiazines). These drugs also have large apparent distribution volumes that prolong their effects. Although chronic uremia often decreases body fat, it is doubtful that such drugs distribute abnormally in acute renal failure.

Metabolic Loads Induced by Drugs

Although the drug itself may be innocuous in renal failure, it may provide an intolerable metabolic load (Table 3.1). The most quoted

Table 3.1
Metabolic Effects of Drugs

Effect	Example
Potassium excess	Penicillin
Sodium load	Kayexalate
Magnesium load	Laxatives
Calcium load	Vitamin D
Acidosis	Phenformin
Alkalosis	Carbenicillin
Nitrogen load	Tetracycline
Water retention	Morphine
Dehydration	Lithium
Cation depletion	Cis-platinum

example is hyperkalemia due to the potassium content of penicillin. Metabolic effects of drugs include depletion as well as solute excess. For example, a cation must be excreted with carbenicillin. When sodium intake is limited and homeostatic mechanisms promote sodium conservation, potassium or hydrogen ion must be excreted with carbenicillin, potentially causing hypokalemic alkalosis.

Alterations in Substrate and Target Organs

Gastrointestinal irritability in uremic patients increases the likelihood that vomiting will complicate the use of mucosal irritants. The resultant extracellular fluid volume depletion can adversely affect vital organ perfusion. Myocardial irritability also increases in uremic patients. Hence, arrhythmia is a more frequent drug complication than occurs when renal function is normal. The action of central nervous system depressants is augmented, not immediately after binephrectomy, but once azotemia has occurred. Regrettably, drug-induced sedation continues to occur in such patients and is often misinterpreted as uremia.

Many adverse drug effects in uremic patients present as dermal reactions. These may be misinterpreted as uremic dermatitis, may exaggerate uremic pruritus, and often lead to excoriation and hemorrhage.

Renal failure itself connotes the inability to achieve high renal or urinary concentrations of drugs except at the expense of high plasma levels. Thus, adequate urinary levels of antimicrobials cannot be achieved without the use of toxic doses, and often diuretics are minimally effective despite doses that cause a high incidence of toxic effects such as deafness.

Drug Elimination

Drugs are eliminated only via a few routes. Although some are eliminated by the lung (e.g., paraldehyde), and losses through the skin, gastrointestinal tract, and drainage fluids can sometimes be substantial, the kidney and the liver are the major organs of drug elimination. Artificial methods such as dialysis often add substantially to drug elimination. Hepatic elimination is usually a biotransformation process. The drug metabolite ordinarily depends on renal elimination. Such biotransformed drugs may be inactive, but active metabolites can be retained in uremia (e.g., N-acetylprocainamide) or toxic metabolites may persist (e.g., normeperidine). Thus, hepatic elimination of a drug does not assure freedom from "retention" toxicity in patients with acute renal failure.

It is a common misconception that the renal clearance of drugs decreases comparably with the decline in glomerular filtration rate. Few drugs are handled exclusively by glomerular filtration. Many undergo tubular secretion, the rate of decrement of which may differ from the fall in filtration rate. Other drugs are filtered and reabsorbed. Fractional reabsorption of many solutes decreases as renal failure progresses, maintaining excretion rates relatively well compared to glomerular filtration rate. These concepts are appreciated by recalling that potassium and phosphate excretion do not decrease as much as creatinine excretion, and without a change in production rates these solutes do not accumulate in plasma to the same extent as creatinine. Of course, in the anuric patient such compensatory mechanisms do not apply. Elimination rates are dose dependent when excretion involves a rate-limited transport mechanism for tubular secretion or reabsorption. Moreover, when drugs accumulate in uremic patients, metabolic clearance rates may decline because of enzyme saturation.

Elimination Rate, Half-life

The rate of elimination of a drug can be quantified as a clearance, expressed in units of volume/time. Conventionally, creatinine clearance is expressed in milliliters per minute, but drug clearances are often expressed as liters per kilogram per hour. The clearance indicates functional efficiency of the pertinent organ of elimination, but as an isolated parameter does not guide drug therapy. When a given clearance, e.g., 100 ml/min, removes a drug from a large distribution volume, e.g., 400 liters, the drug disappears slowly. In contrast, the same clearance value removing a drug from a 15-liter space would cause a rapid decrement in concentration. Hence, it may be preferable to express the elimination rate as a coefficient that defines the fractional removal of a drug in a given time, e.g., in 1 hour.

When half of the total quantity of the drug is removed in 1 hour and the plasma concentration (equilibrated with extravascular concentrations) decreases by 50%, the half-life of the drug is defined. The half-life is an inverse function of the removal rate and is calculated as $t_{1/2} = 0.7 \ V_d/Cl$, where V_d equals the distribution volume and Cl equals the clearance. Total body clearance cannot be measured as readily as renal clearance, which derives from the Fick principle. When neither arteriovenous difference nor the quantity excreted is available, half-life is estimated by plotting the decay slope of plasma concentrations determined serially.

Following a bolus injection, the rapid decrease in peak plasma concentration (α phase) does not represent elimination, but rather drug distribution. Unless serial sampling is done in the postdistributive phase, a falsely short half-life is estimated, a frequent error. The half-life of a drug in plasma is the major determinant of the appropriate interval for maintenance doses.

Because of their inverse relationship, halving the clearance doubles the half-life, a decrease in the clearance to one-tenth of normal causes a 10-fold increase in the half-life, and so forth. Because the margin of safety of most drugs is not very narrow (cardiac glycosides and aminoglycosides are notable exceptions), drug accumulation is only important clinically when the organ of elimination is severely impaired. When two organs contribute importantly to elimination, functional loss of one is usually insufficient to affect the half-life substantially. However, enzyme saturation kinetics or other transport ceilings may limit the adaptive increase in elimination by the healthy organ.

Dosage Adjustment in Renal Failure

Usually, maintenance doses are 50–100% of the loading dose given after one to several half-life intervals have elapsed. Administration of half the loading dose at intervals of one half-life should allow plasma concentrations to vary approximately from the peak to half that level. When the half-life is prolonged but the usual dosing interval is used, the drug accumulates in plasma, equilibrating after about six half-lives at a concentration about as many-fold increased as the extent of prolongation of the half-life.

Either the dose should be reduced or the dosing interval prolonged to adjust for impaired elimination. Because it is difficult to fractionate pills accurately, it is customary to prolong the dosing interval. Moreover, by administering a small dose, for example after the plasma level has decreased to only 90% of the peak level, the mean concentration is higher than if a 50% repletion is given after one half-life. This higher mean concentration can increase toxicity, whereas for many drugs an intermittent peak concentration achieves the desired therapeutic effect.

Drug clearance is ordinarily not measured clinically. When available, sequential plasma drug concentrations can be used to monitor therapy. Attention should be paid to the trough (predose) level, and also to the rate of decrease in concentration, a reflection of elimination efficiency. Often, dosing must be guided by a measure of organ function such as creatinine clearance. The plasma level of the endogenous metabolite, creatinine, which relates inversely to the elimination rate, is often used but is not a good estimate of renal function in patients with acute renal failure because equilibrium has not been reached. Indeed, under any circumstance of rapidly changing renal function the plasma creatinine concentration lags behind the increase or decrease in clearance. With stable chronic renal failure the plasma creatinine concentration correlates directly with the prolongation of the half-life and inversely with the elimination rate of many drugs. Because creatinine production also determines the concentration, it is not as high as anticipated for the severity of functional loss in the elderly or those with malnutrition and muscle wasting. Nevertheless, it is customary to prolong the dosing interval according to the level of plasma creatinine. For example, multiplying the serum creatinine concentration by four approximates the appropriate dosing interval in hours for gentamicin. However, it may be inadvisable to prolong the interval between doses of antibiotics more than 24 hours because of the loss of antibacterial activity. A combination of dosage reduction and interval prolongation is preferable.

Removal of Drugs and Poisons by Dialysis

The dialysis of drugs can also be considered kinetically. Solute (drug) removal rates or clearances are determined by concentration gradients and are inversely proportional to molecular mass. Blood flow rate, dialysis fluid flow rate, membrane area, and permeability determine the transfer rate of a given solute. Because of higher flow rates, hemodialysis is much more efficient than peritoneal dialysis despite a less permeable membrane. With intermittent peritoneal dialysis the urea clearance should be about 20 ml/min. For an unbound solute of undetermined transport properties, the clearance can be estimated by multiplying urea clearance by the ratio of the square root of the weight of urea to the square root of the other solute's weight. For example, a drug with a molecular mass of 400 daltons has an expected clearance of $20 \times \sqrt{60}/\sqrt{400}$ ($20 \times 7.75/20$) or 7.75 (76). Clearances by continuous ambulatory peritoneal dialysis are lower and never exceed the dialysate exchange rate, maximally 8.0 ml/min. The urea clearance with hemodialysis is usually about 150 ml/min and the decrease in clearance that occurs as solute size increases is estimated more closely as (mass urea/mass larger solute) × urea clearance than by a ratio of mass roots. With either technique, large drugs such as vancomycin and polymyxin are cleared slowly.

Protein binding limits the transport rate of many drugs (111). To adjust for binding, the clearance (estimated by solute size) should be reduced by multiplying by the ratio of unbound to total plasma drug concentration. The considerable difference in barbiturate clearances by dialysis correlates with the extent of protein binding, not the small difference in molecular mass. For drugs such as cloxacillin and furosemide that are more than 90% protein bound in plasma, removal by dialysis is negligible. This observation does not apply to reverse dialysis; rapid absorption from dialysate is not impeded by binding. There is also considerable difference in efficiency of various hemodialyzers and techniques.

Hemoperfusion is not limited appreciably by membrane transport resistance or by protein binding. Thus, when a procedure is specifically indicated for drug removal, hemoperfusion is often preferred; however, it does not correct urea retention, fluid and electrolyte abnormalities, or acid-base imbalance. Hence, dialysis continues to be preferred for some intoxications such as salicylism.

Hemofiltration clears solutes, without discrimination by size, until membrane sieving occurs as the solute size approaches that of the membrane pore. It is an effective method of removing large solutes, but not as efficient as hemodialysis in clearing small solutes. Continuous arteriovenous hemofiltration clears most drugs at a rate close to the ultrafiltration rate multiplied by the unbound fraction.

Dialysis has little impact on the course of some intoxications, not because the drug is impermeable, but rather because the distribution volume is so large. In general, this guideline is more likely to apply to those drugs eliminated by the liver; digoxin, excreted by the kidney from a very large distribution volume, is a notable exception, however. Only a small fraction of the drug circulates at any given time and is available for removal by the dialyzer.

For some drugs, removal by dialysis or hemoperfusion is faster than the intercompartmental transfer rate. This fast removal rate causes a rapid decrease in concentration within a small compartment, followed by a rebound increase as reequilibration occurs. During the procedure the quantity removed may be overestimated. Intoxicated patients often show marked clinical improvement, albeit temporary, when plasma concentrations decrease appreciably; there is little evidence to suggest that toxins sequestered in body fat stores contribute directly to toxicity.

The role of dialysis and hemoperfusion in removing poisons must also be considered in relation to pharmacodynamics (140). Intoxication by those drugs having an immediate action that does not persist (so-called hit-and-run toxins) does not respond to removal after the fact. Toxicity must be concentration dependent and sufficiently gradual to allow successful intervention.

Removal by dialysis must add significantly to the usual mode of elimination under the circumstances encountered. Aminoglycoside removal from the anuric patient by dialysis is much faster than endogenous elimination. The same removal rate has much less of an impact on the half-life of the acutely (single dose) overdosed patient who still has normal renal function. Similarly, the very slow removal rate of heavy metals by dialysis may contribute appreciably to the overall elimination rate in the anuric patient. In contrast, very rapid removal of bromide by hemodialysis is usually not necessary, since forced diuresis corrects bromism rapidly enough in most patients. In general, removal of 25% of the body burden of a drug is considered clinically significant.

PHARMACOKINETICS OF INDIVIDUAL DRUGS

The generalizations outlined above indicate that the data shown here must be interpreted thoughtfully. In the individual patient, physiologic derangements may cause deviations from the anticipated pharmacokinetics. Clinical judgment must supersede specific guidelines. The pharmacokinetic parameters listed are only approximations based on available published values. Tables 3.2 to 3.8 list data for patients with normal elimination kinetics, those with anuria, and those undergoing dialysis. For patients with renal failure and some residual function, values may be interpolated between those for anephric and normal subjects for approximations.

Penicillins (Table 3.2)

The major side effect of penicillins, hypersensitivity, is not dose dependent and may involve the kidney as an acute interstitial nephritis. Massive dosage of penicillins in patients with renal failure (or when tubular secretion is blocked, e.g., by probenecid) causes neurotoxicity with myoclonic seizures and coma. Hepatotoxicity and coagulation abnormalities are less frequent. Potassium (1.7 mEq/million units of penicillin) accumulation can also occur. Synthetic penicillins contain as much sodium as 5 mEq/g, contributing to sodium retention or inducing hypokalemic alkalosis.

The molecular mass of the penicillins ranges from about 350 to 470 daltons. Their relatively slow removal by dialysis results more from 18–95% protein binding in plasma, however. The distribution volume of the penicillins ranges from 0.13 to 0.33 liters/kg and most are eliminated predominantly by the kidney. Fortunately, there is a wide margin of safety for these very useful drugs. Knowledge of the pharmacokinetic data of penicillins (Table 3.2) may help guide therapy. Penicillin clearance is reduced considerably by acute renal failure, prolonging the half-life appreciably. Clearance by hemodialysis is somewhat more than ex-

Table 3.2
Penicillin Pharmacokinetics[a,b]

| Drug | Clearance (ml/min) | | Half-life (hr) | | | | Dose (% N)[c] |
	N	A	N	A	H	P	A
Penicillin	420	36	0.5	1.2	4.0	11	15
Ampicillin	270	30	1.3	14	5.0	12	50
Amoxicillin	310	40	1.2	12	3.0	10	50
Methicillin	425	50	0.6	4.0	—	—	30
Nafcillin	410	200	0.8	2.0	2.0	2.0	100
Oxacillin	400	200	0.5	1.5	1.4	—	100
Cloxacillin	150	—	0.5	1.5	—	—	75
Carbenicillin	100	11	1.2	20	8.0	14	20
Ticarcillin	120	16	1.2	14	3.5	8.8	25
Azlocillin	180	60	1.1	5.0	2.8	—	40
Piperacillin	260	60	1.2	3.5	1.9	—	75
Mecillinam	380	70	1.0	4.0	2.4	3.7	30
Temocillin	44	10	4.5	24	8.3	—	50
Mezlocillin	450	50	0.9	6.0	2.1	5.5	30

[a] Data from references 1, 2, 9, 10, 14, 18, 26, 28, 57, 68, 82, 90, 99, 115.
[b] N, normal values; A, values in anephric patients; H, values with hemodialysis; P, values with peritoneal dialysis. Interpolate values for renal failure with some residual function. For example, with 10% function add 10% of elimination rate (for penicillin $(420 - 36) = 384 \times 0.1 = 38$). This doubles clearance, decreases half-life to 6 hours, and should allow dosing at 30% of normal.
[c] Dose = percentage of normal 24-hour total dose for anephric patients.

trarenal clearance, and the combination reduces the half-life by more than 50%, but not to normal values. Penicillin toxicity may occur despite regular dialysis, and more rapid removal of this protein-bound antibiotic occurs with hemoperfusion.

The phenoxymethyl derivative, penicillin V, is absorbed better, but elimination kinetics are similar to those of penicillin G. Hetacillin, pivampicillin, bacampicillin, talampicillin, cyclacillin, and epicillin have pharmacokinetics similar to those of ampicillin (68). The isoxazolyl penicillins, oxacillin, dicloxacillin, and floxacillin, have pharmacokinetics (Table 3.2) similar to those for cloxacillin (99). Little, if any, dosage modification of these drugs is required in acute renal failure or during dialysis treatment. Ticarcillin, azlocillin, and mezlocillin have pharmacokinetics similar to those of carbenicillin (82). Clavulanic acid, an adjunct to penicillin therapy, is retained in renal failure, prolonging the half-life from 1.0

to 4.0 hours, but hemodialysis restores the elimination rate to normal (26, 57).

Cephalosporins (Table 3.3)

The cephalosporins are chemically similar to the penicillins, are excreted predominantly by the kidney by filtration and secretion, and have a broad antibacterial spectrum. Hypersensitivity reactions to cephalosporins are similar to those of penicillins, and neurotoxicity can occur with excessive accumulation. Coagulopathy correlates with a cephalosporin side chain that accumulates in uremic patients. Nephrotoxicity occurs with some congeners, especially when the drugs accumulate or there is concurrent exposure to other nephrotoxins or potent diuretics. Cephaloridine nephrotoxicity is sufficiently frequent to recommend its abandonment.

The cephalosporins have molecular masses

Table 3.3
Cephalosporin Pharmacokinetics[a]

| Drug | Clearance (ml/min) | | Half-life (hr) | | | | Dose (% N) |
	N	A	N	A	H	P	A
Cephalothin	450	30	0.6	12	3.0	5.1	30
Cefaclor	240	90	0.8	2.6	1.7	2.4	50
Cefadroxil	170	12	1.4	24	3.2	17	25
Cefamandole	320	20	1.0	12	5.5	10	25
Cefazolin	70	5.0	2.0	35	9.0	30	20
Cefixime	165	40	3.2	14.9	8.2	—	50
Cefmetazole	110	—	0.8	15	—	—	20
Cefonicid	23	2.0	5.5	65	65	—	25
Cefoperazone	80	64	2.0	2.6	2.1	2.4	80
Ceforanide	46	6.0	3.0	24	12	22	30
Cefotetan	40	16	3.6	30	6.5	16	20
Cefotiam	300	—	0.6	8.0	—	—	30
Cefotaxime	230	85	1.1	3.5	1.8	3.0	50
Cefoxitin	350	15	0.8	18	4.0	14	25
Cefroxadine	200	5.0	0.9	32	3.4	20	15
Cefsulodin	120	15	1.9	12	1.9	10	30
Ceftazidime	125	11	1.8	32	3.6	8.7	30
Ceftezole	220	—	0.6	11	—	—	30
Ceftizoxime	160	12	1.6	28	—	12	20
Ceftriaxone	15	8.0	7.0	15	10	12	80
Cefuroxime	165	10	1.4	17	3.3	12	25
Cephacetrile	330	—	1.4	25	2.0	—	20
Cephalexin	250	17	0.9	28	5.2	8.5	15
Cephapirin	270	70	0.8	2.4	1.8	2.3	80
Cephradine	360	25	1.0	15	—	13	20
Cefmenoxime	232	21	0.8	7.6	4.2	—	30
Aztreonam	90	24	1.7	8.0	2.7	7.1	50
Moxalactam	90	12	2.6	19	3.2	16	25

[a]Data from references 1, 2, 6, 9, 10, 22, 24, 25, 38, 40, 50, 59, 61, 63, 64, 70, 74, 77, 90, 97, 100, 142. See footnotes b and c of Table 3.2.

that range from about 350 to 500 daltons. Protein binding of cephalosporins in plasma, ranges from 10% to 90%, and distribution volumes are between 0.13 and 0.33 liters/kg. Renal excretion of these drugs represents 50–96% of total elimination (Table 3.3).

Peritoneal dialysis removes cephalosporins at less than half the rate of hemodialysis, so the supplemental dose should be no more than half of that following hemodialysis. Hemoperfusion clears cephalosporins much faster. Cephradine is only minimally bound to plasma proteins, so it should be removed rapidly by dialysis. Cephaloglycin, ceftotetan, and cephanone are retained in uremic patients and require dosage reduction, as do most cephalosporins. Cephoperazone and cefotaxime have the lowest fractional elimination by the kidney and are least affected by dialysis. All other cephalosporins require major dose reduction when renal failure has occurred, and an appreciable supplemental dose should be given after hemodialysis. The deacetyl metabolite of cefotaxime is active and retained in renal failure. Cephaloridine should be avoided because of the high incidence of nephrotoxicity.

Aminoglycosides (Table 3.4)

The aminoglycosides are very effective antibiotics, the use of which is limited by dose-dependent ototoxicity, nephrotoxicity, and neuromuscular blockade. Aminoglycoside nephrotoxicity is more likely with some congeners (e.g., neomycin), advancing age, prior renal dysfunction, exposure to other nephrotoxins, or prior extracellular volume depletion. Nephrotoxicity follows renal cortical accumulation of the aminoglycosides of which the half-life is usually several days (4, 60, 69, 116). The introduction of slightly less nephrotoxic aminoglycoside congeners has not lowered the incidence of acute renal failure because of somewhat more liberal dosing of these drugs. High dosage for 1 or 2 days is not likely to cause toxicity; it is persistent administration and drug accumulation between the 10th and 20th day of treatment that usually precedes overt toxicity.

Most aminoglycosides are poorly absorbed from the gastrointestinal tract, are negligibly bound to plasma proteins (except streptomycin, which is about 30% bound), and distribute in volumes of 0.2–0.28 liters/kg. Molecular mass ranges from about 440 to 620 daltons, and excretion of aminoglycosides is more than 90% renal.

Table 3.4 lists pharmacokinetic data for most of the aminoglycosides. As a guideline, the 24-hour maintenance dose for anuric patients should be about 10% of that recommended for those with normal renal function and an additional 20% or 25% should be given after hemodialysis. Intermittent peritoneal dialysis achieves clearances of about 8 ml/min and reduces the half-life in anuric patients to about 20 hours; thus supplemental dosage, if any, should be less than half of that after hemodialysis. Continuous ambulatory peritoneal dialysis clears aminoglycosides at about 4 ml/min, so the half-life is about 30 hours. Hemoperfusion removes aminoglycosides somewhat faster than hemodialysis, but the supplemental

Table 3.4
Aminoglycoside Pharmacokinetics[a]

| Drug | Clearance (ml/min) | | Half-life (hr) | | | | Dose (% N) |
	N	A	N	A	H	P	A
Amikacin	85	1.6	2.0	60	5.0	30	15
Gentamicin	90	2.0	2.2	50	7.0	36	8
Kanamycin	78	4.0	2.4	55	6.0	30	10
Netilmicin	70	5.0	2.5	45	6.0	22	8
Streptomycin	80	2.0	2.3	70	5.0	30	10
Tobramycin	79	4.0	2.2	55	5.0	35	10
Dibekacin	96	4.3	2.3	42	3.7	—	—
Sisomicin	—	—	2.7	50	—	—	—
Lividomycin	—	—	2.0	44	—	—	—
Paromomycin[b]	—	—	2.0	40	—	—	—
Neomycin[b]	—	—	2.0	24	9.0	—	—

[a] Data from references 1, 9, 10, 23, 27, 88, 90, 102, 110, 116. See footnotes b and c of Table 3.2.
[b] Restricted to oral use.

Table 3.5
Half-lives of Miscellaneous Antibiotics and Antimicrobials[a]

Drug	Half-life (hr)			Dose (% N)
	N	A	H	A
Tetracycline	8.0	70	>30	10
Chlortetracycline	6.0	8.0	—	60
Demeclocycline	13	70	>30	15
Doxycycline	18	21	—	80
Minocycline	16	24	—	80
Oxytetracycline	9.0	60	>30	15
Colistimethate	4.0	15	14	20
Polymyxin B	4.0	36	35	10
Sulfisoxazole	6.0	12	6.0	50
Sulfamethoxazole	11	25	12	40
Sulfadiazine	10	22	11	50
Trimethoprim	12	27	25	50
Chloramphenicol	3.0	4.5	4.2	80
Clindamycin	3.0	3.2	3.2	100
Lincomycin	4.5	12	10	60
Vancomycin	6.0	200	120	10
Erythromycin	1.6	5.0	4.5	80
Imipenim	1.0	3.7	2.5	30
Fosfomycin	1.5	15	3.0	25
Ciprofloxacin	4.5	11	3.2	50
Ethambutol	3.0	10	5.0	30
Isoniazid[b]	1.0, 3.5	5.0, 12	1.5, 5.0	60
Rifampin	3.5	4.0	4.0	100
p-Aminosalicylate	1.0	20	18	10
Amphotericin B	24	24	24	90
Flucytosine	4.0	120	10	10
Ketoconazole	2.4	2.1	—	100
Miconazole	22	22	—	100
Acyclovir	2.4	20	5.5	20
Amantadine	12	200	—	10
Metronidazole	7.0	9.0	3.0	80
Ornidazole	12	11	6.0	100
Tinidazole	13	14	4.3	100

[a] Data from references 1, 9, 10, 15, 19, 23, 33, 40, 42, 45, 49, 52, 54, 56, 65, 69, 77, 84, 90, 95, 96, 103, 112, 113, 123, 127, 137. See footnotes b and c of Table 3.2.
[b] Data are given for rapid and slow isoniazid acetylators.

dose can be the same after this briefer procedure. Despite dosage adjustment there is an appreciable incidence of nephrotoxicity, but it is usually milder. Netilmicin appears to be the safest drug for uremic patients.

Other Antibiotics (Table 3.5)

The tetracyclines should be avoided, if possible, in patients with renal failure (124). Doxycycline is the least likely to aggravate azotemia. Molecular masses of tetracyclines average about 450 daltons. Most are more than 60% bound in plasma, predicting low clearances by dialysis. Distribution volumes of tetracyclines are high (1.0–1.9 liters/kg), and renal excretion varies from 10% to 50% of the total elimination rate (54). Demeclocycline inhibits renal tubular free water reabsorption, potentially causing dehydration or removing retained water in patients with inappropriate antidiuretic hormone secretion. Hemoperfusion can remove toxic accumulations of tetracyclines.

Renal and neural toxicity are major drawbacks to therapy with the polymyxins, a group of polypeptides of which colistimethate and polymyxin B are the least toxic (56). Dosage should be kept below 2.0 mg/kg/day in anuric patients. Because of their large molecular size, these drugs are removed slowly by dialysis.

Most sulfonamides are well absorbed from the gastrointestinal tract, bind highly to proteins in plasma (50–90%), and distribute in volumes that can range from 0.15 to 0.60 liters/kg. Elimination of both free and acetylated sulfonamides is predominantly renal, so half-lives are prolonged in uremic patients (137). Alkalinization of the urine increases the renal clearance and decreases the likelihood of nephrotoxicity due to crystalline precipitates. Sulfonamides and their numerous chemical derivatives are important causes of acute interstitial nephritis. Uremia decreases protein binding of sulfonamides, hence hemodialyzer clearance in patients with renal failure decreases the half-life appreciably.

Chloramphenicol is eliminated predominantly by hepatic conjugation. The glucuronide conjugate persists in renal failure with a half-life of about 100 hours but is not considered toxic to the bone marrow. Protein binding in plasma (55%), albeit decreased in uremia, inhibits removal by dialysis (127). Chloramphenicol distributes in a volume of 0.9 liters/kg. The dose must be reduced substantially with hepatic failure.

Clindamycin is about 95% bound in plasma and distributes in 0.7 liters/kg from which it is rapidly cleared, mostly by the liver. Neither renal failure nor dialysis affects the half-life appreciably (103). The clearance by hemoperfusion may exceed 100 ml/min. Lincomycin has similar pharmacokinetics.

Imipenim accumulates in renal failure and is rapidly removed by dialysis (42). Cilastin, which inhibits the enzymatic catabolism of imipenim, is even more dependent on renal elimination and readily dialyzed.

Vancomycin, a large solute (molecular mass about 1800 daltons), is about 10% bound in plasma and distributes slowly into a volume of about 0.6 liters/kg. Elimination is almost exclusively renal, and the dose should be decreased in anuric patients from 1.0 g every 12 hours to 1.0 g every 7 days to avoid nephrotoxicity (84). Dialysis removes vancomycin very slowly.

Erythromycin (734 daltons) is moderately absorbed when given orally, distributes in 0.7 liters/kg, and is 70% bound in plasma. Elimination is mostly hepatic and neither renal failure nor dialysis should affect pharmacokinetics appreciably; ototoxicity correlates with modest accumulation (96).

Novobiocin pharmacokinetics are not changed substantially by renal failure or dialysis. Fosfomycin is retained in renal failure but removed by dialysis. The dose in anuric patients should be reduced (113). Bacitracin is too nephrotoxic for systemic use. When absorbed, it is cleared mostly by the kidney and is poorly dialyzable.

Long-term use of tuberculostatic drugs can be complicated in renal failure. Isoniazid is biotransformed by acetylation, and elimination is only modestly affected by renal failure (45). Hemodialysis doubles the elimination rate, so a supplement is required thereafter. Rifampin is highly protein bound and distributes in a large volume. Neither renal failure nor dialysis affects elimination kinetics sufficiently to warrant dosage modification (112). Ethambutol distributes in a large volume, is minimally bound in plasma, and is rapidly excreted by the kidney. The dose should be reduced when renal failure occurs, and a supplemental dose given after dialysis. Cycloserine is excreted by the kidney and removed by dialysis. P-Aminosalicylate should be avoided in anuric patients; it is retained in uremic patients and removed by dialysis. Both pyrazinamide and viomycin depend on renal elimination whereas ethionamide does not.

In general, urinary antiseptics should be avoided in patients with advanced renal failure. Nitrofurantoin accumulates in uremic patients and can cause peripheral neuropathy (32). Methenamine mandelate, nalidixic acid, norfloxacin, pipemidic acid, and ascorbic acid are each retained somewhat with renal failure and exaggerate metabolic acidosis. Phenazopyridine is potentially nephrotoxic and depends on renal elimination. Elimination of cinoxacin is delayed in patients with renal failure, decreasing efficacy and potentially causing toxicity.

Miscellaneous Antimicrobials (Table 3.5)

The fungicide, amphotericin B, causes dose-dependent nephrotoxicity but does not depend on the kidney for elimination. Dose reduction is not required with preexistent renal failure, but often the dose is somewhat limited because there is no leeway for a further renal functional loss. The development or progression of azotemia warrants dose reduction or cessation if possible. Because acute renal failure induced by amphotericin B can be irreversible, the drug should be continued only for serious fungal infection once renal failure occurs. The normal half-life is several days and negligible amounts of amphotericin are removed by dialysis.

Renal failure prolongs the half-life of 5-fluorocytosine from 5 to 100 hours, so the maintenance dose in anuric patients should be curtailed sharply. Because dialysis removes this drug rapidly, a supplement of about 15% of the usual daily maintenance dose should be given thereafter (13). Miconazole is eliminated mainly by the liver and is about 90% bound in plasma (130). Neither renal failure nor dialysis appreciably alters the pharmacokinetics of miconazole or ketoconazole.

Chloroquine normally has a long half-life and is eliminated predominantly by the liver, but somewhat slower in uremic patients (112). Modest dosage reduction is required with severe renal failure. The elimination of chloroguanide is delayed somewhat in uremic patients. Primaquine is rapidly biotransformed but the metabolite is active. Guidelines for dosage reduction are not established. Pyrimethamine has a long half-life and may be retained in anuric patients. The half-life of trimethoprim increases in uremic patients, and modest dosage reduction is advisable (10). The liver hydroxylates quinine and the 6-hour half-life is not prolonged in uremic patients. Hemodialysis improves quinine intoxication (34).

Dapsone and other sulfones used for leprosy are excreted mostly by the kidney, so dosage reduction is advisable (1). Clofazimine (another antileprosy agent) has a large distribution volume and a long half-life minimally affected by renal failure.

Pentamidine distributes rapidly into tissues, where it persists for months (10). Chronic use should be at a lower dosage in uremic patients but short-term therapy is probably unaffected by renal failure.

Amantidine, an antiviral agent, accumulates in uremic patients and can induce arrhythmias and neuropsychiatric toxicity (143). Hemodialysis reduces the half-life toward normal. Acyclovir is excreted in the urine, retained in uremia, and rapidly removed by dialysis (123).

Thiabendazole (used for strongyloidiasis) and mebendazole (for echinococcosis) are eliminated mainly by the liver. Neither renal failure nor dialysis affects their pharmacokinetics appreciably (118).

Sedatives, Tranquilizers, and Psychotherapeutic Drugs (Table 3.6)

The long-acting barbiturates are excreted by the kidney and rapidly cleared by hemodialysis. Barbital accumulates in uremic patients, distributes into a small volume, binds minimally in plasma, and is removed rapidly by hemodialysis. Renal excretion of phenobarbital is increased by alkaline diuresis and ac-

Table 3.6
Half-lives of Sedatives and Analgesics[a]

Drug	Half-life (hr)		
	N	A	H
Phenobarbital	80	110	9
Secobarbital	25	30	18
Pentobarbital	30	35	18
Chloral hydrate[b]	30/7	—	4
Chlordiazepoxide	10	12	11
Diazepam	40	65	60
Oxazepam	10	25	24
Nortriptyline	23	25	23
Metoclopramide	4.2	14	13.6
Bromide	24	—	2
Lithium	22	50	4
Salicylate	12	—	4
Acetaminophen	2.5	2.5	1.6
Ibuprofen	2	2	2
Naproxen	17	17	17
Phenylbutazone	80	60	—
Piroxicam	45	44	—
Sulfinpyrazone	25	95	—
Propoxyphene	12	12	11
Morphine	2.0	1.8	—

[a]Data from references 3, 7, 8, 9, 10, 17, 39, 40, 55, 90, 117, 120, 140, 141. See footnotes b and c of Table 3.2.
[b]Trichlorethanol, the active metabolite of chloral hydrate, has a 7-hour half-life.

counts for about 25% of total elimination. The dosage of phenobarbital should be limited with renal failure. Intoxication can mimic uremic coma and responds to hemodialysis or more slowly to peritoneal dialysis (120). Elimination is impeded by 20% protein binding and a distribution volume of 0.9 liters/kg. Secobarbital and pentobarbital (preferentially distributed in body fat and about 35% bound in plasma) are short-acting and eliminated predominantly by hepatic biotransformation, but can aggravate uremic lethargy and coma. Removal by either forced diuresis or dialysis is relatively slow. Thiopental, which is ultra-short-acting, rapidly distributes in body fat. Although eliminated by metabolism, thiopental narcosis is prolonged by uremia, and protein binding decreases. Amobarbital and butabarbital are intermediate in their elimination rates by dialysis, protein binding, lipid partition, and duration of action. Lipid-soluble, protein-bound barbiturates are cleared faster by hemoperfusion through resin or charcoal columns (140). Decreased protein binding, saturation of metabolic biotransformation processes, and retention of conjugates argue for some dosage reduction of all barbiturates in uremic patients, and careful observation for signs of oversedation.

The benzodiazepines are all highly bound to proteins in plasma and undergo hepatic biotransformation. Although the metabolites have long half-lives and depend on renal elimination, most of these drugs are well tolerated by uremic patients (112). Chlordiazepoxide, diazepam, and flurazepam have active metabolites whereas the metabolites of lorazepam and oxazepam are inactive. Multiple dosing prolongs the half-life of benzodiazepines. Uremia decreases protein binding of benzodiazepines, and may increase the large distribution volumes and impair the rate of hepatic biotransformation. Although dosage does not usually have to be restricted, the patients should be observed for signs of metabolic encephalopathy. Hemoperfusion should remove the benzodiazepines at clearances of 100–150 ml/min, which is faster than achieved by hemodialysis, 5–60 ml/min.

Chloral hydrate circulates about 50% bound to plasma proteins and is biotransformed to trichlorethanol, an active metabolite eliminated by the liver and the kidney (17). Hemodialysis rapidly clears both chloral hydrate and trichlorethanol.

Glutethimide is about 50% bound in plasma, distributes into a large volume (about 3 liters/kg), and is eliminated mainly by saturable hepatic metabolism (89). Hemodialysis decreases the half-life appreciably but hemoperfusion clears glutethimide more rapidly (140). Neither forced diuresis nor peritoneal dialysis affects pharmacokinetics appreciably.

Ethchlorvynol, about 40% bound in plasma and distributed in a volume of 4 liters/kg, is also eliminated mainly by hepatic metabolism. Removal by hemodialysis or peritoneal dialysis can decrease the normal 25-hour half-life, but hemoperfusion clears it even faster (132, 140).

Meprobamate is only about 20% bound in plasma, and has a distribution volume approximating total body water and a half-life of about 10 hours. About 20% is excreted unchanged by the liver, while the remainder is biotransformed. Modest reduction of dosage is warranted with renal failure, and overdosage responds to dialysis or hemoperfusion (85, 140).

Methyprylon undergoes predominantly extrarenal elimination, so dosage reduction is not required in uremic patients. Intoxication responds to either dialysis or hemoperfusion (101).

Methaqualone intoxication responds well to hemoperfusion. Clearances by dialysis are considerably lower because 80% is bound in plasma (140). Elimination is hepatic from a volume of about 6 liters/kg with a 25-hour half-life.

Uremia increases susceptibility to paraldehyde acidosis, but elimination is mostly hepatic and some unchanged drug is expired (51). Paraldehyde intoxication responds to dialysis.

The phenothiazines, such as chlorpromazine, avidly bind to plasma and tissue proteins and are highly lipophilic. Elimination is slow by hepatic metabolism (9). Uremic patients have increased susceptibility to extrapyramidal myoclonus and toxic psychosis from these drugs. Because distribution volumes may be as high as 20 liters/kg, neither dialysis nor hemoperfusion removes appreciable quantities of phenothiazines.

Amitriptyline, nortriptyline, imipramine, and their congeners also avidly bind to plasma proteins, are highly lipophilic, and distribute in volumes of about 10 liters/kg. Elimination of the tricyclic antidepressants is by hepatic metabolism and only a small fraction is removed by dialysis of hemoperfusion, although transient clinical improvement may occur (9). Active conjugated hydroxymetabolites are retained in uremic patients (83).

The pharmacologic effects of monoamine oxidase inhibitors such as phenelzine persist after the drugs or their active metabolites are eliminated. These drugs are not retained in uremic patients. Although clinical improvement has occurred with dialysis, there is no pharmacokinetic rationale for such treatment (140).

The central dopaminergic antagonist, metoclopramide, is an antiemetic that is retained in renal failure because of decreased renal and nonrenal clearance. Haloperidol (another dopaminergic antagonist) has a long half-life that depends only moderately on renal function.

Sodium bromide is eliminated from extracellular fluid by the kidney at a clearance below 2 ml/min. It accumulates in patients retaining salt, e.g., in heart failure, cirrhosis, or nephrotic syndrome, and is eliminated faster in salt-losing nephritis, with diuretics, and possibly in patients with polyuric renal failure. When administered to anuric patients it accumulates and can cause psychosis, and is rapidly removed by dialysis (117).

Lithium salts accumulate in renal failure and are eliminated rapidly by forced diuresis or dialysis. Toxicity correlates with total body lithium, not with the plasma concentration, and includes neuromuscular irritability and nephrogenic diabetes insipidus with distal tubular necrosis. With chronic excess, the distribution volume expands and reequilibrates slowly with plasma as dialysis rapidly lowers concentrations (62).

Analgesics (Table 3.6)

Salicylates are small solutes, distributed in a volume of 15% of body weight and as much as 50% bound in plasma (9). Their pharmacokinetics are complex. The kidney excretes salicylate and several metabolites and accumulation can occur with renal failure, causing such problems as prolonged bleeding. Dialysis removes salicylates rapidly and corrects the metabolic abnormalities of salicylism. The half-life of salsalate, a salicylate precursor, increases from 1.2 to 2.1 hours with renal failure. Diflunisal, a difluorophenyl salicylate, is more than 99% bound in plasma and thus is poorly filtrable and not dialyzable. Its metabolite is unstable and depends on renal elimination.

Phenacetin and its major metabolite, acetaminophen, are biotransformed by the liver, but the conjugates accumulate in uremic plasma (44). Hemodialysis and hemoperfusion remove these drugs rapidly, but not as fast as hepatic clearance (139). Acute overdosage should be treated by N-acetylcysteine infusion to prevent hepatic necrosis.

Most nonsteroidal antiinflammatory drugs are highly bound to plasma proteins, do not depend on renal elimination, and have inactive metabolites. With renal failure, fractional protein binding may decrease, raising the metabolic clearance and shortening the half-life. Toxic renal syndromes include acute renal ischemia, hyperkalemic acute interstitial nephritis, nephrotic syndrome, tubular necrosis, and papillary necrosis (21). Inhibition of prostaglandin synthetase and hypersensitivity contribute to these lesions. Indomethacin has biphasic elimination with half-lives of 1–9 hours, unaffected by renal failure. Tolmetin, ibuprofen, fenoprofen, and mefenamic acid have short half-lives negligibly influenced by renal failure or dialysis. Naproxen, piroxicam, and phenylbutazone have long half-lives that decrease somewhat with renal failure. Sulfinpyrazone is excreted by the kidney and accumulates in patients with renal failure.

Propoxyphene is eliminated by the liver and dosage adjustment is not necessary in uremic patients. The distribution volume is large (10–25 liters/kg). Dialysis and hemoperfusion remove some propoxyphene, but hepatic metabolism is faster (39).

The half-life of antipyrine is shorter in uremic patients than in normal subjects, a paradox attributed to hepatic microsomal induction since the distribution volume does not change.

Pentazocine is oxidized and conjugated in the liver. Uremic patients do not require dosage modification.

The opiates rapidly distribute into a large volume and are eliminated by hepatic biotransformation (136). Although opiates are not retained in uremic patients, increased sensitivity to standard dosage often occurs. Morphine intolerance relates to a decreased distribution volume raising plasma levels and to retention of active glucuronide metabolites (141). Morphine is partially removed by dialysis. Methadone is used in uremic patients without complications since it is about 85% bound in plasma and eliminated by the liver. Caution is advised with codeine since standard doses can cause narcosis in patients with renal failure. About 10% of meperidine is excreted by the kidney, while most of the drug degrades rapidly in the liver to normeperidine, which accumulates in uremic patients and induces convulsions (131).

Cardiovascular Drugs (Table 3.7)

Digitalis toxicity is a frequent, serious problem in patients with renal failure. Emphasis should be on control of salt and water intake in patients with renal failure rather than on liberal use of digitalis.

Ouabain is rapidly excreted by the kidney and accumulates in uremic patients (119). Plasma protein binding is negligible and the large distribution space decreases with uremia. Dialysis removes a modest fraction of ouabain. Digitalis is excreted more slowly from a large volume and accumulates in uremic patients.

Digoxin is well absorbed, is about 25% bound in plasma, and distributes in a volume of 9 liters/kg. Absorption is slower and delayed by aluminum hydroxide in uremic patients, but peak concentrations are higher because the distribution space is about 50% smaller. The number of binding sites and their affinity for digoxin are decreased in patients with renal failure. Excretion is predominantly renal and the maintenance dose should be decreased in uremic patients to 20–35% of the usual. Digoxin dosage based on formulas depending on

Table 3.7
Half-lives of Cardiovascular Drugs[a]

Drug	Half-life (hr)		
	N	A	H
Ouabain	16	60	45
Digoxin	40	120	100
Digitoxin	155	165	160
Hydralazine	4.0	11	10
Methyldopa	6.0	15.6	9.5
Clonidine	12	40	24
Minoxidil	4	4	—
Propranolol	3.9	3.6	3.6
Nadolol	19	45	28
Sotalol	7	50	8
Practolol	9	60	14
Atenolol	6	60	6
Metoprolol	3.5	3.5	2.5
Labetalol	4.5	5.5	5.0
Lidocaine	1.7	2.0	—
Procainamide	3	13	6
Quinidine	7	10	9.0
Disopyramide	7	18	13
Bretylium	8	32	13
Thiazides	1.5	5.0	—
Furosemide	0.7	3.0	2.3
Amiloride	6.0	80	—
Diltiazem	5.0	3.4	3.4
Nifedipine	2.5	2.6	2.6
Verapamil	5.0	3.7	3.7

[a] Data from references 9, 10, 31, 36, 41, 48, 58, 63, 71, 73, 90, 93, 107, 119, 122, 134. See footnote b of Table 3.2.

creatinine clearance, body weight, and distribution volume are not fully reliable, so therapy should be guided by plasma level determinations (36). Toxicity is frequent at concentrations about 3.0 ng/ml, or lower if hypercalcemia or hypokalemia is present. Removal by dialysis is too slow to improve intoxication, but hemoperfusion can be useful (43). (Dialysis may precipitate digitalis intoxication by correcting protective metabolic abnormalities.)

Digitoxin is extensively metabolized by hepatic microsomal enzymes, the kidney excreting mostly inactive metabolites. It is highly bound in plasma and normally has a long half-life that is affected only slightly by renal failure or dialysis (63). Hemoperfusion removes appreciable amounts of digitoxin (121).

ANTIHYPERTENSIVE AGENTS

Uremic patients often require antihypertensive agents despite control of salt and water balance by limiting intake and by ultrafiltration. The blood pressure response is generally the best guide to dosage of antihypertensives,

but complications may accompany accumulation of drugs or metabolites.

Reserpine distributes in a large volume and is eliminated partly unchanged by the kidney and partly after metabolic hydrolysis. The long half-life (80 hours) doubles in renal failure but dialysis has little effect (144). Reserpine toxicity can mimic uremia.

Hydralazine is about 85% bound in plasma, distributes in a volume of 1.6 liters/kg, and is eliminated mainly by hepatic acetylation (9). Increased concentrations in uremic patients may represent a retained metabolite. The effect of dialysis appears to be minimal.

Prazosin distributes in a volume of 1.6 liters/kg and protein binding in plasma exceeds 90%. The half-life of about 3 hours increases modestly with renal failure and should not be influenced by dialysis, but the blood pressure response may be increased in uremic patients (87).

Methyldopa undergoes hepatic conjugation, and the metabolite is eliminated by the kidney (98). This biphasic elimination occurs with half-lives of 2 hours and 6 hours. In uremic patients, the metabolite is retained but hepatic biotransformation accelerates. Dialysis removes 30–40% of an administered dose, decreasing the half-life appreciably.

Clonidine distributes in a volume of about 3.0 liters/kg and is about 30% bound in plasma. Elimination is predominantly renal, but usually only modest dosage reduction to 25–50% of normal is necessary in patients with renal failure (58).

Guanfacine has properties similar to clonidine, but is biotransformed and does not accumulate in uremic patients. The half-life is about 15 hours in normal subjects and in uremic patients. The hemodialyzer clearance of 53 ml/min adds only 15% of the elimination rate (72).

Guanethidine distributes into a large space from which it is slowly removed by both hepatic metabolism and renal excretion. The normal half-life of several days is prolonged in anuric patients. The effects of renal failure and dialysis require further quantification.

The ganglionic blockers, hexamethonium, mecamylamine, and tetraethylammonium, depend primarily on the kidney for elimination. Blood pressure reduction should be titrated using lower doses than usual when patients have renal failure.

Minoxidil is cleared from a distribution volume approaching 3 liters/kg by hepatic conjugation, with a half-life of 3–4 hours (48). Accumulation is not expected in uremic patients and the effects of dialysis are unknown. Minoxidil is often effective for patients with renal failure who have resistant hypertension.

Diazoxide effectiveness correlates with the level of the unbound drug. Protein binding occurs rapidly and normally exceeds 90%, a value that decreases in uremic patients. Renal failure, however, does not appreciably change the long half-life in plasma, but dialysis may decrease it (106).

Nitroprusside is rapidly metabolized to thiocyanate, which depends on renal elimination, can cause psychosis and hypothyroidism, and is eliminated rapidly by dialysis.

Captopril is eliminated by the liver and the kidney with a half-life of about 2 hours, which increases appreciably with renal failure, prolonging the antihypertensive effect (29). Hemodialysis decreases the half-life to 4 hours. Captopril may decrease renal blood flow, aggravating uremia and hyperkalemia. The half-life of enalapril is normally 8.4 hours and increases to 10.9 hours in renal failure (125). Its antihypertensive effects are comparable with those of captopril but it has a more salutary effect on renal blood flow. Saralasin has a very short half-life since it is metabolized by aminopeptidases. The α-adrenergic blockers, phentolamine and phenoxybenzamine, depend on both hepatic and renal elimination. Doxazosin has a half-life of 9.5 hours, minimally prolonged by renal failure and uninfluenced by dialysis (20).

The β-adrenergic blockers do not have uniform pharmacokinetics (31, 73, 134). Propranolol is more than 90% bound in plasma, distributes in a large volume, and is eliminated by hepatic metabolism. In uremic patients the half-life is slightly shorter because of a decreased distribution volume, but active hydroxy-metabolites persist in plasma and are cleared rapidly by dialysis. Nadolol is removed by the kidney and by dialysis. The dose for anuric patients is 25% of the normal. Pindolol, only partially eliminated by the kidney with a 3.5-hour half-life, does not accumulate in uremic patients. Sotalol accumulates in patients with renal failure but is removed rapidly by dialysis. Atenolol also depends on renal elimination; it accumulates in uremic patients, mandating a dose reduction to 25% of normal, and is cleared rapidly by hemodialysis. Practolol has similar pharmacokinetics. Acebutolol and metoprolol are eliminated by hepatic bio-

transformation, but their metabolites accumulate in uremic patients and are removed by dialysis. Labetolol is rapidly biotransformed by the liver. The elimination half-lives of several other β-blockers (alprenolol, bufuralol, mepindolol, terazosin, timolol, and tolamolol) are not prolonged by renal failure.

ANTIARRHYTHMIC AGENTS

The antiarrhythmic, lidocaine, is eliminated from a large distribution volume almost entirely by the liver. Its half-life is not appreciably affected by uremia or dialysis (133). Tocainamide, a longer acting lidocaine analogue, is retained somewhat in renal failure and is cleared by dialysis (138). Lorcainide does not accumulate in uremic patients.

Procainamide is eliminated by both hepatic acetylation and renal excretion. The half-life is prolonged with renal failure and the active N-acetyl metabolite is retained as well, so the dose should be reduced to about 20% of the normal, or the drug avoided (41). A small supplement is warranted after dialysis. N-Acetyl procainamide may accumulate despite modest removal by hemodialysis, and hemoperfusion can be required to treat toxicity.

Quinidine distributes in a large space and is about 75% bound in plasma. Hepatic elimination is not delayed in uremic patients, but metabolites accumulate (71). Hemodialysis clears quinidine slowly, but has induced improvement in intoxicated patients.

Disopyramide, about 30% bound in plasma and distributed in a volume approaching 1.0 liter/kg, is partly eliminated by the kidney, accumulates with renal failure, and is modestly affected by dialysis (66). Bretylium depends mostly on renal excretion. It has a low molecular weight, is minimally bound, and is rapidly removed by dialysis (67). Mexiletine elimination is mostly independent of renal function. The half-life increases from about 11 to 15 hours with renal failure and is not reduced by dialysis because of 70% plasma protein binding and a large distribution volume. The half-life of cibenzoline is approximately doubled with renal failure, whereas amiodarone elimination is not affected by uremia or by dialysis.

The calcium channel blocking agents, diltiazem, nifedipine, and verapamil, are all highly protein bound in plasma, distribute in large volumes, and are rapidly metabolized by the liver. Dialysis does not remove these drugs or their metabolites appreciably.

DIURETICS

As renal failure progresses, diuretics become less effective but tend to be given in higher doses, causing more toxicity. Mannitol accumulates in uremic patients and can precipitate circulatory congestion with pulmonary edema, hyperosmolality, hypernatremia, and intracellular dehydration. Organic mercurials depend on renal elimination and are contraindicated in patients with renal failure. Acetazolamide is tightly bound to carbonic anhydrase in tissues and is excreted by the kidney (112). It is retained in uremic patients and may aggravate metabolic acidosis. Thiazides are not effective when renal failure is moderate or severe and are eliminated by the kidney (9). Chlorthalidone has a long half-life and is eliminated by both renal and nonrenal mechanisms. Ethacrynic acid may induce saluresis but often only after high doses with the risk of ototoxicity (81). Elimination is partly hepatic and partly renal. Like other loop diuretics, ethacrynic acid is highly protein bound. Furosemide can also induce a clinically effective diuresis, despite renal failure and potential ototoxicity (81). It accumulates in patients with renal failure or cirrhosis and is not readily removed by dialysis because of high fractional protein binding, which is reduced somewhat by uremia. Piretanide is eliminated in part by the kidney; the half-life is prolonged from 0.7 to 2.8 hours with renal failure (11). Bumetanide accumulation is minimal in renal failure, however, because decreased protein binding accelerates nonrenal clearance (104). Torazemide is not retained in renal failure or removed by dialysis (86). The major problem with these potent diuretics is their overzealous use in an attempt to achieve diuresis in depleted patients who instead should be repleted. Spironolactone is less effective in patients with renal failure, but the risk of hyperkalemia is increased (1). It is rapidly biotransformed by the liver to active metabolites that may accumulate in uremic patients. Triamterene also is a less effective saluretic in uremic patients but may cause hyperkalemia. Elimination is predominantly hepatic but hydroxy-metabolites accumulate and may be pharmacologically active. Amiloride depends on renal elimination and accumulates in uremic patients (37). Protein binding limits the removal of most diuretics by dialysis.

Table 3.8
Half-lives of Miscellaneous Drugs[a]

Drug	Half-life (hr)		
	N	A	H
Theophylline	6.2	7.3	2.6
Dyphylline	2.0	11.9	5.5
Cortisone	1.3	3.5	3.4
Prednisolone	3.2	4.2	4.2
Cyclophosphamide	6.0	7.0	2.5
Bleomycin	3.0	22	—
Tolbutamide	5.0	5.0	5.0
Chlorpropamide	30	200	150
Phenytoin	16	8.0	7.6
Valproic acid	12	10	8.3
Propylthiouracil	17	50	—
Methimazole	2.0	9.0	—
Organic iodides	1.0	30	4.2
Cimetidine	1.9	4.3	2.5
Ranitidine	2.0	7.0	4.3
Clofibrate	17	100	—
Gallamine	2.2	12.5	6.0
Atracurium	0.3	0.4	—
Vecuronium	1.3	1.6	—
Pancuronium	2.2	4.3	—
Metocurine	6.0	11.4	—

[a] Data from references 1, 9, 12, 16, 44, 53, 78, 79, 90, 105, 114, 135. See footnote b Table 3.2.

Miscellaneous Drugs (Table 3.8)

Theophylline is eliminated mainly by the liver and does not accumulate with renal failure. Despite appreciable protein binding it is rapidly removed by hemodialysis, which doubles the elimination rate, and by peritoneal dialysis. Hemoperfusion clears theophylline even faster than dialysis. Dyphylline has a high renal clearance, accumulates in uremic patients, and is rapidly cleared by dialysis (79). Terbutaline is metabolized by the liver with a normal half-life of about 1.2 hours.

Allopurinol is rapidly metabolized to oxipurinol, which inhibits xanthine oxidase. Oxipurinol is slowly excreted by the kidney and accumulates in uremic patients, so the allopurinol dose should not exceed 300 mg/day (30). Oxipurinol is readily dialyzable. Colchicine is very rapidly eliminated even in uremic patients. Probenecid is more slowly eliminated. Although it is metabolized before excretion, this drug should be avoided in uremic patients.

Adrenal corticosteroids are removed metabolically and dosage does not have to be restricted in uremic patients, although azotemia is aggravated by inhibition of anabolism by these drugs.

Cyclophosphamide is mostly biotransformed in the liver, yet with renal failure its half-life increases slightly. Dosage reduction is usually required because of the potential severity of toxicity and because of active metabolites rather than concern for retention of the parent compound (135). Cyclophosphamide is cleared rapidly by dialysis. Other alkylating agents, such as chlorambucil, mechlorethamine, melphalan, and busulfan, are metabolized and uninfluenced by renal failure or dialysis.

Azathioprine is rapidly cleaved nonenzymatically to 6-mercaptopurine and oxidized (44). Although not retained in patients with renal failure, other considerations often warrant dosage reduction in uremic patients. Dialysis increases azathioprine elimination minimally.

Methotrexate is eliminated mainly by renal excretion (9, 44). This drug accumulates in renal failure, and binding in plasma decreases. Hence, both peak and trough concentrations increase, so the dose must be decreased and the dosing interval prolonged. Methotrexate is not effectively removed by dialysis, but hemoperfusion rapidly lowers plasma levels. The nitrosoureas, carmustine, lomustine, and streptozocin, can be nephrotoxic. Their elimination is hepatic but active metabolites can be retained in uremic patients. The pyrimidine analogues, 5-fluorouracil and cytosine arabinoside, are rapidly metabolized. Renal failure does not delay elimination and the large distribution spaces limit removal by dialysis. Bleomycin accumulates in uremic patients, causing increased cutaneous and gastrointestinal toxicity (105). It is not removed by dialysis. Doxorubicin and daunorubicin are eliminated by the liver, do not accumulate in uremic patients, but can cause renal injury (44). Mithramycin is eliminated by the kidney and can be nephrotoxic.

Cyclosporine is a large, highly bound solute that distributes into body fat. Renal elimination is minimal and removal by dialysis is insignificant (109). The normal half-life is 7 hours. Bredinin is another new immunosuppressive drug used for transplants, which depends on renal elimination and is rapidly removed by dialysis.

Many organic compounds of heavy metals accumulate in patients with renal functional impairment and cause further renal injury. Such compounds include arsenicals, antimonials, gold compounds, bismuth preparations, iron-dextran, and cis-platinum. Chelates accelerate removal of some of these metals, which are normally highly bound in plasma and tissue (91, 108). Chelates can accumulate and can also be nephrotoxic.

Uremic patients have delayed elimination of insulin and peripheral resistance to its action (35). They have increased sensitivity to the oral hypoglycemic agents. Tolbutamide is the preferred oral hypoglycemic agent because it does not depend on renal elimination and is not removed appreciably by dialysis (128). The metabolites of tolazamide and acetohexamide cause hypoglycemia and depend on renal elimination. Chlorpropamide, about 90% bound in plasma, accumulates in uremic patients causing recurrent hypoglycemia and is not removed appreciably by dialysis (128). The biguanides, phenformin and buformin, are rapidly excreted by the kidney. Phenformin is no longer recommended because it causes lactic acidosis.

Phenytoin is eliminated by oxidation, conjugation, and renal excretion of the metabolite. Uremia decreases protein binding, reducing the distribution space and accelerating elimination. Phenytoin is well tolerated in uremic patients, and usually no dosage adjustment is required. Excessive phenytoin can be slowly removed by dialysis since binding is decreased. This slow removal helps clinically, because saturation kinetics limit metabolic removal at high concentrations (16).

Trimethadione and paramethadione are eliminated by the liver. Valproic acid undergoes β oxidation. Dosage modification is not required for any of these drugs. Carbamazepine is normally eliminated slowly, and hemodialyzer clearance exceeds the endogenous removal rate (80). Ethosuximide has similar pharmacokinetics, including a relatively high clearance by dialysis.

Neither heparin nor the oral anticoagulants, bishydroxycoumarin, warfarin, or phenindione, depends on renal elimination; dialysis does not augment their elimination (9, 44). Caution is advised with anticoagulant use, not because of abnormal pharmacokinetics, but because of the bleeding diathesis and lesions of uremia. Dipyridamole elimination is not influenced by uremia or dialysis. Thrombolytic agents are inactivated in circulation and are not known to be affected by uremia.

Propylthiouracil is excreted in part by the kidney and accumulates in uremic patients, hence dosage reduction is warranted (1). Methimazole is also retained in the plasma of uremic patients. The effect of dialysis on these antithyroid drugs is unknown.

Iodide is excreted by the kidney in competition with thyroidal uptake. Povidone-iodine absorbed locally can contribute to iodine retention. Iodinated radiographic contrast media accumulate in patients with renal failure, can accelerate renal functional loss, and can be removed by dialysis (53).

Cimetidine is eliminated mostly by the kidney, excretion correlating with creatinine clearance. In patients with severe renal failure, the dose must be reduced by 50% to prevent toxic symptoms that mimic uremic encephalopathy (75). Hemodialysis removes cimetidine (and its sulphoxide metabolite) rapidly, but hemoperfusion clears it even faster, while peritoneal clearance does not accelerate elimination appreciably. Cimetidine inhibits renal secretion of creatinine, raising plasma levels acutely. Ranitidine has similar pharmacokinetics (114). The dose of either histamine blocker should be reduced about 50% with renal failure.

Clofibrate is excreted by the kidney partly unchanged and partly after hepatic conjugation. Dosage reduction is mandatory in uremic patients, and removal by dialysis is slow because of extensive protein binding (46). Bezafibrate and fenofibrate are new hypolipemic drugs that are retained in patients with renal failure and are highly protein bound, preventing removal by dialysis.

Preexisting renal functional impairment predisposes to further nephron injury by the fluorinated anesthetics, enflurane and methoxyflurane (126). Atropine also depends in part on renal elimination, and caution is advised in prescribing it to uremic patients (47). Dialysis has negligible effects on its elimination kinetics.

The neuromuscular relaxant, gallamine, depends on renal excretion; it accumulates in renal failure, prolonging neuromuscular blockade, and can be removed by dialysis. Vecuronium and atracurium have short half-lives that are not prolonged with renal failure (12). Laudanosine, a metabolite of atracurium, accumulates in uremic patients, however, and stimulates the central nervous system. Pancuronium and metocurine accumulate to a moderate extent with renal failure. D-Tubocurarine also depends on renal elimination. Fazadinium and norcuron are metabolized.

Pyridostigmine depends on renal excretion. The metabolites of neostigmine and of succinylcholine are active and accumulate in patients with renal failure.

Even vitamins must be considered pharma-cokinetically in uremic patients (94, 129). Vitamin C depletion can occur with renal failure, and losses are accelerated by dialysis. However, excessive supplementation of ascorbic acid leads to accumulation and metabolic breakdown that can contribute to the oxalosis of uremia. The B vitamins are water soluble and removed by dialysis. Only modest reduction in plasma concentrations occur (5–30%) with hemodialysis, and because of its large molecular size vitamin B_{12} traverses dialysis membranes slowly. Pyridoxine is the only B vitamin that requires supplementation in nourished uremic patients, the need arising from incomplete activation or a retained inhibitor. Folic acid is low in plasma but usually normal in erythrocytes, and plasma riboflavin levels are variably low. Chronic uremia often requires 1,25-dihydroxycholecalciferol supplements because of inadequate renal metabolic activation of vitamin D. Toxicity can ensue from excessive supplements. Vitamin A supplements can also cause toxicity, although much of the increment in measured levels represents retinol-binding protein.

CONCLUSIONS

When selecting a drug for the uremic patient, it is preferable to choose an agent that does not depend mainly on renal excretion, is minimally affected by changes in protein binding, distribution volume, or receptor sensitivity, and does not have active or toxic metabolites.

Critically ill patients often have hemodynamic abnormalities that impair metabolic clearance, as well as renal excretion. Accordingly, in these patients drug use should be restricted to definite indications, dosing must be monitored carefully following pharmacokinetic principles, and patients must be monitored carefully for drug toxicity, which must be considered whenever unexplained abnormalities occur. Those who rely blindly on nomograms and "cookbook" guidelines for dosing have no business administering potentially toxic drugs to patients with abnormal elimination mechanisms.

References

1. Anderson RJ, Bennett WM, Gambertoglio JG, Schrier RW: Fate of drugs in renal failure. In Brenner BM, Rector FC Jr (eds): *The Kidney.* Philadelphia, WB Saunders, 1981, pp 2659–2708.

2. Andrassy K, Ritz E: Antimicrobial therapy in dialysis patients. I. Penicillins and cephalosporins. *Blood Purif* 3:94–103, 1985.
3. Anttila M, Haataja M, Kasanen A: Pharmacokinetics of naproxen in subjects with normal and impaired renal function. *Eur J Clin Pharmacol* 18:263–268, 1980.
4. Appel GV, Neu HC: The nephrotoxicity of antimicrobial agents. *N Engl J Med* 296:663–670, 722–728, 784–787, 1977.
5. Atkinson AJ Jr, Kushner W: Clinical pharmacokinetics. *Annu Rev Pharmacol Toxicol* 19:105–127, 1979.
6. Balant L, Dayer P, Rudhardt M, Allaz AF, Fabre J: Cefoperazone: pharmacokinetics in humans with normal and impaired renal function and pharmacokinetics in rats. *Clin Ther* 3:50–59, 1980.
7. Balogh A, Funfstuck R, Demme U, Kangas L, Sperschneider H, Traeger A, Stein G, Pekkarinen A: Dialysability of benzodiazepines of haemodialysis and controlled sequential ultrafiltration (CSU) in vitro. *Arch Pharmacol Toxicol* 49:174–180, 1981.
8. Bateman DN, Gokal R, Dodd TRP, Blain PG: The pharmacokinetics of single doses of metoclopramide in renal failure. *Eur J Clin Pharmacol* 19:437–441, 1981.
9. Benet LZ, Sheiner LB: Design and optimization of dosage regimens; pharmacokinetic data. In Gilman AG, Goodman LS, Rall TW, Murad F (eds): *Goodman and Gilman's The Pharmacological Basis of Therapeutics*, ed 7. New York, MacMillan, 1985, pp 1663–1733.
10. Bennett WM, Muther RS, Parker RA, Feig P, Morrison G, Golper TA, Singer I: Drug therapy in renal failure: dosing guidelines for adults. *Ann Intern Med* 93:62–89, 286–325, 1980.
11. Berg KH, Walstad RA, Bergh K: The pharmacokinetics and diuretic effects of piretanide in chronic renal insufficiency. *Br J Clin Pharmacol* 15:347–353, 1983.
12. Bevan DR, Donati F, Gyasi H, Williams A: Vecuronium in renal failure. *Can Anaesth Soc J* 31:491–496, 1984.
13. Block ER, Bennett JE, Levoti LG, Klein WJ, MacGregor RR, Henderson L: Flucytosine and amphotericin B: hemodialysis effects on the plasma concentration and clearance. *Ann Intern Med* 80:613–617, 1974.
14. Boelaert J, Daneels R, Schurgers M, Mellows G, Suaisland AJ, Lambert AM, Van Landuyt HW: Effects of renal functions and dialysis on temocillin pharmacokinetics. *Drugs* 29(suppl 5):109–113, 1985.
15. Boelaert J, Valcke Y, Schurgers M, Daneels M, Rosseel MT, Bogaert MG: The pharmacokinetics of ciprofloxacin in patients with impaired renal function. *J Antimicrob Chemother* 16:87–93, 1985.
16. Borgå O, Hoppel C, Odar-Cederlof I, Garle M: Plasma levels and renal excretion of phenytoin and its metabolites in patients with renal failure. *Clin Pharmacol Ther* 26:306–314, 1979.
17. Breimer DD: Clinical pharmacokinetics of hypnotics. *Clin Pharmacokinet* 2:93–109, 1977.
18. Brogard JM, Comte F, Spach MO, Lavillaureix J: Pharmacokinetics of mezlocillin in patients with kidney failure: special reference to hemodialysis and dosage adjustments in relation to renal function. *Chemotherapy* 29:318–326, 1982.
19. Bunke CM, Aronoff GR, Brier ME, Sloan RS, Luft FC: Vancomycin kinetics during continuous ambulatory peritoneal dialysis. *Clin Pharmacol Ther* 334:631–637, 1983.
20. Carlson RV, Bailey RR, Begg EJ, Cowlishaw MG, Sharman JR: Pharmacokinetics and effect on blood pressure of doxazosin in patients with renal failure. *Clin Pharmacol Ther* 40:561–566, 1986.
21. Carmichael J, Shankel SW: Effects of nonsteroidal antiinflammatory drugs on prostaglandins and renal function. *Am J Med* 78:992–1000, 1985.
22. Chodos J, Francke EL, Saltzman M, Neu HC: Pharmacokinetics of intravenous cefotaxime in patients undergoing chronic hemodialysis. *Ther Drug Monitor* 3:71–74, 1981.
23. Christopher TG, Blair AD, Forrey AW, Cutler RE: Hemodialyzer clearances of gentamicin, kanamycin, tobramycin, amikacin, ethambutol, procainamide, and flucytosine with a technique for planning therapy. *J Pharmacokinet Biopharm* 4:427–441, 1976.
24. Cohen D, Appel GB, Scully B, Neu HC: Pharmacokinetics of ceftriaxone in patients with renal failure and in those undergoing hemodialysis. *Antimicrob Agents Chemother* 24:529–432, 1983.
25. Craig WA, Welling PG, Jackson TC, Kunin CM: Pharmacology of cephazolin and other cephalosporins in patients with renal insufficiency. *J Infect Dis* 128:S347–S353, 1973.
26. Dalet F, Amado E, Cabrera E, Donate T, del Rio G: Pharmacokinetics of the combination of ticarcillin with clavulanic acid in renal insufficiency. *J Antimicrob Chemother* 17(suppl C):57–64, 1986.
27. Danish M, Schultz R, Jusko WJ: Pharmacokinetics of gentamicin and kanamycin during hemodialysis. *Antimicrob Agents Chemother* 6:841–847, 1974.
28. De Schepper PJ, Tjandramaga TB, Mullie A, Verbesselt R, van Hecken A, Verbeckmoes R, Verbist L: Comparative pharmacokinetics of piperacillin in normals and in patients with renal failure. *J Antimicrob Chemother* 9(suppl B):49–57, 1982.
29. Duchin KL, Pierides AM, Heald A, Singhvi SM, Rommel AJ: Elimination kinetics of captopril in patients with renal failure. *Kidney Int* 25:942–947, 1984.
30. Elion GB, Benezra FM, Beardmore TD, Kelley WN: Studies with allopurinol in patients with impaired renal function. *Adv Exp Med Biol* 122A:263–267, 1980.
31. Fabre J, Fox HM, Dayer P, Balant L: Differences in kinetic properties of drugs: implications as to the selection of a particular drug for use in patients with renal failure with special emphasis on antibiotics and β-adrenoceptor blocking agents. *Clin Pharmacokinet* 5:441–464, 1980.
32. Felts JH, Hayes DM, Gergen JA, Toole JF: Neural, hematologic and bacteriologic effects of nitrofurantoin in renal insufficiency. *Am J Med* 51:331–339, 1971.
33. Flouvat BL, Imbert C, Dubois DM, Temperville BP, Roux AF, Chevalier GC, Humbert G: Pharmacokinetics of tinidazole in chronic renal failure and in patients on haemodialysis. *Br J Clin Pharmacol* 15:735–741, 1983.
34. Floyd M, Hill AVL, Ormston BJ, Menzies R, Porter R: Quinine amblyopia treated by hemodialysis. *Clin Nephrol* 2:44–46, 1974.
35. Fuss M, Bergans A, Brauman H, Toussaint C, Vereerstraeten P, Franckson M, Corvilain J: ^{125}I-insulin metabolism in chronic renal failure treated by renal transplantation. *Kidney Int* 5:372–377, 1974.
36. Gault MH, Jeffrey JR, Chiruto E, Ward LL: Studies of digoxin dosage, kinetics and serum concentrations in renal failure and review of the literature. *Nephron* 17:161–187, 1976.
37. George CF: Amiloride handling in renal failure. *Br J Clin Pharmacol* 9:94–95, 1980.
38. Gerig JS, Bolton N, Swabb EA, Scheld WM, Bolton WK: Effect of hemodialysis and peritoneal dialysis on aztreonam pharmacokinetics. *Kidney Int* 26:308–318, 1984.
39. Giacomini KM, Gibson TP, Levy G: Effect of hemodialysis on propoxyphene and norpropoxyphene concentrations in blood of anephric patients. *Clin Pharmacol Ther* 27:508–514, 1980.
40. Gibson TP: Renal disease and drug metabolism: an overview. *Am J Kidney Dis* 8:7–17, 1986.
41. Gibson TP, Atkinson AJ Jr, Matusik E, Nelson LD, Briggs WA: Kinetics of procainamide and N-acetylprocainamide in renal failure. *Kidney Int* 12:422–429, 1977.
42. Gibson TP, Demetriades JL, Bland JA: Imipenem/cilastin pharmacokinetic profile in renal insufficiency. *Am J Med* 78(suppl 6A):54–61, 1985.

43. Gibson TP, Lucas SV, Nelson HA, Atkinson AJ Jr, Okita GR, Ivanovich P: Hemoperfusion removal of digoxin from dogs. *J Lab Clin Med* 91:673–682, 1978.

44. Gibson TP, Nelson HA: Drug kinetics and artificial kidneys. *Clin Pharmacokinet* 2:403–426, 1977.

45. Gold CH, Buchanan N, Tringham V, Viljoen M, Strickwold B, Moodley GP: Isoniazid pharmacokinetics in patients in chronic renal failure. *Clin Nephrol* 6:365–369, 1976.

46. Goldberg AP, Sherrard DJ, Haas LB, Brunzell JD: Control of clofibrate toxicity in uremic hypertriglyceridemia. *Clin Pharmacol Ther* 21:317–325, 1977.

47. Gosselin RE, Gabourel JD, Wills JH: Fate of atropine in man. *Clin Pharmacol Ther* 1:597–603, 1960.

48. Gotlieb TB, Thomas RC, Chidsey CA: Pharmacokinetic studies of minoxidil. *Clin Pharmacol Ther* 13:436–441, 1972.

49. Guay DR, Meatherall RC, Baxter H, Jacyk WR, Penner B: Pharmacokinetics of metronidazole in patients undergoing continuous ambulatory peritoneal dialysis. *Antimicrob Agents Chemother* 25:306–310, 1984.

50. Guay DRP, Meatherall RC, Harding GK, Brown GR: Pharmacokinetics of cefixime (CL 284, 635; FK 027) in healthy subjects and patients with renal insufficiency. *Antimicrob Agents Chemother* 30:485–490, 1986.

51. Gutman RA, Burnell MJ, Solak F: Paraldehyde acidosis. *Am J Med* 42:440–455, 1967.

52. Halstenson CE, Blevins RB, Salem NG, Matzke GR: Trimethoprim-sulfamethoxazole pharmacokinetics during continuous ambulatory peritoneal dialysis. *Clin Nephrol* 22:239–243, 1984.

53. Hansson R, Lindholm T: Elimination of hypaque (sodium 3,5 diacetamido-2,4,6 triiodobenzoate) and the effect of hemodialysis in anuria. A clinical study and an experimental investigation on rabbits. *Acta Med Scand* 174:611–626, 1963.

54. Heaney D, Eknoyan G: Minocycline and doxycycline kinetics in renal failure. *Clin Pharmacol Ther* 24:233–239, 1978.

55. Held H, Enderle C: Elimination and serum protein binding of phenylbutazone in patients with renal insufficiency. *Clin Nephrol* 6:388–393, 1976.

56. Hoeprich PD: The polymyxins. *Med Clin North Am* 54:1257–1265, 1970.

57. Horber FF, Frey FJ, Descoludres C, Murray AT, Reubi FC: Differential effects of impaired renal function on the kinetics of clavulanic acid and amoxicillin. *Antimicrob Agents Chemother* 29:614–619, 1986.

58. Hulter HN, Licht JH, Ilnicki LP, Singh S: Clinical efficacy and pharmacokinetics of clonidine in hemodialysis and renal insufficiency. *J Lab Clin Med* 94:223–231, 1979.

59. Humbert G, Fillastre JP, Leroy A, Godin M, Van Winzum C: Pharmacokinetics of cefoxitin in normal subjects and in patients with renal insufficiency. *Rev Infect Dis* 1:118–126, 1979.

60. Humes HD, Weinberg JM, Knauss TC: Clinical and physiologic aspects of aminoglycoside toxicity. *Am J Kidney Dis* 2:5–29, 1982.

61. Jacobson EJ, Zahrowski JJ, Nissenson AR: Moxalactam kinetics in hemodialysis. *Clin Pharmacol Ther* 30:487–490, 1981.

62. Jaeger A, Sauder P, Kopferschmitt J, Jaegle ML: Toxicokinetics of lithium intoxication treated by hemodialysis. *J Toxicol Clin Toxicol* 23:501–517, 1986.

63. Jeliffe RW, Buell J, Kalaba R, Sridhar R, Rockwell R, Wagner JG: An improved method of digitoxin therapy. *Ann Intern Med* 72:453–464, 1970.

64. Johnson CA, Zimmerman SW, Rogge M: The pharmacokinetics of antibiotics used to treat peritoneal dialysis-associated peritonitis. *Am J Kidney Dis* 4:3–17, 1984.

65. Johnson RJ, Blair AD, Ahmad S: Ketoconazole kinetics in chronic peritoneal dialysis. *Clin Pharmacol Ther* 37:325–329, 1985.

66. Johnston A, Henry JA, Warrington SJ, Hamer NAJ: Pharmacokinetics of oral disopyramide phosphate in patients with renal impairment. *Br J Clin Pharmacol* 10:245–248, 1980.

67. Josselson J, Narang PK, Adir J, Yacobi A, Sadler JH: Bretylium kinetics in renal insufficiency. *Clin Pharmacol Ther* 33:144–150, 1983.

68. Jusko WJ, Lewis GP, Schmitt GW: Ampicillin and hetacillin pharmacokinetics in normal and anephric subjects. *Clin Pharmacol Ther* 14:90–99, 1973.

69. Keller F, Lode H, Offerman G: Antimicrobial therapy in dialysis patients. II. Remaining antibiotics and antimicrobial agents. *Blood Purif* 3:104–108, 1985.

70. Keller F, Offerman G, Lode H: Supplementary dose after hemodialysis. *Nephron* 30:220–227, 1982.

71. Kessler KM, Lowenthal DT, Warner H, Gibson T, Briggs W, Reidenberg MM: Quinidine elimination in patients with congestive heart failure or poor renal function. *N Engl J Med* 290:706–709, 1974.

72. Kirch W, Kohler H, Axthelm T: Pharmacokinetics of guanfacine in patients undergoing haemodialysis. *Eur J Drug Metab Pharmacokinet* 7:277–280, 1982.

73. Klooker P, Bommer J, Ritz E: Treatment of hypertension in dialysis patients. *Blood Purif* 3:15–26, 1985.

74. Konishi K: Pharmacokinetics of cefmenoxime in patients with impaired renal function and in those undergoing hemodialysis. *Antimicrob Agents Chemother* 30:901–905, 1986.

75. Larsson R, Erlanson P, Bodemar G, Walan A, Bertler A, Fransson L, Norlander B: The pharmacokinetics of cimetidine and its sulphoxide metabolites in patients with normal and impaired renal function. *Br J Clin Pharmacol* 13:163–170, 1982.

76. Lasrich M, Maher JM, Hirszel P, Maher JF: Correlation of peritoneal transport rates with molecular weight: a method for predicting clearances. *asaio J* 2:107–113, 1979.

77. Lee CS, Marbury TC: Drug therapy in patients undergoing haemodialysis. Clinical pharmacokinetic considerations. *Clin Pharmacokinet* 9:42–66, 1984.

78. Lee CS, Peterson JC, Marbury TC: Comparative pharmacokinetics of theophylline in peritoneal dialysis and hemodialysis. *J Clin Pharmacol* 23:274–280, 1983.

79. Lee CS, Wang LH, Majeske BL, Marbury TC: Pharmacokinetics of dyphylline elimination by uremic patients. *J Pharmacol Exp Ther* 217:340–344, 1981.

80. Lee CS, Wang LH, Marbury TC, Bruni J, Perchalski RJ: Hemodialysis clearance and total body elimination of carbamazepine during chronic hemodialysis. *Clin Toxicol* 17:429–438, 1980.

81. Levin NW: Furosemide and ethacrynic acid in renal insufficiency. *Med Clin North Am* 55:107–119, 1971.

82. Libke RD, Clarke JT, Ralph ED, Luthy RP, Kirby WMM: Ticarcillin vs carbenicillin: clinical pharmacokinetics. *Clin Pharmacol Ther* 17:441–446, 1975.

83. Lieberman JA, Cooper TB, Suckow RF, Steinberg H, Borenstein M, Brenner R, Kane JM: Tricyclic antidepressant and metabolite levels in chronic renal failure. *Clin Pharmacol Ther* 37:301–307, 1985.

84. Lindholm DD, Murray JS: Persistence of vancomycin in the blood during renal failure and its treatment by hemodialysis. *N Engl J Med* 274:1047–1051, 1966.

85. Lobo PI, Spyler D, Surratt P, Westervelt FB Jr: Use of hemodialysis in meprobamate overdosage. *Clin Nephrol* 7:73–75, 1977.

86. Loute G, Adam A, Ers P, Heremans C, Willems B: The influence of haemodialysis and haemofiltration on the clearance of torazemide in renal failure. *Eur J Clin Pharmacol* 31(suppl):53–55, 1986.

87. Lowenthal DT, Hobbs D, Affrime MB, Twomey TM, Martinez EW, Onesti G: Prazosin kinetics and effectiveness in renal failure. *Clin Pharmacol Ther* 27:779–783, 1980.

88. Luft FC, Brannon DR, Stropes LL, Costello RJ, Sloan RS, Maxwell DR: Pharmacokinetics of netilmicin in patients with renal impairment and in patients on dialysis. *Antimicrob Agents Chemother* 14:403–407, 1978.

89. Maher JF: Determinants of serum half life of gluteth-imide in intoxicated patients. *J Pharmacol Exp Therap* 174:450–455, 1970.

90. Maher JF: Pharmacological aspects of renal failure and dialysis. In Drukker W, Parsons FM, Maher JF (eds): *Replacement of Renal Function by Dialysis*. The Hague, Martinus Nijhoff, 1983, pp 749–797.

91. Maher JF: Toxic and irradiation nephropathies. In Earley LE, Gottschalk CW (eds): *Strauss and Welt's Diseases of the Kidney*. Boston, Little, Brown & Co, 1979, pp 1431–1474.

92. Manuel MA, Paton TW, Cornish WR: Drugs and peritoneal dialysis. *Peritoneal Dial Bull* 3:117–125, 1983.

93. Martre H, Sari R, Taburet AM, Jacobs C, Singlas E: Haemodialysis does not affect the pharmacokinetics of nifedipine. *Br J Clin Pharmacol* 20:115–158, 1985.

94. Marumo F, Kamata K, Okubo M: Deranged concentrations of water-soluble vitamins in the blood of undialyzed and dialyzed patients with chronic renal failure. *Int J Artif Intern Organs* 9:17–24, 1986.

95. Merdjan H, Baumelou A, Diquet B, Chick O, Singlas E: Pharmacokinetics of ornidazole in patients with renal insufficiency; influence of haemodialysis and peritoneal dialysis. *Br J Clin Pharmacol* 19:211–217, 1985.

96. Mery A, Kanfer A: Ototoxicity of erythromycin in patients with renal insufficiency. *N Engl J Med* 301:944, 1979.

97. Moellering RC Jr, Swartz MN: The newer cephalosporins. *N Engl J Med* 294:24–28, 1976.

98. Myhre E, Rugstad HE, Arnold E, Stenback O, Hansen T: Pharmacokinetics of methyldopa in renal failure and bilaterally nephrectomized patients. *Scand J Urol Nephrol* 16:257–263, 1982.

99. Nauta EH, Mattie H: Dicloxacillin and cloxacillin pharmacokinetics in healthy and hemodialysis subjects. *Clin Pharmacol Ther* 20:98–108, 1976.

100. Ohkawa M, Kuroda K: Pharmacokinetics of ceftezole in patients with normal and impaired renal function. *Chemotherapy* 26:242–247, 1980.

101. Pancorbo AS, Palagi PA, Piecoro JJ, Wilson HD: Hemodialysis in methyprylon overdose; some pharmacokinetic considerations. *JAMA* 237:470–471, 1977.

102. Pechere J, Dugal R: Pharmacokinetics of intravenously administered tobramycin in normal volunteers and in renal-impaired and hemodialyzed patients. *J Infect Dis* 134:S118–S124, 1976.

103. Peddie BA, Dann E, Bailey RR: The effect of impairment of renal function and dialysis on the serum and urine levels of clindamycin. *Aust NZ J Med* 5:198–202, 1975.

104. Pentikäinen PJ, Pasternak A, Lampainen E, Neuvonen PJ, Penttila A: Bumetanide kinetics in renal failure. *Clin Pharmacol Ther* 37:582–588, 1985.

105. Pitrilli ES, Castaldo TW, Matutat RJ, Ballon SC, Gutierrez ML: Bleomycin pharmacology in relation to adverse effects and renal function in cervical cancer patients. *Gynecol Oncol* 14:350–354, 1982.

106. Pohl JEF, Thurston H: Use of diazoxide in hypertension with renal failure. *Br Med J* 4:142–145, 1971.

107. Pozet N, Brazier JL, Hadj Aissa A, Khenfer G, Apoil E, Traeger J: Pharmacokinetics of diltiazem in severe renal failure. *Eur J Clin Pharmacol* 24:635–638, 1983.

108. Prestayko AW, Luft FC, Einhorn L, Crooke ST: Cisplatin pharmacokinetics in a patient with renal dysfunction. *Med Pediatr Oncol* 5:183–188, 1978.

109. Ptachcinski RJ, Venkataramanan R, Burckart GJ: Clinical pharmacokinetics of cyclosporin. *Clin Pharmacokinet* 11:107–132, 1986.

110. Regeur L, Golding H, Jensen H, Kaupmann JP: Pharmacokinetics of amikacin during hemodialysis and peritoneal dialysis. *Antimicrob Agents Chemother* 11:214–218, 1977.

111. Reidenberg MM: The binding of drugs to plasma proteins and the interpretation of measurements of plasma concentrations of drugs in patients with poor renal function. *Am J Med* 62:467–474, 1977.

112. Reidenberg MM: *Renal Function and Drug Action*. Philadelphia, WB Saunders, 1971, p 113.

113. Revert L, Lopez J, Pons J, Olag T: Fosfomycin in patients subjected to periodic hemodialysis. *Chemotherapy* 23(suppl 1):204–209, 1977.

114. Roberts AP, Harrison C, Dixon GT, Curtis JR: Plasma ranitidine concentrations after intravenous administration in normal volunteers and haemodialysis patients. *Postgrad Med J* 59:25–27, 1983.

115. Schapira A: Single dose kinetics and dosage of mecillinam in renal failure and haemodialysis. *Clin Pharmacokinet* 9:364–370, 1984.

116. Schentag JJ, Cerra FB, Plaut ME: Clinical and pharmacokinetic characteristics of aminoglycoside toxicity in 201 critically ill patients. *Antimicrob Agents Chemother* 21:721–726, 1982.

117. Schmitt GW, Maher JF, Schreiner GE: Ethacrynic acid enhanced bromuresis. A comparison with peritoneal and hemodialysis. *J Lab Clin Med* 68:913–922, 1966.

118. Schumaker JD, Band JD, Lensmeyer GL, Craig WA: Thiabendazole treatment of severe strongyloidiasis in a hemodialyzed patient. *Ann Intern Med* 89:644–645, 1978.

119. Selden R, Haynie G: Ouabain plasma level kinetics and removal by dialysis in chronic renal failure. A study in fourteen patients. *Ann Intern Med* 83:15–19, 1975.

120. Setter JG, Freeman RB, Maher JF, Schreiner GE: Factors influencing the dialysis of barbiturates. *Trans Am Soc Artif Intern Organs* 10:340–344, 1964.

121. Shah G, Nelson HA, Atkinson AJ Jr, Okita GT, Ivanovich P, Gibson TP: Effect of hemoperfusion on the pharmacokinetics of digitoxin in dogs. *J Lab Clin Med* 93:370–380, 1979.

122. Shah GM, Winer RL: Verapamil kinetics during maintenance hemodialysis. *Am J Nephrol* 5:338–341, 1985.

123. Shah GM, Winer RL, Krasny HC: Acyclovir pharmacokinetics in a patient on continuous ambulatory peritoneal dialysis. *Am J Kidney Dis* 7:507–510, 1986.

124. Shils ME: Renal disease and the metabolic effects of tetracycline. *Ann Intern Med* 58:389–408, 1963.

125. Shionoiri H, Miyazaki N, Yasuda G, Sugimoto K, Uneda S, Kaneko Y: Blood concentration and urinary excretion of enalapril in patients with chronic renal failure. *Nippon Jinzo Gakkai Shi* 27:1291–1297, 1985.

126. Sievenpiper TS, Rice SA, McClendon F, Kosek JC, Mazze RI: Renal effects of enflurane anesthesia in Fischer rats with preexisting renal insufficiency. *J Pharmacol Exp Ther* 211:36–41, 1979.

127. Slaughter RL, Cerra FB, Koup JR: Effect of hemodialysis on total body clearance of chloramphenicol. *Am J Hosp Pharm* 37:1083–1086, 1980.

128. Smith DL, Vecchio TI, Forist AA: Metabolism of antidiabetic sulfonylureas in man. *Metabolism* 14:229–240, 1965.

129. Stein G, Sperschneider H, Koppe S: Vitamin levels in chronic renal failure and need for supplementation. *Blood Purif* 33:52–62, 1985.

130. Stevens DA, Levine HB, Deresinski SC: Miconazole in coccidioidomycosis. II. Therapeutic and pharmacologic studies in man. *Am J Med* 60:191–202, 1976.

131. Szeto HH, Inturrisi CE, Houde R, Saal S, Cheigh J, Reidenberg MM: Accumulation of normeperidine, an active metabolite of meperidine, in patients with renal failure or cancer. *Ann Intern Med* 86:738–741, 1977.

132. Teehan BP, Maher JF, Carey JJH, Flynn PD, Schreiner

GE: Acute ethchlorvynol (Placidyl[R]) intoxication. *Ann Intern Med* 72:875–882, 1970.

133. Thomson PD, Melmon KL, Richardson JA, Cohn K, Steinbrunn W, Cudihee R, Rowland M: Lidocaine pharmacokinetics in advanced heart failure, liver disease and renal failure in humans. *Ann Intern Med* 78:499–508, 1973.

134. Tjandramaga TB: Altered pharmacokinetics of β-adrenoreceptor blocking drugs in patients with renal insufficiency. *Arch Int Pharmacodyn Ther* 248(suppl):38–53, 1980.

135. Wang LH, Lee CS, Majeske BL, Barbury TC: Clearance and recovery calculations in hemodialysis: application to plasma, red blood cell and dialysate measurements for cyclophosphamide. *Clin Pharmacol Ther* 29:365–372, 1981.

136. Wang T, Wuellner D, Woosley RL, Stone WJ: Pharmacokinetics and nondialyzability of mexilitine in renal failure. *Clin Pharmacol Ther* 37:649–653, 1985.

137. Weinstein L, Madoff MA, Samet CM: The sulfonamides. *N Engl J Med* 263:793–800, 842–849, 1960.

138. Wiegers U, Hanrath P, Kuck KH, Pottage A, Graffner C, Augustin J, Runge M: Pharmacokinetics of tocainide in patients with renal dysfunction and during haemodialysis. *Eur J Clin Pharmacol* 24:503–507, 1983.

139. Winchester JR, Gelfand MC, Helliwell M, Vale JA, Goulding R, Schreiner GE: Extracorporeal treatment of salicylate or acetaminophen poisoning—is there a role? *Arch Intern Med* 141:370–374, 1981.

140. Winchester JF, Gelfand MC, Knepshield JH, Schreiner GE: Dialysis and hemoperfusion of poisons and drugs update. *Trans Am Soc Artif Intern Organs* 23:762–842, 1977.

141. Woolner DF, Winter D, Frendin TJ, Begg EJ, Lynn KL, Wright GJ: Renal failure does not impair the metabolism of morphine. *Br J Clin Pharmacol* 22:55–59, 1986.

142. Wright N, Wise R, Hegarty T: Ceftotetan elimination in patients with varying degrees of renal dysfunction. *J Antimicrob Chemother* 11(suppl A):213–216, 1983.

143. Wu MJ, Ing TS, Soung LS, Daugirdas JT, Hano JE, Gandhi VC: Amantidine pharmacokinetics in patients with impaired renal function. *Clin Nephrol* 17:19–23, 1982.

144. Zsoter TT, Johnson GE, DeVeber GA, Paul H: Excretion and metabolism of reserpine in renal failure. *Clin Pharmacol Ther* 14:325–330, 1973.

4

Alterations in Pharmacology Caused by Congestive Heart Failure in the Critically Ill Patient

Rodney W. Savage, M.D., F.A.C.C.
Timothy P. Blair, M.D., F.A.C.C., F.A.C.P.

GENERAL CONSIDERATIONS

Heart failure may lead to important alterations in drug absorption, distribution, biotransformation, action, interaction, and excretion in the critically ill patient. Unfortunately, systematic study of many of the pharmacologic alterations remains incomplete. In this chapter, we discuss a variety of pharmacotherapeutic considerations that are pertinent in patients with heart failure.

Pathophysiology and Etiologies of Congestive Heart Failure

Congestive heart failure in the critically ill patient results from several pathophysiologic states. Arterial hypertension causes pressure overload with resulting left ventricular hypertrophy, decreased diastolic compliance, and increased left ventricular end diastolic pressure. Later, left ventricular dilatation with decreased ejection fraction and increased wall stress may occur. Coarctation of the aorta and aortic stenosis lead to a similar response by the left ventricle. Mitral stenosis causes increased left atrial pressure leading to pulmonary hypertension and right heart failure. Other causes of pulmonary hypertension include (a) left-sided heart failure (the most common situation); (b) chronic obstructive, restrictive, or interstitial lung disease; (c) recurrent pulmonary emboli; (d) primary pulmonary hypertension; and (e) obliterative pulmonary vascular disease from congenital heart disease (Eisenmenger's syndrome). The right ventricle responds to pressure overload in the same fashion as the left ventricle. The acute onset of pulmonary hypertension to pressures greater than 50 mm Hg, however, is poorly tolerated by the less muscular normal right ventricle and may precipitate acute right-sided failure (53).

Volume overload commonly results from regurgitant valvular lesions such as aortic insufficiency and mitral regurgitation. When acute and severe, pulmonary edema and low output shock rapidly ensue. Emergency valve repair or replacement is required. Chronic volume overload, on the other hand, may be surprisingly well tolerated until the patient suffers progressive dilatation of the left ventricle resulting in reduced contractility. In addition, the physiologic stress of another illness may precipitate left ventricular failure in previously compensated situations. Although clinically less common, pulmonary insufficiency and tricuspid regurgitation may lead to similar difficulties in the right heart. These lesions are often well tolerated, but may lead to a low output state, hepatic congestion, ascites, and malnutrition due to malabsorption from bowel edema. High output states represent a type of volume overload that may also precipitate congestive heart failure in a previously compensated, diseased heart. When severe (acute or chronic), high output states may lead to heart failure even with an otherwise previously normal heart (114).

Decreased contractility may result from damage imposed by chronic pressure or volume overload, as discussed above. It may also result from primary muscle loss or dysfunction as seen in dilated cardiomyopathies. Finally, ischemia leads to a reduction in ventricular function (29). Myocardial infarction results in scar and the potential for aneurysm formation, increased wall stress of remaining muscle, and decreased ventricular compliance. Cardiogenic shock results when more than 40% of the left ventricular myocardium is lost (113).

Restricted filling leads to increased filling pressure and limited, then reduced, cardiac output. Pericardial tamponade from a variety of causes must be considered in the critically ill patient with elevated right-sided filling pressures. Ventricular hypertrophy with decreased diastolic compliance is a more frequent cause of restricted filling (102). Although usually secondary to arterial hypertension, left ventricular hypertrophy may also be due to aortic stenosis, idiopathic hypertrophic cardiomyopathy, or infiltrative disease such as amyloidosis. Endomyocardial fibrosis is a rare cause of restrictive cardiomyopathy.

Profound bradyarrhythmias can lead to a low cardiac output, pulmonary congestion, and systemic venous congestion—even in the presence of an otherwise normal heart. Tachyarrhythmias from atrial fibrillation, atrial flutter, paroxysmal supraventricular tachycardia, and ventricular tachycardia can also lead to congestive heart failure. Although sinus tachycardia is usually compensatory, in the face of a reduced stroke volume it may occasionally represent an overcompensation, and clinical improvement may occur following careful use of β blockade (136).

Hemodynamic Alterations and Effects on the Periphery

Heart failure is defined as "the pathophysiological state in which an abnormality of cardiac function is responsible for the failure of the heart to pump blood at a rate commensurate with the requirements of the metabolizing tissues" (21). Restated, this definition implies a relative mismatch between the metabolic needs of the periphery and the heart's ability to deliver nourishing blood flow. Although cardiac output is often reduced in absolute terms, it may be reduced in only relative terms. This reduction results in clinical fatigue and frequently leads to prerenal azotemia. Plasma levels of norepinephrine and vasopressin increase (47, 52). The renin-angiotensin-aldos-

terone axis is activated (3). Ultimately, the tissues shift to anaerobic metabolism with the production of lactic acid. These changes may occur with or without hypotension and with increased, normal, or decreased systemic vascular resistance. In the usual case, left ventricular end diastolic pressure increases lead to pulmonary congestion, which may dominate the clinical picture. Secondary pulmonary hypertension may or may not occur. In its presence, right heart failure may develop with increased central venous pressure, hepatic congestion, and edema. Primary right heart failure may occur in certain disease states with "right-sided" changes occurring earlier in the clinical presentation and followed by signs of decreased output as left-sided filling limitations occur. In all of the above situations, an increase in the basal heart rate is common, perhaps representing a maladaptive overcompensation in some cases (3).

Alterations in the Periphery and Pharmacologic Effects

Heart failure alters both pharmacokinetics and pharmacodynamics. Furthermore, with the use of multiple drugs, drug interactions demand the clinician's constant attention. The disturbances in normal drug metabolism, however, can be quite complex since the physiology of congestive heart failure may vary considerably from patient to patient. The clinician, then, must consider not only the drug, but also how the specific peripheral effects of congestive heart failure alter that drug by affecting its absorption, distribution, biotransformation, actions, interactions, and excretion.

Increased central venous pressure causing gut edema may cause decreased gastrointestinal absorption of medications as demonstrated with quinidine sulfate (35). Drug absorption improves with diuretic therapy, necessitating both clinical monitoring and drug level reevaluation with clinical improvement. The transcutaneous route of administration becomes less efficient with decreased skin blood supply, which often accompanies the increased systemic vascular resistance of congestive heart failure. Studies using transdermal nitroglycerin in heart failure patients show a significant but variable reduction in absorption (56, 105). For similar reasons, intramuscular absorption of lidocaine is also reduced in heart failure (91). Although sublingual and pulmonary absorption probably remain rapid, these routes of administration have not, to our knowledge, been systematically studied in any of the various pathophysiologic subtypes of congestive heart failure. The same may be said for the rectal and subcutaneous routes of drug administration. The intravenous route, of course, circumvents these difficulties of absorption and remains the most direct and reliable pathway for drug administration.

Drug distribution to various body compartments also changes with congestive heart failure. Total body water increases in congestive heart failure, resulting in an increased volume of distribution for highly water-soluble medications. Similarly, lowering the extracellular fluid pH causes an increase in the intracellular concentration of weak acids and a decrease in that of weak bases, provided that intracellular pH also does not change (14). Altered binding of acidic drugs to albumin and basic drugs to α-1-acid-glycoprotein may also alter drug distribution. Delivery of nonpolar drugs to fat stores may be reduced as a result of shunting of blood away from such areas in severe congestive heart failure.

As a general rule, weak organic acids or bases that are lipid soluble are not easily eliminated until biotransformed. Most such reactions occur in the liver via microsomal and nonmicrosomal enzyme systems (68, 83). Other tissues active in this process include plasma, kidney, lung, and gastrointestinal tract. Decreased hepatic blood flow may significantly reduce the rate of metabolism of drugs cleared by the liver, such as lidocaine, leading to overt clinical toxicity at relatively normal clinical doses (38). Furthermore, a reduced capacity to eliminate drugs in congestive heart failure may not be accompanied by abnormalities in routine liver function tests. The aminopyrine breath test has been found to be helpful in such cases, but is not readily available to the clinician (62). β-Blockers can cause a decrease in hepatic blood flow, especially when given during congestive heart failure (110). Competitive inhibition between most substrates for microsomal enzymes usually does not occur since most agents are inactivated by exponential (first order) rather than linear (zero order) kinetics. Some drugs, however, normally exhibit saturable inactivation in the presence of another drug. For example, dicumerol inhibits the metabolism of phenytoin (14), an inhibition possibly exaggerated by decreased hepatic blood flow and hepatic congestion.

Heart failure alters drug excretion by reducing renal blood flow, altering the acid-base balance, and increasing extravascular volume. Renal clearance of digoxin decreases dramatically as glomerular filtration rate falls (42, 106), predisposing to drug-induced toxicity. If liver dysfunction coexists, however, digoxin-like immunoreactive substance may be measured with the same digoxin assay (107). Quinidine, highly protein bound and largely metabolized by the liver, is also excreted by the kidneys (20% of administered drug) and may well exhibit decreased excretion in congestive heart failure secondary to either hepatic or renal function alterations (31, 75). Renal excretion of this weak base is enhanced by an acidic urine.

Changes in drug action in congestive heart failure may occur because of alterations in number or affinity of drug receptors. Acidosis, for example, can blunt the effectiveness of various sympathomimetic amines (145). In chronic congestive heart failure, decreased β-adrenergic receptor number and affinity occur as a result of increased levels of norepinephrine (22, 138), leading to decreased effect for any dose of drug. Furosemide also shows decreased effectiveness for any given dose as a result of decreases in glomerular filtration rate and tubular blood flow induced by heart failure (127).

Finally, the clinician must always consider drug interactions. These are made more likely by the many drugs often required by critically ill patients and are potentially accentuated by altered renal clearance, decreased hepatic function, and altered electrolyte or acid-base status.

SPECIFIC DRUGS

Unfortunately, many of the drugs used in treating critically ill patients have not been well studied in terms of their effects in patients with congestive heart failure. The clinician must apply available knowledge to the specific hemodynamic situation of each patient, anticipating possible alterations in drug metabolism. The patient should be observed carefully using bedside, electrocardiographic, hemodynamic, and laboratory methods. Circulating drug levels can be followed as the state of heart failure changes, in an effort to minimize drug-induced toxicity and optimize drug effectiveness. In the following sections we shall explore what is known about the metabolism of a number of drugs commonly used in critically ill patients with congestive heart failure.

Digoxin

Digoxin is widely used for rate control of atrial fibrillation and as a weak inotrope in chronic congestive heart failure. Oral administration of the tablet form results in 60–75% absorption from the gastrointestinal tract (70). A new capsule formulation is approximately 20% more bioavailable (17). A peak serum concentration in either case is reached 45–60 minutes after ingestion. Elimination, mostly by renal excretion of unconjugated drug, leads to a half-life of 31.3 hours (41). Normal absorption may be distorted in critically ill patients due to ileus, gut edema, decreased perfusion, changes in bowel flora, and the presence of other drugs. These changes remain difficult to quantitate from patient to patient, but seem less dramatic with the capsule preparation. Intravenous administration, of course, avoids these vagaries and achieves tissue distribution and binding in 30 minutes (41).

Once absorbed, digoxin is only 20–25% protein bound (95), allowing for excellent glomerular filtration of the predominantly unmetabolized, polar drug. Hyperkalemia and hyponatremia may reduce myocardial binding. Hypomagnesemia increases the risk of toxicity (43). Reduced digoxin excretion occurs in renal failure. Glomerular filtration plays the predominant role in excretion, but tubular secretion is also involved. Sodium depletion, however, results in increased reabsorption of sodium in the proximal tubule causing a decrease in digoxin clearance even in the presence of a stable creatinine clearance (55). To further complicate the picture, plasma digoxin levels may be falsely elevated in congestive heart failure patients with severe renal dysfunction because of the presence of digoxin-like immunoreactive substance (107).

With or without congestive heart failure, digoxin has many drug interactions. The quinidine-digoxin interaction reduces the volume of distribution of digoxin by 30–40% and reduces renal clearance by 30–50% (24). The increased rate of digoxin absorption with concomitant quinidine therapy is too small to be of clinical importance. Reduced nonrenal clearance also produces only minimal changes in circulating digoxin levels. Recent work shows a near doubling of serum digoxin concentrations five weeks after starting amiodarone, an increase due to a change in volume of distribution since urinary digoxin clearance was unchanged (122). Verapamil may cause a 70% increase in serum digoxin concentration. This increase is dose-dependent and thought to occur secondary to reduced renal excretion without a reduction in glomerular filtration (77). As renal secretion of digoxin declines with hypokalemia (134), any diuretic that causes kaliuresis would be expected to increase digoxin levels. This rule holds true with furosemide but not bumetanide (60). Triamterene (115) and spironolactone (133) both cause decreased renal tubular secretion of digoxin. Amiloride, in contrast, increases tubular secretion of digoxin, but decreases extrarenal clearance, yielding only a slight decline in total body clearance (142). Antacids and kaolin-pectin each reduce peak serum digoxin concentrations, but not the time to peak concentration or completeness of absorption (5). Digoxin tablet absorption is increased by propantheline, which reduces gut motility (98). Finally, in approximately 10% of patients, antibiotic therapy changes gut flora and may result in a doubling of serum digoxin concentrations (92). Other interactions certainly exist, some of which are indirect. For example, rifampin increases the elimination of quinidine, which in turn may lead to a reduction of serum digoxin (4).

Dobutamine and Dopamine

Dobutamine and dopamine are rapidly metabolized, titratable intravenous sympathomimetic inotropes that are frequently used in critically ill patients. Dobutamine differs from dopamine in that it has less chronotropic effect and is devoid of dopaminergic renal vasodilation and peripheral vasoconstriction. Both drugs are rapidly distributed and metabolized by monoamine oxidase and catechol-O-methyltransferase in the periphery (88). This metabolism is not apparently altered in congestive heart failure, although the volume of distribution increases with edema (73). Sequestration of β-adrenergic receptors occurs rapidly in congestive heart failure (97), causing down regulation of β-receptors and diminished β-adrenergic effects (129). Dobutamine and dopamine may improve hemodynamics in congestive heart failure (93) and alter the pharmacokinetics of other agents. Dobutamine infusion, in addition, may lead to statistically significant reductions in serum potassium and magnesium concentrations (51).

Nitroprusside

Nitroprusside, a balanced arteriolar and venous vasodilator, possesses a rapid intravenous onset of action and is rapidly metabolized and excreted. It is used to lower systemic resistance in the setting of arterial hypertension, dissection of the aorta, and congestive heart failure. The pharmacokinetics and pharmacodynamics of the agent have not been studied in normal subjects versus congestive heart failure patients. However, these parameters are probably minimally affected, except for the occurrence of reduced thiocyanate excretion when prerenal azotemia complicates the clinical picture. Initial decomposition of nitroprusside involves the nonenzymatic conversion to cyanide, which is then rapidly converted to mitochondrial rhodanese to thiocyanate, a reaction requiring a sulfur donor (29). This enzyme is thought to be deficient in patients with tobacco amblyopia or Leber's optic atrophy (147). Dosages considerably above 3 μg/min may lead to toxicity, especially when used for longer than 3 days. In this situation, free cyanide ion combines with cytochromes, leading to anaerobic metabolism and lactate production. Such metabolic acidosis is followed by confusion, hyperreflexia, and coma. Toxicity from nitroprusside can be minimized by monitoring blood thiocyanate levels, with concentrations of less than 10 mg/dl considered safe (29). Also, prophylactic infusion of hydroxycobalamin, which reacts with cyanide to form cyanocobalamin, may avoid toxicity (32). Other than discontinuation of the infusion and dialysis, toxicity may be treated with the administration of thiosulfate (a sulfur donor) and sodium nitrate (which induces methemoglobin to combine with cyanide forming cyanomethemoglobin). Finally, variable hypoxemia secondary to increased pulmonary shunting may occur with nitroprusside administration.

Nitrates

The nitrates show great flexibility in routes of administration—topical, sublingual, buccal, oral, and intravenous. Mucosal absorption of nitroglycerin is excellent. Transdermal absorption varies with dose, vehicle, and place of application. Once absorbed, the drug is rapidly distributed, bound, and metabolized in the periphery to 1,2- and 1,3-glyceryl dinitrate and subsequently excreted in the urine. Isosorbide dinitrate tablets are more slowly absorbed via the oral mucosa or gastrointestinal tract; this drug exhibits a high level of first pass hepatic metabolism (20–25% bioavailability) by glutathione organic reductase to 2- and 5-isosorbide mononitrate, both active metabolites. All related compounds are excreted in the urine. The mechanism of action of nitroglycerin and isosorbide dinitrate remains unknown, but resides in the vascular smooth muscle (i.e., does not involve the neuroendocrine system) (2). Veins show greater avidity for nitrates than arteries, and veins dilate at lower nitroglycerin doses (67). Tolerance to nitrate therapy is more common with sustained blood levels and frequently repeated large doses (1). Nitrate-free periods restore normal responsiveness (112), but are difficult to employ in the critically ill patient. No significant alteration in nitrate pharmacokinetics occurs in patients with congestive heart failure (48).

Furosemide

Furosemide continues to fill a vital role in the treatment of congestive heart failure. Its immediate effect is to increase venous capacitance, which is followed by a brisk diuresis (39). The potential side effects of such therapy are hypokalemia, hypomagnesemia, metabolic alkalosis, and hypovolemia. Serum digoxin levels are increased with furosemide therapy (42, 106, 134). Time to peak serum concentration is increased and peak serum concentrations are reduced with oral furosemide in decompensated congestive heart failure compared with the compensated state. The total amount of furosemide absorbed, however, does not differ between the two states (11). Furosemide is less excreted by the kidneys, is less effective, and has a longer half-life in patients with renal insufficiency (141). The drug is secreted into the proximal tubule and initiates a diuresis from the luminal side of the ascending loop of Henle (23). Since patients with heart failure often have reduced renal blood flow, it is not surprising that less drug is delivered to its site of action and results in diminished diuresis. Hydralazine (an arteriolar vasodilator) increases both urinary sodium excretion and furosemide excretion in this setting (108). Whether other vasodilators show similar effects is unknown.

Bumetanide

Bumetanide demonstrates much greater potency than furosemide in heart failure. Drug absorption is more rapid and bioavailability improved. Although quantitative absorption is not affected by congestive heart failure, time of peak concentration is increased and peak concentration is diminished through undetermined mechanisms (20). The diuretic action of bumetanide is diminished with renal insufficiency (15). The drug's activity results from effects on both the blood and luminal sides of the nephron, instead of solely on the luminal side, as with furosemide (19).

Lidocaine

Lidocaine was originally synthesized in 1943 and was utilized for two decades as a local anesthetic (135). Its antiarrhythmic properties were noted in the 1960s, and it quickly became the primary therapy for treatment and prophylaxis of ventricular rhythm disturbances in intensive care units (59). Lidocaine is a class I drug and acts by shortening duration of the action potential, shortening the effective refractory period, and decreasing automaticity (148). When administered by a continuous infusion, it requires several hours before a steady state is achieved; therefore, lidocaine is usually administered as a bolus of 50–100 mg followed by a continuous infusion at 1–4 mg/min. Serum therapeutic levels are considered to be 2–6 μg/ml. Toxic side effects include paresthesis, slurred speech, somnolence, psychosis, apnea, and convulsions, and occur frequently when serum levels are above 9 μg/ml (150).

Lidocaine disposition after an intravenous bolus is described by a two-compartment model with a fast distribution phase (half-life, 8 minutes) and a slower distribution phase (half-life, 100 minutes). Seventy percent of lidocaine clearance is by hepatic metabolism and its clearance varies directly with hepatic blood flow (135, 139). The site of the remainder of lidocaine metabolism has not been identified (139), but less than 5% is excreted in the urine. The rate of lidocaine metabolism is exten-

sively altered in congestive heart failure. Thomson and associates (139) noted a decreased volume of distribution and a 37% decrease in plasma lidocaine clearance in patients with heart failure. Plasma clearance of lidocaine was also reduced in patients with liver disease. Patients receiving dialysis did not have abnormalities in lidocaine clearance. However, metabolites that undergo renal clearance might accumulate with prolonged infusion. It takes 5–8 hours to reach a new steady state in normal subjects following a change in lidocaine infusion rate. This time is prolonged in patients with heart failure.

The elimination phase for lidocaine may be considerably longer when the infusion is continued beyond 12 hours and in patients with acute myocardial infarction. Le Lorier and associates (89) found a mean half-life of 3.2 hours in patients with acute myocardial infarction. Furthermore, the patients had a serum lidocaine level of more than twice the predicted level. Prescott and colleagues (119) found the clearance half-life of lidocaine to be increased from 1.4 hours in normal volunteers to 4.3 hours in patients with uncomplicated acute myocardial infarction and 10.2 hours in heart failure. One patient in cardiogenic shock demonstrated no fall in serum lidocaine levels over 8 hours. The authors postulated a decrease in hepatic blood flow and other contributory factors, such as stress, hypoxia, hepatic venous congestion, competitive inhibition caused by accumulation of lidocaine metabolites, and administration of other drugs, as the cause for the decreased drug metabolism. They recommended limiting lidocaine infusions, after a loading bolus, to 2 mg/min unless persistent arrhythmias occur.

Zito and associates (151) studied the effects of a 1 mg/kg bolus of lidocaine followed by a constant infusion of 35 μg/kg/min. Both normal volunteers and patients with coronary artery disease (without heart failure) developed an early dip in plasma lidocaine levels, which fell below a therapeutic level of 2.4 μg/ml and lasted for 90 minutes. However, in patients with chronic heart failure (New York heart class IV), or acute myocardial infarction (Killip class II or III), the dip did not occur. The authors hypothesized that the higher plasma lidocaine levels resulted from decreased hepatic extraction.

Zito and Reid (150) subsequently extended their observations by showing that the clearance of lidocaine was directly proportional to the clearance of indocyanine green dye. Nineteen percent of their patients had toxic levels; all of these patients had heart failure and 15% had clinical evidence of toxicity. The authors recommended a lidocaine infusion rate of 35–38 μg/kg/min for New York class I failure, 12–35 μg/kg/min for class II, and 5–12 μg/kg/min for class III–IV. They also found that lidocaine infusion rates could be calculated from the indocyanine green clearance as follows: lidocaine rate = 0.3 + 1.07 (indocyanine green clearance) × desired lidocaine level.

Although Bax and colleagues (9) did not find a linear correlation between indocyanine clearance and lidocaine clearance, Lopez and associates (94) compared the dosage recommended by Zito and Reid (150) in New York heart class I–II heart failure with a control group that received a bolus followed by a 1–4 mg/min infusion. In the control group, 30% of the drug levels were in the toxic range and 12% were subtherapeutic. In the group that received the dose recommended by Zito and Reid, 81% of the drug levels were in the therapeutic range and none were in the toxic range.

These data indicate that adjustments in lidocaine administration must be made in patients with acute myocardial infarction, heart failure, or hepatic disease. Furthermore, constant adjustments in lidocaine infusions must be made as the hemodynamic status of the patient fluctuates.

Procainamide

Procainamide is a class I drug with properties similar to quinidine, and has been in clinical use since 1950. It is a second-line drug for treatment of ventricular rhythm disturbances (130).

Therapeutic plasma concentrations range from 4 to 8 mg/liter. Toxicity is frequently seen with serum levels above 8 mg/liter and almost universal toxicity occurs above 16 mg/liter (80).

Gastrointestinal absorption of procainamide ranges from 72 to 94% (83). Peak serum levels occur in 1–2 hours. The mean circulating half-life is 3.5 hours and does not change with prolonged administration, suggesting that there is no induction of metabolizing enzymes. About 48% of procainamide is excreted unchanged in the urine. The renal clearance ranges from 179 to 309 ml/min, whereas plasma clearance is 396–680 ml/min; therefore, active renal secretion occurs.

A major metabolite is N-acetylprocainamide (NAPA), which also possesses antiarrhythmic

properties. Impaired renal function due to either primary renal disease or low cardiac output states results in a marked rise in serum NAPA levels (81). The dosage of procainamide should be adjusted based on serum procainamide and NAPA levels.

In acute myocardial infarction, the time of absorption after an oral dose of procainamide can vary greatly: only four of 15 patients had peak levels at 1 hour, and in six, levels were still rising at 3 hours (80). The delay in procainamide absorption may be secondary to delayed gastric emptying, decreased intestinal motility, food, altered gastric pH, or decreased splanchnic blood flow. Since plasma concentrations after oral administration are unpredictable, a parenteral route of administration should be used in the first hours after myocardial infarction.

Early work suggested that procainamide had a reduced volume of distribution and prolonged half-life during congestive heart failure. This finding has been recently challenged. Kessler and associates (74) assessed procainamide kinetics in controls, patients with acute myocardial infarction, and patients with congestive heart failure. They found no difference in half-life, volume of distribution, peak NAPA levels, or percentage of unbound procainamide in the various groups. Patients with acute infarction had lower thresholds for suppression of premature ventricular contractions. The investigators thought this difference in response to procainamide was due to variation in the electrophysiologic properties of the heart during acute infarction. Administration of procainamide does not alter serum digoxin levels.

Quinidine

Quinidine is a membrane stabilizing drug. Peak levels occur 2 hours after oral administration, and the circulating half-life is 6.5–7.0 hours (35, 75). Side effects include diarrhea, nausea, vomiting, and prolongation of the QRS and QT intervals.

In congestive heart failure, the absorption of quinidine after oral administration is slower and results in peak plasma quinidine levels at 4 hours after dosing (12). Compared with normal subjects, only half as much orally administered quinidine is absorbed from the gut. A decreased volume of distribution is suggested in heart failure patients by the finding that plasma levels were 41% higher than in controls (12, 35). The circulating half-life is only slightly increased to 8.2 hours in heart failure (75). However, in patients with renal failure, quinidine's half-life after oral administration is 11.7 hours (12, 75). Quinidine may be given by the intramuscular route (75); however, the very slow absorption makes this route a poor choice.

The risk of adverse effects from quinidine is increased in the setting of hypokalemia (126, 149). Roden and coworkers (126) examined 22 patients with quinidine-induced torsade de pointes and found that 80% were taking diuretics. Hypokalemia was present in six patients, and 12 had serum potassium levels in the low-normal range (3.5–3.9 μg/liter). The investigators recommended maintaining the serum potassium level above 4 mEq/liter before initiating quinidine therapy.

Although intravenous quinidine, in experimental animals, decreases heart rate and blood pressure, the effect on left ventricular contractility is variable. Echocardiographic study of patients with cardiomyopathy did not reveal any change of left ventricular function as measured by end diastolic dimension, percentage fractional shortening, or posterior wall velocity (34). The same study could not eliminate the possibility that quinidine may have a mild depressant effect in normal subjects that is masked by its vagolytic effects.

The addition of quinidine may result in elevated serum digoxin concentrations (40, 54) and clinical toxicity (64, 86). Garty and associates (50) reported that quinidine produced a 63% reduction in total body digitoxin clearance without causing a change in the apparent volume of distribution of the central compartment. These quinidine-induced changes resulted in a 2.5-fold increase in the digitoxin elimination half-life.

Disopyramide

Disopyramide is a class I antiarrhythmic agent with electrophysiologic properties similar to those of quinidine (decreased rate of phase IV diastolic depolarization, decreased upstroke velocity of phase 0, and increased action potential duration) (79, 117). It is generally regarded to be as effective as quinidine, with fewer side affects. It has little effect on PR, QRS, and QT intervals in normal therapeutic doses (79). The major side effects of disopyramide are due to its anticholinergic effects and are manifested by dry mouth, blurred vision,

and urinary retention. It is almost completely absorbed from the gastrointestinal tract. Excretion is predominantly by glomerular filtration: 55% as the unchanged drug; 15–25% as the N-monodealkylated metabolite, which has weak antiarrhythmic properties; and 10% as minor metabolites (79, 85). The normal circulating half-life of disopyramide is 4.4–7.0 hours (79). In congestive heart failure, the rate of absorption is slower than normal, but the peak serum concentration is higher than in normal subjects, probably because of decreased volume of distribution (79). There is no change in serum digoxin levels when disopyramide is initiated.

Intravenous disopyramide has prominent negative inotropic effects (100, 146). Cardiac output is decreased 10% by an intravenous infusion of 1–2 mg/kg, 22% by 5 mg/kg, and 49% by 10 mg/kg (146). The basis for the cardiac depression is not known. Chronic therapy with oral disopyramide also possesses negative inotropic properties. Podrid and coworkers (117) noted the development of congestive heart failure in patients given disopyramide. Most patients were also taking digitalis and diuretics. These investigators employed a loading dose of 300 mg and maintenance doses of 300–800 mg/day, which would now be considered large. Sixteen percent of their patients developed heart failure: a minority of these (19%) had the onset of heart failure within 48 hours of initiation of therapy; the remainder developed failure during longer therapy (up to 9 months). In the absence of a history of cardiac failure, the chance of developing heart failure was less than 5%. Although effective in suppressing arrhythmias, this medication should be avoided if there is a history of heart failure.

Tocainide

Tocainide is a primary amine analogue of lidocaine. It produces shortening of both the action potential duration and the effective refractory periods and depresses the maximal upstroke phase 0 (96). It has relatively low hepatic extraction and may be administered orally (96). Therapeutic plasma concentrations (compared with 2–6 μg/ml for lidocaine) range from 3 to 4 μg/ml (96, 125). The clearance half-life is 11 hours in normal subjects. About 38–50% of the drug is excreted unchanged by the kidneys and the remainder undergoes hepatic glucuronidation before renal excretion (44, 78).

The mean renal clearance rate of tocainide is 104–154 ml/min. Side effects are similar to those of lidocaine and occur in 38% of patients. These include nausea, vomiting, dizziness, tremor, confusion, and psychosis (44, 78). It is not possible to predict which patients will develop tocainide-induced side effects. Side effects cannot be predicted from serum plasma values; however, central nervous system and gastrointestinal side effects can be decreased by reducing dosage (77). Tocainide is as effective as quinidine (143) or disopyramide (101) in its antiarrhythmic effects and suppresses premature ventricular contractions in about 65% of patients (125, 143).

There are no reports of tocainide interactions with other drugs, in particular, digoxin (125). Tocainide may work synergistically with quinidine (65).

Exacerbation of congestive heart failure is very uncommon with oral tocainide (65). Some investigators have found no differences in elimination half-life, volume of distribution, or total body clearance of tocainide when comparing normal volunteers with patients with acute myocardial infarction. (104) However, intravenous tocainide caused a small decrease in cardiac output and an increase in systemic vascular resistance in patients with heart failure secondary to myocardial infarction (109). Another study of patients with acute myocardial infarction and failure, but not pulmonary edema, found an increase in plasma clearance half-life to 15.6 hours after intravenous administration of 250 mg of tocainide (96). Mean plasma tocainide levels 5 minutes after the infusion were 2.95 μg/ml. The mean cardiac index initially was 2.4 liters/min/m². It decreased to 2.07 liters/min/m² 5 minutes after completion of the infusion, returned to baseline by 90 minutes, and increased to 2.49 liters/min/m² at 24 hours. There was no change in heart rate, blood pressure, or pulmonary artery pressure. Since the negative inotropic effects were seen at levels well below the therapeutic range, the authors urged caution in employing higher doses of the drug in patients with left ventricular dysfunction after acute myocardial infarction.

In renal insufficiency, the clearance of tocainide is markedly reduced to 35–94 ml/min and the elimination half-life prolonged to a mean of 22 hours (144). Therefore, a decrease in dosage or an increase in administration intervals, or both, should be employed in renal failure.

In the setting of concomitant hepatic and renal disease, the reduction of tocainide clearance appears to be largely attributable to renal dysfunction (111). No study of tocainide kinetics in isolated hepatic dysfunction has been performed (44).

Flecainide

Flecainide acetate is a class IC agent that markedly depresses the maximum upstroke of phase 0 of the action potential (33, 84). It shortens the duration of the action potential and effective refractory period in canine Purkinje fibers and prolongs them in ventricular muscle. The PR and QRS intervals are routinely prolonged (124). Twenty-seven percent of the drug is excreted unchanged in the urine by both filtration and active secretion. The remainder undergoes biotransformation to two major metabolites with less antiarrhythmic efficacy. The normal plasma half-life of flecainide is 14 hours; however, it increases by 20% to 19 hours in patients with congestive heart failure (124). In severe renal failure, the clearance of flecainide may be reduced 40% and the half-life increased to 58 hours (124). The decreased clearances of the drug and the increased plasma levels may result in serious cardiac toxicity (30, 46). Therefore, in the setting of cardiac and/or renal insufficiency, flecainide should be administered in lower doses and at longer intervals. Increases in dosage should be made no more often than every 4 days (124).

Flecainide also has multiple drug interactions. The clearance is decreased and prolonged by 13–27% with cimetidine (140). Flecainide interacts with propranolol to raise each drug's plasma concentration and results in additive negative inotropic effects (90). The simultaneous administration of amiodarone results in raised flecainide levels.

Flecainide is effective in the suppression of ventricular ectopy (63), more so than quinidine (45) or disopyramide (76). In one study, flecainide was 92% successful in suppressing premature ventricular contractions whereas disopyramide was only 39% successful (76).

Flecainide's major side effect has been exacerbation of congestive heart failure. In one study, 16% of patients with heart failure had exacerbation of symptoms with flecainide therapy (71). In another study of 32 patients who had nonsustained ventricular tachycardia and had failed previous antiarrhythmic therapy, three patients with left ventricular ejection fractions of 23–36% developed heart failure (84). This adverse effect could be controlled by increasing the dose of diuretics. Proarrhythmic effects occurred in one patient. The authors recommended initiating flecainide therapy with 200 mg/day, increasing dosages every 4 days, avoiding dosages greater than 400 mg/day, and maintaining plasma levels 1 μg/ml or less. Furthermore, caution should be employed in utilizing the drug in patients with severely depressed left ventricular function and in those whose depressed cardiac output results in variations in renal elimination.

In patients with an ejection fraction measured by radionuclide angiography of greater than 45%, an intravenous infusion of flecainide results in an 11% reduction in ejection fraction (72). A 21% ejection fraction reduction occurred in the group with ejection fractions of less than 45%. Furthermore, for the entire group, there was an 8% reduction in cardiac index and an 8% increase in systemic vascular resistance.

In summary, although flecainide has excellent antiarrhythmic properties, it should be used with extreme caution in settings of compromised ventricular function.

Mexiletine

Mexiletine is a lidocaine congener. It is well absorbed after oral administration, although absorption may be impaired in acute myocardial infarction (120).

Mexiletine, like lidocaine, mainly undergoes hepatic metabolism (10). In patients with hepatic or renal disease, mexiletine may accumulate (131). Patients with cirrhosis may have particularly marked prolongation of mexiletene clearance. One study found persistent levels of the drug in the serum of patients with cirrhosis 3 days after administration, but in none of the controls (131). Intravenous mexiletene does not produce myocardial depression at therapeutic levels; however, at toxic levels, myocardial depression has been noted (26).

Orally administered mexiletine does not appear to cause clinically important cardiac depression. Stein and associates (132) evaluated 10 patients with symptomatic ventricular tachycardia or fibrillation who also had ejection fractions of less than 50% by radionuclide angiography. In their 72-hour study of orally administered mexiletine, no change occurred in the mean left ventricular ejection fraction

(28% versus 27%) following the institution of therapy. There was a statistically insignificant fall in right ventricular ejection fraction from 46% to 41%. Mexiletine was effective in suppressing ventricular ectopy in 60% of patients at rest and 80% during exercise. No changes were observed in resting heart rate, exercise duration, or peak exercise heart rate.

The therapeutic effects of mexiletine can be enhanced by quinidine, permitting lower doses of mexiletine to be used and avoiding side effects (128). There is no change in serum digoxin level when mexiletine is initiated.

Another study evaluated mexiletine in patients with congestive heart failure who had no intrinsic hepatic or renal disease after acute myocardial infarction (87). The circulating half-life of the drug was 8.1 hours and the peak serum level occurred 3.2 hours after an oral dose. The renal elimination was 8%, which was not significantly different from normal.

Encainide

Encainide resembles procainamide but differs in having a p-substituted aromatic ring that is bridged to a tertiary amine by an amide (123). Encainide, like lidocaine, shortens the duration of the action potential. However, it also prolongs the effective refractory period. There is a dose-related prolongation of the PR and QRS intervals on the electrocardiogram. It has the advantage of being very effective in nanogram plasma concentrations, with minimal side effects (123). The half-life of encainide is 3–4 hours in normal subjects under steady state conditions. Furthermore, it does not alter radionuclide ejection fractions.

Encainide was evaluated in 19 patients with depressed left ventricular function (36). All patients had ejection fractions of less than 45%, and 63% had congestive heart failure. The mean ejection fraction was 22% before encainide and did not change with encainide therapy. The heart rate, blood pressure, stroke volume, and end diastolic volume did not change. However, a marked variability in plasma encainide levels was observed. Encainide does not alter digoxin levels.

Bretylium Tosylate

Bretylium acts by increasing the ventricular threshold (8). It is useful for treatment of refractory ventricular tachycardia or fibrillation. It is approved only for intramuscular or intravenous injection.

Approximately 70–80% of the drug is excreted unchanged in the urine (82). The half-life is 6–10 hours and increases in renal insufficiency (61). Although bretylium does not decrease myocardial contractility (61), it must be used with caution in critically ill patients since it may cause hypertension, even in the supine position (27). No evaluation of this drug in heart failure has been made. However, if renal function is compromised, the level of administration should probably be decreased.

Amiodarone

Amiodarone is a unique antiarrhythmic agent with excellent therapeutic efficacy for ventricular and supraventricular arrhythmias. Its therapeutic efficacy is offset by pulmonary, hepatic, thyroidal, ocular, and cutaneous toxicity. Amiodarone is predominantly metabolized by the liver and excreted in the bile. It undergoes enterohepatic recirculation (7). If hepatic insufficiency occurs because of heart failure or other etiology, the dosage should be reduced. Amiodarone is neither excreted by the kidney (6, 7, 121) nor removed by hemodialysis (18, 58).

Amiodarone interacts with numerous medications. It may elevate serum levels of the following drugs if administered to patients with previously achieved stable levels: aprindine, digoxin, flecainide, phenytoin, procainamide, quinidine, and warfarin (99). The amiodarone-induced elevations may result in undesirable clinical events, and it is recommended that the dosage of these drugs be decreased and their serum values monitored when amiodarone is initiated. Furthermore, since it may take many days or weeks before a stable state is established after initiation of amiodarone, the serum levels should be measured serially.

Although oral amiodarone is generally well tolerated in congestive heart failure, a study in patients with chagasic cardiomyopathy showed decreases in heart rate and cardiac index, and elevations of right atrial pressure, left ventricular end diastolic pressure, pulmonary artery pressure, and systemic vascular resistance during the 1st hour of intravenous amiodarone infusion. These parameters returned to baseline by 24 hours (13). Careful monitoring of bolus therapy is required when amiodarone is administered to patients with compensated heart failure.

Theophylline

Theophylline is widely used in the intensive care unit in patients with chronic obstructive pulmonary disease, bronchospasm, and occasionally, pulmonary edema. Its beneficial effects are mediated through bronchodilation, augmented diaphragmatic contraction, increased cardiac inotropy, arteriolar vasodilation, and increased venous capacitance. Therapeutic serum theophylline concentrations range from 10 to 20 μg/ml. Theophylline is eliminated by hepatic metabolism and follows first order kinetics. It is not affected by the dose or rate of administration (103). Although beneficial, theophylline is associated with cardiac and neurologic toxicity. Sixty percent of drug-related deaths in one intensive care unit were attributed to theophylline (25). Furthermore, patients with congestive heart failure or hepatic dysfunction are especially prone to seizures while receiving theophylline (152).

Administration of theophylline results in marked variability in serum levels in patients with heart failure. The volume of distribution is not significantly different from that in the normal control group, and the peak theophylline levels are similar after a single dose in patients with heart failure (116). However, patients with heart failure have markedly prolonged plasma half-lives. There is a 20-fold variation in these parameters in patients with pulmonary edema compared with a 4-fold variation in normal patients.

Serum levels may fluctuate during the course of heart failure. Jenne and coworkers (69) reported such an instance in a patient with chronic bronchitis who had near cessation of theophylline clearance when he developed severe heart failure. Following improvement in the heart failure, a marked increase in theophylline removal was observed. A bromosulphalein test also showed marked improvement with resolution of heart failure, suggesting that decreased liver blood flow or hypoxic liver dysfunction, or both, had resulted in decreased hepatic theophylline metabolism.

Marked individual variability in the rate of hepatic metabolism occurs, depending on the degree of pulmonary, hepatic, or cardiac disease. Powell and associates (118) established a standard clearance of 40.9 ml/hr/kg in normal controls. In smokers, theophylline clearance increased by a factor of 1.57 (57%). However, clearance was decreased to 43% of standard in congestive heart failure, to 37% by pneumonia, and to 84% by severe bronchial obstruction. Therefore, an estimate of theophylline clearance would rise to 64.1 ml/hr/kg for a smoker, but fall to 17.6 ml/hr/kg for a patient in heart failure. Furthermore, the logarithmic nature of the regression model makes the effect of multiple variables on theophylline clearance multiplicative rather than additive. In a patient who both smokes and has heart failure, the standard clearance of 40.9 ml/hr/kg is multiplied by both 1.57 and 0.43, resulting in a clearance rate of 27.6 ml/hr/kg, or 68% of standard. This value is close to the mean clearance found in patients with heart failure who also smoke.

Powell and associates (118) have developed a formula to guide infusions of theophylline. They recommend a loading dose of 6 mg/kg, to be infused at a rate of 0.2 mg/kg/min. A maintenance infusion is infused at 0.5 mg/kg/hr. If the patient is a smoker, the rate of infusion should be 0.8 mg/kg/hr; in heart failure and pneumonia, 0.2 mg/kg/hr; and if severe pulmonary obstruction is present, 0.4 mg/kg/hr.

Angiographic Contrast Agents

Critically ill patients frequently undergo angiographic evaluation. Administration of radiographic contrast agents is responsible for 10% of hospital-acquired acute renal failure and follows renal hypoperfusion states and major surgery as the third most common etiology (66). Ninety percent of patients who have acute renal dysfunction after receiving radiocontrast agents have preexisting renal insufficiency (57).

Taliercio and colleagues (137) evaluated 139 patients who underwent cardiac angiography and had a preprocedure serum creatinine of greater than 2 mg/dl. Thirty-two patients developed contrast nephropathy; 13 patients had oliguria or anuria and two patients required dialysis. The mean increment in serum creatinine was 2.6 mg/dl and the peak serum creatinine level occurred 2.8 days after angiography. Renal function returned to baseline in 25 patients. Cardiac events resulted in mortality in six patients 3–7 days after angiography. The most significant variable associated with the occurrence of contrast nephropathy was congestive heart failure. Contrast nephropathy developed in 25% of patients with New York heart class IV heart failure who did not have low cardiac output. However, in patients with New York heart class IV failure and low cardiac output who required continuous intravenous inotropic or vasodilator therapy or an intraaortic balloon pump, the incidence of contrast nephropathy was 71%. Other risk factors included multiple contrast studies within 72 hours, insulin-dependent diabetes mellitus, and radiocontrast dosage of more than 125 ml/study.

In addition to avoiding unnecessary procedures, a reduction in dye load may be achieved by using ultrasonic, nuclear imaging, or digital subtraction angiography when possible. The use of nonionic agents has not been associated with less nephrotoxicity (49).

An infusion of mannitol and furosemide has been utilized when performing angiographic studies (16) in patients with renal insufficiency to decrease the development of contrast-induced nephropathy. An effective regimen is to use a solution of 500 ml of 20% mannitol and add furosemide at a dose of 100 mg for each milligram per deciliter of serum creatinine. One hour before the administration of contrast, the infusion is started at a rate of 20 ml/hr and continued through the procedure and for 6 hours afterward. Urine output is replaced with a solution of 5% dextrose in 0.45% saline with 30 mg of potassium chloride added per liter (16).

SUMMARY

The clinician should use drugs sparingly in patients with heart failure and use clearly defined pharmacologic goals. When possible, an intravenous route of administration is preferable. Titratable drugs with short half-lives, which can be rapidly metabolized and excreted, offer many advantages. Renal function, acid-base balance, and hepatic function should be monitored. It must be remembered, however, that reduced hepatic enzymatic function often exists without abnormalities in standard liver enzyme determinations. The enlightened use of blood drug level determinations often helps avoid significant drug toxicity. Finally, hemodynamic changes mandate reevaluation of drug therapy.

Acknowledgments

Appreciation is expressed to Peter Marghella and Ron Landers for their assistance in preparation of this manuscript.

References

1. Abrams J: The brief saga of transdermal nitroglycerin discs: Paradise lost? *Am J Cardiol* 54:220–224, 1984.
2. Abrams J: Pharmacology of nitroglycerin and long-acting nitrates. *Am J Cardiol* 56:12A–18A, 1985.
3. Ader R, Chatterjee K, Ports T, Brundage B, Hiramatsu B, Parmley WW: Immediate and sustained hemodynamic and clinical improvement in chronic heart failure by an oral angiotensin converting enzyme inhibitor. *Circulation* 61:931–937, 1980.
4. Ahmad P, Mathur P, Ahuja S, Henderson R, Carruthers G: Rifampicin-quinidine interaction. *Br J Dis Chest* 73:409–411, 1979.
5. Allen MD, Greenblatt DJ, Harmatz JS, Smith TW: Effect of magnesium-aluminum hydroxide and kaolin-pectin on absorption of digoxin from tablets and capsules. *J Clin Pharmacol* 21:26–30, 1981.
6. Anastasion-Nana M, Levis GM, Moulopoulos S: Pharmacokinetics of amiodarone after intravenous and oral administration. *Int J Pharmacol Ther Toxicol* 20:524–529, 1982.
7. Andreason F, Agerback H, Bjerregaard P, Gotzsche H: Pharmacokinetics of amiodarone after intravenous and oral administration. *J Clin Pharmacol* 19:293–299, 1981.
8. Bacaner MB: Treatment of ventricular fibrillation and other acute arrhythmias with bretylium tosylate. *Am J Cardiol* 21:530–543, 1968.
9. Bax NDS, Tucker GT, Woods HF: Does indocyanine green predict lidocaine requirements? *N Engl J Med* 299:662–663, 1978.
10. Beckett AH, Chidomere EC: The distribution, metabolism, and excretion of mexiletene in man. *Postgrad Med J* 53(suppl I):60, 1977.
11. Beerman B, Dalen E, Lindstrom B: Elimination of furosemide in healthy subjects and in those with renal failure. *Clin Pharmacol Ther* 22:70–78, 1977.
12. Bellet S, Roman LR, Boza A: Relation between serum quinidine levels and renal function. *Am J Cardiol* 27:368–371, 1971.
13. Bellotti G, Silra LA, Filho AE, Rati M, De Moraes AV, Ramires JAF, da Luz P, Pileggi F: Hemodynamic effects of intravenous administration of amiodarone in congestive heart failure from chronic Chagas' disease. *Am J Cardiol* 52:1046–1049, 1983.
14. Benet LZ, Scheiner LB: Pharmacokinetics: the dynamics of drug absorption, distribution, and elimination. In Gilman AG, Goodman LS, Rall TW, Murad F, (eds): *Goodman and Gilman's The Pharmacological Basis of Therapeutics*, ed 7. New York, Macmillan, 1985, p 11.
15. Berg KJ, Tromsdal A, Wideroe TE: Diuretic action of bumetanide in advanced chronic renal insufficiency. *Eur J Clin Pharmacol* 9:265–275, 1976.
16. Berkseth RO, Kjellstrand CM: Radiologic contrast-induced nephropathy. *Med Clin North Am* 68:351–370, 1984.
17. Binnion PF: A comparison of digoxin bioavailability in capsule, tablet, and solution taken orally with I.V. digoxin. *J Clin Pharmacol* 16:461–467, 1976.
18. Bonati M, Galletti F, Volpi A, Cunnetti C, Rumolo R, Tognoni G: Amiodarone in patients on long-term dialysis. *N Engl J Med* 308:906, 1983.
19. Brater DC: Disposition and response to bumetanide and furosemide. *Am J Cardiol* 57:20A–25A, 1986.
20. Brater DC, Day B, Burdette A, Anderson S: Bumetanide and furosemide in heart failure. *Kidney Int* 26:183–189, 1984.
21. Braunwald E: Pathophysiology of heart failure. In Braunwald E (ed): *Heart Disease*, ed 2. Philadelphia, WB Saunders, 1984, p 447.
22. Bristow MR, Ginsburg R, Minobe W, Cubicciotti R, Sageman WS, Lurie K, Billingham ME, Harrison PC, Stinson EB: Decreased catecholamine sensitivity and β-adrenergic-receptor density in failing human hearts. *N Engl J Med* 307:205–211, 1982.
23. Burg M, Stoner L, Cardindal J, Green N: Furosemide effect in isolated perfused tubules. *Am J Physiol* 225:119–124, 1973.
24. Bussey HI: The influence of quinidine and other agents on digitalis glycosides. *Am Heart J* 104:289–302, 1982.
25. Camarata SJ, Weil MH, Harashiro PK, Shubin H: Cardiac arrest in the critically ill. I: A study of predisposing causes in 132 patients. *Circulation* 44:688–695, 1971.
26. Carlier J: Hemodynamic, electrocardiographic, and toxic effects of the intravenous administration of increasing doses of mexiletene in the dog: comparison with similar effects produced by other antiarrhythmics. *Acta Cardiol* [Suppl] (Brux) 25:81–100, 1980.
27. Chatterjee K, Mandel WJ, Vyden JK, Parmley WW, Forrester JS: Cardiovascular effects of bretylium tosylate in acute myocardial infarction. *JAMA* 223:757–760, 1973.
28. Chatterjee K, Swan HJC, Parmley WW, Sustaita H, Marcus H, Matloff J: Depression of left ventricular function due to acute myocardial ischemia and its reversal following aortocoronary saphenous vein bypass. *N Engl J Med* 286:1117–1122, 1972.
29. Cohn JN, Burke LP: Nitroprusside. *Ann Intern Med* 91:752–757, 1979.
30. Conrad GJ, Oler RE: Metabolism of flecainide. *Am J Cardiol* 53:41B–51B, 1984.
31. Conrad KA, Molk BL, Chidsey CA: Pharmacokinetic studies of quinidine in patients with arrhythmias. *Circulation* 55:1–7, 1977.
32. Cottrell JE, Casthely P, Brodie JO, Patel K, Klein A, Turndorf H: Prevention of nitroprusside-induced cyanide toxicity with hydroxycobalamin. *N Engl J Med* 298:809–811, 1978.
33. Cowan CJC, Williams EMV: Characterization of new oral anti-arrhythmic drug, flecainide (R-818). *Eur J Pharmacol* 73:333–342, 1981.
34. Crawford MH, White DH, O'Rourke RA: Effects of oral quinidine on left ventricular performance in normal subjects and patients with congestive cardiomyopathy. *Am J Cardiol* 44: 714–718, 1979.
35. Crouthamel WG: The effect of congestive heart failure on quinidine pharmacokinetics. *Am Heart J* 90:335–339, 1975.
36. Dami M, Derbekyan VA, Lisbona R: Hemodynamic effects of encainide in patients with ventricular arrhythmia and poor ventricular function. *Am J Cardiol* 52:507–511, 1983.
37. Darbey JT, Thompson KA, Echt DS, Woosley RL, Roder DM: Combination of low dose quinidine and tocainide in the treatment of ventricular arrhythmias in man (abstract). *J Am Coll Cardiol* 7:108–121, 1986.
38. Davison R, Parker M, Atkinson AJ: Excessive serum lidocaine levels during maintenance infusions: mechanisms and prevention. *Am Heart J* 104:203–208, 1982.
39. Dikshit K, Byden JK, Forrester JS, Chatterjee K, Prakosh R, Swan HJC: Renal and extrarenal hemodynamic effects of furosemide in congestive heart failure after acute myocardial infarction. *N Engl J Med* 288:1087–1090, 1973.
40. Doering W: Quinidine-digoxin interaction: pharmacokinetics, underlying mechanism and clinical implications. *N Engl J Med* 301:400–404, 1979.

41. Doherty JE, Perkins WH, Mitchell GK: Tritiated digoxin studies in human subjects. *Arch Intern Med* 108:531–539, 1961.

42. Doherty JE, Perkins WH, Wilson MC: Studies with tritiated digoxin in renal failure. *Am J Med* 37:536–544, 1964.

43. Dyckner T, Webster PO: Ventricular extrasystoles and intracellular electrolytes before and after potassium and magnesium infusions in patients on diuretic treatments. *Am Heart J* 97:12–18, 1979.

44. Elvin At, Keenaghan JB, Byrnes EW: Tocainide conjugation in humans: novel biotransformation pathway for a primary amine. *J Pharmacol Ther* 69:47–49, 1980.

45. Flecainide-Quinidine Research Group: Flecainide versus quinidine for treatment of chronic ventricular arrhythmias: a multicenter clinical trial. *Circulation* 67:1117–1123, 1983.

46. Franciosa JA, Wilen M, Weeks CE, Tanenbaum R, Kuan DC, Miller AM: Pharmacokinetics and hemodynamic effects of flecainide in patients with chronic low output heart failure. *J Am Coll Cardiol* 1:699, 1983.

47. Francis GS, Goldsmith SR, Cohn JN: Relationship of exercise capacity to resting left ventricular performance and basal plasma norepinephrine levels in patients with congestive heart failure. *Am Heart J* 104:725–731, 1982.

48. Fung HL, Ruggirello D, Stone JA, Parker JO: Effects of disease, route of administration, cigarette smoking, and food intake on the pharmacokinetics and circulating effects of isosorbide dinitrate. *Z Kardiol* 72(suppl 3):5–10, 1983.

49. Gale ME, Robbins AH, Hamberger I, Widrich WC: Renal toxicity of contrast agents: iopamidol, iothalamate, diatrizoate. *AJR* 142:333–335, 1984.

50. Garty M, Sood P, Rollins D: Digitoxin elimination reduced during quinidine therapy. *Ann Intern Med* 94:35–37, 1981.

51. Goldenberg IF, Low BT, Olivari MJ, Daniel JA, Nelson RR, VanTassel RA, Ochi R, Levine TB, Cohn JN: Effect of dobutamine infusion on serum electrolytes and arterial oxygenation in congestive heart failure. *J Am Coll Cardiol* 9:34A, 1987.

52. Goldsmith SR, Francis GS, Crawley AW, Levine TB, Cohn JN: Increased plasma arginine vasopressin in patients with congestive heart failure. *J Am Coll Cardiol* 1:1385–1390, 1983.

53. Grossman W, Alpert JJ, Braunwald E: Pulmonary hypertension. In Braunwald E (ed): *Heart Disease*, ed 2. Philadelphia, WB Saunders, 1984, p 827.

54. Hager WD, Fenstar P, Mayersohn M, Perrier D, Graves P, Marcus FI, Goldman S: Digitoxin-quinidine interaction: pharmacokinetic evaluation. *N Engl J Med* 300:1238–1241, 1979.

55. Halkin H, Sheiner LB, Peck CC, Melmon KH: Determinants of the renal clearance of digoxin. *Clin Pharmacol Ther* 17:385–394, 1975.

56. Hansen MS, Woods SL, Willis RE: Relative effectiveness of nitroglycerin ointment according to site of application. *Heart Lung* 8:716–720, 1979.

57. Harkonen S, Kjellstrand CM: Contrast nephropathy. *Am J Nephrol* 1:69–77, 1981.

58. Harris L, Hird CRK, McKenna WJ: Renal elimination of amiodarone and its desethyl metabolite. *Postgrad Med J* 59:440–442, 1983.

59. Harrison DC, Sprous J, Morrow AG: Antiarrhythmic properties of lidocaine and procainamide: clinical and physiological studies on their cardiovascular effects in man. *Circulation* 28:486–491, 1963.

60. Hayes AH Jr, Shiroff RA, Limjuco RA, Schuech DW: Effect of bumetanide on the renal excretion of digoxin (abstract). *Clin Pharmacol Ther* 25:228, 1979.

61. Heissenbuttel RH, Ryger JT Jr: Bretylium tosylate, a newly available drug for ventricular arrhythmias. *Ann Intern Med* 91:229–238, 1979.

62. Hepner GW, Vesell ES, Tantum KR: Reduced drug elimination in congestive heart failure. *Am J Med* 65:271–276, 1978.

63. Hodges M, Haugland JM, Grarud G, Conard GJ, Asinger RW, Mikell FL, Krejci JA: Suppression of ventricular ectopic depolarization by flecainide acetate, a new antiarrhythmic agent. *Circulation* 65:879–885, 1982.

64. Hooymans PM, Merkus FWHM: Effect of quinidine on plasma concentrations (letter). *Br Med J* 2:1022, 1978.

65. Horn HR, Hadidan Z, Johnson JL, Vassallo HG, Williams JH, Young MD: Safety evaluation of tocainide in American Emergency Use Program. *Am Heart J* 100:1037–1040, 1980.

66. Hou SH, Bushinsky DA, Wish JB, Cohen JJ, Harrington JT: Hospital-acquired renal insufficiency: a prospective study. *Am J Med* 74:243–248, 1983.

67. Imhof PR, Ott B, Frankhausser P, Chu LC, Hodler J: Difference in nitroglycerin dose-response in the venous and arterial beds. *Eur J Clin Pharmacol* 18:455–460, 1980.

68. Jeaner P, Testa B (eds): *Concepts in Drug Metabolism, Drugs and the Pharmaceutical Sciences Series*, New York, Marcel Decker, 1981, vol 10, part B.

69. Jenne JW, Chick TW, Miller BA, Strickland RD: Apparent theophylline half-life fluctuations during treatment of acute left ventricular failure. *Am J Hosp Pharm* 34:408–409, 1977.

70. Johnson BF, Grear H, McCreavie J, Fowle A: Rate of dissolution of digoxin tablets as a predictor of absorption. *Lancet* 1:1473–1475, 1973.

71. Josephson MA, Ikeda N, Singh BN: Effects of flecainide on ventricular function: clinical and experimental correlations. *Am J Cardiol* 53:95B–100B, 1984.

72. Josephson MA, Kaul S, Hopkins J, Kra D, Singh BN: Hemodynamic effects of intravenous flecainide relative to the level of ventricular function in patients with coronary artery disease. *Am Heart J* 109:41–45, 1985.

73. Kates RE, Leier CV: Dobutamine pharmacokinetics in severe heart failure. *Clin Pharmacol Ther* 24:537–541, 1978.

74. Kessler KM, Kayder DS, Estes D, Kozlosskis P, Sequira R, Myerbraid RJ: Procainamide pharmacokinetics/pharmacodynamics in acute myocardial infarction or congestive heart failure (abstract). *Circulation* 70(suppl 2):446, 1984.

75. Kessler KM, Lowenthal DT, Warner H, Gibson T, Briggs W, Reidenberg MM: Quinidine elimination in patients with congestive heart failure or poor renal function. *N Engl J Med* 290:706–709, 1974.

76. Kjekshus J, Bathen J, Orning OM, Storsteiin L: A double-blind crossover comparison of flecainide acetate and disopyramide phosphate in the treatment of ventricular premature complexes. *Am J Cardiol* 53:72B–78B, 1984.

77. Klein HO, Long R, Weiss E, DiSegni E, Libhaber C, Guerrero J, Kaplinsky E: The influence of verapamil on serum digoxin concentration. *Circulation* 65:998–1003, 1982.

78. Klein MD, Leveine PA, Ryan TJ: Antiarrhythmic efficacy, pharmacokinetics, and clinical safety of tocainide in convalescent myocardial infarction patients. *Chest* 77:726–730, 1980.

79. Koch-Weser J: Disopyramide. *N Engl J Med* 300:957–962, 1979.

80. Koch-Weser J: Pharmacokinetics of procainamide in man. *Ann NY Acad Sci* 179:370–382, 1971.

81. Koch-Weser J, Klein SW: Procainamide dosage schedules, plasma concentrations, and clinical effects. *JAMA* 214:1454–1460, 1971.

82. Kuntzman R, Tsai I, Chang R, Conney AH: Disposition of bretylium in man and rat. *Clin Pharmacol Ther* 11:829–837, 1970.

83. LaDu BN, Mandel HG, Way EL (eds): *Fundamentals*

of Drug Metabolism and Drug Disposition Baltimore, Williams & Wilkins, 1971.

84. Lal R, Chapman PD, Naccarelli GV, Schectman KB, Rinkerberger RL, Troup PJ, Kim SS, Dougherty AH: Flecainide in the treatment of nonsustained ventricular tachycardia. Ann Intern Med 105:493–498, 1986.

85. Landmark K, Bredesen JE, Thaulow E, Simons S, Amlie JP: Pharmacokinetics of disopyramide in patients with imminent to moderate cardiac failure. Eur J Clin Pharmacol 19:187–192, 1981.

86. Leahey EB, Reiffel JA, Giardina EGV, Bigger JT: The effect of quinidine and other oral antiarrhythmic drugs on serum digoxin: a prospective study. Ann Intern Med 94:34–37, 1981.

87. Leahey GB, Giardina EGU, Bigger JT: Effect of ventricular failure on stady state kinetics of mexiletine (abstract). Clin Res 26:239, 1980.

88. Leier CV, Unverferth DV: Dobutamine. Ann Intern Med 99:490–496, 1983.

89. Le Lorier J, Grenor D, Latour Y, Caille G, Dumont G, Brosseau A, Solignac A: Pharmacokinetics of lidocaine after prolonged intravenous infusions in uncomplicated myocardial infarction. Ann Intern Med 87:700–702, 1977.

90. Lewis GP, Haltzman JL: Interaction of flecainide with digoxin and propranolol. Am J Cardiol 53:52B–57B, 1984.

91. Lie KI, Liem KL, Louridtz WJ, Janse MJ, Willebrands AF, Durrer: Efficacy of lidocaine in preventing primary ventricular fibrillation within one hour after a 300 mg intramuscular injection. Am J Cardiol 42: 486–488, 1978.

92. Lindenbaum J, Rund DG, Butler VP Jr, Tse-Eng D, Saha JR: Inactivation of digoxin by gut flora: reversal by antibiotic therapy. N Engl J Med 305:789–794, 1981.

93. Loeb HS, Bredakis J, Gunnar RM: Superiority of dobutamine over dopamine for augmentation of cardiac output in patients with chronic low output cardiac failure. Circulation 55:375–381, 1977.

94. Lopez I, Mehta JL, Robinson JD, Roberts RJ: Optimal lidocaine dosing in patients with myocardial infarction. Ther Drug Monit 4:271–276, 1982.

95. Lukas DS, DeMartino AG: Binding of digitoxin and some related corderolides to human plasma protein. J Clin Invest 48:1041–1053, 1969.

96. MacMahon B, Bakshi M, Braragan P, Kelly JG, Wash MJ: Pharmacokinetics and hemodynamic effects of tocainide in patients with acute myocardial infarction complicated by left ventricular failure. Br J Clin Pharmacol 19:429–434, 1985.

97. Maisel AS, Motulsky JH, Isnel PA: Sequestration of beta-adrenergic receptors in acute heart failure: comparison of lymphocytes and heart (abstract). Circulation 74(suppl II):81, 1986.

98. Manninen V, Melin J, Apajalahti A, Karesoja M: Altered absorption of digoxin in patients given propantheline and metoclopramide Lancet 1:398–399, 1973.

99. Mason JW: Amiodarone. N Engl J Med 316:455–466, 1987.

100. Mathur PP: Cardiovascular effects of a new antiarrhythmic agent: disopyramide phosphate. Am Heart J 84:764–770, 1972.

101. McLaren CJ, Hassack KF, Mielson GH, Seskied V: Oral tocainide versus disopyramide: a double blind, randomized, cross-over study of outpatients with stable ventricular premature beats. J Cardiovasc Pharmacol 6:657–662, 1984.

102. Mirsky I, Parmley WW: Assessment of passive elastic stiffness for isolated muscle and the intact heart. Circ Res 33:233–243, 1973.

103. Mitenko PA, Ogilvie RI: Rational intravenous doses of theophylline. N Engl J Med 289:600–603, 1973.

104. Mohiuddin SM, Esterbrooks D, Hilleman DE, Aronow WS, Patterson AJ, Mooss AN, Hee TT, Reich JW: Tocainide kinetics in congestive heart failure. Clin Pharmacol Ther 34:596–603, 1983.

105. Muller P, Imhoff PR, Burkart F, Chu LC, Gerodin A: Human pharmacological studies of a new transdermal system containing nitroglycerin. Eur J Pharmacol 22:473–480, 1982.

106. Naafs MAB, Vanderltoek C, vanDuin S, Koorevaar G, Schoman W, Silberbusch J: Decreased renal clearance of digoxin in chronic congestive heart failure. Eur J Clin Pharmacol 29:249–252, 1985.

107. Nanj AA, Greenway DC: Widely differing plasma digoxin levels in patients with congestive heart failure and severe liver dysfunction. Arch Pathol Lab Med 110:75–76, 1986.

108. Nomura A, Yasuda H, Minami M, Akimoto T, Miyazuki K, Arita T: Effect of furosemide in congestive heart failure. Clin Pharmacol Ther 30:177–182, 1981.

109. Nyquist O, Forssell G, Nordlarder R, Schenck-Gustafson K: Hemodynamic and antiarrhythmic effects of tocainide in patients with acute myocardial infarction. Am Heart J 100:1000–1005, 1980.

110. Ochs HR, Carstens G, Greenblatt DJ: Reduction in lidocaine clearance during continuous infusion and by coadministration of propranolol. N Engl J Med 303:333–377, 1980.

111. Oltmans D: Pharmacokinetics of tocainamide in patients with chronic liver disease (abstract). Naunyn Schmiedebergs Arch Pharmacol 321(suppl):R49, 1982.

112. Packer M, Kessler PD, Lee WH, Medina N, Yushak M, Gottlieb SS: Does the intermittent administration of nitroglycerin prevent the development of hemodynamic tolerance in patients with severe heart failure? J Am Coll Cardiol 9:103A, 1987.

113. Page DL, Caufield JB, Kastor JA, DeSanctis RW, Sardeus CA: Myocardial changes associated with cardiogenic shock. N Engl J Med 285:133–137, 1971.

114. Parmley WW: Pathophysiology of congestive heart failure. Am J Cardiol 55:9A–14A, 1985.

115. Pederson KE, Hastrup J, Hvidt S: The effect of quinidine on digoxin kinetics in cardiac patients. Acta Med Scand 207:291–295, 1980.

116. Piafsky KM, Sitar OS, Rangno RE, Ogilvie RI: Theophylline kinetics in acute pulmonary edema. Clin Pharmacol Ther 21:310–316, 1977.

117. Podrid PJ, Schoeneberger A, Lown B: Congestive heart failure caused by oral disopyramide. N Engl J Med 302:614–617, 1980.

118. Powell JR, Vozeh S, Hopewell P, Costello J, Scheiner LB, Reigelman S: Theophylline disposition in acutely ill hospitalized patients: the effect of smoking, heart failure, severe airway obstruction, and pneumonia. Am Rev Respir Dis 118:229–238, 1978.

119. Prescott LF, Adjepon-Yamoah KK, Talbot RG: Impaired lignocaine metabolism in patients with myocardial infarction and cardiac failure. Br Med J 1:939–941, 1976.

120. Prescott LF, Pottage A, Clements JA: Absorption, distribution, and elimination of mexiletene. Postgrad Med 53(suppl 1):50–55, 1977.

121. Riva G, Gerna M, Zatini R, Giani P, Volpi A, Magzioni A: Pharmacokinetics of amiodarone in man. J Cardiovasc Pharmacol 4:264–269, 1982.

122. Robinson KC, Walter S, Johnston A, Mulraw JP, McKenna WJ, Holt DW: The digoxin-amiodarone interaction (abstract). Circulation 74(suppl II):225, 1986.

123. Roden DM, Reele SB, Higgins SB, Mayol RF, Gammans RE, Oates JA, Woosley RL: Total suppression of ventricular arrhythmias by encainide: pharmacokinetics and electrocardiographic characteristics. N Engl J Med 302:877–882, 1980.

124. Roden DM, Woosley RL: Flecainide. N Engl J Med 315:36–41, 1986.

125. Roden DM, Woosley RL: Tocainide. N Engl J Med 315:41–45, 1986.

126. Roden DM, Woosley RL, Bortick D, Bernard Y, Primm RK: Quinidine-induced long QT syndrome; incidence and presenting features (abstract). *Circulation* 68(suppl 3):267, 1983.

127. Rose JH, Pruitt AW, Dayton PG, McNay JL: Relationship of urinary furosemide excretion rate to natriuretic effect in experimental azoteuria. *J Pharmacol Exp Ther* 199:490–497, 1976.

128. Ruff HJ, Roden D, Primm RK, Oates JA, Woosley RL: Mexiletine in the treatment of resistant ventricular arrhythmias: enhancement of efficacy and reduction of dose-related side effects by combination with quinidine. *Circulation* 67:1124–1128, 1983.

129. Ruffolo RR Jr, Kopia GA: Importance of receptor regulation in the pathophysiology and therapy of contive heart failure. *Am J Med* 80(suppl 2B):67–72, 1986.

130. Schneeweiss A: *Drug Therapy in Cardiovascular Disease.* Philadelphia, Lea & Febiger: 1984, p 521.

131. Shelly JH: Harmony and discord; a review of interactions with mexiletine. In Sandoe E et al (eds): *Management of Ventricular Tachycardia: Role of Mexiletine.* Amsterdam, Excerpta Medica, 1978, p 841.

132. Stein J, Podrid P, Lawn B: Effects of oral mexiletine on left and right ventricular function. *Am J Cardiol* 54:575–578, 1984.

133. Steiness E: Renal tubular secretion of digoxin. *Circulation* 50:103–107, 1974.

134. Steiness E: Suppression of renal excretion of digoxin in hypokalemic patients. *Clin Pharmacol Ther* 23:511–514, 1978.

135. Stenson RE, Constantino RT, Harrison DC: Interrelationship of hepatic blood flow, cardiac output, and blood levels of lidocaine in man. *Circulation* 43:205–211, 1971.

136. Swedberg K, Hjalmarsan A, Waagstein F, Wallentin I: Beneficial effects of long-term beta blockade in congestive cardiomyopathy. *Br Heart J* 44:117–133, 1980.

137. Taliercio CP, Vliestra RE, Fisher LP, Burnett JC: Risks for renal dysfunction with cardiac angiography. *Ann Intern Med* 104:501–504, 1986.

138. Thomas JA, Markis BH: Plasma norepinephrine in congestive heart failure. *Am J Cardiol* 41:233–243, 1978.

139. Thomson PP, Melmon KI, Richardson JA, Cohn K, Steinbrunn W, Cudihee R, Rowland M: Lidocaine pharmacokinetics in advanced heart failure, liver disease, and renal failure in humans. *Ann Intern Med* 78:499–508, 1973.

140. Tjarda Maga B, Verbesselt R, Van Hecken Aa, Van Hecken A, Van Melle P, De Schepper PJ: Oral flecainide elimination kinetics: effects of cimetidine (abstract). *Circulation* 68(suppl 3):416, 1983.

141. Vasko MR, Brown-Cartwright D, Knochel JP, Nixon JV, Brater DC: Furosemide absorption altered in decompensated congestive heart failure. *Ann Intern Med* 102:314–318, 1985.

142. Waldorff S, Hansen PB, Kjaergard H, Bach J, Egeblad H, Steiness E: Amiloride-induced changes in digoxin dynamics and kinetics: abolition of digoxin-induced ionotropism with amiloride. *Clin Pharmacol Ther* 30:172–176, 1981.

143. Wasermiller JT, Aronow WS: Effects of tocainide and quinidine on premature ventricular contractions. *Clin Pharmacol Ther* 28:431–435, 1980.

144. Wiegers U, Hanrath P, Kuck KH, Pottage A, Craffner C, Augustin J, Runge M: Pharmacokinetics of tocainide in patients with renal dysfunction and during hemodialysis. *Eur J Clin Pharmacol* 24:503–507, 1983.

145. Williamson JR, Schaffer DW, Ford C, et al: Contribution of tissue acidosis to ischemic injury in the perfused rat heart. *Circulation* 53(suppl I):3–14, 1976.

146. Willis PW, III: The hemodynamic effects of norpace (Part II). *Angiology* 26(suppl 1):102–110, 1975.

147. Wilson J: Leber's hereditary optic atrophy: a possible defect of cyanide metabolism. *Clin Sci* 29:505–515, 1965.

148. Wittig J, Harrison LA, Wallace AG: Electrophysiological effects of lidocaine on distal Purkinje fibers (abstract). *Circulation* 46(suppl II):39, 1972.

149. Woosley RL, Echt DS, Roden DM: Treatment of ventricular arrhythmias in the failing heart: pharmacologic and clinical considerations. *Drug Ther* 19(10):1–7, 1985.

150. Zito RA, Reid PR: Lidocaine kinetics predicted by indocyanine clearance. *N Engl J Med* 299:662–663, 1978.

151. Zito RA, Reid PR, Longstreth JA: Variability of early lidocaine levels in patients. *Am Heart J* 94:292–296, 1977.

152. Zwillich CW, Sutton FD, Neff TA, Cohn WM, Matthay RA, Weinberger MM: Theophylline-induced seizures in adults: correlation with serum concentrations. *Ann Intern Med* 82:784–787, 1975.

5

Adjustment of Medications in Liver Failure

Patricia A. Arns, M.D.
Peter J. Wedlund, Ph.D.
Robert A. Branch, M.D.

Patients with liver disease are commonly treated with one or more different drugs in an effort to alleviate the numerous pathologic changes often associated with this and/or other concurrent disease processes. Commonly used drugs include diuretics, antibiotics, sedatives, and antiinflammatory, cardiovascular, and cancer chemotherapeutic agents. This use of potent and often multidrug therapy is generally considered to be a contributing factor to the frequent and sometimes fatal drug reactions that occur in this patient population (121). Of equal importance are the effects of liver disease on the absorption, distribution, elimination, and pharmacologic response to these drugs. Such changes may require reductions in drug dosage in order to avoid drug toxicity. The understanding of how liver disease can influence drug disposition and dosage requirements entails appreciation for:

1. The various types of functions that the liver performs;
2. The pathologic changes produced by liver disease and how these changes alter hepatic function; and
3. The parameters that influence drug disposition and how they are affected by liver disease.

LIVER FUNCTION IN HEALTH AND DISEASE: IMPLICATIONS FOR DRUG DISPOSITION

Hepatic Function

The strategic location of the liver between the splanchnic and systemic circulations is well suited for the large number of functions that this organ carries out. Included in this list of functions are (a) the synthesis of most plasma proteins (e.g., albumin, transport proteins, α-1-acid glycoproteins, lipoproteins, and clotting factors); (b) the regulation and synthesis of glucose, amino acids, fatty acids, and cholesterol; (c) the removal of ammonia, endotoxins, bilirubin, lactic acid, endogenous hormones, toxic substances, and waste products from the blood; and (d) the synthesis of bile and urea. Although this is a short list of the more than 1500 known functions carried out by the liver, it indicates the diversity and importance of this organ in maintaining homeostasis in the body.

The liver also plays an important role in the metabolism and elimination of drugs that may be too lipophilic to be efficiently removed by the kidneys. This function is carried out by a number of different enzymes located in liver cells. For example, one group of isoenzymes, referred to collectively as the cytochromes P-450, is important for carrying out many of the mixed function oxidative reactions that convert lipophilic compounds into more water-soluble products. Other enzymes in the liver may further transform these metabolites (or other drugs) by conjugating them with sugars, amino acids, sulfates, or acetate to form products that can be more readily eliminated in the bile or removed by the kidney. Still other liver enzymes (i.e., esterases, deaminases, hydrolases, and reductases) are important for the metabolic transformation and elimination of certain drugs and endogenous chemicals.

Many of these homeostatic and metabolic functions are compromised when the liver is damaged by different etiologic agents such as chemicals (including drugs) and diseases. The actual degree of damage to liver hemoperfusion, biliary excretion, and synthetic and metabolic functions in the liver can vary widely and therefore lead to variable changes in drug disposition. Such changes in drug disposition reflect, to some extent, the degree to which the liver is impaired. For example, alcoholic liver disease can range from fatty liver, with little or no change in the disposition of most drugs, to severe cirrhosis, with major changes in the disposition of certain classes of drugs. Hepatic neoplasms also show great variability in the effect on drug disposition, depending on type (primary versus secondary), size, invasiveness, and vascularity of tumor mass. Moreover, certain acute injuries to the liver, as seen in viral hepatitis, may affect the disposition of some drugs, but this effect may be reversible as the injury subsides.

Hepatic reserves may help to maintain liver functions, and changes in drug metabolism may be slight since few if any liver functions are performed at 100% of their capacity. For example, under normal conditions, urea formation from ammonia and amino acids occurs at 60% of capacity. Glucose maintenance requires only 20% of liver function. Bilirubin elimination must fall below 10% of normal before jaundice develops, and albumin and clotting factors are synthesized by only a small percentage of the total liver cells at any one time. Furthermore, these and other liver processes may be increased when there is increased demand. As a result, it is often difficult to determine the extent of liver damage caused by an agent because reserve and repair mechanisms tend to maintain hepatic function.

Such reserve and recuperative properties are obviously advantageous for the liver. This regenerative capability allows the liver to recover completely following acute liver insult. Even when the damage is extensive, if the causative agent is removed, the liver is capable of full recovery. However, if the etiologic agent is not removed so that the liver becomes exposed to chronic damage, then hepatic reserves may become seriously depleted. A limited repertoire of liver responses to such chronic damage will result in a characteristic pathophysiologic state of cirrhosis. Under such circumstances, significant changes in drug disposition may occur. The level of cytochrome P-450 enzymes in the liver, for example, may decline (38, 171, 188) and this change can seriously impair the liver's ability to metabolize endogenous products and drugs (33, 188). Deterioration in other liver functions (i.e., the removal of bilirubin and fatty acids and synthesis of plasma proteins) may lead to further alterations in drug disposition by influencing drug binding and distribution in the body (15, 20, 88, 170, 205).

Architecture and Blood Flow in Cirrhosis

The development of cirrhosis begins with initial hepatocellular damage producing inflammation, followed by phagocytic removal of dead or necrotic cells. This damage stimulates the secretion of collagen by fibroblasts to help maintain the integrity of the liver architecture while the damaged and dead cells are repaired or replaced. As the damage continues, collagen secretion may be further stimulated resulting in its accumulation in liver sinusoidal spaces. This accumulation of collagen in the sinusoids leads to the formation of bands of connective scar tissue characteristic of cirrhosis. In compensation for hepatocellular damage, hepatocyte regeneration may lead to the clustered formation of new hepatocytes, which later form liver nodules. These nodules may increase in size and further distort the normal liver architecture.

As the liver architecture becomes distorted, the resistance to the flow of blood through the liver is increased. This increase in turn causes the portal venous pressure to rise. To alleviate an elevated pressure, portal venous blood is shunted around the liver through collateral channels directly into the systemic circulation. The development of these collateral channels for shunting the portal venous blood occurs primarily where tributaries of the portal venous system lie in close proximity to those of the systemic circulation (i.e., submucosa of the esophagus, stomach, rectum, left renal vein, and abdomen). The increased blood flow and pressure in gastroesophageal varices predispose cirrhotic patients to an increased risk of gastrointestinal hemorrhage; a major cause of death in these patients (45).

The development of collateral channels for shunting of portal venous blood around the liver can alter the effective hepatic blood flow and the amount of drug reaching the systemic circulation after oral administration (60, 143, 150, 184). These and other changes in drug disposition may require the dosage of some drugs to be reduced.

In addition, recent studies have shown that hepatic disease may also alter the microcirculation of the liver. Sinusoidal plasma in the healthy liver has direct access to the hepatocyte. Although the sinusoid is lined by endothelial cells, this is not a continuous layer; there is an incomplete basal lamina, and endothelial cells contain multiple fenestrations.

Between the sinusoidal endothelium and the hepatocyte is the space of Disse, which contains the microvilli of hepatic cells, reticular fibers, and fat storage cells. Alcoholic liver disease is associated with an increase in type III collagen in the space of Disse, formation of a basal lamina, and a decrease in the number of fenestrations and porosity of the endothelial cell as seen with scanning electron microscopy (63, 99, 137, 187). This endothelialization transforms sinusoids into capillary-like channels and limits the access of sinusoidal blood to the hepatocyte. Studies using multiple indicator dilution techniques support the concept that conversion of loose interendothelial cell junctions to tight endothelial cell junctions may provide a barrier to the movement of molecules into the proximity of the hepatocyte (65–67). This could be of importance in the diffusion of albumin and other large molecules, including protein-bound substances such as drugs, which may result in decreased ability for drug metabolism by the liver.

Renal Function

Hemodynamic changes may also be present in the kidneys of patients with liver disease. Renal blood flow has been shown to be decreased in cirrhosis without laboratory evidence of decreased renal function or the development of edema or ascites (159–161). Glomerular filtration rate is variable in early cirrhosis (83), but is usually decreased when ascites develops. Moreover, the handling of electrolytes by the kidneys is disturbed in patients with cirrhosis. Renal sodium retention is a well-known phenomenon associated with this disease and is an important factor in the development of ascites. With progression of liver disease, a number of these factors will further depress kidney function to the point of renal failure (175). It follows that drugs having a major renal route of elimination may have an altered disposition in patients with liver disease, because of the secondary development of functional renal failure.

Ascites Formation and Albumin Concentration

Increased sodium and fluid retention by the kidneys and increased production of lymph both contribute to the formation of ascites. The increased production of lymph is associated with increases in blood pressure in the sinusoidal spaces of the liver. Lymph production in the liver is particularly sensitive to changes in blood pressure because of the very "leaky" extravascular spaces that separate the hepatocytes from the sinusoidal blood. As the production of lymph within the liver is increased, lymph channels enlarge to accommodate the increased production. Unfortunately, these channels have a limited capacity to handle the increased production and may become blocked or overwhelmed. When lymph formation exceeds the ability of lymph channels to return it to the systemic circulation, lymph may weep from the liver into the peritoneal cavity contributing to the formation of ascites.

This lymph carries with it albumin and other plasma proteins, often at a time when the synthesis of new albumin and other proteins by the liver is depressed. In response to both these factors, total serum protein and albumin levels may fall. With the fall in serum protein levels, the binding and retention of drugs within the vascular compartment may decline. These changes may modify drug distribution and/or pharmacologic response by allowing drug to pass from the blood into other tissue compartments of the body.

CHARACTERISTICS OF DRUG DISPOSITION

Whether pathologic changes associated with liver disease require an alteration in a normal drug regimen is determined by the dispositional characteristics of the drug and the biological determinants of the system. Drug disposition, which includes both the distribution and elimination of drug, is determined in part by the physical properties of the drug. Important characteristics include molecular size, charge, pK_a, and lipid solubility. These factors will determine distribution as well as the route of elimination. In general, water-soluble drugs have a small volume of distribution and can be eliminated unchanged in urine, and lipid-soluble drugs have a large volume of distribution and require metabolism to more water-soluble moieties. Depending on the physical characteristics of any given drug, the balance of physiologic factors influencing that drug's disposition will vary. These physiologic factors have the potential to be altered by disease states. Thus, the influence of any one disease process can be complex; it can be mediated by a variety of factors and can influence the disposition of different drugs to a variable extent.

Distribution

The major aspects of distribution affected by liver disease are volume of distribution (V_d) and plasma protein binding. Conceptually, the apparent volume of distribution is the volume into which a drug distributes in the body when it is at equilibrium and is related to the pool from which the drug concentration is measured. It is a theoretical concept and reflects the partitioning of drug between the fluid compartments in the body, e.g., plasma, interstitial fluid, and intracellular fluid. It is calculated by:

$$V_d = \frac{D}{Cp} \qquad (1)$$

where D represents the fraction of the dose absorbed and Cp is drug concentration at equilibrium. One way that liver disease can affect the V_d is by the production of ascites, which may produce an increase in the body's total fluid compartment. For example, propranolol has been shown to exhibit a 2-fold increase in V_d in patients with ascites, regardless of the extent of protein binding (18).

Most drugs in plasma are reversibly bound to proteins, such as albumin, globulin, α-1-acid glycoprotein, lipoproteins, ceruloplasmin, and transferrin. Acidic drugs commonly bind to albumin, whereas basic drugs more commonly bind to α-1-acid glycoprotein. Only unbound drug is available for distribution into tissues and capable of evoking a pharmacologic response (72, 94, 96, 142, 176). The extent of protein binding is therefore important in determining both pharmacologic response and drug disposition.

Cirrhosis causes a number of alterations that can also influence the binding of drugs within the blood, including (a) a decrease in serum albumin levels, (b) the appearance of altered or defective plasma proteins, and (c) the accumulation of endogenous and exogenous compounds that can displace drugs from protein binding sites. For example, acute viral hepatitis or primary biliary cirrhosis can lead to elevated serum bilirubin levels. The strong affinity of bilirubin for protein binding sites on albumin and the elevated levels are in part responsible for the displacement of some acidic drugs from the protein (15, 211). Taken together, these factors can produce alterations in drug binding to proteins and in the unbound serum drug concentrations. As a result, changes may occur in drug distribution and elimination and pharmacologic response.

With a decrease in drug binding to plasma or blood proteins, more drug may become available for distribution into tissues, increasing the drug's apparent volume of distribution. This change can alter the drug's elimination half-life independently of any change in drug metabolism. The reason for this change is apparent from the dependence of the half-life $(t_{1/2})$ on both its total clearance from the blood (Cl) and its apparent volume of distribution (V_d), according to the equation:

$$t_{1/2} = \frac{0.693 \, V_d}{Cl} \qquad (2)$$

As a result of this dependence, the half-life of a drug can be a misleading parameter when attempting to determine the effect(s) of liver disease on drug elimination. For example, an increase in the apparent volume of distribution of a drug may lead to a prolongation in its elimination half-life in the absence of any real change in metabolic drug elimination. The increase in the half-lives of valproic acid (88) and lorazepam (89) in patients with liver disease, in fact, has been explained entirely by an increase in drug distribution secondary to decreased plasma binding rather than by a reduction in clearance.

In addition to influencing drug distribution, changes in protein binding can influence drug elimination. A change in the free fraction of a drug in the blood can lead to an increase in the amount of drug available to the drug-metabolizing enzymes and therefore to an increase in the total clearance of some drugs. This increase can shorten the half-life of a drug in the absence of any change in the activity of drug-metabolizing enzymes. Indeed, the decrease in the half-life of tolbutamide (211) in acute viral hepatitis has been attributed solely to a decrease in its binding to plasma proteins, since it has been shown that even though total (free + bound) clearance of tolbutamide increases, protein binding decreases and free clearance remains unchanged.

These examples indicate that the effect of protein binding on drug disposition is difficult to predict. As shown in Table 5.1, these changes in binding are a function of both type and severity of disease, as well as of the drug itself. Presently, there are no guidelines for predicting the effect of liver disease on drug binding. However, two general rules may provide some

Table 5.1
Changes in the Plasma Protein Binding of Drugs Caused by Liver Disease

Drug	Free Fraction (f_p) in Plasma (%)	Change in f_p with Liver Disease (%)	Significance	Type of Disease	Reference
Amylobarbital	39.3	76	$P<0.005$	Cirrhosis	106
Azapropazone	0.44	377	$P<0.05$	Cirrhosis	70
Caffeine	68.7	8.4	$P<0.01$	Cirrhosis	31
Chlordiazepoxide	3.5	54	$P<0.05$	Cirrhosis	163
Chlordiazepoxide	3.5	131	$P<0.01$	Acute hepatitis	163
Chlormethiazole	35.6	24	$P<0.01$	Cirrhosis	143
Clindamycin	20.8	1	NS	Cirrhosis	11
Clofibrate (CPIB)	2.8	0	NS	Acute hepatitis	50
Clofibrate (CPIB)	2.8	157	$P<0.05$	Cirrhosis	50
Dapsone	18.5	125	—	Cirrhosis	155
Diazepam	2.2	113	$P<0.001$	Cirrhosis	85
Diphenylhydantoin	8.3	41	NS	Cirrhosis	4
Diphenylhydantoin	10.8	44	$P<0.05$	Cirrhosis	62
Diphenylhydantoin	9.9	27	$P<0.05$	Acute hepatitis	15
Diphenylhydantoin	5.8	309	$P<0.005$	Hepatic failure	135
Furosemide	4.0	155	$P<0.001$	Cirrhosis	200
Furosemide	1.9	63	$P<0.01$	Cirrhosis	5
Hexobarbital	53	1.9	NS	Cirrhosis	218
Lorazepam	6.8	68	$P<0.01$	Cirrhosis	89
Meperidine	36	−1.6	NS	Cirrhosis	87
Meperidine	42	5.5	NS	Acute hepatitis	108
Morphine	80.1	3.4	NS	Cirrhosis	140
Morphine	64.9	16	$P<0.05$	Hepatic failure	135
Oxazepam	13.3	6.9	NS	Cirrhosis	178
Oxazepam	13.3	4.9	NS	Acute hepatitis	178
Phenylbutazone	6	67	$P<0.01$	Cirrhosis	205
Prednisolone	46.5	15	$P<0.05$	Chronic liver disease	152
Prednisolone	46.5	6.7	NS	Acute hepatitis	152
Propoxyphene	25	8	NS	Cirrhosis	44
Propranolol	6.6	55	$P<0.05$	Cirrhosis	214
Propranolol	12.2	45	$P<0.05$	Cirrhosis	20
Quinidine	11	18	$P<0.05$	Chronic liver disease	144
Quinidine	14.1	194	$P<0.001$	Cirrhosis	4
Salicylate	27	52	$P<0.005$	Cirrhosis	22
Salicylate	19.9	30	NS	Chronic liver disease	144
Salicylate	27	18.5	NS	Mixture	205
Sulfadiazine	46	46	$P<0.01$	Mixture	205
Theophylline	47	33	—	Cirrhosis	147
Theophylline	35	103	$P<0.001$	Cirrhosis	101
Thiopental	28.0	89	$P<0.01$	Cirrhosis	43
Tolbutamide	2.2	100	$P<0.02$	Alcoholic	195
Tolbutamide	6.8	28	$P<0.01$	Acute hepatitis	211
Triamterene	19.3	71	$P<0.01$	Cirrhosis	4
Valproic acid	11.3	159	$P<0.002$	Cirrhosis	88
Valproic acid	11.3	36	—	Acute hepatitis	88
Warfarin	1.2	0	NS	Acute hepatitis	212

insight into the more important factors influencing the extent of change. (a) If protein binding is altered by a particular liver disease, the degree of liver damage will influence the extent of change in drug binding to plasma proteins. (b) Changes in the extent of binding to plasma proteins will tend to be greater for extensively bound drugs (i.e., >60% bound) than for poorly bound drugs (i.e., <60% bound). Although these are general rules that have

their exceptions, they should provide some appreciation for the effects of liver disease on plasma protein binding.

Elimination

Elimination of drug is defined as the irreversible loss of drug from the site of measurement and includes both metabolism and excretion. Clearance is an important parameter that relates drug concentration to the rate of elimination, thereby providing a measure of efficiency of the elimination process. By definition, total or systemic clearance is a measure of the amount of plasma cleared of drug per unit time. This measure can be obtained from measurements of drug concentration in plasma after single doses (Equation 2) or at steady state:

$$Cl = \frac{\text{rate of drug administration}}{Cp_{ss}} \qquad (3)$$

where Cp_{ss} is the steady state plasma concentration. Clearance is independent of the mechanism of elimination involved, and if multiple routes of elimination occur concurrently, it provides an estimate of the sum of these processes.

When the rate of elimination is proportional to the amount of drug present, this is known as a first order process. Clearance of drug is constant (linear) over a range of concentrations. Not all drugs undergo first order kinetics; however, in some instances dose-dependent elimination occurs. Clearance in these cases is nonlinear and will vary depending on the achieved concentration of drug.

Clearance can also be described as the efficiency of removal of drug across an organ of elimination, the two major organs being liver and kidney. Hepatic clearance, (Cl_H) reflects the efficiency with which the liver irreversibly removes drug from the blood. It is determined by both the fraction of drug removed or extracted (E) from the blood during passage through the liver and the liver blood flow (Q_H). The relationship between these parameters is given by:

$$Cl_H = Q_H E \qquad (4)$$

Drugs that are given orally must first pass through the liver before reaching the systemic circulation. If hepatic enzymes extract drug from the blood as it passes through, then the fraction (F) of the total dose entering the general circulation is reduced. For drugs that are completely absorbed from the gastrointestinal tract, this fraction F (or bioavailability) is determined from the drug's extraction (E) by the liver according to the equation:

$$F = 1 - E \qquad (5)$$

The ability of the liver to extract a drug is in turn dependent on three separate factors: (a) the intrinsic activity of metabolic enzymes

and transport processes within the liver that irreversibly remove drug from the blood, (b) the fraction of total drug in blood that is free to interact with enzymes responsible for its elimination, and (c) the rate at which drug passes or flows through the liver (146, 165, 209).

The irreversible removal of drug from the blood may be carried out by a number of separate enzymes in the liver. For simplicity, however, the elimination process is often considered as if it is due to only a single enzyme system. Thus, metabolic and transport processes responsible for drug removal by the liver, defined as the free intrinsic drug clearance (Cl^u_{int}), can be described by a simple Michaelis-Menten equation as:

$$Cl^u_{int} = \frac{V_{max}}{(K_m + C^u_L)} \qquad (6)$$

where V_{max} represents the maximal rate of irreversible drug elimination by all liver enzymes, K_m is the Michaelis-Menten constant for the overall enzymatic removal process, and C^u_L is the concentration of unbound or free drug in liver.

The second factor that can contribute to the extraction of a drug by the liver is the free fraction of drug in blood (f_B). If the unbound fraction of total drug in blood changes, then the free drug concentration at the site of elimination will also change. For some drugs, changes in binding can alter hepatic extraction by metabolic and transport enzymes in the liver.

Finally, the total amount of drug extracted by the liver is dependent on the rate at which drug is delivered to the enzymes responsible for its elimination. This rate of delivery is determined by the liver blood flow (Q_H) perfusing functional hepatocytes. If intrinsic clearance is high, flow becomes the rate-limiting factor and reductions in flow will not change hepatic extraction, but rather will reduce hepatic clearance. If, on the other hand, intrinsic clearance is low, then as flow is decreased, hepatic extraction will increase and hepatic clearance will not be influenced by blood flow.

The relationship of the extraction (E) of a drug by the liver with its free intrinsic clearance (Cl^u_{int}), free fraction in the blood (f_B), and the total effective liver blood flow (Q_H) is given by:

$$E = \frac{f_B Cl^u_{int}}{(Q_H + f_B Cl^u_{int})} \qquad (7)$$

If Equation 7 is now substituted into Equation 4, which defines hepatic clearance, the expression obtained relates hepatic clearance with three variables—f_B, Q_H and Cl^u_{int}. Thus, hepatic clearance may be written as:

$$Cl_H = Q_H E = Q_H \frac{f_B Cl^u_{int}}{(Q_H + f_B Cl^u_{int})} \qquad (8)$$

Although these relationships may appear complex, it is important to recognize that hepatic clearance is determined by only these three physiologic variables, each of which can be changed independently by liver disease. The effect on drug disposition of any one of these variables can be anticipated by knowing the relative importance of each of these variables to that drug's disposition. This concept has been used to provide a framework for the classification of drugs into a system in which those drugs sharing a rate-limiting characteristic are grouped together.

Drugs Classified by Dispositional Characteristics

FLOW-LIMITED DRUGS

When the total intrinsic clearance ($f_B Cl^u_{int}$) of a drug is large relative to liver blood flow (Q_H), such that $E > 0.6$, hepatic clearance of the drug becomes dependent on liver blood flow (Equation 8). The rate at which the liver is able to remove these drugs from the blood is limited by their rate of presentation to the liver. Metabolism and protein binding, theoretically, should not affect hepatic clearance of these drugs. Accordingly, this class of drugs is referred to as blood flow–limited and is sensitive to factors that can alter only the effective liver blood flow (Table 5.2).

ENZYME-LIMITED DRUGS

When the total intrinsic clearance of a drug is small relative to liver blood flow, such that $E < 0.2$, hepatic clearance becomes essentially dependent on the intrinsic activity of liver enzymes (Equation 8). Factors that influence the ability of the liver enzymes to remove drug become more important in altering drug elimination than changes in liver blood flow. Drugs with this characteristic belong to the class referred to as enzyme-limited. This class is further subdivided according to the extent of protein binding.

Enzyme-limited, Binding-insensitive Drugs

For enzyme-limited drugs with low binding to plasma or blood proteins (i.e., <50% bound), a change in plasma protein binding is not an important factor in altering hepatic drug elimination (Equation 8). This drug class is most affected by factors that change the level or activity of liver enzymes (Cl^u_{int}) responsible for their elimination. Drugs with these characteristics are referred to as enzyme-limited and binding-insensitive (Table 5.2).

Enzyme-limited, Binding-sensitive Drugs

For enzyme-limited drugs that are extensively bound to plasma or blood proteins (i.e., >85% bound), hepatic clearance is sensitive to changes in protein binding in the blood (f_B) and/or liver enzyme activity (Cl^u_{int}). Drugs with these characteristics are referred to as enzyme-limited, binding-sensitive drugs. Factors that may alter binding to proteins in the blood or the activity of liver enzymes responsible for drug elimination influence the hepatic clearance of these drugs (Table 5.2).

FLOW/ENZYME-SENSITIVE DRUGS

A drug may not be extensively bound or poorly extracted by the liver, but fall somewhere between the flow-limited and enzyme-limited classes. The clearance of these drugs from the blood may be sensitive to changes in liver blood flow, intrinsic clearance by the liver, and in some cases, binding to plasma proteins (Equation 8). Drugs with these characteristics are referred to as flow and enzyme sensitive (Table 5.2).

Table 5.2 lists a number of drugs eliminated by the liver according to this classification. The extraction ratios and plasma protein binding reported are approximate values from subjects with normal liver and kidney function. Drugs are classified according to this scheme to help provide a better appreciation for the importance of pathophysiologic changes produced by liver disease in altering drug disposition.

It is important to emphasize, however, that Table 5.2 is based on information about the handling of drugs by normal, healthy subjects and that certain biological determinants of metabolism (i.e., disease or genetic predisposition) may change the classification of a given drug for an individual patient.

Table 5.2
Characterization of Drugs Eliminated Primarily by the Liver

	Approximate Extraction (E)	Protein Binding (%)	Comments on Effects of Liver Disease
Flow-limited drugs			Changes in liver blood flow and intrinsic clearance associated with liver disease affect these drugs. The shunting of blood around the liver has important effects on the bioavailability of these drugs.
Chlormethiazole	0.70	99	
Labetalol	0.85	40	
Lidocaine	0.60	65	
Lorcainide	0.65	70	
Morphine	0.75	35	
Pentazocine	0.60	65	
Propoxyphene	>0.90	75	
Propranolol	0.65	95	
Verapamil	0.80	92	
Flow/enzyme-sensitive drugs			Changes in liver blood flow, free intrinsic clearance, and free fraction of drug in blood may be important for this class of drugs.
Acetaminophen	0.30	20	
Chloramphenicol	0.28	70	
Chlorpromazine	0.30	95	
Erythromycin	0.30	80	
Isoniazid	0.27	10	
Meperidine	0.50	70	
Methohexital	0.53	—	
Metoprolol	0.56	10	
Nafcillin	0.27	90	
Nortriptyline	0.50	95	
Quinidine	0.27	85	
Ranitidine	0.28	15	
Enzyme-limited, binding-insensitive			This class of drugs is most sensitive to changes occurring in the free intrinsic drug clearance with liver disease.
Antipyrine	0.05	10	
Amylobarbital	0.03	60	
Caffeine	0.04	31	
Cyclophosphamide	0.08	14	
Hexobarbital	0.15	47	
Theophylline	0.05	62	
Enzyme-limited, binding-sensitive			This class of drugs will be influenced by changes in free fraction of drug in blood and free intrinsic drug clearance. The overall change in drug clearance will be governed by which one of these factors changes the most as a result of the disease process.
Cefoperazone	0.04	90	
Chlordiazepoxide	0.02	96	
Diazepam	0.02	97	
Diphenylhydantoin	0.03	92	
Fenprofen	0.13	>99	
Indomethacin	0.08	90	
Naproxen	0.005	>99	
Phenylbutazone	0.01	99	
Rifampin	0.11	85	
Tolbutamide	0.02	98	
Valproic acid	0.02	89	
Warfarin	0.005	99	

It is now known that some people have genetic defects in the metabolism of certain drugs. Fast and slow acetylators of isoniazid have been recognized since the 1950s. More recently, independent genetic polymorphisms have been found for a number of other drugs metabolized by different oxidative enzymes. Poor and extensive metabolizers of debrisoquine, an antihypertensive agent, and mephenytoin, an anticonvulsant, are representative examples of two independent routes of oxidative metabolism. Debrisoquine acts as a flow-limited drug in subjects who are extensive metabolizers, but as an enzyme-limited drug in those who are poor metabolizers (182). Not only will the effect of liver disease have a greater effect on the clearance of this drug in extensive metabolizers than in poor metabolizers, but the effect of factors such as development of portal-systemic shunts will have a marked influence in systemic availability in extensive but not poor metabolizer subjects.

INFLUENCE OF LIVER DISEASE ON DRUG DISPOSITION

As previously mentioned, both dispositional characteristics of a drug and biological determinants of the system involved are important in determining the effects of liver disease on ultimate drug disposition. In the following sections, the effects of liver disease on each of these factors are discussed.

Route of Elimination

Since there are multiple routes of elimination, only some of which involve the liver, it is important to determine which route is utilized for a given drug. For a drug that is excreted unchanged by the kidney, liver disease should have no effect on disposition, provided that there is no secondary or concomitant renal disease.

Figure 5.1 shows the relationship between

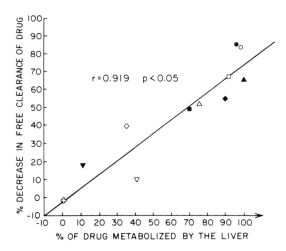

Figure 5.1 Relationship between the percentage of drug eliminated by the liver and the observed percentage decrease in the free clearance of drug in cirrhotic patients. Only drugs that are known or appear to be metabolized via oxidative pathways within the liver have been used for this plot. Each symbol represents the mean percentage change in the free clearance of one, or the average percentage change in free clearance of more than one drug. ✛ = cefuroxime; ▼ = ampicillin; ◇ = furosemide; ▽ = cimetidine; ■ = nafcillin; △ = cefoperazone; ◆ = caffeine and theophylline; □ = antipyrine; ● = meperidine and propranolol; ○ = diazepam, verapamil, amylobarbital, lorcainide, and valproic acid; ▲ = chlordiazepoxide, chlormethiazole, and hexobarbital.

free clearance and extent of metabolism in cirrhotic patients for several drugs known, or assumed, to undergo oxidative metabolism. This plot was constructed from many different studies and, although all were conducted in cirrhotic patients, the severity of liver disease was not controlled for. The significant correlation found in Figure 5.1 implies a strong relationship between the extent of oxidative metabolism of a drug by the liver and the percentage decrease in its free clearance caused by liver cirrhosis. Liver disease has the greatest effect on those drugs that undergo extensive oxidative metabolism.

Route of Metabolism

For drugs that are metabolized by the liver, the route of metabolism is also important in determining the effects of liver disease on drug disposition. All metabolic pathways are not affected equally by liver disease. For example, the elimination of lorazepam, morphine, and oxazepam, which are primarily metabolized by conjugation with glucuronic acid, is unaltered by liver disease (89, 140, 178). The reason for this fact is unknown. It may reflect the sparing of conjugative pathways of drug metabolism in the liver during liver disease, and/or the importance of other organs to the elimination of drugs by this route. This preservation contrasts with reductions in clearance of drugs that are eliminated by oxidative metabolism.

Routes and Duration of Drug Administration

The effect of liver disease on drug disposition is determined by (a) the route of drug administration, (b) the class to which the drug belongs (i.e., flow-limited, flow/enzyme-sensitive, or enzyme-limited), and (c) duration of drug administration.

As noted previously, drugs that are taken orally, unlike those administered intravenously or intramuscularly, must pass through the liver before reaching the systemic circulation and target tissues. This provides an opportunity for presystemic elimination, particularly for flow-limited drugs, with their high hepatic extractions, which normally have a low bioavailability. For flow-limited drugs, liver disease may reduce the efficiency of drug me-

Table 5.3
Influence of Liver Cirrhosis on the Bioavailability of Flow-limited Drugs

Drug	Bioavailability in Controls	Bioavailability in Cirrhotics	Change in Bioavailability (%)	Reference
Labetalol	0.33	0.63	91	60
Lidocaine	0.33	0.65	97	198
Meperidine	0.48	0.87	81	121
Metoprolol	0.50	0.84	68	154
Pentazocine	0.20	0.70	250	150
Pentazocine	0.18	0.68	278	122
Propranolol	0.38	0.54	42	214
Verapamil	0.22	0.52	136	184
Verapamil	0.14	0.30	114	215

tabolism and considerably increase their bioavailability (Table 5.3). This increased bioavailability, however, is only partially explained by a decrease in the efficiency of drug extraction by liver enzymes. Another important factor contributing to this increase is the rerouting of blood from the portal vein through intrahepatic and extrahepatic portal-systemic shunts in response to portal hypertension caused by liver disease. In severely cirrhotic patients, this shunting may involve 60% or more of portal venous blood flow (49, 192, 193). This shunting allows a large amount of an orally administered drug to bypass the liver altogether and enter the systemic circulation directly. As a result of the changes in bioavailability of flow-limited drugs, peak blood concentrations following single oral dose administration are substantially higher in patients with cirrhosis than in normal subjects. (Fig. 5.2). In contrast, the bioavailability of enzyme-limited drugs is high in normal subjects and remains unaffected in liver disease. Thus, peak concentrations following single oral dose administration are the same in cirrhotic and normal subjects (Fig. 5.2).

The case is somewhat different for chronic oral therapy: drug blood levels accumulate to an approximate steady state situation that is dependent on drug clearance, the fraction of the dose that reaches the systemic circulation, and the dosage interval (Equation 3). Reductions in clearance due to liver disease result in the potential for excessive drug accumulation during chronic therapy for both flow-limited and enzyme-limited drugs (Fig. 5.2). This may require dosage reduction in order to obtain the desired therapeutic objective.

In summary, the influence of liver disease on drug disposition is a function of how a drug is handled in healthy subjects. For flow-limited drugs, initial blood concentrations follow-

ing intravenous or intramuscular administration can be expected to be similar in cirrhotic and normal subjects, whereas peak blood concentrations are higher in cirrhotic patients after single oral dose administration or at steady state during chronic therapy. In contrast, enzyme-limited drugs can be expected to have similar initial blood concentrations after both intravenous and single oral dose administration in cirrhotic and normal subjects, but increased blood concentrations at steady state during chronic therapy in cirrhotic subjects.

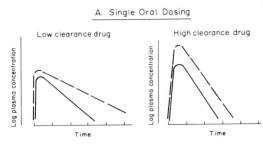

A. Single Oral Dosing

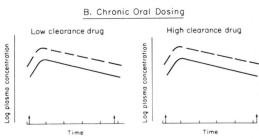

B. Chronic Oral Dosing

Figure 5.2 The effects of single **(A)** and chronic **(B)** oral dosing on low clearance (enzyme-limited) and high clearance (flow-limited) drugs in patients with cirrhosis *(dashed lines)* and in normal subjects *(solid lines)*. *Arrows* indicate dosage interval for chronic dosing graphs.

Severity of Liver Disease

The type and severity of liver disease are one example of the effect of biological determinants on drug disposition. All drugs that undergo extensive oxidative metabolism are not affected to an equal extent by all liver diseases. Acute viral hepatitis, for example, does not have any effect on the metabolic elimination (Cl^u_{int}) of tolbutamide, warfarin, diphenylhydantoin, or antipyrine (15, 37, 90, 211, 212), whereas it does produce changes in metabolic elimination of hexobarbital, meperidine, and chlordiazepoxide (21, 108, 208). These observations might reflect differences in the degree to which different oxidative pathways of drug elimination are affected by liver disease, but more likely reflect the differences in the severity of the disease process in patients used for the separate studies. Thus, it may not be possible to find any change in the metabolic elimination of drugs in patients with mild or moderate forms of hepatitis. Certainly the levels of cytochrome P-450 drug-metabolizing enzymes are not altered in liver biopsies from such patients (38). With more extensive liver damage due to viral hepatitis or other causes, the level of these enzymes declines (38, 171). This decline should cause a decrease in the free intrinsic clearance of those drugs that are oxidatively metabolized in the liver by this enzyme system.

Drug Interactions in Liver Disease

As stated earlier, patients with liver disease are often on a multidrug regimen. Certain drugs are well known to affect drug metabolism either by induction or inhibition of metabolic enzymes.

Phenobarbital, pentobarbital, tolbutamide, and phenytoin act as metabolic inducers, increasing the synthesis of metabolic enzymes. The administration of enzyme-inducing drugs to patients with moderate liver disease may offset the disease-induced decrease in cytochrome P-450 enzymes. This effect, however, is limited. With an increase in the severity of liver damage, liver reserves may become too depressed for drug administration to exert much of an effect on either the level or activity of these enzymes (38, 188).

Cimetidine, on the other hand, a drug commonly used in the treatment of patients with alcoholic liver disease, has been shown to decrease total plasma clearance of theophylline (52) and chlordiazepoxide (123) in both control and cirrhotic subjects. It is believed that cimetidine interferes with oxidative metabolism but does not alter hepatic blood flow (123). Consequently, patients with liver disease may have an additional risk of impaired drug metabolism. The study by Nelson and colleagues (123) showed the decrease in plasma clearance of chlordiazepoxide to be greater in the control group than in the cirrhotic group, suggesting that the greater the initial microsomal function, the greater the effect of an inhibitor. However, it should be emphasized that this further decrease in drug metabolism may still be of importance in a patient with liver disease who may already have decreased metabolic function.

Endogenous substances may also affect drug metabolism. Both interferon and interferon inducers have been shown to decrease drug biotransformation (102, 113, 114, 156, 157, 180, 181). The mechanism for this is not completely understood, although it is thought to involve variable depression of the cytochrome P-450 enzymes. This factor has important implications for patients with viral hepatitis, for not only do interferon levels increase with acute infection, but recently exogenous interferon has been used as a treatment for patients with hepatitis B or non-A, non-B viral hepatitis.

RECOMMENDATIONS FOR DOSAGE ADJUSTMENTS

As seen from the discussion of pharmacokinetic considerations in liver disease, it is not easy to predict the effect of disease on drug disposition in individual patients. Although severity of disease seems to play a major role in distribution and elimination of a drug, there is no good predictor of hepatic function. Despite a considerable effort by a number of investigators (8, 14, 31, 148, 177), there is no useful noninvasive test of liver function to guide dosage adjustments. The best that can be said for most of the so-called liver function tests (i.e., serum albumin, prothrombin time, bilirubin, serum glutamic-oxaloacetic and glutamic-pyruvic transaminases (SGOT and SGPT), alkaline phosphatase, etc.) is that they reflect but do not predict the extent of liver damage.

Measuring cytochrome P-450 enzyme levels from liver biopsies might be expected to provide a better measure of the degree to which oxidative drug metabolism in the liver has been damaged. The level of these enzymes, however, has not been found to be a useful predictor of the metabolic elimination of drugs by this organ (188). One explanation for the poor predictive value is that this measure fails to account for total hepatic size (148).

Some measures do exist that correlate with drug clearance, such as tests of antipyrine, aminopyrine, and indocyanine green clearance; however, these studies are not usually conducted as part of a patient's routine clinical evaluation. Moreover, the correlation coefficients usually only approximate 0.6 in most studies, accounting for only 40% or less of variance. Therefore, a good predictor of hepatic function or drug clearance has not been found; and at the present time, there is not a good hepatic counterpart for glomerular filtration rate, which is a reliable indicator of renal function.

Before considering the influence of liver disease on drug dosage requirements, some mention must be made of the use of drugs in general. There are always risks associated with the use of any drugs, and these risks may become particularly pronounced in patients with liver disease. In a prospective, drug-monitoring study of over 2000 patients, Naranjo and colleagues (120) found the frequency of adverse drug reactions (ADRs) to be higher in patients with cirrhosis than in those with renal disease, other liver diseases, or neither liver nor renal disease. In the group of cirrhotic patients, the frequency of ADRs was significantly correlated with the severity of liver dysfunction as measured by a composite clinical and laboratory index. Thus, consideration should be given as to whether the drug is really needed and whether its benefits outweigh the risks. For example, the use of some drugs in patients with liver disease is associated with a particularly high risk and they should be used with great caution or not at all in these patients (Table 5.4). In general, the drugs listed in Table 5.4 fall into three categories: (a) drugs capable of causing liver damage even in normal patients, (b) drugs that can further compromise depressed liver functions often found in liver disease patients, and (c) drugs that can make the complications of liver disease worse. In the above-cited study, diuretics were found to be the most common cause of ADRs and to cause the most severe reactions.

If drug treatment is required and alternatives are available, it is preferable to use a drug whose disposition is least affected by the liver disease (e.g., a drug that is renally excreted or metabolized by glucuronidation). If a drug must

Table 5.4
Drugs That Should Be Used with Caution or Not at All in Liver Disease Patients

Group I: Drugs capable of causing hepatic damage
    Acetaminophen
    Acetylsalicylic acid
    Chlorpromazine
    Erythromycin estolate
    Methotrexate
    Methyldopa
Group II: Drugs that can compromise liver functions
    Anabolic and contraceptive steroids
    Prednisone (in acute viral hepatitis)
    Tetracycline
Group III: Drugs that may make complications of liver disease worse
    Cyclooxygenase inhibitors (indomethacin)
    Diuretics
    Meperidine and other CNS depressants
    Morphine
    Pentazocine
    Phenylbutazone

be prescribed that may be affected by the disease process, then a number of factors need to be considered, including (a) the extent of liver damage, (b) the degree of hepatic elimination of the drug, (c) the degree of protein binding, (d) the class to which the drug belongs (i.e., enzyme-limited, flow/enzyme sensitive, or flow-limited, (e) the route of administration; and (f) the duration of administration.

A considerable amount of information has been gathered over the years regarding disposition of specific drugs in liver disease. Most of this work has been done in cirrhosis, a lesser amount in acute viral hepatitis, and very little in other types of liver disease. To help the clinician, a compilation has been made of the dispositional characteristics of a number of drugs in normal subjects, the route of elimination of these drugs, the effect of liver disease on their disposition, and the recommendations for adjustment of dose (Table 5.5).

For drugs not listed in Table 5.5, general guidelines for dosage adjustment are given in Table 5.6. While these considerations may not be all inclusive, they should provide some guidance as to the extent of dosage change required with liver disease. It should be kept in mind, however, that these may not be the only variables to consider in patients with this condition. For example, as noted earlier, in moderate liver disease the administration of drugs capable of increasing drug metabolism may offset the decline in the metabolic elimination of drugs due to the disease, and the adminis-

Table 5.5
The Dispositional Characteristics in Normal Subjects and in Patients with Liver Disease, Routes of Elimination, and Recommendations for Dose Adjustment for a Variety of Drugs[a]

Drug	Protein Binding (%)	Volume of Distribution (V_d) (liter/kg)	Half-life ($t_{1/2}$) (hr)	Clearance (Cl) (ml/min)	Class	Hepatic/Renal Elimination	Effect of Liver Disease on Drug Disposition	Adjustment of Dose	References
Antibiotic									
Amantadine	—	4.75	20.0	190	—	<10% Hepatic >90% Renal	Negligible unless renal function decreased	None	
Amikacin	5	0.26	2.5	85	—	<5% Hepatic >95% Renal	Negligible unless renal function decreased	None	
Ampicillin	30	0.28	1.0	340	—	<10% Hepatic >90% Renal	$t_{1/2}$ ↑; V_d ↑; Cl →; f_p? →	None	95
Aztreonam	56	0.15	1.9	70	—	33% Hepatobiliary 66% Renal	$t_{1/2}$ ↑; V_d →; Cl →	Decrease if chronic, high-dosing	98
Carbenicillin	48	0.16	1.0	130	—	<10% Hepatic >90% Renal	Negligible unless renal function decreased	None	59
Cefaclor	24	0.35	1.0	280	—	<10% Hepatic >90% Renal	Negligible unless renal function decreased	None	
Cefamandole	74	0.16	1.0	130	—	<5% Hepatic >95% Renal	Negligible unless renal function decreased	None	
Cefazolin	84	0.15	1.8	68	—	<5% Hepatic >95% Renal	$t_{1/2}$ ↓; f_p ↑	None	130
Cefoperazone	90 non-linear	0.20	1.7	80	Enzyme-limited, binding-sensitive	75% Hepatic 25% Renal	$t_{1/2}$ ↑; V_d →; Cl ↓ 60%; f_p?	Decrease dose	16, 17, 28, 29, 48
Cefotaxime	36	0.24	1.2	94	—	40% Hepatic 60% Renal	$t_{1/2}$ ↑; V_d?; Cl?	Unknown	115
Cefoxitin	73	0.12	1.0	98	—	15% Hepatic 85% Renal	Negligible unless renal function decreased	None	
Ceftazidime	17	0.2	1.7	75	—	10% Hepatic 90% Renal	$t_{1/2}$ ↑; V_d ?; Cl slight ↓	Negligible, unless renal function decreased	139
Ceftriaxone	90	0.14	8.4	16	Enzyme-limited, binding-sensitive	60% Hepatobiliary 40% Renal	$t_{1/2}$ →; V_d ↑ if ascites present; Cl →; f_p ↑	None	190, 191
Cefuroxime	30	0.33	1.2	210	—	<1% Hepatic >99% Renal	Negligible unless renal function decreased	None	133

Table 5.5 (*continued*)

Drug	Protein Binding (%)	Volume of Distribution (V_d) (liter/kg)	Half-life ($t_{1/2}$) (hr)	Clearance (Cl) (ml/min)	Class	Hepatic/Renal Elimination	Effect of Liver Disease on Drug Disposition	Adjustment of Dose	References
Cephalothin	75	0.30	0.60	470	—	30–50% Hepatic 50–70% Renal	$t_{1/2}$ slight ↑; V_d →; Cl ↓	None	130
Chloramphenicol	70	1.0	3.0	170	Enzyme-limited, binding-sensitive	>90% Hepatic <10% Renal glucuronidation of drug	$t_{1/2}$ ↑; V_d slight ↓; Cl ↓ 65%; f_p →?; unknown if f_p changes	Decrease dose	12, 92, 119
Clindamycin	79	0.58	2.0	160	Enzyme-limited, binding-sensitive	90% Hepatic 10% Renal	$t_{1/2}$ slight ↑; V_d →; Cl ↓ 23%; f_p →	Decrease dose in severe cases	11, 58
Doxycycline	82	—	12.0	195	—	<10% Hepatic >90% Renal	Negligible unless renal function decreased	None	
Erythromycin	80	0.77	1.6	600	Enzyme-limited, binding-sensitive	>90% Hepatic <10% Renal	$t_{1/2}$ ↑; no other information	Decrease dose in moderate or severe disease	54, 91
Gentamicin	< 5	0.25	2.0	100	—	<5% Hepatic >95% Renal	Negligible unless renal function decreased	None	
Isoniazid	<10	0.6	2.0 fast 6.0 slow	480 fast 170 slow	Enzyme-limited, binding-insensitive	85% Hepatic 15% Renal Drug acetylated	$t_{1/2}$ ↑; some assume Cl ↓; genetic differences more important than disease	Decrease dose in severe cases	2, 93
Kanamycin	<10	0.20	3.0	55	—	<5% Hepatic >95% Renal	Negligible unless renal function decreased	None	
Metronidazole	10	0.75	8.0	85	—	>90% Hepatic <10% Renal	$t_{1/2}$ ↑; V_d →; Cl ↓	Decrease dose	30, 36
Nafcillin	90	0.4	1.0	580	Enzyme-limited, binding-sensitive	70% Hepatic 30% Renal	$t_{1/2}$ ↑ but little change; V_d ↓; Cl ↓ 50–60%; fp →?	Decrease dose in moderate or severe disease	105
Neomycin	40	—	2.0	—	—	<5% Hepatic >95% Renal	Negligible unless renal function decreased	None	
Rifampin	85	0.4	2.5	180	Enzyme-limited, binding-sensitive	90% Hepatic 10% Renal	$t_{1/2}$ ↑; V_d?; Cl ↓; f_p?	Decrease in severe disease	78, 153
Streptomycin	35	0.26	2.5	85	—	<5% Hepatic >95% Renal	Negligible unless renal function decreased	None	
Sulphamethoxazole	66	0.17	9.0	15	Enzyme-limited, binding-sensitive	70% Hepatic 30% Renal Drug acetylated	Unknown, but probably little change unless there is severe liver disease	Slight decrease	

Tobramycin	<5	0.24	2.5	80	—	<5% Hepatic >95% Renal	Negligible unless renal function decreased	None	
Trimethoprim	45	1.5	12.0	96	—	30% Hepatic 70% Renal	Slight unless renal function decreased	None	
Vancomycin	55	0.4	5.0	80	—	<10% Hepatic >90% Renal	$t_{1/2} \uparrow$; $V_d \rightarrow$; $Cl \downarrow$	Decrease dose	23

Analgesic

Acetaminophen	20	0.9	2.2	350	Flow/enzyme-sensitive	>95% Hepatic <5% Renal Mostly conjugated	$t_{1/2} \uparrow$; V_d?; $Cl \downarrow$ 54%; assume $f_p \rightarrow$; little change in Cl if albumin > 3.5 g/100 ml	Avoid chronic use; single dose—no change	10, 40, 41, 174, 179
Meperidine	65	4.5	4.5	900	Flow/enzyme-sensitive	>95% Hepatic <5% Renal	$t_{1/2} \uparrow$; $V_d \rightarrow$; $Cl \downarrow$ 50%; $f_p \rightarrow$	Decrease oral dose by 50% in cirrhosis or acute viral hepatitis	87, 108, 122, 151
Methadone	80	4.0	28	150	Enzyme-limited, binding-sensitive	80% Hepatic 20% Renal	$t_{1/2} \uparrow$ with severe liver disease; $Cl \rightarrow$; $V_d \uparrow$ slightly	None or decrease	125, 126
Morphine	35	3.7	2.0	1200	Flow-limited	90% GI tract and liver, 10% renal Extensive glucuronidation	$t_{1/2} \rightarrow$; $V_d \rightarrow$; $Cl \rightarrow$; $f_p \rightarrow$, $f_p \uparrow$	None, but avoid in severe liver disease	135, 140, 141
Pentazocine	65	5.4	4.5	1000	Flow-limited	>95% Hepatic <5% Renal	$t_{1/2} \uparrow$; $V_d \rightarrow$; $Cl \downarrow$ 50%	Decrease oral dose by 2/3	122, 150
Propoxyphene	75	16	12	1200	Flow-limited	>95% GI tract and liver; <2% renal	$t_{1/2} \uparrow$ slightly; $Cl \downarrow$ 25%; $f_p \rightarrow$	Decrease oral dose by 50%	44

Anticancer

Adriamycin	50	2.5	20	100	Enzyme-limited, binding-insensitive	>95% Hepatic <5% Renal Most biliary Active metabolite	$t_{1/2} \uparrow$; V_d?; Cl?; f_p?, assume $f_p \rightarrow$	Unknown	13
Bleomycin	0	0.3	2.0	120	—	40% Hepatic 60% Renal	Unknown; probably not altered greatly	None? Perhaps decrease	
Cyclophosphamide	14	0.6	5.0	120	Enzyme-limited, binding-insensitive	90% Hepatic 10% Renal Active metabolite	$t_{1/2} \uparrow$; $V_d \rightarrow$; $Cl \downarrow$ 43%; $f_p \rightarrow$?	Unknown	74, 204

Table 5.5 (*continued*)

Drug	Protein Binding (%)	Volume of Distribution (V_d) (liter/kg)	Half-life ($t_{1/2}$) (hr)	Clearance (Cl) (ml/min)	Class	Hepatic/Renal Elimination	Effect of Liver Disease on Drug Disposition	Adjustment of Dose	References
Cytosine arabinoside	13	2.5	2.5	800	—	Extensive extrahepatic elimination; 40% renal	No data; probably little effect	None	
Etoposide	—	.28	5.6	39	—	65% Hepatic 35% Renal	$t_{1/2} \rightarrow$; $V_d \rightarrow$; $Cl \rightarrow$	None	32, 55
5-Fluorouracil	—	0.5	0.1	—	Flow-limited	Hepatic and extrahepatic; <5% Renal	Some decrease in clearance expected	Probable slight decrease	
Methotrexate	50	0.5	9.0	80	—	15% Hepatic; mostly biliary; 85% Renal	No data; probably little effect. Drug is hepatoxic and should be avoided if possible.	None	
Antiepileptic									
Carbamazepine	75	1.1	18.0 induced	—	Enzyme-limited, binding-sensitive	>98% Hepatic <2% Renal	No data; expect a decrease in clearance and increase in $t_{1/2}$	Probably decrease dose	
Diphenylhydantoin	92	0.65	15.0 non-linear	40	Enzyme-limited, binding-sensitive	>95% Hepatic <5% Renal	AVH $t_{1/2} \rightarrow$; $Cl \rightarrow$; $f_p \uparrow$. Cirrhosis $f_p \uparrow$	Decrease dose in moderate to severe liver disease	15, 62, 135
Phenobarbital	50	0.8	100	8	Enzyme-limited, binding-insensitive	75% Hepatic 25% Renal	$t_{1/2} \uparrow$; presumed $Cl \downarrow$	Decrease with severe liver disease	7
Valproic Acid	89 non-linear	12	0.14	30	Enzyme-limited, binding-sensitive	>98% Hepatic <25% Renal	$t_{1/2} \uparrow$; V_d slightly $\uparrow$; $Cl \downarrow$ 40%; $f_p \uparrow$	Decrease dose	88
Antipyretic/ Antiinflammatory									
Antipyrine	<10	0.58	12	50	Enzyme-limited, binding-insensitive	92% Hepatic 8% Renal	$t_{1/2} \uparrow$; $V_d \uparrow$ or $\rightarrow$; $Cl \downarrow$ 60% or more, but actual decrease in Cl depends on disease	Not used clinically	24, 35, 61, 69, 90, 109, 112, 118, 148, 186, 188, 194
Dexamethasone	68	0.75	3.25	260	Flow/enzyme-sensitive	>97% Hepatic <3% Renal	$f_p \rightarrow$; $V_d \rightarrow$; $t_{1/2} \uparrow$; $Cl \downarrow$	Decrease dose	76
Fenprofen	>99	0.10	1.5	200	Enzyme-limited, binding-sensitive	>98% Hepatic <2% Renal	No data; would expect $fp \uparrow$; $t_{1/2} \uparrow$; $Cl \uparrow$ or $\rightarrow$	Decrease dose	

Drug					Classification	Extent	Changes	Dose adjustment	Ref.
Ibuprofen	>99	0.15 V area/F	2.0	52	Enzyme-limited, binding-sensitive	>99% Hepatic <1% Renal	$t_{1/2}$ slightly ↑ in severe LD; V_d?; Cl?	Decrease in severe liver disease if high doses	73
Indomethacin	90	0.17	8.0	125	Enzyme-limited, binding-sensitive	>98% Hepatic <2% Renal	$t_{1/2}$ ↑; no other information. Assume Cl ↓, f_p ↑	Decrease dose as required	56
Naproxen	99.6	0.10	14.0	5	Enzyme-limited, binding-sensitive	>90% Hepatic <10% Renal	$t_{1/2}$ ↑; V_d →; Cl →; 28%; f_p?	Decrease dose in moderate to severe disease	25, 213
Phenylbutazone	98.5	0.17	70	2	Enzyme-limited, binding-sensitive	>99% Hepatic <1% Renal	$t_{1/2}$ ↑ or →; f_p ↑; V_d?; Cl? Assume Cl ↓ with liver disease	Decrease dose	22, 68, 93, 207
Prednisolone	80	0.6	3.0	180	Enzyme-limited, binding-sensitive	>85% Hepatic <15% Renal	$t_{1/2}$ →; V_d →; Cl →; f_p → or ↑. Drug little affected by liver disease.	None	76, 152, 168, 199
Salicylic acid	80–95 dose dependent	0.17 dose dependent	2.4–19	13 in therapeutic range	—	2–30% Renal; dose dependent	$t_{1/2}$ →; V_d →; Cl?; f_p ↑	None	162
Sulfinpyrazone	99	0.06	6.0	23	Enzyme-limited, binding-sensitive	65% Hepatic 35% Renal	No data; would expect some decrease in Cl with liver disease	Sight decrease in dose	
Cardiovascular									
Atenolol	<5	0.55	6.5	55–130	—	10% Hepatic 90% Renal	$t_{1/2}$ →; V_d →; Cl →	None	81
Digitoxin	95	0.60	180	2.5	Enzyme-limited, binding-sensitive	70% Hepatic 30% Renal	$t_{1/2}$ → or ↓; Cl ↑ or →; f_p ↑	None	80, 127, 145
Digoxin	30	6.0	35	150	—	30% Hepatic 70% Renal	Appears negligible	None	100, 104, 219
Disopyramide	80 non-linear	1.0	8	100	—	45% Hepatic 55% Renal	No data; would not expect a tremendous change in liver disease	Probably slight decrease	
Labetalol	50	11.5	3.0	1600	Flow-limited	>95% Hepatic <5% Renal	$t_{1/2}$ →; V_d ↓; Cl → or ↓; f_p?, assume ↑	Decrease oral dose; decrease i.v. dose to much smaller extent	60

Table 5.5 (continued)

Drug	Protein Binding (%)	Volume of Distribution (V_d) (liter/kg)	Half-life ($t_{1/2}$) (hr)	Clearance (Cl) (ml/min)	Class	Hepatic/Renal Elimination	Effect of Liver Disease on Drug Disposition	Adjustment of Dose	References
Lidocaine	65 nonlinear	1.1	2.0	1000	Flow-limited	97% Hepatic 3% Renal	$t_{1/2}$ ↑; V_d ↑ or →; Cl ↓ ~50%; f_p? Low therapeutic ratio. Decrease in Cl depends on severity of disease	Decrease dose by 50% in severe liver disease	3, 41, 64, 196–198, 210
Lorcainide	70	12.9	8.0	1700	Flow-limited	98% Hepatic 2% Renal	$t_{1/2}$ ←; V_d →; Cl ↓ 29%; f_p ↑ slightly. Cl_{Int} exhibits a very large decrease	Decrease dose	86
Metoprolol	10	3.2	4.0	800	Flow-limited	95% Hepatic 5% Renal	$t_{1/2}$ ↑; V_d ↑ slightly; Cl ↓ slightly; f_p? assumed unaffected	Decrease dose slightly	154
N-Acetyl procainamide	10	1.4	8.0	210	—	20% Hepatic 80% Renal	No data; expect little change unless renal function altered	None	
Nifedipine	98	1.0	3.0	600	Flow-limited, binding-sensitive	100% Hepatic	$t_{1/2}$ ↑; V_d →; Cl ↓; f_p ↑	Decrease dose	82
Pindolol	57	6.2	3.5	300	Enzyme-limited, binding-insensitive	70% Hepatic 30% Renal	Not affected by AVH. Cirrhosis Cl ↓ slightly and renal excretion of drug is increased	Some decrease in severe liver disease	131
Prazosin	97	1.3	3.0	450	Flow-limited	95% Hepatic 5% Renal	No data—would expect $t_{1/2}$ ↑; Cl ↓; f_p ↑	Decrease dose	
Procainamide	15	2.2	3.0	600	—	45% Hepatic 55% Renal Drug acetylated	$t_{1/2}$ ↑; V_d? Cl? probably decreased slightly	Some minor decrease in dose	34
Propranolol	95	4.0	4.0	850	Flow-limited	>95% Hepatic <5% Renal	$t_{1/2}$ ↑; V_d ↑; Cl ↓ ~60%; f_p ↑. Tremendous decrease in Cl_{Int}. Flow/enzyme-limited in cirrhosis	Decrease dose depending on extent of damage	20, 146, 214
Quinidine	85	3.0	6.0	330	Flow/enzyme-sensitive	80% Hepatic 20% Renal	$t_{1/2}$ ↑; V_d ↑; Cl →; f_p ↑; Cl_{Int} decreased significantly	Decrease dose	4, 79, 144

Drug	%				Classification	Hepatic/Renal	Disposition changes	Recommendation	References
Tocainide	10	3.0	13	150	Enzyme-limited	60% Hepatic 40% Renal	$t_{1/2} \uparrow$; V_d ?; $Cl \downarrow$	Decrease dose	136
Verapamil	92	6.7	3.5	1570	Flow-limited	95% Hepatic 5% Renal	$t_{1/2} \uparrow$; $V_d \uparrow$; $Cl \downarrow$ 60%; $f_p \rightarrow$; Cl_{int} decreases even more than 60%	Decrease dose by 50% in severe liver disease	184, 215
Diuretic									
Bumetanide	?	9.45	1.0	129	—	36% Hepatic 64% Renal	$t_{1/2} \uparrow$; $V_d \downarrow$; $Cl \downarrow$	Minor decrease in dose	103
Furosemide	95	0.15	1.0	170	—	35% Hepatic 65% Renal	$t_{1/2} \downarrow$ or $\rightarrow$; $V_d \uparrow$ or $\rightarrow$; $Cl \rightarrow$; $f_p \uparrow$; the change in f_p compensates for decrease in Cl_{int} of liver	None or slight decrease in severe cases	5, 42, 46, 77, 167, 200, 203
Hydrochlorothiazide	95	1.5	2.5	480	—	<10% Hepatic >90% Renal	No data; probably little affected unless renal function altered	None	
Spironolactone	98	—	20	—	Enzyme-limited, binding-sensitive, and extrahepatic metabolism	>85% Hepatic <15% Renal	No apparent change in drug disposition with liver disease; $t_{1/2} \rightarrow$	None	1, 166
Triamterene	50	2.5	2.0	1000	Flow-limited	95% Hepatic 5% Renal	$Cl \downarrow$; $f_p \rightarrow$; expect $t_{1/2} \uparrow$	Decrease dose	202
Sedative/hypnotic									
Amylobarbital	60	1.2	21	35	Enzyme-limited, binding-insensitive	>95% Hepatic <5% Renal	$t_{1/2} \uparrow$; $V_d \rightarrow$; $Cl \downarrow$ 55%; $f_p \uparrow$. Little change if albumin > 3.5 g/100 ml	Decrease dose	106
Chlordiazepoxide	96	0.3	12 age-dependent	20	Enzyme-limited, binding-sensitive	>99% Hepatic <1% Renal	$t_{1/2} \uparrow$; $V_d \rightarrow$; $Cl \downarrow$ 60%; $f_p \uparrow$. Both AVH and cirrhosis affect drug	Decrease dose	110, 116, 163, 164, 172
Diazepam	99	1.2	45	28	Enzyme-limited, binding-sensitive	>97% Hepatic <3% Renal	$t_{1/2} \uparrow$; $V_d \uparrow$; $Cl \downarrow$ 50%; $f_p \uparrow$. AVH and cirrhosis increase $T_{1/2}$. Large therapeutic index—safe	Single dose, no change; chronic, decrease dose	9, 19, 57, 84, 85, 107, 128
Hexobarbital	47	1.2	6.0	232	Enzyme-limited, binding-insensitive	>99% Hepatic <1% Renal	$t_{1/2} \uparrow$; $V_d \downarrow$; $Cl \downarrow$ 62% (Cl decreased in AVH and cirrhosis, $Cl \rightarrow$ in cholestasis); $f_p \rightarrow$	Decrease during chronic dosing	21, 158, 218

Table 5.5 (continued)

Drug	Protein Binding (%)	Volume of Distribution (V_d) (liter/kg)	Half-life ($t_{1/2}$) (hr)	Clearance (Cl) (ml/min)	Class	Hepatic/Renal Elimination	Effect of Liver Disease on Drug Disposition	Adjustment of Dose	References
Lorazepam	90	1.3	12.0	53	Enzyme-limited, binding-sensitive	>98% Hepatic <2% Renal Extensive glucuronidation	$t_{1/2}$ ↑; V_d ↑; Cl →; f_p ↑. Neither AVH nor cirrhosis affects drug dosing	None	89
Methohexital	—	61	2.0	829	Flow/enzyme-sensitive	>90% Hepatic <10% Renal	No data; assume Cl ↓, $t_{1/2}$ ↑	Probably decrease dose	
Midazolam	—	1.3	1.6	624	Flow-limited	>95% Hepatic <5% Renal	$t_{1/2}$ ↑; V_d slightly ↑; Cl ↓	Decrease dose	6, 97
Nitrazepam	87	1.9	26	63	Enzyme-limited	>99% Hepatic <1% Renal Mainly nitro-reduction	$t_{1/2}$ →; V_d →; Cl →; f_p ↑	None	71
Oxazepam	90	1.6	6.0	140	Enzyme-limited, binding-sensitive	>99% Hepatic <1% Renal Extensive glucuronidation	$t_{1/2}$ →; V_d →; Cl →; f_p →. Neither AVH nor cirrhosis alters disposition significantly	None	172, 178
Pentobarbital	65	1.0	30	30	Enzyme-limited, binding-sensitive	99% Hepatic <1% Renal	No data; expect Cl ↓, $t_{1/2}$ ↑	Single dose, no change; chronic, lower dose	173
Primidone	19	0.86	17	41	—	60% Hepatic 40% Renal (in children)	$t_{1/2}$ →; V_d slight ↑; Cl slight ↑ in hepatitis	None	149
Temazepam	98	1.2	14	80	—	>98% Hepatic <2% Renal Mainly glucuronidation	$t_{1/2}$ →; V_d →; Cl →; f_p →	None	129
Others									
Alfentanil	90	0.28	1.5	200	Flow/enzyme-sensitive	99% Hepatic 1% Renal	$t_{1/2}$ ↑; V_d →; Cl ↓; f_p ↑ (dose-dependent)	Decrease dose	39
Atracurium	—	0.16	0.33	385	—	Hofmann elimination; auto-metabolism	$t_{1/2}$ →; V_d ↑; Cl →; long $t_{1/2}$ of metabolite	Decrease dose if long-term use	206
Caffeine	31	0.54	6.0	63	Enzyme-limited, binding-insensitive	95% Hepatic 5% Renal	$t_{1/2}$ ↑ slightly; V_d →; Cl ↓ 40%; f_p ↑; large therapeutic ratio	None	31

Drug								Dose recommendation	
Chlormethiazole	64	0.12	7.0	1100	Flow-limited; vitamin B substitute	>99% Hepatic <1% Renal	$t_{1/2}$ ↑; V_d →; Cl ↓ 28%; f_p ↑	Probably not necessary	143
Cimetidine	20	1.1	2.3	550	—	40% Hepatic 60% Renal	$t_{1/2}$ →; V_d ↑ or ↓ or →; Cl → or ↓; f_p changes assumed unimportant. Drug associated with increased incidence of mental confusion in cirrhotics	Decrease dose in severe liver disease	27, 47, 51, 52, 123, 124, 132, 170, 185, 201, 217
Clofibrate (CPIB)	95	0.15	18.0	8	Enzyme-limited, binding-sensitive	90% Hepatic <10% Renal Glucuronidation of metabolite	$t_{1/2}$ →; V_d ↑ slightly; Cl →; f_p ↑. AVH does not alter Cl; cirrhosis does have an effect on Cl_{int} ↓ 50%	Decrease dose in cirrhosis by 50%	49
Diphenhydramine	78	6.5	9.5	696	Flow-limited	>98% Hepatic <2% Renal	$t_{1/2}$ ↑; free Cl ↓; total Cl →; f_p ↑	Decrease dose	111
Fentanyl	80	3.5	4.0	750	—	92% Hepatic 8% Renal	$t_{1/2}$ →; V_d →; Cl →	None	53
Ranitidine	15	1.5	2.3	600	—	30% Hepatic 70% Renal	$t_{1/2}$ →; V_d →; Cl → or ↓	None	117, 134, 183, 216
Sulfisoxazole	92	0.15	6.6	20	Enzyme-limited, binding-sensitive	50% Hepatic 50% Renal Acetylation	$t_{1/2}$ →; V_d ↑; Cl ↑; f_p ↑	None	26
Theophylline	52	0.5	8.0	45	Enzyme-limited, binding-insensitive	91% Hepatic 9% Renal	$t_{1/2}$ ↑; V_d → cirrhosis, ↑ hepatitis and cholestasis; Cl ↓ 55%; f_p ↑. Low therapeutic index caution	Decrease dose by 50%	75, 101, 147, 189
Thiopental	85	2.3	9.0	275	Enzyme-limited	>99% Hepatic <1% Renal	$t_{1/2}$ →; V_d →; Cl →; f_p ↑	Uncertain; may need to decrease dose	138
Tolbutamide	98	0.15	5.0	20.0	Enzyme-limited, binding-sensitive	95% Hepatic 5% Renal	$t_{1/2}$ slightly ↑ or →; V_d →; Cl ↑; f_p ↑. AVH has been reported to increase rate of elimination	None; probably not used in liver disease	211
Warfarin	99	0.20	23	8.0	Enzyme-limited, binding-sensitive	99% Hepatic 1% Renal	$t_{1/2}$ →; V_d →; Cl →; f_p →. AVH no effect, but may be related to extent of liver damage	None; probably not used in liver disease	212

[a] GI, gastrointestinal; AVH, acute viral hepatitis; LD, liver disease.

Table 5.6
Considerations for Drug Dosage Adjustments in Liver Disease Patients

Extent of Change in Drug Dose	Conditions or Requirements to Be Satisfied
No change or minor change in dose	1. Mild liver disease 2. Extensive elimination of drug by kidneys and no renal dysfunction 3. Elimination by pathways of metabolism spared by liver disease 4. Drug is enzyme-limited and given acutely 5. Drug is flow/enzyme-sensitive and only given acutely by i.v. route 6. No alteration in drug sensitivity
Decrease in dose up to 25%	1. Elimination by the liver does not exceed 40% of the dose; no renal dysfunction 2. Drug is flow-limited and given by i.v. route, with no large change in protein binding 3. Drug is flow/enzyme-limited and given acutely by oral route 4. Drug has a large therapeutic ratio
Decrease in dose of greater than 25%	1. Drug metabolism is affected by liver disease; drug administered chronically 2. Drug has a narrow therapeutic range; protein binding altered significantly 3. Drug is flow-limited and given orally 4. Drug is eliminated by kidneys and renal function severely affected 5. Altered sensitivity to drug due to liver disease

tration of drugs that inhibit drug metabolism may further decrease an already depressed level of metabolic function. Age, genetic factors, or smoking can also influence drug disposition and make it difficult to accurately predict dosage requirements. Faced with such a wide array of variables influencing drug disposition, the best advice is still the following: (a) use caution when dosing, (b) follow blood levels if possible, and (c) be alert for signs of drug toxicity.

Acknowledgment

This work was supported in part by United States Public Health Service Grant GM 31304.

References

1. Abshagen U, Rennekamp H, Luszpinski G: Disposition kinetics of spironolactone in hepatic failure after single doses and prolonged treatment. *Eur J Clin Pharmacol* 11:169–176, 1977.
2. Acocella G, Bonollo L, Garimoldi M, Mainardi M, Tenconi LT, Hicolis FB: Kinetics of rifampin and isoniazid administered alone and in combination to normal subjects and patients with liver disease. *Gut* 13:47–53, 1972.
3. Adjepon-Yamoah KK, Himmo J, Prescott LF: Gross impairment of hepatic drug metabolism in a patient with chronic liver disease. *Br Med J* 4:387–388, 1974.
4. Affrime A, Reidenberg MM: The protein binding of some drugs in plasma from patients with alcoholic liver disease. *Eur J Clin Pharmacol* 8:267–269, 1975.
5. Allgulander C, Beerman B, Sjogren, A: Furosemide

pharmacokinetics in patients with liver disease. *Clin Pharmacokinet* 5:570–575, 1980.
6. Allonen H, Zieglar G, Koltz U: Midazolam kinetics. *Clin Pharmacol Ther* 30:653–660, 1981.
7. Alvin J, Meltorse T, Hoyumpa A, Bush MT, Schenker S: The effect of liver disease in man on the disposition of phenobarbital. *J Pharmacol Exp Ther* 192:224–235, 1975.
8. Andreasen PB, Greisen G: Phenazone metabolism in patients with liver disease. *Eur J Clin Invest* 6:21–26, 1976.
9. Andreasen PB, Hendel J, Greisen G, Hvidberg EF: Pharmacokinetics of diazepam in disordered liver function. *Eur J Clin Pharmacol* 10:115–120, 1976.
10. Andreasen PB, Hutters L: Paracetamol (acetaminophen) clearance in patients with cirrhosis of the liver. *Acta Med Scand [Suppl]* 624:99–105, 1979.
11. Avant GR, Schenker S, Alford RH: The effect of cirrhosis on the disposition and elimination of clindamycin. *Am J Dig Dis* 20:223–230, 1975.
12. Azzollini F, Gazzaniga A, Lodola E, Natangelo R: Elimination of chloramphenicol and thiamphenicol in subjects with cirrhosis of the liver. *Int J Clin Pharmacol Ther Toxicol* 6:13–134, 1972.
13. Benjamin RS: Clinical pharmacology of adriamycin (NSC-123127). *Cancer Chemother Rep* 6:183–185, 1975.
14. Bircher J, Blankart R, Halpern A, Hacki W, Laissue J, Preisig R: Criteria for assessment of functional impairment in patients with cirrhosis of the liver. *Eur J Clin Invest* 3:72–85, 1973.
15. Blaschke TF, Meffin, PJ, Melmon KL, Rowland M: Influence of acute viral hepatitis on phenytoin kinetics and protein binding. *Clin Pharmacol Ther* 17:685–691, 1975.
16. Boscia JA, Korzeniowski OM, Kobasa WD, Rocha H, Levison ME, Kaye D: Pharmacokinetics of cefoperazone in normal subjects and patients with hepatosplenic schistosomiasis. *J Antimicrob Chemother* 12:407–410, 1983.
17. Boscia JA, Korzeniowski OM, Snepar R, Kobasa WD,

Levison ME, Kaye D: Cefoperazone pharmacokinetics in normal subjects and patients with cirrhosis. *Antimicrob Agents Chemother* 23:385–389, 1983.

18. Branch RA, James J, Read AE: A study of factors influencing drug disposition in chronic liver disease, using the model drug (+)-propranolol. *Br J Clin Pharmacol* 3:243–249, 1976.

19. Branch RA, Morgan MH, James J, Read AE: Intravenous administration of diazepam in patients with chronic liver disease. *Gut* 17:975–983, 1976.

20. Branch RA, Shand DG: Propranolol disposition in chronic liver disease: a physiological approach. *Clin Pharmacokinet* 1:264–279, 1976.

21. Breimer DD, Zilly W, Richter E: Pharmacokinetics of hexobarbital in acute hepatitis and after apparent recovery. *Clin Pharmacol Ther* 18:433–440, 1975.

22. Brodie MJ, Boobis S: The effect of chronic alcoholic ingestion and alcoholic liver disease on binding of drugs to serum proteins: *Eur J Clin Pharmacol* 13:435–438, 1978.

23. Brown N, Ho DHW, Fong KL, Bogerd L, Maksymiuk A, Bolivar R, Fainstein V, Bodey GP: Effects of hepatic function on vancomycin clinical pharmacology. *Antimicrob Agents Chemother* 23:603–609, 1983.

24. Burnett DA, Barak AJ, Tuma DJ, Sorrell MF: Altered elimination of antipyrine in patients with acute viral hepatitis. *Gut* 17:341–344, 1976.

25. Calvo MV, Dominguez-Gil A, Macias JG, Dietz JL: Naproxen disposition in hepatic and biliary disorders. *Int J Clin Pharmacol Ther Toxicol* 18:242–246, 1980.

26. Cello JP, Oie S: Binding and disposition of sulfisoxazole in alcoholic cirrhosis. *J Pharmacokinet Biopharm* 13:1–12, 1985.

27. Cello JP, Oie J: Cimetidine disposition in patients with Laennec's cirrhosis during multiple dosing therapy. *Eur J Clin Pharmacol* 25:223–229, 1983.

28. Cochet B, Belaieff J, Allaz AF, Rudhardt M, Balant L, Fabre J: Decreased extrarenal clearance of cefoperazone in hepatocellular diseases. *Br J Clin Pharmacol* 11:389–390, 1981.

29. Cochet B, Belaieff J, Allaz AJ, Rudhardt M, Balant L, and Fabre J: Serum levels and urinary excretion of cefoperazone in patients with hepatic insufficiency. *Infection* 9(suppl 1):537–539, 1981.

30. Daneshmend TK, Homeida M, Kaye CM, Elamin AA, Roberts CJC: Disposition of oral metronidazole in hepatic cirrhosis and in hepatosplenic schistosomiasis. *Gut* 23:807–813, 1982.

31. Desmond PV, Patwardhan RV, Johnson RF, Schenker S: Impaired elimination of caffeine in cirrhosis. *Dig Dis Sci* 25:193–197, 1980.

32. D'Incalci M, Rossi C, Zucchetti M, Urso R, Cavalli F, Mangioni C, Williams Y, Sessa C: Pharmacokinetics of etoposide in patients with abnormal renal and hepatic function. *Cancer Res* 46:2566–2571, 1986.

33. Doshi J, Luisada-Oppe A, Leevy CM: Microsomal pentobarbital hydroxylase activity in acute viral hepatitis. *Proc Soc Exp Biol Med* 140:492–495, 1975.

34. duSouich P, Erill S: Metabolism of procainamide and p-aminobenzoic acid in patients with chronic liver disease. *Clin Pharmacol Ther* 22:588–595, 1977.

35. El-Raghy I, Back DJ, Osman F, Nafeh MA, Orme M L'E: The pharmacokinetics of antipyrine in patients with graded severity of schistosomiasis. *Br J Clin Pharmacol* 20:313–316, 1985.

36. Farrell G, Baird-Lambert J, Cvejic J, Buchanan N: Disposition and metabolism of metronidazole in patients with liver failure. *Hepatology* 4:722–726, 1984.

37. Farrell GC, Cooksley WGE, Hart P, Powell LW: Drug metabolism in liver disease. Identification of patients with impaired hepatic drug metabolism. *Gastroenterology* 75:580–588, 1978.

38. Farrell GC, Cooksley WGE, Powell LW: Drug metabolism in liver disease: Activity of hepatic microsomal metabolizing enzymes. *Clin Pharmacol Ther* 26:483–492, 1979.

39. Ferrier C, Marty J, Bouffard Y, Haberer JP, Levron JC, Duvaldestin P: Alfentanil pharmacokinetics in patients with cirrhosis. *Anesthesiology* 62:480–484, 1985.

40. Forrest JA, Adriaenssens P, Finlayson NDC, Prescott LF: Paracetamol metabolism in chronic liver disease. *Eur J Clin Pharmacol* 15:427–431, 1979.

41. Forrest JAH, Finlayson NDC, Adjepon-Yamoah KK, Prescott LF: Antipyrine, paracetamol, and lidocaine elimination in chronic liver disease. *Br Med J* 1:1384–1387, 1977.

42. Fuller R, Hoppel C, Ingalls ST: Furosemide kinetics in patients with hepatic cirrhosis with ascites. *Clin Pharmacol Ther* 30:461–467, 1981.

43. Ghoneim MM, Pandya H: Plasma protein binding of thiopental in patients with impaired renal or hepatic function. *Anesthesiology* 42:545–549, 1975.

44. Giacomini KM, Giacomini JC, Gibson TP, Levy G: Propoxyphene and norpropoxyphene plasma concentrations after oral propoxyphene in cirrhotic patients with and without surgically constructed portacaval shunt. *Clin Pharmacol Ther* 28:417–424, 1980.

45. Giargcau AJ, Chalmers TC: The natural history of cirrhosis. I. Survival with esophageal varices. *N Engl J Med* 268:469–473, 1963.

46. Gonzalez G, Arancibia A, Rivas MI, Caro P and Antezana C: Pharmacokinetics of furosemide in patients with hepatic cirrhosis. *Eur J Clin Pharmacol* 22:315–320, 1980.

47. Grahnen A, Jameson S, Lööf L, Tyllström J, Lindström B: Pharmacokinetics of cimetidine in advanced cirrhosis. *Eur J Clin Pharmacol* 26:347–355, 1984.

48. Greenfield RA, Gerber AU, Craig WA: Pharmacokinetics of cefoperazone in patients with normal and impaired hepatic and renal function. *Rev Infect Dis* 5(suppl 1):S127–S136, 1983.

49. Groszman R, Kotelanski B, Khatri IM, Cohn JN: Quantitation of portasystemic shunting from the splenic and mesenteric beds in alcoholic liver disease. *Am J Med* 53:715–722, 1972.

50. Gugler R, Kurten JW, Jensen CJ, Klehr U, Hartlapp J: Clofibrate disposition in renal failure and acute and chronic liver disease. *Eur J Clin Pharmacol* 15:341–347, 1979.

51. Gugler R, Muller Liebenau B, Somogyi A: Altered disposition and availability of cimetidine in liver cirrhotic patients. *Br J Clin Pharmacol* 14:421–429, 1982.

52. Gugler R, Wolf M, Hansen HH, Jensen JC: The inhibition of drug metabolism by cimetidine in patients with liver cirrhosis. *Klin Wochenschr* 62:1126–1131, 1984.

53. Haberer JP, Schoeffler P, Couderc E, Duvaldestin P: Fentanyl pharmacokinetics in anaesthetized patients with cirrhosis. *Br J Anaesth* 54:1267–1270, 1982.

54. Hall KW, Nightingale CH, Gibaldi M, Nelson E, Bates TR, Disanto AR: Pharmacokinetics of erythromycin in normal and alcoholic liver disease subjects. *J Clin Pharmacol* 22:321–325, 1982.

55. Hande KR, Wedlund PJ, Noone RM, Wilkinson GR, Greco FA, Wolff SN: Pharmacokinetics of high-dose etoposide (VP-16-213) administered to cancer patients. *Cancer Res* 44:379–382, 1984.

56. Helleberg L: Clinical pharmacokinetics of indomethacin. *Clin Pharmacokinet* 6:245–258, 1981.

57. Hepner GW, Vesell ES, Lipton A, Harvey HA, Wilkinson GR, Schenker S: Disposition of aminopyrine, antipyrine, diazepam and indocyanine green in patients with liver disease or on anticonvulsant drug therapy: diazepam breath test and correlations in drug elimination. *J Lab Clin Med* 90:440–456, 1977.

58. Hinthorn DR, Baker LH, Romig DR, Hassanien K, Liu C: Use of clindamycin in patients with liver disease. *Antimicrob Agents Chemother* 9:498–501, 1976.

59. Hoffman TA, Cestero R, Bullock WE: Pharmacodyn-

amics of carbenicillin in hepatic and renal failure. *Ann Intern Med* 73:173–178, 1970.

60. Homeida M, Jackson L, Roberts CJC: Decreased first-pass metabolism of labetalol in chronic liver disease. *Br Med J* 2:1048–1050, 1978.

61. Homeida M, Roberts CJC, Halliwell M, Read AE, Branch RA: Antipyrine clearance per unit volume liver: an assessment of hepatic function in chronic liver disease. *Gut* 20:596–601, 1979.

62. Hooper WD, Bochner F, Eadie MJ, Tyrer JH: Plasma protein binding of diphenylhydantoin. Effects of sex hormones, renal and hepatic disease. *Clin Pharmacol Ther* 15:276–282, 1974.

63. Horn T, Christofferson P, Henriksen JH: Alcoholic liver injury: defenestration in noncirrhotic livers—a scanning electron microscopic study. *Hepatology* 7:77–82, 1987.

64. Huet P, Lelorier J: Effects of smoking and chronic hepatitis B on lidocaine and indocyanine green kinetics. *Clin Pharmacol Ther* 28:208–215, 1980.

65. Huet P-M, Goresky CA, Villeneuve J-P, Marleau D, Lough JO: Assessment of liver microcirculation in human cirrhosis. *J Clin Invest* 70:1234–1244, 1982.

66. Huet P-M, Pomier-Layrargues G, Villeneuve J-P, Varin F, Viallet A: Intrahepatic circulation in liver disease. *Semin Liver Dis* 6:277–286, 1986.

67. Huet P-M, Villeneuve J-P, Pomier-Layrargues G, Marleau D: Hepatic circulation in cirrhosis. *Clin Gastroenterol* 14:155–168, 1985.

68. Hvidberg EF, Andreasen PB, Ranek L: Plasma half-life of phenylbutazone in patients with impaired liver function. *Clin Pharmacol Ther* 15:171–177, 1974.

69. Ishizaki T, Chiba K, Sasaki T: Antipyrine clearance in patients with Gilbert's syndrome. *Eur J Clin Pharmacol* 27:297–302, 1984.

70. Jahnchen E, Blanck KJ, Breuing KH, Gilfrich HJ, Meinertz T, Trenk D: Plasma protein binding of azapropazone in patients with kidney and liver disease. *Br J Clin Pharmacol* 11:361–367, 1981.

71. Jochemsen R, Van Beusekom BR, Spoelstra P, Janssens AR, Breimer DD: Effect of age and liver cirrhosis on the pharmacokinetics of nitrazepam. *Br J Clin Pharmacol* 15:295–302, 1983.

72. Johannessen SI, Gerna M, Bakke J, Strandjord RE, Morselli PL: CSF concentrations and serum protein binding of carbamazepine and carbamazepine-10gll-epoxide in epileptic patients. *Br J Clin Pharmacol* 3:575–582, 1976.

73. Juhl RP, VanThiel DH, Dittert LW, Albert KS, Smith RB: Ibuprofen and sulindac kinetics in alcoholic liver disease. *Clin Pharmacol Ther* 34:104–109, 1983.

74. Juma FD: Effect of liver failure on the pharmacokinetics of cyclophosphamide. *Eur J Clin Pharmacol* 26:591–593, 1984.

75. Jusko WJ, Gardner MJ, Mangione A, Shentag JJ, Koup JR, Vance JW: Factors affecting theophylline clearances: age, tobacco, marijuana, cirrhosis, congestive heart failure, obesity, oral contraceptives, benzodiazepines, barbiturates and ethanol. *J Pharm Sci* 68:1358–1366, 1979.

76. Kawai S, Ichikawa Y, Homma M: Differences in metabolic properties among cortisol, prednisolone, and dexamethasone in liver and renal diseases. Accelerated metabolism of dexamethasone in renal failure. *J Clin Endocrinol Metab* 60:848–854, 1985.

77. Keller E, Hoppe-Seyler G, Mumm R, Schollmeyer P: Influence of hepatic cirrhosis and end-stage renal disease on pharmacokinetics and pharmacodynamics of furosemide. *Eur J Clin Pharmacol* 20:27–33, 1981.

78. Kenny MT, Strates B: Metabolism and pharmacokinetics of the antibiotic rifampin. *Drug Metab Rev* 12:159–218, 1981.

79. Kessler KM, Humphries WC, Black M, Spann JF: Quinidine pharmacokinetics in patients with cirrhosis or receiving propranolol. *Am Heart J* 96:627–635, 1978.

80. Kirch W, Ohnhaus EE, Dylewicz P, Pabst J, Storstein L: Bioavailability and elimination of digitoxin in patients with hepatorenal insufficiency. *Am Heart J* 111:325–329, 1986.

81. Kirch W, Schäfer-Korting M, Mutschler E, Ohnhaus EE, Braun W: Clinical experience with atenolol in patients with chronic liver disease. *J Clin Pharmacol* 23:171–177, 1983.

82. Kleinbloesem CH, van Harten J, Wilson JPH, Danhof M, van Brummelen P, Breimer DD: Nifedipine: kinetics and hemodynamic effects in patients with liver cirrhosis after intravenous and oral administration. *Clin Pharmacol Ther* 40:21–28, 1986.

83. Klinger EL, Vaamonde CA, Vaamonde LS, Lancestremere RG, Morosi HJ, Frisch E, Papper S: Renal function changes in cirrhosis of the liver. *Arch Intern Med* 125:1010–1015, 1970.

84. Klotz U, Antonin KH, Brugel H, Bieck PR: Disposition of diazepam and its major metabolite desmethyldiazepam in patients with liver disease. *Clin Pharmacol Ther* 21:430–436, 1977.

85. Klotz U, Avant GR, Hoyumpa A, Schenker S, Wilkinson GR: The effects of age and liver disease on the disposition and elimination of diazepam in adult man. *J Clin Invest* 55:347–359, 1975.

86. Klotz U, Fischer C, Muller-Seydlitz P, Schulz J, Mueller WA: Alterations in the disposition of differently cleared drugs in patients with cirrhosis. *Clin Pharmacol Ther* 26:221–227, 1979.

87. Klotz U, McHorse TS, Wilkinson GR, Schenker S: The effect of cirrhosis on the disposition and elimination of meperidine in man. *Clin Pharmacol Ther* 16:667–675, 1974.

88. Klotz U, Rapp T, Müller WA: Disposition of valproic acid in patients with liver disease. *Eur J Clin Pharmacol* 13:55–60, 1978.

89. Kraus JW, Desmond PV, Marshall JP, Johnson RF, Schenker S, Wilkinson GR: Effects of aging and liver disease on disposition of lorazepam. *Clin Pharmacol Ther* 24:411–419, 1978.

90. Krausz Y, Zylber-Katz E, Levy M: Antipyrine clearance and its correlation to routine liver function tests in patients with liver disease. *Int J Clin Pharmacol Ther Toxicol* 18:253–257, 1980.

91. Kroboth PD, Brown A, Lyon JA, Kroboth FJ, Juhl RP: Pharmacokinetics of single-dose erythromycin in normal and alcohol liver disease subjects. *Antimicrob Agents Chemother* 21:135–140, 1982.

92. Kunin CM, Glazko AJ, Finland M: Persistence of antibiotics in blood of patients with acute renal failure. Chloramphenicol and its metabolic products in the blood of patients with severe renal disease or hepatic cirrhosis. *J Clin Invest* 38:1498–1508, 1959.

93. Levi AJ, Sherlock S, Walker D: Phenylbutazone and isoniazid metabolism in patients with liver disease in relation to previous drug therapy. *Lancet* 1:1275–1279, 1968.

94. Levy G: Effect of plasma protein binding of drugs on duration and intensity of pharmacological activity. *J Pharm Sci* 65:1264–1265, 1976.

95. Lewis GP, Jusko WJ: Pharmacokinetics of ampicillin in cirrhosis. *Clin Pharmacol Ther* 18:475–484, 1975.

96. Lima JJ, Boudoulas H, Blanford M: Concentration-dependence of disopyramide binding to plasma protein and its influence on kinetics and dynamics. *J Pharmacol Exp Ther* 219:741–747, 1981.

97. MacGilchrist AJ, Birnie GG, Cook A, Scobie G, Murray T, Watkinson G, Brodie MJ: Pharmacokinetics and pharmacodynamics of intravenous midazolam in patients with severe alcoholic cirrhosis. *Gut* 27:190–195, 1986.

98. MacLeod CM, Bartley EA, Payne JA, Hudes E, Vernam K, Devlin RG: Effects of cirrhosis on kinetics of aztreonam. *Antimicrob Agents Chemother* 26:493–497, 1984.

99. Mak KM, Lieber CS: Alterations in endothelial fenestrations in liver sinusoids of baboons fed alcohol: a scanning electron microscopic study. *Hepatology* 4:386–391, 1984.

100. Malini PL, Sarti F, Dal Monte PR, Grepioni A, Boschi S, Ambrosioni E: Effect of chronic liver disease on plasma levels and metabolism of digoxin and beta-methyl digoxin. *Int J Clin Pharmacol Res* 1:21–27, 1982.

101. Mangione A, Inhoff TE, Lee RV, Shum LY, Jusko WJ: Pharmacokinetics of theophylline in hepatic disease. *Chest* 73:616–622, 1978.

102. Mannering GJ, Renton KW, el Azhary R, Deloria LB: Effects of interferon-inducing agents on hepatic cytochrome P-450 drug metabolizing systems. *Ann NY Acad Sci* 350:314–331, 1980.

103. Marcantonio LA, Auld WHR, Murdock WR, Purohit R, Skellern GG, Howes CA: The pharmacokinetics and pharmacodynamics of the diuretic bumetanide in hepatic and renal disease. *Br J Clin Pharmacol* 15:245–252, 1983.

104. Marcus FI, Kapadia GG: The metabolism of tritiated digoxin in cirrhotic patients. *Gastroenterology* 47:517–524, 1964.

105. Marshall JP, Salt WB, Elam RO, Wilkinson GR, Schenker S: Disposition of nafcillin in patients with cirrhosis and extrahepatic biliary obstruction. *Gastroenterology* 73:1388–1392, 1977.

106. Mawer GE, Miller NE, Turnberg LA: Metabolism of amylobarbitone in patients with chronic liver disease. *Br J Pharmacol* 44:549–560, 1972.

107. McConnell JB, Curry SH, Davis M, Williams R: Clinical effects and metabolism of diazepam in patients with chronic liver disease. *Clin Sci* 63:75–80, 1982.

108. McHorse TS, Wilkinson GR, Johnson RF, Schenker S: Effect of acute viral hepatitis in man on the disposition and elimination of meperidine. *Gastroenterology* 68:775–780, 1975.

109. Mehta MU, Venkataramanan R, Burckart GJ, Ptachcinski RJ, Yang SL, Gray JA, Van Thiel DH, Starzl TE: Antipyrine kinetics in liver disease and liver transplantation. *Clin Pharmacol Ther* 39:372–377, 1986.

110. Mendenhall CL, Robinson JD, Morgan DD: Chlordiazepoxide, librium (L), therapy in hepatic insufficiency. *Gastroenterology* 69:845, 1975.

111. Meredith CG, Christian CD Jr, Johnson RF, Madhavan SV, Schenker S: Diphenhydramine disposition in chronic liver disease. *Clin Pharmacol Ther* 35:474–479, 1984.

112. Miguet J-P, Vuitton D, Deschamps J-P, Allemand H, Joanne C, Bechtel P, Carayon P: Cholestasis and hepatic drug metabolism: comparison of metabolic clearance rate of antipyrine in patients with intrahepatic or extrahepatic cholestasis. *Dig Dis Sci* 26:718–722, 1981.

113. Morahan PS, Munson AE, Regelson W, Commerford SL, Hamilton LD: Antiviral activity and side effects of polyriboinosinic-cytidylic acid complexes as affected by molecular size. *Proc Natl Acad Sci USA* 69:842–846, 1972.

114. Morahan PS, Regelson W, Munson AE: Pyran and polyribonucleotides: differences in biological activities. *Antimicrob Agents Chemother* 2:16–22, 1972.

115. Moreau L, Durand H, Biclet P: Cefotaxime concentrations in ascites. *J Antimicrob Chemother* 6(suppl A):121–122, 1980.

116. Morgan DD, Robinson JD, Mendenhall CL: Clinical pharmacokinetics of chlordiazepoxide in patients with alcoholic hepatitis. *Eur J Clin Pharmacol* 19:279–285, 1981.

117. Morichau-Beauchant M, Houin G, Mavier P, Alexandre C, Dhumeaux D: Pharmacokinetics and bioavailability of ranitidine in normal subjects and cirrhotic patients. *Dig Dis Sci* 31:113–118, 1986.

118. Narang APS, Datta DV, Nath N, Mathur VS: Impairment of hepatic drug metabolism in patients with acute viral hepatitis. *Eur J Drug Metab Pharmacokinet* 7:255–258, 1982.

119. Narang APS, Datta DV, Nath N, Mathur VS: Pharmacokinetic study of chloramphenicol in patients with liver disease. *Eur J Clin Pharmacol* 20;479–483, 1981.

120. Naranjo CA, Busto U, Janecek E, Ruiz I, Roach CA, Kaplan K: An intensive drug monitoring study suggesting possible clinical irrelevance of impaired drug disposition in liver disease. *Br J Clin Pharmacol* 15:451–458, 1983.

121. Naranjo CA, Busto U, Mardones R: Adverse drug reactions in liver cirrhosis. *Eur J Clin Pharmacol* 13:429–434, 1978.

122. Neal EA, Meffin PJ, Gregory PB, Blaschke TF: Enhanced bioavailability and decreased clearance of analgesics in patients with cirrhosis. *Gastroenterology* 77:96–102, 1979.

123. Nelson DC, Avant GR, Speeg KV Jr, Hoyumpa AM Jr, Schenker S: The effect of cimetidine on hepatic drug elimination in cirrhosis. *Hepatology* 5:305–309, 1985.

124. Nouel O, Bernuau J, Lebar M, Rueff B, Benhamou JP: Cimetidine-induced mental confusion in patients with cirrhosis. *Gastroenterology* 79:780–781, 1980.

125. Novick DM, Kreek MJ, Arns PA, Lau LL, Yancovitz SR, Gelb AM: Effect of severe alcoholic liver disease on the disposition of methadone in maintenance patients. *Alcoholism* 9;349–354, 1985.

126. Novick DM, Kreek MJ, Fanizza AM, Yancovitz SR, Gelb AM, Stenger RJ: Methadone disposition in patients with chronic liver disease. *Clin Pharmacol Ther* 30:353–362, 1981.

127. Ochs HR, Greenblatt DJ, Bodem G, Dengler HJ: Disease-related alterations in cardiac glycoside disposition. *Clin Pharmacokinet* 7:434–451, 1982.

128. Ochs HR, Greenblatt DJ, Eckardt B, Harmatz JS, Shader RI: Repeated diazepam dosing in cirrhotic patients: accumulation and sedation. *Clin Pharmacol Ther* 33:471–476, 1983.

129. Ochs HR, Greenblatt DJ, Verburg-Ochs B, Matlis R: Temazepam clearance is unaltered in cirrhosis. *Am J Gastroenterol* 81:80–84, 1986.

130. Ohashi K, Tsunoo M, Tsuneoka K: Pharmacokinetics and protein binding of cefazolin and cephalothin in patients with cirrhosis. *J Antimicrob Chemother* 17:347–351, 1986.

131. Ohnhaus EE, Münch U, Meier J: Elimination of pindolol in liver disease. *Eur J Clin Pharmacol* 22:247–251, 1982.

132. Okolicsanyi L, Venuti M, Orlando R, Lirussi R, Nassuato G, Benvenuti C: Oral and intravenous pharmacokinetics of cimetidine in liver cirrhosis. *Int J Clin Pharmacol Ther Toxicol* 20:482–487, 1982.

133. Okolicsanyi L, Venuti M, Orlando R, Xerri L, Pugina M: Pharmacokinetic studies of cefuroxime in patients with liver cirrhosis. *Arzneimittelforschung* 7:777–782, 1982.

134. Okolicsanyi L, Venuti M, Strazzabosco M, Orlando R, Nassuato G, Iemmolo RM, Lirussi R, Muraca M, Pastorino AM, Castelli G: Oral and intravenous pharmacokinetics of ranitidine in patients with liver cirrhosis. *Int J Clin Pharmacol Ther Toxicol* 22:329–332, 1984.

135. Olsen GD, Bennett WM, Potter GA: Morphine and phenytoin binding to plasma proteins in renal and hepatic failure. *Clin Pharmacol Ther* 17:677–684, 1976.

136. Oltmanns D, Pottage A, Endell W: Pharmacokinetics of tocainide in patients with combined hepatic and renal dysfunction. *Eur J Clin Pharmacol* 25:787–790, 1983.

137. Orrego H, Medline A, Blendis LM, Rankin JG, Kreaden DA: Collagenisation of the Disse space in alcoholic liver disease. *Gut* 20:673–679, 1979.

138. Pandele G, Chaux F, Salvadori C, Farinotti M, Duvaldestin P: Thiopental pharmacokinetics in patients with cirrhosis. *Anesthesiology* 59:123–126, 1983.

139. Pasko MT, Beam TR, Spooner JA, Camara DS: Safety and pharmacokinetics of ceftazidime in patients with chronic hepatic dysfunction. *J Antimicrob Chemother* 15:365–374, 1985.

140. Patwardhan R, Johnson R, Sheehan J, Desmond P, Wilkinson G, Hoyumpa A, Branch R, Schenker S: Morphine metabolism in cirrhosis. *Gastroenterology* 80:1344, 1981.

141. Patwardhan RV, Johnson RF, Hoyumpa A, Sheehan JJ, Desmond PV, Wilkinson GR, Branch RA, Schenker S: Normal metabolism of morphine in cirrhosis. *Gastroenterology* 81:1006–1011, 1981.

142. Pearson RM, Breckenridge AM: Renal function, protein binding and pharmacological response to diazoxide. *Br J Clin Pharmacol* 3:169–175, 1976.

143. Pentikainen PJ, Neuvonen PJ, Jostell K-G: Pharmacokinetics of chlormethiazole in healthy volunteers and patients with cirrhosis of the liver. *Eur J Clin Pharmacol* 17:275–284, 1980.

144. Perez-Mateo M, Erill S: Protein binding of salicylates and quinidine in plasma from patients with renal failure, chronic liver disease and chronic respiratory insufficiency. *Eur J Clin Pharmacol* 11:225–231, 1977.

145. Perrier D, Mayersohn M, Marcus FI: Clinical pharmacokinetics of digitoxin. *Clin Pharmacokinet* 2:292–311, 1977.

146. Pessayre D, Lebrec D, Descatorie V, Peignoux M, Benhamou J-P: Mechanism for reduced drug clearance in patients with cirrhosis. *Gastroenterology* 74:566–571, 1978.

147. Piafsky KM, Sitar DS, Rangno Re, Oglivie RI: Theophylline disposition in patients with hepatic cirrhosis. *N Engl J Med* 296:1495–1497, 1977.

148. Pirttiaho HI, Sotaniemi EA, Ahlqvist J, Pitkanen U, Pelkonen RO: Liver size and indices of drug metabolism in alcoholics. *Eur J Clin Pharmacol* 13:61–67, 1978.

149. Pisani F, Perruca E, Primerano G, D'Agostino AA, Petrelli RM, Fazio A, Oteri G, Di Perri R: Single-dose kinetics of primidone in acute viral hepatitis. *Eur J Clin Pharmacol* 27:465–469, 1984.

150. Pond SM, Tong T, Benowitz NL, Jacob P: Enhanced bioavailability of pethidine and pentazocine in patients with cirrhosis of the liver. *Aust NZ J Med* 10:515–519, 1980.

151. Pond SM, Tong T, Benowitz NL, Jacob P, Rigod J: Presystemic metabolism of meperidine to normeperidine in normal and cirrhotic subjects. *Clin Pharmacol Ther* 30:183–188, 1981.

152. Powell LW, Axelsen E: Corticosteroids in liver disease: studies on the biological conversion of prednisone to prednisolone and plasma protein binding. *Gut* 13:690–696, 1972.

153. Pozzi E, Menghini P: Blood levels of rifampicin in liver diseases. *Int J Clin Pharmacol* 10:44–49, 1974.

154. Regardh, G-G, Jordo L, Ervik M, Lundborg P, Olsson R, Ronn O: Pharmacokinetics of metoprolol in patients with hepatic cirrhosis. *Clin Pharmacokinet* 6:375–388, 1981.

155. Reidenberg MM, Affrime M: Influence of disease on binding of drugs to plasma proteins. *Ann NY Acad Sci* 226:115–126, 1973.

156. Renton KW, Mannering GJ: Depression of hepatic cytochrome P-450–dependent monooxygenase systems with administered interferon inducing agents. *Biochem Biophys Res Commun* 73:343–348, 1976.

157. Renton KW, Mannering GJ: Depression of the hepatic cytochrome P-450 mono-oxygenase system by administered tilorone (2,7-bis (2-(diethylamino) ethoxy) fluoren-9-one dihydrochloride). *Drug Metab Dispos* 4:223–231, 1976.

158. Richter E, Breimer DD, Zilly W: Disposition of hexobarbital in intra- and extrahepatic cholestasis in man and the influence of drug metabolism–inducing agents. *Eur J Clin Pharmacol* 17:197–202, 1980.

159. Ring-Larsen H: Renal blood flow in cirrhosis: relation to systemic and portal haemodynamics and liver function. *Scand J Clin Lab Invest* 37:635–642, 1977.

160. Ring-Larsen H, Birger H, Henriksen JH, Christensen NJ: Sympathetic nervous activity and renal and systemic hemodynamics in cirrhosis: plasma norepinephrine concentration, hepatic extraction, and renal release. *Hepatology* 2:304–310, 1982.

161. Ring-Larsen H, Henriksen JH: Pathogenesis of ascites formation and hepatorenal syndrome: humoral and hemodynamic factors. *Semin Liver Dis* 6:341–352, 1986.

162. Roberts MS, Rumble RH, Wanwimolruk S, Thomas D, Brooks PM: Pharmacokinetics of aspirin and salicylate in elderly subjects and in patients with alcoholic liver disease. *Eur J Clin Pharmacol* 25:253–261, 1983.

163. Roberts RK, Wilkinson GR, Branch RA, Schenker S: Effect of age and parenchymal liver disease on the disposition and elimination of chlordiazepoxide (Librium). *Gastroenterology* 75:479–485, 1978.

164. Robinson JD, Whitney HAK Jr, Guisti DL, Morgan DD, Mendenhall CL: The absorption of intramuscular chlordiazepoxide (Librium) in patients with severe alcoholic liver disease. *Int J Clin Pharmacol Ther Toxicol* 21: 433–438, 1983.

165. Rowland M, Benet LZ, Graham GG: Clearance concepts in pharmacokinetics. *J Pharmacol Biopharm* 1:123–136, 1973.

166. Sadee W, Schroder R, V Leitner E, Dagcioglu M: Multiple dose kinetics of spironolactone and canrenoate-potassium in cardiac and hepatic failure. *Eur J Clin Pharmacol* 7:195–200, 1974.

167. Sawhney VK, Gregory PB, Swezey SE, Blaschke TF: Furosemide disposition in cirrhotic patients. *Gastroenterology* 81:1012–1016, 1981.

168. Schalm SW, Summerskill Wolt J, Go VLW: Prednisone for chronic active liver disease: pharmacokinetics, including conversion to prednisolone. *Gastroenterology* 72:910–913, 1977.

169. Schenker S, Breen KJ, Hoyumpa AM: Hepatic encephalopathy: current status. *Gastroenterology* 66:121–151, 1974.

170. Schentag JJ, Cerra FB, Calleri GM, Leising ME, French MA, Bernhard H: Age, disease, and cimetidine disposition in healthy subjects and chronically ill patients. *Clin Pharmacol Ther* 29:737–743, 1981.

171. Schoene B, Fleischmann RA, Remmer H: Determination of drug metabolizing enzymes in needle biopsies of human liver. *Eur J Clin Pharmacol* 4:65–73, 1972.

172. Sellers EM, Greenblatt DJ, Giles HG, Naranjo CA, Kaplan H, MacLeod SM: Chlordiazepoxide and oxazepam disposition in cirrhosis. *Clin Pharmacol Ther* 26:240–246, 1979.

173. Sessions JT, Minkel HP, Bullard JC, Ingelfinger FJ: The effect of barbiturates in patients with liver disease. *J Clin Invest* 33:1116–1127, 1954.

174. Shamszad M, Soloman H, Mobarhan S, Iber FL: Abnormal metabolism of acetaminophen in patients with alcohol liver disease. *Gastroenterology* 69:865, 1975.

175. Shear L, Kleinerman J, Gabuzda GJ: Renal failure in patients with cirrhosis of the liver. *Am J Med* 39:184–198, 1965.

176. Shoeman DW, Azarnoff DL: Diphenylhydantoin potency and plasma protein binding. *J Pharmacol Exp Ther* 195:84–86, 1975.

177. Shreeve WW, Shoop JD, Ott DG, McInteer BB: Test for alcoholic cirrhosis by conversion of ^{14}C- or ^{13}C-galactose to expired CO_2. *Gastroenterology* 71:98–101, 1976.

178. Shull HJ, Wilkinson GR, Johnson R and Schenker S: Normal disposition of oxazepam in acute viral hepatitis and cirrhosis. *Ann Intern Med* 84:420–425, 1976.

179. Siegers C-P, Oltmanns D, Younes M: Effect of alcohol and chronic liver disease on the metabolic disposal of paracetamol in man. *Hepatogastroenterology* 28:304, 1981.

180. Singh G, Renton KW: Homogeneous interferon from

E. coli depresses hepatic cytochrome P-450 and drug biotransformation. *Biochem Biophys Res Commun* 106:1256–1261, 1982.

181. Singh G, Renton KW: Interferon-mediated depression of cytochrome P-450–dependent drug biotransformation. *Mol Pharmacol* 20:681–684, 1981.

182. Sloan TP, Lancaster R, Shah RR, Idle JR, Smith RL: Genetically determined oxidation capacity and the disposition of debrisoquine. *Br J Clin Pharmacol* 15:443–450, 1983.

183. Smith IL, Ziemniak JA, Bernhard H, Eshelman FN, Martin LE, Schentag JJ: Ranitidine disposition and systemic availability in hepatic cirrhosis. *Clin Pharmacol Ther* 35:487–494, 1984.

184. Somogyi A, Albrecht M, Kliens G, Schafer K, Eichelbaum M: Pharmacokinetics, bioavailability and ECG response of verapamil in patients with liver disease. *Br J Clin Pharmacol* 12:51–60, 1981.

185. Sonne J, Poulsen HE, Dossing M, Larsen NE, Andreasen PB: Cimetidine clearance and bioavailability in hepatic cirrhosis. *Clin Pharmacol Ther* 29:191–197, 1981.

186. Sotaniemi EA, Luoma PV, Jarvensiva PM, Sotaniemi KA: Impairment of drug metabolism in polycystic nonparasitic liver disease. *Br J Clin Pharmacol* 8:331–335, 1979.

187. Sotaniemi EA, Niemälä O, Risteli L, Stenbäck F, Pelkonen RO, Lahtela JT, Risteli J: Fibrotic process and drug metabolism in alcoholic liver disease. *Clin Pharmacol Ther* 40:46–55, 1986.

188. Sotaniemi EA, Pelkonen RO, Puukka M: Measurement of hepatic drug-metabolizing enzyme activity in man. *Eur J Clin Pharmacol* 17:267–274, 1980.

189. Staib AH, Schuppan D, Lissner R, Zilly W, Bomhard GV, Richter E: Pharmacokinetics and metabolism of theophylline in patients with liver diseases. *Int J Clin Pharmacol Ther Toxicol* 18:500–502, 1980.

190. Stoeckel K, Koup JR: Pharmacokinetics of ceftriaxone in patients with renal and liver insufficiency and correlations with a physiologic nonlinear protein. *Am J Med* 19:26–32, 1984.

191. Stoeckel K, Tuerk H, Trueb V, McNamara PJ: Single-dose ceftriaxone kinetics in liver insufficiency. *Clin Pharmacol Ther* 36:500–509, 1984.

192. Syrota A, Paraf A, Gaudebout C, Desgrez A: Significance of intra- and extrahepatic portasystemic shunting in survival of cirrhotic patients. *Dig Dis Sci* 26:878–885, 1981.

193. Syrota A, Vinot J-M, Paraf A, Roucayrol JC: Scintillation splenoportography: hemodynamic and morphological study of the portal circulation. *Gastroenterology* 71:652–659, 1976.

194. Teunissen MWE, Spoelstra P, Koch CW, Weeds B, Van Duyn W, Janssens AR, Breimer DD: Antipyrine clearance and metabolite formation in patients with alcoholic cirrhosis. *Br J Clin Pharmacol* 18:707–715, 1984.

195. Thiessen JJ, Sellers EM, Denbeigh P, Dolman L: Plasma protein binding of diazepam and tolbutamide in chronic alcoholics. *J Clin Pharmacol* 16:345–351, 1976.

196. Thomson PD, Melmon KL, Richardson JA, Cohn K, Steinbrunn W, Cudihee R, Rowland M: Lidocaine pharmacokinetics in advanced heart failure, liver disease, and renal failure in humans. *Ann Intern Med* 78:499–508, 1973.

197. Thomson PD, Rowland M, Melmon KL: The influence of heart failure, liver disease, and renal failure on the disposition of lidocaine in man. *Am Heart J* 82:417–421, 1971.

198. Tschang C, Steiner JA, Hignite CE, Huffman DH, Azarnoff DL: Systemic availability of lidocaine in patients with liver disease (abstract). *Clin Res* 25:609A, 1977.

199. Uribe M, Summerskill WHJ, Go VLW: Comparative serum prednisone and prednisolone concentrations following administration to patients with chronic active liver disease. *Clin Pharmacokinet* 7:452–459, 1982.

200. Verbeeck RK, Patwardhan RV, Villeneuve J-P, Wilkinson GR, Branch RA: Furosemide disposition in cirrhosis. *Clin Pharmacol Ther* 31:719–725, 1982.

201. Villeneuve J-P, Fortunet-Fouin H, Arsene D: Cimetidine kinetics and dynamics in patients with severe liver disease. *Hepatology* 3:923–927, 1983.

202. Villeneuve J-P, Rocheleau F, Raymond G: Triamterene kinetics and dynamics in cirrhosis. *Clin Pharmacol Ther* 35:831–837, 1984.

203. Villeneuve J-P, Verbeeck RK, Wilkinson GR, Branch RA: Furosemide kinetics and dynamics in patients with cirrhosis. *Clin Pharmacol Ther* 40:14–20, 1986.

204. Wagner VT, Heydrich D, Bartels H, Hohorst HJ: The influence of damaged liver parenchyma, renal insufficiency and hemodialysis on the pharmacokinetics of cyclophosphamide and its activated metabolites. *Arzneimittelforschung* 30:1588–1592, 1980.

205. Wallace S, Brodie MJ: Decreased drug binding in serum from patients with chronic hepatic disease. *Eur J Clin Pharmacol* 9:429–432, 1976.

206. Ward S, Weatherley BC: Pharmacokinetics of atracurium and its metabolites. *Br J Anaesth* 58:6S–10S, 1986.

207. Weiner M, Chenkin T, Burns JJ: Observations on the metabolic transformation and effects of phenylbutazone in subjects with hepatic disease. *Am J Med Sci* 228:36–39, 1954.

208. Wilkinson GR: The effects of liver disease and aging on the disposition of diazepam, chlordiazepoxide, oxazepam and lorazepam in man. *Acta Psychiatr Scand* 274:561–573, 1978.

209. Wilkinson GR, Shand DG: A physiological approach to hepatic drug clearance. *Clin Pharmacol Ther* 18:377–390, 1975.

210. Williams RL, Blaschke TF, Meffin PJ, Melman KL, Rowland M: Influence of viral hepatitis on the disposition of two compounds with high clearance: lidocaine and indocyanine green. *Clin Pharmacol Ther* 20:290–299, 1976.

211. Williams RL, Blaschke TF, Meffin PJ, Melmon KL, Rowland M: Influence of acute viral hepatitis on disposition and plasma binding of tolbutamide. *Clin Pharmacol Ther* 21:301–309, 1977.

212. Williams RL, Schary WL, Blaschke TF, Meffin PJ, Melmon KL, Rowland M: Influence of acute viral hepatitis on disposition and pharmacological effect of warfarin. *Clin Pharmacol Ther* 20:90–97, 1976.

213. Williams RL, Upton RA, Cello JP, Jones RM, Blitstein M, Kelly J, Nierenburg D: Naproxen disposition in patients with alcoholic cirrhosis. *Eur J Clin Pharmacol* 27:291–296, 1984.

214. Wood AJJ, Kornhauser DM, Wilkinson GR, Shand DG, Branch RA: The influence of cirrhosis on steady-state blood concentrations of unbound propranolol after oral administration. *Clin Pharmacokinet* 3:478–487, 1978.

215. Woodcock BG, Rietbrock I, Vohringer HF, Rietbrock N: Verapamil disposition in liver disease and intensive care patients: kinetics, clearance and apparent blood flow relationships. *Clin Pharmacol Ther* 29:27–34, 1981.

216. Young CJ, Daneshmend TK, Roberts CJC: Effects of cirrhosis and aging on the elimination and bioavailability of ranitidine. *Gut* 23:819–823, 1982.

217. Ziemniak JA, Bernhard H, Schentag JJ: Hepatic encephalopathy and altered cimetidine kinetics. *Clin Pharmacol Ther* 34:375–382, 1983.

218. Zilly W, Breimer DD, Richter E: Hexobarbital disposition in compensated and decompensated cirrhosis of the liver. *Clin Pharmacol Ther* 23:525–533, 1978.

219. Zilly W, Richter E, Rietbrock E: Pharmacokinetics and metabolism of digoxin- and β-methyl-digoxin-12α-^{3}H in patients with acute viral hepatitis. *Clin Pharmacol Ther* 17:302–309, 1975.

6

Adjustment of Medications in Pulmonary Failure

Charles B. Watson, M.D.

The lung plays an active role in the pharmacokinetics of endogenous compounds and certain drugs. Several new lines of research suggest that the lung's role as a metabolic organ or a determinant of the body's drug response may be important in certain disease states. Information concerning the impact of pulmonary disease on drug requirements in humans continues to be accumulated, although there is no coherent schema for understanding the hypothesized mechanisms for alteration in both the kinetic and dynamic interactions between patients and their drug therapy. The vast majority of this information is derived from animal models of lung injury and studies of drug action in subpopulations of patients with specific lung disease.

Extrapolation of data from clinical case reports and series suggests that the patient with pulmonary failure may have unique problems with drug therapy. The critically ill patient with acute or chronic lung disease is also known to be at increased risk for adverse drug interactions that may increase morbidity and limit the success of therapy. Drug therapy of the pulmonary patient, in particular, should be instituted with a specific endpoint in mind and tracked by frequent monitoring of drug levels, clinical response, and early indications of toxicity.

THE PROBLEM

The lung was first recognized as a metabolic organ in 1953 when Gaddum and associates (41) described the removal of 5-hydroxytryptamine from the pulmonary circulation. Since that time the lung clearance and metabolism of a number of endogenous compounds (norepinephrine, angiotensin, bradykinin, prostaglandins E_2 and $F_{2\alpha}$, steroids, and cyclic nucleotides) have been described, together with some of the metabolic pathways for their biodegradation (15). The active participation of the lung in the uptake, storage, and distribution of exogenous drugs has also been demonstrated in animals and humans. In animals, the basic amines (methadone, chlorphentermine, amphetamine, etc.) are avidly taken up, and a number of other drug classes (adrenergics, antihistaminics, antipsychotics, tricyclic antidepressants, local anesthetics, barbiturates, and antidysrhythmics, etc.) are taken up by the lung to a significant extent (9). Drug interactions affecting lung uptake have also been described in animals. Such a drug interaction has been demonstrated with the local anesthetics lidocaine and mepivacaine in humans (63), but on the whole, very little information is available for humans (15). Both endogenous substances and drugs are metabolized in the lung by mixed function oxidases; however, given the relatively greater quantities of these enzymes in the liver, it is likely that the lung is not normally a major contributor to drug metabolism (15). An exception is presented by some of the adrenergic bronchodilators given by the inhalational route (64). Unfortunately, the clinical significance of the lung's interaction with drug therapy and hormonal homeostasis is uncertain because of the scarcity of human data, although the implications are tantalizing. Areas of ongoing interest to both the acute and chronic care physician include angiotensin-converting enzyme and prostaglandin activity in health and disease.

The diseased lung may have an important impact on drug requirements in the critically ill patient by two mechanisms: first, a direct alteration in the lung uptake, distribution, and metabolism or clearance of pharmacologic agents; second, an indirect alteration of these parameters of pharmacokinetics or drug-receptor response. Various animal models of lung disease categories and speculation surrounding clinical reports suggest that hypoxemia, acidosis, loss of lung vascular surface or reserve, and pulmonary artery or venous hypertension may have far-reaching effects on the determinants of drug kinetics and dynamics in humans (15). In general, pulmonary diseases that affect the endothelial cell or reduce lung perfusion are more likely to have a direct effect on lung uptake and clearance, whereas diseases that present an increased circulatory load and demand, with altered oxygenation and acid-base status, are more likely to cause secondary alterations in pharmacokinetics or dynamics by remote actions. The variable extent to which specific pulmonary disease entities have been shown to affect drug action in differing models may be due to the poorly controlled presence or absence of associated hypoxemia and right heart failure (15). To date, the drugs that have received the most attention and are most important in the clinical setting are those that, like the theophylline compounds, digitalis glycosides, and adrenergic blocking compounds, have an essential role in the management of patients with cardiopulmonary disease and are known to have a poor margin of safety in clinical use.

The problem of drug interaction in critically ill patients is reviewed in Chapter 2; however, the patient with pulmonary disease is at increased risk for adverse drug reactions. According to the Boston Collaborative Drug Surveillance Program, there is an overall 2% incidence of drug toxicity with a 2-fold greater incidence in medical patients than in surgical patients (21). Of the complications reported, the majority are associated with antibiotics, chlorothiazide diuretics, digoxin (88) and aminophylline. Steel and associates (117) reported a 36% incidence of iatrogenic illness on a general medical service in a teaching hospital. Drugs are associated with 17% of the major complications, and theophylline compounds account for a third of these. The probability of drug-related complications of therapy is 5% when five or fewer drugs are prescribed, but 40% when 15 or more drugs are prescribed. Aspirin, digoxin, antibiotics, anticoagulants, steroids, and diuretics are most frequently associated with iatrogenic complications. Intravenous administration of aminophylline is the major cause of drug-related cardiopulmonary arrest in critically ill patients according to Camarata and coworkers (14). They estimate that the chance of cardiac arrest following an appropriate loading dose of aminophylline is 60 times greater than following other high-risk drugs (e.g., intravenous digoxin or penicillin).

Drug therapy for an acute exacerbation of bronchospasm in a patient with obstructive pulmonary disease may include a combination of a selective β_2-adrenergic drug, intravenous aminophylline, a broad spectrum antibiotic, a corticosteroid preparation, and a digoxin-diuretic-oxygen regimen designed to treat cor pulmonale. The addition of a cardiac glycoside to one or several diuretics and antianginal or antihypertensive therapy is not uncommon. The pediatric patient is not excluded from the population at risk—a significant number of infants with bronchopulmonary dysplasia and children with asthma or cystic fibrosis may require similar pharmacologic support (85). Children and adults with acute respiratory failure frequently require a similar pharmacologic regimen in addition to chest physiotherapy, oxygen therapy, and mechanical ventilation. Thus, the combination of multiple medications in pulmonary patients may challenge the clinician's ability to anticipate and avoid drug-related complications.

The patient with overt or impending pulmonary failure rarely has an isolated disease. When a patient with compensated or recurrent pulmonary illness presents with acute decompensation, the clinician should look for associated infection or other systemic causes. The previously well patient who presents with impending or acute respiratory failure generally has either an overwhelming pulmonary infection or a severe systemic illness presenting with pulmonary manifestations. Acute respiratory failure superimposed on intercurrent illness, whether medical or surgical, increases the risk of multiple organ system failure with an increased risk of morbidity and mortality (6, 23).

What makes the critically ill pulmonary patient different from other patients with chronic or acute pulmonary disease is defined by the clinical setting. Critically ill patients require more pharmacologic support and present with rapidly evolving pathology, an uncertain clinical background, a poorly documented laboratory data base, unstable hemodynamics, and a high incidence of associated organ system dysfunction. When such a patient's disease process worsens, it is difficult to determine whether this change is due to drug therapy failure, further pulmonary decompensation (87) or an adverse drug reaction.

In the light of these conditions, it is essential

to understand the determinants of drug uptake, distribution, and excretion in patients with pulmonary disease. Factors that may change drug receptor affinity, density, or responsiveness are important but difficult to quantify. Since the assessment of pharmacokinetic and pharmacodynamic factors is difficult in the acute setting, a knowledge of well-identified management problems will prevent drug misadventures and predict problems with newer drugs as they are introduced. Therefore, putative mechanisms for alteration of pharmacokinetics and pharmacodynamics, and recommendations for the adjustment of medications in the patient with pulmonary disease are reviewed in this chapter.

MECHANISMS OF ALTERED KINETICS IN THE PULMONARY PATIENT

In this section, the effects of pulmonary disease on drug uptake, distribution, metabolism, and excretion, and on drug receptor interaction are examined. Pulmonary disease may alter these determinants by direct or secondary (indirect) means. Most of the time it is the secondary effects of pulmonary failure that alter these parameters.

Administration

Pulmonary disease per se has little impact on traditional routes of drug administration other than the inhalational route. Diseases that disturb the relationship between ventilation and perfusion may have profound effects on pulmonary gas exchange, oxygen therapy requirement, and the uptake of drugs administered as medical gases or vapors. In general, lung disease that presents with large pulmonary-systemic shunt has the greatest effect in slowing uptake, and the effect is greatest for less soluble vapors and gases (119, 140). Equilibrium pressures are not altered, however, so the potency of volatile anesthetics is not altered (33).

Aerosolized drugs are well absorbed by the tracheal and broncheal mucosa, provided that they are water-soluble and the airway is patient (22). Although most of any aerosolized drug dose is deposited in the oropharynx and swallowed, it is an effective means of drug administration in both the intubated and non-

intubated patient and is unlikely to be disturbed by mucosal injuries even so severe as those caused by upper airway burns (10, 52, 131). The inhalational route is used for administration of bronchodilators, corticosteroids, cromolyn sodium, and other drugs. It offers the advantage of direct application of drug to the receptor organ, bypassing other systemic routes and probably reducing systemic toxicity. The efficacy of inhaled anticholinergics and antibiotics is more controversial, but this route has been chosen for critically ill patients (53).

Uptake

Pulmonary disease affects the determinants of drug absorption from other sites by indirect mechanisms. Subcutaneous, transdermal, intramuscular, sublingual, oral, and rectal absorption are all dependent on tissue blood flow, tissue binding, and solubility. Tissue hypoxia and acid-base derangements have marked effects on the distribution of organ blood flow and the absorption of weakly ionized acids and bases. A 0.3 unit decrement in pH may cause a doubling of ionized base in tissue compartments and markedly decrease transport into capillaries. If pH changes protein binding, the quantity of drug available for diffusion out of the capillary and into the tissue may be markedly altered.

The stress imposed by increasing cardiopulmonary work requirements during respiratory decompensation redistributes blood flow away from splanchnic beds and reduces uptake from the gastrointestinal tract (55). As a patient with impending respiratory failure becomes unable to perform respiratory or cardiac work, derangements in tissue blood flow may render all routes of drug administration ineffective other than the intravenous or inhalational routes. Marked decreases in tissue perfusion during stress or shock may isolate the drug administration to any tissue compartment. This can delay drug absorption and cause an apparent "rebound" or resurgence of drug effect when tissue perfusion is restored.

Distribution

Drug distribution is determined by the distribution of blood flow, extent of protein binding, drug ionization, lipid solubility, and kinetics of drug binding to and release from receptor sites. Changes in the volume of distribution alter drug concentration at any given dose and, consequently, affect drug receptor site kinetics unless the drug has an extremely high affinity for the receptor and blood flow to receptor tissue is consistently high. In general, the required loading dose of a drug is a direct function of the volume of distribution, whereas maintenance requirements are determined by receptor affinity, redistribution, metabolism, and clearance.

Pulmonary disease has little direct effect on the volume of distribution. Age, nutritional status, blood volume, and circulatory status are better known factors. Theophylline compounds, probably the best studied model, are 50–60% protein-bound with a volume of distribution of 0.5 liters/kg in the adult (149). Loading dose recommendations per unit mass are the same for adults and children, even in conditions that change the volume of distribution more than does active pulmonary disease (96, 103).

Although pulmonary disease can alter the distribution of blood flow to the lung and respiratory muscles, the most important changes affect drug clearance rather than the volume of distribution.

Clearance

The clearance of theophylline compounds, antibiotics, steroids, β_2-adrenergic agents, digoxin, sedatives, muscle relaxants, and propranolol are affected by acute and chronic pulmonary disease (126, 129, 130), protein binding (88), drug interaction (95, 112, 130), congestive heart failure (97), and the cardiovascular changes associated with controlled mechanical ventilation (7, 76, 107, 147, 148).

Until recently, there was no direct evidence that acute pulmonary disease has any effect on drug clearance. Vozeh and associates (129) reported 2- to 3-fold alterations in theophylline clearance during acute pulmonary decompensation in the absence of heart failure or changes in hepatic function. Subclinical changes in the distribution of the cardiac output associated with hypoxemia or mechanical ventilation were not ruled out in this study, and many investigators cite these factors as probable reasons for the wide variability in steady state aminophylline or antibiotic dose requirements (17, 61, 65, 108).

Individual Variation

Age, malnutrition, and associated hepatic or renal function changes are the most commonly cited reasons for wide variations in theophylline drug kinetics in acutely ill patients and patients with decompensated pulmonary disease (101).

Age-dependent clearance affects most drugs with renal or hepatic clearance. Age and sex variables change rifampin requirements (60). Pharmacokinetic analysis of methicillin clearance in patients with cystic fibrosis shows that the volume of distribution, metabolism, and creatinine clearance are no different from controls; yet renal clearance is more rapid—possibly due to an intrinsic alteration in tubular transport (150). The pharmacogenetics of isoniazid and succinylcholine are well described, and clinical response to the former is thought to relate to this, whereas the clinical response to the latter drug is undoubtedly inherited. Since children clear theophylline compounds more rapidly than do adults (34), it is recommended that a higher steady state dose will be effective and safe (96). More recent data suggest that the kinetics of theophylline compounds can convert from first order to dose-dependent in both children and adults (136). The phenomenon of dose dependency with theophylline is less commonly observed in adult patients who smoke, and although not as common as first supposed, is likely due to the saturation of hepatic enzyme systems (77, 149). This conversion occurs at higher drug levels, as is the case for barbiturates (149). A number of pharmacokinetic variables change during pregnancy, and although the hepatic clearance of theophylline is reduced during the second and third trimester, an increased volume of distribution with decreased protein binding and increased renal clearance tend to compensate for this reduction so that overall unbound clearance does not change significantly (40).

A specific breakdown of the determinants of drug clearance and metabolism is beyond the scope of this chapter. From the preceding discussion it should be clear that a multiplicity of subject-specific and drug-specific variables may markedly alter drug clearance. It is the secondary effects of pulmonary disease that most affect drug clearance; however, interindividual variability may be pronounced and the role of drug level monitoring in clarifying these variations has become increasingly important. Serum drug levels can be obtained for most antiarrhythmic and anticonvulsant drugs. The use of serum concentrations as a guide to therapy is well recognized for antimicrobials such as gentamicin and tobramycin and for the theophylline compounds. Drug levels are only helpful when there is a clear-cut relationship between the serum concentration and the therapeutic efficacy or toxicity. They are essential for monitoring the above drugs because of the narrow therapeutic index of these drugs and the unreliability of clinical signs for prediction of either therapeutic effect or toxicity (17, 128, 151).

PHARMACODYNAMIC FACTORS

Early reports of tachyphylaxis to inhaled bronchodilators and the clinical discovery that, in this setting, multiple drug therapy is more effective and less toxic than single drug therapy alone, focused attention on the second messenger hypothesis and the intracellular modification of adrenergic responsiveness (16, 59, 72, 73, 121). This example of the therapeutic interaction of drugs that alter pharmacodynamic variables is a striking paradigm of drug action for the clinician. It is a key concept in the therapy of bronchospastic disorders as well as a model for other endocrine pharmacotherapy, including the management of the failing heart.

The roles of steroid hormones and phosphodiesterase inhibitors in the "up" or "down" regulation of the β-adrenergic receptor and in the coupling of receptor activation to biological response remain to be clarified. Whether β-receptor blockade, competitive antagonism, down-regulation, antibody formation, or other subcellular interactions play the primary role in modifying any individual subject's response, it is evident that pharmacologic intervention in the treatment of bronchospasm must be directed at multiple levels—especially in the critically ill patient (62). At present, there are no better defined guidelines for therapy than clinical response.

It is not known whether pulmonary disease *per se* changes receptor function in other organs, in addition to general changes associated with chronic hypercapnia, acidosis, and hypoxia. Recent work suggests that chronic administration of β-adrenergic drugs that are less selective may modulate receptor density in several tissues (44), as do endogenous catecholamines (39).

DRUG INTERACTIONS IN THE PULMONARY PATIENT

Pharmacokinetic Interactions

Drugs interact to increase the likelihood of toxicity or failed therapy in several ways. Nausea, a well-recognized prodrome of theophylline or digoxin toxicity, may limit the uptake of other orally administered drugs. Gastrointestinal disturbance following cancer chemotherapy commonly interferes with the dosing of other orally administered drugs.

A common problem with concomitant drug therapy is alteration of the pharmacokinetics of one drug by another. In the preceding examples, the absorption and uptake of one drug may be limited by the toxicity or accepted side effects of another. The acute care setting (emergency room or intensive care unit) presents us with a high risk of drug incompatibility when drugs are administered intravenously in order to eliminate variables that limit the uptake and absorption of drugs administered by other routes. We commonly see antibiotics, calcium, hydrocortisone, isoproterenol, narcotics, and sodium bicarbonate infusions mixed in this setting, although the potential drug incompatibilities with these agents are well documented.

Displacement of one protein-bound drug by another can increase the quantity of the drug at effector sites, or alter the rate of metabolism and excretion. This fact is most important with highly bound drugs such as propranolol, phenytoin, or diazepam but may play a role by altering an individual's drug clearance or raising the likelihood of drug toxicity at dose levels that previously established effective and safe steady state concentrations. The side effects of prednisone and diazepam are increased in hypoproteinemic patients. Carrier protein displacement may also be of concern with antibiotic interactions (149).

Drug interaction caused by enzyme induction or inhibition of metabolism may reduce therapeutic drug levels or increase toxicity. Many postoperative and critically ill patients who require ventilatory support receive a combination of cimetidine and antacids to decrease the incidence of stress-induced gastritis and gastrointestinal bleeding. Cimetidine impairs the elimination and metabolism of diazepam and propranolol (149); it binds to cytochromes P-448 and P-450, thus nonspecifically impairing drug metabolism (24). Theophylline clearance is impaired by cimetidine and not by ranitidine, an H_2-antagonist that has less affinity for the cytochromes (24). Cimetidine evidently does not alter the clearance of methylprednisolone (48). It reduces hepatic blood flow and thus impairs the clearance of intravenous drugs that have high hepatic extraction, such as propranolol and lidocaine.

Erythromycin reduces the clearance of theophylline by an average of 25%. Whether this effect is mediated by a change in hepatic clearance or by converting the first order theophylline kinetics to dose-dependent kinetics through enzymatic inhibition is not known (69).

The quinidine-digoxin interaction presents a model of drug interference at several levels. Quinidine displaces bound digoxin from myocardial and peripheral compartments and thus reduces the volume of distribution of digoxin. Renal clearance of digoxin is also reduced in the absence of a measurable change in the glomerular filtration rate (149).

These examples of pharmacokinetic interaction are by no means exhaustive, but they illustrate possible ways in which combined drug therapy may alter clinical response to drugs. Since the acutely ill patient often receives several new drugs simultaneously, it is difficult to predict or identify specific loci of drug interaction. Frequent assessment of serum drug levels may be the only way to anticipate possible toxicity.

Pharmacodynamic Interactions

The pharmacodynamic interactions of drugs are more difficult to monitor. Several examples will be discussed in more detail elsewhere. The most common interaction involves two drugs with common sites of action. Tachyarrhythmias in the bronchospastic patient who is receiving combined therapy with β-adrenergic agonists and aminophylline may be due to additive effects on the cardiac β-system.

A drug that has a different site of action may cause an intrinsic change in the receptor site or effector mechanism of a second drug and narrow its therapeutic margin of safety. For example, diuretic therapy may potentiate digitalis toxicity and digitalis toxic arrhythmias. These are well-known clinical problems. Less predictable is the alteration in central respiratory drive when lidocaine antiarrhythmic therapy is added to sedation with diazepam in an anxious patient with compensated chronic

obstructive pulmonary disease. Prolonged weakness may occur in an elderly postoperative patient with diuretic-induced hypokalemia who receives polymyxin or aminoglycoside antibiotics. Such are often identified as idiosyncratic drug reactions.

In these situations, the pharmacodynamic factors are less well understood. Close monitoring of clinical parameters indicative of therapeutic response or prodromal toxicity is required even when therapeutic drug levels are known to be safe or optimal.

ADJUSTMENT OF MEDICATIONS IN THE CRITICAL CARE PULMONARY PATIENT (TABLE 6.1)

β-Adrenergic Drugs

A "selective" generation of β-adrenergic drugs (Table 6.2) has been derived from molecular modification of isoproterenol. Those that are catecholamines are metabolized by catechol O-methyltransferase (COMT) and monoamine oxidase and their onset and duration of action is more limited than the longer acting, non-catecholamine compounds (22, 149). For the same reason, the longer acting agents can be administered orally during chronic therapy, and it is doubtful that aerosol therapy with these drugs is more advantageous than oral or subcutaneous therapy (98). The only advantage of inhalational administration is more rapid onset and peak action.

All of the newer agents are labeled "selective" β_2-agonists, but all are nonspecific in the sense that β_1 stimulation occurs with higher doses (121). Tachyarrhythmias, ectopy, angina, tremor, and other peripheral manifestations of β-receptor stimulation become more common as the dose increases, although at equivalent doses the relative incidence of these problems is less common than with isoproterenol (106). The most important toxicity is cardiovascular. Consequently, heart rate, rhythm, and blood pressure are essential monitors of toxicity whenever dose requirements change (as in the acute setting) and drug levels must be increased acutely.

Metaproterenol and terbutaline are longer acting drugs because they are not catecholamines and are not metabolized by COMT. The catecholamines albuterol and isoetharine are shorter acting and, like isoproterenol and epinephrine, are rapidly inactivated when ab-

Table 6.1
Overview of Common Drug Adjustment Problems in the Acutely Ill Pulmonary Patient

Drug Therapy	Problem[a]
Congestive heart failure (CHF)	
Inotropes and vasodilators	Blunt HPV
Relaxants	↓ Clearance
Antiarrhythmics	↓ Respiratory drive, weakness
Aminophylline	↓ Clearance
Chronic obstructive pulmonary disease (COPD)	
β-Adrenergic drugs	Tachyphylaxis, ↓ HPV, cardiotoxicity
β-Blockers	Bronchospasm, pulmonary edema
Dopamine	Blunt hypoxic respiratory drive, ↓ HPV
Theophylline compounds	CNS cardiotoxicity, ↓ HPV, ↓ clearance
Corticosteroids	Infection, gastritis, increased aminophylline levels, mineralocorticoid effects, adrenal suppression
Respiratory stimulants	Neurotoxicity
Nutrition	↑ CO_2 production, hypermetabolism, changes CO_2 response curve
Anticholinergics	Thick secretions, central effects
Muscle relaxants	Respiratory muscle wasting, ↓ hemodynamics
Oxygen	↓ HPV, absorption atelectasis, blunt respiratory drive
Sedatives and narcotics	Respiratory failure, ↓ respiratory drive, ↓ reflexes
Diuretics	Hypovolemia, alkalosis, hypokalemia
Neoplastic disease	
Chemotherapy	↑ Catabolism, malnutrition, oxygen toxicity; GI, hepatic, renal dysfunction
Nutrition	↑ Respiratory quotient, ↑ CO_2 production
Corticosteroids	Mineralocorticoid effects, adrenal suppression, gastritis, ↓ immune function, myasthenic syndrome
Muscle relaxants	Abnormal clearance and metabolism
Oxygen	↑ Toxicity
Adult Respiratory Distress Syndrome (ARDS)	
Corticosteroids	Fluid retention, alkalosis, gastritis, immune suppression
Inotropic agents	↑ QS/QT, ↓ HPV, ↑ O_2 consumption
Vasodilators	↓ HPV
Diuretics	Hypovolemia, alkalosis, hypokalemia
Oxygen	Pulmonary toxicity, absorption atelectasis, ↑ QS/QT
Muscle relaxants	Hypotension, tachycardia, bronchospasm, ↓ clearance
Asthma	
Adrenergic drugs	Cardiotoxicity, ↓ HPV, tachyphylaxis
Aminophylline	Variable clearance, CNS and cardiotoxicity, nausea
Corticosteroids	↑ Theophylline levels, mineralocorticoid effect, adrenal suppression, infection risk, GI bleeding
Erythromycin	↓ Aminophylline clearance
Sedatives and narcotics	Respiratory failure
Muscle relaxants	Variable clearance, hypotension, bronchospasm, tachycardia
Infant respiratory distress syndrome (IRDS)	
β-Adrenergic drugs	↓ Response
Aminophylline	Uncertain clearance
Corticosteroids	Growth retardation, adrenal suppression
Oxygen	Retinal and pulmonary toxicity
Bicarbonate	Hyperosmolar cerebral edema, hemorrhage
Antibiotics	Variable clearance, specific toxicities
Diuretics	Hypovolemia, alkalosis
Cystic fibrosis	
Oxygen	Blunted respiratory drive
Corticosteroids	Growth retardation, adrenal suppression, H_2O retention, mineralocorticoid effects, adrenal suppression and infection

Drug Therapy	Problem[a]
cystic fibrosis (*continued*)	
Nutrition	Malabsorbtion, change $\dot{V}_{CO_2}$ and respiratory drive
Bronchodilators and aminophylline	Only 40% response, ↓ HPV, variable kinetics
Mucolytics	Bronchospasm
Diuretics	Alkalosis, dehydration
Methacillin	Increased clearance
Bronchopulmonary dysplasia	
Oxygen	Lower toxicity threshold
Aminophylline	Clearance, ↓ toxicity threshold
β-Adrenergic agents	↓ Responsiveness < 6 months
Digitalis	Variable clearance ↓
Diuretics	Alkalosis, volume depletion
Pulmonary embolism	
Heparin	Bleeding, ↑ requirement, ↓ clearance
Streptokinase	Monitoring therapy difficult, hemorrhage

[a] HPV, hypoxic pulmonary vasoconstriction; CNS, central nervous system; GI, gastrointestinal.

sorbed from the gastrointestinal tract. The terminal isopropylamine substitution of isoproterenol and alprenolol ensures that they will be taken up by COMT-rich tissues and metabolized (86).

Most of the newer agents have been studied extensively in the outpatient setting. Isoproterenol has been investigated as a primary therapy for refractory asthma in the pediatric intensive care setting, with good results when given by intravenous titration (30). Terbutaline has also been given intravenously, although one comparative study suggests that it loses its selective β_2-agonist predominance when so administered (123). Most clinicians rely on inhalational therapy with these drugs because this route has been most extensively studied. Unfortunately, effective therapy is limited in children because of low inspiratory capacity and flow rates, especially during acute bronchospasm (29, 133).

Opponents of the aerosol therapy approach have pointed out that aerosols may actually trigger bronchospasm (67, 132). Mucous plugging may block aerosol delivery, and the uptake of the aerosolized agents is less predictable (134). In the acute setting, titration to effect is most likely to succeed with minimal toxicity when a short-acting drug is administered intravenously and the cardiovascular system is closely monitored. The common clinical regimen of a long-acting drug with intermittent inhalational boluses of a short-acting, pressurized aerosol is potentially more risky from the pharmacokinetic point of view because variations in blood levels and a changing threshold of toxicity may interact disadvantageously.

Table 6.2
Mixed Adrenergic Agonists

Drug	Route	Starting Dose	Onset	Peak	Duration
Epinephrine	i.v. drip	0.1 μg/kg/min	1–2 min	5–15 min	Evanescent
	i.v. bolus	5–10 μg/kg	Immediate	1–2 min	5–15 min
	Sub-Q	0.2–0.5 mg	5–15 min	15 min	15–30 min
Racemic epinephrine	Inhaled	4–15 mg	5–10 min	½–1 hr	2–4 hr
Isoproterenol	i.v.	0.1% solution 0.1 μg/kg/min	1–2 min	5–15 min	Short
Isoproterenol	Inhaled	0.1–0.3 mg	2–5 min	5–30 min	1–3 hr
Terbutaline	i.v.	0.1%; 0.1 μg/kg/min	1–2 min	5–15 min	Unknown
	Sub-Q	0.25–0.5 mg	5–15 min	½–1 hr	3–4 hr
	Oral	2.5–5 mg	30 min	2–3 hr	4–8 hr
Metaproterenol	Inhaled	1–2 mg	2–10 min	1 hr	1–4 hr
	Oral	10–20 mg	½ hr	2–3 hr	1–5 hr
Albuterol	Inhaled	0.1–0.4 mg	5–10 min	½–1 hr	3–6 hr
	Oral	2–4 mg	½ hr	1–2 hr	3–4 hr

Titration of intravenous isoproterenol has been quite successful in the pediatric age group. Refractory *status asthmaticus* has led to continuous mechanical ventilation in only 8% of children treated this way (28–30). Relative contraindications to high-dose therapy with adrenergic compounds have limited the intravenous approach in adults, although intravenous salbutamol and isoproterenol have both been used for treatment of asthma in adults (125). Coronary artery disease, arrhythmias, cardiac asthma, hyperthyroidism, hypertension, diabetes, and a history of β-adrenergic refractory asthma should suggest the need for a cautious approach to such therapy (26, 57). Appropriate monitoring should permit the use of these valuable agents in high-risk patients, and the extent to which one can "push" β-adrenergic drug administration is a matter for clinical judgment (62).

Oxygen therapy is usually indicated because most of the sympathomimetic agents may cause hypoxemia by blocking hypoxic pulmonary vasoconstrictor responses and increasing the pulmonary shunt fraction (49, 59, 105).

Pharmacodynamic considerations argue strongly for the use of combined drug therapy using several modalities in the critically ill patient with bronchospasm. β-Receptor responsiveness is apparently nonexistent below the age of 6 months and is variable up to 20 months of age (29). The increased likelihood of β-receptor unresponsiveness and "cholinergic rebound" suggests that a polypharmacy approach is efficacious, and this approach has become routine in the treatment of very severe bronchospasm or in status asthmaticus (Chapter 23) (18, 29, 84, 100, 127).

Aminophylline is the water-soluble, ethylenediamine salt of theophylline (1,3-methylxanthine). It is more reliably absorbed after oral and rectal dosing than other methylxanthines and is approximately 80% theophylline by weight. Theophylline was introduced at the beginning of this century for the treatment of heart failure and has become a front-line drug for the treatment of acute and chronic bronchospastic diseases since that time (29, 31, 118, 134). Intravenous aminophylline is the primary drug for the treatment of status asthmaticus in children and remains the most effective preparation for acute therapy of the critically ill bronchospastic patient (29, 86, 96). The clinical response in chronic inflammatory disease is less dramatic but can be predicted based on measured pulmonary variables (142).

Aminophylline and other methylxanthines have a synergistic action with the β-adrenergic drugs (1). Methylxanthines are phosphodiesterase inhibitors—increasing the intracellular concentration of the second messenger cyclic adenosine 3',5'-monophosphate (cAMP). The drugs act on multiple target tissues including the brain, kidney, heart, muscle, and endocrine systems, in addition to the smooth muscle of the airways and pulmonary vasculature. Several additional mechanisms including modulation of presynaptic catecholamine release and manipulation of intracellular calcium transport have been postulated.

Despite aminophylline's recognized toxicity, the key reason for the continued use of this drug is that it provides dose-related bronchodilation even when patient and in vitro tissue models become β-receptor–unresponsive (31).

Target systems for aminophylline toxicity are the brain and cardiovascular systems. The pharmacokinetics of aminophylline are quite variable (128), and despite a well-documented, step dose-response curve that correlates with serum levels about 5–10 pg/ml, the occurrence of seizures and arrhythmias appears with little or no obvious prodrome (61, 120). Consequently, there is strong support for the argument that aminophylline kinetics should be measured on an individual basis (92, 128, 149).

Guidelines are offered for aminophylline dose and infusion rates to achieve steady state concentrations between 10 and 20 pg/ml (Table 6.3). One must anticipate wide variation, since age, acute illness, congestive heart failure, hepatic failure and cirrhosis, and chronic obstructive pulmonary disease (COPD) may increase or decrease clearance. Children with cystic fibrosis evidently have increased aminophylline clearance compared with asthmatics (104). Acute hypoxemia alone does not alter theophylline clearance in adults with COPD (20). Drug interaction possibilities include those with ephedrine, erythromycin, and steroids—all of which may decrease clearance (13, 93, 135). Aminophylline should be titrated in the critically ill patient with pulmonary disease. Since clearance may change dramatically within several half-lives and the clearance may vary 3- to 6-fold in critically ill patients, aminophylline levels should be obtained frequently in order to track changes in dose requirement and adjust dose before levels fall below the therapeutic or rise above the toxic threshold (57, 83, 85). Steady state conditions are achieved within four to five half-

Table 6.3
Guide to Intravenous Aminophylline Therapy in the Acutely Ill Patient[a,b]

Prior Prescription	Patients	Loading Dose[c] (mg/kg)	Steady State Dose (mg/kg/hr)	Mean Half-life (hr)	Level Monitoring Interval[d] (hr)
No	Adults	6	0.9	4.5	8–10
No	Adults/CHF	6	0.4	Quite variable	8
No	Adults/smoking	6	1.3	Decreased	6
Yes	Adults	3	0.9	4.8	8
No	Children	6	1.2	3.6	6
Yes	Children	3	1.2	Variable	6

[a] Data from references 57, 83, 118.
[b] This drug should be infused via peripheral vein in dilute solution. ECG rhythm monitoring is essential.
[c] Loading dose should be diluted and administered over 15–20 minutes (14).
[d] >95% of steady state is predicted at 4–5 multiples of a half-life. Level monitoring interval is defined as 2 half-lives to identify abnormal kinetics.

lives. The author recommends obtaining levels after the loading dose, at one half-life, and at every two predicted half-lives thereafter until the patient is quite stable and no longer requires closely titrated therapy.

Anticholinergic Therapy

A clinical role for manipulation of balance between the sympathetic and parasympathetic systems by blockade of the latter is controversial. Surgical vagotomy and muscarinic blockade have both been used to treat asthma but have been largely abandoned—the first because of the morbidity of surgery and the second because the combination of β-adrenergic drug and aminophylline is quite effective and anticholinergic therapy often causes intolerable tachycardia (43). Drying of secretions and worsening airway obstruction are also frequently suggested as reasons for avoiding anticholinergic therapy.

Inhibition of central and peripheral cholinergic tone is likely to be effective when histamine release, antigen-antibody reactions, or direct airway irritation have caused bronchospasm (86, 149). Although the issue is not settled, recent evidence suggests that some of the earlier work demonstrating no or reduced response to anticholinergic therapy was invalid. (Compare the intravenous doses of atropine (0.01 mg/kg) with the inhalational dose (0.1 mg/kg) (124).) Several long-acting anticholinergic drugs are under investigation for inhalation and intravenous therapy (43). Currently, atropine and other long-acting anticholinergics are not approved by the Food and Drug Administration for the treatment of asthma (86).

Antihistamines

Antihistamines are indicated adjuncts to the therapy of anaphylactoid reactions and bronchospasm in patients with known histamine release problems. Additional mechanisms of action may be subcellular or associated with some mediator other than histamine (8).

Corticosteroid Therapy

Corticosteroids (Table 6.4) play an essential role in the chronic and acute management of severe asthma (99, 122) and a somewhat more controversial role in the acute management of aspiration pneumonitis, noncardiogenic pulmonary edema (adult respiratory distress syndrome (ARDS) or "shock" lung), interstitial lung disease, and chronic bronchospastic diseases such as "asthmatic bronchitis" (111, 143). Several mechanisms of actions have been identified, but a key biochemical effect may be the pharmacodynamic enhancement of β-receptor–mediated catecholamine action (13, 35, 91, 100). Table 6.4 lists preparations that are most often used for the management of patients with pulmonary disease.

Synthetic steroids are rapidly absorbed. They are metabolized in the liver and excreted by renal mechanisms. The plasma half-life correlates very poorly with the pharmacodynamic half-life of glucocorticoid and mineralocorticoid effects (36, 149).

There are two major indications for steroid therapy in the pulmonary patient: (a) stress response coverage for the patient with an abnormal hypothalamic-pituitary-adrenal axis and (b) high or "pharmacologic" dose steroids for

Table 6.4
Corticosteroid Drugs in Pulmonary Disease

Drug	Mineralocorticoid Potency	Antiinflammatory Potency	Plasma Half-life (hr)	Pharmacologic Half-life	Dose Equivalent
Hydrocortisone	+ +	1	1½	12 hr	20
Cortisone	+ +	0.8	½	12 hr	25
Prednisone	+	3.5	5	½–1½ days	5
Methylprednisolone	+	5	5	½–1½ days	4
Dexamethasone	0	30	5	1½–3 days	0.75
Beclomethasone (aerosol)	0	?	Minimal	8 hr	0.1

the acutely ill or relapsed pulmonary patient. In the acute setting, toxicity is not a problem, aside from the sometimes surprising hypotension following massive intravenous doses (32, 70, 74). With more chronic administration, hyperglycemia, gastrointestinal bleeding, osteoporosis, suppression of the immune response, muscle wasting and weakness, and electrolyte or acid-base disturbances due to the mineralocorticoid effects of high doses with most agents become more difficult problems. Since steroid pharmacokinetics have so little effect on pharmacodynamics and there is no precise definition of a therapeutic dose threshold, most clinicians increase doses when in doubt about the effectiveness of therapy. Hepatic enzyme inducers increase steroid clearance, and patients who are receiving barbiturates should have larger steroid doses (149). Very large doses probably eliminate problems such as steroid resistance and diminish the effects of increased clearance on therapeutic efficacy (113).

The aerosol form of beclomethasone has been helpful in the chronic care setting because of its prolonged duration of and reduced suppression of pituitary adrenal responsiveness. Converting from systemic therapy to inhalational therapy has caused deaths due to unrecognized adrenal insufficiency after withdrawal of physiologic replacement. With inhalation of steroids, oropharyngeal candidiasis occurs with distressing frequency, especially in the setting of high-dose systemic antibiotics (79, 149). Despite hypothesized effects on intracellular levels of cAMP, there have been no adverse interactions reported between adrenergic bronchodilators and inhaled steroids (134). Intravenous therapy with large doses has also been remarkably safe (70).

Key guidelines for steroid administration (Table 6.5) recognize that single, large-dose administration of steroids has little or no toxic implications, whereas some possible clinical advantages and putative sites of action exist for the critically ill pulmonary patient. The duration of steroid effect does not correlate with duration of plasma levels, so that deter-

Table 6.5
Pharmacologic Doses of Corticosteroid Preparations for Acute Intravenous Treatment of Lung Disease[a]

Drug	Daily Dose for Adrenal Suppression (mg)	Loading Dose (mg/kg)	Maintenance (mg/kg/day)	Tapering Doses	Biologic Half-life
Hydrocortisone	20–30	7	7	Half dose q 12 hr	12 hr
		4	3 (adult, 1–200 mg q 4 hr)	Stop, or half dose q 12 hr	12 hr
Dexamethasone	1–1.5	0.3–0.5	0.3–0.5	Stop, or taper to half dose q 12–24 hr	1½–2½ days
Methylprednisolone	10	30 (1–2 gm)	15–30 (adult, 20–40 mg q 4 hr)	Stop, or halve consecutive doses	½–1½ days

[a] Data from references 70, 71, 79, 114, 138.

mination of plasma levels is not helpful. Acute therapy is a low-risk proposition, whereas chronic therapy increases the likelihood of side effects and suppression of the hypothalamic-pituitary-adrenal axis. Dosage and tapering protocols vary considerably because clinical assessment of response and relapse varies so greatly. Acute treatment of the chronic steroid-dependent patient may (or may not) require greater doses of drug.

Prostaglandins

Prostaglandins are derived from polyunsaturated eicosanoic fatty acids. Related compounds include prostacyclin, the slow-reacting substance of anaphylaxis, leukotrienes, and monohydroxperoxy and monohydroxy fatty acids (see Chapter 38). They have multiple actions and play the natural role of counteracting substances as part of an autoregulation process in many organ systems. For example, prostaglandin E_1 (PGE_1) is a bronchodilator and prostaglandin F_2 (PGF_2) is a bronchoconstrictor. These drugs have been used in various clinical circumstances, such as the induction of labor or abortion and the hormonal maintenance of a patent ductus arteriosus. Their potential role in the therapy of pulmonary disease, among others, is fascinating (109); however, none of the prostaglandin bronchodilators has yet been approved or marketed commercially. The reader is referred elsewhere for a review of this subject (59).

Antibiotic Therapy

Infection is a cause for the exacerbation of chronic reversible or obstructive pulmonary disease. Appropriate cultures should always be taken. Infection at sites other than the lungs may cause pulmonary decompensation, and consequently, a thorough infectious disease evaluation is indicated. Acute respiratory distress is a common manifestation of systemic sepsis and is often the most remarkable clinical finding until sepsis is quite advanced. When diffuse alveolar disease or symmetrical interstitial infiltrates appear in a patient with no prior cardiac history, sepsis should always top the list of differential diagnoses. Broad spectrum antibiotic coverage of the acutely ill pediatric patient should be effective for *Haemophilus* species as well as the most likely opportunistic organisms (85). The debilitated

patient with chronic obstructive pulmonary disease, whether from cystic fibrosis, bronchopulmonary dysplasia, or "asthmatic bronchitis," should be treated for Gram-negative organisms (17), and in the acutely ill individual the question of mycoplasma pneumonia or Legionnaire's disease should also be raised, pending definitive culture (102). It is well to remember the erythromycin-aminophylline interaction in the latter case and follow theophylline levels carefully when initiating new therapy.

The macrolide and aminoglycoside antibiotics may cause prolonged weakness after anesthesia and surgery by means of a magnesium-like, direct muscular effect. This side effect should be considered in any patient receiving these medications who is slow to recover from anesthesia or paralysis (107, 116, 149).

Sedatives

When patients require ventilator support, sedatives may allow more effective ventilation by decreasing central factors that contribute to bronchospasm or ventilator dyssynchrony. Acute interventions followed by heavy sedation and controlled mechanical ventilation often lead to hypotension because of a combination of the hemodynamic effects of intermittent positive pressure ventilation, a reduction in carbon dioxide levels and endogenous catecholamine release.

The author recommends light to moderate sedation with morphine or a nonhistamine-releasing narcotic such as fentanyl citrate or meperidine. All of these can be reversed with naloxone, whereas drugs such as diazepam, chlorpromazine, or haloperidol may be quite long-acting, especially in the patient whose respiratory work demands are high and whose central respiratory drive is blunted (66).

Local Anesthetics

Reflex bronchoconstriction has been documented following endotracheal intubation in normal awake and anesthetized volunteers (42). This event may be partially blocked by the administration of topical or intravenous local anesthetics (27). Severe bronchospasm may follow the intubation of individuals with hyperreactive airways due to "asthmatic bronchitis," asthma, aspiration, or bronchopneumonia (laryngotracheitis-bronchiolitis in children). Currently, there is some evidence that both the bronchoconstrictor and hypertensive responses to intubation can be blunted with intravenous lidocaine (50).

Muscle Relaxants

Muscle relaxation is the last resort in the management of the agitated bronchospastic patient who does not tolerate sedation well and remains hypercapneic and acidotic despite large tidal volume, low-rate mechanical ventilation, optimal pulmonary toilet, and bronchodilator therapy. These drugs have the advantage of reducing the chest wall component of pulmonary noncompliance by eliminating the active interference caused by dyssynchronous breathing. The cardiovascular impact of mechanical ventilation is diminished by lowering the mean airway pressures of combative patients and by reducing minute oxygen consumption. Concomitantly, carbon dioxide production may be reduced as muscular work, shivering, or tremor are reduced along with oxygen consumption and the work at breathing. Disadvantages include the loss of normal transpulmonary pressure gradients. A decrease in venous return to the right and left heart and increased tissue edema are associated with elimination of the peripheral venous and lymphatic pumping effects of muscular activity. Overenthusiastic use of paralysis for the management of patients on ventilators leads to loss of the patient's active role in chest physiotherapy, blocks the patient's communication with the nursing staff, and obtunds almost all clinical findings associated with the neurologic examination.

If the patient is bronchospastic, a nondepolarizing muscle relaxant with minimal histamine releasing and ganglionic blocking effect should be used (107) (Table 6.6). Pharmacodynamic interactions with these agents are difficult to predict, but the most common are drug interactions, electrolyte imbalance, and the marked variation in individual sensitivity to each drug. Major interactions with antibiotics are important (Table 6.7). Profound hypocalcemia, hypokalemia, hypophosphatemia, and hypermagnesemia all contribute to increased individual sensitivity. Relaxant dosage is best managed by monitoring of the neuromuscular junction with a nerve stimulator. In the absence of this, it is best to redose the patient only after signs of returning muscle function. Otherwise, one cannot avoid prolonged paralysis after the requirement of relaxants has passed.

Depolarizing muscle relaxants are effectively antagonized by the competitive inhibition of acetylcholinesterase only if some muscular receptors are available for normal receptor-transmitter interaction. If reversal of the neuromuscular blockade is not effective after the administration of neostigmine, 0.07 mg/kg, plus atropine, 0.01 mg/kg, or pyridostigmine, 0.21 mg/kg, plus glycopyrrolate, 0.005 mg/kg, it should not be attempted again for several hours. This fact is because the cholinesterase inhibitor may interact with the primary muscle relaxant to augment neuromuscular blockade. Anticholinergic drugs must be combined with cholinesterase-inhibiting compounds so as to avoid a cholinergic crisis at other sites—specifically marked by profound bradycardia, salivation, gastrointestinal cramping, and bronchospasm (116).

Table 6.6
A Guide to Intravenous Administration of Muscle Relaxants in Critical Care[a]

Drug	Loading Dose (mg/kg)	Maintenance Dose (mg/kg)	Duration	Excretion	Complications
d-Tubocurine	0.6	0.2–0.3	1–1½ hr	40% renal, 60% enterohepatic	Releases histamine, hypotension
Dimethylcurarine	0.3	0.1	40 min	Like curare	Mild histamine release, hypotension
Pancuronium bromide	0.12	0.02	40 min	80% renal	Tachycardia, vagolysis
Atracurium	0.5–1	0.25	20 min	Plasma hydrolysis	Weak histamine release
Vecuronium	0.1	0.01	30 min	Hepatic clearance	None

[a] Data from reference 37.

Table 6.7
Antibiotics and Other Drugs That May Interact with Muscle Relaxants[a]

Drugs	Potentiates Succinylcholine	Potentiates d-Tubocurarine
Gentamicin	?	Yes
Neomycin	Yes	Yes
Streptomycin	Yes	Yes
Polymyxins	?	Yes
Tetracycline	No	Yes
Clindamycin	?	Yes
Benzodiazepine	No	Yes
Dantrolene	?	Yes
Ca^{2+} channel blockers	?	Probably
Steroids	?	Possibly
Quinidine	Yes	Yes
Procainamide	Yes	Yes
Phenytoin	Yes	Yes
Propranolol	Yes	Yes
Lidocaine	Yes	Yes

[a] Data from reference 116.

Oxygen

Oxygen is a drug with pharmacokinetics of its own as well as pharmacodynamic tissue interactions. Most pulmonary patients require oxygen therapy when they are critically ill, and some require continuous or intermittent low-flow oxygen therapy as outpatients. Oxygen toxicity is both dose-related and time-related (144).

An interesting pharmacokinetic interaction between steroids and oxygen has been investigated and advanced as one rationale for steroid administration in septic shock and other states in which the oxygen extraction ratio is abnormal. Pharmacologic doses of steroids either improve oxygen unloading by manipulation of the oxyhemoglobin dissociation curve or improve oxygen uptake by changing the distribution of capillary blood flow or the function of the cell membranes (12, 78). A number of other interactions affecting oxygen transport by hemoglobin are probably minor and overshadowed by the profound effects of acid-base changes, anemia, carbon monoxide or cyanide binding to hemoglobin, and circulatory abnormalities of critically ill patients (11).

Oxygen has the property of inducing its own metabolism, possibly by increasing the production of free radical quenching compounds (115, 144, 146). Unfortunately, this is an unpredictable mechanism for prevention of oxygen toxicity (82). Superoxide dismutase (SOD),

an oxygen free-radical scavenger, is entering clinical trials in the United States. If oxygen free radicals prove to be a major mechanism for hyperoxic and reperfusion injury to the lung and other tissues, therapy with SOD may limit oxygen toxicity to a number of systems. The exact site of oxygen toxicity is poorly understood (4, 19, 38, 51), and there is currently no way to prevent or alleviate oxygen toxicity other than to limit duration and magnitude of exposure. In the adult, use of 100% oxygen for no longer than 15–20 hours or more than 50% oxygen for longer periods may cause oxygen toxicity (145). The fetus and premature neonate have a lowered toxicity threshold, and it is as yet unclear what levels are safe to prevent retinal or pulmonary oxygen toxicity in this clinical setting (68, 85). The full-term neonate and the infant are no longer at risk.

An additional pharmacokinetic reaction that may potentiate oxygen toxicity occurs in cancer patients who have experienced prior chemotherapy with bleomycin (46, 139). Other drugs and associated factors affecting tissue oxygen consumption, normal free-radical scavenging mechanisms, and cellular sensitivity to oxygen injury may become better known in the future (45, 47, 90). In the meantime, all measures should be directed toward limiting oxygen dose and exposure by reducing the pulmonary shunt fraction in patients who are critically ill (89). When this approach is not possible (e.g., with cyanotic congenital heart disease), it may be better to use other modes of therapy, since increasing oxygen dose has little effect on systemic tissue oxygenation (54).

Cardiovascular Drugs

Important drug interactions in the patient with pulmonary disease usually relate to the secondary effect of hemodynamic changes or other organ alterations involved in drug metabolism. Several major interactions are worth reviewing here. β-Adrenergic agents, theophylline compounds, and vasodilators may diminish hypoxic pulmonary vasoconstriction, especially in those patients whose pulmonary ventilation-perfusion balance is tenuous (49, 94, 137). Consequently, the patient who receives nitroglycerin and other nitrates for the treatment of angina may become hypoxemic because of this or other effects on pulmonary functions. The response to sodium nitroprusside cannot be blocked by the prior or subsequent administration of a β-blocker (80).

A second potential problem presents when the pulmonary patient receives dopamine infusions. Dopamine blunts the peripheral chemoreceptors' response to hypoxemia (56, 141). Sabol and Ward (110) have recently shown that 3 μg/kg/min of dopamine reduced hypoxic sensitivity by 77% during normocapnia and by as much as 38% during hypercapnia in humans. The same dose reduced the normoxic ventilatory response at all carbon dioxide levels, although the potentiation of hypoxic drive by hypercapnia was still observed during dopamine infusion. In the cat, low doses of dopamine inhibit and high doses increase carotid sinus nerve activity. These findings suggest blood gas monitoring or choice of another inotropic agent when patients with chronic compensated respiratory acidosis need inotropic support.

The pulmonary patients' respiratory muscle work requirements are generally elevated. These patients are rarely able to manage normal gut function. Therefore, parenteral nutrition may be required to maintain respiratory muscle function and to decrease the likelihood of sepsis (5). Overfeeding with solutions containing a high carbohydrate: protein ratio precipitates hypermetabolism and fever in some patients (3) and increases minute carbon dioxide production by elevation of the respiratory quotient (2). Also, hyperalimentation formulas with an increased ratio of neutral amino acids to tryptophan appear to increase central respiratory drive, possibly by inhibiting central nervous system availability of serotonin (140). Nutrition therapy should be tailored for the patient with marginal ventilatory function and respiratory drive mechanisms (75). These potential problems indicate a need for close metabolic monitoring of nutritional support in the acutely ill pulmonary patient.

Diuretic therapy is accepted as a mainstay of support for both the adult and pediatric patient with interstitial lung disease, heart failure, cor pulmonale, and edematous states. Hypokalemic, hypochloremic, or "contraction" alkalosis may be superimposed on the normal compensatory metabolic alkalosis of patients with chronic respiratory acidemia by the combination of fluid restriction and vigorous diuresis with hydrochlorothiazide or more potent loop diuretics such as furosemide (58). Progressive carbon dioxide retention and pulmonary decompensation may complicate the marginal status of acutely ill medical or surgical patients during such therapy. Close attention to electrolyte and acid-base balance during diuresis will prevent this problem. Acetazolamide is a particularly useful agent in combination with potassium-sparing diuretics, aldosterone inhibitors, and careful potassium replacement for maintaining an effective diuresis without producing iatrogenic compensatory hypercapnia (25, 81).

CONCLUSION

The pharmacokinetics and pharmacodynamics of drugs administered to patients with acute or chronic pulmonary disease vary significantly. A number of variables change in pulmonary disease, but the aggregate effect is difficult to predict a priori. Acutely ill pulmonary patients are at high risk for drug toxicity and adverse drug interactions. Pharmacokinetic models have been insufficient in the critically ill patient because of uncertain pharmacokinetics and marked interpatient variation.

An overview of the ways in which drug kinetics are known to be altered by pulmonary disease has demonstrated this to be a poorly understood area. At present, the most important contributors to pharmacokinetic variation appear to operate by secondary, or indirect, means. Intravenous titration of agents with a short, predictable metabolism and clearance is the best way to avoid unexpected interactions or overdose of the acutely ill patient. When this approach is impossible, the logical way to predict changes in clearance is by close monitoring of pharmacokinetic trends and blood levels.

Pharmacodynamic interactions in the pulmonary patient are poorly understood. Clinicians rely on pharmacodynamic interactions in day-to-day care, and some insight into these interactions is required for the optimal management of bronchospastic and infected patients in particular. The drug-effect interaction is an exciting area of research on the threshold of clinically relevant discovery. Close clinical monitoring offers the only practical way to assess these interactions.

Given the potential for drug-related complications in the critically ill pulmonary patient, one must review the drug history periodically and institute therapy with well-defined clinical endpoints in mind. The critical care unit is a setting for frequent monitoring of drug levels and direct, serial observation of the patient's clinical response. Whenever one employs a high-risk pharmacologic intervention it is wise to formulate a treatment strategy before drug toxicity occurs. Each new pharmacologic modality that is proposed must be assessed in the light of what is known about the kinetics and dynamics of similar agents, and must be placed within the clinical context of the specific disease entity and patient situation. Since predictive models of drug action have so often been proven inaccurate in the pulmonary patient, the observation and documentation of patient response is a key aspect of therapy.

Overall recommendations are as follows:

1. Determine drug history in the acute situation.
2. Institute therapy with defined clinical goals.
3. Track drug kinetics by frequent assessment of drug levels.
4. Monitor the patient's clinical response with treatment goals in mind.
5. Anticipate probability of toxicity and prepare treatment strategies.
6. Document patient response and identify new drug problems as they occur.
7. Evaluate each new pharmacotherapeutic modality proposed in the light of what is known about the pharmacokinetics and pharmacodynamics of similar agents.

References

1. Albert RK, Martin TR, Lewis SW: Controlled clinical trial of methylprednisolone in patients with chronic bronchitis and acute respiratory insufficiency. *Ann Intern Med* 92:753–758, 1980.
2. Askanazi J, Elwyn DH, Silverberg PA: Respiratory distress secondary to the high carbohydrate load of TPN: a case report. *Surgery* 87:595–599, 1980.
3. Askanazi J, Nordenstrom J, Rosenbaum SH, et al: Nutrition for the patient with respiratory failure: glucose vs. fat. *Anesthesiology* 54:373–377, 1981.
4. Balantine JD: Pathologic effects of exposure to high oxygen tensions. *N Engl J Med* 275:1038–1040, 1960.
5. Benotti P, Blackburn GL: Protein and caloric or micronutrient management of the critically ill patient. *Crit Care Med* 7:520–525, 1979.
6. Berk JL: Multiple organ failure. In Berk JL, Sampliner JE (eds): *Handbook of Critical Care*, ed 2. Boston, Little, Brown, & Co, 1982, chap 1.
7. Bonnet F, Richard C, Glaser P, et al: Changes in hepatic flow induced by continuous positive pressure ventilation in critically ill patients. *Crit Care Med* 10:703–705, 1982.
8. Branch RA: Histamine and H_1 and H_2 receptor antagonists. In Wood M, Wood AJJ (eds): *Drugs and Anesthesia*. Baltimore, Williams & Wilkins, 1982, chap 23.
9. Brandenburger-Brown EA: The localization, metabolism and effects of drugs and toxicants in lung. *Drug Metab Rev* 3:33–87, 1974.
10. Branscomb BV: Metaproterenol solution in the treatment of asthmatic patients by IPPB. *J Clin Pharmacol* 22:231–235, 1982.
11. Bryan-Brown CW: Gas transport and delivery. In: *Critical Care: State of the Art.* Fullerton, CA, SCCM Press, 1980, vol 1, (E) pp 1–35.
12. Bryan-Brown CW, Makbali G, Baek SM, et al: Hemodynamic responses and oxygen delivery after methylprednisolone sodium succinate. In Gless TM (ed): *Proceedings of Steroids and Shock.* Philadelphia, University Park Press, 1974, pp 361–375.
13. Buchanan N, Harwitz S, Butler P: A possible interaction between hydrocortisone and theophylline (letter to editor). *S Afr Med J* 1147–1148, December 29, 1979.
14. Camarata SJ, Weil MH, Hanashiro PK, et al: Cardiac arrest in the critically ill. *Circulation* 44:688–695, 1971.
15. Camus P, Jeannin L. The diseased lung and drugs. *Arch Toxicol* 7(suppl):66–87, 1984.
16. Cheung WY: Calmodulin plays a pivotal role in cellular regulation. *Science* 207:19–27, 1980.
17. Cipolle RJ, Seifert RD, Zaske DE, et al: Hospital acquired gram-negative pneumonias: response rate and dosage requirements with individualized tobramycin therapy. *Ther Drug Monit* 2:359–363, 1980.
18. Conolly ME, Davies DS, Dollery CT, et al: Resistance to β-stimulants. *Br J Pharmacol* 43:389, 1971.
19. Crapo JD, Tierney DF: Superoxide dismutase and pulmonary oxygen toxicity. *Am J Physiol* 226:1401, 1974.
20. Cusack BJ, Crowley JJ, Mercer GD, Charan NB, Vestel RE. Theophylline clearance in patients with severe chronic obstructive pulmonary disease receiving supplemental oxygen and the effect of acute hypoxemia. *Am Rev Respir Dis* 133:1110–1114, 1986.
21. Danielson DA, Porter JB, Dinan BJ, et al: Drug monitoring of surgical patients. *JAMA* 248:1482–1485, 1982.
22. Davies DS, George CF, Blackwell E, et al: Metabolism of terbutaline in man and dog. *Br J Clin Pharmacol* 1:129–136, 1974.
23. Davis H, Lefrak SS, Mider D, et al: Prolonged mechanically assisted ventilation. *JAMA* 243:43–45, 1980.
24. Del Negro R, Pomari C, Zoccatelli O, Trevisan F, Turco P: Pharmacokinetics of theophylline and the H_2-antagonist drugs cimetidine and ranitidine. *Int J Clin Pharmacol Ther Toxicol* 22:221–226, 1984.
25. Dickenson GE, Myers ML, Goldbach M, et al: Acetazolamide in the treatment of ventilatory failure complicating acute metabolic alkalosis. *Anesth Analg [Cleve]* 60:608–610, 1981.
26. Douglas JS, Lewis AJ, Ridgeway P, et al: Tachyphylaxis to β-adrenoreceptor agonists in guinea pig airway smooth muscle *in vivo* and *in vitro*. *Eur J Pharmacol* 42:195, 1977.
27. Downes H, Hirshman CA: Do lidocaine aerosols reduce allergic bronchoconstriction. *Anesthesiology* 53:S393, 1980.
28. Downes JJ et al: IV isoproterenol infusion in children. *Crit Care Med* 1:63–68, 1973.
29. Downes JJ, Heiser MS: Status asthmaticus in children. In Gregory G (ed): *Respiratory Failure in the Child.* New York, Churchill Livingstone, 1981, chap 9.
30. Downes JJ, Wood DW, Striker TW, et al: Arterial blood gas and acid base disorders in children with status asthmaticus. *Pediatrics* 42:238–249, 1968.
31. Dusdieker L, Green M, Smith G, et al: Comparison of orally administered metaproterenol and theophylline in the therapy of chronic asthma. *J Pediatr* 101:281–287, 1982.
32. Dutton RE, English M, Powers SA: Hypotension with steroid therapy. *Ann Surg* 181:317, 1975.
33. Eger EI: Effect of ventilation-perfusion abnormalities. In *Anesthetic Uptake and Action.* Baltimore, Williams & Wilkins, 1976, chap 8.
34. Ellis EF, Koysooko R, Leay G: Pharmacokinetics of theophylline in children with asthma. *Pediatrics* 58:542–547, 1976.

35. Ellul-Micalley R, French FF: Effect of intravenous prednisolone in asthmatics with diminished adrenergic responsiveness. *Lancet* 2:1269, 1975.

36. Feeley J: Drugs and the endocrine system. In Wood M, Wood AJJ (eds): *Drugs and Anesthesia.* Baltimore, Williams & Wilkins, 1982, chap 20.

37. Feldman SA: Nondepolarizing drugs. In *Muscle Relaxants*, ed 2. Philadelphia, WB Saunders, 1979.

38. Frank L, Bucher JR, Roberts RT: Oxygen toxicity in neonatal and adult animals of various species. *J Appl Physiol* 45:699, 1978.

39. Fraser J, Nadeau J, Robertson D, et al: Regulation of human leukocyte beta receptors by endogenous catecholamines: relationship of leukocyte beta receptor density to the cardiac sensitivity to isoproterenol. *J Clin Invest* 67:1777–1784, 1981.

40. Frederiksen MC, Ruo TI, Chow MJ, Atkinson AJ. Theophylline pharmacokinetics in pregnancy. *Clin Pharmacol Ther* 40:321–328, 1986.

41. Gaddum JH, Hebb CO, Silver A, Swan AAB: 5-Hydroxytryptamine: pharmacological action and destruction in perfused lungs. *J Exp Physiol* 38:255–262, 1953.

42. Gal TJ, Rochester DF: The effects of endotracheal intubation of pulmonary mechanics in man. *In American Society of Anesthesiologists Abstracts.* Chicago, American Society of Anesthesiologists Press, 1977, p 647.

43. Gal TJ, Suratt PM: Bronchomotor effect of glycopyrolate and atropine aerosol inhalation. *Anesthesiology* 57:A479, 1982.

44. Galant SP, Duiseti L, Underwood S, et al: Decreased beta adrenergic receptors on polymorphonuclear leukocyte after adrenergic therapy. *N Engl J Med* 299:933–966, 1978.

45. Goldiner PG, et al: Bleomycin O_2 tox. *Br Med J* 1:1664, 1978.

46. Goldiner PG, Carlon GC, Cvitkovic E, et al: Factors influencing postoperative morbidity and mortality in patients treated with bleomycin. *Br Med J* 1:1664–1667, 1978.

47. Goldiner PG, Schweizer O: The hazards of anesthesia and surgery in bleomycin-treated patients. *Semin Oncol* 6:121, 1979.

48. Green AW, Ebling WF, Gardner MJ, Jusco WJ: Cimetidine-methylprednisolone-theophylline metabolic interaction. *Am J Med* 77:1115–1118, 1984.

49. Hales CA, Kazemi H: Hypoxic vascular response of the lung: effect of aminophylline and epinephrine. *Am Rev Respir Dis* 110:126–132, 1974.

50. Hamill JF, Bedford RF, Weaver DC, et al: Lidocaine before endotracheal intubation: intravenous or laryngotracheal. *Anesthesiology* 55:578–581, 1981.

51. Hangaard N: Poisoning of cellular reactions by oxygen. *Ann NY Acad Sci* 148:736–744, 1968.

52. Hedley-Whyte J, Burgess GE, Feeley T, et al: Burns and respiratory function. In *Applied Physiology of Respiratory Care.* Boston, Little, Brown & Co, 1976, chap 16.

53. Hedley-Whyte J, Burgess GE, Feeley T, et al: Problems of nosocomial pulmonary infection. In *Applied Physiology of Respiratory Care.* Boston, Little, Brown, & Co, 1976, chap 5.

54. Hedley-Whyte J, Burgess GE, Feeley T, et al: Pulmonary oxygen toxicity in respiratory therapy management. In *Applied Physiology of Respiratory Care.* Boston, Little, Brown, & Co, 1976, chap 31.

55. Hedley-Whyte J, Burgess GE, Feeley T, et al: Trauma and respiratory failure. In *Applied Physiology of Respiratory Care.* Boston, Little, Brown, & Co, 1976, chap 3.

56. Heistad DD, Abbond FM: Circulatory adjustments to hypoxia. *Circulation* 61:463–470, 1980.

57. Hendeles L, Weinberger M: Guidelines for avoiding theophylline over dosage. *N Engl J Med* 300:1217, 1979.

58. Hudson HE, Harber PI, Smith TC: Respiratory depression from alkalosis and opioid interaction in man. *Anesthesiology* 40:543–551, 1974.

59. Hyman AL, Spannhake EW, Kadowitz PJ: Prostaglandins and the lung. *Am Rev Respir Dis* 117:111–136, 1980.

60. Iwainsky H, Winsel K, Werner E, et al: On the pharmacokinetics of rifampicin during treatment with intermittent administration. *Scand J Respir Dis* 57:5–11, 1976.

61. Jacobs MH, Senior RM, Kessler G: Clinical experience with theophylline prodrome. *JAMA* 235:1983–1986, 1976.

62. Jenne JW: Beta adrenergic agents—how much is enough? *J Allergy Clin Immunol* 63:74–76, 1979.

63. Jorfeldt L, Lewis DH, Lofstrom JB, Post Cl: Lung uptake of lidocaine in man as influenced by anesthesia mepivicaine infusion on lung insufficiency. *Acta Anesthesiol Scand* 27:5–9, 1983.

64. Junod AF: Metabolism of the intact pulmonary circulation. *Ann NY Acad Sci* 384:66–71, 1982.

65. Kadlec GJ, Ha LT, Jarboe CH, et al: Effect of ampicillin on theophylline half-life in infants and young children. *South Med J* 71:1584, 1978.

66. Kafer ER, Marsh HM: Effect of anesthetic drugs and disease on the chemical regulation of ventilation. *Int Anesthesiol Clin* 15(2):1–38, 1977.

67. Keighley JF: Iatrogenic asthma associated with adrenergic aerosols. *Ann Intern Med* 65:985, 1966.

68. Kinsey VE, Arnold HJ, Kalina RE, et al: PaO_2 levels and retrolental fibroplasia: a report of the cooperative study. *Pediatrics* 60:655–668, 1977.

69. LaForce CF, Miller MM, Chai H: Effect of erythromycin on theophylline clearance in asthmatic children. *J Pediatr* 99:153–156, 1981.

70. Lancet (editorial): The big shot. *Lancet* 1:633–634, 1977.

71. Lancet (letter to editor): Corticosteroids in acute severe asthma. *Lancet*, July 26, 1975.

72. Lefkowitz RJ: Beta-adrenergic receptors: recognition and regulation. *N Engl J Med* 295:323–328, 1976.

73. Lefkowitz RJ: Direct binding studies of adrenergic receptors: biochemical, physiological, and clinical implications. *Ann Intern Med* 91:450–458, 1979.

74. Lorzman J, Dutton RE, English M, et al: Hypotension with steroid Rx. *Ann Surg* 181:317, 1975.

75. Markov AK, Oglethorpe N, Turner MD, et al: Fructose diphosphate: analeptic for a barbiturate. *Anesthesiology* 53:5246, 1980.

76. Marquez JM, Douglas ME, Downes JB, et al: Renal function and cv response during PAP. *Anesthesiology* 50:393, 1979.

77. Massey KL, Gotz VP, Russell WL: Dose-dependent kinetics of theophylline in adults with pulmonary disease. *Ther Drug Monit* 6:284–289, 1984.

78. McConn R, Del Guercio LRM: Respiratory function of blood in the acutely ill patient and the effect of steroids. *Ann Surg* 174:436–450, 1970.

79. *Med Lett Drugs Ther* 20:761, 1977.

80. Miller JR, Benumof JL, Trousdale FR: Combined effects of sodium nitroprusside and propranolol on hypoxic pulmonary vasoconstriction. *Anesthesiology* 57:267–271, 1982.

81. Miller PD, Berns AS: Acute metabolic alkalosis perpetuating hypercapnia: a role for acetazolamide in chronic obstructive pulmonary disease. *JAMA* 238:2400–2401, 1977.

82. Miller WM, Waldhausen JA, Raskkind WJ: Comparison of oxygen poisoning of the lung in cyanotic and acyanotic dogs. *N Engl J Med* 282:943, 1970.

83. Mitenko PA, Ogalvie RI: Rational intravenous doses of theophylline. *N Engl J Med* 289:600–603, 1973.

84. Mithoefer JC, Runser RH, Karetzky MS: The use of sodium bicarbonate in the treatment of acute bronchial asthma. N Engl J Med 272:1200–1203, 1965.

85. Morray JP, Redding GJ: Chronic lung disease. In Gregory GA (ed): *Respiratory Failure in the Child*. New York, Churchill Livingstone, 1982, chap 9.

86. Mueller RA: Recent developments in the physiology of bronchomotor tone and the pharmacology of bronchodilators. Int Anesthesiol Clin 15:140–167, 1977.

87. Mulder DS, Rubush JL, Denbesten L, et al: Tracheopleural fistula: a complication of the cuffed tracheostomy tube. J Thorac Cardiovasc Surg 63:416, 1972.

88. Murphy AM: Clinically significant interaction between digoxin and quinidine. Br Med J December 1, 1979, p 1401.

89. Nunn JF, Williams IP, Jones JG, et al: Detection and reversal of pulmonary absorbtion collapse. Br J Anaesth 50:91–100, 1978.

90. Nygaard K, Smith-Erichsen N, Hatlevoll R, et al: Pulmonary complications after bleomycin, irradiation, and surgery for esophageal cancer. Cancer 41:17–22, 1978.

91. Parker CW, Huber WG, Baumann ML: Alterations in cAMP metabolism in asthma. J Clin Invest 52:1342, 1973.

92. Pessayre D, Allemand H, Benoist C, et al: Effects of surgery under general anesthesia on antipyrine clearance. Br J Clin Pharmacol 6:505–513, 1978.

93. Pfeiffer HF, Greenblatt DJ, Friedman P: Effect of three antibiotics on theophylline kinetics. Clin Pharmacol Ther 26:36–40, 1979.

94. Phelan PD, Williams HE: Sympathomimetic drugs in acute viral bronchiolitis: their effect on pulmonary resistance. Pediatrics 44:493–497.

95. Piafsky KM, Borga O, Odar-Cederlof I, et al: Increased plasma protein binding of propranolol and chloropromazine mediated by disease-induced elevations of plasma and acid glycoprotein. N Engl J Med 299:1435–1439, 1978.

96. Piafsky KM, Ogalvie RI: Dosage theophylline in bronchial asthma. N Engl J Med 292:1218–1222, 1975.

97. Piafsky KM, Sitar DS, Ragno RE, et al: Theophylline kinetics in acute pulmonary edema. Clin Pharmacol Ther 21:310–316, 1978.

98. Pickup ME, May CS, Sendagire R, et al: The pharmacokinetics of ephedrine after oral dosage in asthmatics receiving acute and chronic treatment. Br J Clin Pharmacol 3:123–134, 1976.

99. Pierson WE, Bierman CW, Kelley VC: A double-blind trial of corticosteroid therapy in status asthmaticus. Pediatrics 54:282–288, 1974.

100. Pollet RJ, Levey GS: Principles of membrane receptor physiology and their application to clinical medicine. Ann Intern Med 92:663–680, 1980.

101. Powel JR, Voseh S, Hopewell P, et al: Theophylline disposition in acutely ill hospitalized patients. Am Rev Respir Dis 118:229–238, 1978.

102. Prince AS, Neu HC: Use of piperacillin, a semisynthetic penicillin, in the therapy of acute exacerbations of pulmonary disease in patients with cystic fibrosis. J Pediatr 97:148–151, 1980.

103. Rangno RE, Piafsky KM, Sitar D, et al: The clinical pharmacology of theophylline and its pharmacokinetics in pulmonary edema and cirrhosis. Arzneimittelforschung 21:1268–1269, 1976.

104. Repetto T, Marianelli L, Valenza T, Rosselli P, Messori A. Farmacocinetica della teofilina orale confronto tra pazienti asmatici e pazienti con fibrosi cistica. Pediatr Med Chir 7:823–826, 1985.

105. Reyes A, Sykes MK, Charkabarti MK, et al: Effects of orciprenaline on hypoxic pulmonary vasoconstriction in dogs. Respiration 38:185–193, 1979.

106. Riker JB, Cacace LG: Double-blind comparison of metaproterenol and isoetharine-phenylephrine solutions in IPPB in bronchospastic conditions. Chest 78:723–725, 1980.

107. Roizen MF, Feeley TW: Pancuronium bromide. Ann Intern Med 88:64, 1978.

108. Rothstein RJ: Intravenous theophylline therapy in asthma: a clinical update. Ann Emerg Med 9:327–330, 1980.

109. Rubin LJ, Grover BM, Reeves JT, et al: Prostacyclin-induced pulmonary vasodilatation in primary pulmonary hypertension. Circulation 66:334–338, 1982.

110. Sabol SJ, Ward DS: Effect of dopamine on hypoxic-hypercapnic interaction in humans. Anesth Analg 67:619–624, 1987.

111. Sahn SA: Corticosteroids in chronic bronchitis and pulmonary emphysema. Chest 73:389–396, 1978.

112. Smith NT (ed): *Drug Interactions in Anesthesia*. Philadelphia, Lea & Febiger, 1980.

113. Schwartz HJ, Lowell FC, Melby JC: Steroid resistance in bronchial asthma. Ann Intern Med 69:493, 1968.

114. Shibel M: Respiratory emergencies. In Summer WR, Permutt S (eds): *Acute Lower Airway Obstruction*. St. Louis, CV Mosby, 1977, chap 8.

115. Smith G, Winter PM, Wheelis RF: Delayed rate of development of pulmonary oxygen toxicity following oleic acid induced lung damage. Br J Anaesth 45:641, 1973.

116. Standaert FG: Interactions among neuromuscular blocking agents and other drugs. In *Refresher Courses in Anesthesiology*. Philadelphia: JB Lippincott, 1981, chap 9.

117. Steel K, Gertman PM, Crescenzi C, et al: Iatrogenic illness on a general medicine service at a university hospital. N Engl J Med 304:638–642, 1981.

118. Stirt JA, Sullivan SF: Aminophylline. Anesth Analg [Cleve] 60:587–602, 1981.

119. Stoelting RK, Longnecker DE: Effect of right-to-left shunt on rate of increase in arterial anesthetic concentration. Anesthesiology 36:352–356, 1972.

120. Reference deleted in proof; see reference 151.

121. Swillins S, Dumont JE: A unifying model of current concepts and data on adenylate cyclase activation by β-adrenergic agonists. Life Sci 27:1013–1023, 1980.

122. Tattersfield AE, Holgate ST: Intravenous prednisolone in asthma. Lancet 1:422, 1976.

123. Thiringer G, Svedmyr N: Comparison of infused and inhaled terbutaline in patients with asthma. Scand J Respir Dis 57:17, 1976.

124. Tiakelman DG, Cavanaugh MJ, Copper DM: Inhibition of exercise. Induced bronchospasm by atropine. Am Rev Respir Dis 114:87–94, 1976.

125. Tribe AE, Wong RM, Robinson JS: A controlled trial of intravenous salbutamol and aminophylline in acute asthma. Med J Aust 2:749–752, 1976.

126. Vestal RE, Wood AJJ, Branch RA, et al: Effects of age and cigarette smoking on propranolol disposition. Clin Pharmacol Ther 26:8–15, 1979.

127. Vestal RE, Wood AJJ, Shand DG: Reduced β-adrenoceptor sensitivity in the elderly. Clin Pharmacol Ther 26:181–186, 1979.

128. Vozeh S, Kewitz G, Wenk M, et al: Rapid prediction of steady-state serum theophylline concentration in patients treated with intravenous aminophylline. Eur J Clin Pharmacol 18:473–477, 1980.

129. Vozeh S, Powell RJ, Riegelman, S, et al: Changes in theophylline clearance during acute illness. JAMA 240:1882–1884, 1978.

130. Walker J, Hendeles L: The interaction of erythromycin and theophylline in the asthmatic dental patient. J Am Dent Assoc 99:995–996, 1979.

131. Walker SR, Evans ME, Richards AJ, et al: The clinical pharmacology of oral and inhaled salbutamol. Clin Pharmacol Ther 13:861–867, 1972.

132. Waltman CL, Bergman NA: Increased respiratory re-

sistance provoked by endotracheal administration of aerosols. *Am Rev Respir Dis* 108:520, 1976.

133. Webb-Johnson DC, Andrews JL: Bronchodilator therapy (Part I). *N Engl J Med* 297:476–482, 1977.

134. Webb-Johnson DC, Andrews JL: Bronchodilator therapy (Part II). *N Engl J Med* 297:758, 1977.

135. Weinberger M, Bronsky E: Interaction of ephedrine and theophylline. *Clin Pharmacol Ther* 17:585–592, 1975.

136. Weinberger M, Ginchansky E: Dose dependent kinetics of theophylline disposition in asthmatic children. *J Pediatrics* 91:820–824, 1977.

137. Weir EK, Chidsey CA, Weil JV, et al: Minoxidil reduced pulmonary vascular resistance in dogs and cattle. *J Lab Clin Med* 88:885–894, 1976.

138. Weiss EB, Segal (eds): Status asthmaticus. In *Bronchial Asthma, Mechanisms, and Therapeutics.* Boston, Little, Brown, & Co, 1976, chap 60.

139. Weiss RB, Muggia FM: Cytotoxic drug-induced pulmonary disease: update 1980. *Am J Med* 68:259–266, 1980.

140. Weissman C, Askanazi J, LaSala P, et al: Aminoacids and respiration. *Anesthesiology* 57:A495, 1982.

141. Welsh MJ, Heistad DD, Abboud FM: Depression of ventilation by dopamine: evidence for mediation through arterial chemoreceptors. *J Clin Invest* 61:708, 1978.

142. Whiting B, Kelman AW, Struthers AD: Prediction of response to theophylline in chronic bronchitis. *Br J Clin Pharmacol* 17:1–8, 1984.

143. Wilson JD, Sutherland DC, Thomas AC: Has the change to β-agonists combined with oral theophylline increased cases of fatal asthma. *Lancet,* June 6, 1981, pp 1235–1237.

144. Winter PM: Oxygen toxicity. *Am Soc Anesth Refresher Course* 117:1–7, October 1982.

145. Winter PM, Miller JN: Clinical manifestations of oxygen toxicity. *Int Anesthesiol Clin* 19:179–195, 1981.

146. Winter PM, Smith G, Wheelis RF: The effect of prior pulmonary injury on the rate of development of fatal oxygen toxicity. *Chest* 66:1S–4S, 1974.

147. Wood AJJ, et al Propranolol disposition in renal failure. *Br J Clin Pharmacol* 10:561–566, 1980.

148. Wood AJJ, Kornhauser DM, Wilkinson GR, et al: The influence of cirrhosis on steady state blood concentrations of unbound propranolol after oral administration. *Clin Pharmacokinet* 3:478–487, 1978.

149. Wood M, Wood AJJ: *Drugs and Anesthesia,* ed 1. Baltimore: Williams & Wilkins, 1982.

150. Yaffe SJ, Gerbracht LM, Mosovich LL, et al: Pharmacokinetics of methicillin in patients with cystic fibrosis. *J Infect Dis* 135:828–831, 1977.

151. Zwillich CW, Sutton FD, Neff TA, et al: Theophylline-induced seizures in adults: correlation with serum concentrations. *Ann Intern Med* 82:784–787, 1975.

7

Pediatric Pharmacotherapy

Daniel A. Notterman, M.D., F.A.A.P.

Children develop and grow, and their response to drug therapy is conditioned by age, size, and stage of development. It is axiomatic that the change in body size associated with growth is a factor in determining dosage and response. However, even when the effect of size is accommodated, age and maturity exert a profound effect on response to pharmacotherapy. The influence of developmental factors is modulated, and usually amplified, by the imposition of critical illness, multiple organ system failure, heredity, and coadministration of other drugs. In infants and small children, vagaries of drug delivery systems and administration techniques assume significance (51, 64, 87, 110, 144, 145). This chapter provides a review of selected aspects of pediatric clinical pharmacology. It is not intended as, and does not include, a compendium of pediatric drug dosages. The pharmacology of individual agents is reviewed in greater detail in other chapters. The purpose here is to describe specific features that distinguish pharmacologic responses of children from those of adults, and to indicate, when possible, which observed pharmacologic differences are likely to result in important clinical differences.

Age-related differences in response are both pharmacokinetic and pharmacodynamic in origin (7, 18, 149, 151). The pharmacokinetic description concerns the relationship, over time, between drug *dosage* and drug *concentration*. The pharmacodynamic description concerns the relationship between this concentration and the resulting *response*. Narrowly construed, "pharmacodynamics" means "sensitivity," and applies to the relationship between unbound drug concentration (theoretically at the site of action; in practice, in the plasma) and magnitude of effect. Broadly conceived, pharmacodynamics comprises all of the biochemical and physiologic effects of a substance (149). Sensitivity is graphically represented in several ways (149); most often

as a plot of the log of drug concentration versus intensity of pharmacologic response. Figure 7.1, described in more detail in a subsequent section, is from a study by Driscoll and associates (38), and displays the pharmacodynamic relationship between dopamine concentration and the resulting inotropic effect in puppy ventricles from animals of different ages. Figure 7.2 illustrates an age-related pharmacodynamic effect from a study involving the elderly (139). It indicates that increasing age is associated with a reduction in the concentration of diazepam needed to induce a specified degree of hypnosis. By measuring diazepam concentration (rather than simply dosage), the

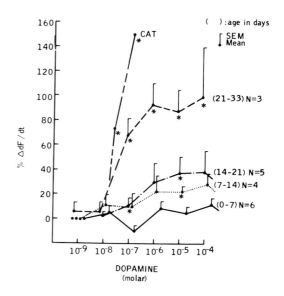

Figure 7.1. Inotropic (% ΔdF/dt) dose-response curves of puppy ventricles and adult cat ventricle treated with dopamine. There is an increasing inotropic responsiveness with age of isolated puppy ventricle to dopamine.* $P < 0.05$ using puppies 0–7 days old as control. (From Driscoll DJ, Gillette PC, Ezrailson EG, et al: Inotropic response of the neonatal canine myocardium to dopamine. *Pediatr Res* 12:42, 1978.)

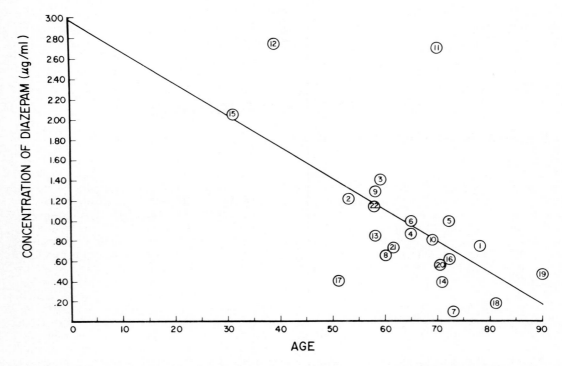

Figure 7.2. Relationship between age (31–90 years) of patient and plasma concentration of diazepam causing failure to respond to vocal but not painful stimuli. $P < 0.01$. (From Reidenberg MM, Levy M, Warner H, et al: Relationship between diazepam dose, plasma level, age and central nervous system depression. *Clin Pharmacol Ther* 23:371, 1978.)

investigators have excluded the hypothesis that a pharmacokinetic difference accounts for lower diazepam dosage requirements. Unfortunately, similar work is quite uncommon in the pediatric age group (7, 18), and experimentally proven differences in sensitivity between adults and children are not well documented.

A fundamental requirement for pharmacodynamic analysis is that there be precise pharmacokinetic information regarding the drug of interest *in the population in question.* Such is gradually becoming available in the pediatric age group.

PHARMACODYNAMIC VARIATION

Pharmacodynamic differences between the responses of pediatric patients and adult patients will be considered in the context of (a) unique effects in children, (b) adverse effects, and (c) therapeutically desired effects. This last category will focus on the catecholamines.

Unique Effects

Drugs may have unique effects in children. Many substances disturb patterns of growth and differentiation that occur only during particular phases of life (94). Notable in this regard are teratogens, which have unique, adverse effects on the fetus (18, 94, 97, 144, 163). To a certain extent, children share this special vulnerability with the fetus until growth and development cease at maturity. Thus, the tetracyclines affect bone growth in the fetus and newborn infant (28), as well as development of the teeth in children less than 6 years of age (66, 194). Corticosteroids, among their other adverse effects, suppress the linear growth of children (93), an effect that cannot occur in adults.

Cartilage toxicity is also a concern with nalidixic acid (170) and related fluoroquinoline antibiotics such as ciprofloxacin and norfloxacin (74, 113). It has been suggested that these newly developed quinoline derivatives, which are likely to have important critical care applications, be avoided in children until skeletal growth is complete (74, 113).

Adverse Effects

INCREASED OCCURRENCE OR SENSITIVITY

Metoclopramide and other dopamine antagonists such as prochlorperazine (Compazine), haloperidol, and chlorpromazine, have a variety of potential critical care indications (82, 100, 141, 183). These drugs produce acute dystonic reactions much more frequently in children and adolescents than in adults (9, 10, 172). A pharmacokinetic basis for this increase in dystonic reactions has been examined and rejected (9). The increase in CNS sensitivity to a variety of dopamine antagonists might be caused by the greater concentration of dopamine-2 receptors in the brains of young subjects (190).

Verapamil, a calcium entry blocking agent, is used to treat supraventricular tachycardia and other atrial dysrhythmias in children (65, 133, 166). There are clinical reports of infants developing acute, severe cardiorespiratory failure following administration of the drug (43, 56, 135). For this reason, verapamil should not be administered to individuals less than 1 year of age (43, 56, 135).

In infants, elastic and resistive properties of the lung entail optimal efficiency at high respiratory rates with low tidal volumes (131). Thus, the resting respiratory rate is higher, and the infant responds to the need for hyperventilation by increasing rate in preference to tidal volume (131). The need to maintain rapid respiratory rates implies greater sensitivity to respiratory depressants. Indeed, some years ago, Way and associates (181) demonstrated that compared with adults, infants required one-third the dose of morphine (on a weight normalized basis) for comparable depression in CO_2 sensitivity. Pharmacokinetic factors were not excluded, and further work on the effect of depressant drugs on the immature respiratory system would be useful.

DECREASED OCCURRENCE OR SENSITIVITY

Children enjoy relative protection from the adverse effects of several drugs. In most cases, the mechanism responsible for the relative immunity of youth has not been determined.

Several drugs cause hepatic injury less frequently in children than in adults. These include isoniazid (6, 41, 49, 116, 167), halothane (20, 24, 45, 96, 99, 180), and acetaminophen (4, 48, 111, 152, 153, 171).

Therapy with isoniazid (INH) is associated with asymptomatic increases in hepatic enzymes in 10–20% of adults (6, 41). In children 9–14 years of age, 17% had elevations of serum glutamic-oxaloacetic transaminase (SGOT) or glutamic-pyruvic transaminase (SGPT), similar to those in adults (167). INH hepatitis, a potentially fatal disorder, develops in some individuals receiving the drug. The risk of developing INH hepatitis increases with age: 0 per 1000 in patients less than 20 years of age, 3 per 1000 for those 20–34 years of age, 12 per 1000 for those 35–49 years old, 23 per 1000 for those 50–65 years of age, and 8 per 1000 for those older than 65 years (49). Despite occasional reports of INH hepatitis in children (167), usually when INH and rifampin are coadministered (116), the incidence is still extremely low, and measurement of SGOT is not routinely performed in children receiving INH alone. Neither the mechanism of INH hepatitis, nor the reason for the relative protection of youth, has been elucidated.

Although there are isolated case reports to the contrary (24, 180), halothane hepatotoxicity appears to be extremely rare in children, even following multiple exposures to the drug, which increases risk in adults (180). Again, the mechanism of protection is unknown.

Acetaminophen produces marked elevation (>1000 IU/liter) of SGOT following ingestion of a substantial overdose (>150 mg/kg) (152). Without administration of an antidote, such as N-acetylcysteine (153), severe hepatitis occurs in 10%, with an associated mortality of 10–20% (48). Of individuals with potentially toxic acetaminophen levels, 5.5% of those less than 12 years of age had SGOT levels above 1000 IU/liter, while 29% of those older than 12 years had an increase of this magnitude (152). The protection conferred by young age has been related to ingestion of relatively small quantities of drug and to early emesis (152, 153). This fact is not the only explanation, since severe hepatotoxicity in children is rare even in the presence of levels associated with severe injury to adults (152). Children younger than about 9 years of age conjugate acetaminophen with sulfate as well as glucuronate (171). It is suggested that this additional pathway of detoxification reduces flux through the mixed function oxidase pathway implicated in acetaminophen hepatotoxicity (152, 171); or, that children have increased availability of glutathione, used to detoxify acetaminophen metabolites (152). These explanations remain speculative. Cases of severe acetaminophen toxicity, and death, have occurred in children (4, 111). Thus, children who ingest a potentially toxic quantity should be fully evaluated and treated with N-acetylcysteine if the concentration of acetaminophen exceeds the "probable risk" line of the Rumack nomogram (153), or if more than 150 mg/kg has been ingested and a serum level cannot be determined within 16 hours of ingestion (152).

Aminoglycoside ototoxicity and nephrotoxicity are probably less common in infants and children than in adults (31, 72, 98, 136). This subject has been recently reviewed (98). There is experimental and clinical evidence that the kidney of the infant or child is more tolerant of aminoglycoside exposure (31, 72). Enzymuria, a marker of renal tubular injury, is less in infants and children following treatment with an aminoglycoside, and there is less renal accumulation of these drugs in infants (72). In an analysis of controlled studies to date, the incidence of cochlear and vestibular toxicity was not found to be greater in infants receiving aminoglycosides than in control subjects (98). The relatively low incidence of aminoglycoside toxicity in infants and children should not be taken as evidence that these drugs are innocuous (98). The usual precautions for minimizing aminoglycoside toxicity, including therapeutic drug monitoring when appropriate, are indicated.

Infants tolerate higher serum concentrations of digoxin than do older children or adults (71, 118, 122), although some investigators dispute this observation (70). Lessened susceptibility to glycoside-induced arrhythmias may be a result of decreased norepinephrine content and sympathetic innervation of ventricular myocardium (54, 70, 80, 122); increased vagal tone (127); and/or a healthier myocardium without superimposed coronary artery disease (122).

Three other points should be mentioned. *First,* the observation that infants tolerate higher concentrations of digoxin without manifesting toxicity does not mean that they require higher concentrations in order to achieve therapeutic benefit. In fact, no therapeutic advantage accrues to maintaining serum digoxin levels greater than those associated with therapeutic efficacy (1–2 ng/ml) in adults (106, 122, 124,

130). Infants with relatively high, and relatively low, digoxin levels have comparable shortening of systolic time intervals (130, 154). An average level of 1.3 ng/ml provides adequate cardiac functional improvement in infants with congestive heart failure (122, 124). *Second,* when normalized by weight, the dose of digoxin needed to achieve a particular digoxin concentration is larger in infants than adults (106, 122, 124). This fact represents a true pharmacokinetic difference between the two populations, and is reflected in different dosage requirements (106, 122). As discussed, this pharmacokinetic observation does not mean that infants are less sensitive to the drug. *Third,* the recent discovery of an endogenous digoxin-like substance that interacts with digoxin assays employing antibody systems (173, 174) means that much of the recent information concerning digoxin pharmacokinetics and dosage in infants and patients with hepatic or renal failure may need revision.

Serious theophylline toxicity is life-threatening and is manifest by seizures and cardiac rhythm disturbances. In adults, these events have been noted at concentrations of less than 50 mg/liter (23, 197). Children seem less sensitive to acute intoxications. In one prospective study, seizures or life-threatening rhythm disturbances did not occur when the concentration was less than 100 mg/liter (57). This observation has been incorporated into guidelines for managing theophylline overdosage in children: aggressive methods for reducing theophylline concentration, such as charcoal hemoperfusion (121) or hemodialysis (84, 132) are avoided in acute intoxications unless the concentration of theophylline exceeds 80–100 mg/liter or a life-threatening event has occurred (1). Peritoneal dialysis is ineffective in removing theophylline (101), and its use is contraindicated.

Therapeutically Desired Effects

CARDIAC GLYCOSIDES

An earlier incorrect belief that infants require higher serum concentrations of digoxin to achieve comparable pharmacologic effect is discussed above.

NEUROMUSCULAR BLOCKING AGENTS

Newborns and infants respond differently from older children and adults to neuromuscular blocking agents. They require smaller dosages of competitive (nondepolarizing) agents such as pancuronium and d-tubocurarine (11, 12, 29, 188, 192). This probably represents a pharmacodynamic increase in sensitivity. Electrophysiologic examination of the young infants' (<12 weeks) neuromuscular junctions indicates similarities to those of adult myasthenics (11). The dose of d-tubocurarine or pancuronium needed to induce paralysis is much lower in young infants: Bennett and associates (12) found that 40 μg/kg of pancuronium produced apnea in the 1-day-old infant, whereas 92 μg/kg was required at one month. Similar results have been reported with d-tubocurarine (11, 188). This difference persists even when d-tubocurarine is prescribed on the basis of surface area (neonate: 4.1 mg/m²; adult: 7.0 mg/m²) (29). The reduced dosage requirement of infants cannot be explained on a pharmacokinetic basis, since clearance is *greater* in infants than in adults (117). In contrast, equal doses of succinylcholine, per unit weight, yield a shorter duration of apnea in infants than in adults (29, 30, 188). On the basis of body weight, infants require twice the adult dose to produce equivalent degrees of blockade (115). The discrepancy is attenuated when dose is normalized to body surface area rather than mass, and a uniform dose of 40 mg/m² produces equivalent duration of effect

Table 7.1
Dosage of Neuromuscular Blocking Drugs in Children[a,b]

Drug	Dose (mg/kg)
Succinylcholine	
Newborns, infants	2
Children, adolescents, adults	1
Pancuronium	
Newborn–1 week	0.03
1–2 weeks	0.06
2–4 weeks	0.09
>4 weeks (continuous infusion 0.1 mg/kg/hr; slightly lower dose may be adequate)	0.1
d-Tubocurarine	
Newborn–1 week	0.2
1–2 weeks	0.3
2–4 weeks	0.4
4–6 weeks	0.5
>6 weeks	0.6

[a] Adapted from Nugent SK, Laravuso R, Rogers MC: Pharmacology and use of muscle relaxants in infants and children. *J Pediatr* 94:481, 1979.
[b] Note that dose of succinylcholine is greater in infants, but doses of pancuronium and d-tubocurarine are smaller.

in infants and adults (29, 188). As discussed in a later section ("Adjustment for Size"), this finding suggests a pharmacokinetic rather than true pharmacodynamic basis for the apparent decrease in sensitivity of infants to succinylcholine. In line with this conclusion, the elimination half-life of succinylcholine is shorter in infants than in older children and adults (188).

Dosage guidelines incorporate these observations, and are summarized in Table 7.1.

SYMPATHOMIMETIC AGENTS

It has been suggested that the immature cardiovascular system responds differently to inotropic agents, including exogenously administered catecholamines. Structural and physiologic cardiovascular differences between the fetus, infant, child, and adult have been summarized (5, 25, 52, 53, 127, 195) and will not be explored in detail. The clinical pharmacology of sympathomimetic agents, particularly the catecholamines, is reviewed in Chapter 31. The following discussion highlights differences between adults, children, and infants that are of particular relevance to the clinical use of catecholamine infusions.

Driscoll and coworkers (38) examined the inotropic response of isolated, perfused ventricles from puppies of different ages as the preparations were exposed to perfusate containing varying concentrations of dopamine and isoproterenol. Figure 7.1 displays the data obtained when dopamine was in the perfusate. Sensitivity increased with increasing puppy age from 0–7 days to 21–33 days. This relationship was ablated by pretreatment with reserpine, and was not noted when isoproterenol was tested. These observations suggested that the blunted inotropic response to dopamine of preparations from younger animals resulted from incomplete sympathetic innervation and reduced norepinephrine stores. Relative deficiencies of sympathetic innervation have been repeatedly demonstrated in newborn animals (52, 54, 58, 127). This fact has not been evaluated in human infants, and the timing of complete myocardial innervation has not been elucidated (54). Others have also observed cardiac subsensitivity to exogenous catecholamines (39, 146). However, results have varied between laboratories, even when the same species was examined. For example, Rockson and associates (146), administered bolus injections of isoproterenol to intact puppies, and unlike

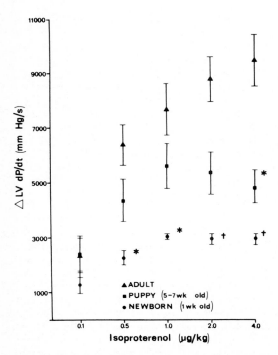

Figure 7.3. Inotropic dose-response curves to isoproterenol for adult, 1-week-old, and 5- to 7-week-old puppies. The mean inotropic response of newborn animals was blunted throughout the dose-response range, and the maximal stimulation was achieved at a much lower dose of isoproterenol at this stage of development. Responses significantly different from adults are noted by *($P < 0.05$) and +($P < 0.01$). (From Rockson SG, Homcy CJ, Quinn P, et al: Cellular mechanisms of impaired adrenergic responsiveness in neonatal dogs. *J Clin Invest* 67:319, 1981.)

Driscoll and associates (38) found that there was a close relationship between age and inotropic response to isoproterenol (Fig. 7.3). Geis and coworkers (58) reported that compared with adult dogs, puppies responded equally well to isoproterenol and exhibited a greater chronotropic response to norepinephrine. Methodologic rather than physiologic differences may play a role in the diversity of these observations. The subtlety of potential experimental artifact was reemphasized by Park and colleagues (123) who showed that the age-dependent difference in inotropic response of right atrial rabbit tissue to isoproterenol disappeared when the preparations were tested at 38°C rather than 26° or 32°C. Thus, the presumed age-dependent difference in inotropic response to β-agonists may be an age-dependent difference in temperature sensitivity.

The immature heart has a greater proportion of noncontractile relative to contractile tissue (52, 53) and has a lower compliance (53, 127, 147, 148). Stroke volume is smaller when normalized to weight (127). Decreased compliance and stroke volume imply that the immature heart has a limited "preload reserve" (53, 127). The increase in stroke volume that follows volume loading is smaller than expected (147, 148). Newborn ventricles exhibit greater interdependence than those from adult animals (147), which is also expected to limit the efficacy of volume loading. A high baseline heart rate (127), coupled with limited ability to augment stroke volume, impairs the ability of the heart to increase cardiac output. Stroke volume may not be augmented by the usual inotropic agents; increases in cardiac output may depend on drug-induced acceleration of heart rate (53, 127). It is in this context that Friedman and George (53) have referred to the limited "total functional reserve" of the infant heart.

The cardiovascular response to catecholamines may also be limited by differences in the number and function of adrenergic receptors. Binding studies of peripheral white blood cells indicate that β-adrenergic receptor number may be reduced in infants and children (140, 143). It is not certain that the number of β-receptors on peripheral white cells reflects the number in the myocardium. Work in the elderly (178) and in patients with heart failure (63) suggests that this fact may be so. Evidence against a role for the adrenergic receptor in neonatal cardiac subsensitization was provided by Rockson and associates (146), who observed that the density of β-adrenergic binding sites was *increased* in immature animals, and that these receptors generated cyclic AMP appropriately, even though the inotropic response to isoproterenol and norepinephrine was reduced. This finding was thought to represent an adaptive response to decreased myocardial innervation, but suggests that diminished number and function of receptors does not play a major role in the limited response of immature animals to catecholamines.

Studies in nonhuman neonates have shown age-related or maturational-related differences in α- and β-adrenergic receptor content of lung, brain, liver, platelets, and fat cells (184). It would not be surprising if these differences produced qualitative and quantitative alterations in noncardiovascular pharmacologic effects of catecholamine infusions. Postnatal changes in vascular responsiveness to adrenergic agents have been extensively explored. Decreased vascular sensitivity to a variety of catecholamines has been a fairly constant (5, 21, 42) but not invariant (42) finding in immature animals. The newborn pig requires a higher dose of isoproterenol than does the adult to reduce vascular resistance (22), and sheep display greater sensitivity to both norepinephrine and isoproterenol with increasing fetal and postnatal age (5). Interestingly, the authors of this study related increasing sensitivity to closure of vascular shunts rather than to maturation of the neuroeffector system. These in vivo experiments are supported by in vitro work with isolated vascular muscle strips and rings, and experiments in which the microvasculature is directly observed. This work has been recently reviewed (42).

In addition to deficiencies in adrenergic innervation and receptor number, the immature cardiovascular system displays limited reflex integration. Hydralazine does not evoke reflex tachycardia in the rat until 14 days of age (8).

In human infants and children, several published clinical studies have evaluated the use of dopamine or dobutamine. Surprisingly, these studies do not provide unambiguous evidence that pediatric patients display a diminished or different response to catecholamines; in fact, the contrary may be true.

Lang and coworkers (86) treated five children (age, 1–24 months; mean age, 8 months) with dopamine following cardiovascular surgery. For the group as a whole, neither heart rate, blood pressure, nor cardiac output increased significantly at infusion rates less than 15 μg/kg/min. Increases in cardiac output were related to higher heart rate rather than greater stroke volume. Adults display increases in blood pressure and cardiac output at infusion rates below 5–10 μg/kg/minute and increases in heart rate below 10 μg/kg/minute (13, 27, 60, 168, 187). Lang's study has been taken to support the view that the cardiovascular system of infants and children is less sensitive to dopamine (53). However, the study was uncontrolled and included a heterogeneous group of patients. Driscoll and associates (40) evaluated dopamine in 24 children (age, 2 days to 18 years; mean age, 39 months) with shock of disparate medical and surgical causes (20 of 24 had congenital heart disease). The infusion was started at 2–10 μg/kg/min and titrated to desired response. More than half of the subjects responded favorably to the infusion ($\geq$15% increase in systolic blood pressure), at a mean dosage in responders of 8.3 $\pm$ 1.5 μg/kg/min. In

this group, blood pressure increased significantly, but heart rate did not. The study design did not permit evaluation of a dose-response relationship. Perez and colleagues (125) observed that a group of five hypotensive newborn infants studied prospectively required a dopamine infusion rate of greater than 20 μg/kg/min to achieve adequate blood pressure, capillary refill, and urine output. The average infusion rate of dopamine required to increase mean arterial pressure from 27 to 54 mm Hg was 25 $\pm$ 10 μg/kg/min, and the highest dosage was 50 μg/kg/min. At this dosage, urine output increased and there was no clinical evidence of cutaneous vasoconstriction. Since infusion rates of this magnitude in adults are often associated with marked peripheral vasoconstriction, Perez and associates interpreted their findings to support the concept of cardiac and peripheral vascular subsensitization to catecholamines during infancy. In contrast, in a placebo-controlled study of infants, DiSessa and associates (35) observed that relatively modest (2.5 μg/kg/min) dosages of dopamine were associated with improvement in blood pressure and myocardial performance, evaluated by echocardiogram; Seri and coworkers (161) made similar observations.

These clinical studies do not permit firm conclusions. The subjects had diverse underlying and coexisting conditions, including structural cardiac disease, recent cardiac operation, asphyxia, pulmonary hypertension, and septicemia. Indications for pressor therapy, volume status, and measure of pharmacologic response were not standardized. A large variety of factors other than age and development, reviewed elsewhere in this text, are known to affect adrenergic receptor function and cardiovascular response to catecholamine infusion (27, 195, 196). These factors were not controlled. Plasma dopamine levels were not measured, and pharmacokinetic data in a population of critically ill children are not available.

Padbury and colleagues (120) incorporated measurement of dopamine concentration with assessment of cardiovascular response in newborn infants. Infusion rates as low as 0.5–1.0 μg/kg/min were associated with important effects on blood pressure and cardiac output. Heart rate increased at infusion rates of 2–3 μg/kg/min. The calculated thresholds for changes in selected hemodynamic functions are listed in Table 7.2. As indicated in Figure 7.4, there was a conventional log-linear relationship between dopamine concentration and several hemodynamic variables. The dopa-

Table 7.2
Concentration of Dopamine and Associated Dopamine Infusion Rate That Produce Threshold Response of Mean Blood Pressure (MBP), Systolic Blood Pressure (SBP), and Heart Rate (HR) in 14 Newborn Infants[a]

Effect	Dopamine Concentration (pg/ml ± SEM)	Infusion Rate (μg/kg/min)
MBP increase	14,000 ± 3500	0.5–1.0
SBP increase	18,000 ± 4500	1–2
HR increase	35,000 ± 5000	2–3

[a]Data from Padbury JF, Agata Y, Baylen BG, et al: Dopamine pharmacokinetics in critically ill newborn infants. *J Pediatr* 294:293, 1987.

mine clearance reported by Padbury and associates was 48–60 ml/kg/min, and did not correlate with age or birth weight. Clearance values of this magnitude have been observed in the pediatric age group by other workers (Notterman, unpublished data; Zaritsky, personal communication, 1987), and are not appreciably different from those recorded in studies of adults (68, 77). This excludes a pharmacokinetic basis for Padbury's observation that newborn infants are as sensitive to dopamine as older children or adults. Table 7.3 summarizes several studies of dopamine pharmacodynamics and pharmacokinetics.

The hemodynamic effects of dobutamine in children have been examined in several studies (15, 37, 126, 156, 169). None contains pharmacokinetic measurements, and such information has not been developed in the pediatric age group. Detailed pharmacodynamic and kinetic information is available for healthy and acutely ill adults (79, 89, 90).

Age-related differences in response to dobutamine have not been consistently observed. In addition to the anticipated increase in cardiac output and stroke volume, Driscoll and Gillette (37) found a fairly consistent increase in systemic vascular resistance, contrary to the behavior of adults with congestive heart failure (81, 89). Driscoll's subjects had structural con-

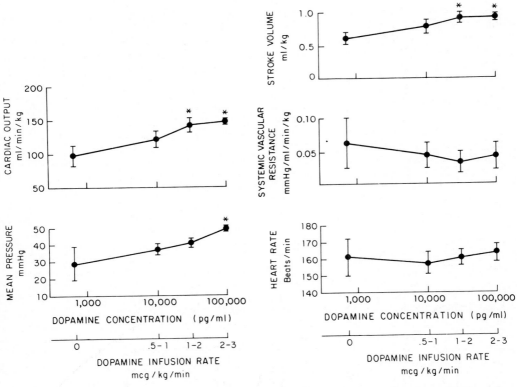

Figure 7.4. Sequential cardiac output, mean arterial pressure, stroke volume, systemic vascular resistance, and heart rate in four infants during dopamine infusions. Dopamine infusion rates are ranges calculated from dopamine clearance values. (Adapted and redrawn from Padbury JF, Agata Y, Baylen BG, et al: Dopamine pharmacokinetics in critically ill newborn infants. *J Pediatr* 294:293, 1987.)

Table 7.3
Dopamine Response Threshold for Heart Rate (HR), Systolic Blood Pressure (SBP), Systemic Vascular Resistance (SVR), and Stroke Volume (SV) in Selected Studies[a,b]

Investigators	No. of Subjects	Age (Condition)	Response Threshold								Clearance (ml/kg/min)
			Infusion Rate (μg/kg/min)				Dopamine Concentration (ng/ml)				
			HR	SBP	SVR	SV	HR	SBP	SVR	SV	
Lang et al (86)	5	1–24 months (post CVS)	15	15	NS	NS (CO-15)	Not measured				NM
Driscoll et al (40)	24	1.7–18 years (20–24 post CVS)	NS	8.3°	NM	NM	Not measured				NM
Seri et al (161)	18	Premature infant (hyaline membrane disease)	8	2	NM	NM	Not measured				NM
Padbury et al (120)	14	Premature/term infants (medical shock)	2–3	0.5–1.0	NM	NM	35	18	NM	NM	48–60
Jarnberg et al (77)	10	32–61 years (post elective surgery)	5†	5†	NM	NM	79	79	NM	NM	70–75
Gundert-Remy et al (68)	5	24–34 years (healthy adults)	6*	6*	NM	NM	74	74	NM	NM	61–85

[a] Data from references 40, 68, 77, 86, 120, 161.
[b] For studies involving adults, only those in which dopamine concentration was measured are included. Response threshold in terms of plasma dopamine concentration and infusion rate is included when available. NS, no significant change at dosage range tested; NM, variable not measured; °, group mean; †, 2 or 5 μg/kg/min tested, no intermediate infusion rate; *, approximate infusion rates calculated from data provided by author; CVS, cardiovascular surgery.

genital heart disease, and most were not in heart failure—these differences, rather than age, probably account for the disparity. Perkin and Levin (126) found dobutamine to be effective in augmenting cardiac output and stroke volume in a variety of conditions associated with shock. Subjects younger than 12 months displayed a trend (not statistically significant) toward an attenuated response to the inotropic effect of the drug. These younger subjects also responded to infusion of dobutamine with an increase in pulmonary capillary wedge pressure. An adverse effect on pulmonary capillary wedge pressure has not been observed in other studies involving children or adults, and would stand as one of the few documented differences between the responses of infants and adults to catecholamine infusion. In newborn infants with "heart failure" of diverse etiology, Stopfkuchen and associates (169) found that abnormal left ventricular systolic time intervals changed significantly during infusion of dobutamine. This change was associated with a significant chronotropic effect. Schranz and coworkers (156) documented a substantial positive inotropic effect with little acceleration of heart rate in 12 children with shock of various etiologies.

In children emerging from cardiopulmonary bypass, dobutamine may not be a desirable agent because of undesirable chronotropy and slight improvement in stroke volume (17). A small left ventricle is thought to limit the inotropic effect of dobutamine in children who are recovering from repair of tetralogy of Fallot (15). In these children, increases in cardiac output depend on dobutamine-associated increases in heart rate. More work will be needed to clarify the relative importance of development, type of structural lesion, and cardiopulmonary bypass in producing these differences.

Work in infants and adults has not as yet documented systematic age-related differences in catecholamine pharmacokinetics or pharmacodynamics. This fact is surprising because of the extensive work in animals that supports reduced responsiveness to catecholamines in the young. The extent of our knowledge in humans, however, is limited by methodologic problems and by the virtual absence of pharmacokinetic data in infants and children. There is detailed pharmacokinetic and pharmacodynamic information concerning each of the clinically employed catecholamines in healthy and, to a limited extent, critically ill adults (32, 33, 47, 62, 88, 89, 165). Recent developments in analytic chemistry presage an exten-

sion of this knowledge to the pediatric age group and to critically ill patients of any age.

PHARMACOKINETIC VARIATION

The weight of the average 18-year-old male, 63 kg, exceeds that of the average term newborn infant, 3.4 kg (94), by a factor of 19. Expressed in terms of surface area, this factor becomes 8.5. Thus, it is not surprising that infants and children require smaller dosages than adults. In this section, the effect of changing size and function on pharmacokinetics will be examined. Such alterations affect each of the major aspects of drug disposition: absorption, distribution (including protein binding), biotransformation, and excretion of changed and unchanged drug (18, 106, 142, 151). Lack of awareness of the need to account for altered function as well as altered size has been responsible for serious therapeutic misadventures such as the "gray syndrome" (182) of the 1960s (neonatal chloramphenicol toxicity) and the "gasping syndrome" (50, 59) of the 1980s (neonatal benzyl alcohol toxicity).

Special Problems in Drug Delivery to Children

Children require and tolerate smaller volumes of intravenous fluid than do adults. This fact limits the volume of intravenously administered fluid in which a drug can be diluted and the maximum rate at which the drug can be infused. These problems are magnified by the imposition of fluid limits associated with critical cardiac, respiratory, or renal disease.

Dilution volumes of intravenous medications can be adjusted, but physical properties of many drugs, as well as concern for safety, place a limit on maximum drug concentration. Current recommendations for dilution of several drugs employed in pediatric critical care are listed in Table 7.4. These recommendations (51, 110) are based on both clinical observation and pharmaceutical information concerning solubility and stability, but may not have been subjected to experimental testing.

Low intravenous flow rates result in a substantial delay before delivery of drug actually starts or is completed. The magnitude of this delay depends on the rate of infusion, the drug dosage volume, and the site of introduction of

Table 7.4
Maximum Drug Concentrations for Intravenous Infusion in Infants and Children[a,b]

Drug	Concentration
Antibiotics	
Acyclovir	7 mg/ml
Amikacin	6 mg/ml
Amphotericin	0.1 mg/ml
Beta-lactam	50–100 mg/ml
Chloramphenicol	50–100 mg/ml
Clindamycin	6 mg/ml
Erythromycin lactobionate	5 mg/ml
Gentamicin	2 mg/ml
Imipenem	5 mg/ml
Kanamycin	6 mg/ml
Metronidazole	8 mg/ml
Penicillin G	50–100,000 units/ml
Sulfamethoxazole/trimethoprim	1 ml/15 ml
Tobramycin	2 mg/ml
Vancomycin	5 mg/ml
Vidarabine	0.45 mg/ml
Miscellaneous	
Aminophylline	1 mg/ml
Bretylium tosylate	10 mg/ml
Catecholamine	Varies
Ethacrynate	1 mg/ml
Lidocaine	Varies
Magnesium sulfate	10 mg/ml
Methyldopa	10 mg/ml

[a] Adapted from Nelson JD: *Pocketbook of Pediatric Antimicrobial Therapy,* ed 7. Baltimore, Williams & Wilkins, 1987; Ford DC, Leist ER, Algren JT: *Guidelines for Administration of Intravenous Medications to Pediatric Patients,* ed 2. Bethesda, American Society of Hospital Pharmacists, 1984; and information provided by manufacturers.
[b] Intravenous push injection, when appropriate, may require different dilution. Information represents literature consensus and may not have been evaluated by appropriate pharmaceutical tests.

the drug into the intravenous tubing. The length of delay can be surprising. For example, when drug is added to the fluid reservoir of a system in which the rate of flow is 25 ml/hr, delivery of drug does not begin for nearly 2 hours and is not complete for 4 hours (145). Delayed drug delivery has several untoward consequences, which were recently summarized by Roberts (125). (a) In one study, 36% of the total daily dose of certain intravenous medications was inadvertently discarded when intravenous sets were routinely changed. (b) Therapeutic drug monitoring becomes inaccurate when the precise time of delivery of drug cannot be determined. (c) When the rate of infusion is less than or equal to the drug's elimination rate, plasma drug levels will be negligible. Clearly,

precise knowledge of the characteristics of drug delivery systems must be an important consideration in devising treatment plans.

Gould, Roberts, and Leff (64, 87, 145) evaluated several methods of intravenous drug delivery; based on their experiments, they developed a plan for the selection of an appropriate drug delivery system (Figs. 7.5 and 7.6). The reader is referred to the original publications for details (64, 87, 145).

Absorption

Absorption of drug occurs from the gastrointestinal tract (mouth, stomach, small intestine, rectum), from intramuscular or subcutaneous sites of injection, from the skin, and from lung. Agents that are administered by vein or artery bypass the process of absorption.

The effect of age on enteral absorption is not uniform and is difficult to predict. Newborns absorb drugs more slowly, but not necessarily less completely than older children and adults (18, 105, 106, 144). Drugs known to be well absorbed when given orally to adults may not be available in a form suitable for administration to young children. For example, when isoniazid tablets are crushed and administered with applesauce, as some recommend, the INH is poorly absorbed. This practice has led to failed treatment of tuberculous meningitis (114). Untested, extemporaneous forms of medication should not be administered to children.

Absorption from intramuscular sites has not been broadly examined in children, although some antibiotics display excellent bioavailability (78, 109). This route is not recommended for use with critically ill children.

In the past, rectal suppository administration was frequently prescribed for drugs such as phenobarbital, aspirin, acetaminophen, aminophylline, belladonna, opium, and others. Rectal suppository administration is generally not desirable in the critical care setting, and many substances are slowly and unpredictably absorbed by this route (18). Therapeutic failure and severe intoxication have occurred with rectal administration of aminophylline (18, 112). Recently, however, rectal administration of solutions of diazepam or sodium valproate (104, 176) has been suggested for control of status epilepticus.

Transdermal drug delivery has not been exploited in therapy of children. Since percutaneous absorption is facilitated by the relatively thin stratum corneum of the infant and child

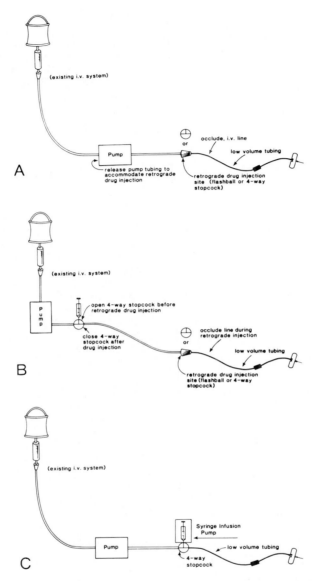

Figure 7.5. A, Construction of an intravenous system for manual retrograde injection. An injection site (flashball or stopcock) and low-volume extension tubing are located at the distal end of the existing intravenous set-up. **B,** Construction of intravenous system for retrograde injection modified for a volume infusion pump device unable to accept retrograde injection. System consists of existing intravenous set-up to which is attached an extension set with a proximal four-way stopcock and distal flashball injection site. A large-volume syringe is attached to the four-way stopcock and acts as an overflow reservoir for the intravenous fluid displaced by the dose volume. **C,** Construction of mechanical (syringe) infusion system. A four-way stopcock and low-volume extension tubing are attached distal to the existing intravenous system. The dosing syringe is attached directly to the four-way stopcock before placement on the syringe infusion device. For details see original sources. (Adapted from Leff RD, Roberts RJ: Methods of intravenous drug administration in the pediatric patient. *J Pediatr* 98:681, 1981; and Roberts RJ: Intravenous administration of medications in pediatric patients: problems and solutions. *Pediatr Clin North Am* 28:23, 1986.)

Steps

#1.   On admission establish only a "basic" I.V. set-up which includes I.V. fluid container, volume control device (Metriset) and associated I.V. tubing connected directly to venous catheter (butterfly, abocath, etc.).

#2.   On the basis of **I.V. FLOW RATE** and **DOSE VOLUME** select the appropriate system (retrograde or syringe infusion).

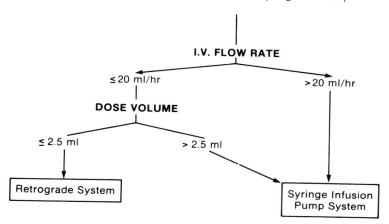

Figure 7.6.   Selection of an appropriate method (retrograde versus syringe infusion pump system) for intravenous drug administration based on intravenous flow rate and dose volume. (From Roberts RJ: Intravenous administration of medications in pediatric patients: problems and solutions. *Pediatr Clin North Am* 28:23, 1986.)

(106), both therapeutic and toxic effects of topically applied substances will be greater than in adults. Numerous examples of inadvertent systemic absorption and toxicity in infants have been recorded (26, 46, 61, 76, 107, 150, 155, 162, 189). The pediatric intensive care physician should be cautious about application of presumably innocuous substances to the integument of these patients. Viscous lidocaine has produced seizures following topical application to the oral mucosa (150), and delirium has been reported after administration of aerosolized tripelennamine, an antihistamine (155).

Intraosseous administration of emergency medications has been reintroduced (14, 75, 119, 164). The technique is simple, rapid, and is not associated with major complications. Following intraosseous administration, brisk appearance in the bloodstream has been documented for several emergency drugs: catecholamines, calcium, bicarbonate, blood, colloid, and saline (119, 164). Intraosseous administration permits continuous infusion of catecholamines and resuscitation fluid, and permits bolus injection of most standard emergency medications. This is an important advantage over the intratracheal route (179). Con-

sidering the difficulty in securing vascular access during a cardiorespiratory or hemodynamic emergency, intraosseous administration is the method of choice for administration of emergency drugs and fluids when intravenous access cannot be secured within a few minutes. This method is preferred over intracardiac administration (119).

Distribution

Distribution refers to the movement of drug from the central compartment to peripheral compartments and ultimately, to the site of action and elimination. Changes in volume of distribution (V_d) result in reciprocal changes in the drug concentration (C) following a single drug dose or during repetitive drug dosing (see Chapter 1).

Distribution is affected by several parameters, including the cardiac output, individual organ blood flow, composition and relative size of body compartments, pH of body fluids, and extent of drug binding to plasma proteins and peripheral tissues (79, 83, 106, 151). Important age-related changes include differ-

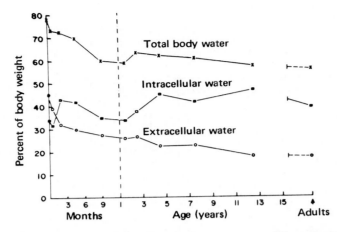

Figure 7.7. Developmental changes in total body, intracellular, and extracellular water in infants and children. The changes are expressed as percentages of body weight. (From Rane A, Wilson JT: Clinical pharmacokinetics in infants and children. In Gibaldi M, Prescott L (eds): *Handbook of Clinical Pharmacokinetics.* New York, ADIS Health Science Press, 1983. Data from Friis-Hansens B: *Pediatrics* 28:169, 1961.)

ences in body composition and protein binding.

BODY COMPOSITION

In the neonate, infant, and child, the various body compartments have a different absolute and relative size than in adults. The size and composition of these compartments vary continuously. As indicated in Figure 7.7, total body water (expressed as percentage of body weight) decreases from about 80% in the newborn infant to 60% in the adult, whereas extracellular water (ECW) decreases from 45% to 20% during the same interval (138). Conversely, expressed as a function of body surface area, ECW is relatively constant (7, 18). As a percentage of body mass, adipose tissue doubles during the first year of life. In the infant, skeletal muscle mass is reduced, and the brain and liver are much larger in relation to body weight than they are in the adult (106).

PROTEIN BINDING

Many drugs are less avidly bound to plasma proteins in the neonate and infant than they are in the older patient (18, 106, 144, 191). Decreased binding affects acidic drugs (e.g., phenytoin), which are bound to albumin (175), as well as basic drugs (e.g., lidocaine), which are bound to α_1-glycoprotein (16, 128, 191). Reduced binding to plasma proteins is associated with at least three potentially important effects: (a) increase in apparent volume of distribution (V_d) (144); (b) decrease in the total

plasma drug concentration following a standard dosage (151, 185); and (c) decrease in the range of total plasma drug concentrations associated with both therapeutic efficacy and toxicity. These effects are important for extensively protein-bound drugs that have a low hepatic extraction ratio (151, 185).

Although the protein binding of many drugs is reduced in the newborn, these observations have not been extended into later infancy (105, 106, 144). Reduced binding is of definite clinical importance for drugs that are both extensively bound and subject to therapeutic drug monitoring. Phenytoin (91, 175) is the usual example. When an infant or young child is treated with this anticonvulsant, the free rather than the total phenytoin concentration should be monitored. Other extensively bound drugs with reduced binding in early infancy include quinidine (129), diazepam (108), furosemide (108), some antibiotics (18, 106), propranolol, and thiopental (18). However, the effect on therapy has not been delineated, and it would be incorrect to assume that these alterations in protein binding must be clinically important. Further investigation is warranted. Protein binding of certain neuromuscular blocking agents is reduced in infancy (188, 192), but the substances are so weakly bound in adults (192) that this observation is not likely to have clinical significance.

Changes in protein binding affect other kinetic functions and calculations, including clearance and volume of distribution. These are reviewed in Chapter 1 and in several publications (106, 144, 151, 175, 177, 185), which include a discussion of the manner in which efficiency of hepatic extraction interacts with the extent of protein binding to affect total and unbound drug clearance. The net effect of greater ECW, diminished protein binding, and the relatively large brain and liver in the infant is to increase, on a weight-normalized basis, the V_d of most drugs (106, 151). This change in V_d does not necessarily entail a larger dosage of these drugs, because of the countervailing influence of reduced elimination.

Binding of unconjugated bilirubin to plasma proteins is affected by drug therapy (18). This subject has been extensively reviewed, and is not considered in this chapter.

Elimination

Elimination of drug from the body occurs by two processes: biotransformation (metabolism) and excretion (91, 151). Age-related differences in both processes are well described and are of clinical importance.

BIOTRANSFORMATION

Drug biotransformation is divided into two phases: phase 1 and phase 2 (186). Phase 1 reactions are catalyzed by oxidoreductases and hydroxylases, which produce carboxyl, epoxide, hydroxyl, amino, and sulfur groups (36, 95). These reactive groups promote elimination and permit phase 2 conjugation reactions with moieties such as acetate, amino acids, glucuronic acid, sulfate, and glutathione. Conjugation leads to more polar products that are readily eliminated via the kidney or gastrointestinal tract. The hepatic contribution to biotransformation is the largest and best characterized (177). Hepatic phase 1 and phase 2 reactions are both depressed in the neonate, but increase during later infancy and childhood, often to rates much greater than those seen in the adult (106).

Phase 1 Reactions

Phase 1 biotransformation of many drugs is slow in newborn infants (105, 106, 144). At birth, the cytochrome P-450 content of the liver is only 28% of the adult level. Activity of a variety of monooxygenases is depressed to less than 50% of adult activity (177). Depressed rates of metabolism persist for a variable but substantial period of time. Table 7.5 indicates selected compounds that display im-

Table 7.5
Selected Drugs That Undergo Oxidation: Plasma Half-lives in Full-term Newborns and Adults[a]

Drug	Elimination Half-life (hr)	
	Newborns	Adults
Aminopyrine	30–40	2–4
Bupivacaine	25	1.3
Caffeine	95	4
Carbamazepine	8–28	21–36
Diazepam	25–100	15–25
Indomethacin	14–20	2–11
Lidocaine	2.9–3.3	1.0–2.2
Meperidine	22	3–4
Mepivacaine	8.7	3.2
Nortriptyline	56	18–22
Phenobarbital	28–43	36–38
Phenylbutazone	21–34	12–30
Phenytoin	21	11–29
Theophylline	24–36	3–9
Tolbutamide	10–40	4.4–9

[a] Adapted from Rane A: Basic principle of drug disposition and action. In Yaffe SJ (ed): *Pediatric Pharmacology*. New York, Grune & Stratton, 1980; and Morselli PL, Franco-Morselli R, Bossi L: Clinical pharmacokinetics in newborns and infants. *Clin Pharmacokinet* 5:485, 1980.

paired oxidation reactions. This category of reaction is most consistently impaired in the newborn period (95, 137). In contrast, demethylation reactions, as illustrated by diazepam, are relatively intact (18, 106), indicating that each class of compound must be individually evaluated.

As expected, the newborn and young infant display reduced oxidative activity toward theophylline and caffeine. Instead of undergoing N-demethylation as in adults, theophylline is N-methylated to caffeine (69), a compound with similar biologic activity. By 7–9 months of age, the adult metabolic pattern is attained (69). This fact illustrates that not only is biotransformation slower, as a rule, in early infancy, but the end products may be different.

Deficient phase 1 activity is not limited to the mixed function oxidase system. Other enzymes known to be deficient in the newborn are reviewed elsewhere (95, 106, 107), and include (with their substrates in parentheses) alcohol dehydrogenase (ethyl alcohol, methyl alcohol, chloral hydrate), plasma esterase (local anesthetics), and N-acetyltransferase (INH, hydralazine) (102).

Phase 2 Reactions

Conjugation reactions are also limited at birth. Glucuronic acid conjugation is severely im-

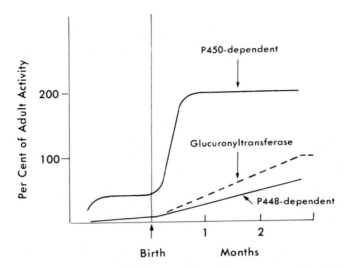

Figure 7.8. Developmental pattern of cytochrome P-450– and P-448–dependent reactions and of UDP-glucuronyltransferase in human liver. (From Vessey DA: Hepatic metabolism of drugs and toxins. In Zakim D, Boyer TD (eds): *Hepatology.* Philadelphia, WB Saunders, 1982.)

paired for some (not all) compounds; this is implicated in intoxication with chloramphenicol (182). Sulfate and glycine conjugation are well preserved in the neonate, and sulfonation of steroids occurs at near adult rates (95). Thus, as with phase 1 reactions, generalization regarding the effect of immaturity on phase 2 reactions can be misleading. Each reaction must be individually evaluated.

Maturation of Biotransformation

Concurrent with the maturation of hepatic biotransformation (Fig. 7.8), there is a dramatic acceleration of the elimination rates of many compounds (106, 151). Beyond early infancy, children metabolize many substances more rapidly than do adults. As Morselli and associates (106) indicate, disposition rates that are less than 30% of adult values in the newborn become several-fold greater than adult values by the end of the first year of life. The intensive care physician caring for infants and children thus encounters a heterogeneous population of subjects with regard to drug elimination. Figures 7.9 and 7.10 vividly illustrate the effect of age on elimination half-life ($t_{1/2}$) and maintenance dosage requirement. Detailed information about maturation of hepatic biotransformation is available (18, 95, 106, 144, 151, 177).

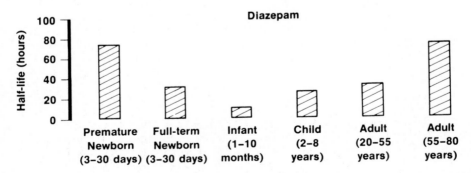

Figure 7.9. The elimination half-life of diazepam is shortest in the infant and longest in the newborn and the elderly. (From Rowland M, Tozer TN: *Clinical Pharmacokinetics.* Philadelphia, Lea & Febiger, 1980. Adapted from the data of Morselli PL: *Drug Disposition During Development.* New York, Spectrum Publications, 1977; and Klotz U, Avant GR, Hoyumpa A, et al: The effect of age and liver disease on the disposition and elimination of diazepam in adult man. *J Clin Invest* 55:347, 1975.)

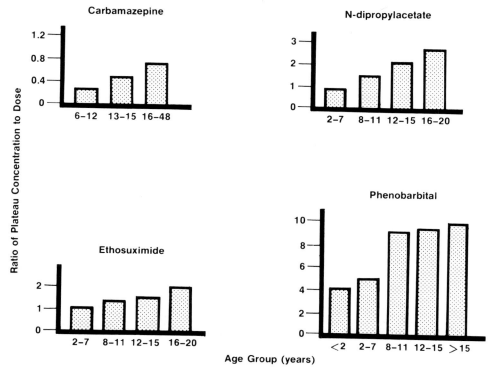

Figure 7.10. Plateau plasma drug concentrations of several antiepileptic drugs after chronic oral medication in children. An increased clearance per kilogram of body weight explains the lower ratio of concentration:dose per kilogram in the youngest children. (From Rowland M, Tozer TN: *Clinical Pharmacokinetics.* Philadelphia, Lea & Febiger, 1980. Adapted from the data of Morselli PL: Antiepileptic drugs. In Morselli PL (ed): *Drug Disposition During Development.* New York, Spectrum Publications, 1977.)

RENAL ELIMINATION

At birth, many aspects of renal function are reduced, even when normalized to body weight or to surface area. In full-term neonates, the glomerular filtration rate (GFR) is 2–4 ml/min (15 ml/min/1.73 m^2) (3, 67). It doubles during the first 2 weeks of life. When normalized to surface area, adult rates of filtration (90–130 ml/min/1.73 m^2) are achieved by 6 months of age (3). Thereafter, there is a linear relation between GFR and body surface area (Fig. 7.11). Tubular function is also reduced in the newborn, and maturation of tubular function is slower than maturation of glomerular filtration (18). Neonates display decreased transport capacity for a variety of substances, including acids, bases, glucose, protein, and bicarbonate (3, 67, 106).

Many substances are eliminated by the kidney in unchanged form. Whether it be due to immaturity or to disease, reduced renal function decreases clearance and prolongs elimination half-life. This may entail a reduction in

dosage. Rane and Wilson (138) have elegantly shown how reduced glomerular filtration or tubular secretion in the infant can affect drug $t_{1/2}$. They examined two drugs—p-aminohippurate, assumed to be eliminated exclusively by tubular secretion, and inulin, assumed to be eliminated exclusively by glomerular filtration. Based on age-appropriate V_d and measured total body clearances (Cl) for these substances, it is simple to calculate resulting elimination half-life, since:

$$t_{1/2} = \frac{0.693 \times V_d}{Cl} \tag{1}$$

The calculations are shown in Table 7.6. Inulin, representing drugs that are cleared by filtration (e.g., aminoglycosides), displays a 50% increase in its $t_{1/2}$ in the infant compared with the adult. p-Aminohippurate, representing drugs cleared by tubular secretion (e.g., penicillin), displays a 3-fold increase in its $t_{1/2}$. These theoretic calculations conform reasonably well to measured values (134). As renal

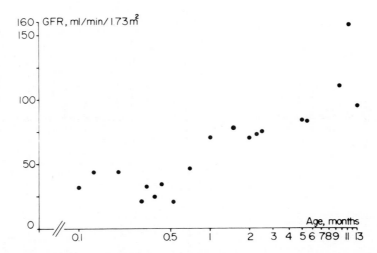

Figure 7.11. Glomerular filtration rate *(GFR)* during the first year of life, related to the logarithm of age. Determined by inulin disappearance curve. (From Aperia A, Broberger O, Thodenius K, et al: Development of renal control of salt and fluid homeostasis during the first year of life. *Acta Paediatr Scand* 64:393, 1975.)

function matures (Fig. 7.11), these values approach those seen in adults.

Generalization is problematic, since renal elimination of some drugs is either unchanged in infancy (e.g., colistin) (134) or actually greater than in adults. The latter is the case for lidocaine (103) and digoxin (122), and may represent maturation of filtration prior to tubular reabsorptive function (124).

Digoxin elimination provides an interesting example of maturation of renal function. In neonates, clearance of this drug is lower than in older infants and children, reflecting immature rates of filtration and elimination (106, 122). Clearance of digoxin increases between the 2nd and 3rd month of life, to the extent that it is greater in children than in adults (92, 106, 122). A portion of this increase in clearance can be attributed to the fact that the V_d of digoxin is 1.5–2 times greater in the child than the adult ($Cl = K_e \times V_d$, where K_e is elimi-

nation rate constant). An additional factor is that in children, but not adults, glomerular filtration of digoxin is augmented by secretion (92). During adolescence, net tubular secretion and total renal clearance of digoxin decrease toward adult values. This decrease is correlated with sexual maturity stage (Tanner stage 4–5) rather than chronologic age (92). A relationship between sexual maturity (rather than size or age) and drug elimination rate may also have significance for drugs other than digoxin.

Impairment of Renal Drug Elimination by Disease

Serum creatinine is lower in the pediatric age group than in healthy adults. By the 5th day of life, the plasma creatinine is 0.40 ± 0.02 mg/dl (67). During the balance of childhood (up to 18 years of age), creatinine values are

Table 7.6
Calculation of Half-life for a Proposed Drug with the Same Clearance as Inulin (Glomerular Filtration) or p-Aminohippuric Acid (PAH) (Tubular Secretion) in an Infant (1.5 months old) and Adult[a,b]

Weight (kg)	ECW			Inulin		PAH	
	% of Weight	Total Volume (ml)		Clearance (ml/min)	$t_{1/2}$ (min)	Clearance (ml/min)	$t_{1/2}$ (min)
4.5	32	1,440		10	100	25	40
70.0	18	12,600		130	67	650	13

[a] From Rane EM, Gilman AG: Pharmacodynamics: mechanisms of drug action and the relationship between drug concentration and effect. In Gilman AG, Goodman LS, Roll TW, Murad F (eds): *The Pharmacological Basis of Therapeutics*, ed 7. New York, Macmillan, 1985.
[b] The drug distributes in the extracellular water space (ECW). Calculation is based on $t_{1/2} = 0.693 \times V_d \times Cl^{-1}$.

Table 7.7
Method for Calculating Cl_{cr} in Children Aged 1 Week to 21 Years[a,b]

Cl_{cr} (ml/min/1.73 m^2) = length (cm) × k/P_{cr} (mg/dl)	
Age	k
Infant (1–52 weeks)	0.45
Child (1–13 years)	0.55
Adolescent (14–21 years)	
Male	0.7
Female	0.55

[a]Based on Schwartz and associates (157–159).
[b]This method is valid for individuals without severe muscle wasting and with stable plasma creatinine (P_{cr}) values.

lower than 0.8 mg/dl in healthy individuals (160), reflecting lesser muscle mass. Creatinine values that would be considered normal in young and middle-aged adults can represent significant degrees of renal dysfunction in the child.

Modifying drug dosage to account for impaired renal function depends on an estimate of the extent of impairment. This usually involves measurement or estimation of creatinine clearance. Timed urine collection is difficult in the child, and may not be complete before therapeutic decisions are necessary. However, unless age is taken into account, an isolated serum creatinine measurement does not provide an accurate estimate of renal function. For example, at 6 months of age, a serum creatinine value of 1.0 mg/dl is associated with a clearance of approximately 30 ml/min/1.73 m^2. At 20 years, the same creatinine level indicates a clearance of approximately 115 ml/min/1.73 m^2. Fortunately, it is possible to accurately estimate creatinine clearance from knowledge of the patient's age, sex, length, and plasma creatinine (157–159). The equation and appropriate constants are indicated in Table 7.7.

Adjustment of dosage in renal failure is discussed in detail in Chapter 3, and is briefly considered here. The creatinine clearance is estimated using the method indicated in Table 7.7. The following equation is used to estimate corrected dosage:

$$D_r = D_n \times [1 - f(1 - R)] \qquad (2)$$

where R, the fraction of remaining renal function, is given by

$$R = \frac{\text{estimated } Cl_{cr} \text{ of patient (per 1.73 m}^2)}{\text{normal } Cl_{cr} \text{ for age (per 1.73 m}^2)} \qquad (3)$$

During the first year of life, normal Cl_{cr} for age is estimated as shown in Table 7.7. Subse-

quently, it is assumed to be 100 ml/min/1.73 m^2. Other terms in Equation 2 are as follows: f, fraction of drug excreted unchanged by the kidney in a normal subject (Table 7.8); D_r, daily dose during renal failure; and D_n, daily dose in a normal subject (of the same age). D_r, the total daily dose during renal failure, can be delivered by administering the usual dose at an extended interval, or by offering a reduced dose at the usual interval. It may be most appropriate both to reduce individual dose and to extend dosing interval. Further details are available in a number of publications (2, 34, 44, 142, 151).

EXAMPLE: A 3-year-old child (weight, 15 kg; length, 96 cm) with a serum creatinine of 1.2 mg/dl requires gentamicin ($f = 1.0$). The usual dosage for this age is 5 mg/kg/day (75

Table 7.8
Fraction of Dose Excreted Unchanged in Urine (f) with Normal Renal Function[a,b]

Drug	f
Antibiotics	
*Acyclovir	0.9
*Aminoglycosides	1.0
*Ampicillin	0.9
Amphotericin	0
Erythromycin	0.1
*Cefazolin	0.7
Cefoperazone	0.3
*Cefoxitin	0.9
*Ceftazidime	0.9
*Cefuroxime	0.9
Chloramphenicol	0
*Ganciclovir	1.0
*Imipenem/cilastin	0.7
*Methicillin	0.9
Nafcillin	<0.2
*Oxacillin	0.8
*Penicillin	0.9
Rifampin	0
*Sulfamethoxazole	0.9
*Trimethoprim	0.7
*Vancomycin	1.0
Miscellaneous	
*Cimetidine	0.8
*Digoxin	0.7
*Lithium	1.0
*Ranitidine	0.7

[a]From Rowland M, Tozer TN: *Clinical Pharmacokinetics*. Philadelphia, Lea & Febiger, 1980; Nelson JD: *Pocketbook of Pediatric Antimicrobial Therapy*, ed 7. Baltimore, Williams & Wilkins, 1987; and manufacturers' information.
[b]f may change in the presence of renal or hepatic disease. *Indicates that dosage reduction may be necessary with clinically significant renal dysfunction. Individual product information should be consulted.

mg), divided into three 8-hourly doses. The corrected dosage for this child is calculated as follows:

1. Creatinine clearance of patient:

$$Cl_{cr} = \frac{0.55 \times 96 \text{ cm}}{1.2 \text{ mg/dl}}$$

$$= 44 \text{ ml/min/m}^2$$

2. Calculation of dosage:

$$R = \frac{44 \text{ ml/min/m}^2}{100 \text{ ml/min/m}^2}$$

$$= 0.44$$

$$D_r = 75 \text{ mg/day} \times [1 - 1.0 \ (1 - 0.44)]$$

$$= 33 \text{ mg/day}$$

This dosage can be given at the usual (8-hour interval, 11 mg every 8 hours, or at an extended interval, 33 mg every 24 hours. The 8-hourly schedule prevents prolonged subtherapeutic concentrations, whereas the 24-hourly schedule permits the usual peak, trough, and mean drug concentrations.

This presentation does not take into account excretion of products of hepatic drug metabolism by the kidney or the effect of altered renal function on drug metabolism in the liver and other organs. These subjects are reviewed in Chapters 1–6 and elsewhere (2, 144, 151).

Exchange Transfusion

Exchange transfusion is performed in neonates for control of hyperbilirubinemia. In older infants and children, this procedure is occasionally advocated for therapy of diverse hematologic and metabolic conditions. Usually, a double volume exchange is performed, although "partial" exchange transfusions employing lesser volumes are occasionally employed. Exchange of the blood volume represents an additional mode of elimination and perturbs distribution. Lackner (85) presented the following equation for estimating the fraction of drug removed (f_x) as a result of an exchange transfusion:

$$f_x = 1 - e^{-V/V_d} \qquad (4)$$

In most instances, the amount of drug loss is trivial (<20%). With the possible exception of theophylline ($f_x = 32.4\%$), specific drug replacement is not necessary unless exchanges are numerous or greater than two blood volumes.

Adjustment for Size

Adjusting dosage to body size can be complex: Ritschel (142) was able to count no less than 23 separate approaches, employing a total of 52 different equations! Most methods involve adjustment for body weight or adjustment for body surface area.

Adjustments for body weight have the advantage of simplicity and familiarity. In most reference sources, pediatric dosages are presented in terms of body weight. The theoretic and practical objection to this method is that the weight-normalized dosage of many drugs increases as weight decreases. If a constant per unit weight dosage is employed, small individuals (children) will receive too small a dose.

Basing dosage on surface area has the apparent advantage of *approximating* constant dosage over a wide range of body size and age. This supposition is illustrated in Figure 7.12 for theophylline (193), and was discussed earlier in connection with succinylcholine. It is true of a variety of drugs used in critical care (18, 55).

The relative linearity between surface area

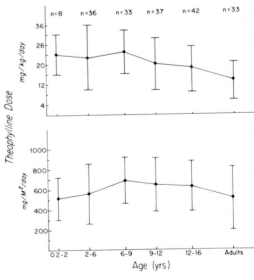

Figure 7.12. Weight-adjusted *(upper)* and body surface area–adjusted *(lower)* theophylline dose requirements (mean ± 2 SD). Dosage was adjusted to maintain peak serum theophylline concentrations between 10 and 20 μg/ml during chronic therapy. (From Wyatt R, Weinberger M, Hendeles L: Oral theophylline dosage for the management of chronic asthma. *J Pediatr* 92:125, 1978.)

and dosage is predicated on the pharmacokinetic observation that clearance (Cl) is determined by both elimination rate constant (K_e) and volume of distribution (V_d): $Cl = K_e \times V_d$. For many drugs, V_d is related to the volume of the extracellular water. ECW increases relative to mass as size decreases (Fig. 7.11). However, ECW remains nearly constant relative to surface area as size decreases. Thus, relative to mass, clearance increases with decreasing size; relative to surface area, clearance remains constant. Recall that clearance determines dosage (dosage = clearance × concentration). Thus, per kilogram dosage increases with decreasing size, while per meter squared dosage remains *relatively* constant.

Other physiologic processes that affect drug disposition are also directly related to surface area rather than mass. These include cardiac output, GFR, intestinal surface area, and hepatic blood flow (18, 55).

The apparently constant relationship between surface area and dosage leads many to advocate this method of normalization. While there are compelling reasons to employ surface area normalization—(a) during new drug development trials (55); (b) for extrapolation from dosages in adults; and (c) at extremes of weight (obesity, malnutrition) (142)—there appears to be no intrinsic advantage in routine clinical practice. Calculation of surface area is laborious and many nomograms are inaccurate (19). For theophylline, use of surface area–normalized dosages does not reduce interpatient variability (193).

The relative constancy of surface area–normalized dosages should not obscure the real increases in elimination rate that are typical in the preadolescent child (Figs. 7.9 and 7.10). In these individuals, more rapid elimination is signified by a shorter $t_{1/2}$, and will be manifest whether the dosage is calculated on the basis of surface area or weight. For example, the $t_{1/2}$ of theophylline is 3.4 hours at 2.5 years of age and 8.2 hours in healthy, nonsmoking adults (mean, 26 years) (73). The $t_{1/2}$ of phenytoin ranges from 2 to 7 hours in later infancy and from 12 to 40 hours in the adult (138). Drugs such as these also have a narrow therapeutic range, and large fluctuations around the mean steady state concentration should be avoided. This approach requires administration at intervals equal to or less than the $t_{1/2}$. Hence the need, in children, for more frequent division of daily dose, or for formulation of sustained release preparations.

CONCLUSION

The axiom that children are not merely small adults is nowhere more manifest than in consideration of pediatric pharmacotherapy. Pharmacodynamic and pharmacokinetic differences between children and adults are common and important; these differences are derived from the significant changes in human physiology that attend growth and development. Knowledge of basic pharmacological principles guides the clinician in adapting information derived from experience in adults to children; but, these basic (and general) principles must be supplemented by rigorous and detailed knowledge of specific drugs and their application to children.

References

1. Albert S: Aminophylline toxicity. *Pediatr Clin N Am* 34:61, 1987.
2. Anderson RJ: Drug prescribing for patients in renal failure. *Hosp Pract*, February 1983.
3. Aperia A, Broberger O, Thodenius K, et al: Development of renal control of salt and fluid homeostasis during the first year of life. *Acta Paediatr Scand* 64:393, 1975.
4. Arena JM, Rourk MH Jr, Sibrack CD: Acetaminophen: report of an unusual poisoning. *Pediatrics* 61:68, 1978.
5. Assali NS, Brinkman CR, Woods JR, et al: Development of neurohumoral control of fetal, neonatal, and adult cardiovascular functions. *Am J Obstet Gynecol* 129:748, 1977.
6. Bailey WC, Weill H, DeRoven, et al: The effect of isoniazid on transaminase levels. *Ann Intern Med* 81:200, 1974.
7. Barthels H: Drug therapy in childhood: what has been done and what has to be done. *Pediatr Pharmacol* 3:31, 1983.
8. Bartolome J, Mills E, Lau C, et al: Maturation of sympathetic neurotransmission in the rat heart. V. Development of baroceptor control of sympathetic tone. *J Pharmacol Exp Ther* 215:596, 1980.
9. Bateman DN, Croft AW, Nicholson E, et al: Dystonic reactions and the pharmacokinetics of metoclopramide in children. *Br J Clin Pharmacol* 15:557, 1983.
10. Bateman DN, Rawlins MD, Simpson JM: Extrapyramidal reactions to prochlorperazine and haloperidol in the United Kingdom. *Q J Med* 59:549, 1986.
11. Bennett EJ, Ignacio A, Patel K, et al: Tubocurarine and the neonate. *Br J Anaesth* 48:687, 1976.
12. Bennett EJ, Ramamurthy S, Dalal FY, et al: Pancuronium and the neonate. *Br J Anaesth* 47:75, 1975.
13. Beregovich J, Bianchi C, Rubler S: Dose-related hemodynamic and renal effects of dopamine in congestive heart failure. *Am Heart J* 87:550, 1974.
14. Berg RA: Emergency infusion of catecholamines into bone marrow. *Am J Dis Child* 138:810, 1984.
15. Berner M, Rouge JC, Friedli B: The hemodynamic effect of phentolamine and dobutamine after open heart operations in children: influence of the underlying heart defect. *Ann Thorac Surg* 35:643, 1983.
16. Bienvenu J, Sann L, Bienvenu F, et al: Laser nephelometry of orosomucoid in serum of newborns: refer-

ence intervals and relation to bacterial infections. *Clin Chem* 27:721, 1981.

17. Bohn DJ, Poirier CS, Edmonds JF, et al: Hemodynamic effects of dobutamine after cardiopulmonary bypass in children. *Crit Care Med* 8:367, 1980.

18. Boreus LO: *Principles of Pediatric Pharmacology.* New York, Churchill Livingstone, 1982.

19. Brion L, Fleischman AR, Schwartz GJ: Evaluation of four length-weight formulas for estimating body surface area in newborn infants. *J Pediatr* 107:801, 1985.

20. Brown BR Jr: Halothane hepatitis revisted. *N Engl J Med* 313:1347, 1985.

21. Buckley NM, Brazeau P, Gootman P: Maturation of circulatory responses to adrenergic stimuli. *Fed Proc* 42:1643, 1983.

22. Buckley NM, Gootman PM, Yellin EL, et al: Age related cardiovascular effects of catecholamines in anesthetized piglets. *Circ Res* 45:282, 1979.

23. Bukowsky M, Nakatsu K, Munt PW: Theophylline reassessed. *Ann Intern Med* 101:63, 1984.

24. Carney FT, Van Dyke RA: Halothane hepatitis: a critical review. *Anesth Analg* 51:135, 1972.

25. Casella ES, Rogers MC, Zahka KG: Developmental physiology of the cardiovascular system. In Rogers MC (ed): *Textbook of Pediatric Intensive Care.* Baltimore, Williams & Wilkins, 1987.

26. Chabrolle JP, Rossier A: Goitre and hypothyroidism in the newborn after cutaneous absorption of iodine. *Arch Dis Child* 53:495, 1978.

27. Chernow B, Rainey TG, Lake CR: Endogenous and exogenous catecholamines in critical care medicine. *Crit Care Med* 10:409, 1982.

28. Cohlan SQ, Bevelander G, Tiamsic T: Growth inhibition of prematures receiving tetracycline: clinical and laboratory investigation. *Am J Dis Child* 105:453, 1963.

29. Cook DR: Muscle relaxants in infants and children. *Anesth Analg* 60:335, 1981.

30. Cook DR, Fischer CG: Neuromuscular blocking effects of succinylcholine in infants and children. *Anesthesiology* 42:662, 1975.

31. Cowan RH, Jukkola AF, Arant BS: Pathophysiologic evidence of gentamicin nephrotoxicity in neonatal puppies. *Pediatr Res* 14:1204, 1980.

32. Cryer PE: Physiology and pathophysiology of the human sympathoadrenal neuroendocrine system. *N Engl J Med* 303:436, 1980.

33. Cryer PE, Rizza RA, Haymond MW, et al: Epinephrine and norepinephrine are cleared through beta-adrenergic, but not alpha-adrenergic, mechanisms in man. *Metabolism* 29:1114, 1980.

34. Dettli L: Drug dosage in renal disease. In Gibaldi M, Prescott L (eds): *Handbook of Clinical Pharmacokinetics.* New York, ADIS Health Science Press, 1983.

35. DiSessa TG, Leitner M, Ching CT, et al: The cardiovascular effects of dopamine in the severely asphyxiated neonate. *J Pediatr* 99:772, 1981.

36. Drayer DE: Pathways of drug metabolism in man. *Med Clin North Am* 58:927, 1974.

37. Driscoll DJ, Gillette PC: Hemodynamic effects of dobutamine in children. *Am J Cardiol* 43:581, 1979.

38. Driscoll DJ, Gillette PC, Ezrailson EG, et al: Inotropic response of the neonatal canine myocardium to dopamine. *Pediatr Res* 12:42, 1978.

39. Driscoll DJ, Gillette PC, Lewis RM, et al: Comparative hemodynamic effects of isoproterenol, dopamine, and dobutamine in the newborn dog. *Pediatr Res* 13:1006, 1979.

40. Driscoll DJ, Gillette PC, McNamara DG: The use of dopamine in children. *J Pediatr* 92:309, 1978.

41. Drugs for tuberculosis. *Med Lett Drugs Ther* 24:17, 1982.

42. Duckles SP, Banner W Jr: Changes in vascular smooth muscle reactivity during development. *Annu Rev Pharmacol Toxicol* 24:65, 1984.

43. Epstein ML, Kiel EA, Victorica BE: Cardiac decompen-

sation following verapamil therapy in infants with supraventricular tachycardia. *Pediatrics* 75:737, 1983.

44. Fabre J, Balant L: Renal failure. In Gibaldi M, Prescott L (eds): *Handbook of Clinical Pharmacokinetics.* New York, ADIS Health Science Press, 1983.

45. Farrell G, Prendergast D, Murray M: Halothane hepatitis. Detection of a constitutional susceptibility factor. *N Engl J Med* 313;1310, 1985.

46. Filloux F: Toxic encephalopathy caused by topically applied diphenhydramine. *J Pediatr* 108:1018, 1986.

47. Fitzgerald GA, Barnes P, Hamilton CA, et al: Circulating adrenaline and blood pressure: the metabolic effects and kinetics of infused adrenaline in man. *Eur J Clin Invest* 10:401, 1980.

48. Flower RJ, Moncada S, Vane JR: Analgesic-antipyretics and anti-inflammatory agents; drugs used in the treatment of gout. In Gilman AG, Goodman LS, Roll TW, Murad F (eds): *The Pharmacological Basis of Therapeutics,* ed 7. New York, Macmillan, 1985.

49. Food and Drug Administration: *FDA Drug Bull* 8:11, 1978.

50. Food and Drug Administration: *FDA Drug Bull* 12:10, 1982.

51. Ford DC, Leist ER, Algren JT: *Guidelines for Administration of Intravenous Medications to Pediatric Patients,* ed 2. Bethesda, American Society of Hospital Pharmacists, 1984.

52. Friedman WF: The intrinsic physiologic properties of the developing heart. *Prog Cardiovasc Dis* 15:87, 1972.

53. Friedman WF, George BL: New concepts and drugs in the treatment of congestive heart failure. *Pediatr Clin North Am* 31:1197, 1984.

54. Friedman WF, Pool PE, Jacobiwitz D, et al: Sympathetic innervation of the developing rabbit heart. Biochemical and histochemical comparisons of fetal, neonatal, and adult myocardium. *Circ Res* 23:25, 1968.

55. Garson A: Dosing the newer antiarrhythmic drugs in children: considerations in pediatric pharmacology. *Am J Cardiol* 57:1405, 1986.

56. Garson A: Medicolegal problems in the management of cardiac arrhythmias in children. *Pediatrics* 79:84, 1987.

57. Gaudreault P, Wason S, Lovejoy FH Jr: Acute pediatric theophylline overdose: a summary of 28 cases. *J Pediatr* 102:474, 1983.

58. Geis WP, Tatooles CJ, Priola DV: Factors influencing neurohumoral control of the heart in the newborn dog. *Am J Physiol* 228:1685, 1975.

59. Gershanik J, Boecler B, Ensley H, et al: The gasping syndrome and benzyl alcohol poisoning. *N Engl J Med* 307:1384, 1982.

60. Goldbloom LI: Dopamine—clinical use of an endogenous catecholamine. *N Engl J Med* 291:707, 1974.

61. Goldbloom RB, Goldbloom A: Boric acid poisoning, *J Pediatr* 43:631, 1953.

62. Goldstein DS, Zimlichman R, Stull R, et al: Plasma catecholamine and hemodynamic responses during isoproterenol infusions in humans. *Clin Pharmacol Ther* 40:233, 1986.

63. Gordon EP, Bristow MR, Laser JA, et al: Correlation between beta-adrenergic receptors in human lymphocytes and heart. *Circulation* 68:99, 1983.

64. Gould T, Roberts RJ: Therapeutic problems arising from the intravenous route for drug administration. *J Pediatr* 95:465, 1979.

65. Greco R, Musto B, Arienzo V: Treatment of paroxysmal supraventricular tachycardia in infancy with digitalis, adenosine-5-triphosphate, and verapamil: a comparative study. *Circulation* 66:504, 1982.

66. Grossman ER, Walchek A, Freedman H, et al: Tetracycline and permanent teeth: the relation between dose and tooth color. *Pediatrics* 47:567, 1971.

67. Guignard JP: Renal function in the newborn infant. *Pediatr Clin North Am* 29:777, 1982.

68. Gundert-Remy U, Penzien J, Hildebrandt R, et al: Cor-

relation between the pharmacokinetics and pharmacodynamics of dopamine in healthy subjects. *Eur J Clin Pharmacol* 26:163, 1984.

69. Haley TJ: Metabolism and pharmacokinetics of theophylline in human neonates, children, and adults. *Drug Metab Rev* 14:295, 1983.

70. Halkin H, Radomsky M, Blieden L, et al: Steady state serum digoxin concentration in relation to digitalis toxicity in neonates and infants. *Pediatrics* 61:184, 1978.

71. Hayes GJ, Butler VP Jr, Gersony WM: Serum digoxin studies in infants and children. *Pediatrics* 52:561, 1973.

72. Heimann G: Renal toxicity of aminoglycosides in the neonatal period. *Pediatr Pharmacol* 3:251, 1983.

73. Hendeles L, Massanari M, Weinberger M: Theophylline. In Evans WE, Schentag JJ, Jusko WJ (eds): *Applied Pharmacokinetics: Principles of Therapeutic Drug Monitoring*, ed 2. Spokane, Applied Therapeutics, 1986.

74. Hooper DC, Wolfson JS: The fluoroquinolones: pharmacology, clinical uses and toxicities in humans. *Antimicrob Agents Chemother* 28:716, 1985.

75. Iserson KV, Criss E: Intraosseous infusions: a usable technique. *Am J Emerg Med* 4:540, 1986.

76. James LS: Hexachlorophene. *Pediatrics* 49:492, 1972.

77. Jarnberg PO, Bengesson L, Erstrand J, et al: Dopamine infusion in man. Plasma catecholamine levels and pharmacokinetics. *Acta Anaesthesiol Scand* 25:334, 1981.

78. Kaplan JM, McCracken GH Jr, Horton CJ, et al: Pharmacologic studies in neonates given large dosages of ampicillin. *J Pediatr* 84:571, 1974.

79. Kates RE, Leier CV: Dobutamine pharmacokinetics in severe heart failure. *Clin Pharmacol Ther* 24:537, 1978.

80. Kelliher GJ, Roberts J: Effect of age on the cardiotoxic action of digitalis. *J Pharmacol Exp Ther* 197:10, 1976.

81. Kho TL, Henquet JW, Punt R, et al: Influence of dobutamine and dopamine on hemodynamics and plasma concentrations of noradrenaline and renin in patients with low cardiac output following acute myocardial infarction. *Eur J Clin Pharmacol* 18:213, 1980.

82. Kittinger JW, Sandler RS, Heizer WD: Efficacy of metoclopramide as an adjunct to duodenal placement of small bore feeding tubes: a randomized, placebo-controlled, double-blind study. *J Parenter Enteral Nutr* 11:33, 1987.

83. Klotz U: Pathophysiology and disease-induced changes in drug distribution volume. In Gibaldi M, Prescott L (eds): *Handbook of Clinical Pharmacokinetics*. New York, ADIS Health Science Press, 1983.

84. Krishna GG, Zahrowski JJ, Nissenson AR, et al: Hemodialysis for theophylline overdose. *Dial Transplant* 12:40, 1983.

85. Lackner TE: Drug replacement following exchange transfusion. *J Pediatr* 100:811, 1982.

86. Lang P, Williams RG, Norwood WI, et al: Hemodynamic effects of dopamine in infants after corrective cardiac surgery. *J Pediatr* 96:630, 1980.

87. Leff RD, Roberts RJ: Methods of intravenous drug administration in the pediatric patient. *J Pediatr* 98:631, 1981.

88. Legan E, Chernow B: Catecholamine response to acute illness. *Semin Respir Med* 7:88, 1985.

89. Leier CV, Unverferth DV, Kates RE: The relationship between plasma dobutamine concentrations and cardiovascular responses in cardiac failure. *Am J Med* 66:238, 1979.

90. Leier CV, Unverferth DV: Dobutamine. *Ann Intern Med* 99:490, 1983.

91. Levy RH, Bauer LA: Basic pharmacokinetics. *Ther Drug Monit* 8:47, 1986.

92. Linday LA, Drayer DE, Kahn MAA, et al: Pubertal changes in net renal tubular secretion of digoxin. *Clin Pharmacol Ther* 35:438, 1984.

93. Leob JN: Corticosteroids and growth. *N Engl J Med* 295:547, 1976.

94. Lowrey GH: *Growth and Development of Children*, ed 7. Chicago, Year Book, 1978.

95. Mannering GJ: Drug metabolism in the newborn. *Fed Proc* 44:2302, 1985.

96. Marshall BE, Wollman H: General anesthetics. In Gilman AG, Goodman LS, Roll TW, Murad F (eds): *The Pharmacological Basis of Therapeutics*, ed 7. New York, Macmillan, 1985.

97. McBride WG: Thalidomide and congenital abnormalities. *Lancet* 2:1358, 1961.

98. McCracken GH Jr: Aminoglycoside toxicity in infants and children. *Am J Med* 80:172, 1986.

99. McLain GE, Sipes IG, Brown BR Jr: An animal model of halothane hepatotoxicity: roles of enzyme induction and hypoxia. *Anesthesiology* 91:321, 1979.

100. Metoclopramide for gastroesophageal reflux. *Med Lett Drugs Ther* 27:21, 1985.

101. Micelli JN, Bidani A, Aronow R: Peritoneal dialysis of theophylline. *Clin Toxicol* 14:539, 1979.

102. Miceli JN, Olson, WA, Cohen SN: Elimination kinetics of isoniazid in the newborn infant. *Dev Pharmacol Ther* 2:225, 1981.

103. Mihaly GW, Moore RG, Thomas JW, et al: The pharmacokinetics and metabolism of the anilide local anesthetics in neonates. *Eur J Clin Pharmacol* 13:143, 1978.

104. Milligan N, Dhillon S, Richens A, et al: Rectal diazepam in the treatment of absence status: a pharmacodynamic study. *J Neurol Neurosurg Psychiatry* 44:914, 1981.

105. Morselli PL: Clinical pharmacokinetics in neonates. *Clin Pharmacokinet* 1:81, 1976.

106. Morselli PL, Franco-Morselli R, Bossi L: Clinical pharmacokinetics in newborns and infants. *Clin Pharmacokinet* 5:485, 1980.

107. Mullick FC: Hexachlorophene toxicity. Human experience at the Armed Forces Institute of Pathology. *Pediatrics* 51:395, 1973.

108. Nau H, Luck W, Kuhnz W, et al: Serum protein binding of diazepam, desmethyldiazepam, furosemide, indomethacin, warfarin, and phenobarbital in human fetus, mother, and newborn infant. *Pediatr Pharmacol* 3:219, 1984.

109. Nelson JD: Antimicrobial drugs. In Yaffe SJ (ed): *Pediatric Pharmacology*. New York, Grune & Stratton, 1980.

110. Nelson JD: *Pocketbook of Pediatric Antimicrobial Therapy*, ed 7. Baltimore, Williams & Wilkins, 1987.

111. Nogen AG, Bremner JE: Acetaminophen overdosage in a young child. *J Pediatr* 92:832, 1978.

112. Nolke AC: Severe toxic effects from aminophylline and theophylline suppositories in children. *JAMA* 161:693, 1956.

113. Norfloxacin. *Med Lett Drugs Ther* 29:25, 1987.

114. Notterman DA, Nardi M, Saslow JG: Effects of dose formulation on isoniazid absorption in two young children. *Pediatrics* 77:850, 1986.

115. Nugent SK, Laravuso R, Rogers MC: Pharmacology and use of muscle relaxants in infants and children. *J Pediatr* 94:481, 1979.

116. O'Brien RJ, Long MW, Cross FS, et al: Hepatotoxicity from isoniazid and rifampin among children treated for tuberculosis. *Pediatrics* 72:491, 1983.

117. O'Keefe, Gregory GA, Stanski DR, et al: d-Tubocurarine: pharmacodynamics and kinetics in children. *Anesthesiology* 51:S270, 1979.

118. O'Mally K, Coleman EN, Doig WB, et al: Plasma digoxin levels in infants. *Arch Dis Child* 48:99, 1973.

119. Orlowski JP: My kingdom for an intravenous line. *Am J Dis Child* 138:803, 1984.

120. Padbury JF, Agata Y, Baylen BG, et al: Dopamine pharmacokinetics in critically ill newborn infants. *J Pediatr* 294:293, 1987.

121. Papadopoulou AL, Novello AC: The use of hemoper-

fusion in children. *Pediatr Clin North Am* 29:1039, 1982.

122. Park MK: Use of digoxin in infants and children with specific emphasis on dosage. *J Pediatr* 108:871, 1986.

123. Park MK, Johnson JM, Hayashi S: Is age dependent difference in inotropic responses to isoproterenol temperature dependent? *Pediatr Res* 20:208A, 1986.

124. Park MK, Ludden T, Arom KV, et al: Myocardial vs serum digoxin concentrations in infants and adults. *Am J Dis Child* 136:418, 1982.

125. Perez CA, Reimer JM, Schreiber MD, et al: Effect of high dose dopamine on urine output in newborn infants. *Crit Care Med* 14:1045, 1986.

126. Perkin RM, Levin DL: Dobutamine: a hemodynamic evaluation in children with shock. *J Pediatr* 100:97, 1982.

127. Perloff WH: Physiology of the heart and circulation. In Swedlow DB, Raphaely RC (eds): *Cardiovascular Problems in Pediatric Critical Care*. New York, Churchill Livingstone, 1986.

128. Piafsky, KM: Disease induced changes in the plasma binding of basic drugs. *Clin Pharmacokinet* 5:246, 1980.

129. Pikoff AS, Kessler KM, Singh S, et al: Age related differences in the protein binding of quinidine. *Dev Pharmacol Ther* 3:108, 1981.

130. Pinsky WW, Jacobsen JR, Gillette PC, et al: Dosage of digoxin in premature infants. *J Pediatr* 96:639, 1976.

131. Polgar G, Weng TR: The functional development of the respiratory system. *Am Rev Respir Dis* 120:625, 1979.

132. Pond AM: Diuresis, dialysis, and hemoperfusion. *Emerg Med Clin North Am* 2:29, 1984.

133. Porter CJ, Garson A, Gillette PC: Verapamil: an effective calcium blocking agent for pediatric patients. *Pediatrics* 71:748, 1983.

134. Prandota J: Clinical pharmacokinetics of changes in drug elimination in children. *Dev Pharmacol Ther* 8:311, 1985.

135. Radford D: Side effects of verapamil in infants. *Arch Dis Child* 58:465, 1983.

136. Rajchgot P, Prosber CG, Soldins S, et al: Aminoglycoside related nephrotoxicity in the premature newborn. *Clin Pharmacol Ther* 35:394, 1984.

137. Rane A: Basic principle of drug disposition and action. In Yaffe SJ (ed): *Pediatric Pharmacology*. New York, Grune & Stratton, 1980.

138. Rane A, Wilson JT: Clinical pharmacokinetics in infants and children. In Gibaldi M, Prescott L (eds): *Handbook of Clinical Pharmacokinetics*. New York, ADIS Health Science Press, 1983.

139. Reidenberg MM, Levy M, Warner H, et al: Relationship between diazepam dose, plasma level, age and central nervous system depression. *Clin Pharmacol Ther* 23:371, 1978.

140. Reinhardt D, Zehmisch T, Becker B, et al: Age dependency of alpha and beta-adrenoreceptor on thrombocytes and lymphocytes of asthmatic and nonasthmatic children. *Eur J Pediatr* 142:111, 1984.

141. Ricci DA, Saltzman MB, Meyer C, et al: Effect of metoclopramide in diabetic gastroparesis. *J Clin Gastroenterol* 7:25, 1985.

142. Ritschel WA: *Handbook of Basic Pharmacokinetics*, ed 2. Hamilton, Drug Intelligence Publications, 1980.

143. Roan Y, Galant SP: Decreased neutrophil beta adrenergic receptors in the neonate. *Pediatr Res* 16:591, 1982.

144. Roberts RJ: *Drug Therapy in Infants*. Philadelphia, WB Saunders, 1984.

145. Roberts RJ: Intravenous administration of medications in pediatric patients: problems and solutions. *Pediatr Clin North Am* 28:23, 1986.

146. Rockson SG, Homcy CJ, Quinn P, et al: Cellular mechanisms of impaired adrenergic responsiveness in neonatal dogs. *J Clin Invest* 67:319, 1981.

147. Romero T, Covell J, Freidman WF: A comparison of pressure volume relations of the fetal, newborn and adult heart. *Am J Physiol* 222:1285, 1972.

148. Romero T, Friedman WF: Limited left ventricular response to volume overload in the neonatal period: a comparative study with the adult animal. *Pediatr Res* 13:910, 1979.

149. Ross EM, Gilman AG: Pharmacodynamics: mechanisms of drug action and the relationship between drug concentration and effect. In Gilman AG, Goodman LS, Roll TW, Murad F (eds): *The Pharmacological Basis of Therapeutics*, ed 7. New York, Macmillan, 1985.

150. Rothstein P, Dornbusch J, Shaywitz BA: Prolonged seizures associated with the use of viscous lidocaine. *J Pediatr* 101:461, 1982.

151. Rowland M, Tozer TN: *Clinical Pharmacokinetics*. Philadelphia, Lea & Febiger, 1980.

152. Rumack BH: Acetaminophen overdose in young children. *Am J Dis Child* 138:428, 1984.

153. Rumack BH, Peterson RC, Koch G, et al: Acetaminophen overdose. *Arch Intern Med* 141:380, 1981.

154. Sandor GGS, Bloom KR, Izukawa T, et al: Noninvasive assessment of left ventricular function related to serum digoxin levels in neonates. *Pediatrics* 65:541, 1980.

155. Schipioe PG: An unusual case of antihistamine poisoning. *J Pediatr* 71:589, 1967.

156. Schranz D, Stopfkuchen H, Jungst BK, et al: Hemodynamic effects of dobutamine in children with cardiovascular failure. *Eur J Pediatr* 139:4, 1982.

157. Schwartz GJ, Feld LG, Langford DJ: A simple estimate of glomerular filtration rate in full term infants during the first year of life. *J Pediatr* 104:849, 1984.

158. Schwartz GJ, Haycock GB, Edelmann CM Jr, et al: A simple estimate of glomerular filtration rate in children derived from body length and plasma creatinine. *Pediatrics* 58:259, 1976.

159. Schwartz GJ, Haycock GB, Gauthier B: A simple estimate of glomerular filtration rate in adolescent boys. *J Pediatr* 106:522, 1985.

160. Schwartz GJ, Haycock GB, Spitzer A: Plasma creatinine and urea concentration in children: normal values for age and sex. *J Pediatr* 88:828, 1976.

161. Seri I, Tulassay T, Kiszel J, et al: Cardiovascular response to dopamine in hypotensive preterm neonates with severe hyaline membrane disease. *Eur J Pediatr* 142:3, 1984.

162. Shawn DH, McGuigan MA: Poisoning from dermal absorption of promethazine. *Can Med Assoc J* 130:1460, 1984.

163. Shaywitz SE, Caparulo BK, Hodgson ES: Developmental language disability as a consequence of prenatal exposure to ethanol. *Pediatrics* 68:850, 1981.

164. Shoor PM, Berryhill RE, Benumof JL: Intraosseous infusion: pressure-flow relationship and pharmacokinetics. *J Trauma* 19:772, 1979.

165. Silverberg AB, Shah SD, Haymond MW, et al: Norepinephrine: hormone and neurotransmitter in man. *Am J Physiol* 234:E252, 1978.

166. Singh BN, Nademanee K, Baky SH: Calcium antagonists. Clinical use in the treatment of arrhythmias. *Drugs* 25:125, 1983.

167. Spyridis P, Sinaniotis C, Papadea I, et al: Isoniazid liver injury during chemoprophylaxis in children. *Arch Dis Child* 94:65, 1979.

168. Stoner JD, Bolen JL, Harrison DC: Comparison of dobutamine and dopamine in treatment of severe heart failure. *Br Heart J* 39:536, 1977.

169. Stopfkuchen H, Schranz R, Huth R, et al: Effects of dobutamine on left ventricular performance in newborns as determined by systolic time intervals. *Eur J Pediatr* 146:135, 1987.

170. Tatsumi H, Senda H, Yatera S, et al: Toxicological studies on pipemidic acid. V. Effect on diarthrodial

joints of experimental animals. *J Toxicol Sci* 3:357, 1978.

171. Tenenbein M: Pediatric toxicology: current controversies related to nephrotoxicity in the premature newborn. Clinical and recent advances. *Curr Probl Pediatr* 16:185, 1986.

172. Terrin BN, McWilliams NB, Maurer HM: Side effects of metoclopramide as an antiemetic in childhood cancer chemotherapy. *J Pediatr* 104:138, 1984.

173. Valdes R Jr: Endogenous digoxin-like immunoreactive factors: impact on digoxin measurement and potential physiological implications. *Clin Chem* 31:1985, 1985.

174. Valdes R Jr, Graves SW, Brown BA: Endogenous substance in newborn infants causing false-positive digoxin measurements. *J Pediatr* 152:947, 1983.

175. Vallner JJ: Binding of drugs by albumin and plasma protein. *J Pharm Sci* 66:447, 1977.

176. van-der-Kleijn E, Baars AM, Vree TB, et al: Clinical pharmacokinetics of drugs used in the treatment of status epilepticus. *Adv Neurol* 34:421, 1983.

177. Vessey DA: Hepatic metabolism of drugs and toxins. In Zakim D, Boyer TD (eds): *Hepatology*. Philadelphia, WB Saunders, 1982.

178. Vestal RE, Wood AJJ, Shand DG: Reduced beta-adrenoreceptor sensitivity in the elderly. *Clin Pharmacol Ther* 26:181, 1979.

179. Ward JT: Endotracheal drug therapy. *Am J Emerg Med* 1:71, 1983.

180. Warner LO, Beach TP, Garvin JP: Halothane and children. The first quarter century. *Anesth Analg* 63:838, 1984.

181. Way WL, Costley EC, Way EL: Respiratory sensitivity of the newborn infant to meperidine and morphine. *Clin Pharmacol Ther* 6:454, 1962.

182. Weiss CF, Glazko AJ, Weston JK: Chloramphenicol in the newborn infant. *N Engl J Med* 262:787, 1960.

183. Whately K, Turner WW Jr, Dey M, et al: When does metoclopramide facilitate transpyloric intubation? *J Parenter Enteral Nutr* 8:679, 1984.

184. Whitsett JA, Noguchi A, Moore JJ: Developmental aspects of alpha and beta-adrenergic receptors. *Semin Perinatol* 6:125, 1982.

185. Wilkinson GR, Shand DC: A physiologic approach to hepatic drug clearance. *Clin Pharmacol Ther* 7:377, 1975.

186. Williams RT: *Detoxification Mechanisms*. John Wiley & Sons, New York, 1959.

187. Wilson RF, Sibbald WJ, Jaanimagi JL: Hemodynamic effects of dopamine in critically ill septic patients. *J Surg Res* 20:163, 1976.

188. Wingard LB, Cook DR: Clinical pharmacokinetics of muscle relaxants. *Clin Pharmacokinet* 2:330, 1977.

189. Wolff JA: Methemoglobinemia due to benzocaine. *Pediatrics* 20:915, 1957.

190. Wong DF, Wagner HN, Dannals RF, et al: Effects of age on dopamine and serotonin receptors measured by positron tomography of the living human brain. *Science* 226:1393, 1984.

191. Wood M, Wood AJJ: Changes in plasma drug binding and alpha$_1$-acid glycoprotein in mother and newborn infant. *Clin Pharmacol Ther* 4:522, 1981.

192. Wood M, Wood AJJ: Neuromuscular blocking agents. In Wood M, Wood AJJ (eds): *Drugs and Anesthesia*. Baltimore, Williams & Wilkins, 1982.

193. Wyatt R, Weinberger M, Hendeles L: Oral theophylline dosage for the management of chronic asthma. *J Pediatr* 92:125, 1978.

194. Yaffe SJ, Bierman CW, Cann HM, et al: Requiem for tetracyclines. *Pediatrics* 55:142, 1975.

195. Zaritsky A, Chernow B: Use of catecholamines in pediatrics. *J Pediatr* 105:341, 1984.

196. Zaritsky AL, Eisenberg MG: Ontogenetic considerations in the pharmacotherapy of shock. In Chernow B, Shoemaker W (eds): *Critical Care—State of the Art*. Fullerton, Society of Critical Care Medicine, 1986, vol 7.

197. Zwillich CW, Sutton FD, Neff TA, et al: Theophylline-induced seizures in adults. *Ann Intern Med* 82:784, 1975.

8

Pharmacy Services in the Intensive Care Unit

Harold J. DeMonaco, M.S.

The traditional role of a department of pharmacy has been confined to that of drug supplier. This role is especially true in the intensive care unit (ICU). However, as a result of the initiatives of the American Society of Hospital Pharmacists, a few intensive care physicians, and the dedication of a group of pharmacy practitioners, the role of the pharmacy department in the ICU is expanding to entail teaching, research, and clinical practice (1).

Little has been published about the direct involvement of pharmacy in the care of the critically ill patient. Direct patient care pharmacy services in many ICUs are provided by nurses and physicians. The Committee on Guidelines for the Organization of Critical Care Units of the Society of Critical Care Medicine has previously defined the critical care team as composed of physicians, nurses, biomedical technicians and engineers, and a variety of other technically oriented specialists. The pharmacist was not mentioned as a member of the critical care team. The reasons for this noticeable absence remain obscure and open to speculation. This lack of involvement may be related to administrative, logistic, educational, or motivational hindrances (2).

Critical care medicine has advanced in its ability to provide optimal care to the critically ill patient on a variety of fronts. Newer pharmacologic agents and a better recognition of older agents have enhanced the intensive care physician's abilities and contributed to the decrease in morbidity and mortality associated with critical illness. This increased sophistication, at both the community and teaching hospital level, has not been without its own inherent liabilities. With it has come a bewildering array of drug side effects and interactions previously unrecognized and unforeseen, as well as an unprecedented increase in the cost of medication on a per patient basis. It is common for critically ill patients to incur thousands of dollars per day in expenses. A crucial component to a pharmacy's delivery of services is to ensure cost-effective therapy. This statement does not suggest that expensive therapy is necessarily inappropriate, but rather that the medications used should be the most appropriate ones.

Ideally, a consensus of opinion between the medical staff, nursing service, and pharmacy should be reached prior to the establishment of pharmacy services to the critical care unit. Unfortunately, the pharmacy's involvement is often after the fact—a drug distribution system usually predates any appreciable pharmacy involvement in most intensive care units.

The appropriate level and types of services a pharmacy department should provide are dependent on the setting, but may include:

Accurately preparing and dispensing all medications in as "ready-to-use" a format as is possible, on time and for 24 hours a day.

Maintaining drug security and adequate inventory control.

Detecting and advising of all potential adverse drug reactions, incompatibilities, and drug-laboratory and drug-drug interactions, preferably in a prospective manner.

Providing patient-specific drug-related information to both physicians and nurses, preferably for 24 hours a day.

Evaluating individual patient drug therapy as it relates to efficacy, toxicity, patient clinical status, and organ system function.

DRUG DISTRIBUTION

All established critical care units have an existing drug distribution system. It is incumbent on pharmacy management to determine nurses' level of satisfaction with the system, regardless of planned enhancements in the level of services provided.

The foundation on which pharmacy services are based is the drug distribution system. The

DATE

FILLED BY

DESCRIPTION	UNITS	M	T	W	T	F	S	S	M	T	W	T	F	S	S	Commodity Number	TOTAL
ISOXSUPRINE INJ 5 MG/ML VASODILAN	2 ML															P150490	
KANAMYCIN SULF PED INJ 75 MG KANTREX	2 ML															P151550	
KANAMYCIN SULF INJ 500 MG VIAL KANTREX	2 ML															P151600	
LEVARTERENOL BITAR INJ 1 MG/ML LEVOPHED	4 ML															P158450	
LEVOTHYROXINE SOD INJ 100 MCG SYNTHROID	10 ML															P158790	
LEVOTHYROXINE SOD INJ 500 MCG SYNTHROID	10 ML															P158800	
LIDOCAINE HCL 2% 1 G IV CA AR ESI	25 ML															P160415	
LIDO HCL 4% INJ 2 G XYLO ESI	50 ML															P160420	
LIDO HCL 2% INJ CARD DISPOS SYR	5 ML															P160225	
LIDOCAINE HCL 0.5% INJ XYLO VIAL	50 ML															P159450	
LIDOCAINE HCL 0.5% INJ W/EP XYLO	50 ML															P159500	
LIDOCAINE HCL 1% INJ XYLO AMP	2 ML															P159550	
LIDOCAINE HCL 1% INJ XYLO AMP	5 ML															P159560	
LIDOCAINE HCL 1% INJ XYLO VIAL	20 ML															P159600	
LIDOCAINE HCL 1% W/EP XYLO VIAL	20 ML															P159950	
LIDOCAINE HCL 2% INJ XYLO AMP	2 ML															P159905	
LIDOCAINE HCL 2% INJ W/EP XYLO	2 ML															P160150	
LIDOCAINE HCL 2% INJ XYLO VIAL	20 ML															P160250	
LIDOC HCL 2% INJ W/EPI XYLO VIAL	20 ML															P160300	
LORAZEPAM INJ 2 MG/ML TUBEX ATIVAN	1 ML															P162954	
MAGNES SULF 50% INJ (8 MEQ MG) 1 G AMP	2 ML															P165050	
MANNITOL 25% INJECTION 12.5 G VIAL	50 ML															P165960	
METARAMINOL BITART INJ 10 MG/ML ARAMINE	10 ML															P172300	
METHOCARBAMOL INJECTION 1 G ROBAXIN	10 ML															P174250	
METHOHEXITAL SOD INJ 500 MG BREVITAL	EA															P174400	

Figure 8.1. Representative page of floor stock consignment book. Pharmacy personnel indicate amount of drug stocked per day. The book runs for a 2-week period. At the end of the period, consignments to nursing units are tallied and charged.

type and level of sophistication of a drug distribution system to an intensive care unit are dependent on a variety of factors. In addition to pharmacy-related issues, such factors as the type of patient treated, type of medical coverage, medication order turnover rate, and institutional resources must be kept in mind. The acutely traumatized patient consumes resources, both supplies and personnel time, in a manner different from that of a patient who has suffered an acute myocardial infarction. As a result, specialty critical care units devoted to specific types of patients require entirely different levels of service.

Some critical care pharmacists suggest that one must provide for full drug distribution systems encompassing unit-dose drug delivery and intravenous solution additive programs from a "critical care pharmacy satellite" (1). However, this approach is beyond the scope of many institutions and may be an inappropriate consumption of resources for all but the largest medical centers. It is possible to provide an adequate drug distribution system for an ICU using a floor stock method. While not an ideal situation, the realities of resource limits and priority allocation make a floor stock system a pragmatic reality for many institutions. The design of the floor stock system is contingent on a host of factors. Whatever method is used, it should be developed from a consensus opinion among the nursing staff, medical director, and pharmacy management (4).

Although many floor stock systems are maintained by the nursing staff of the unit,

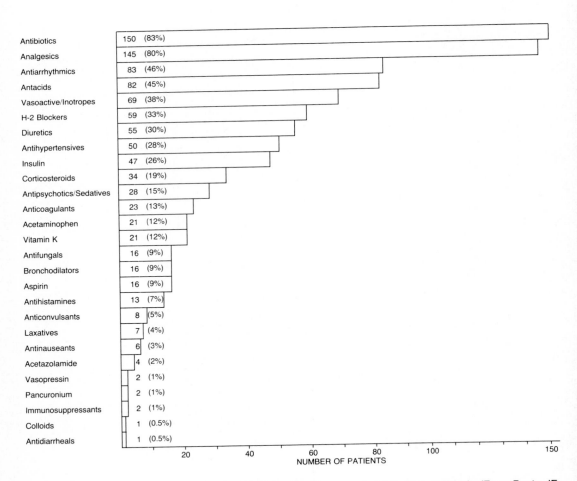

Figure 8.2.   Distribution histogram of drug classes utilized in a surgical intensive care unit. (From Dasta JF: Drug use in a surgical intensive care unit. *Drug Intell Clin Pharm* 20:752–756, 1986.)

this method is probably not ideal. If a floor stock system is to be used, it should be maintained by the pharmacy staff.

A standardized list of the types of medications and the number of doses to be maintained should be developed and known to all parties. This list should be updated with some regularity and should only include those drugs that have been approved for use within the institution. Figure 8.1 is a representative page of the floor stock book used at Massachusetts General Hospital. This page is a standardized format, which includes the majority of medications stocked by the pharmacy. With the advent of premixed solutions of many of the commonly used critical care agents, as well as antibiotics, the pharmacy is in a position to offer better drug distribution without extensive expenditures of personnel time and other resources. These agents can and should be added to the floor stock list of the critical care unit, if a full unit-dose/intravenous additive program is not available.

Floor stock systems are very useful for those critical care units having either a high turnover rate for medication orders or a short length of stay for patients. This usefulness is especially true for institutions that do not have the services of a pharmacist for 24 hours a day. A floor stock system is not without its liabilities, however. Turnaround time for medication and intravenous additive orders can be excessive unless an automated delivery system, such as a pneumatic tube system, is available or the ICU is close to the pharmacy. Lost charges for medications administered from floor stock supplies and the inventory value of the floor stock represent financial liabilities that are frequently overlooked. Floor stock systems inappropriately place nurses in the role of a surrogate in the performance of pharmaceutic functions.

Support for the broadening of pharmacy services to the ICU has been growing over the past several years. A significant component of this broader role is the establishment of a specialized and dedicated ICU satellite pharmacy. The specific objectives of an ICU satellite pharmacy vary from institution to institution. There are several common themes, however, which may include the following (5):

1. Reduction of turnaround time for medications and intravenous admixtures.
2. Reduction in the number of lost charges due to inadequate charting of medications administered.
3. Reduction in the value of inventory and an increase in the pharmacy inventory turnover rate.
4. Provision of clinical pharmacy services.
5. Reduction or elimination of nursing time spent in pharmacy-related functions.

Critical care satellite pharmacies, while components of an overall drug distribution system, face unique challenges related to the severity of patient illnesses and the intensity of drug therapy. The number of patients, length of stay, number of medications used per patient, and type of drugs used all play important roles in facility design and location. In addition, physical plant design of the institution, the proposed satellite location, and the intensive care unit must be considered.

Few studies have documented the number of medications used daily on patients treated in an intensive care unit. Recent estimates suggest that between five and six drugs are

Table 8.1
Minimal Floor Stock Requirements for the ICU

Aminophylline injection	250 mg/ml
Atropine sulfate injection	0.4 mg/ml
Bretylium tosylate injection	500 mg/10 ml
Calcium chloride injection (10%)	10 mg/ml
Dexamethasone injection	4 mg/ml
Diazepam injection	5 mg/ml
Digoxin injection	0.25 mg/ml
Diphenhydramine injection	50 mg/ml
Dobutamine injection	250 mg
Dopamine injection	200 mg/5 ml
Ephedrine sulfate injection	25 mg/ml
Epinephrine injection, 1:1000	1 ml
Epinephrine injection, 1:10,000	10 ml
Furosemide injection	10 mg/ml
Furosemide injection	100 mg/ml
Hydrocortisone injection	100 mg
Hydrocortisone injection	250 mg
Isoproterenol injection	0.2 mg/ml
Lidocaine injection	100 mg/5 ml
Lidocaine for injection	1 g
Magnesium sulfate injection	1 g/2 ml
Methyldopa injection	250 mg
Naloxone injection	0.4 mg/ml
Neostigmine injection	1 mg/ml
Nitroglycerin injection	
Nitroglycerin tablets	0.3 mg
Nitroprusside injection	50 mg
Norepinephrine injection	1 mg/ml
Phenylephrine injection	1 mg/ml
Phenytoin injection	50 mg/ml
Physostigmine injection	
Phytonadione injection	10 mg/ml
Procainamide injection	250 mg/ml
Propranolol injection	1 mg/ml
Vasopressin injection	20 units/ml

Pharm. No. 237 Rev. 6/85

MASSACHUSETTS GENERAL HOSPITAL PHARMACY
INTRAVENOUS PIGGY-BACK COMPATIBILITY CHART

N.B.: THESE ARE GUIDELINES ONLY. CONDITIONAL COMPATIBILITIES EXIST. FOR FURTHER INFORMATION, CHECK WITH PHARMACY FIRST.

Column headers (1–20):
1. ACETATE (POTASSIUM OR SODIUM)
2. AMIKACIN SULFATE
3. AMINOPHYLLINE
4. AMPICILLIN SODIUM
5. BRETYLIUM TOSYLATE
6. CALCIUM CHLORIDE
7. CALCIUM GLUCONATE
8. CEFAMANDOLE NAFTATE
9. CEFAZOLIN SODIUM
10. CEPHAPIRIN SODIUM
11. CEFOPERAZONE SODIUM
12. CEFOTAXIME SODIUM
13. CEFOXITIN SODIUM
14. CEFTRIAXONE SODIUM
15. CHLORAMPHENICOL SODIUM SUCCINATE
16. CIMETIDINE HCl
17. CLINDAMYCIN PHOSPHATE
18. DEXTRAN$_{40}$ IN DEXTROSE 5% WATER
19. DIPHENHYDRAMINE HCl
20. DOBUTAMINE HCl

#	DRUG	pH	1	2	3	4	5	6	7	8	9	10	11	12	13	14	15	16	17	18	19	20
1	ACETATE (POTASSIUM OR SODIUM)	6.2–6.5		C	C	C		C	C		C						C	C		C		
2	AMIKACIN SULFATE	3.5–5.5			X			C	C		X	X	X	X		X		C			C	
3	AMINOPHYLLINE	8.6–9.0	C		C			C	C	C	C			X	C		C	X	X	C	C	X
4	AMPICILLIN SODIUM	8.0–10.0	C	X	C													X	C	X	C	
5	BRETYLIUM TOSYLATE	5.0–7.0	C					C	C									C		C		C
6	CALCIUM CHLORIDE *	6.0–7.5	C	C			C					C					C		X			C
7	CALCIUM GLUCONATE	6.0–8.2	C	C	C		C			X	X	C					C		X	X		C
8	CEFAMANDOLE NAFTATE	6.0–8.5			C				X										X		C	
9	CEFAZOLIN SODIUM	4.8–5.5	C	X	C				X										C		C	
10	CEPHAPIRIN SODIUM	6.5–8.5		X	C			C	C									C			C	
11	CEFOPERAZONE SODIUM	4.5–6.5		X															C			
12	CEFOTAXIME SODIUM	4.5–6.5		X	X													C	C			
13	CEFOXITIN SODIUM	4.5–7.0			C														C			
14	CEFTRIAXONE SODIUM	6.0–7.0		X															C			
15	CHLORAMPHENICOL SODIUM SUCCINATE	6.4–7.0	C		C	X		C	C			C							C			C
16	CIMETIDINE HCl	3.8–6.0	C	C	X	C	C			X	C				C				C	C		C
17	CLINDAMYCIN PHOSPHATE	6.0–6.3		X	X			X	X										C	C		
18	DEXTRAN$_{40}$ IN DEXTROSE 5% WATER	4.5–5.1	C		C	C	C			X	C	C				C	C	C	C	C		C
19	DIPHENHYDRAMINE HCl	5.0–6.0		C	C								C									
20	DOBUTAMINE HCl *	2.5–5.0			X			C	C	C								C	C	C		C
21	DOPAMINE HCl*	3.0–4.5			C			C	C	C					C		C	C	C	C		C
22	DOXYCYCLINE HYCLATE	2.0–6.0			X			X	X	X								C		C	C	X
23	DROPERIDOL	3.0–3.8																				
24	EPINEPHRINE HCl*	2.5–5.0		C	X	X	C			X			C				X	C		C		C
25	ERYTHROMYCIN LACTOBIONATE	6.0–8.0		X	C	X			C				C			X		C			C	
26	FUROSEMIDE	8.9–9.3			C										X							X
27	GENTAMICIN SULFATE	3.0–5.5			X	X	X		X	X	X		X	X			X	C	C	C		C
28	HEPARIN SODIUM	5.0–7.5	C	X	C	C			C	C	C	C			C		C	C	C	C	C	C
29	HYDROCHLORIC ACID (CENTRAL LINE ONLY)	0.1–0.4			X	X			C	X	X	X					X	C	X			C
30	HYDROCORTISONE SODIUM SUCCINATE	7.0–8.0	C	C	C	C	C	C	C	C	C						C	C	C	C	X	C
31	INSULIN (CZI)	7.0–7.8	C		X			C	C	C		C	C			C						
32	ISOPROTERENOL HCl	3.5–4.5	C		X				C									C	C		C	C
33	LEVARTERENOL BITARTRATE * (NOREPINEPHRINE)	3.0–4.5		C	X			C	C	C			X					C	C			C
34	LIDOCAINE HCl	6.0–7.0	C		C	C	C	C	C	C	C	C	C	C	C	C		C	C	C	C	C
35	MAGNESIUM SULFATE	5.5–7.0	C	X		X				C	C	C	C	C	C		C	C	X			C
36	MANNITOL	4.5–7.0	X		X	X				C					C							C
37	METHYLDOPATE HCl	3.5–4.2	C		C		C											C	C		C	C
38	METHYLPREDNISOLONE SODIUM SUCCINATE	7.0–8.0							X	C	C						C	C	C	C	X	C
39	METOCLOPRAMIDE HCl	3.0–5.0	C	X	C			X	X	X	X	C		X		X	X		C	C	C	C
40	METRONIDAZOLE	5.0–7.0			C																	X
41	MORPHINE SULFATE	2.5–6.0			C																C	C
42	NAFCILLIN SODIUM	5.0–8.0			C													C		C	C	
43	NITROGLYCERIN	5.5			C	C																C
44	NITROPRUSSIDE SODIUM	3.5–6.0			X													X				C
45	OXACILLIN SODIUM	8.0			X	X												C		C		C
46	PENICILLIN G (POTASSIUM OR SODIUM)	6.0–7.0	C		X		X	C	C										C	C	C	C
47	PHENYLEPHRINE HCl*	3.0–5.5			X													C	C		C	C
48	PHOSPHATE (POTASSIUM OR SODIUM)	6.5	C		X			X	X													C
49	POTASSIUM CHLORIDE	4.0–8.0	C	C	C	C	C	C	C	C	C	C	C	C	C	C	C	C	C	C	C	C
50	PROCAINAMIDE HCl	4.0–6.0			X	X	C			X	X						X	C	X	C	C	C
51	SODIUM BICARBONATE	7.0–8.5		C	C	X	X	X	X	C	C	C			X	C		C	C	C	C	X
52	THEOPHYLLINE PRE-MIX	4.0																				
53	TICARCILLIN DISODIUM	6.0–8.0																C		C		
54	TOBRAMYCIN SULFATE	3.5–7.0			X	X	X	X	X	X	X		X	X			X	C	C	C		C
55	TUBOCURARINE HCl	2.5–5.0				C												C		C	C	
56	VANCOMYCIN HCl	2.8–4.5			X		X	C	C		X						X	C		C	C	
57	VASOPRESSIN, AQUEOUS*	2.5–4.5			X	X	X			X	X						X		X			X

*CENTRAL LINE PREFERRED

Figure 8.3. Intravenous drug piggyback compatibility chart. *C* indicates drugs are compatible: *X*, incompatible.

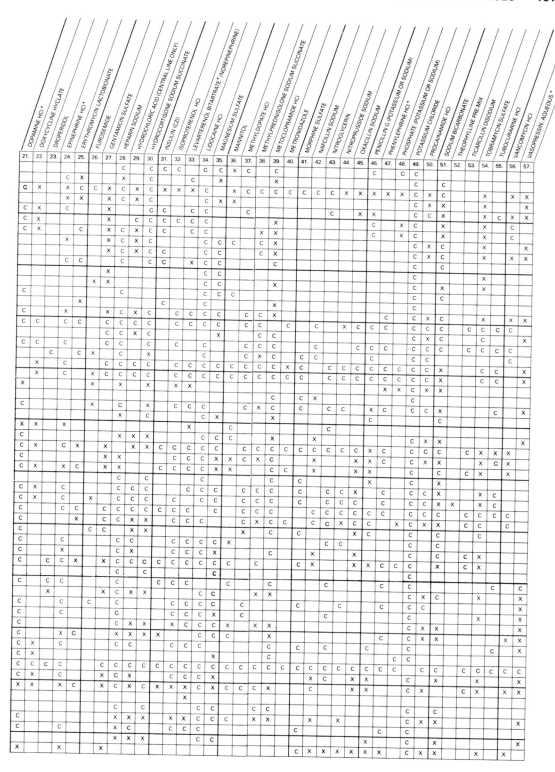

Figure 8.3. *(continued)*

administered per patient in surgical intensive care units. In one recent study, the number of drugs administered per patient-day ranged from one to 16 (3). Figure 8.2 depicts drug use by class or specific type of drug reported. The few studies that have examined the average length of stay for patients treated in either a medical or surgical intensive care unit suggest that the average patient spends between 3 and 3.7 days in the ICU. These factors have an impact on both the size and staffing levels of a critical care pharmacy.

There is little consensus in the literature on the best drug distribution system for the intensive care unit (3, 5). Given the diversity of institutional needs and opinions, it is unlikely that one system design can and will fulfill all needs. One could argue that hybridization is a logical solution.

Regardless of the type of distribution system established, specific medications must be readily available in the ICU. Table 8.1 provides a proposed listing of these drugs. Wherever possible, these medications should be available in as "ready-to-use" a format as possible and in sufficient quantities to allow for multiple patients' needs.

CLINICAL SERVICES

The critical care pharmacist should be recognized as a drug therapy expert by the staff of the critical care unit. This recognition comes not necessarily through specialized education or by degree, but rather by demonstrated excellence. The timely and accurate dissemination of information is intended to inform rather than confuse the desired goal. In order to completely fulfill this role, the critical care pharmacist must monitor the drug therapy of all patients treated (6, 7, 9).

An examination of the patient's medication administration record or nursing flow sheet is as adequate as a pharmacist's drug profile. Since the patient's chart contains all that is known about the patient's history and current progress, it is the best possible source of information. Drug therapy–monitoring forms, while useful under certain circumstances, are by their very nature incomplete since they do not contain information provided by the primary care givers.

The pharmacist practicing in a critical care environment must be proficient in both the prevention and detection of drug-drug incompatibilities. A greater percentage of drug ad-

ministration in the critically ill patient is by the intravenous route than in the general (non-ICU) hospital population. Although many textbooks and computer programs are available to assist in the determination of compatibilities, they are limited in their appreciation of the specialized needs of the critically ill patient (10). At Massachusetts General Hospital, we rely heavily on charts prepared by our staff that use a number of reference sources as well as locally conducted research. These charts may be specialized according to the needs of the individual critical care unit or may be useful throughout the hospital (Figs. 8.3 and 8.4). Critically ill patients are more susceptible to drug incompatibility problems simply because more of their drugs are administered intravenously than in the general hospital population, and because of their injuries they have less physiologic reserve.

The pharmacist's role is that of consultant to the primary physician, not primary care giver. This role may be fulfilled in many different ways depending on the setting. In the teaching center where formal teaching and work rounds are undertaken, the critical care pharmacist should become part of the team. Sufficient time should regularly be allocated to the pharmacist by the pharmacy's administrative personnel. Haphazard or intermittent services should never be allowed. This goal requires a commitment on the part of the staff pharmacist as well as the director of pharmacy. For those practicing in a community setting in which formal rounds are not conducted, the pharmacist should be present during change of shift reports. Highlights of the patient's progress are presented, as well as pertinent information concerning the patient's history and future treatments. This forum is very informative and should not be ignored. Information obtained during these presentations should be included in the pharmacist's data base on the patient and directly related to the drug therapy in use. The sudden development of supraventricular arrhythmias in a patient receiving aminophylline or dopamine should raise the suspicion of a drug toxicity that may otherwise go undetected until more serious arrhythmias develop.

QUALITY ASSURANCE

The development of a quality assurance program for pharmacy services to the ICU depends on a clear definition of both the role of the

MGH PHARMACY
SYRINGE COMPATIBILITY CHART

Drug	Atropine sulfate	Butorphanol tartrate	Chlordiazepoxide HCL	Chlorpromazine HCL	Diazepam	Diphenhydramine HCL	Droperidol	Glycopyrrolate	Hydromorphone HCL	Hydroxyzine HCL	Lorazepam	Meperidine HCL	Metoclopramide HCL	Morphine sulfate	Nalbuphine HCL	Pentazocine lactate	*Pentobarbital sodium	Perphenazine	Prochlorperazine edisylate	Promethazine HCL	Scopolamine HBr
Atropine sulfate	—	C	X	C	X	C	C	C	C	C	X	C	C	C	C	C	C	C	C	C	C
Butorphanol tartrate	C	—	X	C	X	C	C	N	N	C	X	C	C	C	N	C	X	C	C	C	C
Chlordiazepoxide HCL	X	X	—	X	X	X	X	X	X	X	X	X	X	X	X	X	X	X	X	X	X
Chlorpromazine HCL	C	C	X	—	X	C	C	C	C	C	X	C	C	C	N	C	X	C	C	C	C
Diazepam	X	X	X	X	—	X	X	X	X	X	X	X	X	X	X	X	X	X	X	X	X
Diphenhydramine HCL	C	C	X	C	X	—	C	C	C	C	X	C	C	C	N	C	X	C	C	C	C
Droperidol	C	C	X	C	X	C	—	C	N	C	X	C	C	C	C	C	X	C	C	C	C
Glycopyrrolate	C	N	X	C	X	C	C	—	C	C	X	C	N	C	N	X	X	N	C	C	C
Hydromorphone HCL	C	N	X	C	X	C	N	C	—	C	X	N	N	N	N	C	C	N	X	C	C
Hydroxyzine HCL	C	C	X	C	X	C	C	C	C	—	X	C	C	C	C	C	X	N	C	C	C
Lorazepam	X	X	X	X	X	X	X	X	X	X	—	X	X	X	X	X	X	X	X	X	X
Meperidine HCL	C	C	X	C	X	C	C	C	N	C	X	—	C	X	N	C	X	C	C	C	C
Metoclopramide HCL	C	C	X	C	X	C	C	N	N	C	X	C	—	C	N	C	N	C	C	C	C
Morphine sulfate	C	C	X	C	X	C	C	C	N	C	X	X	C	—	N	C	N	C	C	C	C
Nalbuphine HCL	C	N	X	N	X	N	C	N	N	C	X	N	C	N	—	N	X	N	C	C	C
Pentazocine lactate	C	C	X	C	X	C	C	X	C	C	X	C	C	C	N	—	X	C	C	C	C
*Pentobarbital sodium	C	X	X	X	X	X	X	X	C	X	X	X	N	X	X	X	—	X	X	X	C
Perphenazine	C	C	X	C	X	C	C	N	N	N	X	C	C	C	N	C	X	—	C	C	C
Prochlorperazine edisylate	C	C	X	C	X	C	C	C	X	C	X	C	C	C	C	C	X	C	—	C	C
Promethazine HCL	C	C	X	C	X	C	C	C	C	C	X	C	C	C	C	C	X	C	C	—	C
Scopolamine HBr	C	C	X	C	X	C	C	C	C	C	X	C	C	C	C	C	C	C	C	C	—

Physical compatibilities of medications in syringes for 15 minutes
C = Compatible   X = Incompatible   N = No Documented Information

*compatibility profile is characteristic of most barbiturate salts, such as secobarbital and thiopental

Discard **any** unused portions of mixed drugs.

Figure 8.4. Drugs in syringe compatibility chart. (Data from Trissel LA: *Handbook on Injectable Drugs*, ed 3. American Society of Hospital Pharmacists, 1983; and Parker WA: Physical compatibility update of preanesthetic medications. *Hosp Pharm* 19:475–478, 1984.)

pharmacy staff and an objective measure of quality. If the pharmacist's role is limited to that of drug supplier, quality assurance need only examine how well this process is undertaken. Missing doses in a unit-dose distribution system or order turnaround time are frequently used as measures of quality control in determining the level of service. On the other hand, if the pharmacist's role is broadened to include the monitoring of patient drug therapy, outcome measures should be directed by the effects of therapy on the patient.

An adequate quality assurance program for pharmacy services in the critical care setting should include both drug distribution and clinical services, including drug information. Drug information questions encountered on the general patient floors as well as the critical care areas should be documented (Fig. 8.5). Ideally, these forms should be collected and analyzed by the quality assurance coordinator. The information provided is reviewed weekly with the staff in a formal setting. Frequently occurring questions or those that require additional research and clarification are slated for pharmacy inservices. Although many institutions use a centralized drug information center to maintain standardization, it is possible to conduct a high quality program using a decentralized approach. Since many individ-

MGH PHARMACY
DRUG INFORMATION REQUEST

DATE: _____   FLOOR: _____

QUESTION: _____

_____

_____

CHECK OFF WHERE APPLICABLE

_____ Pharmacology   _____ Dose/Dosing
_____ Administration   _____ Use Precautions
_____ Use/Indication   _____ Drug Interactions
_____ Overdose   _____ Side Effect/Toxicity
_____ Stability   _____ Alternative Therapy
_____ Kinetics   _____ Incompatibilities
_____ Research Use   _____ Other

RESPONSE: _____

_____

_____

_____

_____

REFERENCE(S): _____

_____

_____

PHARMACIST: _____

FOR OFFICE USE ONLY

_____ analgesics   _____ antiarrhythmics
_____ anticoagulants   _____ antiinfectives
_____ autonomics   _____ diuretics
_____ foreign   _____ hormone/endocrine
_____ vasodilators   _____ inotropes/vasopressors
_____ IV therapy   _____ pulmonary
_____ psychotropes   _____ sedative/hypnotics
_____ GI   _____ nutrition/electrolytes
_____ cardiac   _____ neurologics
_____ non-therapeutic   _____ miscellaneous

Figure 8.5. Drug information request form. This form is used by pharmacists in documenting questions posed or answered during daily activities. Forms are submitted daily to the Coordinator of Drug Information/Staff Development.

uals are involved in this process, standardization of responses to questions is difficult, but not impossible. If a decentralized system of drug information is used, quality assurance becomes all the more important.

EDUCATIONAL PROGRAMS

Educational programs for the department of pharmacy are of two types: internal for mem-

bers of the staff and external for members of the nursing and medical staff. Education is a key factor to the successful fulfillment of the critical care pharmacist's responsibilities.

In addition to having a clear understanding of drug therapy, the pharmacist must be educated as to the types of invasive and noninvasive monitoring performed on patients, and their interpretation. Rapid interpretation of the electrocardiogram and basic/advanced life support are minimal requirements for the critical care pharmacist. A basic understanding of nutritional support, fluid and electrolyte maintenance, and the nature and extent of a patient's injuries/disease state must be within the critical care pharmacist's grasp. This information may be obtained through the nursing service's and medical staff's educational programs. The critical care pharmacist should also be a participant in these programs. Educational programs specifically related to drug therapy should be conducted by the pharmacist for the nursing and medical staff. This recommendation is especially important for the introduction of new drugs to the critical care environment.

CONCLUSIONS

The role of the pharmacist in the critical care unit is expanding. It is within the scope of most pharmacists, regardless of their age or educational background, to participate in the management of the care of the most critically ill patients in the hospital as well as those treated on the general medical/surgical units. The exclusion of this patient population from the services of the pharmacist is inexcusable, for it is this population that can benefit the most.

References

1. Caldwell RD, Tuck BA: Justification and operation of a critical care satellite pharmacy. *Am J Hosp Pharm* 40:2141–2145, 1983.
2. Dasta JF: Critical care therapeutics: a frontier for clinical pharmacy. *Drug Intell Clin Pharm* 16:398–399, 1982.
3. Dasta JF: Drug use in a surgical intensive care unit. *Drug Intell Clin Pharm* 20:752–756, 1986.
4. Einarson TR, McGhan WF, Bootman JL: Decision analysis applied to pharmacy practice. *Am J Hosp Pharm* 42:364–371, 1985.
5. Ellinoy BR, Clarke JE, Wagers PW, Swinney RS: Comprehensive pharmaceutical services in a medical intensive care unit. *Am J Hosp Pharm* 41:2335–2342, 1984.

6. Helper CD: Pharmacy as a clinical profession. *Am J Hosp Pharm* 42:1298–1306, 1985.
7. Koda-Kimble MA, Katcher BS, Young LY (eds): *Applied Therapeutics for Clinical Pharmacists.* San Francisco, Applied Therapeutics, 1978.
8. Parker P: Reflections on clinical pharmacy's first 20 years. *Am J Hospital Pharm* 42:364–371, 1985.
9. Smith MC, Brown TR (eds): *Handbook of Institutional Pharmacy Practice.* Baltimore, Williams & Wilkins, 1979.
10. Zeller FP, Anders RJ: Compatibility of intravenous drugs in a coronary intensive care unit. *Drug Intell Clin Pharm* 20:349–352, 1986.

9

Cardiovascular Adrenoceptors: Physiology and Critical Care Implications

Robert R. Ruffolo, Jr., Ph.D.

The cardiovascular system is regulated by α- and β-adrenoceptors. The neurotransmitter, norepinephrine, influences cardiovascular function under normal homeostatic conditions and in a variety of pathophysiologic conditions. In addition, the actions of the circulating bloodborne hormone, epinephrine, and exogenously administered catecholamines are largely mediated through interaction with α- and β-adrenoceptors in the major effector organs of the cardiovascular system, such as the heart, vasculature, and kidney. An understanding of these receptors, in terms of their function, location, and distribution, is of primary importance in treating the critically ill patient inasmuch as the best available pharmacologic treatments for these patients involve the stimulation or blockage of α- and β-adrenoceptors in the cardiovascular system.

There have been many recent developments in our understanding of α- and β-adrenoceptors and the functions they subserve in the regulation of the cardiovascular system. It is the intent of this chapter to review these major recent developments, with emphasis on the clinical setting and the use of drugs currently available or being developed that perturb the cardiovascular system through stimulation or blockade of α- and β-adrenoceptors.

CONTROL OF THE CARDIOVASCULAR SYSTEM

Organization of the Autonomic Nervous System

The cardiovascular system is under the control and regulation of the autonomic nervous system. Although effector organs of the cardiovascular system (heart, vasculature, kidneys)

function in the absence of autonomic nerves, the sympathetic and parasympathetic divisions of the autonomic nervous system provide a delicate balance involving closed reflex loops to maintain these organs in an optimal functional state.

The autonomic nervous system is composed of the parasympathetic division, in which the neurotransmitter at the effector organ is acetylcholine, and the sympathetic division, in which the neurotransmitter is norepinephrine. The parasympathetic division exits the central nervous system from the brain stem (vagus) and the sacral region of the spinal cord. These nerves are characterized by long preganglionic neurons and short postganglionic neurons, the latter innervating the effector organs. The neurotransmitter in the parasympathetic ganglia is acetylcholine. The heart receives a dense cholinergic innervation from the vagus, and cholinergic "tone" in the heart predominates over adrenergic tone. In general, there is no significant parasympathetic innervation to the vasculature, although blood vessels nonetheless contain muscarinic cholinergic receptors that are stimulated by acetylcholine and mediate vasodilation through release of an endothelial derived relaxant factor (43).

The sympathetic division of the autonomic nervous system originates from the intermediolateral cell column of the thoracic and lumbar portions of the spinal cord. The relatively short preganglionic fibers characteristic of sympathetic nerves terminate in the sympathetic ganglia chain, where the neurotransmitter is acetylcholine. The postganglionic sympathetic neurons are long and liberate norepinephrine, which interacts postsynaptically with adrenoceptors in the heart, vasculature, and kidney. The innervation to the vasculature is almost exclusively adrenergic where the end organ response is vasoconstriction.

Although the sympathetic and parasympathetic components of the autonomic nervous system originate in the spinal cord and are considered peripheral nerves, both divisions are under the control of nuclei located in the brain stem, which in turn receive input from higher centers in the brain. Most of the cardiovascular reflex loops consist of afferent nerves from various peripheral chemoreceptors and baroreceptors, which travel to the regulatory nuclei in the brain stem where the information is integrated. The efferent component of the reflex loop involves descending pathways originating from the brain stem nuclei, which ultimately recruit the sympathetic and parasympathetic divisions of the autonomic nervous system to make the necessary alterations in the functional state of the various effector organs of the cardiovascular system.

Cardiovascular Reflexes

Cardiovascular reflexes maintain cardiovascular function, in particular blood pressure, within a relatively narrow optimal range. A sensitive and highly efficient series of positive and negative feedback loops detect deviations from normal cardiovascular function and then "up-regulate" or "down-regulate" the function of peripheral organs of the cardiovascular system after integration in the central nervous system. Pressure receptors in the carotid sinus and aortic arch sense changes in peripheral arterial blood pressure and initiate the cardiovascular reflex. Afferents from the carotid sinus and aortic arch enter the central nervous system through cranial nerves IX (glossopharyngeal) and X (vagus), respectively, and form in part the solitary tract in the medulla. The first synapse in the cardiovascular reflex loop occurs in the nucleus tractus solitarii, where the neurotransmitter appears to be L-glutamate (109). Synapses are made within the nucleus tractus solitarii, both with inhibitory neurons that course to the ventrolateral medulla, which ultimately regulates sympathetic outflow, and with excitatory neurons that send connections to the dorsal motor nucleus of the vagus, which in turn regulates parasympathetic outflow.

Increases in systemic arterial blood pressure activate the afferent component of the cardiovascular reflex loop. As a result, the inhibitory neurons originating in the nucleus tractus solitarii and terminating in the ventrolateral medulla are activated, reducing sympathetic outflow to the heart, vasculature, and kidney.

As a direct consequence, heart rate, stroke volume (and therefore cardiac output), and total peripheral vascular resistance are reduced, and blood pressure is reduced to within normal limits. In addition, the excitatory neurons that originate from the nucleus tractus solitarii and terminate in the dorsal motor nucleus of the vagus are activated, and cholinergic outflow is increased, further decreasing heart rate and cardiac output (74) and thus augmenting the reduction in arterial blood pressure. This reduction restores the afferent input to a near-normal level such that the "error signal" becomes small, and the system achieves a new steady state.

α-ADRENOCEPTORS

Adrenoceptors may be subdivided into the α type and β type (114). β-Adrenoceptors are selectively activated by epinephrine, norepinephrine, and isoproterenol. α-Adrenoceptors are also stimulated by epinephrine and norepinephrine, but are resistant to isoproterenol. β-Adrenoceptors may be subdivided further into the β_1 and β_2 subtypes; isoproterenol and epinephrine stimulate both subtypes, and norepinephrine stimulates only the β_1 subtype. Likewise, α-adrenoceptors have been subdivided into the α_1 and α_2 subtypes, and epinephrine and norepinephrine stimulate both. Although the naturally occurring catecholamines cannot distinguish between α_1- and α_2-adrenoceptors, many synthetic drugs do. Thus, phenylephrine and methoxamine are potent and highly selective α_1-adrenoceptor agonists, whereas clonidine and α-methylnorepinephrine (the latter being the active metabolite of α-methyldopa) are potent and selective α_2-adrenoceptor agonists (116).

Central α-Adrenoceptors

Stimulation of central α_2-adrenoceptors in the ventrolateral medulla induces a reduction in sympathetic outflow to the periphery, manifested as a reduction in arterial blood pressure accompanied by bradycardia. This response has been studied extensively over the past two decades, and several comprehensive reviews are available (74, 112, 122, 143). Quantitative structure-activity studies have shown excellent correlation between the α_2-adrenoceptor agonist potency of a series of clonidine analogues and blood pressure reduction, provided a lipophilicity term is included to correct for penetration through the blood-brain barrier, which is required in order to gain access to the site of action within the central nervous system (119).

The characteristic response to intravenous administration of an α_2-adrenoceptor agonist in a normotensive or hypertensive animal is an immediate pressor response, due to stimulation of peripheral arterial postjunctional α_1- and α_2-adrenoceptors (119). This response is also seen in human subjects following intravenous administration of clonidine (100). This pressor response is relatively short-lived and is followed by a slow decline in arterial blood pressure to levels lower than those observed prior to drug administration. This long-lasting depressor/antihypertensive response is a result of central α_2-adrenoceptor stimulation. Heart rate declines immediately following administration and continues to be reduced for the duration of drug action. If the α_2-adrenoceptor agonist is administered directly into the central nervous system, or via the vertebral artery, which allows for easy access to the central nervous system, the initial pressor response is not observed (140). High oral doses of centrally acting α_2-adrenoceptor agonists, such as clonidine or guanfacine, can also transiently increase blood pressure via peripheral arterial α-adrenoceptor stimulation (29), and this may provide an explanation for the "therapeutic window" seen with clonidine in antihypertensive therapy (42).

The antihypertensive action of α_2-adrenoceptor agonists results from stimulation of postsynaptic α_2-adrenoceptors in the brain stem. A brain stem site appears likely based on the inability of transection at the intercollicular level or at the pontomedullary junction to attenuate the antihypertensive activity of clonidine (123). Many experiments have been performed in an attempt to locate more precisely the site of action of α_2-adrenoceptor agonists within the brain stem. Although the nucleus tractus solitarius has often been considered as the principal site of action of central α_2-adrenoceptor agonists (122), recent studies using microinjections of clonidine suggest the lateral reticular nucleus in the ventrolateral medulla as a more likely candidate (46). This nucleus is readily accessible from the ventral surface of the medulla, where α_2-adrenoceptor agonists have been shown to be effective following local application (13, 46).

In addition to a reduction in sympathetic outflow, central α_2-adrenoceptor stimulation can enhance parasympathetic outflow. This has usually been demonstrated as a potentiation of the reflex bradycardia induced by intravenous injection of a pressor agent such as angiotensin II (74). This action also requires penetration of the α_2-adrenoceptor agonist into the central nervous system (74), but the precise site of action has not yet been determined (46).

Central α_2-adrenoceptor stimulation is utilized clinically for antihypertensive therapy. In addition to the directly acting central α_2-adrenoceptor agonists discussed above, α-methyldopa, which has been extensively employed for nearly two decades, is now known to stimulate central α_2-adrenoceptors following metabolic conversion to α-methylnorepinephrine (142), which has much greater α_2-adrenoceptor selectivity than norepinephrine (115). Following chronic treatment with α-methyldopa in rats, medullary norepinephrine stores are almost completely replaced by α-methylnorepinephrine (25), which is available for interaction with medullary α_2-adrenoceptors to inhibit sympathetic outflow. The therapeutic and side effect profile of α-methyldopa is similar to that observed with the directly acting central α_2-adrenoceptor agonists (143).

In addition to clonidine and α-methyldopa, guanfacine is now in general use as an antihypertensive drug. This compound has an in vitro pharmacologic profile similar to that of clonidine (125), but appears to have a longer duration of action (108). Clinical trials have been conducted with several other α_2-adrenoceptor agonists, including St 600 (73), tiamenidine (22), monoxidine, lofexidine (126), and B-HT 933 (azapexole) (108). The latter compound is more selective than clonidine for α_2 vis-à-vis α_1-adrenoceptors (141), and its antihypertensive activity confirms an α_2-adrenoceptor–mediated mechanism. As in animal studies, the clinical cardiovascular profiles of the various α_2-adrenoceptor agonists are relatively similar (107). Besides their antihypertensive indication, the sympatholytic action of the centrally active α_2-adrenoceptor agonists may offer clinical benefit in congestive heart failure and angina pectoris, again through a centrally mediated reduction in sympathetic outflow. Although extensive evaluation for efficacy in these conditions has not yet been performed, preliminary trials in patients are encouraging (46).

One important issue associated with antihypertensive therapy with centrally acting α_2-adrenoceptor agonists is the "rebound hypertension" or "withdrawal" phenomenon that often occurs when treatment is abruptly terminated (55). This phenomenon is characterized by tachycardia and abrupt rises in blood pressure, sometimes to levels greater than that observed before initiation of therapy (54). Studies in animals have confirmed the presence of a hyperadrenergic state following abrupt termination of chronic clonidine therapy (54). Administration of an α_2-adrenoceptor antagonist, such as yohimbine, can also precipitate this withdrawal phenomenon (54).

The withdrawal phenomenon observed following abrupt cessation of α_2-adrenoceptor agonist therapy bears some similarity to opiate withdrawal (55), and appears to involve overactivity of locus ceruleus neurons (37). This may represent a rebound phenomenon following chronic suppression of the firing rate of these neurons during chronic antihypertensive treatment. In view of the similarities and possible receptor interactions between α_2-adrenoceptors and opiate receptors, it is not surprising that morphine can suppress, via a naloxone-sensitive mechanism, some of the cardiovascular rebound effects observed following termination of clonidine infusion in rats (139).

Peripheral Arterial α-Adrenoceptors

SYSTEMIC CIRCULATION

It is now widely accepted that arterial vasoconstriction may be mediated by a mixed population of postjunctional vascular α_1- and α_2-adrenoceptors. We are now beginning to understand the physiologic function and/or distribution of these receptors. It appears that in the arterial circulation, postjunctional vascular α-adrenoceptors located at the neuroeffector junction (i.e., junctional receptors) are of the α_1 subtype, whereas those located away from the neuroeffector junction (i.e., extrajunctional receptors) are of the α_2 subtype. Support for this concept of junctional α_1- and extrajunctional α_2-adrenoceptors in the arterial circulation has been obtained in many arterial test systems (80, 81, 144, 145).

The physiologic role of the postsynaptic junctional arterial α_1-adrenoceptors appears to be in maintaining resting vascular tone. Presumably, these receptors, which are located in the vicinity of the neurovascular junction, interact with endogenous norepinephrine liberated from sympathetic nerves. The physiologic role of the extrajunctional α_2-adrenoceptors is

not fully understood, but a number of proposals have been made. The extrajunctional α_2-adrenoceptors would not normally interact with liberated norepinephrine since they are located at some distance from the adrenergic nerve terminal, and the highly efficient neuronal uptake pump keeps synaptic levels of norepinephrine sufficiently low, preventing diffusion of the neurotransmitter to the extrajunctional sites (80). The extrajunctional α_2-adrenoceptors may respond to circulating epinephrine liberated from the adrenal gland and acting as a bloodborne hormone (81). Although circulating catecholamines may be below the levels required to exert a physiologic effect, in times of stress these levels may be elevated to threshold levels at which postsynaptic vascular α_2-adrenoceptors are activated (27). The contribution made by arterial extrajunctional α_2-adrenoceptors to total peripheral vascular resistance may be greater in certain hypertensive states than in normotensive patients (11, 69), implying that postjunctional vascular α_2-adrenoceptors may play an important role in pathophysiologic states such as hypertension and possibly congestive heart failure, in which circulating catecholamine levels are high (24, 84). It is unclear at the present time whether epinephrine is in fact responsible for stimulating the extrajunctional α_2-adrenoceptors in these states, since circulating levels of norepinephrine are also particularly high and could account, at least in part, for α_2-adrenoceptor activation in disease states such as hypertension and congestive heart failure.

CORONARY CIRCULATION

Although the precise role of α-adrenoceptor stimulation in the dynamic regulation of coronary blood flow is still unclear, it has been known for some time that following β-adrenoceptor blockade, α-adrenoceptor agonists or cardiac sympathetic nerve stimulation can produce coronary artery vasoconstriction leading to an increase in coronary arterial resistance and a decrease in coronary artery blood flow. α-Adrenoceptor agonists, such as phenylephrine (105), methoxamine (56), and norepinephrine (56), produce coronary artery vasoconstriction in the dog as well as in other species. In animals pretreated with β-adrenoceptor blocking agents, cardiac sympathetic nerve stimulation produces a fall in coronary artery blood flow that can be blocked by α-adrenoceptor antagonists, demonstrating that α-adrenoceptors can mediate vasoconstrictive response to endogenous as well as exogenous norepinephrine in the coronary circulation (38).

It has recently been suggested that α_2-adrenoceptors may play a role in the α-adrenoceptor–mediated regulation of coronary artery blood flow. In the presence of β-adrenoceptor blockade, intracoronary administration of the selective α_1-adrenoceptor agonist, phenylephrine, and the selective α_2-adrenoceptor agonist, B-HT 933, produces a rapid decrease in coronary artery blood flow, and these effects are blocked by the α_1- and α_2-adrenoceptor antagonists, prazosin and rauwolscine, respectively (63). These same investigators have demonstrated that the reduction in coronary artery blood flow elicited by exogenously administered norepinephrine is antagonized to a greater degree by rauwolscine than by prazosin, thus suggesting a more prominent role of α_2-adrenoceptors in the regulation of coronary artery blood flow. The presence of α_1-adrenoceptors on the large, epicardial coronary arteries has recently been demonstrated (60), whereas α_2-adrenoceptors appear to be located primarily on the smaller subendocardial resistance vessels of the coronary vascular bed (75). In addition, it has been found that the pressure of a flow-limiting coronary artery stenosis can unmask a vasoconstrictor response mediated by sympathetic nerve stimulation, and that this response can be antagonized by the nonselective α-adrenoceptor antagonist, phentolamine, as well as by the selective α_2-adrenoceptor antagonist, rauwolscine, but not by the selective α_1-adrenoceptor antagonist, prazosin (59). These results suggest that α_2-adrenoceptor–mediated coronary artery vasoconstriction may occur in the coronary circulation under pathologic conditions (i.e., coronary artery disease, angina, or coronary artery vasospasm), and that α_2-adrenoceptors might therefore represent a novel therapeutic target.

The selective α_2-adrenoceptor antagonist, idazoxan, has recently been shown to produce a greater degree of blockade of the coronary vasoconstrictor response to sympathetic nerve stimulation than does the selective α_1-adrenoceptor antagonist, prazosin. It thus appears that α_1- and α_2-adrenoceptors coexist in the coronary circulation, and that both α-adrenoceptor subtypes mediate coronary artery vasoconstriction. Furthermore, the data suggest that postjunctional vascular α_2-adrenoceptors may play a more important functional role than postjunctional vascular α_1-adrenoceptors in the coronary circulation, and that α_2-adre-

noceptors may be preferentially innervated (i.e., junctional), since they may be selectively activated by endogenous norepinephrine liberated from sympathetic nerves on electrical stimulation.

PULMONARY CIRCULATION

Postjunctional vascular α_1- and α_2-adrenoceptors mediate vasoconstriction in the pulmonary circulation of the dog (129). This fact is evidenced by the dose-related increase in pulmonary perfusion pressure produced by the selective α_1-adrenoceptor agonist, methoxamine, which is highly sensitive to blockade by the α_1-adrenoceptor antagonist, prazosin, and resistant to blockade by the α_2-adrenoceptor antagonist, rauwolscine. Accordingly, the pulmonary pressor effects mediated by the selective α_2-adrenoceptor agonist, B-HT 933, are sensitive to blockade by rauwolscine and are resistant to prazosin. The results indicate that postjunctional vascular α_1- and α_2-adrenoceptors coexist in the pulmonary circulation, and that both α-adrenoceptor subtypes mediate vasoconstriction (65, 129).

Prazosin and rauwolscine both antagonize the increases in pulmonary perfusion pressure elicited by exogenously administered norepinephrine, indicating that norepinephrine has the capacity to stimulate both postjunctional α_1- and α_2-adrenoceptors in the pulmonary circulation (129). Pulmonary pressor responses to endogenous norepinephrine released from sympathetic nerves are antagonized primarily by prazosin, with little or no effect of rauwolscine. It appears, therefore, that endogenous norepinephrine acts primarily on α_1-adrenoceptors in the pulmonary vascular bed of the dog (130), and that endogenously released norepinephrine stimulates predominantly junctional α_1-adrenoceptors, whereas exogenously administered norepinephrine stimulates both junctional α_1-adrenoceptors as well as extrajunctional α_2-adrenoceptors in the canine pulmonary vascular bed. Similar conclusions have been made regarding the peripheral arterial circulation of the dog, in which preferential innervation of postjunctional vascular α_1-adrenoceptors has been demonstrated (82).

The ability of selective α_2-adrenoceptor agonists and exogenously administered norepinephrine to elicit increases in pulmonary perfusion pressure may indicate that, under some conditions, circulating catecholamines play a role in maintaining or elevating pulmonary vascular tone by a mechanism involving, at least in part, postsynaptic vascular α_2-adrenoceptors. Hyman and associates (66) have infused epinephrine into the perfused pulmonary circulation of the cat (after propranolol treatment) to elicit a large rise in pulmonary perfusion pressure (10–20 mm Hg). Recently, Sawyer and colleagues (121) have demonstrated that circulating catecholamines are responsible for α_2-adrenoceptor–mediated pressor effects in the spontaneously hypertensive rat. Therefore, in certain disease states, such as congestive heart failure, in which pulmonary pressure is elevated and circulating catecholamine levels are high (24), α_2-adrenoceptor–mediated increases in pulmonary vascular resistance may possibly be secondary to the elevated circulating catecholamines.

When pulmonary vascular tone is elevated even slightly with a vasoconstrictor agent, responses to the selective α_2-adrenoceptor agonist, B-HT 933, are markedly potentiated (130). Furthermore, the enhanced responsiveness of α_2-adrenoceptors is tone-dependent and highly selective for α_2-adrenoceptors, since responses to the α_1-adrenoceptor agonist, methoxamine, or to angiotensin II are not potentiated by elevating pulmonary vascular tone (130). The nature of the vasoconstrictor agent used to elevate pulmonary vascular tone does not influence the enhanced α_2-adrenoceptor responsiveness, although the manner in which pulmonary vascular pressure is elevated is critically important. When pulmonary perfusion pressure is elevated by increased pulmonary blood flow as opposed to pulmonary vasoconstriction, responses to α_2-adrenoceptor agonists are not potentiated as they are when vasoconstrictor agents are utilized to elevate pulmonary pressure (130). This observation indicates that pulmonary vascular smooth muscle tone, and not pulmonary pressure per se, is the major determinant of the potentiation in α_2-adrenoceptor responsiveness in the pulmonary vasculature. The selective potentiation of α_2-adrenoceptor–mediated vasoconstriction in the pulmonary circulation under conditions of high pulmonary vascular tone may be relevant to certain pathophysiologic conditions such as congestive heart failure, in which pulmonary vascular resistance is elevated and circulating catecholamine levels are high. Both of these factors may predispose the patient to a further exacerbation of the elevation in pulmonary vascular resistance by this selective potentiation mechanism.

RENAL CIRCULATION

The kidneys receive approximately 20% of the cardiac output and provide a significant contribution to total systemic vascular resistance. Their dense adrenergic innervation extends to both the afferent and efferent arterioles (7). Stimulation of the renal nerves and administration of α-adrenoceptor agonists produce an increase in renal vascular resistance with redistribution of blood flow from the cortical to the medullary areas. This response is blocked by phenoxybenzamine or phentolamine (26, 101), indicating the activation of α-adrenoceptors. Initial in vivo studies of the α-adrenoceptor subtype mediating renal vascular responses to exogenously administered agonists suggested an almost exclusive role of α_1-adrenoceptors in the renal vasculature of the rat (124), cat (34), and dog (64). More recent studies show that α_2-adrenoceptor activation may also produce an increase in renal vascular resistance (58). However, despite evidence demonstrating the presence of postjunctional α_2-adrenoceptors in the renal arterial vasculature, it does appear that postjunctional α_1-adrenoceptors predominate.

MESENTERIC CIRCULATION

The splanchnic circulation receives approximately 20–25% of the cardiac output and contains a similar proportion of the blood volume. The major part of the splanchnic blood supply is received by the mesenteric circulation, which supplies the small intestine and the upper two-thirds of the large intestine via the superior mesenteric artery. Consequently, the mesenteric circulation has the potential to play a major role in the determination of total systemic vascular resistance. Sympathetic nerve stimulation and exogenous administration of norepinephrine produce mesenteric arteriolar vasoconstriction by activation of α-adrenoceptors (52). Studies using the in situ autoperfused superior mesenteric arterial bed of the rat suggest that only α_1-adrenoceptors are present in the mesenteric vasculature, since vasoconstrictor responses to norepinephrine are blocked exclusively by low doses of prazosin and are relatively unaffected by yohimbine (97). However, Hiley and Thomas (62) have recently shown that the mesenteric vasculature of the rat does indeed possess postjunctional vascular α_2-adrenoceptors in addition to the previously identified α_1 subtype, with an apparent greater density of α_1-adrenoceptors relative to α_2-adrenoceptors. Similarly, studies in the cat (34) and the dog (131) have demonstrated a significant population of postjunctional vascular α_2-adrenoceptors in the superior mesenteric arterial bed. Neuronally released norepinephrine, which presumably acts exclusively on α_1-adrenoceptors in the resistance vessels, does not produce a significant redistribution of blood flow within the intestinal wall. Thus, α_1-adrenoceptors appear to be relatively uniformly distributed throughout the arterial circulation in the gut wall.

CEREBRAL CIRCULATION

The arteries supplying blood to the brain clearly have different pharmacologic characteristics from peripheral arteries. A marked decrease in sensitivity to norepinephrine is seen just prior to the entry of the vessel into the subarachnoid space (10). This point of transition corresponds to the change in embryologic origin of the proximal and distal portions of each of these blood vessels.

Although cerebral blood vessels have extensive and active sympathetic innervation (35), the α-adrenoceptor–mediated responses of these vessels to sympathetic nerve stimulation are small compared with peripheral vessels (92). This difference may be related either to insensitivity of the α-adrenoceptor or to reduced α-adrenoceptor number (9). Nevertheless, there is evidence that the sympathetic nervous system can modulate cerebral blood flow in the conscious animal through an α-adrenoceptor–mediated effect, as measured by hypothalamic washout of radioactive xenon in the rabbit (110).

In vitro characterization of α-adrenoceptors on cerebral blood vessels has not yet yielded a uniform picture. Radioligand binding studies show the presence of both α_1- and α_2-adrenoceptors in membranes from human and monkey cerebral arteries.

Much information on the role of the α-adrenoceptor subtypes in mediating vasoconstriction of cerebral arteries still remains to be elucidated. Nevertheless, in certain species, including humans, both α_1- and α_2-adrenoceptors can be demonstrated in radioligand binding studies; by vasoconstriction induced by α_1- and α_2-adrenoceptor agonists; and by blockade of the response to the physiologic neurotransmitter, norepinephrine, by selective α_1- and α_2-adrenoceptor antagonists.

ENDOTHELIUM

It has recently been demonstrated that vascular endothelial cells mediate relaxation of arterial smooth muscle in response to certain vasodilators, such as acetylcholine, bradykinin, and substance P, by the release of the so-called endothelial derived relaxing factor (EDRF) (43). Activation of α_2-adrenoceptors on endothelial cells is thought to stimulate the release of EDRF (23, 36, 91), an action that would tend to antagonize vasoconstriction produced by activation of postjunctional vascular α-adrenoceptors. Thus, removal of endothelial cells from arteries produces an increase in responsiveness to α-adrenoceptor agonists (36). Removal of endothelium enhances the vasoconstrictor response produced by norepinephrine in canine and porcine circumflex coronary artery; and after blockade of α_1-adrenoceptors, norepinephrine can produce yohimbine-sensitive and idazoxan-sensitive relaxation of precontracted arteries only in the presence of an intact endothelium (23). Additional studies have shown that α_2-adrenoceptors mediate the release of EDRF from carotid, mesenteric, renal, and femoral arteries of dogs and pigs, although there do appear to be species differences in the magnitude of this response (3). Furthermore, endothelial α_2-adrenoceptors may mediate release of EDRF in coronary microvessels (3). Thus, α_2-adrenoceptor agonists do indeed appear to have the capability of modulating vascular responsiveness via stimulation of EDRF release in large arteries and the microcirculation, but this effect does not occur uniformly in all blood vessels. Recent evidence suggests that EDRF may be chemically identical to nitric oxide (102).

Peripheral Venous α-Adrenoceptors

SAPHENOUS VEIN

The most commonly studied vein is the canine saphenous vein. De Mey and Vanhoutte (31) first reported the potent vasoconstrictor activity of clonidine in this tissue. Additional studies have shown that highly selective α_2-adrenoceptor agonists, such as B-HT 920, B-HT 933, and UK 14,304, produce a vasoconstrictor response that is resistant to antagonism by prazosin and sensitive to blockade by rauwolscine (120). In the canine saphenous vein, norepinephrine, which can activate both α_1-

and α_2-adrenoceptors, appears to activate preferentially the α_2 subtype.

Experiments in isolated human saphenous vein (96) show results similar to those reported for the canine saphenous vein. The response to low concentrations of norepinephrine are essentially unaffected by prazosin but potently antagonized by yohimbine, suggesting that α_2-adrenoceptors may be more important than α_1-adrenoceptors.

The venous circulation resembles the arterial circulation in that postjunctional vascular α_1- and α_2-adrenoceptors coexist, with each α-adrenoceptor subtype mediating vasoconstriction (32, 39). However, in contrast to the arterial circulation, postjunctional vascular α_2-adrenoceptors in veins appear to be preferentially innervated, and postjunctional vascular α_1-adrenoceptors are innervated to a lesser degree and are possibly located predominantly extrajunctionally (39).

PULMONARY VEIN

Assessment of postjunctional α-adrenoceptor activity in the pulmonary vasculature in vitro provides some interesting correlates to what is observed in canine and human saphenous vein. Intralobar pulmonary veins have been reported to contract in response to the selective α_2-adrenoceptor agonist, B-HT 933, and this response is sensitive to inhibition by the selective α_2-adrenoceptor antagonist, rauwolscine (99, 130). In contrast, intralobar pulmonary arteries are relatively unresponsive to B-HT 933 in vitro. These results indicate that postjunctional vascular α_2-adrenoceptors may be preferentially located on the venous side of the pulmonary circulation, as also appears to be the case in the peripheral circulation (113).

HEPATIC PORTAL SYSTEM

A situation similar to that described in the saphenous vein also exists in vivo in the intestinal venous circulation (103). In addition, in the hepatic venous circulation of the cat in vivo, blood volume responses to norepinephrine are mediated by postjunctional vascular α_2-adrenoceptors, as is the hepatic venous response to sympathetic nerve stimulation (128). These results are suggestive of a dominance of α_2- over α_1-adrenoceptors in the hepatic venous circulation, as well as a preferential, if not exclusive, junctional location of vascular α_2-adrenoceptors (128). Furthermore, α_2-adre-

noceptor–mediated responses in the venous circulation appear to be more marked than those in the arterial circulation, consistent with the notion that postjunctional vascular α_2-adrenoceptors may play a more important functional role in venous than in arterial blood vessels (113).

OTHER VEINS

Most other veins have less of an α_2-adrenoceptor contribution relative to that observed in the saphenous vein. Shoji and associates (132) compared the responsiveness of many canine veins to norepinephrine, phenylephrine, and clonidine. The saphenous and cephalic veins have the greatest response to the α_2-adrenoceptor agonist, clonidine, followed by the femoral vein. Interestingly, longitudinal but not helical strips of portal vein, mesenteric vein, and vena cava readily respond to clonidine. Evidence for postjunctional α_2-adrenoceptors in human femoral vein has been provided by the failure of prazosin to antagonize the response to low concentrations of norepinephrine in this tissue, and by the potent contractile effect observed with guanfacine, a moderately selective α_2-adrenoceptor agonist (47).

In a quantitative analysis of α_1- and α_2-adrenoceptor characteristics in femoral and saphenous veins, the selective α_2-adrenoceptor agonist, UK 14,304, was much less effective in inducing contraction in the femoral vein (22% of norepinephrine maximum) than in the saphenous vein (86% of norepinephrine maximum) (40). As seen in some arteries, the response to norepinephrine in certain veins, such as the canine splenic vein, may be sensitive to blockade by both rauwolscine and prazosin, even though the tissue is unresponsive to highly selective α_2-adrenoceptor agonists (61).

PHYSIOLOGIC SIGNIFICANCE OF VENOUS α_2-ADRENOCEPTORS

The physiologic significance of venous α_2-adrenoceptors is unclear. In vivo studies with α_2-adrenoceptor agonists in the rat (45) or dog (146) cannot demonstrate a significant hemodynamic effect clearly attributable to effects on venous capacitance vessels. Since venous α_2-adrenoceptors are sensitive to temperature changes (41) and α_2-adrenoceptors are most prominent in the cutaneous veins (39), the venous α_2-adrenoceptor may be involved in blood flow redistribution to optimize the thermoregulatory process. It has recently been reported that α_2-adrenoceptor–mediated venoconstriction can significantly reduce venous capacitance and thereby increase venous return to the heart, resulting in an increase in cardiac output (70).

Myocardial α-Adrenoceptors

The predominant postsynaptic adrenoceptor in the heart is the β_1-adrenoceptor, which mediates a positive inotropic and chronotropic response (16). However, in the hearts of most mammalian species, including humans, there are postsynaptic α_1-adrenoceptors that mediate a positive inotropic response without notably changing heart rate (127). The mechanism by which cardiac α_1-adrenoceptors increase force of contraction has not been established, but it appears not to be associated with accumulation of cyclic AMP (cAMP) or stimulation of adenylate cyclase (17). In this respect, α_1-adrenoceptors differ from β_1-adrenoceptors in the myocardium. Other differences between myocardial α_1- and β_1-adrenoceptors are the longer rate of onset and longer duration of action of α_1-adrenoceptor–mediated inotropic responses (127). Differences among electrophysiologic actions mediated by α_1- and β_1-adrenoceptors have also been observed (50). β_1-Adrenoceptor–mediated inotropic responses occur at all rates of contraction, but the effect mediated by α_1-adrenoceptors is most prominent at lower rates (16).

Renal α-Adrenoceptors

The presence of α-adrenoceptors in the kidney has been known for many years, and α-adrenergic drugs produce a variety of renal effects. Only now are we beginning to understand the functions and locations of the renal α-adrenoceptors (137). Radioligand binding studies indicate that α_1- and α_2-adrenoceptors coexist in the kidneys of a variety of mammalian species; however the number, proportion, and distribution of each α-adrenoceptor subtype may vary from one species to another (137).

α_1-Adrenoceptors are believed to predominate in the human renal vasculature and to mediate a vasoconstrictor response, thereby modulating renal blood flow (57). α_2-Adrenoceptors have been identified in the juxtaglomerular apparatus and appear to inhibit renin release (137). Recently it has been demonstrated that stimulation of renal α_2-adrenoceptors can inhibit the effects of vasopressin on water and sodium excretion (133). This effect mediated by α_2-adrenoceptors appears to involve inhibition of adenylate cyclase and reductions in cellular cAMP, and may occur at the level of the cortical collecting tubule (78). The α_2-adrenoceptor–mediated enhancement in sodium and water excretion occurs simultaneously with a decrease in potassium secretion (44). α-Adrenoceptors, possibly of the α_1 subtype, may enhance sodium and water reabsorption in the proximal convoluted tubules. Gluconeogenesis in the proximal convoluted tubule has been shown to be under α_1-adrenoceptor control (72).

The density of renal α_2-adrenoceptors is higher in spontaneously hypertensive and Dahl salt-sensitive hypertensive rats than in normotensive controls, and high sodium diets may increase α_2-adrenoceptor number even further (51, 104). Thus, renal α_2-adrenoceptors may be involved in certain forms of genetic hypertension.

Cardiovascular Effects of α-Adrenergic Drugs

PERIPHERAL α-ADRENOCEPTOR BLOCKING AGENTS AS ANTIHYPERTENSIVES

Since vascular tone is mediated predominantly by α-adrenoceptors, it is logical to assume that pharmacologic antagonists of α-adrenoceptors abate hypertension. Indeed, the α-adrenoceptor antagonists, tolazoline (Priscoline) and phentolamine (Regitine), were introduced as clinical antihypertensive agents many years ago. These competitive α-adrenoceptor antagonists do, in fact, lower blood pressure, but their clinical efficacy has been unaccountably low. One explanation for their ineffectiveness is their ability to potentiate neuronal norepinephrine release (136). Both tolazoline and phentolamine are nonselective α-adrenoceptor antagonists and therefore have potent antagonist activity at prejunctional α_2-adrenoceptors in addition to their postjunctional α-adrenolytic effects. Their prejunctional α_2-adrenoceptor antagonist activity appears to interrupt the inhibitory negative feedback loop that regulates neurotransmitter release, increasing synaptic levels of norepinephrine. The elevated levels of norepinephrine in the synaptic cleft may partially overcome the post-junctional α_1-adrenoceptor antagonist effects and thus limit antihypertensive efficacy. This hypothesis has been widely accepted, primarily in the light of the high antihypertensive efficacy observed with prazosin (Minipress), a selective α_1-adrenoceptor antagonist (28). Since prazosin possesses only weak antagonist activity at presynaptic α_2-adrenoceptors, the neuronal negative feedback loop remains intact to prevent elevation of synaptic concentrations of norepinephrine (28).

In human forearm, yohimbine, a selective α_2-adrenoceptor antagonist, produces arterial vasodilation and increases blood flow (12). This finding suggests that, at least in this vascular bed, the postsynaptic extrajunctional α_2-adrenoceptor may also play a significant role, along with the junctional α_1-adrenoceptor, in maintaining vascular tone. Vasoconstrictor activity mediated by postsynaptic extrajunctional α_2-adrenoceptors may play more of a role in the hypertensive state, as shown both in animal studies (90, 93) and in clinical studies in which increased vasodilatory activity of yohimbine has been observed in patients with essential hypertension (12).

Circulating catecholamines are known to be elevated in a major subpopulation of patients with essential hypertension (49), and these high plasma catecholamine levels have been suggested as contributors to the increased vascular resistance characteristic of essential hypertension (2). Since circulating catecholamines appear to be the endogenous agonists for the extrajunctional vascular α_2-adrenoceptors, in this subgroup of patients, postjunctional α_2-adrenoceptors may, in fact, contribute to the elevated peripheral vascular resistance. As such, α_2-adrenoceptor blockade may prove to be beneficial in some forms of hypertension.

α-ADRENOCEPTOR ANTAGONISTS IN CONGESTIVE HEART FAILURE

Vasodilators have assumed a more prominent role in the treatment of congestive heart failure during the past decade. In most patients with congestive heart failure, the optimal vasodilator is one that acts relatively equally on the arterial and venous beds. Sodium nitroprusside acts in this way, but must be administered intravenously. Prazosin, an orally active selective α_1-adrenoceptor antagonist, has been shown to mimic the hemodynamic effects of nitroprusside in congestive heart failure,

increasing cardiac output, decreasing left ventricular filling pressure and systemic and pulmonary vascular resistance, and maintaining heart rate (6). Although acute tolerance has been observed after multiple doses of prazosin over a period of 24–72 hours (5), the beneficial effect often returns with continued therapy, and long-term clinical trials with prazosin show chronic efficacy in patients with congestive heart failure (135). Prazosin improves symptoms most during exercise (111).

Since there is evidence that the degree of sympathetic tone is proportional to the severity of heart failure (98, 138), and the level of plasma catecholamines has been implicated as a primary risk factor in patients with congestive heart failure (24), the use of α-adrenoceptor antagonists in low output cardiac failure may have a rational advantage over other vasodilators. An additional benefit may be that anginal frequency decreases with reduced afterload, and cardiac oxygen needs may be diminished (8).

The factor that best correlates with mortality in patients with heart failure is a high level of circulating catecholamines (24). Since, as discussed earlier, circulating catecholamines may be the natural substrates for postsynaptic extrajunctional α_2-adrenoceptors in the arterial circulation, and since high plasma catecholamine levels may contribute to the increased total peripheral vascular resistance characteristic of congestive heart failure (14, 98), the evaluation of an α_2-adrenoceptor antagonist in low output cardiac failure is indicated.

β-ADRENOCEPTORS

Central β-Adrenoceptors

β-Adrenoceptors have been identified on many neurons of the central nervous system (67), but their role in cardiovascular regulation is unclear. Activating central β-adrenoceptors has been shown to elevate blood pressure and heart rate (30). This observation is supported by the finding that injecting β-adrenoceptor antagonists into the central nervous system decreases blood pressure and heart rate (30). In addition, systemically administering β-adrenoceptor antagonists produce decreases in resting splanchnic sympathetic nerve discharges that correlate with reductions in arterial blood pressure (85). Intravenously administered propranolol has been reported to interrupt the cardiovascular reflex loop in the central nervous system and inhibit sympathetic outflow (33). Increases in blood pressure and heart rate evoked by sinoaortic denervation may be attenuated by injecting small doses of propranolol into the central nervous system (95). These results are highly suggestive of a centrally mediated tonic β-adrenoceptor influence to increase blood pressure, and of a possible central mechanism for the antihypertensive effects of β-blockers (77). However, β-adrenoceptor antagonists that do not penetrate the blood-brain barrier, such as atenolol, are also highly effective antihypertensive agents, suggesting that the peripheral antihypertensive effects of β-adrenoceptor antagonists are also significant.

Peripheral β-Adrenoceptors

PRESYNAPTIC β-ADRENOCEPTORS

The best understood presynaptic adrenoceptor is the α_2-adrenoceptor that inhibits neurotransmitter liberation. More recently, presynaptic β_2-adrenoceptors have been identified and shown to facilitate neurotransmitter release. It has been shown that presynaptic β_2-adrenoceptors enhance stimulus-evoked norepinephrine release, suggesting that prejunctional β_2-adrenoceptors mediate a positive feedback effect on sympathetic neurotransmission. The prejunctional β_2-adrenoceptor has been found in a variety of species, including humans (20, 87, 89).

Most experiments characterizing the prejunctional β_2-adrenoceptor have used either epinephrine or isoproterenol as agonists. Norepinephrine is not a potent presynaptic β_2-adrenoceptor agonist (88), acting instead on the presynaptic α_2-adrenoceptor to inhibit neurotransmitter release. It is therefore logical to assume that epinephrine is the physiologic ligand for the presynaptic β_2-adrenoceptor. This has led to the "epinephrine hypothesis" of essential hypertension, which suggests that activation of prejunctional β_2-adrenoceptors by neuronally released epinephrine may initiate the disease process.

EPINEPHRINE HYPOTHESIS OF ESSENTIAL HYPERTENSION

Epinephrine, synthesized and released by the adrenal gland, has a short half-life in the systemic circulation. Although circulating epinephrine levels during stress are equivalent to the threshold concentration for in vitro activation of prejunctional β_2-adrenoceptors (79), any β_2-adrenoceptor–mediated effect of circulating epinephrine on neuronal norepinephrine release should be transient. However, circulating epinephrine is readily accumulated by sympathetic nerve terminals via the neuronal uptake pump for sympathomimetic amines (uptake$_1$). In the sympathetic nerve terminal, epinephrine can be costored and coreleased with norepinephrine (88). Increases in the epinephrine content of tissues with dense sympathetic innervation are observed after stimulation-induced adrenal epinephrine secretion (106). Since epinephrine, but not norepinephrine, will activate the prejunctional β_2-adrenoceptor, epinephrine coreleased with norepinephrine will shift the balance toward increased β_2- relative to α_2-adrenoceptor–mediated prejunctional effects, thus increasing the net efficiency of sympathetic neurotransmission. Increased norepinephrine release in response to neuronally released epinephrine has been demonstrated in vitro in guinea pig and rat atrial tissue (89) and in vivo in humans (18).

Continuous infusion of low doses of epinephrine induces hypertension in rats (89). This effect is not mimicked by norepinephrine infusion and can be blocked by propranolol, suggesting an action on prejunctional β_2-adrenoceptors. Tachycardia is often an additional consequence of epinephrine infusion; this tachycardia is attenuated by neuronal uptake blockade and is much more persistent after epinephrine infusion than after isoproterenol, the latter not being a substrate for neuronal uptake (19).

The results of a large-scale clinical study in Great Britain correlating blood pressure and plasma catecholamines in hypertensive and prehypertensive subjects support the role of epinephrine in the development of the hypertensive state (18). Although the mechanism(s) of the antihypertensive activity of β-adrenoceptor blocking agents has not been established, the blockade of presynaptic facilitative β-adrenoceptors and the resulting inhibition of neurotransmitter liberation must be considered.

MYOCARDIAL β-ADRENOCEPTORS

The postsynaptic β-adrenoceptor of the heart that mediates an increase in both the rate and force of contraction is predominantly the β_1-subtype (16). Biochemical studies indicate that the positive inotropic and chronotropic responses to catecholamines are mediated by β_1-adrenoceptor activation of adenylate cyclase, with the ultimate generation and accumulation of cAMP (16).

Recent studies have shown that myocardial β_2-adrenoceptors may be present in the sinoatrial node in some mammalian species, including humans. The functional significance of these β_2-adrenoceptors is not known, and they appear to be noninnervated (16). It has been proposed that noninnervated extrajunctional β_2-adrenoceptors in the heart may represent "hormonal" adrenoceptors that are responsive to circulating bloodborne epinephrine (4).

Available data indicate that in congestive heart failure, myocardial β-adrenoceptors undergo "down-regulation," a cellularly mediated decrease in surface receptor number (15). This decrease in β-adrenoceptor number is proportional to the degree of myocardial dysfunction and the loss of contractility that occurs in congestive heart failure. Myocardial β-adrenoceptor down-regulation is chamber-specific, occurring to the greatest degree in the most severely affected ventricular chamber, and is specific to the β_1-adrenoceptor subtype. β-Adrenoceptor down-regulation may be the result of the excessively high levels of plasma catecholamines seen in congestive heart failure, inasmuch as a similar phenomenon of β-adrenoceptor down-regulation is seen in animals treated with high doses of catecholamines. The specific down-regulation in cardiac β-adrenoceptors may be, in part, the cause of the decrease in myocardial function observed during long-term β-adrenoceptor stimulation, and an actual decrease in β-adrenoceptor number has been observed in myocardial tissue from patients with congestive heart failure (117). Down-regulation of β-adrenoceptors in congestive heart failure results in a decrease or loss of efficacy of β-adrenoceptor agonists on long-term administration. Although β-adrenoceptors are down-regulated in congestive heart failure, myocardial α_1-adrenoceptors and histamine H_2-receptors do not appear to be subject to this same regulatory process.

VASCULAR β-ADRENOCEPTORS

Postsynaptic vascular β_2-adrenoceptors mediate vasodilation. The vascular β_2-adrenoceptors, like the vascular α_2-adrenoceptors, appear to be noninnervated (i.e., are located extrajunctionally) (4). It has been proposed, therefore, that extrajunctional vascular β_2-adrenoceptors are "hormonal" receptors that mediate vasodilation in response to circulating epinephrine in certain vascular beds at times of stress, when plasma levels of epinephrine are elevated. As recently shown, the vasodilatory response mediated by vascular β_2-adrenoceptors after ganglionic stimulation is abolished by bilateral adrenalectomy, indicating that this response results from the action of circulating epinephrine liberated by the adrenal glands (4).

RENAL β-ADRENOCEPTORS

The kidney is also heavily under adrenergic control. Probably the most important adrenergic effect in the kidney is the regulation of renin release from the juxtaglomerular apparatus (71). Renin release from the juxtaglomerular cells is enhanced by β_1-adrenoceptor stimulation and/or stimulation of renal adrenergic nerves (71). The increase in renin release evoked by the exogenous administration of β-adrenoceptor agonists or by adrenergic nerve stimulation is antagonized by β-adrenoceptor blocking agents such as propranolol. The juxtaglomerular cells appear to be under a constant adrenergic tone since β-adrenoceptor blocking agents also inhibit basal renin release (71). It has been suggested that the magnitude of the antihypertensive response to β-adrenoceptor antagonists depends on the initial plasma renin activity and the degree of its suppression by β-adrenoceptor blockade (21). However, the relevance of the decrease in renin release mediated by β-adrenoceptor antagonists to the antihypertensive effects of these compounds has been questioned, since the reduction in blood pressure does not always parallel the reduction in renin release. In addition, some β-adrenoceptor blockers with intrinsic sympathomimetic activity may themselves promote renin release by their inherent β-adrenoceptor agonist properties (71), yet these compounds nonetheless are effective antihypertensive agents in humans.

Renal β-adrenoceptors also appear to regulate renal blood flow at the vascular level. β_2-Adrenoceptors in the vasculature have been identified pharmacologically and mediate the expected vasodilatory response, resulting in an increase in renal blood flow.

β-Adrenoceptors may also affect renal salt and water metabolism, but these effects are controversial and the results are often contradictory (71).

Cardiovascular Effects of β-Adrenergic Drugs

β-ADRENOCEPTOR ANTAGONISTS USED IN THE MANAGEMENT OF HYPERTENSION

β-Adrenoceptor blocking agents are commonly used to treat hypertension. Several β-adrenoceptor antagonists are available and differ significantly. Certain β-adrenoceptor antagonists, such as propranolol, are nonselective in that they antagonize both β_1- and β_2-adrenoceptors. Other β-adrenoceptor antagonists, such as atenolol, are termed "cardioselective," preferentially antagonizing myocardial β_1-adrenoceptors. Finally, a class of β-adrenoceptor antagonists with intrinsic sympathomimetic activity is now available; the prototype is pindolol. These different classes of β-adrenoceptor antagonists produce qualitatively and quantitatively distinct hemodynamic responses in humans, and therefore should not be considered as one homogeneous class of drugs possessing similar pharmacologic activities.

As indicated earlier, the mechanism of action of β-adrenoceptor antagonists in hypertension is still a matter of controversy. From the previously discussed effects that may be attributed to central β-adrenoceptors, and peripheral presynaptic and postsynaptic β-adrenoceptors in the heart, vasculature, and kidneys, four logical mechanisms for the antihypertensive activity of β-blocking agents may be postulated: (a) an action within the central nervous system that antagonizes the central β-adrenoceptor–mediated increases in blood pressure and heart rate; (b) presynaptic β-adrenoceptor blockade that inhibits the β-adrenoceptor–mediated positive feedback effect on neurotransmitter (norepinephrine) liberation in the heart, vasculature, and kidneys; (c) blockade of postsynaptic cardiac β_1-adrenoceptors that decreases the rate and force of myocardial contraction and thereby decrease cardiac output; and (d) inhibition of renin release, which is stimulated by β_1-adrenoceptor activation.

All classes of β-adrenoceptor antagonists lower blood pressure, regardless of β-adrenoceptor subtype selectivity or the presence of intrinsic sympathomimetic activity. Furthermore, no one mechanism will adequately account for the antihypertensive activity of β-adrenoceptor antagonists in general. Thus, some β-adrenoceptor blockers do not penetrate the blood-brain barrier whereas others with intrinsic sympathomimetic activity may enhance renin release. In addition, β-adrenoceptor antagonists decrease heart rate and cardiac output acutely, yet the antihypertensive effect of β-adrenoceptor blockers may take days to develop. Thus, several of these mechanisms may contribute to the antihypertensive activity of any one β-adrenoceptor blocker.

When β-adrenoceptor antagonists (without intrinsic sympathomimetic activity) are first administered, there is an acute decrease in heart rate and cardiac output and a reflex increase in total peripheral vascular resistance, such that no net change in blood pressure results. After a period of latency, total peripheral vascular resistance begins to decrease toward initial values in the face of continued reduced cardiac output, and the net effect is a decrease in blood pressure (76). At times, total peripheral resistance may only return to normal levels, but cardiac output remains low and the net effect is still a reduction in blood pressure (94).

In spite of the initial elevation in total peripheral vascular resistance, the antihypertensive effect of propranolol follows closely the secondary fall in peripheral vascular resistance that occurs with time, even when there is some restoration in cardiac output.

β-ADRENOCEPTOR BLOCKING AGENTS IN ANGINA

The β-adrenoceptor blocking agents are useful in angina pectoris because they decrease myocardial oxygen demand. There are three determinants of myocardial oxygen demand: (a) myocardial wall tension, which is a function of ventricular pressure and the radius of the left ventricle; (b) heart rate; and (c) contractility. β-Adrenoceptor antagonists produce a decrease in heart rate and contractile force, simply by β-adrenoceptor blockade. The chronic antihypertensive effect of β-adrenoceptor blockers also serves to reduce myocardial wall tension by decreasing ventricular systolic developed pressure. Therefore, the utility of β-adrenoceptor antagonists in treating angina pectoris results from the ability of these compounds to decrease the myocardial oxygen demand by affecting each of the three factors known to determine oxygen demand (53).

β-ADRENOCEPTOR AGONISTS IN CONGESTIVE HEART FAILURE

In heart failure, the goal of therapy is usually to increase cardiac output, and this is often done by increasing the contractile state of the myocardium. One mechanism that may be used to augment cardiac function is activation of myocardial β_1-adrenoceptors, which increases heart rate and contractility and therefore increases cardiac output. The increase in heart rate that occurs with isoproterenol may be undesirable since it increases myocardial work and oxygen demand. With certain inotropic agents, myocardial contractility can be selectively increased with little or no increase in heart rate.

Intravenous infusion of dobutamine generally increases cardiac output by augmenting stroke volume (1) through enhanced left ventricular contractility (dp/dt_{max}) (68). Total peripheral vascular resistance (afterload) is reduced in part by reflex withdrawal of sympathetic tone (86) and in part by direct arterial vasodilation (118). The reduction in afterload produced by dobutamine further increases left ventricular stroke volume by reducing the impedence to left ventricular ejection. Furthermore, the decrease in total peripheral vascular resistance offsets the contribution made by cardiac output to blood pressure, such that mean arterial pressure is only minimally affected while cardiac output is significantly increased (83).

Dobutamine infusion is generally associated with decreases in central venous pressure, right and left atrial pressures, pulmonary artery pressure and resistance, and pulmonary capillary wedge pressure (83). Consequently, left ventricular end-diastolic volume (preload, represented by left ventricular end-diastolic pressure) is lowered, allowing the enlarged myocardium characteristic of congestive heart failure to reduce to a more efficient size (134). The decrease in left ventricular end-systolic volume also decreases myocardial wall tension, an important determinant of myocardial oxygen consumption (53).

For doses of isoproterenol and dobutamine that produce comparable increases in cardiac output, larger decreases in total peripheral vascular resistance, and hence greater reductions in blood pressure, are observed with isoproterenol (134). In addition, tachycardia is more pronounced with isoproterenol (5), resulting from a greater direct positive chronotropic effect and an additional reflex increase in cardiac rate secondary to the greater reduction in vascular tone. The more profound increase in cardiac rate observed with isoproterenol than with dobutamine, at doses that produce equivalent increases in cardiac output, indicates that a smaller contribution to cardiac output is derived from augmentation of stroke volume with isoproterenol than with dobutamine.

When dopamine and dobutamine are infused at doses that produce equivalent increases in cardiac output, dobutamine is generally associated with greater reductions in left ventricular filling pressure and pulmonary capillary wedge pressure (83). Quite commonly, dopamine is associated with no change or even an increase in pulmonary artery pressure, pulmonary capillary wedge pressure, and left ventricular end-diastolic pressure. Whereas dobutamine tends to have minimal effects on blood pressure, dopamine is more likely to produce an increase in total peripheral vascular resistance and mean arterial blood pressure (83). At low doses, dopamine has been shown to produce a selective increase in renal blood flow, secondary to a decrease in renal vascular resistance (48). This action of dopamine, which is lacking with dobutamine, has been ascribed to selective renal vasodilation resulting from activation of renal DA_1-dopamine receptors. In contrast, the improvement in renal function observed with dobutamine appears to be secondary to an increase in cardiac output and a reflex decrease in total peripheral vascular resistance (83).

At doses that produce comparable increases in cardiac output, epinephrine and norepinephrine cause more tachycardia and greater increases in total peripheral vascular resistance than dobutamine. Consequently, dobutamine tends to increase stroke volume while not greatly affecting blood pressure or heart rate, whereas epinephrine and norepinephrine may cause a smaller increase in stroke volume because of the increased impedence to left ventricular ejection resulting from elevation of afterload, the latter serving to limit increases in stroke volume elicited by improved myocardial contractility.

References

1. Akhtar N, Mikulik E, Cohn JN, Chaudhry MH: Hemodynamic effect of dobutamine in patients with severe heart failure. *Am J Cardiol* 36:202, 1975.

2. Amann FW, Bolli P, Kiowski W, Buhler FR: Enhanced α-adrenoceptor–mediated vasoconstriction in essential hypertension. *Hypertension* 3(suppl 1):I–119, 1981.
3. Angus JA, Cocks TM, Satoh K: The α-adrenoceptors on endothelial cells. *Fed Proc* 45:2355–2359, 1986.
4. Ariens EJ: The classification of α-adrenoceptors. 2. *Trends Pharmacol Sci* 2:170, 1981.
5. Arnold SB, Williams RL, Ports TA, Benet LZ, Parmley WW, Chatterjee K: Attenuation of prazosin effect on cardiac output in chronic heart failure. *Ann Intern Med* 91:345, 1979.
6. Awan NA, Miller RR, Maxwell KS, Mason DJ: Effects of prazosin on forearm resistance and capacitance vessels. *Clin Pharmacol Ther* 22:79, 1977.
7. Barajas L, Wang P: Localization of tritiated norepinephrine in the renal arteriolar nerves. *Anat Rec* 195:525, 1979.
8. Bertel O, Burkart R, Buhler FR: Sustained effectiveness of chronic prazosin therapy in severe chronic congestive heart failure. *Am Heart J* 5:529, 1981.
9. Bevan JA: Autonomic pharmacologist's guide to the cerebral circulation. *Trends Pharmacol Sci* 5:234–236, 1986.
10. Bevan JA: Sites of transition between functional systemic and cerebral arteries of rabbits occur at embryological junctional sites. *Science* 204:635–637, 1979.
11. Bolli P, Erne P, Ji BH, Block LH, Kiowski W, Buhler FR: Adrenaline induces vasoconstriction through postjunctional alpha₂-adrenoceptors and this response is enhanced in patients with essential hypertension. *J Hypertens* 2(suppl 3):115–118, 1984.
12. Bolli P, Erne P, Kiowski W, Ji BH, Amann FW, Buhler FR: Important contribution of post-junctional α₂-adrenoceptor–mediated vasoconstriction to arteriolar tone in man. *J Hypertens* 1(suppl 2):257, 1983.
13. Bousquet P, Guertzenstein PG: Localization of the central cardiovascular action of clonidine. *Br J Pharmacol* 49:573–579, 1973.
14. Bristow MR: The adrenergic nervous system in heart failure. *N Engl J Med* 311:850, 1984.
15. Bristow MR, Ginsberg R, Minobe WA, Harrison DC, Reitz BA, Stinson EB: β-Adrenergic receptor measurements in normal and failing human right and left ventricule. *Circulation* 66(suppl II):II-207, 1982.
16. Broadley KJ: Cardiac adrenoceptors. *J Auton Pharmacol* 2:119–145, 1982.
17. Brodde O-E, Motomura S, Endoh M, Schumann HJ: Lack of correlation between the positive inotropic effect evoked by α-adrenoceptor stimulation and the levels of cyclic AMP and/or cyclic GMP in the isolated ventricle strip of the rabbit. *J Mol Cell Cardiol* 10:207–219, 1978.
18. Brown MJ: The role of adrenaline in essential hypertension in man. In Bevan JA, Godfraind T, Maxwell RA, Worcel M (eds): *Proceedings of the 5th Vascular Neuroeffector Symposium*. 1985.
19. Brown MJ, Brown DC, Murphy MB: Hypokalemia from β₂-receptor stimulation by circulating epinephrine. *N Engl J Med* 309:1414, 1983.
20. Brown MJ, Macquin I: Is adrenaline the cause of essential hypertension? *Lancet* 2:1079, 1981.
21. Buhler FR, Laragh JH, Baer JH, Vaughn ED, Brunner HR: Propranolol inhibition of renin secretion. A specific approach to the diagnosis and treatment of renin-dependent hypertensive disease. *N Engl J Med* 287:1209, 1972.
22. Clifton CG, O'Neill WM, Wallin JD: Tiamenidine, a new antihypertensive agent: efficacy, safety and rebound hypertension. *Curr Ther Res* 30:397–404, 1981.
23. Cocks TM, Angus JA: Endothelium-dependent relaxation of coronary arteries by noradrenaline and serotonin. *Nature* 305:627–630, 1983.
24. Cohn JN, Levine TB, Olivari MM, Garberg V, Luva D, Francis GS, Simon AB, Rector T: Plasma norepineph-

rine as a guide to prognosis in patients with chronic congestive heart failure. *N Engl J Med* 311:819, 1984.
25. Conway EL, Louis WJ, Jarrott B: The effect of acute α-methyldopa administration on catecholamine levels in anterior hypothalamic and medullary nuclei in rat brain. *Neuropharmacology* 18:279–286, 1979.
26. Cooke JH, Johns EJ, MacLeod JH, Singer B: Effect of renal nerve stimulation, renal blood flow and adrenergic blockade on plasma renin activity in the cat. *J Physiol* 226:15–36, 1972.
27. Cutter WE, Bier DM, Shah SD, Cryer PE: Epinephrine plasma clearance rates and physiologic thresholds for metabolic and hemodynamic actions in man. *J Clin Invest* 66:94–101, 1980.
28. Davey MJ: Relevant features of the pharmacology of prazosin. *J Cardiovasc Pharmacol* 2(suppl 3):S287, 1980.
29. Davis DS, Wing LMH, Reid JL, Neill E, Tippett P, Dollery CT: Pharmacokinetics and concentration-effect relationships of intravenous and oral clonidine. *Clin Pharmacol Ther* 21:593–600, 1977.
30. Day MD, Roach AG: Cardiovascular effects of dopamine after central administration into conscious cats. *Br J Pharmacol* 58:505, 1976.
31. De Mey J, Vanhoutte PM: Uneven distribution of postjunctional α₁ and α₂-like adrenoceptors in canine arterial and venous smooth muscle. *Circ Res* 48:875–884, 1981.
32. Docherty JR, Hyland L: Neuro-effector transmission through postsynaptic α₂-adrenoceptors in human saphenous vein. *Br J Pharmacol* 83:362P, 1984.
33. Dorward PK, Korner PI: Effect of dl-propranolol on renal sympathetic baroreflex properties and aortic baroreceptor activity. *Eur J Pharmacol* 52:61, 1978.
34. Drew GM, Whiting SB: Evidence for two distinct types of postsynaptic α-adrenoceptor in vascular smooth muscle in vivo. *Br J Pharmacol* 67:207–215, 1979.
35. Duckles SP: Functional activity of the noradrenergic innervation of large cerebral arteries. *Br J Pharmacol* 69:193–199, 1980.
36. Egleme C, Godfraind T, Miller RC: Enhanced responsiveness of isolated rat aorta to clonidine after removal of the endothelial cells. *Br J Pharmacol* 81:16–18, 1984.
37. Engberg G, Elam M, Svensson TH: Clonidine withdrawal: activation of brain noradrenergic neurons with specifically reduced α₂-receptor sensitivity. *Life Sci* 30:235–243, 1982.
38. Feigl EO: Sympathetic control of coronary circulation. *Circ Res* 20:262–270, 1967.
39. Flavahan NA, Rimele TJ, Cooke JP, Vanhoutte PM: Characterization of postjunctional α-1 and α-2 adrenoceptors activated by exogenous or nerve-released norepinephrine in the canine saphenous vein. *J Pharmacol Exp Ther* 230:699–705, 1984.
40. Flavahan NA, Vanhoutte PM: Alpha₁ and α₂-adrenoceptor: response coupling in canine saphenous and femoral veins. *J Pharmacol Exp Ther* 238:131–138, 1986.
41. Flavahan NA, Vanhoutte PM: The effect of cooling on α₁ and α₂-adrenergic responses in canine saphenous and femoral veins. *J Pharmacol Exp Ther* 238:139–147, 1986.
42. Frisk-Holmberg M, Paalzow L, Wibell L: Relationship between the cardiovascular effects and steady-state kinetics of clonidine in hypertension. *Eur J Clin Pharmacol* 26:309–313, 1984.
43. Furchgott RF, Zawadzki JV: The obligatory role of endothelial cells in the relaxation of arterial smooth muscle by acetylcholine. *Nature* 288:373, 1980.
44. Gellai M, Ruffolo RR Jr: Renal effects of selective α₁ and α₂-adrenoceptor agonists in conscious, normotensive rats, *J Pharmacol Exp Ther* 240:723–728, 1987.
45. Gerold M, Haesler G: Alpha₂-adrenoceptors in rat re-

sistance vessels. *Naunyn Schmiedebergs Arch Pharmacol* 322:29–33, 1983.

46. Giles TD, Thomas MG, Sander GE, Quiroz AC: Central α-adrenergic agonists in chronic heart failure and ischemic heart disease. *J Cardiovasc Pharmacol* 7(suppl 8):S51–S55, 1985.

47. Glusa E, Markwardt F: Characterization of α_2-adrenoceptors on blood platelets from various species using ^{3}H-yohimbine. *Haemostasis* 13:96–101, 1983.

48. Goldberg LI, Hsieh YY, Resnekov L: Newer catecholamines for treatment of heart failure and shock: an update on dopamine and a first look at dobutamine. *Prog Cardiovasc Dis* 19:327, 1977.

49. Goldstein DS: Plasma catecholamines and essential hypertension: an analytical review. *Hypertension* 5:86, 1983.

50. Govier WC: A positive inotropic effect of phenylephrine mediated through α-adrenergic receptors. *Life Sci* 6:1361–1365, 1967.

51. Graham RM, Pettinger WA, Sagalowsky A, et al: Renal α-adrenergic receptor abnormality in the spontaneously hypertensive rat. *Hypertension* 4:881, 1982.

52. Granger DN, Richardson PDI, Kvietys PR, Mortillaro NA: Intestinal blood flow. *Gastroenterology* 78:837–863, 1980.

53. Gross GJ, Urquilla PR: Antianginal drugs. In Craig CR, Stitzel RE (eds): *Modern Pharmacology.* Boston, Little, Brown & Co, 1982, pp 283–294.

54. Hansson L: Clinical aspects of blood pressure crisis due to withdrawal of centrally acting antihypertensive drugs. *Br J Clin Pharmacol* 15:485S–489S, 1973.

55. Hansson L, Hunyor SN, Julius S, Hoobler SW: Blood pressure crisis following withdrawal of clonidine, with special reference to arterial and urinary catecholamine levels and suggestions for acute management. *Am Heart J* 85:605–610, 1973.

56. Hashimoto K, Shigel T, Imai S, Saito Y, Yago N, Uei I, Clark RE: Oxygen consumption and coronary vascular tone in the isolated fibrillating dog heart. *Am J Physiol* 198:965–970, 1960.

57. Hepburn ER, Bentley GA: The effects of α-agonists on various vascular beds. In Bevan JA, Godfraind T, Maxwell RA, Vanhoutte PM (eds): *Vascular Neuroeffector Mechanisms.* New York, Raven Press, 1980, pp 249–251.

58. Hesse IFA, Johns EJ: An in vivo study of the α-adrenoceptor subtypes on the renal vasculature of the anaesthetised rabbit. *J Auton Pharmacol* 4:145–152, 1984.

59. Heusch G, Deussen A: The effects of cardiac sympathetic nerve stimulation on perfusion of stenotic coronary arteries in the dog. *Circ Res* 53:8–15, 1983.

60. Heusch G, Deussen A, Schipke J, Thamer V: Alpha$_1$- and alpha$_2$-adrenoceptor–mediated vasoconstriction of large and small canine coronary arteries *in vivo*. *J Cardiovasc Pharmacol* 6:961–968, 1984.

61. Hieble JP, Woodward DF: Different characteristics of postjunctional α-adrenoceptors on arterial and venous smooth muscle. *Naunyn Schmiedebergs Arch Pharmacol* 328:44–50, 1984.

62. Hiley CR, Thomas GR: Effects of alpha-adrenoceptor agonists on cardiac output and its regional distribution in the pithed rat. *Br J Pharmacol* 90:61–70, 1987.

63. Holtz J, Saeed M, Sommer O, Bassenge E: Norepinephrine constricts the canine coronary bed via postsynaptic α_2-adrenoceptors. *Eur J Pharmacol* 82:199–202, 1982.

64. Horn PT, Kohli JD, Listinsky JJ, Goldberg LI: Regional variation in the α-adrenergic receptors in the canine resistance vessels. *Naunyn Schmiedebergs Arch Pharmacol* 318:166–172, 1982.

65. Hyman AL, Kadowitz PJ: Evidence for existence of postjunctional α_1- and α_2-adrenoceptors in cat pulmonary vascular bed. *Am J Physiol* 249:H891–H898, 1985.

66. Hyman AL, Lippton HL, Kadowitz PJ: Autonomic regulation of the pulmonary circulation. *J Cardiovasc Pharmacol* 7:S80–S95, 1985.

67. Iversen LL: Catecholamine-sensitive adenylate cyclases in nervous tissue. *J Neurochem* 29:5, 1977.

68. Jewitt D, Mitchell A, Birkhead J, Dollery C: Clinical cardiovascular pharmacology of dobutamine. *Lancet* 2:363, 1974.

69. Jie K, van Brummelen P, Vermey P, Timmermans PBMWM, van Zwieten PA: Alpha$_1$- and alpha$_2$-adrenoceptor mediated vasoconstriction in the forearm of normotensive and hypertensive subjects. *J Cardiovasc Pharmacol* 8:190–196, 1986.

70. Kalkman HO, Thoolen MJMC, Timmermans PBMWM, van Zwieten PA: The influence of α_1 and α_2-adrenoceptor agonists on cardiac output in rats and cats. *J Pharm Pharmacol* 36:265–268, 1984.

71. Keeton TK, Campbell WB: The pharmacologic alteration of renin release. *Pharmacol Rev* 32:81, 1980.

72. Kessar P, Saggerson ED: Evidence that catecholamines stimulate renal gluconeogenesis through an α_1-type of adrenoceptor. *Biochem J* 190:119, 1980.

73. Kho TL, Schalekamp MADH, Zaal GA, Wester A, Birkenhager WH: Comparison between the effects of St 600 and clonidine. *Arch Int Pharmacodyn* 217:162–169, 1975.

74. Kobinger W: Central α-adrenergic system as targets for hypotensive drugs. *Rev Physiol Biochem Pharmacol* 81:39, 1978.

75. Kopia GA, Kopaciewicz LJ, Ruffolo RR Jr: α-Adrenoceptor regulation of coronary artery blood flow in normal and stenotic canine coronary arteries. *J Pharmacol Exp Ther* 239:641–647, 1986.

76. Korner PI: Discussion to: Systemic hemodynamic effects of centrally acting antihypertensive agents. In Onesti G, Fernandes M, Kim E (eds): *Regulation of Blood Pressure by the Central Nervous System.* New York, Grune & Stratton, 1976, p 412.

77. Korner PI, Angus JA: Central nervous control of blood pressure in relation to antihypertensive drug treatment. *Pharmacol Ther* 13:321, 1981.

78. Krothapalli RK, Suki W: Functional characterization of the α-adrenergic receptor modulating the hydroosmotic effect of vasopressin on the rabbit cortical collecting tubule. *J Clin Invest* 73:740, 1984.

79. Langer SZ: Presynaptic receptors and their role in the regulation of transmitter release. *Br J Pharmacol* 60:481, 1977.

80. Langer SZ, Shepperson NB: Postjunctional α_1- and α_2-adrenoceptors: preferential innervation of α_1-adrenoceptors and the role of neuronal uptake. *J Cardiovasc Pharmacol* 4:S8–S13, 1982.

81. Langer SZ, Shepperson NB: Recent developments in vascular smooth muscle pharmacology: the postsynaptic α_2-adrenoceptor. *Trends Pharmacol Sci* 3:440–444, 1982.

82. Langer SZ, Shepperson NB, Massingham R: Preferential noradrenergic innervation of α_1-adrenergic receptors in vascular smooth muscle. *Hypertension* 3(suppl I):I-112–I-118, 1981.

83. Leier CV, Unverferth DV: Dobutamine. *Ann Intern Med* 99:490, 1983.

84. Levine TB, Francis GS, Goldsmith SR: Activity of the sympathetic nervous system assessed by plasma hormone levels and their relation to hemodynamic abnormalities in congestive heart failure. *Am J Cardiol* 49:1659–1666, 1982.

85. Lewis PJ, Haeusler G: Reduction in sympathetic nervous activity as a mechanism for hypotensive effect of propranolol. *Nature* 256:440, 1975.

86. Liang CS, Hood WB: Dobutamine infusion in conscious dogs with and without autonomic nervous system inhibition: effects of systemic hemodynamics, regional blood flows and cardiac metabolism. *J Pharmacol Exp Ther* 211:698, 1979.

87. Majewski H, Hedler L, Starke K: The noradrenaline release rate in the anesthetized rabbit: facilitation by adrenaline. *Naunyn Schmiedebergs Arch Pharmacol* 321:20, 1982.

88. Majewski H, Rand MJ, Tung LH: Activation of prejunctional β-adrenoceptors in rat atria by adrenaline applied exogenously or released as a co-transmitter. *Br J Pharmacol* 73:669, 1981.

89. Majewski H, Tung LH, Rand MJ: Adrenaline activation of prejunctional β-adrenoceptors and hypertension. *J Cardiovasc Pharmacol* 4:99, 1982.

90. Majewski H, Tung LH, Rand MJ: Adrenaline-induced hypertension in rats. *J Cardiovasc Pharmacol* 3:179, 1981.

91. Matsuda H, Kuon E, Holtz J, Busse R: Endothelium-mediated dilations contribute to the polarity of the arterial wall in vasomotion induced by α_2-adrenergic agonists. *J Cardiovasc Pharmacol* 7:680–688, 1985.

92. McCalden TA: Sympathetic control of the cerebral circulation. *J Auton Pharmacol* 1:421–431, 1981.

93. Medgett IC, Hicks PE, Langer SZ: Smooth muscle α_2-adrenoceptors mediate vasoconstrictor responses to exogenous norepinephrine and to sympathetic stimulation to a greater extent in spontaneously hypertensive than in Wistar Kyoto rat tail arteries. *J Pharmacol Exp Ther* 231:159, 1984.

94. Meier M, Orwin J, Rogg H, Brunner H: β-Adrenoceptor antagonists in hypertension. In Scriabine A (ed): *Pharmacology of Antihypertensive Drugs*. New York, Raven Press, 1980, pp 179–94.

95. Montastruc J-L, Montastruc P: Effect of intracisternal application of 6-hydroxydopamine on the antihypertensive action of propranolol in the dog. *Eur J Pharmacol* 63:103, 1980.

96. Muller-Schweinitzer E: Alpha-adrenoceptors, 5-hydroxytryptamine receptors and the action of dihydroergotamine in human venous preparations obtained during saphenectomy procedures for varicose veins. *Naunyn Schmiedebergs Arch Pharmacol* 327:299–303, 1984.

97. Nichols AJ, Hiley CR: Identification of adrenoceptors and dopamine receptors mediating vascular responses in the superior mesenteric arterial bed of the rat. *J Pharm Pharmacol* 37:110–115, 1985.

98. Ogasawara B, Ogawa K, Hayashi H, Sassa H: Plasma renin activity and plasma concentration of norepinephrine and cyclic nucleotides in heart failure after prazosin. *Clin Pharmacol Ther* 29:464, 1981.

99. Ohlstein EH, Shebuski RJ, Ruffolo RR Jr: Localization of α_2-adrenoceptors in the canine pulmonary vasculature. *Pharmacologist* 28:141, 1986.

100. Onesti G, Schwartz AB, Kim KE: Antihypertensive effect of clonidine. *Circ Res* 28(suppl 2):53–69, 1971.

101. Oswald H, Greven J: Effects of adrenergic activators and inhibitors on kidney function. In Syekeres L (ed): *Handbook of Experimental Pharmacology*. Springer-Verlag, Berlin, 1981, vol 54, pp 241–288.

102. Palmer RMJ, Ferrige AG, Moncade S: Nitric oxide release accounts for the biological activity of endothelium derived relaxing factor. *Nature* 327:524–526, 1987.

103. Patel P, Bose D, Greenway C: Effects of prazosin and phenoxybenzamine on α- and β-receptor mediated responses in intestinal resistance and capacitance vessels. *J Cardiovasc Pharmacol* 3:1050–1059, 1981.

104. Pettinger WA, Gandler T, Sanchez A, et al: Dietary sodium and renal α-adrenoceptors in Dahl hypertensive rats. *Clin Exp Hypertension* A4(4 and 5):819, 1982.

105. Pitt B, Elliot EC, Gregg DE: Adrenergic receptor activity in the coronary arteries of the unanesthetized dog. *Circ Res* 21:75–84, 1967.

106. Raab W, Gigee W: Die Katecholamine des Herzens. *Naunyn Schmiedeberg's Arch Pharmacol* 219:248, 1953.

107. Reid JL: Central α_2 receptors and the regulation of

blood pressure in humans. *J Cardiovasc Pharmacol* 7(suppl 8):S45–S50, 1985.

108. Reid JL, Rubin PC, Howden CW. Central α_2-adrenoceptors and blood pressure regulation in man: studies with guanfacine (BS 100–141) and azapexole (BHT 933). *Br J Clin Pharmacol* 15(suppl 4):463–469, 1983.

109. Reis DJ: The brain and hypertension: reflections on 35 years of inquiry into the neurobiology of the circulation. *Circulation* 70:III-31, 1984.

110. Rosendorff C, Mitchell G, Scriven DR, Shapiro C: Evidence for a dual innervation affecting local blood flow in the hypothalamus of the conscious rabbit. *Circ Res* 38:140–145, 1976.

111. Rubin SA, Chatterjee K, Gelberg HJ, Ports TA, Brundage BH, Parmley WW: Paradox of improved exercise but not resting hemodynamics with short term prazosin in chronic heart failure. *Am J Cardiol* 43:810, 1979.

112. Ruffolo RR Jr: α-Adrenoceptors. *Monogr Neural Sci* 10:224–253, 1984.

113. Ruffolo RR Jr: Distribution and function of peripheral α-adrenoceptors in the cardiovascular system. *Pharmacol Biochem Behav* 22:827–833, 1985.

114. Ruffolo RR Jr: Relative agonist potency as a means of differentiating α_2-adrenoceptors and α-adrenergic mechanisms. *Clin Sci* 68(suppl 10):9S–14S, 1985.

115. Ruffolo RR Jr: Stereochemical requirements for activation and blockade of α_1 and α_2-adrenoceptors. *Trends Pharmacol Sci* 5:160–164, 1984c.

116. Ruffolo RR Jr: Structure-activity relationships of α-adrenoceptor agonists. In Kunos G (ed): *Adrenoceptors and Catecholamine Action*, Part B. New York, John Wiley & Sons, 1983, pp 1–50.

117. Ruffolo RR Jr, Kopia GA: The importance of receptor regulation in the pathophysiology and therapy of congestive heart failure. *Am J Med* 80(suppl 2B):67–72, 1986.

118. Ruffolo RR Jr, Morgan EL: Interaction of novel inotropic agent, ASL-7022, with α- and β-adrenoceptors in the cardiovascular system of the pithed rat: comparison with dobutamine and dopamine. *J Pharmacol Exp Ther* 229:364, 1984.

119. Ruffolo, RR Jr, Nichols, AJ Hieble JP: Functions mediated by α_2-adrenergic receptors. In Limbird L (ed): *The α-Adrenergic Receptors*. Clifton, NJ, Humana Press, in press, 1988.

120. Ruffolo RR, Jr, Zeid RL: Relationship between α-adrenoceptor occupancy and response for the α-adrenoceptor agonist, cirazoline, and the α_2-adrenoceptor agonist, B-HT 933, in canine saphenous vein. *J Pharmacol Exp Ther* 235:636–643, 1985.

121. Sawyer R, Warnock P, Docherty JR: Role of vascular α_2-adrenoceptors as targets for circulating catecholamines in the maintenance of blood pressure in anesthetized spontaneously hypertensive rats. *J Cardiovasc Pharmacol* 7:809–812, 1985.

122. Schmitt H: Action des α-sympathomimetiques sur les structures nerveuses. *Actual Pharmacol* 24:93–131, 1971.

123. Schmitt H, Schmitt H: Localization of the hypotensive effect of 2-(2,6-dichlorophenylamino)-2-imidazoline hydrochloride. *Eur J Pharmacol* 6:8–12, 1969.

124. Schmitz JM, Graham KM, Saglowsky A, Pettinger WA: Renal α_1- and α_2-adrenergic receptors: biochemical and pharmacological correlations. *J Pharmacol Exp Ther* 219:400–406, 1981.

125. Scholtysik G. Pharmacology of guanfacine. *Br J Clin Pharmacol* 10:21S–24S, 1980.

126. Schultz HS, Chertien SD, Brewer DD, Eltorai MT, Weber MA: Centrally acting antihypertensive agents: a comparison of lofexidine with clonidine. *J Clin Pharmacol* 21:65–71, 1981.

127. Schumann HJ, Endoh M, Brodde O-E: The time course of the effects of β- and α-adrenoceptor stimulation by

isoprenaline and methoxamine on the contractile force and cAMP level of the isolated rabbit papillary muscle. *Arch Pharmacol* 289:291–302, 1975.

128. Segstro R, Greenway C: α-Receptor subtype mediating sympathetic mobilization of blood from the hepatic venous system in anesthetized cats. *J Pharmacol Exp Ther* 236:224, 1986.

129. Shebuski RJ, Fujita T, Ruffolo RR Jr: Evaluation of α_1- and α_2-adrenoceptor-mediated vasoconstriction in the *in situ*, autoperfused, pulmonary circulation of the anesthetized dog. *J Pharmacol Exp Ther* 238:217–223, 1986.

130. Shebuski RJ, Ohlstein EH, Smith JM Jr, Ruffolo RR Jr: Enhanced pulmonary α_2-adrenoceptor responsiveness under conditions of elevated pulmonary vascular tone. *J Pharmacol Exp Ther* 242:158–165, 1987.

131. Shepperson NB, Langer SZ: The effects of the 2-aminotetrahydronaphthalene derivative, M7, a selective α_2-adrenoceptor agonist in vitro. *Naunyn Schmiedebergs Arch Pharmacol* 318:10–13, 1981.

132. Shoji T, Tsuru H, Shigei T: A regional difference in the distribution of postsynaptic α-adrenoceptor subtypes in canine veins. *Naunyn Schmiedebergs Arch Pharmacol* 324:246–255, 1983.

133. Smyth DD, Umemura S, Pettinger WA: α_2-Adrenoceptors and sodium reabsorption in the isolated perfused rat kidney. *Am J Physiol* 247:F680–F685, 1985.

134. Sonnenblick EH, Frishman WH, LeJemtel TH: Dobutamine: a new synthetic cardioactive sympathetic amine. *N Engl J Med* 300:17, 1979.

135. Stanaszek WF, Kellerman D, Brogden RN, Romankiewicz JA: Prazosin update—a review of its pharmacological properties and therapeutic use in hypertension and congestive heart failure. *Drugs* 25:339, 1983.

136. Stokes GS, Marwood JF: Review of the use of α-adrenoceptor antagonists in hypertension. *Methods Find Exp Clin Pharmacol* 6:197, 1984.

137. Summers RJ, McPherson GA: Radioligand studies of α-adrenoceptors in the kidney. *Trends Pharmacol Sci* 3:291, 1982.

138. Thomas JA, Marks BH: Plasma norepinephrine in congestive heart failure. *Am J Cardiol* 41:233, 1978.

139. Thoolen JMC, Timmermans PBMWM, van Zwieten PA: Cardiovascular effects of withdrawal of some centrally acting antihypertensive drugs in the rat. *Br J Clin Pharmacol* 15:491S–505S, 1983.

140. Timmermans PBMWM, Hoefke W, Stahle H, van Zwieten PA: Structure-activity relationships in clonidine-like imidazolidines and related compounds. *Prog Pharmacol* 3:1–104, 1980.

141. van Meel JCA, deJonge A, Timmermans PBMWM, van Zwieten PA: Selectivity of some alpha adrenoceptor agonists for peripheral alpha-1 and alpha-2 adrenoceptors in the normative pithed rat. *J Pharmacol Exp Ther* 219:760–767, 1981.

142. van Zwieten PA: Pharmacology of centrally acting hypotensive drugs. *Br J Clin Pharmacol* 10:13S–20S, 1980.

143. van Zwieten PA: Thoolen, MJMC Timmermans, PBMWM: The pharmacology of centrally acting antihypertensive drugs. *Br J Clin Pharmacol* 15:455S–462S, 1983.

144. Wilffert B, Timmermans PBMWM, van Zwieten PA: Extrasynaptic location of α_2- and noninnervation β_2-adrenoceptors in the vascular system of the pithed normotensive rat. *J Pharmacol Exp Ther* 221:762–768, 1982.

145. Yamaguchi I, Kopin IJ: Differential inhibition of α_1- and α_2-adrenoceptor–mediated pressor responses in pithed rats. *J Pharmacol Exp Ther* 214:275–281, 1980.

146. Zandberg P, Timmermans PBMWM, van Zwieten PA: Hemodynamic profiles of methoxamine and B-HT 933 in spinalized ganglion-blocked dogs. *J Cardiovasc Pharmacol* 6:256–262, 1984.

Resuscitation Pharmacology

10

Resuscitation Pharmacology

Arno L. Zaritsky, M.D.
Allan S. Jaffe, M.D.

The goals of cardiopulmonary resuscitation are (a) to restore stable circulatory and ventilatory function, and (b) to maintain vital critical organ function until such stabilization can be achieved. Early definitive care (usually defibrillation in adults and ventilatory support in infants) whenever possible is the first priority. Thereafter, the maintenance of circulatory and ventilatory function (with chest compression and assisted ventilation) and pharmacologic interventions aimed at facilitating the reestablishment of more normal cardiopulmonary functioning may improve the success of subsequent efforts. Treatment with pharmacologic agents has the potential to:

1. Suppress ventricular tachycardia and/or fibrillation;
2. Maintain coronary and cerebral perfusion until the restoration of more normal cardiopulmonary function;
3. Evoke a rhythm more apt to be associated with an adequate blood pressure in patients with asystole or electromechanical dissociation;
4. Correct hypoxemia and acidosis;
5. Improve hemodynamics.

These goals are similar in all arrest situations, although there may be some unique circumstances (e.g., trauma) in which additional therapies may also be required. This chapter provides a review of the pharmacology, indications, dosages, and potential complications of each agent used during resuscitation. Indications and dosage recommendations are consistent with recently published guidelines (120).

GENERAL GUIDELINES FOR ADMINISTERING MEDICATIONS

During cardiac arrest, intravenous drug administration is preferred. Central venous drug administration produces higher and more rapid peak drug concentrations than peripheral injections during resuscitations (40). This is a potentially important factor for agents with dose-dependent effects on the arterial circulation, such as epinephrine (100).

However, the placement of a central "line" is time consuming, requires the discontinuation of compressions and ventilations, usually for a potentially deleterious duration, and is associated with substantial morbidity to adjacent structures. In the past, an advocacy for the placement of central lines via the femoral vein obviated some of these considerations. However, unless a long catheter can be advanced into the chest (this is more easily accomplished in pediatric than adult patients), this route should not be used since blood flow below the diaphragm is much lower than blood flow above the diaphragm (31). In adults the brachial vein (120) is the site of choice for the placement of an intravenous line. To enhance delivery to the central circulation, each peripheral venous injection should be followed by a bolus of 50 ml of normal saline.

In pediatric patients, rapid intravenous access can be difficult in general (108), and cannulation of the superior vena caval system is particularly difficult. It has not been established that the difference in blood flow between the upper and lower parts of the body during chest compression in adults also occurs in infants, in whom higher cardiac outputs are induced in part by direct cardiac compression (112). Therefore, in infants any venous access site is acceptable. The administration of intravenous drugs should be followed, as in the adult, with an injection of saline (a smaller amount is required). Intraosseous injection (usually via the tibia) also can be used to provide an access site for the administration of fluids and drugs (109) including catecholamines (89).

If intravenous access is not readily available, endotracheal administration of certain drugs (e.g., epinephrine and atropine) can be utilized (135). Optimal endotracheal doses have not been totally defined. In some animal studies as much as 10 times the intravenous dose of epinephrine is required to produce the same hemodynamic effects (103). However, in general, the upper range of the intravenous dose is chosen for endotracheal use (120). Although it may be possible to administer other agents endotracheally, such as lidocaine, bretylium, isoproterenol, and/or propranolol (81, 102, 113), because they are generally used relatively late during the resuscitation sequence, intravenous access is usually available by that time. When utilizing the endotracheal route, medications should be instilled deeply into the trachea either using a catheter positioned beyond the end of the endotracheal tube or by discontinuing compressions and ventilations during the instillation and thereafter hyperventilating the patient (102).

Pressors are often used to support the circulation once a stable rhythm has been restored. Catecholamines are compatible with many intravenous solutions (normal saline, 0.45N saline, Ringer's lactate and 10% dextrose and water), but 5% dextrose and water usually is preferred. Post arrest, catecholamine infusions should be initiated at a sufficiently rapid rate to clear the intravenous tubing of other solutions; otherwise a substantial delay may occur before a drug effect is observed, particularly in pediatric patients in whom lower

infusion rates are typical. Toxicity is avoided by using the lowest possible dose that achieves the desired effect and decreasing the infusion rate as rapidly as possible. Catecholamines should not be mixed in the same intravenous solution bag with alkaline solutions (e.g., bicarbonate, phenytoin, or aminophylline) because catecholamines are autooxidized by basic solutions (89).

ESSENTIAL RESUSCITATION MEDICATIONS

Oxygen

PHARMACOLOGY

Many factors contribute to severely impaired oxygenation during cardiac arrest. Exhaled gas delivered during mouth-to-mouth rescue breathing provides only 16–17% oxygen, which at best produces an alveolar oxygen tension of 80 torr (normal oxygen tension in room air is approximately 104 torr, depending in part on altitude). Cardiopulmonary resuscitation is accompanied by right-to-left intrapulmonary shunting, mismatches between ventilation and perfusion (96) impairing oxygen delivery, and often by aspiration and/or pulmonary edema inhibiting oxygen transport across the alveolus. Because properly performed chest compression only delivers 25–35% of a normal cardiac output (133), oxygen delivery to the tissues is additionally impaired. To compensate, tissue extraction increases, and mixed venous oxygen tension is low. The admixture of this highly desaturated venous blood with poorly oxygenated "arterial" blood further decreases arterial oxygen tension. The net result is that oxygen delivery is markedly compromised during cardiac arrest and resuscitation.

Hypoxemia at the tissue level leads to anaerobic metabolism, lactic acid production, and local acidosis, augmenting intracellular acidosis and cellular dysfunction and eventually leading to cell death. Acidosis also results in vasodilation locally, which may compromise further vital organ perfusion by leading to peripheral pooling and by lowering central aortic pressures and thus diastolic coronary perfusion pressure (see "Epinephrine" below). Acidosis may antagonize the action of catecholamines (87); however, the applicability of this concept to the cardiac arrest setting and the doses of epinephrine utilized is unclear (1, 63, 128). For all of these reasons, aggressive attempts to maximize tissue oxygenation are essential. If the baseline oxygen tension is on the steep portion of the oxyhemoglobin saturation curve, even small increments in oxygen tension may markedly improve the delivery of oxygen to the tissues.

INDICATIONS AND DOSE

Oxygen should be provided in the highest concentration possible (usually 100%) during cardiopulmonary resuscitation. There should be no concern about the development of oxygen toxicity during the short exposure that occurs during resuscitation. Oxygen should not be withheld in any patient with hypoxemia, even if chronic lung disease and carbon dioxide retention is present. By increasing arterial oxygen tension, oxygen content in blood and therefore tissue oxygen delivery may be enhanced.

Although the administration of oxygen improves arterial oxygen tension and content, it does not guarantee adequate oxygen delivery to the tissues. Animal (104) and clinical (137) studies have demonstrated that during cardiopulmonary resuscitation there is a progressive fall in mixed venous oxygen tension, probably the best indicator of the adequacy of tissue oxygen delivery, even when arterial oxygen tension is well maintained. Accordingly, additional therapy is needed to improve tissue oxygen delivery.

Epinephrine

PHARMACOLOGY

The pharmacologic actions of epinephrine are complex and dose related (see Chapter 31). The large doses used during a cardiopulmonary resuscitation produce both α-adrenergic and β-adrenergic effects. During cardiopulmonary resuscitation, epinephrine's α-adrenergic effects on vascular tone are of primary importance because aortic diastolic pressure is a critical determinant of the success or failure of resuscitative efforts in animals (90, 110). During compression, aortic and right atrial pressure are equal and there is little or no coronary blood flow. During diastole, there is a small gradient favoring flow. By increasing arterial vasoconstriction via its effects on α-adrenergic tone, epinephrine elevates aortic diastolic pressure and therefore coronary perfusion pressure, increasing coronary blood flow (143). It is unclear whether the concomitant venoconstriction that increases central vol-

umes diminishes or enhances coronary blood flow (39, 93).

In animals, epinephrine also augments cerebral perfusion. Cerebral blood flow can be maintained at approximately 70% of normal levels with a continuous infusion of epinephrine combined with simultaneous ventilation and compression cardiopulmonary resuscitation in some experimental models (85). The increased cerebral blood flow is related in part to increased blood flow to the upper body due to the thoracic pump mechanism of blood flow during chest compression, and occurs at the expense of blood flow to structures below the diaphragm, including the renal and splanchnic beds (62, 85). This action is augmented by the effects of α-adrenergic stimulation, which improve the rigidity of the arterial system so that pressure and therefore flow are enhanced.

The impact of the β-adrenergic effects of epinephrine is more controversial. The inotropic and chronotropic effects increase myocardial oxygen demand, and many have argued that the increased demand may obviate the benefits of increased coronary flow (38). Furthermore, recent data suggest that it is the α-adrenergic rather than the β-adrenergic effects of epinephrine that enhance the susceptibility of ventricular fibrillation from defibrillation (99). These contentions, along with the possible adverse effects of hypertension and/or arrhythmias that may be induced synergistically by the β- plus α-adrenergic effects of epinephrine following restoration of spontaneous circulation (these effects tend to be worse following intrapulmonary injection of epinephrine when the lungs serve as a depot for epinephrine, which is then released during the postresuscitation period (12, 103)), have led some investigators to advocate the replacement of epinephrine with a more pure α-adrenergic agent such as phenylephrine or methoxamine. Although these agents seem equally effective in supporting coronary perfusion and enhancing the restoration of spontaneous circulation and survival, they do not appear to support cerebral blood flow to the same extent as epinephrine (15–18, 62). Epinephrine therefore remains the drug of choice during cardiopulmonary resuscitation.

INDICATIONS AND DOSE

Epinephrine is indicated in the treatment of cardiac arrest, regardless of mechanism, in infants, children, and adults (120). The optimal dose is undefined. In animals, doses in the range of those recommended during resuscitation in humans (7.5–15 μg/kg) do not increase diastolic blood pressure. Doses of 45, 75, and 150 μg/kg must be used to induce a diastolic pressure of 30 mm Hg or more for up to 5 minutes (76). Nonetheless, concentrations of endogenous catecholamines are quite high during cardiopulmonary resuscitation in humans (well beyond the range usually achieved with infusions in patients with shock (142)) and may be synergistic with exogenous infusions. Thus, although the proper dose in patients is speculative, present recommendations are probably low rather than high, and epinephrine in the recommended dose of 7.5–15 μg/kg should be administered at least every 5 minutes during resuscitation. Estimations of dose should be biased toward greater rather than lesser amounts when exact data are unavailable. The upper range of doses (15 μg/kg) should be utilized with endotracheal administration in which absorption is delayed and therefore peak levels are less (57). Epinephrine should not be injected directly into the heart if it can be avoided, since morbidity has been associated with this procedure, including interruption of compressions and ventilation, coronary artery laceration, cardiac tamponade, pneumothorax, and intractable ventricular fibrillation (57).

Epinephrine, like other catecholamines, should not be mixed with bicarbonate since alkaline solutions autooxidize the drug (89).

Atropine

PHARMACOLOGY

Atropine has predominant parasympatholytic effects at clinically relevant doses. It accelerates sinus or atrial pacemakers, and enhances atrioventricular conduction (37) by competitively antagonizing muscarinic receptors and therefore inhibiting vagal tone. Its use in cardiac arrest is based on its cardiac vagolytic actions. At low doses, atropine has central and peripheral parasympathomimetic actions that may induce paradoxical vagotonic effects (32, 74). Atropine is excreted renally and has a half-life in normal individuals of about 2.5 hours (138). Prolonged elimination should be expected during arrest and the postresuscitation period. Thus, doses of more than 2 mg of atropine, which is a totally vagolytic dose for most individuals (97), should not be used during cardiopulmonary arrest.

INDICATIONS AND DOSE

Atropine is the drug of choice for the treatment of bradycardia, regardless of its mechanism, when it is accompanied by hemodynamic compromise or ventricular ectopy. Its benefit in ventricular asystole is based on the supposition that asystole is the end stage of a spectrum of bradycardias and on the apparent benefit observed in small numbers of patients (19) especially those in a hospital setting where there is a very rapid initiation of resuscitation. There is also some enthusiasm for the use of atropine for asystole in the management of outpatient cardiac arrest, but benefit in the outpatient setting is even more speculative (71, 125). Atropine should be used cautiously in the presence of myocardial ischemia or infarction since excessive increases in heart rate may increase the extent of infarction (97) and can on occasion induce ventricular tachycardia or fibrillation (30). Bradycardia in pediatric cardiac arrest patients and in many adult patients with severe pulmonary disease is due most often to hypoxemia and shock, and is best treated by supporting ventilation and circulation.

The recommended doses of atropine are 1.0 mg for asystole and 0.5 mg for symptomatic bradycardia (120), with a minimal dose of 0.5 mg. A total dose of 2.0 mg generally results in full vagal blockage (97). In pediatric patients, the dose is 0.02 mg/kg intravenously or endotracheally, with a minimum dose of 0.1 mg. The dose may be repeated in 5 minutes, up to 1.0 mg in a child and 2.0 mg in an adolescent. As noted above, smaller doses of atropine, less than 0.5 mg in adults and less than 0.1 mg in pediatric patients, can induce paradoxical vagotonic effects (32, 74).

Lidocaine

PHARMACOLOGY

Lidocaine is a class 1 antiarrhythmic agent. Its primary mode of action is by its membrane-stabilizing effects (131), mediated predominantly by blockade of sodium channels (51). Slowing the slope of phase 4 depolarization, reducing automaticity, is one of lidocaine's important modes of antiarrhythmic action (29). Lidocaine has different effects on the duration of the action potential and the effective refractory period in normal and ischemic tissue, which narrow the differences between these tissues and thus may inhibit the propagation of reentrant arrhythmias (78). In normal tissue lidocaine tends to slightly shorten these intervals, whereas in ischemic tissue it prolongs them. Lidocaine also increases the energy required to induce ventricular fibrillation (the ventricular fibrillation threshold) (78, 119), but high plasma levels appear to be required (2, 25). However, lidocaine does not reduce the energy required to terminate ventricular fibrillation (the ventricular defibrillation threshold). Recent data suggest that it may even increase the energy needed, though only modestly (41, 68). Lidocaine has proven to be as effectives as other agents heralded as having antifibrillatory effects (58, 95). This may be because of the lack of true antifibrillatory effects of the agents with which lidocaine was compared; or because most apparent failures of defibrillation are due to the immediate recurrence of ventricular fibrillation, which is inhibited by the effects of lidocaine on the ventricular fibrillation threshold. At high concentrations, lidocaine can depress myocardial contractility (80) and induce hypotension by peripheral vasodilation (134).

Lidocaine is highly protein bound (14) and is cleared by the liver (29). In normal subjects, its volume of distribution is 0.5 liters/kg. Its elimination has both an α-distributive and a β half-life. In normal subjects, the half-life of lidocaine after a bolus injection (its α-distributive half-life) is 8.3 minutes, and its half-life after achieving a steady state with a constant infusion (the β half-life) is 86–108 minutes. Thus, bolus doses of lidocaine are required to obtain therapeutic blood levels until a steady state concentration (reached after five half-lives) is achieved with a constant infusion. One half of the steady state concentration is reached at one half-life. If the therapeutic range is 2–5 μg/ml, a 4 mg/min infusion will achieve a concentration of approximately 2 μg/ml in 86–108 minutes, assuming normal pharmacokinetics. Clinical circumstances in which hepatic blood flow or cardiac output is reduced and those in which the volume of distribution is altered (older patients) will lead to increased levels of lidocaine for any given dose (7). Accordingly, dose adjustments are required in patients with reduced cardiac output to the liver (e.g., those with shock), in those with congestive heart failure or hepatic dysfunction in which hepatic metabolism is reduced, and in those over the age of 70 in whom the volume of distribution and clearance is decreased (7). In addition, after a 24-hour infusion, the ability of the liver to clear lidocaine appears to de-

crease, mandating a reduced infusion rate if toxicity is to be avoided (33). Although renal disease does not affect the clearance of lidocaine or its volume of distribution, metabolites of lidocaine will accumulate after prolonged infusions (129). There is little information concerning lidocaine levels or pharmacodynamics during cardiopulmonary resuscitation. However, probably as a consequence of the marked reduction in cardiac output, levels after conventional bolus doses are above or within the therapeutic range for at least 20 minutes (26).

Toxic effects of lidocaine usually occur when levels are above the therapeutic range or when the drug is infused very rapidly (26, 33). These effects include central nervous system manifestations such as drowsiness, confusion, numbness and tingling, muscle twitching, and (predominantly) agitation. Seizures requiring treatment can occur.

INDICATIONS AND DOSE

The prophylactic use of lidocaine to prevent ventricular fibrillation in patients highly suspected of having acute myocardial infarction has been widely recommended (10, 120) because of data suggesting that it reduces the incidence of ventricular fibrillation (36, 77). However, many have questioned the risk-benefit ratio on which this recommendation is based, in part because there have been few data to suggest that primary ventricular fibrillation itself is associated with an adverse prognosis (23, 43). Recent data suggest that ventricular fibrillation is indeed associated with an adverse prognosis (132), which should strengthen the advocacy for the drug's routine prophylactic use. If therapy is not initiated prophylactically, traditional indications for the use of lidocaine in suspected acute myocardial infarction include ventricular premature complexes that are more frequent than 6/min, are multiform, encroach on the T wave of the QRS complex, or occur in bursts of two or more in succession (118). In this circumstance, a loading dose of lidocaine can be administered as multiple, slow boluses of 50 mg, every 5 minutes to a total dose of 200–300 mg or at a rate of 20 mg/min to a total dose of 3–5 mg/kg followed by a continuous infusion of 2–4 mg/min for 24 hours (10). The initial doses and the infusion rate should be decreased (many empirically reduce them by 50%) in the presence of congestive heart failure, hepatic dysfunction, patient age above 70 years, or hypotension (41). If the infusion is continued for more than 24 hours, the rate should be reduced by one-half (58).

A similar regimen can also be used in more emergent situations, e.g., when rapid ventricular tachycardia is present, to achieve and maintain therapeutic levels as quickly as possible. In general, lidocaine is the drug of choice for most malignant ventricular arrhythmias, including those induced by digitalis toxicity. Patients with ventricular tachycardia who fail to respond to lidocaine and those severely compromised usually require cardioversion.

During cardiopulmonary resuscitation when an antiarrhythmic agent is required (when ventricular tachycardia or ventricular fibrillation is present), a bolus of 1 mg/kg of lidocaine will provide levels in or above the therapeutic range for at least 20 minutes (80), during which time defibrillation should be reattempted. Since levels are high for so long, only one dose is generally required, although some may prefer to use repetitive doses of 0.5 mg/kg every 8–10 minutes before changing to bretylium (120).

Similar doses of lidocaine, 1 mg/kg, followed by defibrillation are appropriate for pediatric patients with ventricular tachycardia and ventricular fibrillation, although these rhythm disturbances occur in less than 10% of pediatric cardiac arrests and usually as an end result of a primary respiratory disturbance (44). If ventricular tachycardia/fibrillation is not reversed, a second 1 mg/kg bolus of lidocaine is recommended, followed by an infusion of 20–50 μg/kg/min and repeated attempts at defibrillation or cardioversion. The infusion rate of lidocaine for children who have received loading doses of lidocaine and require maintenance infusions should be reduced by at least 50% if shock, congestive heart failure, or hepatic dysfunction is present (120).

Bretylium Tosylate

PHARMACOLOGY

Bretylium is a quarternary ammonium compound with both adrenergic and direct myocardial effects (72, 101). It is classified as a type 3 antiarrhythmic agent. Class 3 antiarrhythmics generally prolong the duration of the action potential and the refractory period by increasing repolarization time. They have little effect on the rate of rise of phase zero or on the resting membrane potential (117). However, these antiarrhythmic effects are observed with more chronic administration. Acute ef-

fects in vivo are probably accounted for by adrenergic stimulation, which will shorten refractory periods. Bretylium's adrenergic effects are biphasic. It initially causes the release of norepinephrine from adrenergic nerve terminals, inducing transient (approximately 20 minutes) hypertension, tachycardia, and in some patients increases in cardiac output. Once norepinephrine is depleted, release is inhibited, and by 45–60 minutes hypotension may be present (59, 83). Since bretylium blocks the uptake of norepinephrine, it may potentiate the effects of exogenously administered catecholamines (72). For some time it was thought that the adrenergic effects of bretylium have little to do with its effects on ventricular fibrillation since neither reserpine nor sympathectomy changes the ventricular fibrillation threshold (24). However, more recent data support the hypothesis that bretylium's effects may be critically dependent on the adrenergic milieu (46). Recently it has been proposed that an increased upstroke velocity of phase zero of the action potential due to catecholamine stimulation, in concert with direct myocardial effects of lengthening of the effective refractory period, are essential to the antiarrhythmic mechanism of the agent (94). Bretylium reduces disparities in refractory periods and conduction velocities between ischemic and normal tissues, and delays the conduction of premature impulses into normal tissue contiguous with ischemic zones ("border zones") (49). In experimental animals and in anecdotal reports in patients, bretylium is capable of terminating ventricular fibrillation (4, 11). Bretylium also has been reported to markedly increase the fibrillation threshold (the amount of energy necessary to induce ventricular fibrillation) even when ischemia or reperfusion is present (3, 61, 70). Recently it has been suggested that the effect on ventricular fibrillation threshold may be unique to certain types of models in which ventricular fibrillation is induced and may be nonapplicable to others (46) and/or of a lesser magnitude than initially described (51). Bretylium either does not change or lowers defibrillation threshold (the energy required to terminate ventricular fibrillation) (68, 75, 127). Despite a pharmacologic profile suggesting that bretylium should be more effective than lidocaine in the treatment of ventricular fibrillation, controlled clinical trials have not been able to discern any differences in efficacy of these drugs in treating ventricular fibrillation (58, 95). Possibly, late administration of antiarrhythmic agents during cardiac arrest sequences is responsible for the lack of difference, or additional factors, as yet undetermined, may modulate the effects of these agents during cardiac arrest.

Bretylium is only utilized intravenously. Its effects generally are delayed for 10–15 minutes when used in conventional doses, which usually are diluted and administered slowly or via an infusion to reduce adverse adrenergic effects. The delay is likely due to the need to concentrate the drug in myocardium (3, 49, 111). Higher doses administered as a bolus without dilution are warranted during emergencies such as cardiac arrest and have more immediate effects. Bretylium is excreted unchanged in the urine. When renal function is normal, 72% is excreted within the first 24 hours and 100% by 72 hours (88). Elimination is similar from myocardium and plasma, with an elimination half-life in humans of 4–17 hours (3, 106). Accordingly, dosage adjustments are required for patients with renal failure.

The principal side effect of bretylium is hypotension, especially orthostatic hypotension, and the nausea and vomiting that are frequently associated. It occurs in 50–75% of patients, depending on dose and rapidity of administration (72). Because bretylium impairs the reuptake of catecholamines, it can potentiate the effects of exogenously administered pressors and/or inotropes (72). Other side effects include negative synergism with other antiarrhythmic agents, but the clinical importance of these interactions in critically ill patients is unclear (5, 34, 72); there is also the possibility that digitalis toxicity could be exacerbated by adrenergic stimulation (59). The treatment for severe hypotension due to bretylium relies on tricyclic antidepressants, which block the access of bretylium to sympathetic neurons but do not affect its antiarrhythmic effects (141).

INDICATIONS AND DOSE

Bretylium is indicated for the treatment of ventricular arrhythmias resistant to other treatments or when other treatments are for some reason contraindicated. For ventricular tachycardia with a pulse, bretylium is usually used after lidocaine, and in most instances procainamide, in a dose of 5–10 mg/kg diluted 1:4. Good results have been obtained even in patients with digitalis toxicity despite concerns about catecholamine stimulation (59). Bretylium is administered slowly, over 8–10 min-

utes, and the dose can be repeated once or twice, followed by intermittent bolus doses every 6–8 hours or a continuous infusion of 1–2 mg/min (72). For ventricular tachycardia without a pulse or ventricular fibrillation, bretylium should be used only if lidocaine has been ineffective or is contraindicated, since in clinical trials lidocaine has proven equally effective (58, 95) and avoids the potentially adverse hemodynamic effects of bretylium (45). In general, a trial of only one dose of lidocaine should precede the use of bretylium in adults. The required dose of bretylium is 5 mg/kg given as a bolus, followed by 10 mg/kg if ventricular fibrillation does not respond to defibrillation. Repeated doses of 10 mg/kg can be given every 15–30 minutes to a maximum dose of 30 mg/kg (72). The indications and doses for pediatric arrests are identical to those for adults.

Intravenous Procainamide

PHARMACOLOGY

Procainamide is a type 1A antiarrhythmic agent. It reduces the rate of phase 4 depolarization in isolated ventricular muscle and Purkinje fibers (60), slows ventricular conduction (115), and increases the refractory period of ventricular tissue (114). How these mechanisms prevent ventricular arrhythmias is not totally clear, but the effects on normal tissue and at the site of impulse formation may be important to procainamide's efficacy (116).

The clearance of procainamide is dependent on both hepatic and renal function. Approximately 60% of any given dose is excreted unchanged in the urine (82) if normal renal function is present, and the remainder undergoes N-acetylation in the liver (42). Thus, elimination is reduced during renal failure or in congestive heart failure if renal and/or hepatic perfusion is impaired (73). In addition, patients may be rapid or slow hepatic acetylators of the agent, which can have clinically important effects on plasma levels (21). The N-acetylated derivative has antiarrhythmic properties that are somewhat different from those of the parent compound (64) and is also excreted renally (42).

Although the metabolism of procainamide is complex, the measurement of both the parent compound and the N-acetyl derivative is routinely available, facilitating more chronic treatment. Difficulties in rapidly obtaining therapeutic blood levels make the agent difficult to use in the emergency setting. Procainamide is a ganglionic blocker with significant vasodilating effects, and at high doses some negative inotropic effects (55). These effects limit the rapidity with which procainamide can be administered (55). Accordingly, the agent must be administered cautiously to patients with hypotension and heart failure or to those whose clearance of procainamide may be impaired (those with hepatic and/or renal dysfunction). Since procainamide slows conduction and increases the refractory period, it can induce heart block, widening of the QRS complex (140), and QT_c prolongation and associated arrhythmias (13).

INDICATIONS AND DOSE

Procainamide is indicated for the treatment of malignant ventricular arrhythmias that do not respond to lidocaine or when treatment with lidocaine is contraindicated. It also may be used intravenously to treat supraventricular arrhythmias (50), but is rarely used to treat ventricular fibrillation because it takes too long to achieve therapeutic levels.

The intravenous loading dose is 50 mg every 5 minutes unless hypotension occurs, the QRS complex has widened by more than 50%, 1 g has been administered, or the arrhythmia has been suppressed. In urgent circumstances, up to 20 mg/min have been given, titrated to the same endpoints (50). An alternative regimen utilizes a loading dose of 17 mg/kg given over 1 hour, followed by a maintenance infusion of 2.8 mg/kg/hr. In patients who might clear the agent slowly, the loading dose is reduced to 12 mg/kg and the infusion rate to 1.4 mg/kg/hr. With this regimen, some patients have therapeutic levels by 15 minutes (66). There are no unique considerations concerning the use of procainamide in children other than to appreciate that ventricular arrhythmia is a rare cause of cardiac arrest, which more commonly develops secondary to acute respiratory failure (44).

OTHER MEDICATIONS OF POTENTIAL USE

Sodium Bicarbonate

PHARMACOLOGY

During cardiopulmonary arrest, metabolic and respiratory acidosis are inevitable. Respiratory acidosis results from inadequate ventilation and is effectively antagonized by providing assisted ventilation. Metabolic acidosis is due to inadequate tissue oxygenation, which leads to anaerobic metabolism and the production of lactic acid (136). Acute respiratory and acute metabolic acidosis have very different effects on intracellular pH. Acute increases in $Paco_2$ acutely decrease intracellular pH because carbon dioxide diffuses rapidly into cells, whereas acute increases in the extracellular hydrogen ion concentration depress intracellular pH less rapidly because both H^+ and HCO_3^- diffuse across cell membranes relatively slowly. In addition, the production of carbon dioxide via the reaction $H^+ + HCO_3^- \leftrightharpoons H_2O + CO_2$ favors the formation of bicarbonate over carbonic acid by a ratio of 20:1 (107, 122).

The adverse effects of acidosis appear to be related to changes in the intracellular and extracellular pH and carbon dioxide concentration. Ischemia, which is a likely occurrence during cardiopulmonary resuscitation given the poor coronary perfusion and high myocardial oxygen consumption, induces increases in intracellular Pco_2 to as high as 300 mm Hg or greater, and a decrease in intracellular pH to below 6 (47, 48). Intracellular acidosis and hypercarbia have been related to diminished contractile performance and an elevated end-diastolic pressure (27, 28). This effect is accentuated by increases in Pco_2 even when extracellular pH is held constant (28). In addition, acidosis blunts the myocardial and peripheral response to exogenous catecholamines, increases pulmonary vascular resistance, vasodilates systemic vascular beds, and decreases glycolytic pathway activity, thus impairing ATP synthesis (1, 107, 122). There also is concern that a high Pco_2 will reduce diaphragmatic function and exacerbate respiratory distress, especially in infants (65). An appreciation of the effects of intracellular acidosis and the differences in diffusion between CO_2 and H^+ and HCO_3^- ions has led to a substantial rethinking of the use of buffers during cardiopulmonary resuscitation.

Originally, sodium bicarbonate in combination with epinephrine was reported to improve the success of defibrillation and survival during resuscitation. Sodium bicarbonate alone was no better than placebo (105). More recently, in a careful study in which coronary perfusion pressure was maintained near the critical level between poor and good outcome, sodium bicarbonate (1 mEq/kg) failed to affect the success of defibrillation or improve the chances for spontaneous circulation or survival (54). Other studies have also failed to observe a beneficial effect from sodium bicarbonate administration (86, 128). This is thought in part to be because sodium bicarbonate solutions already have a high carbon dioxide content (260–280 mm Hg for each 50 ml) (92). In addition, sodium bicarbonate buffers metabolic acids through the reaction $HCO_3^- + H^+ \rightleftharpoons H_2O + CO_2$. Thus, in the presence of H^+ ion, more carbon dioxide is formed. The combination of the intrinsic CO_2 concentration plus that formed by the above reaction will diminish both extracellular and intracellular pH (98). Thus, it should not be surprising that rapid administration of bicarbonate transiently increases PCO_2 and diminishes left ventricular performance even in the absence of cardiac arrest (69). Similar adverse effects have been observed in the presence of lactic acidosis with hypoxemia. In this setting, sodium bicarbonate (2.5mEq/kg administered over 1 hour) diminished blood pressure, impaired splanchnic blood flow, and markedly decreased liver intracellular pH compared with animals who received saline alone (53). Blood lactate and lactic acid production were substantially augmented in animals treated with bicarbonate. In a model of cardiac arrest, administration of bicarbonate raises arterial pH, but depresses cerebrospinal fluid pH because CO_2 diffuses into the central nervous system more rapidly than H^+ or HCO_3^- ions (8). The diminished mental status observed after resuscitations may be partly due to this acute rise in cerebrospinal fluid PCO_2 and fall in pH. When metabolic acidosis is produced by administration of acid (HCl), or experimental diabetic ketoacidosis, bicarbonate impairs cerebral oxygen availability, probably by decreasing cerebral blood oxygen content and/or tissue oxygen release (20). This fact appears to result from a shift in the oxyhemoglobin dissociation curve to the left due to arterial alkalosis, which impairs tissue oxygen delivery; and/or a reduction in cardiac output due to hypoxic lactic acidosis exacerbated by bicarbonate (20), with concomitant tissue acidosis secondary to organ ischemia. The effects of excess CO_2 cannot be overcome by hyperventilation alone because of the limited pulmonary blood flow induced during compression and ventilation. Because of the low cardiac output (25–33% of normal) (69) only a modest percentage of the CO_2 generated reaches the lungs for elimination by ventilation. Thus, although oxygenated blood may have a low or normal PCO_2, venous blood will have a high PCO_2 and a much lower pH.

This event has been termed the "venous paradox" and is observed during cardiopulmonary resuscitation in patients and experimental animals (137).

In addition to the adverse effects due to a high venous PCO_2, administration of sodium bicarbonate during cardiac arrest may cause hyperosmolarity and hypernatremia (84) and extracellular alkalosis (126). Alkalosis induced by excessive bicarbonate administration may reduce the concentration of ionized calcium, decrease plasma potassium concentration, shift the oxyhemoglobin dissociation curve to the left (inhibiting the release of oxygen), and induce malignant arrhythmias (79). Precipitation of calcium carbonate occurs when bicarbonate is mixed with calcium.

INDICATIONS AND DOSE

Because of the lack of information documenting benefit of bicarbonate during cardiopulmonary resuscitation and the concerns discussed above about the potential morbidity of its use, the most recent American Heart Association guidelines deemphasize the role of sodium bicarbonate in both pediatric and adult resuscitation (120). Bicarbonate should not be used until the airway is secured, adequate ventilation and chest compressions have been administered, and the patient fails to respond to defibrillation, antiarrhythmic therapy, and epinephrine. Acidosis, if present, should be treated with vigorous hyperventilation. Attention to airway management is particularly important in pediatric patients since respiratory failure is a major cause of cardiopulmonary arrest (44).

Following the restoration of spontaneous circulation, the role of bicarbonate is more controversial. Lactate may be "washed out" of reperfused tissue beds with an acute exacerbation of metabolic acidosis. Bicarbonate should only be administered if an adequate pH cannot be achieved with hyperventilation. It is probably unnecessary to treat mild-to-moderate metabolic acidosis (pH > 7.20), especially when due to correctable hemodynamic causes.

When used, the dose of bicarbonate is 1 mEq/kg by slow intravenous infusion, for both adult and pediatric patients. Subsequent doses of 0.5 mEq/kg may be given every 10 minutes as needed. In infants, it is preferable to dilute the bicarbonate 1:1 with sterile water to decrease the hyperosmolarity of the 8.4% solution (120).

Calcium

PHARMACOLOGY

Calcium is essential to the process of excitation-contraction coupling. It enters the cell through voltage-dependent channels and stimulates the intracellular release of calcium from the sarcoplasmic reticulum. The transient increase in intracellular calcium concentration results in activation of actin-myosin coupling through interaction with regulatory proteins. Contraction terminates when calcium is pumped out of the cell or back into the sarcoplasmic reticulum. Normally there is approximately a 10,000-fold concentration gradiant between extracellular and intracellular calcium concentration maintained by energy-requiring mechanisms. Calcium has variable effects on systemic vascular resistance, which in part determine the extent to which increased inotropy induced by calcium affects systemic arterial pressure. If the intracellular calcium concentration becomes elevated, such as following ischemic insults, cell death results, in part through calcium-mediated mechanisms (67).

Hypercalcemia may precipitate or exacerbate digitalis toxicity, leading to severe arrhythmias including life-threatening bradycardias (52). Calcium forms an insoluble precipitate (calcium carbonate) if mixed with bicarbonate, it is sclerosing to peripheral veins, and if it infiltrates into the subcutaneous tissues, can produce a severe chemical burn.

INDICATIONS AND DOSE

Advocacy of the use of calcium in cardiopulmonary arrest was stimulated by the observation that calcium administration resulted in positive inotropic effects in patients after cardiopulmonary bypass (126). These patients may have been rendered hypocalcemic by transfusion. In recent clinical studies, calcium has been ineffective in the treatment of refractory electromechanical dissociation (56, 123) and/or asystole (124).

In addition to lack of data concerning the efficacy of calcium in cardiac arrest, there is also concern that postischemic cell injury (so-called reperfusion injury) is exacerbated by the excessive plasma calcium concentrations known to occur when calcium is administered during cardiopulmonary resuscitation (22, 35). Thus, calcium should be used during cardiopulmonary resuscitation only to correct suspected hypocalcemia, to reverse the adverse effects of hyperkalemia and/or hypermagnesemia, or to treat calcium channel blocker toxicity (120). There is little information as to the optimal dose. A dose of 2 ml of 10% calcium chloride (elemental calcium, 2–4 mg/kg) is recommended in adults (120). In pediatric patients, a larger dose (10% calcium chloride, 20 mg/kg; elemental calcium, 5–7 mg/kg) is recommended. The dose should be infused slowly, and may be repeated after 10 minutes if required.

Isoproterenol

PHARMACOLOGY

Isoproterenol is a potent, very short-acting synthetic catecholamine with nearly pure β-adrenergic stimulating properties. As such, isoproterenol induces marked changes in heart rate and contractility centrally and is a potent peripheral and coronary vasodilator. It also markedly increases myocardial work (139).

Isoproterenol may induce or exacerbate ischemia in patients with coronary artery disease (130, 139). Because it lowers perfusion pressure, it increases mortality during experimental resuscitation (91). Isoproterenol can induce ventricular arrhythmias, especially in patients with digitalis toxicity (6).

INDICATIONS AND DOSE

Isoproterenol is not indicated during the management of cardiac arrest since it appears to increase mortality (91), and has been supplanted as a pressor/inotrope by dopamine and dobutamine. Its only role at present is for the temporary treatment of life-threatening bradycardia until a pacemaker can be inserted. With the advent of reliable external pacemakers (144) even this indication may be of less importance in the future. When used to treat bradycardia, the dose of isoproterenol required usually is quite low because it has such potent chronotropic effects. Accordingly, the initial dose should be 2 μg/min. Doses as high as 10 μg/min may be needed to maintain an adequate heart rate (usually approximately 60 beats/min).

In pediatric patients, bradycardia is usually due to hypoxia. Attention to ventilation should precede isoproterenol administration. Epinephrine may be preferable to isoproterenol in pediatric patients since it does not induce vasodilation and thus should better maintain coronary perfusion pressure (120). The infusion dose of isoproterenol is 0.1–1.0 μg/kg/min.

References

1. Andersen MN, Borden JR, Mouritzen CV: Acidosis, catecholamines, and cardiovascular dynamics: when doses of acidosis require correction. *Ann Surg* 166:344, 1967.
2. Anderson JL: Antifibrillatory versus antiectopic therapy. *Am J Cardiol* 54:7A, 1984.
3. Anderson JL, Patterson E, Corlon M, et al: Kinetics of antifibrillatory effects of bretylium: correlation with myocardial drug concentrations. *Am J Cardiol* 46:583, 1980.
4. Bacaner M: Bretylium tosylate for suppression of induced ventricular fibrillation. *Am J Cardiol* 17:528, 1966.
5. Bacaner MB: Treatment of ventricular fibrillation and other acute arrhythmias with bretylium tosylate. *Am J Cardiol* 21:530, 1968.
6. Becker DJ, Nonkin PM, Bennett LD, et al: Effect of isoproterenol in digitalis cardiotoxicity. *Am J Cardiol* 12:242, 1962.
7. Benowitz NL: Clinical applications of the pharmacokinetics of lidocaine. In Melmon K (ed): *Cardiovascular Drug Therapy*. Philadelphia, FA Davis, 1974, p 77.
8. Berenyi KJ, Wolk M, Killip T: Cerebrospinal fluid acidosis complicating therapy of experimental cardiopulmonary arrest. *Circulation* 52:319, 1975.
9. Berg RA: Emergency infusion of catecholamines into bone marrow. *Am J Dis Child* 138:810, 1984.
10. Bethesda Conference Report: Thirteenth Bethesda conference: emergency cardiac care. *Am J Cardiol* 50:365, 1982.
11. Bigger JT, Jr, Jaffe CC: The effect of bretylium tosylate on the electrophysiologic properties of ventricular muscle and Purkinje fibers. *Am J Cardiol* 27:82, 1971.
12. Bleyaert AL, Sands PA, Safar P, et al: Augmentation of post-ischemic brain damage by severe intermittent hypertension. *Crit Care Med* 8:41, 1980.
13. Boccardo D, Pitchon R, Weiner I: Adverse reactions and efficacy of high-dose procainamide therapy in resistant tachyarrhythmias. *Am Heart J* 102:797, 1981.
14. Boyes RN, et al: Pharmacokinetics of lidocaine in man. *Clin Pharmacol Ther* 12:105, 1971.
15. Brillman JA, Sanders AB, Otto CW, et al: Outcome of resuscitation from fibrillatory arrest using epinephrine and phenylephrine in dogs. *Crit Care Med* 13:912, 1985.
16. Brown CG, Werman HA, Davis EA, et al: Comparative effects of epinephrine and phenylephrine on regional cerebral blood flow during cardiopulmonary resuscitation (abstract). *Ann Emerg Med* 15:635, 1986.
17. Brown CG, Werman HA, Davis EA, et al: Effect of high-dose phenylephrine versus epinephrine on regional cerebral blood flow during cardiopulmonary resuscitation (abstract). *Ann Emerg Med* 15:14, 1986.
18. Brown CG, Werman HA, Hamlin R, et al: The comparative effects of methoxamine and epinephrine on regional cerebral blood flow in a swine model (abstract). *Crit Care Med* 14:333, 1986.
19. Brown DC, Lewis AJ, Criley JM: Asystole and its treatment: the possible role of the parasympathetic nervous system in cardiac arrest. *J Am Coll Emerg Phys* 8:448, 1979.
20. Bureau MA, Begin R, Berthiaume Y, et al: Cerebral hypoxia from bicarbonate infusion in diabetic acidosis. *J Pediatr* 96:968, 1980.
21. Campbell W, Tilstone WJ, Lawson DH, et al: Acetylator phenotype and the clinical pharmacology of slow release procainamide. *Br J Clin Pharmacol* 3:1023, 1976.
22. Carlon GC, Howland WS, Kahn RC, et al: Calcium chloride administration in normal calcemic critically ill patients. *Crit Care Med* 8:209, 1980.
23. Carruth JE, Silverman ME: Ventricular fibrillation complicating acute myocardial infarction: reasons against the routine use of lidocaine. *Am Heart J* 104:545, 1985.
24. Cervoni P, Ellis CH, Maxwell RA: The antiarrhythmic action of bretylium in normal reserpine-pretreated and chronically denervated dog hearts. *Arch Int Pharmacodyn* 190:91, 1971.
25. Chow MSS, Kluger J, Dipersio DM, et al: Antifibrillatory effects of lidocaine and bretylium immediately post cardiopulmonary resuscitation. *Am Heart J* 110:938, 1985.
26. Chow MMS, Ronsfeld RAA, Hamilton RA, et al: Effect of external cardiopulmonary resuscitation on lidocaine pharmacokinetics in dogs. *J Pharmacol Exp Ther* 224:531, 1983.
27. Cingolani HE, Faulkner SL, Mattiazzi AR, et al: Depression of human myocardial contractility with "respiratory" and "metabolic" acidosis. *Surgery* 77:427, 1975.
28. Cingolani HE, Mattiazzi AR, Blesa ES, et al: Contractility in isolated mammalian heart muscle after acid base changes. *Circulation* 26:269, 1970.
29. Collinsworth KA, Kalman SM, Harrison DC: The clinical pharmacology of lidocaine as an anti-arrhythmic drug. *Circulation* 50:1217, 1974.
30. Cooper MJ, Abinader EG: Atropine-induced ventricular fibrillation: case report and review of the literature. *Am Heart J* 97:225, 1979.
31. Dalsey WC, Barsan WG, Joyce SM, et al: Comparison of superior vena caval and inferior vena caval access using a radioisotope technique during normal perfusion and cardiopulmonary resuscitation. *Ann Emerg Med* 13:881, 1984.
32. Dauchot P, Gravenstein JS: Bradycardia after myocardial ischemia and its treatment with atropine. *Anesthesiology* 44:501, 1976.
33. Davidson R, Parker M, Atkinson AJ Jr: Excessive serum lidocaine levels during maintenance infusion: mechanisms and prevention. *Am Heart J* 104:203, 1982.
34. De Azevedo IM, Wantanabe Y, Dreifus LS: Electrophysiologic antagonism of quinidine and bretylium tosylate. *Am J Cardiol* 33:633, 1974.
35. Dembo DH: Calcium in advanced life support. *Crit Care Med* 9:358, 1981.
36. DeSilva RA, Hennekens CH, Lown B, et al: Lignocaine prophylaxis in acute myocardial infarction. An evaluation of randomized trials. *Lancet* 2:855, 1981.
37. Dhingia R, Amat-y-Leon F, Wyndham C: Electrophysiologic effects of atropine on human sinus node and atrium. *Am J Med* 38:492, 1976.
38. Ditchey RV: High dose epinephrine does not improve the balance between myocardial oxygen supply and demand during cardiopulmonary resuscitation in dogs (abstract). *J Am Coll Cardiol* 3:596, 1984.
39. Ditchey RV, Lindenfeld J: Potential adverse effects of volume loading on perfusion of vital organs during closed-chest resuscitation. *Circulation* 69:181, 1984.
40. Doan LA: Peripheral versus central delivery of medications during CPR. *Ann Emerg Med* 13(part 2):784, 1984.
41. Dorian P, Fain ES, Davy JM, et al: Lidocaine causes a reversible concentration-dependent increase in defibrillation energy requirements. *J Am Coll Cardiol* 8:327, 1986.
42. Dreyfuss J, Bigger JR, Jr., Cohen AI, et al: Metabolism of procainamide in rhesus monkey and man. *Clin Pharmacol Ther* 13:366, 1972.

43. Dunn HM, McComb JM, Kinney CD, et al: Prophylactic lidocaine in the early phase of suspected acute myocardial infarction. *Am Heart J* 110:353. 1985.
44. Eisenberg M, Bergner L, Hallstrom A: Epidemiology of cardiac arrest and resuscitation in children. *Ann Emerg Med* 12:672, 1983.
45. Euler DE, Leman TW, Wallock ME, et al: Deleterious effects of bretylium on hemodynamic recovery from ventricular fibrillation. *Am Heart J* 112:25, 1986.
46. Euler DE, Scanlon PJ: Mechanism of the effect of bretylium on the ventricular fibrillation threshold in dogs. *Am J Cardiol* 55:1396, 1985.
47. Flaherty JT, Schaff HV, Goldman R, et al: Metabolic and functional effects of progressive degrees of hypothermia during global ischemia. *Am J Physiol* 236:H839, 1979.
48. Flaherty JT, Weisfeldt ML, Bulkley BH, et al: Mechanisms of ischemic myocardial cell damage assessed by phosphorus-31 nuclear magnetic resonance. *Circulation* 65:561, 1982.
49. Fujimoto T, Hamamoto H, Peter T, et al: Electrophysiologic effects of bretylium on canine ventricular muscle during acute ischemia and reperfusion. *Am Heart J* 105:966, 1983.
50. Giardina EGV, Heissenbuttel RH, Bigger JT: Intermittent intravenous procaine amide to treat ventricular arrhythmias. *Ann Intern Med* 78:183, 1973.
51. Gintant GA, Hoffman BF, Naylor RE: The influence of molecular form of local anesthetic-type antiarrhythmic agents on reduction of the maximum upstroke velocity of canine cardiac Purkinje fibers. *Circ Res* 52:735, 1983.
52. Gold H, Edward D: The effects of ouabain on the heart in the presence of hypercalcemia. *Am Heart J* 3:45, 1927.
53. Graf H, Leach W, Arieff AI: Metabolic effects of sodium bicarbonate in hypoxic lactic acidosis in dogs. *Am J Physiol* 2249:F630, 1985.
54. Guerci AD, Chandra N, Johnson E, et al: Sodium bicarbonate does not improve resuscitation from ventricular fibrillation in dogs. *Circulation* 74(suppl 4):75, 1986.
55. Harison DC, Sprouse JH, Morrow AG: The antiarrhythmic properties of lidocaine and procaine amide. Clinical and physiologic studies of their cardiovascular effects in man. *Circulation* 28:486, 1963.
56. Harrison FE, Amey BD: Use of calcium in electromechanical dissociation. *Ann Emerg Med* 13:844, 1984.
57. Hasegawa EA: The endotracheal administration of drugs. *Heart Lung* 15:60, 1986.
58. Haynes RE, Chinn TL, Copan MK, et al: Comparison of bretylium tosylate and lidocaine in management of out-of-hospital ventricular fibrillation. A randomized clinical trial. *Am J Cardiol* 48:353, 1981.
59. Heissenbuttel RH, Bigger JT: Bretylium tosylate: a newly available antiarrhythmic drug for ventricular arrhythmias. *Ann Intern Med* 91:229, 1979.
60. Hoffman BG: The action of quinidine and procainamide on single fibers of dog ventricle and specialized conducting systems. *An Acad Bras Cienc* 29:365, 1958.
61. Holland K, Patterson E, Lucches BR, et al. Prevention of ventricular fibrillation in a conscious canine model of sudden coronary death. *Am Heart J* 105:711, 1983.
62. Holmes HR, Babbs CF, Voorhees WD, et al: Influence of adrenergic drugs upon vital organ perfusion during CPR. *Crit Care Med* 8:137, 1980.
63. Houle DB, Weil MH, Brown EB, et al: Influence of respiratory acidosis on ECG and pressor response to epinephrine, norepinephrine and metaraminol. *Proc Soc Exp Biol Med* 94:561, 1957.
64. Jaillon P, Winkle RA: Electrophysiologic comparative study of procainamide and N-acetyl-procainamide in anesthetized dogs: concentration response relationships. *Circulation* 58:1385, 1979.
65. Juan G, Calverley P, Talamo C, et al: Effect of carbon dioxide on diaphragmatic function in human beings. *N Engl J Med* 310:874, 1984.
66. Kastor JA, Josephson ME, Guss SB, et al: Human ventricular refractoriness. II: Effects of procainamide. *Circulation* 56:462, 1977.
67. Katz A, Tenter M: Cellular calcium and cardiac cell death. *Am J Cardiol* 44:188, 1979.
68. Kerber RE, Pandian NG, Jensen SR, et al: Effect of lidocaine and bretylium on energy requirement for transthoracic defibrillation. Experimental studies. *J Am Coll Cardiol* 7:397, 1986.
69. Kindig NB, Filley GF: Intravenous bicarbonate may cause transient intracellular acidosis. *Chest* 83:712, 1983.
70. Kniffen FJ, Lomas TE, Counsell RE, et al: The antiarrhythmic and antifibrillatory actions of bretylium and its o-iodobenzyltrimethylammonium analog. UM-360. *J Pharmacol Exp Ther* 192:120, 1975.
71. Knoebel SB, McHenry PL, Phillips JF, et al: Atropine-induced cardioacceleration and myocardial blood flow in subjects with and without coronary artery disease. *Am J Cardiol* 33:327, 1974.
72. Koch-Weser J: Drug therapy: bretylium. *N Engl J Med* 300:473, 1979.
73. Koch-Weser J: Pharmacokinetics of procainamide in man. *Ann NY Acad Sci* 179:370, 1971.
74. Koltmeier CA, Gravenstein JS: The parasympathomimetic activity of atropine and atropine methylbromide. *Anesthesiology* 29:1125, 1968.
75. Koo CC, Allen JD, Pantridge JF: Lack of effect of bretylium on electrical defibrillation in a controlled study. *Cardiovasc Res* 18:762, 1984.
76. Kosnik JW, Jackson RE, Keats S, et al: Dose-related response of centrally administered epinephrine on the change in aortic diastolic pressure during closed chest massage in dogs. *Ann Emerg Med* 14:204, 1985.
77. Koster RW, Dunning AJ: Intramuscular lidocaine for prevention of lethal arrhythmias in the prehospital phase of acute myocardial infarction. *N Engl J Med* 313:1105, 1985.
78. Kupersmith J: Electrophysiological and antiarrhythmic effects of lidocaine in canine acute myocardial ischemia. *Am Heart J* 97:360, 1979.
79. Lawson NW, Butler GH III, Roy CT: Alkalosis and cardiac arrhythmias. *Anesth Analg* 52:951, 1973.
80. Lown B, Vassaux C: Lidocaine in acute myocardial infarction. *Am Heart J* 76:685, 1968.
81. Mace SE: Effect of technique of administration on plasma lidocaine levels. *Ann Emerg Med* 15:552, 1986.
82. Mark LC, Kayden HJ, Steele JM, et al: The physiological disposition and cardiac effects of procainamide. *J Pharmacol Exp Ther* 102:5, 1951.
83. Markis JE, Koch-Weser J: Characteristics and mechanisms of inotropic and chronotropic actions of bretylium tosylate. *J Pharmacol* 178:94, 1971.
84. Mattar JA, Weil MH, Shubin H, et al: Cardiac arrest in the critically ill: II. Hyperosmolar states following cardiac arrest. *Ann J Med* 56:162, 1974.
85. Michael JR, Guerci AD, Koehler RC, et al: Mechanisms by which epinephrine augments cerebral and myocardial perfusion during cardiopulmonary resuscitation in dogs. *Circulation* 69:822, 1984.
86. Minuck M, Sharma GP: Comparison of THAM and sodium bicarbonate in resuscitation of the heart after ventricular fibrillation in dogs. *Anesth Analg* 56:38, 1977.
87. Mitchell JH, Wildenthal D, Johnson LR Jr. The effects of acid-base disturbance on cardiovascular and pulmonary function. *Kidney Int* 1:375, 1972.
88. Narang PK, Adir J, Josselson J, et al: Pharmacokinetics of bretylium in man after intravenous administration. *J Pharmacokinet Biopharm* 8:363, 1980.
89. Newton DW, Fung EF, Williams DA: Stability of five

catecholamines and terbutaline sulfate in 5% dextrose injection in the absence and presence of aminophylline. *Am J Hosp Pharm* 38:1314, 1981.

90. Niemann JT, Criley JM, Rosborough JP, et al: Predictive indices of successful cardiac resuscitation after prolonged arrest and experimental cardiopulmonary resuscitation. *Ann Emerg Med* 14:521, 1985.

91. Niemann JT, Haynes KS, Garner D, et al: Post countershock pulseless rhythms: response to CPR, artificial cardiac pacing and adrenergic agonists. *Ann Emerg Med* 15:112–120, 1985.

92. Niemann JT, Rosborough JP: Effects of academia and sodium bicarbonate therapy in advanced cardiac life support. *Ann Emerg Med* 13(part 2):781, 1984.

93. Niemann JT, Rosborough JP, Ung S, et al: Hemodynamic effects of continuous abdominal binding during cardiac arrest and resuscitation. *Am J Cardiol* 53:269, 1984.

94. Nishimura M, Wantanabe Y: Membrane action and catecholamine release action of bretylium tosylate in normoxic and hypoxic canine Purkinje fibers. *J Am Coll Cardiol* 2:287, 1983.

99. Oldson DW, Thompson BM, Dairn JL, et al: A randomized comparison study of bretylium tosylate and lidocaine in resuscitation of patients from out of hospital ventricular fibrillation in a paramedic system. *Ann Emerg Med* 13:807, 1984.

96. Ornato JP, Bryson BL, Farqualharson RR, et al: Measurement of ventilation during cardiopulmonary resuscitation. *Crit Care Med* 11:79, 1983.

97. O'Rourke GW, Greene NM: Autonomic blockade and the resting heart rate in man. *Am Heart J* 80:469, 1970.

98. Ostrea EM, Odell GB: The influence of bicarbonate administration on blood pH in a "closed system": clinical implications. *J Pediatr* 80:671, 1972.

99. Otto CW, Yakaitis RW: The role of epinephrine in CPR: a reappraisal. *Ann Emerg Med* 13(part 2):840, 1984.

100. Otto CW, Yakaitis RW, Blitt CD: Mechanism of action of epinephrine in resuscitation from asphyxial arrest. *Crit Care Med* 9:321, 1981.

101. Patterson E, Lucchesi BR: Bretylium: a prototype for future development of antidysrhythmic agents. *Am Heart J* 106:426, 1983.

102. Raehl CL: Endotracheal drug therapy in cardiopulmonary resuscitation. *Clin Pharmacol* 5:573, 1986.

103. Ralston SH, Tacker WA, Showen L, et al: Endotracheal versus intravenous epinephrine during electromechanical dissociation with CPR in dogs. *Ann Emerg Med* 14:1044, 1985.

104. Ralston SH, Voorhees WD, Showen L, et al: Venous and arterial blood gases during and after cardiopulmonary resuscitation in dogs. *Am J Emerg Med.* 3:132, 1985.

105. Redding JS, Pearson JW: Resuscitation from ventricular fibrillation: drug therapy. *JAMA* 203:255, 1968.

106. Romhilt DW, Bloomfield SS, Lipicky RJ, et al: Evaluation of bretylium tosylate for the treatment of premature ventricular contractions. *Circulation* 45:800, 1972.

107. Roos A, Boron WF: Intracellular pH. *Physiol Rev.* 61:296, 1981.

108. Rosetti VA, Thompson BM, Aprahamian C, et al: Difficulty and delay in intravascular access in pediatric patients. *Ann Emerg Med* 13:406, 1984.

109. Rosetti VA, Thompson BM, Miller J, et al: Intraosseous infusion: an alternative route of pediatric intravascular access. *Ann Emerg Med* 14:885, 1985.

110. Sanders AB, Ewy GA, Taft TV: Prognostic and therapeutic importance of the aortic diastolic pressure in resuscitation from cardiac arrest. *Crit Care Med* 12:871, 1984.

111. Sanna G, Arcidiacono R: Chemical ventricular fibrillation of the human heart with bretylium tosylate. *Am J Cardiol* 32:982, 1973.

112. Schleien CL, Dean JM, Koehler RC, et al: Effect of epinephrine on cerebral and myocardial perfusion in an infant animal preparation of cardiopulmonary resuscitation. *Circulation* 73:809, 1986.

113. Scott B, Martin FG, Matchett J, Whites S: Canine cardiovascular responses to endotracheally and intravenously administered atropine, isoproterenol and propranolol. *Ann Emerg Med* 16:1/17, 1987.

114. Shechter JA, Caine R, Friehling T, et al: Effect of procainamide on dispersion of ventricular refractoriness. *Am J Cardiol* 52:279, 1983.

115. Shensa TD, Gilbert CJ, Schmidt DH, et al: Procainamide and retrograde atrioventricular nodal conduction in man. *Circulation* 65:355, 1982.

116. Singer DH, Strauss HC, Hoffman BF: Biphasic effects of procainamide on cardiac conduction. *Bull NY Acad Med* 43:1194, 1968.

117. Singh BN, Vaughn Williams EM: Local anesthetic and antiarrhythmic actions of alprenolol relative to its effect on intracellular action potentials and other properties of isolated cardiac muscle. *Br J Pharmacol* 38:749, 1970.

118. Sobel BE, Braunwald E: The management of acute myocardial infarction. In Braunwald E (ed): *Heart Disease: A Textbook of Cardiovascular Medicine*, ed 2. Philadelphia, WB Saunders, 1984, vol 2, p 1308.

119. Spear JR, Moore EN, Gerstenblith G: Effect of lidocaine on the ventricular fibrillation threshold in the dog during acute ischemia and premature ventricular contractions. *Circulation* 46:65, 1972.

120. Standards and guidelines for cardiopulmonary resuscitation and emergency cardiac care. *JAMA* 255:2841, 1986.

121. Stargel WW, Shand DG, Routledge PA, et al: Clinical comparison of rapid infusion and multiple injection methods for lidocaine loading. *Am Heart J* 102:872, 1981.

122. Steenbergen C, Deleeuw G, Rich T, et al: Effects of acidosis and ischemia on contractility and intracellular pH of rat heart. *Circ Res* 41:849, 1977.

123. Steuven HA, Thompson B, Aprahamian C, et al: The effectiveness of calcium chloride in refractory electromechanical dissociation. *Ann Emerg Med* 14:626, 1985.

124. Steuven HA, Thompson B, Aprahamian C, et al: Lack of effectiveness of calcium chloride in refractory asystole. *Ann Emerg Med* 14:630: 1985.

125. Steuven HA, Tonsfeldt DJ, Thompson BM, et al: Atropine in asystole: human studies. *Ann Emerg Med* 13(part 2):815, 1984.

126. Stulz PM, Scheidegger D, Drop LJ, et al: Ventricular pump performance during hypocalcemia. *J Thorac Cardiovasc Surg* 78:185, 1979.

127. Tacker WA, Niebauer MJ, Babbs CR, et al: The effect of newer antiarrhythmic drugs on defibrillation threshold. *Crit Care Med* 8:177, 1980.

128. Telivuo L, Maamies T, Siltanen P, et al: Comparison of alkalizing agents in resuscitation of the heart after ventricular fibrillation. *Ann Chir Gynaecol Fenn* 57:221, 1968.

129. Thomson PD, Melmon K, Richardson JA, et al: Lidocaine pharmacokinetics in advanced heart failure, liver disease, and renal failure in humans. *Ann Intern Med* 78:872, 1973.

130. Vatner SR, Baig H: Comparison of the effects of ouabain and isoproterenol on ischemic myocardium of conscious dogs. *Circulation* 58:654, 1978.

131. Vaughan, Williams EM: Classification of antiarrhythmic drugs. In Sandoe E, et al (eds): *Arrhythmias*. Sweden, Sodertalje, 1970, p 449.

132. Volpi A, Maggioni A, Franzosi MG, et al: In-hospital prognosis of patient with acute myocardial infarction complicated by primary ventricular fibrillation. *N Engl J Med* 317:257, 1987.

133. Voorhees WD, Jaeger CS, Babbs CR, et al: Regional

blood flow during cardiopulmonary resuscitation in dogs. *Crit Care Med* 8:134, 1980.

134. Vyden JK, et al: The effect of lidocaine on peripheral hemodynamics. *J Clin Pharmacol* 15:506, 1975.

135. Ward JT Jr: Endotracheal drug therapy. *Ann J Emerg Med* 1:71, 1983.

136. Weil MH, Afifi AA: Experimental and clinical studies on lactate and pyruvate as indicators of the severity of acute circulatory failure (shock). *Circulation* 41:989, 1970.

137. Weil MH, Rackow EC, Trevino R, et al: Difference in acid-base state between venous and arterial blood during cardiopulmonary resuscitation. *N Engl J Med* 315:153, 1986.

138. Weiner N: Atropine, scopolamine, and related antimuscarinic drugs. In Gilman AG, Goodman LS, Rall TW, Murad F (eds): *Goodman and Gilman's, The Pharmacologic Basis of Therapeutics.* New York, Macmillan, 1985, pp 130–144.

139. Weiner N: Norepinephrine, epinephrine and the sympathomimetic amines. In Gilman AC, Goodman LS, Rall TW, Murad F (eds): *Goodman and Gilman's, The Pharmacological Basis of Therapeutics.* New York, Macmillan, 1985, pp 160–161.

140. Wellens, JJH, Durrer DL: Effect of procaine amide, quinidine and ajmaline in the Wolff-Parkinson-White syndrome. *Circulation* 50:114, 1974.

141. Woosely RL, Reele SB, Roden DM, et al: Pharmacologic reversal of hypotensive effect complicating antiarrhythmic therapy with bretylium. *Clin Pharmacol Ther* 32:313, 1982.

142. Wortsman J, Frank S, Cryer PE: Adrenomedullary response to maximal stress in humans. *Am J Med* 77:779, 1984.

143. Yakaitis RW, Otto CW, Blitt CD: Relative importance of alpha and beta adrenergic receptors during resuscitation. *Crit Care Med* 7:293, 1979.

144. Zoll PM, Zoll RH, Falk RH, et al: External noninvasive temporary cardiac pacing: clinical trials. *Circulation* 71:937, 1985.

11

Cerebral Protection

Donald S. Prough, M.D.
Douglas S. DeWitt, Ph.D.

The past three decades have been exciting but frustrating for those involved in neurologic intensive care. Investigators have clarified the pathophysiology of central nervous system (CNS) injury, and scientists and industry have expanded the range of clinical neurophysiologic monitoring. However, new therapeutic approaches have progressed slowly, many initially promising therapeutic possibilities having failed at the preclinical or clinical level.

The development of a comprehensive pathophysiologic understanding of cerebral edema and brain ischemia has been a major milestone (40, 76, 162). The introduction by Lundberg (88) of intraventricular pressure monitoring and the subsequent development of the subarachnoid bolt by Vries et al (160) have provided the initial, important steps toward physiologic monitoring. The introduction by Lassen et al (81) of regional cerebral blood flow measurement has led to the development of effective portable cerebral blood flow monitoring systems, and the development of computed tomography (CT), magnetic resonance imaging (MRI), and positron emission tomography (PET) has permitted increasingly detailed—albeit increasingly expensive—insights into intracranial structural and physiologic derangements. Electrophysiologic monitoring has progressed from the cumbersome technique of continuous electroencephalography (EEG) to the provision of much more manageable data in the form of processed EEG, evoked potential, and brain mapping procedures.

Pharmacologically, neurologic intensive care has focused on the search for clinical situations in which to apply the extensive basic information regarding the neuroprotective effects of interventions such as glucocorticoids and barbiturates. In some instances the results have been gratifying, as in the demonstration by Nussmeier and colleagues (110) that sodium thiopental could, under carefully defined conditions, limit neurologic injury during valvular heart surgery. However, the theory that barbiturates might protect against the neurologic injury that commonly follows cardiac arrest has finally and conclusively been disproven (124), and the utility of corticosteroids in the management of closed head injury has been seriously questioned (132). Currently, calcium entry blockers are arousing intense interest. Calcium entry blockers have improved outcome following experimental focal cerebral ischemia (100) and global cerebral ischemia (147). Clinically, they have provided effective prophylaxis of ischemic neurologic deficits due to subarachnoid hemorrhage (6) and are currently being studied in a broad variety of experimental neurologic injuries.

This chapter reviews the pathophysiology of cerebral ischemia and intracranial hypertension, the normal physiologic regulation of cerebral blood flow, the pharmacologic basis of cerebral protective therapy, and several specific diseases that produce neurologic injury.

PATHOPHYSIOLOGY OF CEREBRAL ISCHEMIA AND INTRACRANIAL HYPERTENSION

Cerebral Ischemia

Cerebral ischemia refers to the inadequate delivery of oxygen to brain tissue, whether due to decreased arterial oxygen content, decreased cerebral blood flow, increased cerebral metabolic demand, or impaired tissue uptake. Cerebral ischemia is a fundamental mechanism of injury in many neurologic insults. Even following closed head trauma, in which the mechanical injury seems to be an adequate explanation for neurologic damage, histopathologic changes due to cerebral ischemia frequently can be demonstrated post mortem (5).

Table 11.1
Normal Cerebral Oxygen Supply and Utilization[a]

Cerebral blood flow (CBF)	50 ml/100 g/min
$CMRo_2 = CBF \times C(a-jv)o_2$	3.5 ml/100 g/min
$C(a-jv)o_2$	7.0 ml/100 ml
Cao_2	20 ml/100 ml
$Cjvo_2$	13 ml/100 ml
$Sjvo_2$	65%
$Pjvo_2$	35 mm Hg
$CDo_2 = CBF \times Cao_2$	10 ml/100 g/min

[a] $CMRo_2$, metabolic consumption of oxygen; Cao_2, arterial oxygen content; $Cjvo_2$, jugular bulb oxygen content; $C(a-jv)o_2$, cerebral arteriovenous oxygen content difference; $Sjvo_2$, jugular bulb oxygen saturation; CDo_2, cerebral oxygen delivery.

Insufficient delivery of oxygen to the brain must be viewed in comparison with normal values for cerebral oxygen supply and demand (Table 11.1). The normal brain, representing about 2% of body mass, receives 15% of the cardiac output, and a greater amount of oxygen is extracted from blood perfusing the brain than from blood perfusing most other tissues. Consequently, jugular venous oxygen content ($Cjvo_2$), tension ($Pjvo_2$), and saturation ($Sjvo_2$) are lower than systemic mixed venous oxygen content ($C\bar{v}o_2$), tension ($P\bar{v}o_2$), and saturation ($S\bar{v}o_2$). The cerebral arteriovenous oxygen content difference is approximately 7.0 ml/100 ml of blood. Each 100 g of brain tissue receives 50 ml of blood per minute; therefore each 100 g of brain tissue consumes approximately 3.5 ml/100 g/min of oxygen.

The brain is highly sensitive to oxygen deprivation for several reasons, including a high resting energy requirement, the absence of oxygen stores, and the absence of unperfused "reserve" capillaries (125). Consequently, even a transient reduction in oxygen supply rapidly depletes high-energy phosphate stores, thereby setting in motion a cascade of events that leads to neuronal and vascular injury (Table 11.2). Neuronal injury is characterized by intracellular acidosis, cell membrane dysfunction, intracellular calcium overload, and cytotoxic edema. Vascular injury, associated with an increase in vascular resistance due to platelet

Table 11.2
Pathogenesis of Ischemic Injury

Neuronal Injury	Vascular Injury
Intracellular acidosis	Platelet aggregation
Membrane injury	Vasospasm
Intracellular calcium overload	Vasogenic edema
Intracellular (cytotoxic) edema	

aggregation or vasospasm and with disruption of the blood-brain barrier, results in plasma extravasation (vasogenic edema). All of the above are major features of ischemic injury to which many biochemical events contribute (Fig. 11.1).

The failure of ATP and phosphocreatine production occurs quickly after oxygen tension declines because of the cessation of perfusion; rapid consumption leads to depletion of high-energy substrates (125, 138). Subsequently, because of dysfunction of the ATP-dependent Na^+/K^+ transport system, intracellular K^+ leaks from the cell and Na^+ enters the cell (81, 47, 125, 155). At a critical level of extracellular K^+, Ca^{2+} floods the cell (31, 47, 55, 125, 155). Increasing concentrations of intracellular Ca^{2+} activate phospholipase A_2, which subsequently releases free fatty acids, including arachidonic acid, from cell membranes (138, 172). The release of free fatty acids increases intracellular acidosis. If oxygen is available (as in incomplete ischemia or following reperfusion of ischemic tissue), arachidonate is metabolized, producing thromboxane A_2, leukotrienes, and free radicals (32, 73, 75, 120, 165). (Fig. 11.2). Thromboxane A_2 is a potent vasoconstrictor, and the leukotrienes and free radicals cause further cell membrane and vessel wall damage (32, 73, 75, 165).

The failure of aerobic ATP production leads to an increase in anaerobic glycolysis. Although insufficient to maintain cell energy needs, anaerobic glycolysis nevertheless results in a rapid accumulation of lactic acid and a precipitous decline in intracellular pH (99). Acidosis further enhances free radical formation (139). If hyperglycemia is present, it may worsen intracellular acidosis and neurologic outcome by providing additional substrate for anaerobic glycolysis (45, 89, 171).

Even if flow is restored to neural tissue after a period of ischemia, prolonged postischemic hypoperfusion typically follows (Fig. 11.3). This state, associated with a profound increase in cerebral vascular resistance, was first described by Ames and associates (7). Pathogenetically, the profound vasoconstriction is associated with edema of surrounding tissue, increased intracellular Ca^{2+}, and evidence of increased tissue and intravascular levels of thromboxane A_2 (73, 120). The no-reflow phenomenon appears not to be due to microvascular obstruction (87), although sludging of cellular blood elements may contribute to decreased flow during the initial ischemic event (103). Both the severity of postischemic vaso-

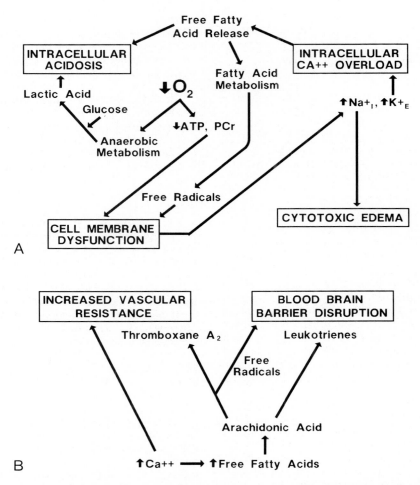

Figure 11.1. A, Biochemical events associated with ischemic injury to neural cells. A reduction in oxygen availability results in a decline in high-energy phosphate metabolites, ATP and phosphocreatine *(PCr)* and a shift to anaerobic metabolism. Cell membrane dysfunction results in ionic shifts, intracellular calcium overload, and the production of free radicals and free fatty acids. **B**, Biochemical events associated with ischemic injury to neural vascular tissue.

constriction and the severity of cerebral edema are directly related to the duration of ischemia (157, 158).

Brain tissue is not homogeneously vulnerable to ischemic damage. Certain regions, especially the arterial boundary zones, the cerebellum, the basal ganglia, and parts of the hippocampus, are especially prone to damage (47). Figure 11.4 displays *experimental* thresholds at which ischemic dysfunction and injury occur. Electrophysiologic evidence of brain ischemia occurs in animals when cerebral blood flow declines to 15–20 ml/100 g/min (31, 47). Below a level of 8–10 ml/100 g/min, the pathophysiologic events described above occur. Clinical thresholds have been less well established because clinical techniques lack the resolution of experimental techniques. However, the thresholds based on data acquired during carotid endarterectomy appear to be similar to those observed in animals (Fig. 11.5) (135).

The deficit produced by an ischemic insult is dependent not only on the magnitude of flow reduction but also on the regionality and the duration of the event. Magnitude refers to whether the ischemia is complete, as in cardiac arrest, or partial, as in shock states or intracranial hypertension. Regionality describes whether the insult is focal, as in stroke, or generalized, as in cardiac arrest. Describing ischemia in these terms helps to predict the

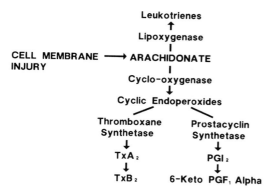

Figure 11.2. Partial scheme of arachidonate metabolism. Arachidonate is metabolized by lipoxygenase and cyclooxygenase. The lipoxygenase pathway results in formation of the leukotrienes. Two particularly important cyclooxygenase metabolites are thromboxane A_2 *(TxA$_2$)* and prostaglandin I_2 (prostacyclin) *(PGI$_2$)*. Thromboxane B_2 *(TxB$_2$)* and 6-keto PGF$_1$ alpha are the stable metabolic products of thromboxane A_2 and prostacyclin.

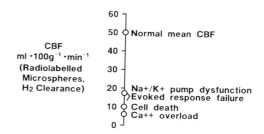

Figure 11.4. Experimental thresholds (severity) for electrophysiologic dysfunction and permanent neurologic injury. *CBF,* cerebral blood flow.

likely response to therapeutic interventions. For instance, focal cerebral ischemia often involves an area of cell death surrounded by an ischemic penumbra of viable but nonfunctional tissue, much of which may be salvageable by appropriate treatment. In experimental focal ischemia, hyperventilation increases cerebral vascular resistance in noninvolved areas, thereby redirecting flow to areas of viable but nonfunctioning tissue—a process termed an "inverse steal." Conversely, hypercapnia may "steal" flow from ischemic tissue.

The duration of cerebral ischemia exerts an important effect on outcome. When cerebral blood flow declines abruptly and severely, reversible neurologic dysfunction develops within seconds, and the insult becomes irreversible after a critical threshold of duration. Although

conventional wisdom states that the human brain is irreversibly damaged if flow is completely interrupted for more than 4 minutes, recent studies in a primate model suggest that the brain can recover function after complete ischemia of 17 minutes or longer (79, 147).

Intracranial Hypertension

Normal intracranial pressure (ICP) is less than 15 mm Hg (200 mm H_2O). ICP reflects the volume of the three compartments—tissue, blood, and cerebrospinal fluid (CSF)—within the noncompliant skull. A small, gradual increase in any one of these compartments is partially compensated for by modest decreases in the volume of one or both of the other components (Fig. 11.6), and ICP remains within normal limits. Once a critical volume is reached, however, any further increments in intracranial volume produce large increments in ICP. Common causes of intracranial hypertension include intracranial neoplasms, subdural and epidural hematomas, intracerebral hemorrhage, acute hydrocephalus, and cerebral edema (40).

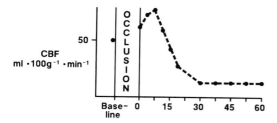

Figure 11.3. Following relief of global cerebral ischemia (represented by termination of a period of vascular occlusion), blood flow *(CBF)* typically increases, then declines to a fraction of its preischemic value. Similar events occur following regional ischemia.

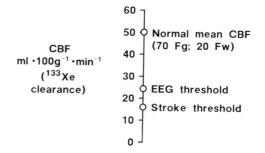

Figure 11.5. Clinical thresholds (severity) for electrophysiologic dysfunction and permanent neurologic injury. *CBF,* cerebral blood flow; *Fg,* flow to cerebral gray matter; *Fw,* flow to cerebral white matter.

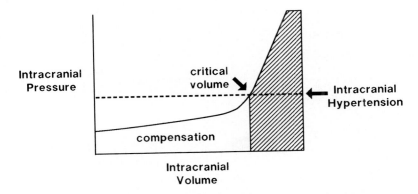

Figure 11.6. Relationship between intracranial volume and intracranial pressure. As the volume of one compartment (tissue, cerebrospinal fluid, or blood) increases, compensation initially is adequate; however, once a critical volume is obtained, intracranial pressure rapidly increases.

Intracranial hypertension may produce cerebral ischemia by reducing cerebral perfusion pressure (CPP). Normally, CPP = MAP − JVP, where MAP is mean arterial pressure and JVP is jugular venous pressure. If ICP exceeds JVP, the equation becomes CPP = MAP − ICP. A sufficient reduction in CPP produces global cerebral ischemia, whereas herniation produces localized ischemic brain damage.

The therapy of intracranial hypertension must, then, address either a decrease in the volume of the component that caused the original problem (e.g., tumor removal) or a decrease in the volume of one of the other components (Fig. 11.7). On an emergent basis,

intracranial hypertension is most quickly treated by reducing cerebral blood volume, usually by intentionally using acute hyperventilation to decrease cerebral blood flow (CBF).

PHYSIOLOGIC REGULATION OF CEREBRAL BLOOD FLOW

The rate of CBF is tightly regulated in normal physiologic states. The major determinants of CBF include the level of neural activity, Pao_2, $Paco_2$, and the phenomenon of pressure autoregulation, a term applied to the

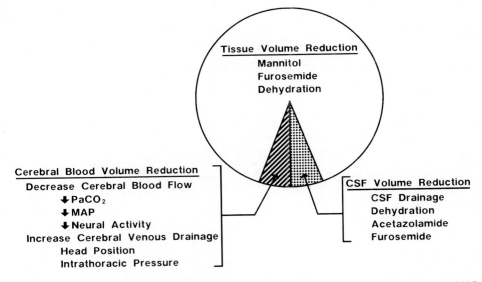

Figure 11.7. Strategies for reducing intracranial pressure based on intracranial compartments. *MAP,* mean arterial pressure; *CSF,* cerebrospinal fluid.

preservation of a constant CBF across a broad range of cerebral perfusion pressures.

Neural Activity

Brain tissue consumes oxygen in order to maintain cellular integrity and to perform electrophysiologic work, and CBF increases in response to increased cerebral metabolic consumption of oxygen ($CMRo_2$). Although seizures most dramatically illustrate the effects of an increase in $CMRo_2$ on CBF, simple motor activity, sensory stimulation, eye movement, reading, and thinking are also associated with demonstrable increases in CBF in appropriate brain regions (94, 127, 130). The mechanism of flow-metabolism coupling remains controversial. It may be accomplished by the local release of adenosine, according to data acquired in experimental studies of adenosine antagonism with caffeine or theophylline or inhibition of adenosine reuptake by dipyridamole or papaverine (13).

Arterial Oxygen Tension, Pao_2

Decreases in arterial oxygen saturation (Sao_2) and tension (Pao_2) cause reciprocal changes in CBF. Cerebral blood flow increases rapidly as Sao_2 is decreased below 90% (Fig. 11.8A) or as Pao_2 is decreased below 60 mm Hg (Fig. 11.8B). The mechanism by which decreased oxygen availability increases CBF may be the same as that by which neural activation increases CBF, specifically the local release of adenosine (66, 113). Recent data suggest that

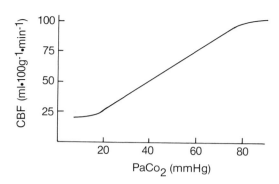

Figure 11.9. Response of cerebral blood flow *(CBF)* to changes in $Paco_2$.

adenosine antagonism by caffeine and theophylline may decrease CBF and perhaps limit the ability of the cerebral vasculature to respond to oxygen lack (16, 93). Increases in Pao_2 produce modest decreases in CBF (about 15% below normal at a Pao_2 of 600 mm Hg).

Arterial Carbon Dioxide Tension, $Paco_2$

The mechanism by which changes in $Paco_2$ influence CBF is alteration of the brain extracellular hydrogen ion concentration. As $Paco_2$ is acutely decreased from 40 to 20 mm Hg, CBF is halved (51, 80) (Fig. 11.9). As $Paco_2$ increases from 40 to 80 mm Hg, CBF doubles (51, 80). On the average, CBF increases 4% for every 1.0 mm Hg increase in $Paco_2$ (51). Because rapid changes in $Paco_2$ produce rapid changes in both CBF and cerebral blood volume, acute hypercapnia may precipitate severe

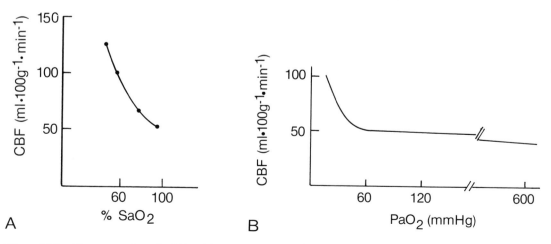

Figure 11.8. Response of cerebral blood flow *(CBF)* to changes **A**, in arterial oxygen saturation *(Sao₂)*, and **B**, in Pao₂.

intracranial hypertension in patients with decreased intracranial compliance. Acute therapeutic hypocapnia may be used to manage intracranial hypertension. If $Paco_2$ is changed acutely and then maintained at a new level for 24–36 hours, CBF returns toward normal values as the brain extracellular hydrogen ion concentration returns to normal (134).

Autoregulation

Autoregulation is the term applied to the process by which cerebral vascular resistance varies directly with changes in MAP (or CPP) to maintain a constant CBF. Under normal circumstances, autoregulation results in a nearly constant CBF over a range from 50 to at least 130 mm Hg (153) (Fig. 11.10). The most widely accepted mechanism explaining autoregulation is the myogenic theory, which states that an increase in wall tension within a cerebral arteriole produces a reflex increase in smooth muscle tone. The lower limit of autoregulation is, in part, determined by the type of physiologic or pharmacologic change that produces the reduction in CPP. In hemorrhagic shock, for instance, the lower limit of autoregulation is shifted toward higher pressures, an effect that is abolished acutely by cervical sympathectomy (41). In addition, the response to regulatory stimuli such as changes in $Paco_2$ may be blunted or abolished when CPP is near the lower threshold for autoregulation (8).

Cerebral autoregulation is impaired by coexistent cerebral vasodilatory stimuli. Hypercapnia severely impairs autoregulation (37, 54), an effect that diminishes as hypercapnia becomes more chronic (123). Cerebral vasodilators, such as the potent inhalational anesthetic halothane, also impair autoregulation (82).

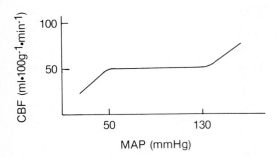

Figure 11.10. Response of cerebral blood flow *(CBF)* to changes in mean arterial pressure *(MAP)*.

PHARMACOLOGY OF CEREBRAL PROTECTION

Numerous drugs are used clinically or are under investigation for the treatment of cerebral ischemia and intracranial hypertension. This section summarizes the CNS effects of drugs that may limit the development of ischemic injury or are used to control intracranial hypertension.

Pharmacologic Management of Cerebral Ischemia

Table 11.3 summarizes the potential abilities of a variety of drugs to limit intracellular acidosis, cell membrane injury, intracellular calcium overload, and cerebral edema, or to limit the severity of ischemia by increasing CBF or decreasing $CMRo_2$.

REVERSAL OF INTRACELLULAR ACIDOSIS

Brain intracellular acidosis, produced by cerebral ischemia, may lead to protein denaturation and enzymatic dysfunction (103). Bicarbonate, the buffer most commonly employed to increase systemic pH, crosses the intact blood-brain barrier to a minimal extent and is therefore ineffective for the management of brain intracellular acidosis. In addition, exogenous bicarbonate increases $Paco_2$ if minute ventilation remains constant; because CO_2 does cross the blood-brain barrier, intracellular acidosis may be aggravated. The buffer tris-hydroxymethylaminomethane (THAM), or tromethamine, penetrates the blood-brain barrier and may produce intracellular alkalinization following neural injury (129). Further studies are needed to characterize the potential efficacy of THAM in a variety of neurologic insults. In areas of low flow due either to pathologic vasoconstriction or to obstructive vascular lesions, adequate delivery of the intracellular buffer might require combination with cerebral vasodilator therapy to improve local flow.

ANTAGONISM OF INTRACELLULAR CALCIUM OVERLOAD

The cerebral effects of calcium entry blockers are undergoing extensive investigation, suggesting that this promising class of drugs may ultimately be widely employed in neurologic disease. The calcium entry blockers are

Table 11.3
Therapeutic Strategies for Reduction of Ischemic Injury

Decrease intracellular acidosis
  THAM
  Dextrose-free fluids
Decrease cell membrane injury
  Inhibit phospholipase
    Glucocorticoids
  Inhibit free radical production
    Superoxide dismutase
Increase cerebral blood flow
  Hemodilution
    Dextran, albumin
  Alter blood rheology
    Pentoxifylline
  Decrease cerebral vascular tone
    Calcium entry blockers
  Inhibit thromboxane production
    Thromboxane synthetase inhibitors
    Cyclooxygenase inhibitors
    Glucocorticoids
	Antagonize intracellular calcium overload
	  Calcium entry blockers
	Decrease cerebral edema (or decrease ICP)
	  Vasogenic edema
	    Glucocorticoids
	  Decrease water in normal brain
	    Mannitol
	  Decrease CSF production
	    Furosemide
	Decrease $CMRo_2$
	  Seizure control
	    Barbiturates
	    Phenytoin
	  Electrophysiologic suppression
	    Barbiturates

a diverse group of drugs, some of which exert prominent intracellular calcium-blocking effects, some of which exert potent blocking effects on calcium entry in the peripheral vasculature or the cardiac conducting system, and some of which exert selective cerebrovascular effects. The calcium entry blocker, nimodipine, appears to have a substantially greater vasodilatory effect on the cerebral vasculature than on the peripheral vasculature (57, 95, 100). The potential therapeutic effects of calcium entry blockers may be related to nonspecific cerebral vasodilation, to blockade of some of the cellular toxicity of calcium (such as activation of phospholipase A_2), or to antagonism of the vascular effects of increased calcium release (postischemic hypoperfusion). Consequently, nimodipine has therapeutic potential for managing focal stroke, cerebral vasospasm associated with subarachnoid hemorrhage, and the reduction in cerebral blood flow that occurs following cardiac arrest. Nimodipine is also undergoing clinical trials as an agent for the reduction of neurologic deficits after cardiopulmonary bypass. The use of nimodipine for this purpose may be particularly promising since, unlike barbiturates, nimodipine should interfere much less with postbypass hemodynamic and ventilatory management.

DECREASE IN CELL MEMBRANE INJURY

Glucocorticoids are commonly given in an attempt to decrease cell membrane injury or to stabilize ischemic cell membranes. The proposed mechanisms of action of glucocorticoids include facilitated clearance of vasogenic edema, stabilization of cellular membranes, and inhibition of the release of arachidonate from cell membranes. The most clearly established use of glucocorticoids is to treat the vasogenic edema associated with brain tumors and brain abscesses (126). On the other hand, glucocorticoids appear to be ineffective in the management of closed head injury (132) and of cellular, or cytotoxic, edema (40), and thus in the management of focal and global cerebral ischemia (65, 83).

Research into antiinflammatory drugs has produced a variety of agents that limit the production of the by-products of arachidonic acid metabolism. In vitro, glucocorticoids inhibit phospholipase A_2. Cyclooxygenase inhibitors, such as indomethacin and ibuprofen, can virtually eliminate the production of the cyclic endoperoxides, the precursor molecules from which many endogenous prostaglandins are synthesized. Recent data suggest that, following experimental ischemic injury, ibuprofen, 12.5 mg/kg administered intravenously, suppresses the release of thromboxane A_2 in the cerebral vasculature, an effect that is associated with increased postischemic blood flow (49). In rats subjected to four-vessel occlusion, the cyclooxygenase inhibitor, zomepirac sodium, 5 mg/kg intravenously, improved postischemic blood flow and EEG recovery (150). Since cyclooxygenase inhibitors also inhibit the production of prostacyclin, an extremely potent cerebral vasodilator, Hallenbeck and Furlow (53) have combined indomethacin with prostacyclin and heparin and have thereby markedly improved regional cerebral blood flow following an experimental ischemic insult. In theory, specific thromboxane synthetase inhibitors should prevent the production of thromboxane A_2, while permitting continued production of vasodilator prostaglandins such as prostacyclin. However, thromboxane synthetase inhibitors have failed to improve cerebral blood flow following either global or regional ischemic insults (106, 120), possibly because the cyclic endoperoxides, which also exert cerebral vasoconstrictive and platelet aggregatory effects, accumulate if the more distal enzymatic pathway is blocked (Fig. 11.2) (42, 133). Finally, investigators have speculated that nimodipine or other calcium entry blockers might act, in part, by inhibiting the activation of phospholipase A_2 by calcium. To date, there are no data that demonstrate a decrease in cerebral venous, brain tissue, or CSF levels of thromboxane metabolites following treatment of cerebral ischemia with a calcium entry blocker.

DECREASE IN CEREBRAL EDEMA

Brain injury due to ischemia, tumor, trauma, inflammation, or metabolic causes, if sufficiently severe, may produce cerebral edema. Diuretics are commonly used to reduce the intracranial hypertension associated with cerebral edema. Mannitol and other osmotic diuretics acutely reduce brain volume, primarily by osmotically removing water from uninjured brain. Clinically, to achieve an acute reduction in intracranial volume, e.g., to reduce ICP in a patient with a mass lesion awaiting surgical decompression, mannitol in an intravenous dose of 1.0–1.5 g/kg is usually employed. For more chronic therapy, e.g., the management of patients with closed head injury and intracranial hypertension, intravenous doses of 0.25–0.5 g/kg may be used. The smaller doses are associated with less risk of rebound intracranial hypertension and of severe fluid and electrolyte depletion. Mannitol and other osmotic diuretics also reduce blood viscosity and may improve microcirculatory flow (65, 108). This effect, in conjunction with the reduction in ICP produced by osmotic diuretics, limits the extent of infarction in animal models of focal ischemia (65, 86). Furosemide, 20–40 mg intravenously, reduces ICP acutely in animal models and in patients (27, 126). The initial

effect of furosemide is to reduce brain water. However, furosemide also inhibits the elaboration of CSF, thereby reducing another of the three components of intracranial volume.

DILATION OF CEREBRAL VESSELS

A variety of agents, such as papaverine and isoxsuprine, dilate intact cerebral vessels (25, 26, 96), but no clinically available agent demonstrates an unequivocal benefit in the acute or chronic management of reduced flow in the diseased cerebral circulation.

As noted above, the calcium entry blocker, nimodipine, appears to dilate preferentially the cerebral vasculature in intact animals and in animals with focally ischemic brain regions (57, 95, 100). This action of nimodipine may provide the possibility for its use in stroke and in clinical states associated with pathologic cerebral vasoconstriction.

Another promising agent that may improve cerebral ischemia is pentoxifylline, which recently became the first drug to receive approval from the Food and Drug Administration for the symptomatic treatment of intermittent claudication due to peripheral arterial occlusive disease (146). Pentoxifylline alters blood rheology, thereby improving flow in tissue perfused by partially occluded vessels. An oral dose of 400 mg three times daily appears to limit the incidence of recurrent transient ischemic attacks (64). Several clinical studies of the acute and chronic oral and intravenous administration of pentoxifylline have demonstrated an improvement in CBF in small numbers of patients with chronic cerebrovascular disease (56, 154), but as yet no data document clinical neuropsychologic improvement associated with the increase in flow.

CEREBRAL METABOLIC DEPRESSION

Barbiturates decrease CBF and blood volume in patients with intracranial hypertension and may decrease CMR_{O_2} in patients with partial cerebral ischemia. In large intravenous doses (sodium thiopental, 20–30 mg/kg; sodium pentobarbital, 30 mg/kg; phenobarbital, 60 mg/kg), by profoundly suppressing the electrical activity of the brain, barbiturates reduce both the CMR_{O_2} and CBF by approximately 50% (104). They have been proposed as possibly effective medical adjunctive therapy for intracranial hypertension associated with closed head trauma, Reye's syndrome, and near-drowning (24, 92, 137). At the present time, however, despite the unequivocal observation that barbiturate loading reduces ICP, there is little evidence that barbiturates materially affect survival in any of those disorders (15, 34, 161).

Although depression of CMR_{O_2} by barbiturates provides protection in animal models of incomplete focal cerebral ischemia (105, 141), barbiturate therapy in human stroke has been unsuccessful. This finding may reflect the poor tolerance of elderly patients with cardiovascular disease to the hemodynamic depression produced by high doses of barbiturates. Recently, however, barbiturates have been shown to decrease the neurologic sequelae associated with valvular heart surgery (see below) (110).

Pharmacologic Management of Intracranial Hypertension

When intracranial hypertension becomes sufficiently severe that global cerebral hypoperfusion, or herniation, or both become a threat, therapeutic reduction of ICP may reduce morbidity and mortality. The potential efficacy of ICP reduction in any neurologic disease process can best be conceptualized by dividing the consequences of the neurologic disease process into the effects of the primary injury and the subsequent secondary injury. The primary injury consists of neuronal damage following trauma, infection, ischemia, or a cytotoxic insult. Secondary injury refers to the effects of subsequent events, such as hypoxemia or hypotension, that may compound the injury. Intracranial hypertension is a particularly important cause of secondary neural injury, because it is possible to monitor ICP and to reduce it effectively in most patients. However, very aggressive control of ICP does not reverse the effects of the primary injury. Severe, irreversible primary insults usually result in an unfavorable neurologic outcome, regardless of how well ICP has been controlled.

Control of increased ICP depends on effective control of cerebral tissue volume, cerebral blood volume, and CSF volume (Fig. 11.7).

REDUCTION OF CEREBRAL TISSUE VOLUME

Reduction in brain tissue volume can be accomplished medically or surgically. Medical control is conventionally based on fluid restriction and the use of osmotic diuretics. Fluid restriction, on a chronic basis, is a relatively ineffective means of reducing brain tissue vol-

ume. Osmotic diuretics, on the other hand, effectively reduce brain tissue volume by dehydrating normal brain tissue. Following a dose of mannitol, ICP is reduced for 3–4 hours. As noted above, an intravenous bolus of 1.0–1.5 g/kg provides brain decompression in anticipation of surgical mass removal, i.e., tumor removal or hematoma drainage. Smaller doses have been used effectively for maintenance reduction of ICP in patients with closed head trauma. Because the effects of mannitol depend on the integrity of the blood-brain barrier, mannitol may be relatively ineffective in patients with severe, diffuse brain injury.

REDUCTION OF CEREBRAL BLOOD VOLUME

Cerebral blood volume may be reduced by reducing CBF or by facilitating cerebral venous drainage. Hypocarbia is commonly employed to reduce CBF, both as a sustained therapeutic measure and as an acute response to sudden increases in ICP. Endotracheal intubation and mechanical ventilation facilitate maintenance of adequate gas exchange, thereby limiting the incidence of inadvertent increases in CBF due to hypoxemia or hypercarbia. Adequate sedation and analgesia, by limiting the effects of brain stimulation on CMR_{O_2} and CBF, are useful in the control of ICP. Patients with multiple injuries, including closed head trauma, may require potent narcotic analgesic agents in sufficient doses to control pain if intracranial hypertension is to be managed effectively. In such narcotized patients, control of ventilation is essential.

Systemic hypertension represents a particularly difficult problem in patients with intracranial hypertension. Autoregulation is attenuated or abolished in areas of injured brain. Consequently, an increase in systemic blood pressure results in an undesirable increase in CBF and cerebral blood volume in those areas. On the other hand, pharmacologic reduction of systemic blood pressure may have adverse effects on intracranial hemodynamics. Nitroprusside has been associated both with cerebral ischemia due to rapid blood pressure reduction (52) and with intracranial hypertension (21, 91). In awake individuals, sodium nitroprusside reduces MAP, CBF, and Pjv_{O_2} (62, 63). Although sodium nitroprusside may decrease CBF, it increases ICP, apparently by increasing cerebral blood volume. Rapid administration of nitroprusside is likely to cause an untoward increase in ICP when intracranial compliance is reduced (21, 91). Nitroglycerin, like nitroprusside, may increase ICP (20). When nitroprusside or nitroglycerin is used to reduce blood pressure in patients with intracranial lesions, the net effect on ICP is the result of (a) a reduction in cerebral blood volume in areas that do not autoregulate because of injury and (b) an increase in cerebral blood volume that is likely in regions where the drug therapy itself inhibits autoregulation.

Other antihypertensive drugs also influence CBF. The calcium entry blocker nifedipine maintains or increases CBF (14). Labetalol, a combination β- and α-antagonist, causes little change in blood flow in hypertensive patients (112).

REDUCTION OF CEREBROSPINAL FLUID VOLUME

Intracranial pressure may also be decreased by reducing the volume of CSF. Dehydration and furosemide decrease the production of CSF. Other drugs such as acetazolamide, 250 mg orally or intravenously, or digoxin also reduce CSF production. CSF can also be withdrawn through an intraventricular catheter. Intraventricular drainage catheters are placed more commonly in cases of intraventricular hemorrhage and less commonly in other situations involving intracranial hypertension.

SPECIFIC DISEASE STATES

Many neurologic diseases, particularly those involving cerebral ischemia, have resisted attempts at therapy. Today, there is reason for cautious optimism regarding the possibility that the extent of neurologic injury produced by a given insult may ultimately be reduced. Much of that optimism is based on the introduction of new drugs, such as the calcium entry blockers, and on increasing research into the biochemical basis of neural injury produced by ischemia and reperfusion. Intense interest has been focused on the neurologic sequelae of cardiopulmonary bypass and of cardiac arrest, on the management of cerebral vasospasm after subarachnoid hemorrhage, and on the mechanisms of permanent neurologic dysfunction following closed head injury. In addition, promising progress has been accomplished experimentally in the management of stroke. The effects of hemorrhagic shock and resuscitation on CBF and cerebral metabolism have received attention, at least in part, because of the common association between closed head injury and hypovolemia in patients who have sustained vehicular trauma.

Cardiopulmonary Bypass

The neurologic sequelae of cardiopulmonary bypass and open heart surgery represent an iatrogenic problem of considerable magnitude, primarily because of the 300,000 coronary revascularization procedures that are performed in the United States each year. Clinically demonstrable neurologic insults can be divided into gross permanent deficits and transient focal and diffuse deficits. Although their cause remains unclear, the percentage of these complications is decreasing. However, the occurrence of more subtle, neuropsychiatric dysfunction is frequent. Studies of subclinical neurologic injury, as manifested by release of adenylate kinase into the CSF, suggest that it is 50% or greater (4). Clearly, further investigations of these subtle but potentially devastating effects of cardiopulmonary bypass on memory, learning, and emotional stability are required.

Nevertheless, permanent, disabling neurologic damage is rare. Branthwaite (17) identified neurologic deficits in 19% of patients in a series published in 1972. A follow-up series in 1975 identified only a 7.0% incidence (18). Aberg (2), employing sophisticated neuropsychiatric testing, found a predictable impairment in intellectual function in 113 patients undergoing open heart surgery between 1972 and 1974. Subsequently, Aberg and Kihlgren (3) described a substantial improvement, apparently due to aggressive attempts to reduce embolic phenomena, in 124 additional patients described in 1977. The incidence of neurologic deficits was higher in patients undergoing valvular heart surgery than in those undergoing coronary artery bypass surgery. Slogoff and associates (140) in 1982 reported 204 patients undergoing a variety of open heart procedures. They identified a 16.2% incidence of transient neurologic sequelae and a 6.4% incidence of permanent neurologic sequelae. The current incidence of discrete, permanent stroke following coronary artery bypass surgery is 1–2% (19, 23). Active investigation of the neuropsychologic sequelae of cardiac surgery is continuing in many centers (136, 142, 145).

The risk factors for neurologic sequelae remain controversial. Stockard and coworkers (151) found an increasing incidence of neurologic sequelae if MAP during cardiopulmonary bypass was less than 50 mm Hg for extended periods of time. They quantitated the risk in terms of "torr-minutes," defined as the number of minutes during which MAP was less than 50 mm Hg multiplied by the number of torr by which MAP was less than 50 mm Hg. However, subsequent investigators have failed to find a correlation between the degree of hypotension during bypass and subsequent neurologic deficits (77). Most investigators report that advanced age, open cardiac procedures, and prolonged cardiopulmonary bypass correlate with postoperative neurologic sequelae. One critical piece of information that is lacking is the relationship between intraoperative CBF and postoperative subtle and overt neurologic deficits.

The cause of postcardiac surgical cerebral injury may be either embolic or related to a global reduction in cerebral perfusion. An embolic cause is supported by the dramatic reduction in neurologic injury that followed the introduction of more effective filtration techniques and improved oxygenator design (3). On the basis of his contention that CBF is increased during cardiopulmonary bypass as a consequence of periischemic hyperemia, Henriksen and colleagues (61) have suggested that embolism is the more likely cause. Other investigators have failed to document an increase in CBF during cardiopulmonary bypass. In fact, they have demonstrated a substantial reduction in CBF, consistent with the extent of metabolic depression that should occur with hypothermia (46, 121). The discrepancy between the data reported by Henriksen and colleagues and those reported by other investigators appears to be related to differences in the technique of measuring CBF and in the management of $Paco_2$ during cardiopulmonary bypass (121). Nussmeier and associates (110) demonstrated that the administration of large doses of sodium thiopental during open cardiac procedures protects against subsequent neurologic deficits. However, that study was conducted during normothermic cardiopulmonary bypass; therefore, the applicability of those conclusions to hypothermic cardiopulmonary bypass is questionable. In addition, the large doses of sodium thiopental employed necessitated a substantial increase in the duration of postoperative ventilation and in the need for postbypass cardiovascular support (110). Smaller doses of sodium thiopental might well be appropriate during hypothermic bypass, since Quasha and coworkers (122) noted

that small doses of thiopental (8.0 mg/kg intravenously) given under these conditions produced marked EEG depression.

Cardiac Arrest

Following the global cerebral ischemic insult that occurs during cardiac arrest, many patients recover adequate cardiovascular, pulmonary, and renal function, but are left with profound neurologic deficits (84, 124). Recent experimental work has emphasized the likely occurrence of reperfusion injury—damage that occurs *after* restoration of flow in neural tissue or in the cerebral vasculature. The therapeutic implications of progressive injury during reperfusion are obvious. Therapeutic interventions could perhaps decrease the neurologic morbidity following cardiac arrest if the mechanisms underlying progressive injury could be identified. Although many biochemical abnormalities are present following complete global cerebral ischemia (Fig. 11.1), postischemic hypoperfusion has generated the greatest investigational interest.

Figure 11.3 schematically depicts the typical sequence of transient hyperemia followed by profound oligemia that occurs after complete experimental cerebral ischemia. This complete sequence has yet to be documented in human beings; however, in one small clinical series, CBF was reduced to a greater extent than $CMRo_2$ immediately following cardiac arrest (12). Animal models of global cerebral ischemia demonstrate a consistent postischemic reduction in CBF (74, 143, 148). In such models, antagonism with nimodipine of the postischemic hypoperfusion state is associated with improved neurologic outcome (147, 149), an observation that has prompted clinical trials of nimodipine currently underway in Europe. Optimism regarding the applicability of this new treatment must be tempered by the recent conclusive demonstration in a large clinical series that barbiturate loading, long an enthusiastically supported form of therapy following global cerebral ischemia, proved not to improve neurologic recovery (124).

Other therapeutic interventions in animal models have been directed toward biochemical changes that occur in association with global ischemia, such as release of free radicals and accumulation of the by-products of fatty acids released from injured brain cell membranes. One such fatty acid derivative is thromboxane A_2, a potent vasoconstrictor that promotes platelet aggregation and is released from brain tissue following global ischemia (120). Postischemic flow is substantially enhanced by inhibiting thromboxane A_2 generation (49, 53), and is improved to a greater extent by a combination of cyclooxygenase inhibition, prostacyclin infusion, and heparinization (53). Short-term neurologic outcome is also enhanced by combination therapy (53). However, the hypotensive effects of prostacyclin are poorly tolerated by patients. The usefulness of multimodal therapy should be tested further, perhaps by combining a cyclooxygenase inhibitor with a calcium entry blocker. One critical requirement for a treatment regimen following cardiac arrest must be that it produces few adverse effects on blood pressure or cardiac output.

Subarachnoid Hemorrhage

Each year, 19,000 patients in the United States die or are disabled as a consequence of subarachnoid hemorrhage (SAH) (69, 70). Neurologic deficits following SAH frequently are secondary to reversible cerebral ischemia due to cerebral vasospasm (22, 156, 163). The more severe the reduction in CBF, the worse the neurologic outcome (44, 156). Older patients are particularly likely to develop cerebral ischemia after SAH (97).

The mechanism of vasospasm following SAH is unclear (71). Considerable experimental evidence supports the likelihood that at least part of the reduction in vessel caliber is due to active smooth muscle contraction in response to spasmogenic substances released from blood in the CSF. A related hypothesis is that vascular relaxation is impaired by abnormalities of vessel wall metabolism or substances present in bloody CSF. The involved vessels ultimately undergo structural changes, such as smooth muscle hypertrophy, inflammation, and fibroblastic infiltration (71).

Therapeutic attempts to improve CBF in patients with cerebral vasopasm have been partially successful. Intravascular volume expansion and induced systemic hypertension return CBF toward normal values (107, 117). Recently, Finn and associates (39) have reported encouraging, though uncontrolled, clinical results, in which the perioperative treatment of vasospasm with volume expansion and, where appropriate, elevation of systemic blood pressure were associated with a favorable outcome in a high percentage of patients.

Calcium entry blockers antagonize the cerebral vasospasm associated with experimental subarachnoid hemorrhage, perhaps in part due to greater sensitivity of the cerebral vessels than the peripheral vessels to calcium antagonists. An extensive multicenter study has demonstrated a prophylactic effect of nimodipine (0.35 mg/kg orally every 4 hours) on the subsequent development of vasospasm in patients entering the hospital with acute SAH but with minimal neurologic deficits (6); however, nimodipine may be less suitable for the treatment of established vasospasm. Because of its potent cerebral vasodilatory effects, nimodipine could increase ICP in patients with brain edema secondary to cerebral ischemia. An alternative approach may be to antagonize calmodulin, the substance that activates the actin-myosin complex as a final step in smooth muscle contraction (109).

Closed Head Injury

Closed head injury related to vehicular trauma represents a pressing social problem. Closed head injury occurs frequently in young, productive, and otherwise healthy persons who, because of their residual disability, may require years of custodial care. The clinical concept that governs the present management of closed head injury is that the ultimate extent of disability is due to the cumulative effects of both the primary mechanical injury and the secondary injuries produced by associated physiologic derangements. The histopathologic evidence of cerebral ischemia frequently seen in fatal closed head injury illustrates the potential importance of recognizing and limiting secondary injury (5).

Much of the current clinical strategy for the management of acute closed head injury is directed toward a reduction in ICP, since the control of intracranial hypertension appears to improve outcome (131). Hyperventilation, which reduces ICP by reducing cerebral blood volume, is most commonly used; however, limited attention has been paid to the maintenance of adequate CBF during therapeutic hyperventilation. During mechanical hyperventilation, patients with closed head trauma frequently have reductions in $Sjvo_2$ below acceptable average levels (28). Further studies are required to determine if monitoring of $Sjvo_2$, in conjunction with monitoring of ICP, can be used to further limit the incidence of secondary injury.

Therapeutic reduction of both CBF and CMRo$_2$, which can be accomplished with barbiturates, appears to be a physiologically sound strategy for the reduction of ICP without adversely affecting brain oxygenation. Marshall and associates (92) have reported good results in a pilot study in which sodium pentobarbital, 3–5 mg/kg followed by an infusion of 100–200 mg every 30–60 minutes, was given to patients with severe closed head injury. Nevertheless, the overall response to barbiturate therapy following closed head trauma has been disappointing (161), perhaps reflecting the variability in CBF responsiveness to barbiturates in this heterogeneous population, as well as variability in the extent of primary injury.

The development of sound animal models of closed head injury should facilitate the development of more effective clinical strategies. The feline fluid percussion model developed at the Medical College of Virginia is a well-characterized model that duplicates many of the electrophysiologic (48), vascular (85), and systemic physiologic (128) features of human closed head injury. Fluid percussion injury produces transient increases in CBF that return to control levels within 30 minutes without evidence of posttraumatic ischemia (33). This finding is consistent with reports that CBF is reduced in some patients, but seldom to ischemic levels in the absence of extensive mass lesions (78). The observed absence of posttraumatic ischemia may seem difficult to reconcile with reports of regional ischemic cell changes on postmortem examination of brain tissue from trauma patients (128). One explanation is that the normal tight coupling between CBF and metabolism may be impaired after injury. Changes in the relationship between CBF and metabolism in discrete brain regions (hippocampus) occur after low-level fluid percussion injury in cats, and these changes may affect regional energy metabolism (170). Thus, animal models can provide important information contributing to a better understanding of the mechanisms that underlie human brain injury. Other studies of the effects of fluid percussion injury on cerebral metabolic activity using the autoradiographic 2-deoxyglucose technique (144) led Hayes and coworkers (59) to the hypothesis that a cholinergic site in the feline brain stem, when activated by fluid percussion injury, produces transient posttraumatic unconsciousness. This region was subsequently shown to be a complex group of nuclei that may also mediate spinal motor and sensory function (72).

The fluid percussion injury model has recently been adapted for use in rats (35), allowing metabolic and physiologic effects to be correlated with behavioral effects of closed concussive brain injury. Fluid percussion injury has been found to suppress reflexes and to impair motor activity (i.e., balancing and walking on a narrow wooden beam) (60). The cholinergic antagonist, scopolamine, whether administered before or after injury, appears to reverse these traumatic effects on reflexes and motor activity (58, 90). Animal models are frequently used for preclinical testing of new therapies. The observation that buffering of posttraumatic acidosis decreased mortality and morbidity in cats (129) led to an ongoing clinical trial of the efficacy of THAM in the treatment of posttraumatic acidosis in patients sustaining severe head injury (11).

The Richmond fluid percussion model is one of several good experimental models used in the study of closed head injury (78). Studies using these models will likely provide a better understanding of mechanisms of traumatic brain damage, yield promising new pharmacologic approaches to the treatment of closed head injury, and serve as a method for testing new therapies before their utilization in controlled clinical trials.

Stroke

Recent advances suggest that the neurologic morbidity produced by stroke may be effectively modified. Many of the proposed therapeutic approaches are based on the concept of the "ischemic penumbra," an area of brain surrounding an area of infarct, in which flow has been reduced to a level that produces ischemic dysfunction without producing cell death. In such a penumbral zone, measures designed to increase CBF or to decrease CMRo$_2$ in dysfunctional but viable tissue might help to preserve neurologic function. Possible forms of therapy include induced hypertension, hypervolemic hemodilution, the use of calcium entry blockers, and the use of pentoxifylline.

Potentially, induced hypertension increases CBF in areas of focal ischemia distal to partially obstructed cerebral arteries. Since ischemia abolishes autoregulation in the involved areas, flow may be increased by an increase in MAP, although autoregulation prevents an increase in flow in nonischemic tissue. Anecdotally, administration of vasopressor drugs improves neurologic status in some patients following an ischemic event (164). However, conclusive evidence of the clinical efficacy of induced hypertension requires additional study.

Hypervolemic hemodilution with dextran produces small, statistically insignificant increases in CBF in animals with normal cerebral vasculature (168). However, in brain tissue distal to an experimental middle cerebral artery occlusion, dextran significantly improves CBF (167, 169). In patients with acute stroke, normovolemic hemodilution increases CBF and improves EEG activity (166). If initiated early, hemodilution therapy appears to improve clinical outcome (152), but the results may not be duplicated easily in a community hospital setting (9). Treatment of stroke with hemodilution carries two physiologic risks. First, hypervolemia may produce cardiac failure or myocardial ischemia in patients who have coexisting cerebrovascular and coronary occlusive disease. Second, although flow may be slightly improved by moderate hemodilution, the reduction in oxygen-carrying capacity may prevent any improvement in local oxygen delivery.

Calcium entry blockers appear to improve CBF and to exert a protective effect on focally ischemic brain distal to mechanically occluded blood vessels (98, 100). Both CBF and intracellular pH are improved by nimodipine, suggesting a possible therapeutic role in human stroke. Following initial clinical evaluation of nimodipine (43), larger clinical trials are now in progress. The major potential drawbacks of nimodipine relate to its systemic hypotensive effects and its tendency to increase ICP. Grotta (50) suggests that combining calcium entry blockers with other therapeutic interventions may be useful.

Because of the extensive experimental results suggesting that prostaglandin I_2 antagonizes the adverse effects of thromboxane A_2 on cerebral vascular tone and platelet aggregation, an extensive study was performed to determine whether the infusion of prostacyclin would ameliorate acute stroke (67). The data suggest that prostacyclin is not efficacious, a finding in concert with the lack of efficacy of prostacyclin alone in experimental cerebral ischemia.

Osmotherapy may well become a key component of combination therapy. Bayer and associates (10) recently reported a double-blind randomized clinical trial in which 173 patients received either 500 ml of 10% glycerol in normal saline or 500 ml of normal saline daily for 6 days following acute stroke (10). The treatment with glycerol reduced acute mortality, but did not significantly change the degree of neurologic disability in survivors. Since potentially useful treatments such as nimodipine may increase ICP, the reduction in ICP produced by osmotherapy could permit more aggressive utilization.

Perhaps, ultimately, therapy designed to interrupt the biochemical cascade of ischemic events may be combined with medical thrombolysis or surgical revascularization. Thrombolysis using tissue plasminogen activator has been effective in experimental studies of stroke (174) and in preliminary clinical studies (173). Emergency surgical revascularization, if performed sufficiently soon after the onset of ischemia, could result in reperfusion of potentially viable brain tissue (103). Antiischemic medical therapy could stabilize injured neurons until surgical therapy could be performed, perhaps for as long as 6 hours or more (103). Both emergency carotid endarterectomy (101) and middle cerebral embolectomy (102) have been performed with promising results. Meyer and colleagues (103) suggest that the success of revascularization represents clinical evidence of the existence of a penumbral zone of electrophysiologically dysfunctional but viable tissue.

In patients with chronic stroke, the rheologic agent pentoxifylline increases CBF acutely in low-flow areas and improves cerebral vasomotor responsiveness (56). Clinical trials are underway to determine whether pentoxifylline improves focal flow in acute stroke and thus whether it can be used to improve the outcome of acute stroke.

Hemorrhagic Shock

Cerebral blood flow is reduced during hemorrhagic shock, an effect apparently due in part to massive sympathetic nervous system activation by the hemorrhage (41). The ultimate extent of CNS damage due to the shock-induced partial cerebral ischemia depends on the magnitude and duration of the hypotensive insult. The effects of hypotension may be the most critical in patients with coexistent neurologic injury, since in these patients the morbidity from partial cerebral ischemia may be added to the primary insult.

Recent studies have focused not only on the effects of shock on CBF, but also on the effects of resuscitation on CBF and ICP. The evidence to date suggests that volume resuscitation from shock, if it does not include red blood cells, may actually result in a reduction in cerebral oxygen delivery ($C\dot{D}o_2$, the product of Cao_2 and CBF) below the levels associated with shock (115, 116, 119). This reduction is due to two factors. First, during volume resuscitation from experimental hemorrhage, CBF rises transiently as MAP improves during expansion of intravascular volume, but then quickly falls to levels no greater than those present during the shock state. These hemorrhage-related changes in CBF are strikingly different from the predictable increase in CBF that accompanies blood-free volume infusion in the absence of shock. Second, the concentration of hemoglobin is reduced if major blood loss is replaced with crystalloid or colloid. Further studies are necessary to determine the implications of reduced $C\dot{D}o_2$ following volume expansion in cases of craniocerebral trauma or intracranial mass lesions.

Catecholamines are often administered with fluid resuscitation for the clinical treatment of circulatory shock. The effects of α-, β-, and dopaminergic receptor agonists consist both of their direct pharmacologic actions and of the indirect effects due to the drug-induced increases in blood pressure, cardiac output, or both. Pure β-agonists, such as isoproterenol, cause no change in CBF (30, 111). Epinephrine and norepinephrine increase both $CMRo_2$ and CBF under specific conditions. CBF is increased only if blood pressure is increased beyond the upper limit of autoregulation, and $CMRo_2$ is increased only if the blood-brain barrier is disrupted (1, 29, 36). Dopamine dilates cerebral vessels independently of changes in blood pressure (159), but increases $CMRo_2$ only if the blood-brain barrier is disrupted (38). The effects on coexistent injury of catecholamines used during resuscitation from shock require further study.

BRAIN PROTECTION: TITRATED CEREBROVASCULAR MONITORING AND THERAPY

In many critically ill patients, long-term neurologic outcome may depend on the adequacy of regional or global CBF. Despite this possibility, useful clinical algorithms regarding appropriate management of the cerebral circulation have developed slowly. To date, clinical protocols have been developed for the management of acute closed head trauma, SAH,

cardiopulmonary bypass, stroke, and cardiac arrest. Although these protocols are based in part on cerebral circulatory considerations, they are primarily derived from physiologic inference rather than data obtained by monitoring.

Although CBF has been measured and to some extent manipulated in patients with intracranial hypertension, the only commonly monitored variable in such patients is ICP. ICP is the outflow pressure for the cerebral circulation in the presence of intracranial hypertension. However, ICP measurements alone, in the absence of measurements of CBF or $CMRo_2$, provide the same potential for erroneous interpretation of the adequacy of cerebral circulation that one would expect if pulmonary capillary wedge pressure were used as the sole measure of the adequacy of systemic circulation.

Two recent developments suggest that cerebral circulatory monitoring might soon become feasible on a wider scale. First, the introduction of continuous monitoring of $Sjvo_2$ as a research tool suggests that this parameter might be employed clinically to monitor the net balance of cerebral oxygen supply and demand for the whole brain (28). Since blood in either jugular bulb represents a "mixed" sample from the entire brain, a reduction in $Sjvo_2$ can only be due to a reduction in $C\dot{D}o_2$ or an increase in $CMRo_2$ (Fig. 11.11). In turn, a reduction in $C\dot{D}o_2$ can only be due to a reduction in either Cao_2 or CBF, and a reduction in Cao_2 can only be due to a reduction in Sao_2 or hemoglobin. Consequently, continuous monitoring of $Sjvo_2$ in patients at risk for global cerebral ischemia may provide a mechanism for early detection of insufficient oxygen availability, following which a rapid, sequential analysis can be made of the factors that may have produced it. Alternatively, niroscopy, a technique that detects changes in cerebral arteriovenous hemoglobin saturation differences by transcranial penetration of near-infrared light, might noninvasively provide qualitative evidence that CBF is insufficient to meet metabolic demand (68, 114, 118).

The second major development that promises to improve the monitoring of cerebral circulation is the use of portable systems for measuring CBF based on the clearance of ^{133}xenon. Such systems have been described recently and are undergoing continuing development (121). They provide discrete focal information about cortical flow and, in combination with Cao_2 and $Cjvo_2$ values, allow a rough approximation of cerebral oxygen con-

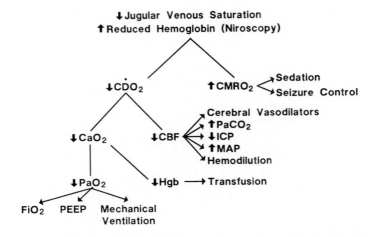

Figure 11.11. Schematic depiction of possible factors contributing to a decrease in jugular venous saturation. *Hgb,* hemoglobin; *Fio₂,* fractional inspired oxygen concentration; *PEEP,* positive end-expiratory pressure. Other abbreviations explained in the text.

sumption. Consequently, in the near future perhaps all of the factors that contribute to cerebral oxygen balance can be estimated quickly at the bedside of the critically ill patient. Rapid evaluation of CaO_2 may be performed with arterial blood gas analysis and cooximetry, or may be monitored on-line with pulse oximetry. Together, CBF and CaO_2 constitute CDO_2. Continuous monitoring of the processed electrocardiogram may permit detection and management of increased electrophysiologic activity (suggesting seizures) or decreased activity (suggesting ischemia). Prompt and effective recognition and management of hypoxemia, cerebral hypoperfusion, and increased metabolic demand should improve the rate of successful neurologic recovery.

References

1. Abdul-Rahman A, Dahlgren N, Johansson BB, Siesjo BK: Increase in local cerebral blood flow induced by circulating adrenaline: involvement of blood-brain barrier dysfunction. *Acta Physiol Scand* 107:227–232, 1979.
2. Aberg T: Effect of open heart surgery on intellectual function. *Scand J Thorac Cardiovasc Surg [Suppl]* 15:1–63, 1974.
3. Aberg T, Kihlgren M: Cerebral protection during open-heart surgery. *Thorax* 32:525–533, 1977.
4. Aberg T, Ronquist G, Tyden H, Brunnkvist S, Hultman J, Bergstrom K, Lilja A: Adverse effects on the brain in cardiac operations as assessed by biochemical, psychometric, and radiologic methods. *J Thorac Cardiovasc Surg* 87:99–105, 1984.
5. Adams JH, Graham DI, Gennarelli TA: Contemporary neuropathological considerations regarding brain damage in head injury. In Becker DP, Povlishock JT (eds): *Central Nervous System Trauma Status Report.* Bethesda, MD, National Institutes of Health, 1985, pp 65–77.
6. Allen GS, Ahn HS, Preziosi TJ, Battye R, Boone SC, Chou SN, Kelly DL, Weir BK, Crabbe RA, Lavik PJ, Rosenbloom SB, Dorsey FC, Ingram CR, Mellits DE, Bertsch LA, Boisvert DPJ, Hundley MB, Johnson RK, Strom JA, Transou CR: Cerebral arterial spasm—a controlled trial of nimodipine in patients with subarachnoid hemorrhage. *N Engl J Med* 308:619–624, 1983.
7. Ames A III, Wright RL, Kowada M, Thurston JM, Majno G: Cerebral ischemia. II. The no-reflow phenomenon. *Am J Pathol* 52:437–453, 1968.
8. Artru AA, Colley PS: Cerebral blood flow responses to hypocapnia during hypotension. *Stroke* 15:878–883, 1984.
9. Asplund K: Hemodilution in acute ischemic stroke—a randomized multicenter trial (abstract). *Stroke* 17:143, 1986.
10. Bayer AJ, Pathy MSJ, Newcombe R: Double-blind randomised trial of intravenous glycerol in acute stroke. *Lancet* 1:405–408, 1987.
11. Becker DP: Brain acidosis in head injury: a clinical trial. In Becker DP, Povlishock JT (eds): *Central Nervous System Trauma Status Report.* Bethesda, MD, National Institutes of Health, NIH/NINCDS, 1985, pp 229–242.
12. Beckstead JE, Tweed WA, Lee J, MacKeen WL: Cerebral blood flow and metabolism in man following cardiac arrest. *Stroke* 9:569–573, 1978.
13. Berne RM, Winn HR, Rubio R: The local regulation of cerebral blood flow. *Prog Cardiovasc Dis* 24:243–260, 1981.
14. Bertel O, Conen D, Radu EW, Muller J, Lang C, Dubach UC: Nifedipine in hypertensive emergencies. *Br Med J* 286:19–21, 1983.
15. Bohn DJ, Biggar WD, Smith CR, Conn AW, Barker GA: Influence of hypothermia, barbiturate therapy, and intracranial pressure monitoring on morbidity and mortality after near-drowning. *Crit Care Med* 14:529–534, 1986.
16. Bowton DL, Alford PT, McLees BD, Prough DS, Stump DA, Hinshelwood L: The effect of aminophylline on cerebral blood flow in patients with chronic obstructive pulmonary disease. *Chest* 91:874–877, 1988.
17. Branthwaite MA: Neurological damage related to open-heart surgery. A clinical survey. *Thorax* 27:748–753, 1972.
18. Branthwaite MA: Prevention of neurological damage during open-heart surgery. *Thorax* 30:258–261, 1975.
19. Breuer AC, Furlan AJ, Hanson MR, Lederman RJ, Loop

FD, Cosgrove DM, Greenstreet RL, Estafanous FG: Central nervous system complications of coronary artery bypass graft surgery: prospective analysis of 421 patients. *Stroke* 14:682–687, 1983.

20. Burt DER, Verniquet AJW, Homi J: The response of canine intracranial pressure to systemic hypotension induced with nitroglycerine. *Br J Anaesth* 54:665–671, 1982.

21. Candia GJ, Heros RC, Lavyne MH, Zervas NT, Nelson CN: Effect of intravenous sodium nitroprusside on cerebral blood flow and intracranial pressure. *Neurosurgery* 3:50–53, 1978.

22. Chyatte D, Sundt TM Jr: Cerebral vasospasm after subarachnoid hemorrhage. *Mayo Clin Proc* 59:498–505, 1984.

23. Coffey CE, Massey EW, Roberts KB, Curtis S, Jones RH, Pryor DB: Natural history of cerebral complications of coronary artery bypass graft surgery. *Neurology* 33:1416–1421, 1983.

24. Conn AW, Edmonds JE, Barker GA: Cerebral resuscitation in near drowning. *Pediatr Clin North Am* 26:691, 1979.

25. Cook P, James I: Cerebral vasodilators (first of two parts). *N Engl J Med* 305:1508–1513, 1981.

26. Cook P, James I: Cerebral vasodilators (second of two parts). *N Engl J Med* 305:1560–1564, 1981.

27. Cottrell JE, Robustelli A, Post K, Turndorf H: Furosemide- and mannitol-induced changes in intracranial pressure and serum osmolality and electrolytes. *Anesthesiology* 47:28–30, 1977.

28. Cruz J, Allen SJ, Miner ME: Hypoxic insults in acute brain injury (abstract). *Crit Care Med* 13:284, 1985.

29. Dahlgren N, Rosen I, Sakabe T, Siesjo BK: Cerebral functional, metabolic and circulatory effects of intravenous infusion of adrenaline in the rat. *Brain Res* 184:143–152, 1980.

30. Davis DH, Sundt TM Jr: Relationship of cerebral blood flow to cardiac output, mean arterial pressure, blood volume, and alpha and beta blockade in cats. *J Neurosurg* 52:745–754, 1980.

31. Dearden NM: Ischaemic brain. *Lancet* 2:255–259, 1985.

32. Demopoulos HB, Flamm ES, Pietronigro DD, Seligman ML: The free radical pathology and the microcirculation in the major central nervous system disorders. *Acta Physiol Scand [Suppl]* 492:91–119, 1980.

33. DeWitt DS, Jenkins LW, Wei EP, Lutz H, Becker DP, Kontos HA: Effects of fluid-percussion brain injury on regional cerebral blood flow and pial arteriolar diameter. *J Neurosurg* 64:787–794, 1986.

34. Diagnosis and treatment of Reye's syndrome. *JAMA* 246:2441–2444, 1981.

35. Dixon CE, Lyeth BG, Povlishock JT, Findling RL, Hamm RJ, Marmarou A, Young HF, Hayes RL: A fluid percussion model of experimental brain injury in the rat. *J Neurosurg* 67:110–119, 1987.

36. Edvinsson L, Lacombe P, Owman C, Reynier-Rebuffel A-M, Seylaz J: Quantitative changes in regional cerebral blood flow of rats induced by alpha- and beta-adrenergic stimulants. *Acta Physiol Scand* 107:289–296, 1979.

37. Ekstrom-Jodal B, Haggendal E, Linder L-E, Nilsson NJ: Cerebral blood flow autoregulation at high arterial pressures and different levels of carbon dioxide tension in dogs. *Eur Neurol* 6:6–10, 1971/72.

38. Ekstrom-Jodal B, Larsson LE: Effects of dopamine on cerebral circulation and oxygen metabolism in endotoxic shock: an experimental study in dogs. *Crit Care Med* 10:375–377, 1982.

39. Finn SS, Stephensen SA, Miller CA, Drobnich L, Hunt WE: Observations on the perioperative management of aneurysmal subarachnoid hemorrhage. *J Neurosurg* 65:48–62, 1986.

40. Fishman RA: Brain edema. *N Engl J Med* 293:706–711, 1975.

41. Fitch W, MacKenzie ET, Harper AM: Effects of decreasing arterial blood pressure on cerebral blood flow in the baboon. Influence of the sympathetic nervous system. *Circ Res* 37:550–557, 1975.

42. FitzGerald GA, Reilly IAG, Pedersen AK: The biochemical pharmacology of thromboxane synthetase inhibition in man. *Circulation* 72:1194–1201, 1985.

43. Gelmers HJ, Gorter K, de Weerdt CJ, Wiezer JHA: Effect of nimodipine on clinical outcome in patients with acute ischemic stroke (abstract). *Stroke* 17:145, 1986.

44. Geraud G, Tremoulet M, Guell A, Bes A: The prognostic value of noninvasive CBF measurement in subarachnoid hemorrhage. *Stroke* 15:301–305, 1984.

45. Ginsberg MD, Welsh FA, Budd WW: Deleterious effect of glucose pretreatment on recovery from diffuse cerebral ischemia in the cat. I. Local cerebral blood flow and glucose utilization. *Stroke* 11:347–354, 1980.

46. Govier AV, Reves JG, McKay RD, Karp RB, Zorn GL, Morawetz RB, Smith LR, Adams M, Freeman AM: Factors and their influence on regional cerebral blood flow during nonpulsatile cardiopulmonary bypass. *Ann Thorac Surg* 38:592–600, 1984.

47. Graham DI: The pathology of brain ischaemia and possibilities for therapeutic intervention. *Br J Anaesth* 57:3–17, 1985.

48. Greenberg RP, Hyatt MS, Becker DP: Transient electrical dysfunction in head-injured cats: a mechanism for loss of consciousness. *Surg Forum* 32:492–494, 1981.

49. Grice SC, Chappell ET, Prough DS, Watkins WD, Whitley JM: Ibuprofen improves cerebral blood flow after global cerebral ischemia in dogs. *Stroke* 18:787–791, 1987.

50. Grotta JC: Can raising cerebral blood flow improve outcome after acute cerebral infarction? *Stroke* 18:264–267, 1987.

51. Grubb RL Jr, Raichle ME, Eichling JO, Ter-Pogossian MM: The effects of changes in PaCO$_2$ on cerebral blood volume, blood flow, and vascular mean transit time. *Stroke* 5:630–639, 1974.

52. Haas DC, Streeten DHP, Kim RC, Naalbandian AN, Obeid AI: Death from cerebral hypoperfusion during nitroprusside treatment of acute angiotensin-dependent hypertension. *Am J Med* 75:1071–1076, 1983.

53. Hallenbeck JM, Furlow TW Jr: Prostaglandin I$_2$ and indomethacin prevent impairment of post-ischemic brain reperfusion in the dog. *Stroke* 10:629–637, 1979.

54. Harper AM: The inter-relationship between PaCO$_2$ and blood pressure in the regulation of blood flow through the cerebral cortex. *Acta Neurol Scand [Suppl]* 14:94–103, 1965.

55. Harris RJ, Symon L, Branston NM, Bayhan M: Changes in extracellular calcium activity in cerebral ischaemia. *J Cereb Blood Flow Metab* 1:203–209, 1981.

56. Hartmann A: Effect of pentoxifylline on regional cerebral blood flow in patients with cerebral vascular disorders. *Eur Neurol* 22(suppl 1):108–115, 1983.

57. Haws CW, Heistad DD: Effects of nimodipine on cerebral vasoconstrictor responses. *Am J Physiol* 247:H170–H176, 1984.

58. Hayes RL, Lyeth BG: Neuropharmacological mechanisms of mild and moderate head injury: implications for treatment. In Levin HS, Eisenberg H (eds): *Mild Head Injury*. Oxford, England, Oxford University Press, in press, 1988.

59. Hayes RL, Pechura CM, Katayama Y, Povlishock JT, Giebel ML, Becker DP: Activation of pontine cholinergic sites implicated in unconsciousness following cerebral concussion in the cat. *Science* 223:301–303, 1984.

60. Hayes RL, Stonnington HH, Lyeth BG, Dixon CE, Yamamoto T: Metabolic and neurophysiological sequelae of brain injury: a cholinergic hypothesis. *CNS Trauma* 3:163–173, 1986.

61. Henriksen L, Hjelms E, Lindeburgh T: Brain hyperperfusion during cardiac operations. Cerebral blood flow measured in man by intra-arterial injection of

[133]xenon: evidence suggestive of intraoperative microembolism. *J Thorac Cardiovasc Surg* 86:202–208, 1983.

62. Henriksen L, Paulson OB: The effects of sodium nitroprusside on cerebral blood flow and cerebral venous blood gases. II. Observations in awake man during successive blood pressure reduction. *Eur J Clin Invest* 12:389–393, 1982.

63. Henriksen L, Paulson OB, Lauritzen M: The effects of sodium nitroprusside on cerebral blood flow and cerebral venous blood gases. I. Observations in awake man during and following moderate blood pressure reduction. *Eur J Clin Invest* 12:383–387, 1982.

64. Herskovits E, Famulari A, Tamaroff L, Gonzalez AM, Vasquez A, Dominguez R, Fraiman H, Vila J: Preventive treatment of cerebral transient ischemia: comparative randomized trial of pentoxifylline versus conventional antiaggregants. *Eur Neurol* 24:73–81, 1985.

65. Hoff JT: Cerebral protection. *J Neurosurg* 65:579–591, 1986.

66. Hoffman WE, Albrecht RF, Miletich DJ: The role of adenosine in CBF increases during hypoxia in young vs aged rats. *Stroke* 15:124–129, 1984.

67. Hsu CY, Faught RE Jr, Furlan AJ, Coull BM, Huang DC, Hogan EL, Linet OI, Yatsu FM: Intravenous prostacyclin in acute nonhemorrhagic stroke: a placebo-controlled double-blind trial. *Stroke* 18:352–358, 1987.

68. Jobsis FF: Noninvasive, infrared monitoring of cerebral and myocardial oxygen sufficiency and circulatory parameters. *Science* 198:1264–1267, 1977.

69. Kassell NF, Drake CG: Review of the management of saccular aneurysms. *Neurol Clin* 1:73–86, 1983.

70. Kassell NF, Drake CG: Timing of aneurysm surgery. *Neurosurgery* 10:514–519, 1982.

71. Kassell NF, Sasaki T, Colohan ART, Nazar G: Cerebral vasospasm following aneurysmal subarachnoid hemorrhage. *Stroke* 16:562–572, 1985.

72. Katayama Y, DeWitt DS, Becker DP, Hayes RL: Behavioral evidence for a cholinoceptive pontine inhibitory area: descending control of spinal motor output and sensory input. *Brain Res* 296:241–262, 1984.

73. Kempski O, Shohami E, von Lubitz D, Hallenbeck JM, Feuerstein G: Postischemic production of eicosanoids in gerbil brain. *Stroke* 18:111–119, 1987.

74. Kirsch JR, Dean JM, Rogers MC: Current concepts in brain resuscitation. *Arch Intern Med* 146:1413–1419, 1986.

75. Kiwak KJ, Moskowitz MA, Levine L: Leukotriene production in gerbil brain after ischemia insult, subarachnoid hemorrhage, and concussive injury. *J Neurosurg* 62:865–869, 1985.

76. Klatzo I: Neuropathological aspects of brain edema. *J Neuropathol Exp Neurol* 26:1–14, 1967.

77. Kolkka R, Hilberman M: Neurologic dysfunction following cardiac operation with low-flow low-pressure cardiopulmonary bypass. *J Thorac Cardiovasc Surg* 79:432–437, 1980.

78. Langfitt TW, Obrist WD: Cerebral blood flow and metabolism after intracranial trauma. In Krayenbuhl H, Maspes PE, Sweet WH (eds): *Craniocerebral Trauma* (Progress in Neurologic Surgery, vol 10). Basel, S Karger, 1981, pp 14–48.

79. Lanier WL, Stangland KJ, Scheithauer BW, Milde JH, Michenfelder JD: The effects of dextrose infusion and head position on neurologic outcome after complete cerebral ischemia in primates: examination of a model. *Anesthesiology* 66:39–48, 1987.

80. Lassen NA: Cerebral and spinal cord blood flow. In Cottrell JE, Turndorf H (eds): *Anesthesia and Neurosurgery*. St Louis, CV Mosby, 1980, pp 1–24.

81. Lassen NA, Høedt-Rasmussen K, Sørensen SC, Skinhø E, Cronquist S, Bodforss B, Ingvar DH: Regional cerebral blood flow in man determined by [85]krypton. *Neurology* 13:719–727, 1963.

82. Lassen NA, Tweed WA: Anaesthesia and cerebral blood flow. In Gordon E (ed): *A Basis and Practice of Neuroanaesthesia* (Monographs in Anaesthesiology, vol 2). Amsterdam, Excerpta Medica, 1975, pp 113–133.

83. Lee MC, Mastri AR, Waltz AG, Loewenson RB: Ineffectiveness of dexamethasone for treatment of experimental cerebral infarction. *Stroke* 5:216–218, 1974.

84. Levy DE, Caronna JJ, Singer BH, Lapinski RH, Frydman H, Plum F: Predicting outcome from hypoxic-ischemic coma. *JAMA* 253:1420–1426, 1985.

85. Lewelt W, Jenkins LW, Miller JD: Autoregulation of cerebral blood flow after experimental fluid-percussion injury of the brain. *J Neurosurg* 53:500–511, 1980.

86. Little JR: Modification of acute focal ischemia by treatment with mannitol and high-dose dexamethasone. *J Neurosurg* 49:517–524, 1978.

87. Little JR, Kerr FWL, Sundt TM Jr: Microcirculatory obstruction in focal cerebral ischemia. Relationship to neuronal alterations. *Mayo Clin Proc* 50:264–270, 1975.

88. Lundberg N: Continuous recording and control of ventricular fluid pressure in neurosurgical practice. *Acta Psychiatr Neurol Scand* 36(suppl 149):1–193, 1960.

89. Lundy EF, Kuhn JE, Kwon JM, Zelenock GB, D'Alecy LG: Infusion of five percent dextrose increases mortality and morbidity following six minutes of cardiac arrest in resuscitated dogs. *J Crit Care* 2:4–14, 1987.

90. Lyeth BG, Dixon CE, Giebel ML, Robinson SE, Hamm RJ, Stonnington HH, Young HF, Hayes RL: The effects of scopolamine pre- and post-treatment on the responses to concussive brain injury in the rat (abstract). *Soc Neurosci Abstr* 12:967, 1986.

91. Marsh ML, Aidinis SJ, Naughton KVH, Marshall LF, Shapiro M: The technique of nitroprusside administration modifies the intracranial pressure response. *Anesthesiology* 51:538–541, 1979.

92. Marshall LF, Smith RW, Shapiro HM: The outcome with aggressive treatment in severe head injuries. Part II: Acute and chronic barbiturate administration in the management of head injury. *J Neurosurg* 50:26–30, 1979.

93. Mathew RJ, Wilson WH: Caffeine induced changes in cerebral circulation. *Stroke* 16:814–817, 1985.

94. Maximilian VA, Prohovnik I, Risberg J: Cerebral hemodynamic response to mental activation in normo- and hypercapnia. *Stroke* 11:342–347, 1980.

95. McCalden TA, Nath RG, Thiele K: The effects of a calcium antagonist (nimodipine) on basal cerebral blood flow and reactivity to various agonists. *Stroke* 15:527–530, 1984.

96. McHenry LC Jr, Stump DA, Howard G, Novack TT, Bivans DH, Nelson AO: Comparison of the effects of intravenous papaverine hydrochloride and oral Pavabid HP capsulets on regional cerebral blood flow in normal individuals. *J Cereb Blood Flow Metab* 3:442–447, 1983.

97. Meyer CHA, Lowe D, Meyer M, Richardson PL, Neil-Dwyer G: Subarachnoid haemorrhage: Older patients have low cerebral blood flow. *Br Med J* 285:1149–1153, 1982.

98. Meyer FB, Anderson RE, Sundt TM Jr, Sharbrough FW: Selective central nervous system calcium channel blockers—a new class of anticonvulsant agents. *Mayo Clin Proc* 61:239–247, 1986.

99. Meyer FB, Anderson RE, Sundt TM Jr, Yaksh TL: Intracellular brain pH, indicator tissue perfusion, electroencephalography, and histology in severe and moderate focal cortical ischemia in the rabbit. *J Cereb Blood Flow Metab* 6:71–78, 1986.

100. Meyer FB, Anderson RE, Yaksh TL, Sundt TM Jr: Effect of nimodipine on intracellular brain pH, cortical blood flow, and EEG in experimental focal cerebral ischemia. *J Neurosurg* 64:617–626, 1986.

101. Meyer FB, Piepgras DG, Sandok BA, Sundt TM Jr, Forbes G: Emergency carotid endarterectomy for patients with acute carotid occlusion and profound neurological deficits. *Ann Surg* 203:82–89, 1986.

102. Meyer FB, Piepgras DG, Sundt TM Jr, Yanagihara T: Emergency embolectomy for acute occlusion of the middle cerebral artery. *J Neurosurg* 62:639–647, 1985.

103. Meyer FB, Sundt TM Jr, Yanagihara T, Anderson RE: Focal cerebral ischemia: pathophysiologic mechanisms and rationale for future avenues of treatment. *Mayo Clin Proc* 62:35–55, 1987.

104. Michenfelder JD: The interdependency of cerebral functional and metabolic effects following massive doses of thiopental in the dog. *Anesthesiology* 41:231–236, 1974.

105. Michenfelder JD, Milde JH: Influence of anesthetics on metabolic, functional and pathological responses to regional cerebral ischemia. *Stroke* 6:405–410, 1975.

106. Moufarrij NA, Little JR, Skrinska V, Lucas FV, Latchaw JP, Slugg RM, Lesser RP: Thromboxane synthetase inhibition in acute focal cerebral ischemia in cats. *J Neurosurg* 61:1107–1112, 1984.

107. Muizelaar JP, Becker DP: Induced hypertension for the treatment of cerebral ischemia after subarachnoid hemorrhage. Direct effect on cerebral blood flow. *Surg Neurol* 25:317–325, 1986.

108. Muizelaar JP, Lutz HA III, Becker DP: Effect of mannitol on ICP and CBF and correlation with pressure autoregulation in severely head-injured patients. *J Neurosurg* 61:700–706, 1984.

109. Nakano M, Tani E, Fukumori T, Yokota M: Effects of chlorpromazine on experimental delayed cerebral vasospasm. *J Neurosurg* 61:857–863, 1984.

110. Nussmeier NA, Arlund C, Slogoff S: Neuropsychiatric complications after cardiopulmonary bypass: cerebral protection by a barbiturate. *Anesthesiology* 64:165–170, 1986.

111. Olesen J, Hougard K, Hertz M: Isoproterenol and propranolol: ability to cross the blood-brain barrier and effects on cerebral circulation in man. *Stroke* 9:344–349, 1978.

112. Pearson RM, Griffith DNW, Woollard M, James IM: Comparison of effects on cerebral blood flow of rapid reduction in systemic arterial pressure by diazoxide and labetalol in hypertensive patients: preliminary findings. *Br J Clin Pharmacol* 8:195S–198S, 1979.

113. Phillis JW, Preston G, DeLong RE: Effects of anoxia on cerebral blood flow in the rat brain: evidence for a role of adenosine in autoregulation. *J Cereb Blood Flow Metab* 4:586–592, 1984.

114. Piantadosi CA, Hemstreet TM, Jobis-Vandervliet FF: Near-infrared spectrophotometric monitoring of oxygen distribution to intact brain and skeletal muscle tissues. *Crit Care Med* 14:698–706, 1986.

115. Poole GV Jr, Johnson JC, Prough DS, Stump DA, Stullken EH: Cerebral hemodynamics after hemorrhagic shock: effects of the type of resuscitation fluid. *Crit Care Med* 14:629–633, 1986.

116. Poole GV Jr, Prough DS, Johnson JC, Stullken EH, Stump DA, Howard G: Effects of resuscitation from hemorrhagic shock on cerebral hemodynamics in the presence of an intracranial mass. *J Trauma* 27:18–23, 1987.

117. Pritz MB, Giannotta SL, Kindt GW, McGillicuddy JE, Prager RL: Treatment of patients with neurological deficits associated with cerebral vasospasm by intravascular volume expansion. *Neurosurgery* 3:364–368, 1978.

118. Proctor HJ, Cairns C, Fillipo D, Palladino GW, Rosner MJ: Brain metabolism during increased intracranial pressure as assessed by niroscopy. *Surgery* 96:273–279, 1984.

119. Prough DS, Johnson JC, Stump DA, Stullken EH, Poole GV Jr, Howard G: Effects of hypertonic saline versus lactated Ringer's solution on cerebral oxygen transport during resuscitation from hemorrhagic shock. *J Neurosurg* 64:627–632, 1986.

120. Prough DS, Kong D, Watkins WD, Stout R, Stump DA, Beamer WC: Inhibition of thromboxane A_2 production does not improve post-ischemic brain hypoperfusion in the dog. *Stroke* 17:1272–1276, 1986.

121. Prough DS, Stump DA, Roy RC, Gravlee GP, Williams T, Mills SA, Hinshelwood L, Howard G: Response of cerebral blood flow to changes in carbon dioxide tension during hypothermic cardiopulmonary bypass. *Anesthesiology* 64:576–581, 1986.

122. Quasha AL, Tinker JH, Sharbrough FW: Hypothermia plus thiopental: prolonged electroencephalographic suppression. *Anesthesiology* 55:636–640, 1981.

123. Raichle ME, Stone HL: Cerebral blood flow autoregulation and graded hypercapnia. *Eur Neurol* 6:1–5, 1971/72.

124. Randomized clinical study of thiopental loading in comatose survivors of cardiac arrest. Brain Resuscitation Clinical Trial I Study Group. *N Engl J Med* 314:397–403, 1986.

125. Rehncrona S, Siesjo BK: Hypoxia, ischemia and cerebral metabolism. In Gordon E (ed): *A Basis and Practice of Neuroanaesthesia*, ed 2 (Monographs in Anaesthesiology, vol 2). Amsterdam, Excerpta Medica 1981, pp 51–97.

126. Reulen HJ: Vasogenic brain oedema. New aspects in its formation, resolution and therapy. *Br. J Anaesth* 48:741–752, 1976.

127. Roland PE, Friberg L: Localization of cortical areas activated by thinking. *J Neurophysiol* 53:1219–1243, 1985.

128. Rosner MJ: Systemic response to experimental brain injury. In Becker DP, Povlishock JT (eds): *Central Nervous System Trauma Status Report*. Bethesda, MD, National Institutes of Health, NIH/NINCDS, 1985, pp 405–415.

129. Rosner MJ, Becker DP: Experimental brain injury: successful therapy with the weak base, tromethamine. With an overview of CNS acidosis. *J Neurosurg* 60:961–971, 1984.

130. Rozenfeld D, Wolfson LI: The effects of activation procedures on regional cerebral blood flow in humans. *Sem Nucl Med* 11:172–185, 1981.

131. Saul TG, Ducker TB: Effect of intracranial pressure monitoring and aggressive treatment on mortality in severe head injury. *J Neurosurg* 56:498–503, 1982.

132. Saul TG, Ducker TB, Salcman M, Carro E: Steroids in severe head injury. A prospective randomized clinical trial. *J Neurosurg* 54:596–600, 1981.

133. Saussy DL Jr, Mais DE, Knapp DR, Halushka PV: Thromboxane A_2 and prostaglandin endoperoxide receptors in platelets and vascular smooth muscle. *Circulation* 72:1202–1207, 1985.

134. Severinghaus JW, Chiodi H, Eger EI II, Brandstater B, Hornbein TF: Cerebral blood flow in man at high altitude. Role of cerebrospinal fluid pH in normalization of flow in chronic hypocapnia. *Circ Res* 19:274–282, 1966.

135. Sharbrough FW, Messick JM Jr, Sundt TM Jr: Correlation of continuous electroencephalograms with cerebral blood flow measurements during carotid endarterectomy. *Stroke* 4:674–683, 1973.

136. Shaw PJ, Bates D, Cartlidge NEF, French JM, Heaviside D, Julian DG, Shaw DA: Early intellectual dysfunction following coronary bypass surgery. *Q J Med* 58(225):59–68, 1986.

137. Shaywitz BA, Rothstein P, Venes JL: Monitoring and management of increased intracranial pressure in Reye syndrome: results in 29 children. *Pediatrics* 66:198–204, 1980.

138. Siesjo BK: Cell damage in the brain: a speculative synthesis. *J Cereb Blood Flow Metab* 1:155–185, 1981.

139. Siesjo BK, Bendek G, Koide T, Westerberg E, Wieloch T: Influence of acidosis on liquid peroxidation in brain tissues in vitro. *J Cereb Blood Flow Metab* 5:253–258, 1985.

140. Slogoff S, Girgis KZ, Keats AS: Etiologic factors in

neuropsychiatric complications associated with cardiopulmonary bypass. *Anesth Analg* 61:903–911, 1982.

141. Smith AL, Hoff JT, Nielsen SL, Larson CP: Barbiturate protection in acute focal cerebral ischemia. *Stroke* 5:1–7, 1974.

142. Smith PLC, Treasure T, Newman SP, Joseph P, Ell PJ, Schneidau A, Harrison MJG: Cerebral consequences of cardiopulmonary bypass. *Lancet* 1:823–825, 1986.

143. Snyder JV, Nemoto EM, Carroll RG, Safar P: Global ischemia in dogs: intracranial pressures, brain blood flow and metabolism. *Stroke* 6:21–27, 1975.

144. Sokoloff L, Reivich M, Kennedy C, Des Rosiers MH, Patlak CS, Pettigrew KD, Sakurada O, Shinohara M: The ^{14}C deoxyglucose method for the measurement of local cerebral glucose utilization: theory, procedure, and normal values in the conscious and anesthetized albino rat. *J Neurochem* 28:897–916, 1977.

145. Sotaniemi KA, Mononen H, Hokkanen TE: Long-term cerebral outcome after open-heart surgery. A five-year neuropsychological follow-up study. *Stroke* 17:410–416, 1986.

146. Spittell JA Jr: Pentoxifylline and intermittent claudication. *Ann Intern Med* 102:126–127, 1985.

147. Steen PA, Gisvold SE, Milde JH, Newberg LA, Sheithauer BW, Lanier WL, Michenfelder JD: Nimodipine improves outcome when given after complete cerebral ischemia in primates. *Anesthesiology* 62:406–414, 1985.

148. Steen PA, Michenfelder JD, Milde JH: Incomplete versus complete cerebral ischemia: improved outcome with a minimal blood flow. *Ann Neurol* 6:389–398, 1979.

149. Steen PA, Newberg LA, Milde JH, Michenfelder JD: Nimodipine improves cerebral blood flow and neurologic recovery after complete cerebral ischemia in the dog. *J Cereb Blood Flow Metab* 3:38–43, 1983.

150. Stevens MK, Yaksh TL, Hansen RB II, Anderson RE: Effect of preischemia cyclooxygenase inhibition by zomepirac sodium on reflow, cerebral autoregulation, and EEG recovery in the cat after global ischemia. *J Cereb Blood Flow Metab* 6:691–702, 1986.

151. Stockard JJ, Bickford RG, Schauble JF: Pressure-dependent cerebral ischemia during cardiopulmonary bypass. *Neurology* 23:521–529, 1973.

152. Strand T, Asplund K, Eriksson S, Hagg E, Lithner F, Wester P-O: A randomized controlled trial of hemodilution therapy in acute ischemic stroke. *Stroke* 15:980–989, 1984.

153. Strandgaard S, Paulson OB: Cerebral autoregulation. *Stroke* 15:413–415, 1984.

154. Stump DA, Prough DS, Lefkowitz DS, Toole JF, Hinshelwood L: Pentoxifylline improves global and regional cerebral blood flow in patients with chronic stroke (abstract). *Anesthesiology* 65:A458, 1986.

155. Symon L: Flow thresholds in brain ischaemia and the effects of drugs. *Br J Anaesth* 57:34–43, 1985.

156. Thie A, Spitzer K, Kunze K: Spontaneous subarachnoid hemorrhage: assessment of prognosis and initial management in the intensive care unit. *J Intensive Care Med* 2:103–115, 1987.

157. Todd NV, Picozzi P, Crockard HA, Russell RR: Duration of ischemia influences the development and res-

olution of ischemic brain edema. *Stroke* 17:466–471, 1986.

158. Todd NV, Picozzi P, Crockard HA, Russell RR: Reperfusion after cerebral ischemia: influence of duration of ischemia. *Stroke* 17:460–466, 1986.

159. von Essen C: Effects of dopamine on the cerebral blood flow in the dog. *Acta Neurol Scand* 50:39–52, 1974.

160. Vries JK, Becker DP, Young HF: A subarachnoid screw for monitoring intracranial pressure. Technical note. *J Neurosurg* 39:416–419, 1973.

161. Ward JD, Becker DP, Miller DJ, Choi SC, Marmarou A, Wood C, Newlon PG, Keenan E: Failure of prophylactic barbiturate coma in the treatment of severe head trauma. *J Neurosurg* 62:383–388, 1985.

162. Wieloch T, Siesjo BK: Ischemic brain injury: The importance of calcium, lipolytic activities, and free fatty acids. *Pathol Biol* 30:269–277, 1982.

163. Wilkins RH: Attempts at prevention or treatment of intracranial arterial spasm: an update. *Neurosurgery* 18:808–825, 1986.

164. Wise G, Sutter R, Burkholder J: The treatment of brain ischemia with vasopressor drugs. *Stroke* 3:135–140, 1972.

165. Wolfe LS: Eicosanoids: prostaglandins, thromboxanes, leukotrienes, and other derivatives of carbon-20 unsaturated fatty acids. *J Neurochem* 38:1–14, 1982.

166. Wood JH, Polyzoidis KS, Epstein CM, Gibby GL, Tindall GT: Quantitative EEG alterations after isovolemic-hemodilutional augmentation of cerebral perfusion in stroke patients. *Neurology* 34:764–768, 1984.

167. Wood JH, Simeone FA, Fink EA, Golden MA: Hypervolemic hemodilution in experimental focal cerebral ischemia. Elevation of cardiac output, regional cortical blood flow, and ICP after intravascular volume expansion with low molecular weight dextran. *J Neurosurg* 59:500–509, 1983.

168. Wood JH, Simeone FA, Kron RE, Snyder LL: Experimental hypervolemic hemodilution: physiological correlations of cortical blood flow, cardiac output, and intracranial pressure with fresh blood viscosity and plasma volume. *Neurosurgery* 14:709–723, 1984.

169. Wood JH, Snyder LL, Simeone FA: Failure of intravascular volume expansion without hemodilution to elevate cortical blood flow in region of experimental focal ischemia. *J Neurosurg* 56:80–91, 1982.

170. Yang MS, DeWitt DS, Becker DP, Hayes RL: Regional brain metabolite levels following mild experimental head injury in the cat. *J Neurosurg* 63:617–621, 1985.

171. Yatsu FM, McKenzie JD, Lockwood AH: Cardiopulmonary arrest and intravenous glucose. *J Crit Care* 2:1–3, 1987.

172. Yoshida S, Inoh S, Asano T, Sano K, Kubota M, Shimazaki H, Ueta N: Effect of transient ischemia on free fatty acids and phospholipids in the gerbil brain. Lipid peroxidation as a possible cause of postischemic injury. *J Neurosurg* 53:323–331, 1980.

173. Zeumer H, Hacke W, Ringelstein EB: Local intraarterial thrombolysis in vertebrobasilar thromboembolic disease. *AJNR* 4:401–404, 1983.

174. Zivin JA, Fisher M, DeGirolami U, Hemenway CC, Stashak JS: Tissue plasminogen activator reduces neurological damage after cerebral embolism. *Science* 230:1289–1292, 1985.

12

Pharmacology of Colloids and Crystalloids

Thomas G. Rainey, M.D.
James F. English, M.D.

In this chapter we review the use of colloids and crystalloids in the therapy of shock. Controversy exists as to the changes in body compartment composition in critical illness. Some investigations show depletion of extracellular fluid in shock from hemorrhage (with intravascular and interstitial fluid volumes both depleted) and an increase in intracellular water secondary to cell membrane and sodium-potassium pump dysfunction (25, 142–144). On the other hand, in surgical patients post trauma, extracellular fluid is found not to be decreased but actually increased, whereas intravascular volume is depleted (42, 135). Despite this controversy, one thing is agreed upon—intravascular volume is depleted in many types of critical illness. Prompt restoration of intravascular volume depletion is essential to reestablish cellular perfusion and accomplish successful resuscitation.

A thorough knowledge of the distribution and pharmacokinetics of plasma expanders allows the clinician to promptly and efficiently resuscitate patients in shock from various causes, including trauma, sepsis, hemodilution, and burns. An understanding of this pharmacologic subject helps the physician to minimize side effects associated with overaggressive volume resuscitation (respiratory failure, peripheral edema) or inadequate resuscitation (renal failure, refractory shock). The chapter begins with a discussion of the general principles of fluid distribution within the body, and then reviews the pharmacology of common plasma volume–expanding agents and their application in various clinical situations.

BODY FLUID DISTRIBUTION BY COMPARTMENTS

The total body water (TBW) ranges from 45% to 65% of total body weight in the human adult. The average adult man's TBW equals 60% of total body weight (55, 104) or 48 liters for an 80-kg man (125) (Table 12.1). Body water is distributed into two main compartments, the intracellular fluid (ICF) space, and the extracellular fluid (ECF) space. Two-thirds (32 liters) of the TBW resides in the ICF space and one-third (16 liters) in the ECF space (Fig. 12.1). The ECF space is further subdivided into the intravascular space and the interstitial space. Normally, approximately one-fourth of ECF resides in the intravascular compartment (4 liters) and three-fourths in the interstitial compartment (12 liters). The membranes separating these compartments are freely permeable to water, which moves under the force of osmotic drive until the osmolality in each compartment is equivalent.

When water is added into one compartment it distributes evenly throughout the TBW, and the amount of volume added to any given compartment is proportional to its fractional representation of TBW. As an example, if 3 liters of "free" water (no osmotically active particles) is added to the intravascular space (assuming none of that water exists in the body), the compartment volumes change from 16 to 17 liters in the ECF space and 32 to 34 liters in the ICF space (Fig 12.2). Note that 3

Table 12.1
Total Body Water as Percentage of Body Weight[a]

	Total Body Water (% of Body Weight)	
Build	Male	Female
Thin	65	55
Average	60	50
Obese	55	45

[a] Modified from Scribner BH (ed): *University of Washington Teaching Syllabus for the Course on Fluid and Electrolyte Balance.* Seattle, University of Washington Press, 1969.

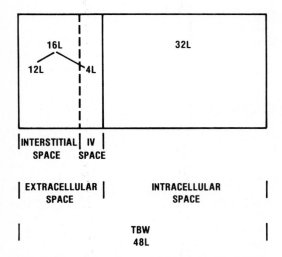

Figure 12.1   Distribution of total body water *(TBW)* in an 80-kg man. *IV,* intravascular.

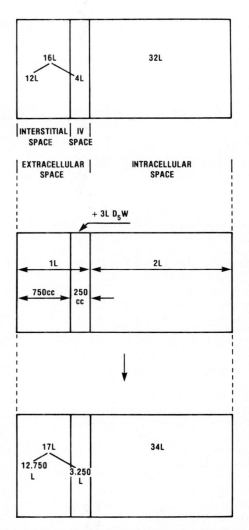

Figure 12.2.   Distribution of 3 liters of free water (5% dextrose in water, *D₅W*) in an 80-kg man with total body water of 48 liters. *IV,* intravascular.

liters of free water placed in the intravascular space results in a net increase of only 250 ml in the intravascular volume after equilibration takes place. Approximately 30 minutes after a rapid volume infusion, less than one-tenth of the volume infused remains in the intravascular space (156)! If the 3 liters of infused solution is isotonic with plasma (Ringer's lactate, normal saline), a different fluid distribution occurs (Fig. 12.3). Since there is no difference in osmolality between the infused fluid and the body fluids, there is no driving force to cause water to diffuse into the intracellular compartment. The intact membrane between the interstitial space and the intravascular space is permeable to ions and small particles, whereas the membrane surrounding the ICF space functionally is not. Consequently, the ECF space is the distribution space for isotonic fluids such as normal saline and Ringer's lactate. Note also that knowledge of the distribution space for isotonic fluid has important practical applications for resuscitation. Only one-fourth of the volume of isotonic fluid infused remains in the intravascular space after 30 minutes.

Application of these basic concepts allows one to predict the space of distribution for any standard intravenous solution since they are all some combination of free water and isotonic fluid. For example, 1000 ml of 0.45% saline can be thought of as 500 ml of normal (0.9%) saline plus 500 ml of free water. The portion that is isotonic (saline) distributes through the ECF space, and the portion that is

water distributes through the TBW. If one tries to expand the intravascular volume of a hypotensive patient by giving 1000 ml of 0.45% saline over 1 hour, the resultant increase in intravascular volume is only 165 ml! After distribution, the 500 ml of free water adds only 40 ml and the 500 ml of normal saline adds approximately 125 ml to the intravascular volume. What initially appears to be a large volume of fluid adds very little to the intravascular volume of 4–5 liters. Writing intravenous fluid prescriptions and predicting the outcome of therapy becomes simple when fluid balance and distribution are thought of in these terms.

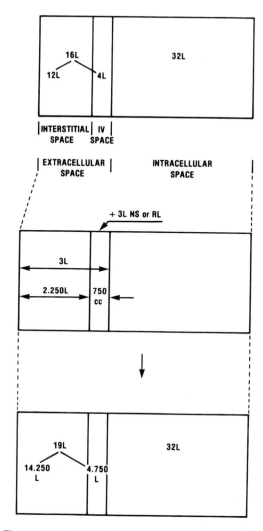

Figure 12.3. Distribution of 3 liters of normal saline *(NS)* or Ringer's lactate *(RL)* in an 80-kg man with total body water of 48 liters. *IV*, intravascular.

CRYSTALLOIDS

The term crystalloid as used here refers to solutions, isotonic with human plasma, that contain sodium as their major osmotically active particle. Ringer's lactate and normal saline are the only solutions considered.

Physiology and Pharmacokinetics

As described in the previous section, isotonic fluids such as Ringer's lactate and normal saline distribute evenly throughout the extracellular space. In normal healthy adults, approximately one-fourth of the volume infused remains in the intravascular space after 1 hour. Equilibration with the extracellular space occurs within 20–30 minutes after infusion. In the critically ill or injured patient, only one-fifth (54) or less (23) may remain in the circulation 1–2 hours after infusion. The "dwell time" in the circulation is the same in shock as in nonshock states (54).

In experimental acute blood loss leading to circulatory collapse, plasma volume becomes reduced and returns to normal over 3–4 days. As this equilibration occurs, hematocrit progressively falls. It takes 24 hours or longer for the hematocrit to stabilize as intravascular volume is restored at the expense of interstitial and ICF volume. By 2 hours, 14–36% of the ultimate change in hematocrit occurs; 36–50% occurs in 8 hours and 63–77% in 24 hours (40). When any plasma expander, including crystalloid, is infused (exogenous fluid), a more immediate fall in hematocrit occurs. However, as redistribution of resuscitation fluid out of the intravascular space occurs, the hematocrit again rises. The apparently erratic changes in serial hematocrit values seen during large-volume crystalloid resuscitations are often the result of these fluid shifts rather than repeated episodes of bleeding.

The total serum protein levels show similar changes. Endogenous restoration of depleted intravascular volume occurs through movement of interstitial fluid into the intravascular space. Catecholamines mediate arteriolar vasoconstriction, which diminishes capillary bed hydrostatic pressure favoring influx of interstitial fluid into the vascular tree distal to the arteriolar constriction. Subsequently, lymphatic flow returns plasma proteins to the intravascular space. Increases in interstitial pressure caused by crystalloid distribution into the interstitial space may augment lymphatic flow and thus the "protein-refill" mechanism (81). This process, combined with increased albumin synthesis and spontaneous diuresis secondary to volume repletion, explains the return of serum protein levels to normal within days after crystalloid resuscitation (143, 166).

Normal saline and Ringer's lactate can be used interchangeably (see prescribing information). The lactate load in Ringer's lactate solution does not potentiate the lactic acidemia associated with shock (161). Rather, as circulating blood volume is restored, diminished lactic acid production and decreased serum lactate levels are found (22, 115). The use of Ringer's lactate does not alter the reliability of blood lactate measurements (85).

The theoretical concern that large volumes of normal saline produce a "dilution acidosis" is not a problem clinically. Normal saline, like Ringer's lactate, causes no acidosis when studied in traumatic shock for which large volumes are administered (85). Saline resuscitation provides an excess of circulating chloride ion, which is normally excreted by the kidney without problem. In patients with acidosis caused by an organic acid (ketoacidosis or lactic acidosis), hyperchloremic acidosis may be seen during the postresuscitation period (101). However, this acidosis is due to loss of the bicarbonate substrate (ketones) in the urine rather than secondary to the administered chloride load.

Indications

Crystalloid solutions are indicated for plasma volume expansion (84, 96). They are inexpensive (Table 12.2), readily available, easily stored, reaction free, and help to correct extracellular electrolyte and volume deficits. In hemorrhagic shock, crystalloids can be used to replace plasma volume immediately (while blood is being crossmatched) and can limit the total amount of blood required for resuscitation. Crystalloids decrease blood viscosity as the blood volume is expanded. In the oliguric patient, a diagnostic "volume challenge" with crystalloid may safely help to distinguish between intravascular volume depletion and acute renal failure.

Side Effects

Crystalloid solutions are nontoxic and free from side effects if used appropriately. Excessive crystalloid administration may cause peripheral and pulmonary edema.

PERIPHERAL EDEMA

Edema is expected from crystalloid use since three-quarters or more of the volume administered distributes in the interstitial compartment of the extracellular space. Edema can be limited by appropriate monitoring of the adequacy of resuscitation to prevent volume overload.

PULMONARY EDEMA

Crystalloid resuscitation lowers colloid oncotic pressure by reducing the serum protein concentrations (53, 166). Whether the reduction in plasma proteins and consequent lowering of plasma colloid oncotic pressure decreases lung function is a controversial issue (54, 57, 112, 123, 136, 142, 167). "Edema safety factors," such as increased lymphatic flow, diminished pulmonary interstitial oncotic pressure, and increased interstitial hydrostatic pressure, limit the effect of lowered colloid oncotic pressure to increase fluid transudation from the vascular space (81). When the total crystalloid volume administered is controlled to prevent volume overload, there is no difference in lung function in resuscitation of shock using crystalloid or colloid solutions (54, 84, 96, 98, 166). The development of the adult respiratory distress syndrome (ARDS) is associated more closely with the presence of sepsis than with the type of fluid used in shock resuscitation.

Table 12.2
Comparative Prices of Volume-Expanding Agents[a]

Agent	Amount (ml)	Average Cost ($)	Cost per 400–500 ml of i.v. Expansion ($)
Albumin 5%	500	130.00	130.00
Albumin 25%	100	125.00	125.00
Hydroxyethyl starch	500	41.11	
Dextran 40	500	33.00	15.00–30.00
Dextran 70	500	21.00	10.00–20.00
Ringer's lactate	1000	4.50	6.00–12.00
Normal saline	1000	3.35	4.40– 8.80

[a] Adapted from Knipping WJ (ed): *Drug Topics Redbook*, ed 90. Oradell, NJ, Medical Economics, 1986.

Recommendations for Use

SHOCK

Crystalloid solutions are used in shock of various etiologies for the restoration of intravascular volume and repletion of interstitial water and electrolyte deficits (98, 130, 154, 166). The volume of crystalloid required to attain adequate volume repletion varies from three (37, 54, 98, 144) to 12 (34) times the volume of colloid solution required to reach the same hemodynamic endpoint. The patient in shock, whether from trauma, hemorrhage, or sepsis, should receive immediate volume replacement with crystalloid solutions during evaluation of the clinical situation. Two to three liters administered promptly may restore blood pressure and peripheral perfusion. If the hematocrit is greater than 30% and hemodynamic stability remains, further aggressive fluid resuscitation may be unnecessary. Acute blood loss of 10–20% of the blood volume may be adequately replaced with crystalloid if given in a quantity of three to four times the blood lost (13, 161, 166). If continued fluid resuscitation is required and the hematocrit remains above 30%, the authors recommend the use of crystalloid in conjunction with 5–10% colloid solutions in a ratio of 4:1 (crystalloid: colloid by volume). If the hematocrit falls below 30%, packed red blood cells should be transfused. If the serum albumin level falls below 2–2.5 g/dl, albumin or another colloid should be added to maintain the colloid oncotic pressure. Other blood components should be administered as necessitated by serial measurement of platelet count, prothrombin time, and partial thromboplastin time.

The major pitfall to avoid in crystalloid resuscitation is inadequate fluid administration. Five liters of crystalloid may be needed to replenish a 1-liter blood loss (134). Edema is to be expected and should not be interpreted as intravascular volume overload. Adequacy of intravascular volume repletion must be assessed by the usual parameters that indicate adequacy of peripheral perfusion—stable mean arterial pressure of 70–80 torr, heart rate less than 100 beats/min, warm extremities with good capillary refill, adequate CNS function, urine volume of 0.5–1 ml/kg/hr, and absence of advancing acidosis. In massive resuscitation or other critical situations, pulmonary artery wedge pressure, cardiac output, mixed venous oxygen content, and arteriovenous oxygen concentration difference (AVD_{O_2}) must supplement these other parameters in guiding fluid administration. A more detailed discussion of hemodynamic monitoring in resuscitation of shock may be found elsewhere (134).

DIAGNOSIS OF OLIGURIA

Oliguria (urine output <0.5 ml/kg/hr) may indicate prerenal hypoperfusion due to intravascular volume depletion or congestive heart failure (CHF). In the critically ill patient (often with underlying chronic obstructive pulmonary disease, ARDS, edema due to large volume resuscitation, hypoproteinemia, or sepsis with capillary leak) it may be impossible to distinguish volume depletion from CHF by physical examination. A volume challenge (500 ml over 5 minutes) with crystalloid solution can be helpful. If after an adequate volume challenge the patient's urine output increases, the diagnosis of intravascular volume depletion is confirmed and subsequent fluid management can be appropriately altered. If the oliguria is not due to intravascular volume depletion, no increase in urine output occurs with volume challenge. Since crystalloid fluids distribute out of the intravascular space rapidly, only a transient increase in intravascular volume results from a fluid challenge, and the patient with CHF does not experience a prolonged increase in vascular volume.

An adequate fluid challenge consists of no less than 500 ml of Ringer's lactate or normal saline given over 5 minutes. A smaller volume or a longer time for infusion will not expand the intravascular volume significantly. Only 100–150 ml of the 500 ml administered will remain in the intravascular space after 30 minutes. If the volume challenge is given over 30 minutes, the intravascular volume (5 liters for a 70-kg man) would be expanded 100–150 ml, thereby providing no information on the etiology of the oliguria since the intravascular volume was never expanded. Similarly, increasing the infusion rate of an oliguric patient from 100 ml/hr to 200 or 300 ml/hr provides no answer to the question of etiology of the oliguria, nor does it adequately treat volume depletion.

Prolonged prerenal hypoperfusion can lead to renal failure. The timely diagnosis and treatment of oliguria secondary to volume depletion is essential to avoid this disastrous consequence. If crystalloid volume challenge does not provide the answer, invasive diagnosis with a pulmonary artery catheter may be required. Colloid solutions should not be used to differentiate between intravascular volume depletion and CHF since their dwell time in the intravascular space is much longer and osmotic diuresis occurs immediately with some preparations (dextran, hydroxyethyl starch).

Prescribing Information

The contents of normal saline and Ringer's lactate solutions are shown in Table 12.3, and their costs in relation to other volume-expanding agents are listed in Table 12.2.

Ringer's lactate contains 28 mEq of lactate, which must undergo hepatic metabolism to bicarbonate to release 28 mEq of free base per liter of solution. In patients with renal failure, this bicarbonate source may be useful as an acid buffer; however, when hyperkalemia is a problem, use of normal saline avoids the 4 mEq/liter potassium content of Ringer's lactate. Similarly, normal saline is preferred in hypercalcemic or hyponatremic states. In the presence of established hyperchloremic metabolic acidosis, Ringer's lactate is preferred to provide a bicarbonate source and to diminish the administered chloride load.

ALBUMIN

Human serum albumin is effective in restoring blood volume in intravascular volume depletion (147). Its clinical indications are controversial, and it costs more than other plasma volume–expanding agents.

Pharmacology and Pharmacokinetics

ENDOGENOUS ALBUMIN

Albumin is produced in the liver and represents 50% of hepatic protein production (119). Its molecular weight is 65,000 (range, 66,300–69,000) (163). In health, approximately 12–14 g/day or 130–200 mg/kg/day are produced by the body (82, 119, 164). Albumin is the major oncotically active plasma protein, contributing about 80% of the plasma colloid oncotic pressure (81, 156). A 50% reduction of the serum albumin concentration decreases the colloid oncotic pressure to one-third of normal (156). Albumin binds cations and anions despite its strong negative charge and is a major transport protein for metals, drugs, fatty acids, hormones, and enzymes (163).

In the adult, 4–5 g of albumin per kilogram of body weight is available in the extracellular space, and 30–40% is present in the intravascular compartment. Albumin is secreted directly from the hepatocyte into the sinusoidal plasma. The final serum concentration of 3.5–5.0 g/dl results from the combination of albumin secretion, volume of distribution, rate of loss from the intravascular space, and ultimate degradation. In cirrhosis with portal hypertension, a large portion of the albumin produced enters directly into the peritoneal space (ascites) rather than the intravascular space, contributing to hypoproteinemia despite a normal or even elevated synthetic rate.

Approximately 50–60% of endogenous albumin is in the interstitial space. Some is tissue-bound and unavailable to the circulation. Free interstitial space albumin returns to the intravascular compartment by lymphatic drainage. This return of non–tissue-bound al-

Table 12.3
Ionic Composition of Various Volume-Expanding Agents

Agent	Component (mEq/liter)				
	Na$^+$	Cl$^-$	K$^+$	Ca^{2+}	Lactate
Ringer's lactate	130	109	4	3	28
Normal saline	154	154	—	—	—
Albumin 5%	130–160	130–160	<1	—	—
Albumin 25%	130–160	130–160	<1	—	—
Dextran 40					
10% in normal saline	154	154	—	—	—
10% in water	0	0	—	—	—
Dextran 70					
6% in normal saline	154	154	—	—	—
6% in water	0	0	—	—	—
Hydroxyethyl starch (hetastarch)	154	154	—	—	—

bumin increases during intravascular volume depletion, as does the synthesis and secretion of new albumin (82, 142). Interstitial space albumin that is tissue-bound is subsequently incorporated into the intracellular space where it is metabolized to amino acids, which return to the liver in a cycle similar to the Cori cycle (136). Catabolism increases albumin metabolism, perhaps accounting for part of stress-induced hypoalbuminemia. Decreases in the degradation of albumin and increases in its distribution in the interstitial space help to compensate for hypoalbuminemia due to loss (nephrotic syndrome, hemorrhage, bowel ob-

Table 12.4
Potential Albumin Losses in Pathologic States

Fluid	Albumin
Edema	
Congestive heart	
failure	1 g/dl
Renal disease	
Cirrhosis	
Lymphedema	>2 g/dl
Ascites	1–2 g/dl
Urine—nephrosis[a]	Usually 100–400 mg/kg/day, but may be more or less

[a] Requires proteinuria of ≥3 g/24 hours.

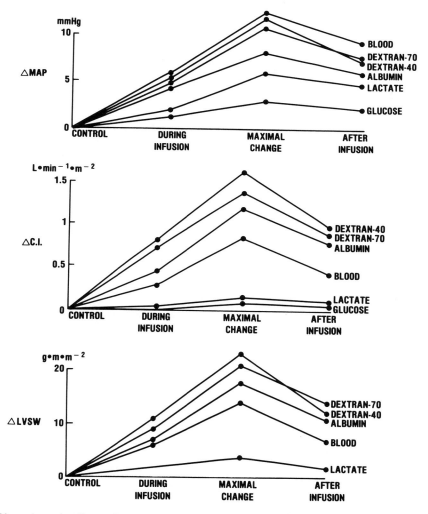

Figure 12.4. Hemodynamic effects of 500 ml of whole blood, 5% albumin, 10% dextran 40, dextran 70, and 1000 ml of 5% glucose or Ringer's lactate all infused over 1 hour. *MAP,* mean arterial pressure; *C.I.,* cardiac index; *LVSW,* left ventricular stroke work. (Modified from Shoemaker WC: Comparison of the relative effectiveness of whole blood transfusions and various types of fluid therapy in resuscitation. *Crit Care Med* 4:71–78, 1976.)

struction) or diminished production (starvation) (61, 116, 119). In injury or stress, albumin synthesis falls acutely whereas the production and serum levels of acute phase reactants (such as globulins, fibrinogen, haptoglobin) increase. In such situations, a 50% depletion of albumin can be corrected by translocation of interstitial albumin into the intravascular space (97). Subsequently, albumin synthesis can increase if hepatic function and the supply of nutrients are adequate (116). For instance, albumin synthesis increases after hemorrhage and burns,

although acutely, serum levels and synthesis fall (119). When appropriate nutrients are provided, albumin synthesis increases in the critically ill patient (116, 144). Albumin synthesis is increased by thyroid hormone and cortisone (81, 117) through stimulation of RNA production, is decreased by malnutrition, and is finely regulated by the oncotic environment of the hepatocytes (119). The serum albumin level exerts no feedback control on albumin synthesis except through albumin's contribution to colloid oncotic pressure (119).

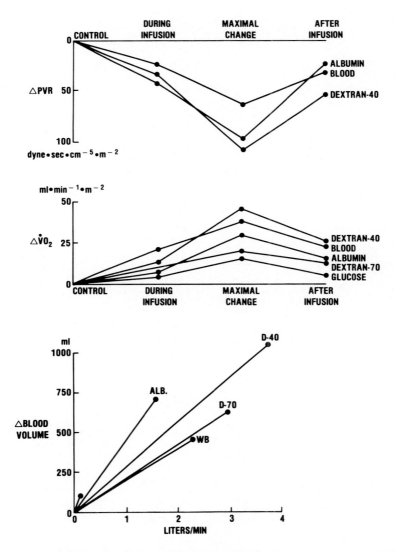

Figure 12.5 Hemodynamic effects of 500 ml of whole blood, 10% dextran 40, dextran 70, and 1000 ml of 5% glucose or Ringer's lactate all infused over 1 hour. *PVR*, pulmonary vascular resistance; $\dot{V}O_2$, oxygen consumption. (Modified from Shoemaker WC: Comparison of the relative effectiveness of whole blood transfusions and various types of fluid therapy in resuscitation. *Crit Care Med* 4:71–78, 1976.)

Albumin loss can occur through various body fluids (Table 12.4).

EXOGENOUS ALBUMIN

The major clinical use of albumin is as a plasma volume expander, and there are 50 years of experimental evidence to document its effectiveness. The reader is referred elsewhere for specific data concerning albumin use in human shock, trauma, or major surgery (6, 19, 32, 54, 70–74, 103, 127, 133, 143, 166) and animal shock (20, 34, 36, 37, 57, 58, 97, 105, 106). The increase in plasma volume resulting from infusion of albumin solutions is associated with hemodynamic improvement (133) (Figs. 12.4 and 12.5).

Administered albumin distributes itself throughout the extracellular space. It is a commonly held, but false, assumption that albumin distributes solely in the intravascular space. It is only a transient passenger in this compartment, although its length of stay is long compared with that of crystalloid fluids. The plasma half-life of albumin is 16 hours, the same as that of endogenously produced albumin. After 2 hours, 90% remains in the intravascular space. In health, the half-life of albumin in the body is approximately 20 days (81). One gram of intravascular albumin binds 18 ml of water by its oncotic activity (57, 81, 123).

Albumin is clinically available as a 5% or 25% solution in isotonic saline. When 100 ml of 25% albumin solution (25 g albumin) are infused, an increase in the intravascular volume occurs over 30–60 minutes to a final volume of 450 ml (54). The intravascular volume is expanded by the translocation of 350 ml of interstitial fluid into the intravascular space (Fig. 12.6). In the face of extracellular volume depletion, this equilibration is not sufficiently brisk or complete unless supplemental isotonic fluid is provided as part of the resuscitation regimen (81, 82, 174). A 500-ml solution of 5% albumin contains 25 g of albumin and increases the intravascular space by 450–500 ml; however, in this instance the albumin is administered in conjunction with the fluid to be retained.

Indications

Albumin is most widely used for its oncotic properties in the resuscitation of patients with an acutely diminished intravascular volume. It has beneficial effects on viscosity and is used for pump-priming in cardiopulmonary bypass and hemodialysis. Its properties as a transport protein have been used advantageously in binding bilirubin during therapy of hemolytic disease of the newborn.

Side Effects

PULMONARY EDEMA

The "colloid-crystalloid debate" has produced conflicting animal and human studies, some showing adverse effects (32, 60, 70, 86, 87, 140, 170) and others showing beneficial effects of albumin (19, 24, 46, 71–74, 84, 96, 97, 105, 127, 143, 166). The method of resuscitation, overall volume used, and the presence or absence of sepsis affects pulmonary function to a far greater extent than does the type of resuscitation fluid used (43, 105, 168).

DEPRESSED IONIZED CALCIUM LEVELS

Albumin may lower the serum ionized calcium concentration, producing a negative inotropic effect on the myocardium (32, 70, 86, 87, 170) and coagulopathy (28); however, these data are controversial.

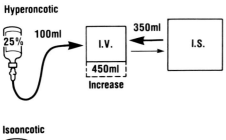

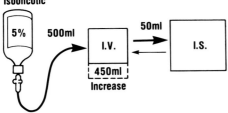

Figure 12.6. Schematic drawing of the influence of albumin solutions on the distribution of water to the intravascular *(I.V.)* and interstitial *(I.S.)* fluid compartments of the body. (Modified from Lamke LO, Liljedahl SO: Plasma volume expansion after infusion of 5%, 20%, and 25% albumin solutions in patients. *Resuscitation* 5:85–92, 1976.)

ANAPHYLAXIS

The incidence of albumin-induced anaphylaxis is between 0.47% and 1.53% (119). Such reactions are short-lived and include urticaria, chills, fever, and very rarely hypotension. Purified protein fraction has an increased incidence of associated hypotension (compared with albumin), perhaps secondary to the presence of kinins or prekallikrein activator (4, 15, 30, 52).

HEPATITIS RISK

There is no hepatitis risk with albumin. The preparations are heated during processing to 60°C for 10 hours—sufficient time to inactivate the hepatitis virus.

AIDS RISK

There is no known risk of acquired immune deficiency syndrome with albumin.

COST

Albumin is expensive. Hospital units have shown albumin to account for 10–30% of pharmacy budgets (164). The cost per liter of albumin is more than for other colloid solutions and 30 times the cost for the intravascular volume–equivalent amount of crystalloid solution (Table 12.2).

Recommendations for Use

In 1975 a National Institutes of Health task force examined the appropriate use of albumin in the light of increasing cost and apparent indiscriminate use (163). The authors' recommendations for albumin utilization are similar (Table 12.5). Albumin is used for its oncotic activity in the resuscitation of shock. In shock therapy, a major goal is prompt repletion of the intravascular volume in order to restore tissue perfusion. For major volume resuscitation (replacement of greater than 30% of the blood volume) colloids such as albumin or hydroxyethyl starch should be used as part of the resuscitation regimen. If colloids are used early, peripheral perfusion may be restored more promptly than with crystalloid alone. Blood component therapy is dictated by the

Table 12.5
Appropriate Albumin Utilization

Clinical Situations	Guidelines for Use (See Text)
1. Acute intravascular volume depletion, including hemorrhage, trauma, acute hemodilution, acute vasodilation.	In conjunction with crystalloid to limit edema from massive crystalloid volume resuscitation in the elderly or in patients with cardiopulmonary impairment or acute blood loss of >30% blood volume. To keep serum albumin >2.5 g/dl in acute resuscitation. Albumin 5% if patient is not edematous. Albumin 25% if patient is edematous.
2. "Third space" fluid loss, including acute peritonitis, mediastinitis, postoperative radical surgery.	Same guidelines as above.
3. Burns.	Greater than 50% surface area burn. Use after first 24 hours when capillary leak has diminished. Maintain serum albumin >2.5 g/dl. Use in conjunction with hyperalimentation.
4. Chronic disease (cirrhosis, nephrotic syndrome) associated with acute volume depletion (post paracentesis, dialysis, or overaggressive diuresis).	For acute intravascular volume resuscitation. Same guidelines as #1 above.
5. Post cardiopulmonary bypass with hemodilution.	Albumin ≥2.5 g/dl.
6. Adult respiratory distress syndrome.	Maintain lowest PAW that provides a CO adequate for tissue perfusion. Use only after capillary leak has resolved. Albumin >2.5 g/dl. T protein ≥5 g/dl. Colloid osmotic pressure >20 mm Hg. To correct intravascular volume depletion associated with diuretic use.

coagulation profile, hemoglobin concentration, and platelet count. The total volume of crystalloid administered, and thus the potential interstitial space fluid distribution, can be limited by using 5% albumin solution as part of the resuscitation treatment. If the patient is edematous, 25% albumin should be used to mobilize the patient's own interstitial volume. A solution of 100 ml of 25% albumin becomes 400–500 ml of intravascular volume over the course of 30–60 minutes. The greatest problem with its use is avoiding unintentional volume overload and pulmonary edema. Because of albumin's long "dwell time" in the intravascular space, volume overload persists unless diuresis or preload reduction is instituted.

A colloid osmotic pressure (COP) of ≥20 mm Hg, a serum albumin of ≥2.5 g/dl, or a total serum protein of ≥5 g/dl indicates adequate plasma oncotic activity in most situations. Large volumes of crystalloid fluids decrease COP whereas colloids (including albumin) increase COP (53). "Edema safety factors" limit the effect of decreased COP on the development of pulmonary edema; these factors include decreased interstitial oncotic pressure, increased lymphatic flow, and increased interstitial tissue pressure. The importance of decreased COP in pulmonary edema development remains unsettled (121, 136, 167).

Shock is associated with loss of capillary wall integrity ("capillary leak"), especially in the lung with subsequent development of ARDS. The use of albumin in the presence of capillary leak (ARDS, sepsis, intestinal obstruction) must be limited, since albumin crosses the capillary wall and exerts its oncotic influence in the interstitial rather than the intravascular space. The authors recommend that colloid use during capillary leak be minimized. Crystalloid fluids should be used until the capillary leak has resolved. Colloids, including albumin, may then be useful in supporting plasma volume during spontaneous or forced diuresis. Unfortunately, determining when capillary leak is present or has resolved is difficult. In burns (119) and intestinal obstruction (121) capillary integrity is restored after approximately 24 hours. In sepsis or ARDS the "leak" may persist.

In ARDS, as in shock, it is skillful fluid management rather than the type of fluid used that is important. In the complicated postshock patient with ARDS, the goal of supportive therapy is to minimize further fluid accumulation in the lung while perfusing body tissues. To do this requires adequate monitoring with pulmonary artery, arterial, and bladder catheters. A cardiac output adequate to support tissue perfusion must be obtained, but at the lowest possible capillary hydrostatic pressure to minimize fluid extravasation into the lung. In the presence of a capillary leak, the higher the capillary hydrostatic pressure, the greater the loss of fluid from the intravascular space into the interstitium of the lung.

There are a few clinical situations in which albumin is commonly but inappropriately used. Infusion of albumin to normalize a marginally lowered serum albumin concentration in the face of chronic disease such as malnutrition, cirrhosis, or nephrotic syndrome is unjustified. The serum albumin level is simply an indicator of some more basic underlying problems, and infusing albumin does not solve the problem. Rosenoer and associates (116) make this analogy: "If one's gas gauge points to empty, one simply need smash the glass and move the indicator up to full." Appropriate nutrition, even in cirrhosis, replenishes albumin stores more efficiently than does albumin infusion. Using albumin as a protein nutrient source is inefficient and more expensive than other forms of parenteral nutrition. Albumin does not contain all the essential amino acids (118, 144), and those it does have are unavailable for immediate protein synthesis because of albumin's long half-life (81).

In cirrhosis, infused albumin equilibrates with ascites and may decrease endogenous albumin synthesis (81). In nephrosis, endogenous albumin synthesis is increased, and there is no evidence that chronic edema or the underlying disease is improved by albumin infusion. Rather, infused albumin is lost in the urine. Although inappropriate for chronic use in each of these situations, the use of albumin for plasma volume support is appropriate, e.g., post paracentesis, dialysis, acute blood loss, and diuretic-induced hypotension.

Prescribing Information

Albumin is provided as three distinct preparations (Table 12.6) (12): normal serum albumin (NSA), 5% and 25%, and purified protein fraction (PPF). None of these products contains coagulation components, and hemodilution of the cellular and protein components of blood occurs with albumin use in large volume. Red blood cells and fresh frozen plasma should be added as appropriate to the resuscitation fluids. NSA has a shelf life of 3–

Table 12.6
Human Serum Albumin Products for Clinical Use[a]

Normal serum albumin (human)(NSA)
  25 ± 1.5% protein
    or
  5 ± 0.3% protein

Purity:	At least 96% of the total protein in the final product must be albumin
pH:	6.9 ± 0.5
Sodium:	25% NSA: not more than 160 mEq/liter
	5% NSA: 130–160 mEq/liter
Dating:	When stored at 2–10°C: 5 years
	When stored at room temperature, no warmer than 37°C: 3 years

Plasma protein fraction (human) (PPF)
  5 ± 0.3% protein

Purity:	At least 83% of the total protein in the final product must be albumin; no more than 17% shall be globulins; no more than 1% of globulins shall be γ-globulin
pH:	7.0 ± 0.3
Sodium:	100–160 mEq/liter
Potassium:	No more than 2 mEq/liter
Dating:	When stored at 2–8°C: 5 years
	When stored at no warmer than 30°C: 3 years

Applicable to NSA and PPF
  Heated at 60°C ± 0.5°C for 10 hours
  No preservatives
  Pass standard tests for sterility and for pyrogenic substances

Stabilizers:	0.16 mmol sodium acetyltryptophanate
	or 0.08 mmol sodium acetyltryptophanate and
	0.08 mmol sodium caprylate

---

[a] From Barker LF: *Proceedings of the Workshop on Albumin,* February 12–13, 1975. Washington, DC, Department of Health, Education and Welfare, DHEW Publication No. (NIH) 76-925, 1976.

5 years, depending on the storage conditions. A 25% solution of NSA is hyperoncotic with an osmolality of 1500 mosm, resulting in its expansion to four to five times the administered volume (of 18 ml/g albumin). A 5% solution of NSA is isotonic with plasma. The protein content of NSA preparations is 96% albumin. PPF preparations contain only 83% albumin, with the remainder being α- and β-globulins. PPF is associated with an increased incidence of hypotension, thought to be secondary to kinins or prekallikrein activator activity present among these other proteins (4, 15, 30, 52).

A 25% albumin solution is often referred to as "salt-poor" albumin. This terminology dates from World War II when albumin preparations had to be stabilized with a "salt-rich" Na^+ content of 300 mEq/liter. Improved stabilization methods have now reduced the Na^+ content of all albumin preparations to 145 ± 15 mEq/liter (12). The "salt-poor" label has persisted although "salt-rich" solutions are no longer made (52). Selection among the albumin solutions can alter the amount of Na^+ a patient receives. Expansion of the intravascular space by 500 ml can be accomplished by using 100 ml of 25% albumin, adding 14.5 mEq of Na^+ (100 ml of a solution with 145 mEq/liter), or 500 ml of 5% albumin, adding 72.5 mEq of Na^+ (500 ml of a solution with 145 mEq/liter).

DEXTRAN

Dextran is a large glucose polymer, isolated originally from sugar beets contaminated with bacteria. In its native form it is a branched polysaccharide of 200,000 glucose units (Fig. 12.7). Partial hydrolysis produces polysaccharides of smaller size, which are available commercially as preparations having average molecular weights of 40,000 (dextran 40; D-40) or 70,000 (dextran 70; D-70). Dextran is

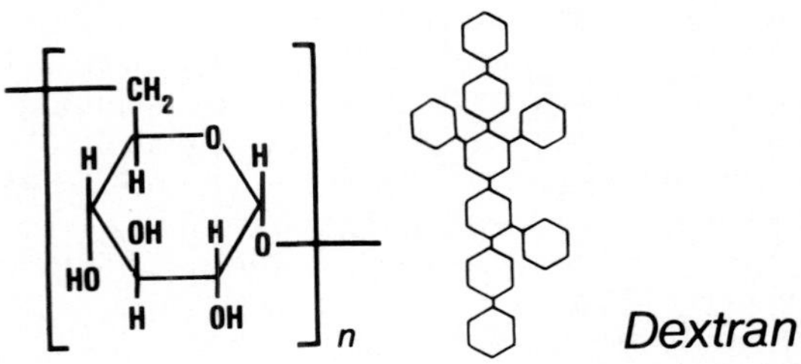

Dextran

Figure 12.7   Dextran: glucose subunit and polymer.

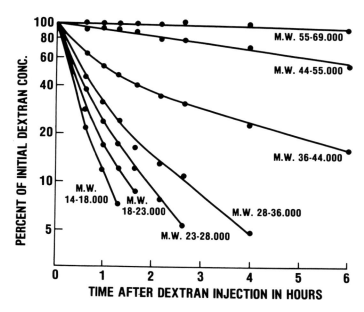

Figure 12.8 The disappearance rate of dextrans of different molecular weights from plasma. (From Arthurson G: *Scand J Clin Lab Invest* 16:76–80, 1964.)

used clinically as a volume-expanding agent; however, it is also used in the prevention of thromboembolism and to increase peripheral blood flow.

Pharmacology and Pharmacokinetics

Dextran molecules distribute in the extracellular space, mainly in the intravascular compartment. The particle size of the various dextrans affects the "dwell time" in the intravascular space and the duration of volume expansion accomplished. The major route of loss of dextran from the intravascular space is through the kidney. Smaller particles (<15,000 molecular weight) are rapidly filtered, not reabsorbed, and lost in the urine; however, while in the circulation, they exert osmotic activity. Larger particles remain in the circulation longer but exert less osmotic activity. D-40 and D-70 contain particles with molecular weights ranging from 10,000 to 80,000 (33) and 40,000 to 100,000, respectively. The circulating half-life of dextran varies with its particle size (37). The half-life for particles with molecular weights of 14,000–18,000 is 15 minutes, whereas for those greater than 55,000 it is several days (Fig. 12.8). Sixty to seventy percent of D-40 and 30–40% of D-70 is cleared in 12 hours (160). Since smaller particles are

cleared more rapidly than larger ones, and D-40 contains smaller particles than does D-70, D-40 is lost from the circulation faster than D-70. As a general rule, only 20% of D-40 dose and 30% of a D-70 dose remains in the circulation after 24 hours, and accumulation of large particles occurs over days of administration. For each preparation, after 24 hours the particles that accumulate have an average molecular weight of more than 80,000. With renal impairment small species accumulate. The larger particles are taken up by the reticuloendothelial system and are eventually metabolized to carbon dioxide and water. Other particles cross into the interstitial space and are recirculated through the lymphatic system.

Indications

VOLUME EXPANSION

Dextran has ideal properties as a plasma volume expander: a long dwell time and ultimate biodegradability. In shock, dextran increases survival (34, 36, 37, 139, 142, 153) and improves hemodynamic parameters (29, 35, 75, 113, 133). Dextran infusion is associated with increased renal plasma flow and a fall in plasma antidiuretic hormone levels when used in hypovolemia (160). It has favorable hemodynamic effects in restoring intravascular volume in shock when compared with other volume expanders (94, 133) (Figs. 12.4 and 12.5).

The reported degree of dextran-induced volume expansion varies, based on the type and concentration of solution used and the experimental setting. Dextran infusion increases the intravascular volume by an amount greater than or equal to that infused; however, the subsequent osmotic diuresis limits the duration of the volume expansion. One gram of dextran obligates 20–30 ml of water to the intravascular space (37, 50, 160). A 500-ml bolus of D-40 produces a 750-ml expansion of intravascular volume at 1 hour and 1050 ml at 2 hours (133). Some volume expansion may persist up to 8 hours in hypovolemic patients. (69). Studies of shock in dogs show similar volume expansion, with 47% of the bolus infused remaining in the intravascular space after 4 hours (37). Four to six hours after the infusion of either D-40 or D-70, the degree of intravascular volume expansion is similar and approximately equal to the amount infused (160).

PROMOTION OF PERIPHERAL BLOOD FLOW

In addition to increasing plasma volume, dextran has other effects on blood flow that potentiate flow in the microvasculature (5). By coating endothelial surfaces, dextran reduces interaction with the cellular elements in blood (160). Sludging and cellular aggregation seen in shock are reduced by reduction of blood viscosity (29) and coating of cellular elements. Altered platelet function, including diminished adherence and degranulation, limits thrombus formation and activation of the clotting cascade mechanism (1, 80, 171). Dextran is also reported to copolymerize with fibrin monomer, resulting in a less stable clot that is more susceptible to endogenous lysis (1).

PREVENTION OF THROMBOEMBOLISM

Dextran is effective in reducing the incidence of thromboembolic disease (115, 122). It is beneficial, compared with controls, for the prevention of deep venous thrombosis in general surgery patients and following total hip replacement. However, data for use of heparin in this same group are as good or better (47, 61), without the attendant risks of dextran.

OTHER USES

Dextran has been used in the therapy of ichemic ulceration of the skin, arterial occlusion, frostbite, and stroke, and in cell harvest in plasmapheresis and priming for extracorporeal circulation.

Side Effects

RENAL FAILURE

Dextran-induced renal failure may occur (45, 89, 90), especially in the face of unrecognized hypovolemia. The mechanism for the renal failure is tubular obstruction secondary to concentration and precipitation of dextran in the tubules with cast formation (26). Three conditions are necessary to cause this side-effect: (a) decreased renal perfusion pressure, (b) dextran in the tubule, and (c) a continued stimulus for water reabsorption. Unfortunately, these conditions exist in intravascular volume depletion and its resuscitation with dextran.

ANAPHYLAXIS

The incidence of anaphylactic reactions to dextran is between 1% (111) and 5.3% (156). Reactions occur early, within one-half hour after the infusion is begun, and may include urticaria, rash, nausea, bronchospasm, shock, and death. Dextran is a potent antigen and has cross-reactivity with bacterial polysaccharide antigens. Patients with *Streptococcus pneumoniae* or *Salmonella* infections may therefore be more prone to dextran reactions. Gut flora make endogenous dextran from dextrose, and a small portion of the patient population has never received dextran yet has circulating precipitins to the dextran molecule.

OSMOTIC DIURESIS

As previously noted, osmotic diuresis occurs almost immediately on infusion of any dextran preparation as smaller species are filtered and not reabsorbed. The effect is greater with D-40 than D-70 because of the prevalence of small species in D-40. In the face of this obligate osmotic diuresis, urine volume cannot serve as a guide to the adequacy of intravascular volume repletion. If blood volume is inadequately restored in the patient receiving dextran, the stage is set for all the conditions to be met to produce renal failure.

BIOCHEMICAL ALTERATIONS

Blood glucose levels can be falsely elevated in patients receiving dextran if the glucose measurement is done by analysis using acid, which converts dextran to dextrose. Dextran may also cause false elevations of the total protein concentration. Total protein measurements can be checked using a refractometer. The refractometer reading is within 1 g/dl of the true value.

Dextran can interfere with the cross-matching of blood. The coating action of dextran on red blood cells causes cells to aggregate, mimicking a (nonexistent) cross-match problem. This is a problem especially when blood is drawn from a site proximal to the dextran intravenous infusion site, and is simply handled by drawing blood prior to dextran infusion or notifying the blood bank that the patient is receiving dextran. Other biochemical alterations include false elevation of the serum bilirubin level and alteration of colloid oncotic pressure measurements (52).

BLEEDING DIATHESIS

Dextran inhibits erythrocyte aggregation in vivo (29). It adheres to vessel walls and cellular elements of the blood (16, 80); decreases platelet adhesiveness (80, 172), serum fibrinogen, and other factor levels (33); and increases Ivy bleeding time and incisional bleeding (156). In dogs, clinical bleeding is not observed until 80% replacement of plasma volume has been achieved (154). At doses less than 1.5 g/kg/day, clinical bleeding is not encountered (160).

RETICULOENDOTHELIAL BLOCKADE

Dextran temporarily impairs reticuloendothelial system function (76), and by so doing may diminish immune competence.

Recommendations for Use

Dextran is an effective agent for intravascular volume expansion and has some specific beneficial effects on blood flow through the microvasculature that makes its use in shock very attractive. In addition, it is ultimately biodegradable. Its side effects, as described above, are noteworthy in the critically ill population. Dextran can cause a bleeding diathesis and interfere with blood cross-matching in a patient suffering from hemorrhagic shock. Its use can produce renal failure whenever renal perfusion is impaired, i.e., in any shock situation. Dextran causes an immediate osmotic diuresis, which if misinterpreted may potentiate volume depletion and ultimately renal failure, especially in critically ill patients with underlying diseases such as diabetes mellitus.

Prescribing Information

PREPARATIONS

Dextran 40 is commercially available as a 10% solution in normal saline or 5% dextrose in water. Dextran 70 is commercially available as a 6% solution in normal saline or 5% dextrose in water or in 10% invert sugar. These preparations require no mixing and can be "hung" just as supplied.

DOSAGE

To avoid bleeding diathesis, the total administered dosage should remain less than 1.5 g/kg/day of D-40 and 2 g/kg/day of D-70. For restoration of blood volume in shock, this amount (approximately 1000 ml of 10% D-40 for a 70-kg man) may be given acutely in conjunction with crystalloid, packed red blood cells, and plasma as necessary. The *Medical Letter on Drugs and Therapeutics* recommends using less than 1000 ml/day of D-40 (3). For use in prophylaxis of thromboembolic disease or peripheral vascular disease, dosage should be increased to 50 ml/hr in 5 ml increments of D-40, with monitoring of urine output and specific gravity. Infusion should be discontinued for specific gravity greater than 1.030 and urine volume less than 0.5 ml/kg/hr (155).

HYDROXYETHYL STARCH

Hydroxyethyl starch is a synthetic starch molecule closely resembling glycogen. Its development is the result of a concerted effort to find a colloidal volume-expanding agent that is free from the toxicities of previously developed plasma expanders. Its similarity to glycogen may account for its relative freedom from immune reactions (Fig. 12.9).

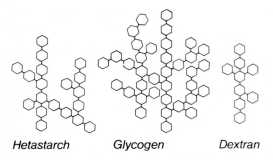

| Hetastarch | Glycogen | Dextran |

Figure 12.9 Two-dimensional representations of hydroxyethyl starch (hetastarch), glycogen, and dextran molecules. (Modified from Thompson WL: Proceedings from a Symposium: Hespan (Hetastarch): Historical Perspective and Development. Toronto, February 1982.)

Physiology and Pharmacokinetics

Hydroxyethyl starch (hetastarch) is available for clinical use as a 6% solution in normal saline. The average molecular weight of the particles is 69,000, with a range of 10,000–1,000,000. Glucose subunits are linked in α-1,4 and α-1,6 linkages to form a polymer that is more branched than dextran and is globular rather than linear. In addition, hydroxyethyl groups are substituted on the glucose subunits, which slows degradation in vivo (Figs. 12.9 and 12.10).

After intravenous infusion there is an almost immediate appearance of smaller particles in the urine (molecular weight, 50,000) (93). Studies in normal human volunteers show that 46% of an administered dose is excreted in the urine by 2 days and 64% by 8 days (108, 176). Larger particles remain in the circulation longer. Their rate of disappearance depends on their absorption by tissues (notably liver and spleen), gradual return to the circulation, uptake by the reticuloendothelial system, and subsequent degradation to smaller particles cleared through urine and bile. Blood α-amylase also degrades larger particles to smaller species. The rate of amylase degradation of hetastarch is slow compared with the rate for naturally occuring starches, probably because of the presence of hydroxyethyl groups substituted on 70% of the glucose subunits. Less than 1% of infused hetastarch can be recovered as exhaled CO_2.

As with dextran, the half-life of hetastarch represents a composite of the half-lives of various sized particles. Ninety percent of a single infusion of hetastarch leaves the circulation in 42 days, with a half-life of 17 days (176). The remaining 10% has a half-life of 48 days. Small amounts of hetastarch have been measured in the circulation as long as 17 weeks after a single infusion. The uptake of hetastarch molecules by the cells of the reticuloendothelial system has caused concern that the immune function of the patient could be compromised. However, clinically significant reticuloendothelial system dysfunction has not been demonstrated (78, 128, 149).

Plasma volume expansion after infusion of hetastarch is equal to or greater than that produced by D-70 (79, 92, 146, 154, 157, 158) or 5% albumin. Studies in humans show an increase in blood volume from 2.3 liters/m² to

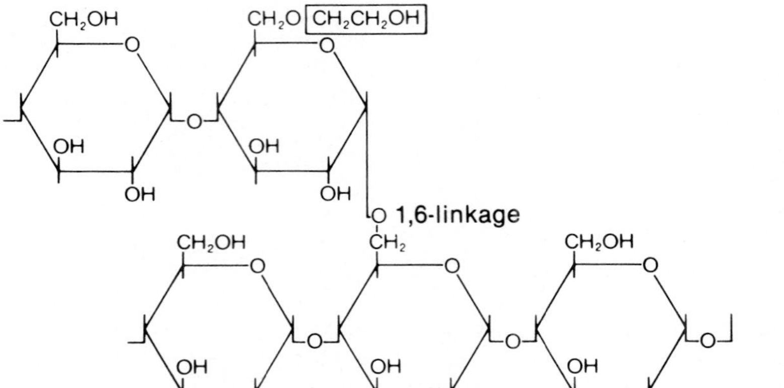

Figure 12.10 The hydroxyethyl starch molecule. Note the α-1,6-linkage and hydroxyethyl groups in *boxes.* (Modified from *Answers to Frequently Asked Questions About Hespan (Hetastarch).* McGraw Park, IL, American Critical Care Publications, 1981, p. 1.

2.9 liters/m², with a duration of at least 3 hours (77). Although there is some variability, infusions of hetastarch increase intravascular volume by an amount equal to or greater than the volume infused (11, 62, 75, 77, 92, 146, 159). The increase in intravascular volume is associated with improvement in hemodynamic parameters in critically ill patients (38, 63, 77, 88, 108, 129). The increase in colloid pressure is similar to that seen with albumin (53, 63).

Indications

Hydroxyethyl starch is indicated for use as a plasma volume–expanding agent in shock from hemorrhage, trauma, sepsis, or burns. It has adjunctive application in leukapheresis, and as a pump prime and volume expander in cardiopulmonary bypass.

Side Effects

COAGULOPATHY

Hetastarch is associated with minor alterations in laboratory measurements, but not with clinical bleeding when used in doses below 1500 ml/day (79, 145); doses greater than 1500 ml/day have been administered without bleeding complications (129). Dilutional effects on cellular and protein elements of the blood clotting cascade are produced secondary to the blood volume–expanding effect. However, the laboratory abnormalities are not explained by dilution alone. Coagulation profile discrepancies include a transient decrease in platelet count, prolonged prothrombin and partial thromboplastin times, and a decrease in the tensile clot strength (114, 145, 150–152, 169). In clinical series bleeding is a problem in only a small minority of cases (79, 145). Experience with hetastarch in leukapheresis is extensive, with bleeding complications occurring only rarely (44, 148).

PULMONARY EDEMA

Hetastarch has been used successfully in critically ill patients with various forms of shock without production of pulmonary edema or change in pulmonary function (77, 108).

ANAPHYLAXIS

The incidence of anaphylactic reactions to hetastarch (molecular weights > 16,000) in-

fusions is less than 0.085%. The incidence of severe reactions including shock or cardiopulmonary arrest is 0.008% (111). Hetastarch is not immunogenic (91, 112) and does not induce histamine release (83).

HYPERAMYLASEMIA

Serum amylase levels are elevated following hetastarch administration (67). Complexes of amylase and hetastarch molecules create macroamylase particles, which undergo urinary excretion at a much slower rate than the solitary amylase molecule. Serum amylase levels commonly reach twice normal after hetastarch infusion. There is no alteration of normal pancreatic function.

Recommendations for Use

Hetastarch may be used whenever colloid is required to restore plasma volume. Its properties as a volume-expanding agent are similar to those of 5% albumin solutions. At doses of 1500 ml/day or less, bleeding complications are avoided; doses greater than 1500 ml/day have been administered without bleeding complications (129). Hetastarch, like other colloid solutions, does not carry oxygen and must be administered in conjunction with packed red blood cells to maintain adequate oxygen content of the blood. Although rare, clinical bleeding has been associated with its use. Fresh frozen plasma and platelets should be replaced as indicated by clinical bleeding and the results of serial coagulation profiles. Hetastarch should be used with extreme caution in the presence of a known bleeding diathesis.

Adequate monitoring for detection of volume overload is crucial in hetastarch as with infusion of all other volume expanders. Volume overload pulmonary edema may be unwittingly produced despite careful monitoring of left heart filling pressures as the osmotic action of the infused hetastarch draws interstitial space water into the circulation. The immediate osmotic diuresis associated with its use protects somewhat from this phenomenon. Urine volume must be expected to increase acutely secondary to the osmotic diuresis, and this must not be misinterpreted as a sign of adequate peripheral perfusion. Patients with renal impairment are particularly subject to initial volume overload and to accumulation of hetastarch in the circulation and tissues with repeated administration. In these patients, initial volume resuscitation accomplished with hetastarch should be maintained with another plasma volume expander such as albumin or crystalloid.

Serum amylase values will be approximately twice normal after hetastarch infusion and are not indicative of pancreatitis. When serum amylase measurements are important (as in pancreatitis, bowel obstruction, parotitis), serum levels should be measured prior to infusion of hetastarch. Elevations of serum amylase may persist for 5 days postinfusion.

Hetastarch costs about one-fourth as much as an equivalent amount of 5% albumin (Table 12.2). Although dextran preparations cost even less than hetastarch, their use is associated with more side effects, such as anaphylactoid reactions, interference with blood typing and cross-matching, antigenicity, coagulopathy, and renal failure.

Prescribing Information

PREPARATIONS

Hetastarch is available as a 6% solution of 0.9% sodium chloride. The pH is 5.5 and the osmolarity 310 mosm/liter. It is bottled ready for infusion in 500-ml bottles.

DOSAGE

Usual total dosage is 20 ml/kg/day, but this is not an absolute upper limit. The total volume may be administered over 1 hour if the clinical situation demands adequate volume resuscitation.

For leukapheresis, 250–700 ml may be infused in the ratio of 1:8 with venous blood. Ten repetitions over the course of 5 weeks have been reported to be safe; however, hetastarch accumulation in the tissues will occur. Safety beyond this duration and frequency of administration is not known.

References

1. Aberg M, Hedner V, Bergentz S: Effect of dextran on factor VIII and platelet function. Ann Surg 189:243–247, 1979.
2. Abramowicz M (ed): Hetastarch (Hespan) a new plasma expander. Med Lett Drugs Ther 23(4):16, 1981.
3. Abramowicz M (ed): Med Lett Drugs Ther 10(1):3,1968.
4. Alving BM, Hojima Y, Pisano JJ: Hypotension associated with prekallikrein activator (Hageman-factor fragments) in plasma protein fraction. N Engl J Med 299:66–70, 1978.
5. Amundson B. Jennische E, Haljamae H: Skeletal muscle microcirculatory and cellular metabolic effects of whole blood. Ringer's acetate and dextran-70 infusions in hemorrhagic shock. Circ Shock 7:111–120, 1980.
6. Appel PL, Shoemaker WC: Evaluation of fluid therapy in adult respiratory failure. Crit Care Med 9:862–869, 1981.
7. Arthurson G. Granath K, Thoren L, Wallenius G: The renal excretion of LMW dextran. Acta Clin Scand 127:543–551, 1964.
8. Arthurson G, Wallenius G: The renal clearance of dextran of different molecular sizes in normal humans. Scand J Clin Lab Invest 16:81–86, 1964.
9. Atik M: Dextran-40 and dextran-70, a review. Arch Surg 94:664–672, 1967.
10. Atik M: The uses of dextran in surgery: a current evaluation. Surgery 65:548–562, 1969.
11. Ballinger WF: Preliminary report on the use of hydroxyethyl starch solution in man. J Surg Res 6:180–183, 1966.
12. Barker LF: Albumin products and the Bureau of Biologics. In Proceedings of the Workshop on Albumin, February 12–13, 1975. Washington, DC, Department of Health, Education and Welfare, DHEW Publication No. (NIH) 76–925, 1976, pp 22–27.
13. Baue AE, Tragus ET, Wolfson SK: Hemodynamic and metabolic effects of Ringer's lactate solution in hemorrhagic shock. Ann Surg 166:29–38, 1967.
14. Bergentz SE: Dextran prophylaxis of pulmonary embolism. World J Surg 2:19–24, 1978.
15. Bland JHL, Laver MB, Lowenstein E: Vasodilation effect of commercial 5% plasma protein fraction solutions. JAMA 224:1721–1724, 1973.
16. Bloom WL, Harmer J, Bryant MF: Coating of blood vessel surfaces and blood cells: a new concept in the prevention of intravascular thrombosis. Proc Soc Exp Biol Med 115:384–386, 1964.
17. Bogan RK, Gale GR, Walton RP: Fate of ^{14}C labelled hydroxyethyl starch in animals. Toxicol Appl Pharmacol 15:206–211, 1969.
18. Boon JC, Jesch F, Ring J, Messmer K: Intravascular persistence of hydroxyethyl starch in man. Eur Surg Res 8:497–503, 1976.
19. Boutros AR, Ruess R, Olson L: Comparison of hemodynamic, pulmonary and renal effects of use of 3 types of fluid after major surgical procedures on abdominal aorta. Crit Care Med 7:9–13, 1979.
20. Brinkmeyer DO, Safar P, Motoyama E: Superiority of colloid over electrolyte solution for fluid resuscitation (severe normovolemic hemodilution). Crit Care Med 9:369–371, 1981.
21. Browse NL, Clemeson G, Bateman NT: Effect of IV dextran-70 and pneumatic leg compression on incidence of post-op pulmonary embolism. Br Med J 2:1281–1284, 1976.
22. Canizaro PC, Prager MC, Shires GT: The influence of Ringer's lactate solution during shock: changes in lactate, excess lactate and pH. Am J Surg 122:494–501, 1971.
23. Carey JS, Scharschmidt BF, Culliford AT: Hemodynamic effectiveness of colloid and electrolyte solutions for replacement of simulated operative blood loss. Surg Gynecol Obstet 131:679–686, 1970.
24. Carey LC, Lowery BD, Cloutier CT: Hemorrhagic shock. Curr Probl Surg 1:3–48, 1971.
25. Carrico CJ, Canizaro PC, Shires GT: Fluid resuscitation following injury; rationale for the use of balanced salt solutions. Crit Care Med 4:46–54, 1976.
26. Chinitz JL: Pathophysiology and prevention of dextran-40 induced anuria. J Lab Clin Med 77:76–87, 1971.
27. Christensen EI, Moundsback AB: Effects of dextran on lysosomal ultrastructure and protein digestion in renal proximal tubule. Kidney Int 16:301–311, 1979.
28. Coghill TH, Moore EE, Dunn EI: Coagulation changes after albumin resuscitation. Crit Care Med 9:22–26, 1981.

29. Cohn JN, Luria MH, Daddario RC: Studies in clinical shock and hypotension. V. Hemodynamic effects of dextran. *Circulation* 35:316–326, 1967.

30. Coleman RW: Paradoxical hypotension after volume expansion with plasma protein fraction. *N Engl J Med* 299:97–98, 1978.

31. Coller FA, Iob B, Vaughn HH, Kalder NM, Moyer CA: Translocation of fluid produced by intravenous administration of isotonic salt solutions in man postoperatively. *Ann Surg* 122:663–677, 1945.

32. Dahn MS, Lucas CE, Ledgerwood AM: Negative inotropic effect of albumin resuscitation for shock. *Surgery* 86:235–241, 1979.

33. Data JL, Nies AS: Dextran 40. *Ann Intern Med* 81:500–504, 1974.

34. Dawidson I, Eriksson B: Statistical evaluations of plasma substitutes based on 10 variables. *Crit Care Med* 10:653–657, 1982.

35. Dawidson I, Eriksson B, Gelin LE: Oxygen consumption and recovery from surgical shock in rats: a comparison on the efficacy of different plasma substitutes. *Crit Care Med* 7:460–465, 1979.

36. Dawidson I, Gelin LE, Haglind E: Plasma volume, intravascular protein content, hemodynamic and oxygen transport changes during intestinal shock in dogs. Comparison of relative effectiveness of various plasma expanders. *Crit Care Med* 8:73–80, 1980.

37. Dawidson I, Gelin LE, Hedman L: Hemodilution and recovery from experimental intestinal shock in rats: a comparison of the efficacy of three colloids and one electrolyte solution. *Crit Care Med* 9:42–46, 1981.

38. Diehl JT, Lester JL, Cosgrove DM: Clinical comparison of hetastarch and albumin in postoperative cardiac patients. *Ann Thor Surg* 34:674–679, 1982.

39. Diomi P: Studies on renal tubular morphology and toxicity after large doses of dextran-40 in the rabbit. *Lab Invest* 22:355–360, 1970.

40. Ebert RV, Stead EA Jr, Gibson JG: Response of normal subjects to acute blood loss with special reference to the mechanism of restoration of blood volume. *Arch Intern Med* 68:578–590, 1941.

41. Elkington JR, Danowski TS: *The Body Fluids: Basic Physiology and Practical Therapeutics.* Baltimore, Williams & Wilkins, 1955.

42. Elwyn DH, Bryan-Brown CW, Shoemaker WC: Nutritional aspects of body water dissociations in postoperative and depleted patients. *Ann Surg* 182:76–85, 1975.

43. Esrig BC, Fulton RL: Sepsis, resuscitated hemorrhagic shock and "shock lung." An experimental correlation. *Ann Surg* 182:218–227, 1975.

44. Farrales FB, Belcher C, Summers T, Bayer WL: Effect of hydroxyethyl starch on platelet function following granulocyte collection using the continuous flow cell separator. *Transfusion* 17:635–637, 1977.

45. Feest TG: Low molecular weight dextran: a continuing cause of acute renal failure. *Br Med J* 2:1300, 1976.

46. Gaisford WD, Pandey D, Jensen CG: Pulmonary changes in hemorrhagic shock. II. Ringer's solution vs. colloid infusion. *Am J Surg* 124:738–743, 1972.

47. Gallus AS, Hirsch J, O'Brien SE: Prevention of venous thrombosis with small, subcutaneous doses of heparin. *JAMA* 235:1980–1984, 1976.

48. Gelin LE, Solvell L, Zederfeldt B: Plasma volume expanding effect of low viscous dextran and macrodex. *Acta Chir Scand* 122:309–322, 1961.

49. Granger DN, Gabel JC, Drahe RE, Taylor AD: Physiologic basis for the clinical use of albumin solutions. *Surg Gynecol Obstet* 146:97–104, 1978.

50. Gruber VF, Messmer K: Colloids for blood volume support. *Prog Surg* 15:49–76, 1977.

51. Guyton AC: *Textbook of Medical Physiology,* ed 4. Philadelphia, WB Saunders, 1971.

52. Habel M: Critical care update. *Crit Care Med* 8:14–21, 1981.

53. Haupt MT, Rackow EC: Colloid osmotic pressure and fluid resuscitation with hetastarch, albumin and saline solutions. *Crit Care Med* 10:159–162, 1982.

54. Hauser CJ, Shoemaker WC, Turpin I: Oxygen transport responses to colloids and crystalloids in critically ill surgical patients. *Surg Gynecol Obstet* 150:811–816, 1980.

55. Hays RM: Dynamics of body water and electrolytes. In Maxwell MH, Kleeman CR (eds): *Clinical Disorders of Fluid and Electrolyte Metabolism.* New York, McGraw-Hill, 1972.

56. Heye JT, Janeway CA: The use of human albumin in military practice. *US Navy Med Bull* 40:785–791, 1942.

57. Holcroft JW, Trunkey DD: Extravascular lung water following hemorrhagic shock in the baboon: comparison between resuscitation with Ringer's lactate and plasmanate. *Ann Surg* 180:408–417, 1974.

58. Holcroft JW, Trunkey DD: Pulmonary extravasation of albumin during and after hemorrhagic shock in baboons. *J Surg Res* 18:91–97, 1979.

59. Janeway CA, Gibson ST, Woodruff LM: Albumin in the treatment of shock. *J Clin Invest* 23:465–475, 1944.

60. Johnson D, Lucan CE, Gerrick SJ: Altered coagulation after albumin supplements for treatment of oligemic shock. *Ann Surg* 114:379–383, 1979.

61. Kakkar VV: International multicenter trial: prevention of fatal postoperative pulmonary embolism by low doses of heparin. *Lancet* 2:45–51, 1975.

62. Kilian J, Spilker D, Borst R: Effect of 6% hydroxyethyl starch, 4.5% dextran 60 and 5.5% oxypolygelatine on blood volume and circulation in human volunteers. *Anaethesist* 24:193–197, 1975.

63. Kirklin JK, Lell WA, Kouchoukos NT: Hydroxyethyl starch vs. albumin for colloid infusion following cardiopulmonary bypass in patients undergoing myocardial revascularization. *Ann Thorac Surg* 37:40–46, 1984.

64. Klapp D, Harrison WL: Evaluation of albumin use by medical audit. *Am J Hosp Pharm* 36:1205–1209, 1979.

65. Knipping WJ (ed): *Drug Topics Redbook,* ed 90. Oradell, NJ, Medical Economics, 1986.

66. Knopp R, Claypool R, Leonardi D: Use of the tilt test in measuring acute blood loss. *Ann Emerg Med* 9(2):29–32, 1980.

67. Kohler H, Kirch W, Horstmann HJ: Hydroxyethyl starch–induced macroamylasemia. *Int J Clin Pharmacol* 15:428–431, 1977.

68. Kohler H, Kirch W, Klein H: The effect of 6% hydroxyethyl starch 450/0.7, 10% dextran 40 and 3.5% gelatin on plasma volume in patients with terminal renal failure. *Anaesthesist* 24:193–197, 1975.

69. Kohler H, Zschiedrich H, Clasen R: Blutvolumen, kolloidosmotischer Druck un Nierenfunktion von Probanden nach Infusion Mittelmolekularer 10% Hydroxyethylstarke 200/0.5 und 10% Dextran 40. *Anaesthesist* 31:61–67, 1982.

70. Kovalik SG, Ledgerwood AM, Lucas CE: The cardiac effect of altered calcium homeostasis after albumin resuscitation. *J Trauma* 21:275–279, 1981.

71. Laks H, O'Connor NE, Anderson W, et al: Crystalloid versus colloid hemodilution in man. *Surg Gynecol Obstet* 142:506–512, 1976.

72. Laks H, Pilon RN, Anderson W: Intraoperative prebleeding in man: effect of colloid hemodilution on blood volume, lung water, hemodynamics and oxygen transport. *Surgery* 78:130–137, 1975.

73. Laks H, Pilon RN, Anderson W, et al: Acute normovolemic hemodilution with crystalloid vs colloid replacement. *Surg Forum* 25:21–22, 1974.

74. Laks H, Pilon RN, Klovekorn WP: Acute hemodilution; its effects on hemodynamics and oxygen transport in anesthetized man. *Ann Surg* 180:103–109, 1974.

75. Lamke LO, Liljedahl SO: Plasma volume changes after infusion of various plasma expanders. *Resuscitation* 5:93–102, 1976.

76. Lamke LO, Liljedahl SO: Plasma volume expansion after infusion of 5%, 20%, and 25% albumin solutions in patients. *Resuscitation* 5:85–92, 1976.

77. Lazrove S, Waxman K, Shippy C: Hemodynamic blood volume and oxygen transport responses to albumin and hydroxyethyl starch infusions in critically ill post operative patients. *Crit Care Med* 8:302–306, 1980.

78. Lenz G, Hempel V, Jurger H, Worle H: Effect of hydroxyethyl starch, oxypolygelatin and human albumin on the phagocytic function of the reticuloendothelial system in healthy subjects. *Anaesthesist* 35:423–428, 1986.

79. Lee WH, Cooper N, Weidner MG: Clinical evaluation of a new plasma expander; hydroxyethyl starch. *J Trauma* 8:381–393, 1968.

80. Lewis JH, Szetol LF, Beyer WL: Severe hemodilution with hydroxyethyl starch and dextrans. *Arch Surg* 93:941–950, 1966.

81. Lewis RT: Albumin: role and discriminative use in surgery. *Can J Surg* 23:322–328, 1980.

82. Liljedahl JO, Rieger, A: Blood volume and plasma protein. IV. Importance of thoracic duct lymph in restitution of plasma volume and plasma proteins after bleeding and immediate substitution in splenectomized dogs. *Acta Chir Scand [Suppl]* 379:39–51, 1967.

83. Lorenz W, Dolniche A, Freund M: Plasma histamine levels in man following infusion of hydroxyethyl starch: a contribution to the question of allergic or anaphylactoid reactions following administration of a new plasma substitute. *Anesthesist* 24:228–230, 1975.

84. Lowe RJ, Moss GS, Jilek J, et al: Crystalloid vs. colloid in the etiology of pulmonary failure after trauma; a randomized trial in man. *Surgery* 81:676–683, 1977.

85. Lowery BD, Cloutier CT, Carey LC: Electrolyte solutions in resuscitation in human hemorrhagic shock. *Surg Gynecol Obstet* 133:273–284, 1971.

86. Lucas CE, Ledgerwood AM, Higgins RF: Impaired pulmonary function after albumin resuscitation from shock. *J Trauma* 20:446–451, 1980.

87. Lucas CE, Weaver D, Higgins RF: Effects of albumin vs. nonalbumin resuscitation on plasma volume and renal excretory function. *J Trauma* 18:564–570, 1978.

88. Maggio RA, Rha CC, Somberry ED, Praeger PI, Pasley RW, Reed GE: Hemodynamic comparison of albumin and hydroxyethyl starch in post operative cardiac surgery patients. *Crit Care Med* 11:943–945, 1983.

89. Mailoux L, Swartz CD, Capizzi R, et al: Acute renal failure after administration of LMW dextran. *N Engl J Med* 277:1113–1118, 1967.

90. Matheson NA, Diomi P: Renal failure after the administration of dextran-40. *Surg Gynecol Obstet* 131:661–668, 1970.

91. Maurer PH, Berardinelli B: Immunologic studies with hydroxyethyl starch (HES). *Transfusion* 8:265–268, 1968.

92. Metcalf W, Papadopoulos A, Talano R: Clinical physiologic study of hydroxyethyl starch. *Surg Gynecol Obstet* 131:255–267, 1970.

93. Mishler JM, Borberg H, Emerson PM: Hydroxyethyl starch, an agent for hypovolemic shock treatment. II. Urinary excretion in normal volunteers following three consecutive daily infusions. *Br J Pharmacol* 4:591–595, 1977.

94. Modig J: Effectiveness of dextran 70 vs. Ringer's acetate in traumatic shock and adult respiratory distress syndrome. *Crit Care Med* 14:454–457, 1986.

95. Moore FD, Daher FJ, Boyden CM: Hemorrhage in normal man. I. Distribution and dispersal of saline infusions following acute blood loss; clinical kinetics of blood volume support. *Ann Surg* 163:485–504, 1966.

96. Moss GS, Lower RJ, Jilek J, et al: Colloid or crystalloid in the resuscitation of hemorrhagic shock. A controlled clinical trial. *Surgery* 89:434–438, 1981.

97. Moss GS, Proctor JH, Homer LD: A comparison of asanguinous fluids and whole blood in the treatment of hemorrhagic shock. *Surg Gynecol Obstet* 129:1247–1257, 1969.

98. Moss GS, Siegel DC, Cochin A, et al: Effects of saline and colloid solutions on pulmonary function in hemorrhagic shock. *Surg Gynecol Obstet* 133:53–58, 1971.

99. Muller N, Popov-Cenic S, Kladetzky RG: The effect of hydroxyethyl starch on the intra and postoperative behavior of haemostasis. *Bibl Anat* 16:460–462, 1977.

100. Nilsson E, Lamke LO, Liljedahl SO: Is albumin therapy worthwhile in surgery for colorectal cancer? *Acta Chir Scand* 146:619–622, 1980.

101. Oh MS, Carroll HT, Goldstein DA: Hyperchloremic acidosis during the recovery phase of diabetic ketosis. *Ann Intern Med* 89:925–927, 1978.

102. O'Riordan JP: Current concepts in utilization and provision of human albumin. *Haematologia* 13:175–184, 1980.

103. Paul K, Schlesinger RG, Schanfield MS: Reaction to albumin (letter to editor). *JAMA* 245:234–235, 1981.

104. Pitts RF: Volume and composition of the body fluids. In *Physiology of the Kidney and Body Fluids*. Chicago, Year Book, 1974.

105. Poole GV, Meredity JW, Pernell T, et al: Comparison of colloids and crystalloids in resuscitation from hemorrhagic shock. *Surg Gynecol Obstet* 154:577–586, 1982.

106. Proctor HJ, Moss GS, Homer LD, et al: Changes in lung compliance in experimental shock and resuscitation. *Ann Surg* 169:82–92, 1969.

107. Puri VK, Howard M, Paidipaty B: Comparative studies of hydroxyethyl starch and albumin in hypovolemia (abstract). *Crit Care Med* 10:230, 1982.

108. Puri VK, Paidipaty B, White L: Hydroxyethyl starch for resuscitation of patients with hypovolemia in shock. *Crit Care Med* 9:833–837, 1981.

109. Reynolds M: Cardiovascular effects of large volumes of isotonic saline infused intravenously into dogs following severe hemorrhage. *Am J Physiol* 158:418–428, 1949.

110. Rice CL, Moss GS: Blood and blood substitutes: current practice. *Adv Surg* 13:93–114, 1979.

111. Ring J, Messmer K: Incidence and severity of anaphylactoid reactions to colloid volume substitutes. *Lancet* 1:466–469, 1977.

112. Ring J, Siefert J, Messmer K: Anaphylactoid reactions due to hydroxyethyl starch infusion. *Eur Surg Res* 8:389–399, 1976.

113. Risberg B, Miller E, Hughes J: Comparison of the pulmonary effects of rapid infusion of a crystalloid and a colloid solution. *Acta Chir Scand* 147:613–618, 1981.

114. Rock G, Wise P: Plasma expansion during granulocyte procurement. Cumulative effects of hydroxyethyl starch. *Blood* 53:1156–1163, 1979.

115. Rose SD: Prophylaxis of thromboembolic disease. *Med Clin North Am* 63:1205–1224, 1979.

116. Rosenoer VM, Skillman JJ, Hastings PR: Albumin synthesis and nitrogen balance in postoperative patients. *Surgery* 87:305–312, 1980.

117. Rothschild MA, Bauman A, Yalow RS: The effect of large doses of desiccated thyroid on the distribution and metabolism of albumin ^{131}I in euthyroid subjects. *J Clin Invest* 36:422–428, 1957.

118. Rothschild MA, Oratz M, Schreiber SS: Albumin metabolism *Gastroenterology* 64:324–337, 1973.

119. Rothschild MA, Oratz M, Schreiber SS: Albumin synthesis. *N Engl J Med* 286:748–756, 816–820, 1972.

120. Rothschild MA, Schreiber SS, Oratz M: The effects of adrenocortical hormones on albumin metabolism studies with albumin ^{131}I. *J Clin Invest* 37:1229–1235, 1958.

121. Rowe MI, Arango A: Colloid vs. crystalloid resuscitation in experimental bowel obstruction. *J Pediatr Surg* 11:635–643, 1976.

122. Sasahara AA, Sharma GV, Parisi AF: New develop-

ments in the detection and prevention of venous thromboembolism. *Am J Cardiol* 43:1214–1224, 1979.

123. Scattchard G, Batchelder AC, Brown A: Chemical, clinical and immunological studies on the products of human plasma fraction. VI. The osmotic pressure of plasma and serum albumin: *J Clin Invest* 23:458–464, 1944.

124. Schildt B, Bouvang RM, Sollenberg M: Plasma substitute induced impairment of the reticuloendothelial system function. *Acta Chir Scand* 141:7–13, 1975.

125. Scribner BH (ed): *University of Washington Teaching Syllabus for the Course on Fluid and Electrolyte Balance.* Seattle, University of Washington Press, 1969.

126. Sgouris JT, Rene A (eds): *Proceedings of the Workshop on Albumin, February 12–13, 1975.* Washington, DC, Department of Health, Education and Welfare, DHEW Publication No. (NIH) 76–925, 1976.

127. Shah DM, Browner BD, Dutten RE: Cardiac output and pulmonary wedge pressure, use for evaluation of fluid replacement in trauma patients. *Arch Surg* 112:1161–1164, 1977.

128. Shatney CH, Chaudry IH: Hydroxyethyl starch administration does not depress reticuloendothelial function or increase mortality from sepsis. *Circ Shock* 13:21–26, 1984.

129. Shatney CH, Deapiha K, Militello PR. Majerus TC, Dawson RB: Efficacy of hetastarch in the resuscitation of patients with multisystem trauma and shock. *Arch Surg* 118: 804–809, 1983.

130. Shires GT, Canizaro PC: Fluid resuscitation in the severely injured. *Surg Clin North Am* 53:1341–1366, 1973.

131. Shires T, Cohn D, Carrico J: Fluid therapy in hemorrhagic shock. *Arch Surg* 88:688–693, 1964.

132. Shires GT, Williams J, Brown F: Acute changes in extracellular fluids associated with major surgical procedures. *Ann Surg* 154:803–810, 1961.

133. Shoemaker WC: Comparison of the relative effectiveness of whole blood transfusions and various types of fluid therapy in resuscitation. *Crit Care Med* 4:71–78, 1976.

134. Shoemaker WC: Fluids and electrolyte problems in the adult. In Shoemaker WC, Thompson WL: *Critical Care State of the Art.* Fullerton, CA, Society of Critical Care Medicine, 1982.

135. Shoemaker WC, Bryan-Brown CW, Quigley L: Body fluid shifts in depletion and post-stress states and their correction with adequate nutrition. *Surg Gynecol Obstet* 136:371–374, 1973.

136. Shoemaker WC, Hauser CJ: Critique of crystalloid vs colloid therapy in shock and shock lung. *Crit Care Med* 7:117–124, 1979.

137. Shoemaker WC, Montgomery ES, Kaplan E: Physiologic patterns in surviving and nonsurviving shock patients. *Arch Surg* 106:630–636, 1973.

138. Shoemaker WC, Schluchter M, Hopkins JA: Comparison of the relative effectiveness of colloids and crystalloids in emergency resuscitation. *Am J Cardiol* 142:73–84, 1981.

139. Shoemaker WC, Schluchter M, Hopkins JA: Fluid therapy in emergency resuscitation; clinical evaluation of colloid and crystalloid regimens. *Crit Care Med* 9:367–368, 1981.

140. Siegel SC, Moss GS, Cochin A: Pulmonary changes following treatment for hemorrhagic shock; saline vs. colloid infusion. *Surg Forum* 21:17–19, 1970.

141. Skillman JJ: The role of albumin and oncotically active fluids in shock. *Crit Care Med* 4:55–61, 1976.

142. Skillman JJ, Hassan AK, Moore FD: Plasma protein kinetics of the early transcapillary refill after hemorrhage in man. *Surg Gynecol Obstet* 125:983–996, 1967.

143. Skillman JJ, Restall DS, Salzman EW: Randomized trial of albumin vs. electrolyte solutions during abdominal aortic operations. *Surgery* 78:291–303, 1975.

144. Skillman JJ, Rosenoer VM, Smith PC: Improved albumin synthesis in postoperative patients by amino acid infusion. *N Engl J Med* 295:1037–1040, 1976.

145. Solanke TF: Clinical trial of 6% hydroxyethyl starch (a new plasma expander). *Br Med J* 3:783–785, 1968.

146. Solanke TF, Khwaja MS, Madojemu EI: Plasma volume studies with four different plasma volume expanders. *J Surg Res* 11:140–143, 1971.

147. Stead EA Jr, Ebert RV: Studies on human albumin. In Mudd S, Thaliver W (eds): *Blood Substitutes and Blood Transfusion.* Springfield, IL, Charles C Thomas, 1942.

148. Strauss RG, Koepke JA, McGuire LC, et al: Clinical and laboratory effects on donors in intermittent flow centrifugation platelet-leukopheresis performed with hydroxyethyl starch and citrate. *Clin Lab Haematol* 2:1–11, 1980.

149. Strauss RG, Snyder EL, Stuber J, Fick RB: Ingestion of hydroxyethyl starch by human leukocytes. *Transfusion* 26:88–90, 1986.

150. Strauss RG, Stump DC, Henrikson RA: Hydroxyethyl starch accentuates von Willebrand's disease. *Transfusion* 25:235–237, 1985.

151. Strauss RG, Stump DC, Henrikson RA, Saunders R: Effects of hydroxyethyl starch on fibrinogen, fibrin clot formation and fibrinolysis. *Transfusion* 25:230–234, 1985.

152. Stump DC, Strauss RG, Henrikson RA, Peterson RE, Saunders R: Effects of hydroxyethyl starch on blood coagulation, particularly factor VIII. *Transfusion* 25:349–354, 1985.

153. Takaori M, Safar P: Acute severe hemodilution with lactated Ringer's solution. *Arch Surg* 94:67–73, 1967.

154. Takaori M, Safar P: Treatment of massive hemorrhage with colloid and crystalloid solutions. *JAMA* 199:297–302, 1967.

155. Thomas JM, Silva JR: Dextran 40 in the treatment of peripheral vascular diseases. *Arch Surg* 106:138–141, 1973.

156. Thompson WL: Rational use of albumin and plasma substitutes. *Johns Hopkins Med J* 136:220–225, 1975.

157. Thompson WL, Britton JJ, Walton RP: Persistence of starch derivatives and dextran when infused after hemorrhage. *J Pharmacol Exp Ther* 136:125–132, 1962.

158. Thompson WL, Fukushima T, Rutherford RB, et al: Intravascular persistence, tissue shortage and excretion of hydroxyethyl starch. *Surg Gynecol Obstet* 131:965–972, 1970.

159. Thompson WL, Walton RP: Circulatory responses to intravenous infusions of hydroxyethyl starch solutions. *J Pharmacol Exp Ter* 146:359–364, 1964.

160. Thoren L: The dextrans–clinical data. Joint WHO/IABS symposium on the standardization of albumin plasma substitutes and plasmaphoresis, Geneva 1980. *Dev Biol Stand* 48:157–167, 1981.

161. Trinkle JK, Rush BF, Eiseman B: Metabolism of lactate following major blood loss. *Surgery* 63:782–787, 1968.

162. Trudnowski RJ, Goel SB, Lam FT, Evers JT: Effect of Ringer's lactate solution and sodium bicarbonate on surgical acidosis. *Surg Gynecol Obstet* 125:807–814, 1967.

163. Tullis JL: Albumin. I. Background and use. *JAMA* 237:355–360, 1977.

164. Tullis JL: Albumin. 2. Guidelines for clinical uses. *JAMA* 237:460–463, 1977.

165. Virgilio RW: Crystalloid vs. colloid resuscitation (reply to letter to editor). *Surgery* 86:515, 1979.

166. Virgilio RW, Rice CL, Smith DE: Crystalloid vs colloid resuscitation: is one better? A randomized clinical study. *Surgery* 85:129–139, 1979.

167. Virgilio RW, Smith DE, Zarino DK: Balanced electrolyte solutions: experimental and clinical studies. *Crit Care Med* 7:98–106, 1979.

168. Vito L, Dennis RC, Weisel RD: Sepsis presenting as

acute respiratory insufficiency. *Surg Gynecol Obstet* 138:896–900, 1974.

169. Weatherbee L, Spencer HH, Knopp CT: Coagulation studies after the transfusion of hydroxyethyl starch protected frozen blood in primates. *Transfusion* 14:109–115, 1974.

170. Weaver DW, Ledgerwood AM, Lucas CE: Pulmonary effects of albumin resuscitation for severe hypovolemic shock. *Arch Surg* 113:387–392, 1978.

171. Weil MH, Henning RJ, Puri VK: Colloid oncotic pressure: clinical significance. *Crit Care Med* 7:113–116, 1979.

172. Weiss HJ: The effect of clinical dextran on platelet aggregation, adhesion and ADP release in man: in vivo and in vitro studies. *J Lab Clin Med* 69:37–46, 1967.

173. Weissler AM, Roehill JR, Peeler RG: Effect of posture on the cardiac response to increased peripheral demand. *J Lab Clin Med* 59:1000–1007, 1962.

174. Woodruff LM, Gobsin ST: Use of human albumin in military medicine. Clinical evaluation of human albumin. *US Navy Med Bull* 40:791–796, 1942.

175. Wong PY, Carroll RE, Lipinski TL: Studies on the renin-angiotensin-aldosterone system in patients with cirrhosis and ascites: effect of saline and albumin infusion. *Gastroenterology* 77:1171–1176, 1979.

176. Yacobi A, Stoll RG, Sum CY: Pharmacokinetics of hydroxyethyl starch in normal subjects. *J Clin Pharmacol* 22:206–212, 1982.

13

Anesthetic Pharmacology and Critical Care

Joseph P. Coyle, M.D.
David J. Cullen, M.D.

Understanding anesthetic pharmacology is important to those involved in the care of critically ill patients. Many patients are admitted to intensive care units after emergency or elective surgical procedures in which a variety of anesthetic agents have been employed. It is important to understand the kinetics, physiologic actions, and potential toxicities of anesthetic drugs during the recovery period. In addition, many anesthetic drugs are used in the routine management of intensive care patients to control pain, allay anxiety, and facilitate airway control and ventilation, and as therapy in certain clinical states. In this chapter, we describe the basic pharmacokinetics, toxicities, and pharmacodynamics of inhalational anesthetics, muscle relaxants, narcotics, sedative hypnotics, and other related drugs. The subject is vast and the reader is referred to basic texts for more detailed discussions of the subject (14, 48). We hope in this chapter to provide a working familiarity with anesthetics for the nonanesthesiologist involved in intensive care.

INHALATIONAL ANESTHETICS

In the intensive care unit, considerations relating to inhalation anesthesia deal primarily with the emergence phase. Recovery from inhalation anesthesia occurs when the partial pressure of the anesthetic in the brain is reduced to a subanesthetic level. This process occurs in two related stages: first, "washout" of anesthetic from the brain, and second, elimination of anesthetic from the lungs. The uptake, and distribution of anesthetic agents and emergence from anesthesia are described in detail elsewhere (18).

The rate of "washout" of anesthetic from the brain depends on cerebral blood flow and the relative solubility of the anesthetic in the tissue and blood, and on the difference in partial pressure of the drug between tissue and blood. When cerebral blood flow is decreased, less anesthetic is washed out of the central nervous system and emergence is slowed. Anesthetics with higher lipid solubility (halothane and enflurane) accumulate to a larger extent in the brain and take longer to move from the brain to the blood. Anesthetics with lower solubility (for example, nitrous oxide) develop less of a reservoir in the brain and move more readily to the blood. The difference in partial pressure of the anesthetic between tissue and blood is the gradient along which the drug moves. If the partial pressure gradient is small, little anesthetic is transferred from brain to blood, and emergence is slowed. This situation arises if the arterial blood is saturated with anesthetic because the lungs fail to eliminate the drug.

Elimination of inhaled anesthetic from the lungs is governed to a large extent by the same factors that govern uptake during induction of anesthesia (18). These factors include cardiac output, blood:gas solubility, and alveolar ventilation. The alveolar partial pressure of anesthetic determines the amount of anesthetic in the arterial blood perfusing the brain. A lower alveolar partial pressure produces lower arterial saturation and speeds washout from the brain. If cardiac output is reduced, less anesthetic is delivered to the alveoli, alveolar partial pressure decreases, and emergence is facilitated. This effect is more marked for more soluble agents and depends on constant ventilation and cerebral blood flow. The more soluble an anesthetic is in the blood, the longer it takes for emergence (83) (Fig. 13.1). This phenomenon occurs because larger amounts of a more soluble drug are in the tissues and the drug has less tendency to move from the blood to the gas phase. Isoflurane has a lower blood:gas solubility coefficient than halothane or enflurane (Fig. 13.1), thus allowing for quicker emer-

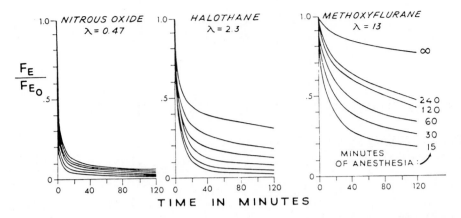

Figure 13.1   Alveolar recovery curves illustrating the effects of duration of anesthesia and solubility on rate of recovery. F_E, fraction of anesthetic in expired air, F_{E_0}, fraction of anesthetic in expired air at time 0; λ, blood:gas solubility coefficient. (From Stoelting RK, Eger EI: The effects of ventilation and anesthetic solubility on recovery from anesthesia: an in vivo and analog analysis before and after equilibration. *Anesthesiology* 30:290–296, 1969.)

gence. Less soluble anesthetics, such as nitrous oxide, have less of a reservoir in the tissues and move readily from the blood to the alveoli, hence emergence is rapid. Finally, the amount of alveolar ventilation is very important in determining the rate of emergence from inhalation anesthesia. The effect of ventilation is more marked for more soluble agents (83) (Fig. 13.2). If the patient hypoventilates while recovering from halothane, as might occur when given a narcotic for pain, emergence is slowed.

Several other factors can affect a patient's rate of recovery from inhalation anesthesia, including (a) duration of anesthesia, (b) ventilation/perfusion abnormalities, (c) changes in

solubility, (d) hypothermia, (e) metabolism, and (f) presence of other drugs.

The longer a patient has been anesthetized, the longer the time for recovery (83) because, as anesthesia proceeds, more anesthetic accumulates in muscle and fat. This fact is particularly true for the more soluble anesthetics. When areas of low ventilation/perfusion matching exist, anesthetic-rich blood is returned to the systemic circulation and emergence is slowed. Clinically, this situation is rarely important because it affects primarily low solubility agents such as nitrous oxide for which emergence is fairly rapid.

Alterations of solubility change the rate of

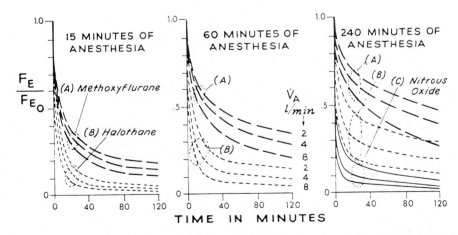

Figure 13.2   Alveolar recovery curves demonstrating the effect of varying alveolar ventilation ($\dot{V}_A$) on recovery from inhalational anesthesia. (From Stoelting RK, Eger EI: The effects of ventilation and anesthetic solubility on recovery from anesthesia: an in vivo and analog analysis before and after equilibration. *Anesthesiology* 30:290–296, 1969.)

emergence. The clearest example of this problem is hypothermia, in which solubility is increased and emergence is slowed. In addition, during hypothermia, anesthetic potency is increased and a lower partial pressure of anesthetic is required for awakening (62). For anesthetics that undergo hepatic metabolism, such as halothane and methoxyflurane, the rate of clearance from the circulation is affected by the rate of metabolism.

All of the above factors affect the rate of change of alveolar partial pressure, which in turn determines anesthetic pressure in the brain. Some factors such as hypothermia can affect the potency of anesthetics and thus delay emergence because a lower partial pressure of anesthetic in the alveoli must be achieved. Sedative/hypnotic drugs, narcotics, lidocaine hydrochloride, and certain antihypertensives such as α-methyldopa hydrochloride and clonidine hydrochloride increase the potency of inhalation anesthetics. In addition, less anesthetic is required in pregnant women and the elderly, and these patients may take longer to recover from anesthesia (28). In summary, emergence from general inhalation anesthesia is a complex process with a rate determined by many variables, including factors that affect washout of the drug, concomitant medications, and preexisting conditions of the patient.

Nitrous Oxide

Nitrous oxide is the only low solubility anesthetic gas in use today. It is nonflammable, has a molecular weight of 44, and is supplied in blue cylinders that contain the vapor over liquid. It has a blood:gas solubility coefficient of 0.47, about one-fifth of that for halothane. Because of the low solubility of nitrous oxide, a higher alveolar partial pressure is quickly achieved since little is taken by the blood. For this reason, induction and recovery from anesthesia are rapid.

Nitrous oxide is much less potent than other anesthetics. Anesthetic potency is described in terms of minimum alveolar concentration (MAC) required to prevent movement response to incision in 50% of patients. The MAC for nitrous oxide is about 105% (37), a figure that can only be achieved in a hyperbaric chamber. Although it can be used alone as an analgesic, nitrous oxide must be supplemented with another volatile anesthetic or intravenous drugs when used for operating room anesthesia.

The cardiovascular effects of nitrous oxide are variable. When used alone, there is an apparent sympathomimetic effect (21, 37, 41), which is associated with elevated circulating catecholamine concentrations, resulting in increased cardiac output and mean arterial and pulmonary artery pressures. When combined with potent inhalational anesthetics or narcotics, nitrous oxide produces moderate decreases in cardiac output and elevates systemic vascular resistence (78). There is little effect of administered nitrous oxide on respiration, although when added to halothane, tidal volume decreases and respiratory rate increases. (31).

The overall toxicity of nitrous oxide is very low, but complications with its use may arise. Diffusion hypoxia can occur during the first few minutes of emergence from nitrous oxide (24). Nitrous oxide moves rapidly from the blood to the alveoli during emergence, diluting the oxygen in the alveoli, and arterial oxygen tension drops (76). Carbon dioxide is also diluted during this period and ventilation may be depressed. Supplemental oxygen is appropriate during this time. Another consequence of the low solubility of nitrous oxide is its tendency to move from the blood into body air cavities (53). For this reason, nitrous oxide is relatively contraindicated in patients with bowel obstruction or pneumothorax, and whenever air embolism is a risk. Finally, prolonged administration of nitrous oxide results in leukopenia and megaloblastic anemia, possibly by binding to vitamin B_{12}, inhibiting methionine and DNA synthesis (56).

The Soluble Anesthetics

Since the introduction of halothane in the 1950s, the halogenated anesthetics (Table 13.1) have gradually replaced diethyl ether and cyclopropane as the most commonly used anesthetics. This trend has occurred because of the decreased toxicity of halothane, lack of explosive risk, and greater patient acceptance of halothane. Because of methoxyflurane's very high solubility, induction and emergence are slow, and because of its renal toxicity (11) it is no longer used. Therefore, our discussion of soluble anesthetics centers on the most commonly employed volatile halogenated anesthetics, halothane, enflurane, and isoflurane.

SYSTEMIC EFFECTS

Systemic arterial blood pressure is decreased by all of the halogenated anesthetics

Table 13.1
Inhalation Anesthetic Agents

Agent	Formula	Minimal Alveolar Concentration (%)	λ^a
Nitrous oxide	N_2O	105	0.47
Enflurane (Ethrane)	(structure)	1.68	1.78
Isoflurane (Forane)	(structure)	1.15	1.41
Halothane (Fluothane)	(structure)	0.76	2.3
Methoxyflurane (Penthrane)	(structure)	0.16	12.0

^{a} Blood:gas solubility coefficient.

in a dose-dependent fashion; however, the mechanism varies for each drug. Both enflurane (13) and isoflurane (79) decrease systemic vascular resistance more than halothane, and increase heart rate through the reflex baroreceptor mechanism (15). With halothane, heart rate usually remains constant or decreases because this anesthetic produces more direct myocardial depression than enflurane, with isoflurane having the least effect on inotropy (13). Patients' cardiovascular response to anesthesia often depends on their preoperative autonomic tone: those with high sympathetic tone have the greatest decrease in blood pressure and cardiac output.

Recently, isoflurane has been shown to reduce coronary vascular resistance by dilating small coronary vessels, leading to the potential for myocardial ischemia in patients with coronary artery disease (3, 6, 61). Reiz and associates (63) have demonstrated electrocardiographic and metabolic evidence of ischemia at 1% isoflurane. Restoration of aortic pressure did not relieve ischemia in three of their patients.

Although all volatile anesthetics cause respiratory depression, enflurane and isoflurane are the worst offenders, whereas halothane causes the least depression. As anesthetic level increases, there is a progressive decrease in tidal volume, with increases in respiratory rate and in $Paco_2$. The ventilatory response to carbon dioxide is decreased with all three halogenated anesthetics. Both the apneic threshold and ventilatory response to carbon dioxide are most affected when the patient is unstimulated (19). Halothane (12), enflurane (34), and isoflurane (32) depress carotid chemoreceptors, and an increase in respiratory rate with hypoxemia is completely ablated at anesthetic levels.

The halogenated anesthetics (halothane in particular) cause bronchodilation and blunt the bronchospastic response to noxious stimuli (30, 77). Halothane, enflurane, and isoflurane have been used in the treatment of refractory bronchospasm in a few select cases (58, 74, 77). The pulmonary vasoconstricting response to hypoxia is also blunted by the halogenated anesthetics, and the rate of mucociliary clearance is decreased (59). Thus, the patient recovering from inhalational anesthesia has a tendency to become hypercapneic and hypoxemic when defense mechanisms to these stresses and airway reflexes are blunted.

Changes in organ blood flow with volatile anesthetics depend on the tissue involved. All halogenated anesthetics can increase cerebral blood flow (54, 86), although the increase with isoflurane is the least, and halothane impairs cerebral autoregulation (75). The increase in cerebral blood flow can be prevented by prior hyperventilation. Renal, splanchnic, and hepatic blood flow are generally decreased by volatile anesthetics.

HEPATIC TOXICITY

Almost all anesthetics have been implicated at some time as being hepatotoxic. Hepatic dysfunction is common in the perioperative period and can range from mild elevations of serum concentration of liver enzymes to frank hepatic necrosis. It may be the result of anesthetics, hypoxia, hypotension, surgical trauma, blood transfusion, exacerbation of chronic liver disease, other drugs, or viral hepatitis, to name a few causes. The anesthetic most commonly associated with hepatic injury is halothane. Reports of postoperative jaundice and hepatic failure after the use of halothane (4, 38) prompted the National Halothane Study (87) to determine the extent of this problem. In this review of 850,000 anesthetic administrations, the incidence of halothane-related hepatotoxicity was less than 1 in 15,000 cases. The study was hampered by the inability to define a specific type of hepatotoxicity associated with halothane and an inability to control for the many other variables that could lead to hepatic injury. Animal models have been used to define and study this phenomenon and show that halothane can cause a centrilobular necrosis when hypoxia is present, hepatic blood flow is decreased, or enzymes are induced (64, 67, 81, 95). Under hypoxic conditions, reductive metabolites bind to liver proteins and membranes, resulting in liver injury (93).

RENAL TOXICITY

All of the inhalational anesthetics cause reductions in renal blood flow and glomerular filtration rate secondary to changes in cardiovascular function. These changes are transient and usually of little clinical importance. Nephrotoxicity was reported with methoxyflurane (11), related to the liberation of fluoride ion during its metabolism. The fluoride ion induces a polyuric, vasopressin-resistant, renal insufficiency. Enflurane also releases fluoride ion when metabolized, but considerably less than methoxyflurane. Mild concentrating defects are reported after prolonged exposure to enflurane (45), and it should be used cautiously in patients with preexisting renal im-

pairment. Both isoflurane and halothane contain fluoride ions, but little fluoride is released during metabolism.

MUSCLE RELAXANTS

Neuromuscular blocking drugs are used in anesthesia to facilitate intubation and to provide surgical relaxation. In the intensive care unit, muscle relaxants may be used for a variety of reasons. In intubated patients with respiratory failure, these drugs may be used to allow ventilation of patients who cannot be ventilated because of coughing or "bucking" and when attempts to match the ventilatory pattern to the patient's needs have failed. In extreme cases of hypoxic respiratory failure, muscle relaxants may be used to decrease oxygen consumption and to prevent shivering when hypothermia is employed for this purpose. Paralysis frequently results in lower peak airway pressures and increased chest wall compliance. Extremely high airway pressure and low compliance interfere with ventilatory support and place the patient at risk for barotrauma. Relaxants are often used during intubation of patients in the intensive care unit when other means of securing the airway have failed or are not possible. Less common indications for neuromuscular blockade include status epilepticus, tetanus, and botulism.

The care of the paralyzed patient presents several challenges to nurses and physicians. Although paralyzed patients do not move, they are not necessarily asleep and deserve adequate sedation and analgesia when possible. Signs of inadequate sedation and analgesia include hypertension, tachycardia, lacrimation, and diaphoresis, particularly in response to painful stimuli. Paralyzed patients require full ventilation; ventilator disconnections or mechanical failure can be fatal. Full monitoring and means to hand-ventilate the patients should be readily available at the bedside. Frequent turning of patients and attention to pressure points is necessary, and appropriate eye care must be used to prevent corneal drying and abrasions. Paralyzed patients cannot cough or swallow, so measures must be employed to ensure adequate clearing of pharyngeal and tracheal secretions. Elements of the medical history and physical examination are lost when patients are paralyzed, and this may be a factor in patients with angina, changing neurologic status, or possible peritonitis. Finally, paralyzed patients may not be able to generate a fever in response to infection, and thus sepsis becomes difficult to detect.

Anatomy and Physiology of Neuromuscular Transmission

The neuromuscular junction (Fig. 13.3) consists of an unmyelinated motor nerve terminal and a specialized area of the skeletal muscle membrane called the motor endplate. Within the nerve terminal are vesicles of acetylcholine, mitochondria, and endoplasmic reticulum. The motor endplate consists of multiple vaginations or clefts lined with acetylcholine receptors and acetylcholinesterase. As a wave of depolarization reaches the motor nerve terminal, acetycholine vesicles, in the presence of calcium, bind to the membrane and empty their contents into the synaptic cleft. The acetylcholine traverses the cleft and binds with receptors causing a miniature endplate potential (MEPP) at the receptor. If enough MEPPs occur, a wave of depolarization is set up in the muscle membrane, ultimately leading to calcium release from the sarcoplasmic reticulum and muscle contraction. Muscle relaxants act by binding to, or competing for, acetylcholine receptors and preventing depolarization of the muscle membrane.

Succinylcholine

Succinylcholine chloride is the only depolarizing relaxant in clinical use today. It acts by binding to the acetylcholine receptor, initially creating a wave of depolarization that manifests clinically as muscle fasciculations. It remains bound to the receptors, preventing subsequent binding of acetylcholine, and neuromuscular blockade results. Succinylcholine is rapidly hydrolyzed by pseudocholinesterase, and normal neuromuscular transmission is restored rapidly. Normally, the duration of apnea after the intubating dose is 10 minutes. Blockade is slightly prolonged (20–30 minutes) when low levels of normal pseudocholinesterase exist, as occurs in liver disease (25), starvation, and pregnancy (57), or in the presence of certain drugs (57) such as echothiophate iodide and cytotoxic drugs. Blockade is also prolonged in the presence of genetically atypical pseudocholinesterase, which occurs in up to 1 in 480 persons in the population (36, 92). With homozygous atypical pseudocholinesterase, blockade may last several hours.

Because of its short duration of action, succinylcholine in doses of 1–2 mg/kg is used primarily to facilitate intubation. The cardiovascular effects of succinylcholine can be explained by its stimulating effect at nicotinic

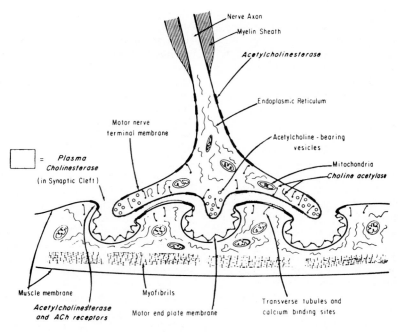

Figure 13.3 Schematic representation of neuromuscular junction. (From Ali HH, Savarese JJ: Monitoring of neuromuscular function. *Anesthesiology* 45:216, 1976).

Table 13.2
Succinylcholine Toxicities

Hyperkalemia
    Major burns
    Massive trauma
    Closed head injuries
    Intraabdominal infection
    Variety of neuromuscular diseases
Increased intragastric pressure
    Regurgitation
Increased intracranial pressure
Bradycardia
Prolonged blockade
    Abnormal pseudocholinesterase
    Overdose (phase II block)
Increased intraocular pressure
Muscle pains

Table 13.3
Muscle Relaxants

Relaxant	Intubating Dose (mg/kg)	Duration of Clinical Effect (min)
Depolarizing		
Succinylcholine	1–2	10–20
Nondepolarizing		
d-Tubocurarine	0.6	60–90
Metocurine	0.3	60–90
Pancuronium	0.1	60–90
Atracurium	0.4	30–60
Vecuronium	0.08	30–60

and muscarinic acetylcholine receptors. Sinus bradycardia frequently results because of the agonist effect of succinylcholine at cardiac muscarinic receptors (84). This effect is most marked with repeated doses of succinylcholine.

The major toxic effects of succinylcholine (Table 13.2) are due to the initial depolarization and subsequent muscle contraction. A small rise in serum potassium (0.5–1 mEq/liter) is noted with routine use of succinylcholine (90), probably due to release from skeletal muscle. Severe hyperkalemia and resultant cardiac arrest have been reported in patients with certain conditions such as major burns (73), trauma (9), closed head injuries (80), intraabdominal infection (35), and a variety of neuromuscular diseases (29). This phenomenon results from denervation hypersensitivity of the endplate due to an increase in the number of acetylcholine receptors (7). When succinylcholine is given, an exaggerated response occurs and potassium leaks from the muscle into the systemic circulation. An increase in intragastric pressure can occur with succinylcholine, probably related to contraction of abdominal muscles. This change in gastric pressure may result in regurgitation, and for that reason, cricoid pressure and pretreatment with small doses of a nondepolarizing agent are advocated to avoid aspiration.

Nondepolarizing Muscle Relaxants

The nondepolarizing muscle relaxants competitively antagonize acetylcholine; they are classified into two groups depending on duration of action (Table 13.3). The long-acting relaxants include d-tubocurarine chloride (curare), metocurine iodide (Metubine), and pancuronium bromide (Pavulon). These long-acting drugs peak 2–5 minutes after an intubating dose, with additional doses required every 45–90 minutes. The intermediate-acting relaxants, atracurium and vecuronium bromide, generally require redosing every 20–40 minutes and are therefore usually given by continuous infusion when used for long-term paralysis. All of these drugs are highly ionized with low lipid solubility, having a volume of distribution roughly equivalent to the extracellular fluid space. The relative potencies of the relaxants are reflected in the doses needed to produce intubating conditions (Table 13.3). Sensitivity to muscle relaxants varies greatly among patients, and therefore it is best to titrate relaxants to effect (71).

The route of elimination of the commonly used nondepolarizing relaxants varies and may have a bearing in selecting an agent for use in the ICU. Metocurine and gallamine rely entirely on renal excretion, resulting in prolonged paralysis in renal failure (47). Hepatic clearance of curare can occur in the presence of renal failure, making it a useful drug in these patients (8). Although pancuronium is 80% eliminated in the urine, the remaining 20% is metabolized in the liver and its duration of action is prolonged in hepatic failure (16). Up to 80% of a dose of vecuronium can be recovered in the bile, both metabolized and unchanged, therefore leading to a prolonged effect in cirrhotic patients. Atracurium is unique among the nondepolarizing relaxants in that its clearance is independent of hepatic and renal function, breakdown of the drug occurring by Hoffman elimination and ester hydrolysis (50). Hoffman elimination can be impaired in severe hypothermia and acidosis, prolonging atracurium's effect in these conditions.

The choice of muscle relaxant often depends on its cardiovascular side effects, which are best understood by knowing the affinity of the relaxants for acetylcholine receptors in autonomic ganglia and muscarinic receptors in the sinus node, and the tendency of the drug to cause histamine release (72). For example, doses of metocurine needed for neuromuscular blockade have little or no effect at sympathetic ganglia or muscarinic receptors. Therefore, metocurine has little hemodynamic effect when given in large boluses that cause mild histamine release (46). Not only does d-tubocurarine cause histamine release at usual doses but in addition, weak blockade occurs at autonomic ganglia and hypotension results (70). Pancuronium causes no ganglionic blockade, but does block muscarinic receptors, resulting in mild to moderate tachycardia. Pancuronium also is thought to have a sympathomimetic effect and often mildly increases blood pressure (82). Gallamine induces a marked tachycardia because of its potent vagolytic action (20). Atracurium can cause some histamine release, resulting in hypotension when given rapidly in large boluses. Vecuronium has no hemodynamic side effects when used in clinical doses.

Many factors affect the degree of neuromuscular blockade (Table 13.4). In terms of acid-base balance, both respiratory acidosis and metabolic alkalosis augment nondepolarizing blockade (49). In a patient recovering from anesthesia with residual neuromuscular blockade, hypoventilation leads to greater neuromuscular blockade and a downhill spiral can ensue, leading to respiratory failure. Electrolyte imbalances such as hypokalemia, hyponatremia, hypocalcemia, and hypermagnesemia

each potentiate neuromuscular blockers (1). Preexisting neuromuscular disease may greatly increase sensitivity to neuromuscular blockers. The most common examples of these diseases are myasthenia gravis and the Eaton-Lambert syndrome (1). A great variety of drugs augment the effect of muscle relaxants. The potent inhalational anesthetics all decrease the need for relaxants, as do most antiarrhythmic drugs. Several types of antibiotics, including aminoglycosides, polymyxins, neomycin, streptomycin, tetracycline, and clindamycin, accentuate relaxant-induced blockade (1). Patients with major burns require larger doses of nondepolarizing relaxants to achieve paralysis (44), as do many patients who have been immobile for prolonged periods.

Reversal of Neuromuscular Blockade

Reversal of neuromuscular blockade is achieved by administering an anticholinesterase, which interferes with hydrolytic breakdown of acetylcholine, thereby shifting the ratio of agonist:antagonist at the receptor in favor of acetylcholine. Considerable reserve for neuromuscular transmission exists such that vital capacity and inspiratory force are normal when 50% of receptors are still blocked (88). It is not known what level of residual neuromuscular blockade allows normal respiratory mechanics and effective cough, but a variety of guidelines exists. A useful clinical assessment of muscle strength is the ability to sustain head lift for 5 seconds. Less sensitive clinical tests include grip strength and tongue protrusion. Measurement of respiratory mechanics such as vital capacity and negative inspiratory force are also used to assess reversal. The most sensitive indicator of residual neuromuscular blockade is the peripheral nerve stimulator. The absolute height of a twitch in response to a single stimulus is insensitive; however, sensitivity is increased when repetitive stimuli are applied and the amount of fade is assessed (1, 2). The "train-of-four" test refers to the application of four impulses at a rate of 2/sec. Fade is evaluated by comparing the height of the fourth twitch with the height of the first twitch. A ratio of greater than 70% implies adequate reversal in most circumstances. The most sensitive test is the application of a tetanic stimulus at 100 Hz observing for fade, but this test is painful to the awake patient.

Table 13.4
Factors Potentiating Neuromuscular Blockade

Respiratory acidosis
Metabolic alkalosis
Electrolyte imbalance
   Hypokalemia
   Hyponatremia
   Hypocalcemia
   Hypermagnesemia
Preexisting neuromuscular disease
   Myasthenia gravis
   Eaton-Lambert syndrome
Drugs
   Inhalation anesthetics
   Antiarrhythmics
   Antibiotics

Rather than rely on any single index of reversal, it is best to correlate the history, clinical strength, respiratory mechanics, and twitch response when assessing residual blockade.

The anticholinesterases used most frequently are neostigmine bromide, pyridostigmine bromide, and edrophonium chloride. Neostigmine is usually given in doses up to 0.07 mg/kg. Onset occurs within 5 minutes and lasts up to 60 minutes (23, 51). Pyridostigmine, given in doses of 0.28 mg/kg, has its onset in 10 minutes and lasts up to 90 minutes (23, 51). Edrophonium can be used in doses that range from 50 to 100 mg for a 70-kg man, and has an onset slightly quicker than that of neostigmine with similar duration (23). By contrast, for supraventricular tachycardias, edrophonium is given in doses of 5–10 mg intravenously.

The major toxicity of anticholinesterases stems from the stimulation of muscarinic receptors. This manifests as excessive salivation; bradycardia, which can be severe, leading to heart block, nodal escape, and premature ventricular contractions; and bronchospasm, which may also result from unopposed muscarinic stimulation. For this reason, anticholinergics (atropine sulfate, 0.4 mg/mg of neostigmine, or glycopyrrolate, 0.2 mg/mg of neostigmine) are given simultaneously with the anticholinesterase drugs.

INTRAVENOUS ANESTHETICS

"Anesthesia" can be viewed as a physical state consisting of several component features including analgesia, amnesia, hypnosis, muscle relaxation, and control of autonomic reflex responses to noxious stimuli. This state can be induced by a single drug such as a volatile anesthetic, but to achieve this goal requires large doses that may have unwanted side effects. A second approach is to use a variety of drugs from different classes directed specifically to the components of anesthesia (i.e., narcotic for analgesia, muscle relaxants, and sedative hypnotics). This approach is termed "balanced anesthesia" and is applicable to how anesthetic drugs can be judiciously used in the ICU.

The use of specific narcotics for pain control is the subject of Chapter 26 and sedative/hypnotic drugs are discussed in Chapter 26. However, several aspects of intravenous anesthetic use warrant further mention.

Narcotics

All of the pure agonist narcotics result in dose-dependent depression of ventilation (17). Minute ventilation is decreased, resulting in an increase in arterial carbon dioxide tension, and the hypercapneic ventilatory response is blunted. Airway reflexes are obtunded, which may facilitate management of intubated patients, but poses a risk to the patient with an unprotected airway. Even small doses of morphine sulfate (7.5 mg) depress the hypoxic ventilatory response (89), and it is likely that this action occurs with other agonist narcotics as well. The agonist/antagonist narcotics have been developed to produce less respiratory depression than the pure agonists. Butorphanol tartrate (10 mg) (55) and nalbuphine hydrochloride (2 mg) (65) have respiratory effects similar to those of 10 mg of morphine; however, no further depression occurs with higher doses. Respiratory depression from narcotics is greater in the elderly (26) and in the presence of other central nervous system depressants.

Chest wall rigidity, which compromises ventilation, is a well-known side effect of rapidly administered fentanyl and sufentanil. This side effect is usually associated with the administration of fentanyl citrate and sufentanil citrate during induction of anesthesia, but it could pose a problem during use of these drugs in the intensive care unit. The rigidity is abolished by the use of muscle relaxants.

CARDIOVASCULAR EFFECTS OF NARCOTICS

The agonist narcotics have hemodynamic effects that differ among drugs. Morphine decreases arterial pressure through venous dilation and decreased central sympathetic output (40) as well as histamine release (66) and a direct effect on vascular smooth muscle. Contractility is not affected (94) and in some cases may be augmented by release of endogenous catecholamines. The undesirable hemodynamic effects of morphine may be minimized by slow administration and, if necessary, by volume infusion. Heart rate usually decreases as a result of increased vagal tone. Meperidine hydrochloride decreases central sympathetic output and has a negative inotropic effect (85), which results in decreased blood pressure. Meperidine can increase heart rate (33), probably by an anticholinergic effect since it is structurally similar to atropine. Fentanyl and sufentanil have gained popularity for use in anesthesia because they have little cardiovascular effect (69). Blood pressure may decrease slightly from a lysis of sympathetic tone manifest in decreased circulating catecholamines. Bradycardia is frequent with both drugs because of an increase in vagal tone.

USE OF NARCOTICS AS ANESTHETICS

Narcotics have traditionally been used in anesthesia to provide analgesia as part of a "balanced" anesthetic with sedative hypnotics, nitrous oxide, and muscle relaxants. Over the past 10 years, an anesthetic technique using only high doses of morphine (1 mg/kg) (39), fentanyl (50–200 µg/kg) (42), or sufentanil (5–20 µg/kg) has gained popularity. The high-dose narcotic technique usually results in smaller cardiovascular changes than traditional balanced or inhalational techniques, and for this reason is used frequently for cardiopulmonary bypass surgery and in certain high-risk patients. Narcotic anesthesia is particularly useful in patients with compromised ventricular function and in septic patients, who often do not tolerate myocardial depression from inhalation anesthesia. Ventilatory depression is prolonged after high-dose narcotics, and postoperative ventilation is mandatory, often for up to 24 hours or more. Awareness can also be a problem with high-dose narcotic techniques if hypnosis and amnesia are not provided.

PERIDURAL NARCOTICS

Considerable attention has recently been directed to peridural administration of narcotics for provision of postoperative analgesia (5, 43). This technique has advantages over systemic narcotic use because much less drug is required and the cardiovascular and respiratory effects are minimal. The resulting analgesia is profound and can last for more than 24 hours with intrathecal morphine. Unlike local anesthetics, there is no loss of motor function with peridural narcotics nor is there sympathetic blockade. Spinal opiates are thought to act on specific opiate receptors in the dorsal horn of the spinal cord, since little narcotic reaches the systemic circulation.

For postoperative pain relief the usual routes of administration are intrathecally in the lumbar subarachnoid space or epidurally in the lumbar or thoracic regions. The drugs most commonly employed are preservative-free morphine (0.01 mg/kg in the cerebrospinal fluid or 5–10 epidurally) or fentanyl (0.1 mg in the epidural space). Morphine has a slow onset (up to 1 hour) and a long duration of action, usually lasting over 24 hours. Fentanyl acts in 15–30 minutes, with clinical pain relief lasting 2–6 hours (10).

Complications of peridural narcotics include acute and delayed respiratory depression, pruritus, urinary retention, and nausea. The delayed respiratory depression is primarily reported with the use of morphine and can occur up to 20 hours after injection. It is thought to result from rostral spread of the drug in the cerebrospinal fluid reaching the respiratory center. The respiratory depression is easily reversed with naloxone hydrochloride titrated to effect, without diminishing the analgesia produced at the spinal cord level. Naloxone is given initially in 0.1-mg increments to reverse respiratory depression, then given as an infusion of 0.1 µg/kg/hr for up to 24 hours after administration of the peridural narcotic.

Thiopental

Sodium thiopental (Pentothal) is an ultra-short-acting barbiturate that is widely used in anesthetic practice as an intravenous induction drug. Sodium thiopental is provided as a 2.5% solution that is strongly basic (pH 10.6). The usual dose for induction of anesthesia is 3–5 mg/kg, although less drug may be needed in sicker patients and in the elderly. At usual doses, loss of consciousness occurs in 1–2 minutes and lasts 20–30 minutes. The rapid decay in blood and brain concentrations of thiopental is a result of rapid redistribution to muscle and fat (68). The elimination of thiopental is slow, with an elimination half-life of about 5 hours (52). Elimination occurs almost entirely via hepatic metabolism. A large fraction of circulating thiopental is bound to serum proteins (60–96%). In patients who are depleted of serum proteins, more free thiopental is available for diffusion into brain and heart, thus prolonging sleep times and enhancing cardiovascular depression (27).

The cardiovascular effects of thiopental include a dose-dependent depression of contractility, venous pooling, decreasing preload, and an increase in systemic vascular resistance (22). All of these effects combine to produce a decrease in cardiac output, which is accentuated in hypovolemic patients and in patients with preexisting myocardial dysfunction. Thiopental, like all barbiturates, is a respiratory depressant frequently inducing apnea in clinical use. Thiopental decreases cerebral metabolism and oxygen consumption and causes a decrease in cerebral blood flow (60), which makes thiopental particularly useful in managing patients with increased intracranial pressure and patients at risk for regional cerebral ischemia.

Ketamine

Ketamine hydrochloride is a "dissociative" anesthetic with limited usefulness in clinical practice because of cardiovascular stimulating properties and its short duration of action. The anesthetic state produced by ketamine is marked by a type of catalepsy in which the eyes may remain open, often with nystagmus and intact corneal reflexes. There may be occasional nonpurposeful movements. In low doses (0.2–0.3 mg/kg) ketamine produces analgesia with little change in the level of consciousness. Ketamine is also used to induce anesthesia in doses of 1–2 mg/kg and results in a rapid onset within 2 minutes, lasting 20–30 minutes. Redistribution accounts for the relatively short duration of action; elimination is almost entirely dependent on hepatic metabolism (96).

Ketamine usually increases heart rate and blood pressure through sympathomimetic actions resulting from central nervous system stimulation (91). In isolated muscle preparations, ketamine has direct myocardial depressant properties. Myocardial depression from ketamine can frequently be seen in critically ill patients when sympathomimetic effects are insufficient to counter the myocardial depression. Ketamine in usual doses does not produce respiratory depression. It decreases airway resistance and blocks bronchospasm, probably because of its sympathomimetic effects (91). Ketamine increases airway secretions and, although airway reflexes are thought to be intact, aspiration can occur. An increase in both cerebral blood flow and oxygen utilization is noted with ketamine, and thus it is contraindicated in patients with elevated intracranial pressure (96).

The most common side effects of ketamine are postanesthetic emergence reactions, which can manifest as vivid dreams, hallucinations, and frank delirium. These adverse actions can be minimized by pretreating the patient with benzodiazepines. The only other major toxicity of ketamine is the tachycardia and hyper-

tension that can result from ketamine-induced sympathetic stimulation.

References

1. Ali HH, Savarese JJ: Monitoring of neuromuscular function. *Anesthesiology* 45:216, 1976.
2. Ali HH, Utting JE, Gray C: Stimulus frequency in the detection of neuromuscular block in humans. *Br J Anesth* 42:967, 1970.
3. Becker LC: Is isoflurane dangerous for the patient with coronary artery disease? *Anesthesiology* 66:259, 1987.
4. Brody GL, Sweet RB: Halothane anesthesia as a possible cause of massive hepatic necrosis. *Anesthesiology* 24:29, 1963.
5. Bromage PR, Camporesi E, Chestnut D: Epidural narcotics for post-operative analgesia. *Anesth Analg* 59:473, 1980.
6. Buffington CW, Romson JL, Levine A, et al: Isoflurane induces coronary steal in a canine model of chronic coronary occlusion. *Anesthesiology* 66:280, 1987.
7. Carter JG, Sokoll MD, Gergis SD: Effect of spinal cord transection on neuromuscular function in the rat. *Anesthesiology* 55:542, 1981.
8. Cohen EN, Brewer HW, Smith D. The metabolism and elimination of d-tubocurarine-H³. *Anesthesiology* 28:309, 1967.
9. Cooperman LH: Succinylcholine-induced hyperkalemia in neuromuscular disease. *JAMA* 213:1867, 1970.
10. Cousins MJ, Mather LE: Intrathecal and epidural administration of opioids. *Anesthesiology* 61:276, 1984.
11. Crandell WB, Pappas SG, MacDonald A: Nephrotoxicity associated with methoxyflurane anesthesia. *Anesthesiology* 27:591, 1966.
12. Davies RO, Edward SMW, Lahiri S: Halothane depresses the response of carotid body chemoreceptors to hypoxia and hypercapnia in the cat. *Anesthesiology* 57:153, 1982.
13. Delaney TJ, Kistner JR, Lake CL, et al: Myocardial function during halothane and enflurane anesthesia in patients with coronary artery disease. *Anesth Analg* 59:240, 1980.
14. Dripps RD, Eckenhoff JE, Vandam LD: *Introduction to Anesthesia—The Principles of Safe Practice.* Philadelphia, WB Saunders, 1972.
15. Duke PC, Fownes D, Wade JG: Halothane depresses baroreflex control of heart rate in man. *Anesthesiology* 46:184, 1977.
16. Duvaldestin P, Agoston S, Henzel D, et al: Pancuronium pharmacokinetics in patients with liver cirrhosis. *Br J Anaesth* 50:1131, 1978.
17. Eckenhoff JE, Oech SR: The effects of narcotics and antagonists upon respiration and circulation in man. *Clin Pharmacol Ther* 1:483, 1960.
18. Eger EI II: *Anesthetic Uptake and Action.* Baltimore, Williams & Wilkins, 1974.
19. Eger EI II, Dolan WM, Stevens WC, et al: Surgical stimulation antagonizes the respiratory depression produced by Forane. *Anesthesiology* 36:544, 1972.
20. Eisele JH, Marta JA, Davis HS: Quantitative aspects of the chronotropic and neuromuscular effects of gallamine in anesthetized man. *Anesthesiology* 35:630, 1971.
21. Eisele JH, Smith NT: Cardiovascular effects of 40% nitrous oxide in man. *Anesth Analg* 51:956, 1972.
22. Etsten B, Li TH: Hemodynamic changes during thiopental anesthesia in humans. Cardiac output, stroke volume, total peripheral resistance and intra-thoracic blood volume. *J Clin Invest* 34:500, 1955.
23. Ferguson A, Egerzegi P, Bevan DR: Neostigmine, pyridostigmine and edrophonium as antagonists of pancuronium. *Anesthesiology* 53:390, 1980.
24. Fink BR: Diffusion anoxia. *Anesthesiology* 16:511, 1955.

25. Foldes FF, Rendell-Baker L, Birch JH: Causes and prevention of prolonged apnea with succinylcholine. *Anesth Analg* 35:609, 1956.

26. Foldes FF, Siverdlow M, Siker SS: *Narcotics and Narcotic Antagonists.* Springfield IL, Charles C Thomas, 1964.

27. Ghoneim MM, Pandya HB, Kelley SE, et al: Binding of thiopental to plasma proteins: effects on distribution in the brain and the heart. *Anesthesiology* 45:635, 1976.

28. Gregory GA, Eger EI II, Munson ES: The relationship between age and halothane requirement in man. *Anesthesiology* 30:488, 1969.

29. Gronert GA, Theye RA: Pathophysiology of hyperkalemia induced by succinylcholine. *Anesthesiology* 43:89, 1975.

30. Hirshman CA, Bergman NA: Halothane and enflurane protect against bronchospasm in an asthma dog model. *Anesth Analg* 57:629, 1978.

31. Hornbein TF, Martin WE, Bonica JJ, et al: Nitrous oxide effects on the circulatory and ventilatory responses to halothane. *Anesthesiology* 31:250, 1969.

32. Kieraszewicz H, Knill RL, Clement JL: Chemical regulation of ventilation during isoflurane sedation and anaesthesia (abstract). *Can Anaesth Soc J* 28:507, 1981.

33. King BD, Elder JD, Dripps RD: The effect of the intravenous administration of meperidine upon the circulation of man and upon the circulatory response to tilt. *Surg Gynecol Obstet* 94:591, 1952.

34. Knill RL, Manninen PH, Clement JL: Ventilation and chemoreflexes during enflurane sedation and anesthesia in man. *Can Anaesth Soc J* 26:353, 1979.

35. Kohlschutter B, Baur H, Roth F: Suxamethonium-induced hyperkalemia in patients with severe intra-abdominal infections. *Br J Anaesth* 48:557, 1976.

36. Lehmann H, Lidell J: Human cholinesterase (pseudocholinesterase): genetic variants and their recognition. *Br J Anaesth* 41:235, 1969.

37. Leighton KM, Koth B: Some aspects of the clinical pharmacology of nitrous oxide. *Can Anaesth Soc J* 20:94, 1973.

38. Lindenbaum J, Leifer E: Hepatic necrosis associated with halothane anesthesia. *N Engl J Med* 268:525, 1963.

39. Lowenstein E, Hallowell P, Levine FH, et al: Cardiovascular response to large doses of intravenous morphine in man. *N Engl J Med* 281:1389, 1969.

40. Lowenstein E, Whiting RB, Bittar DA, et al: Local and neurally mediated effects of morphine on skeletal muscle vascular resistance. *J Pharmacol Exp Ther* 180:359, 1972.

41. Lunn JK, Liu WS, Stanley TH, et al: Peripheral vascular and cardiac effects of nitrous oxide in the bovine. *Can Anaesth Soc J* 24:571, 1977.

42. Lunn JK, Stanley TH, Eisele J, et al: High dose fentanyl anesthesia for coronary artery surgery. *Anesth Analg* 58:390, 1979.

43. Martin R, Salbaing J, Blaise G, et al: Epidural morphine for post-operative pain relief: a dose response curve. *Anesthesiology* 56:423, 1982.

44. Martyn JAJ, Szyfelbein SK, Ali HH, et al: Increased d-tubocurarine requirement following major thermal injury. *Anesthesiology* 52:352, 1980.

45. Mazze RI, Calverley RK, Smith NT: Inorganic fluoride nephrotoxicity: prolonged enflurane and halothane anesthesia in volunteers. *Anesthesiology* 46:265, 1977.

46. McCullough LS, Stone WA, Delaunois AL, et al: The effect of dimethyl tubocurarine iodide on cardiovascular parameters, postganglionic sympathetic activity and histamine release. *Anesth Analg* 51:554, 1972.

47. Meijer DKF, Weitering JG, Vermeer A, et al: Comparative pharmacokinetics of d-tubocurarine and metocurine in man. *Anesthesiology* 51:402, 1979.

48. Miller RD: *Anesthesia,* ed 2. New York, Churchill Livingstone, 1986.

49. Miller RD, Roderick LL: Acid-base balance and neostig-

50. Miller RD, Rupp SM, Fisher DM, et al: Clinical pharmacology of vecuronium and atracurium. *Anesthesiology* 61:444, 1984.

51. Miller RD, Van Nyhuis LS, Eger EI II, et al: Comparative times to peak effect and durations of action of neostigmine and pyridostigmine. *Anesthesiology* 41:27, 1974.

52. Morgan DJ, Blackman GL, Paull JD, et al: Pharmacokinetics and plasma binding of thiopental. I. Studies in surgical patients. *Anesthesiology* 54:468, 1981.

53. Munson ES: Transfer of nitrous oxide into body air cavities. *Br J Anaesth* 46:202, 1974.

54. Murphy FL, Kellell EM, Johnstone RE, et al: The effects of enflurane, isoflurane and halothane on cerebral blood flow and metabolism in man. *Abstracts of Scientific Papers,* American Society of Anesthesiologists Meeting, 1974, pp. 62–63.

55. Nagashima H, Karamanian A, Malovany R, et al: Respiratory and circulatory effects of intravenous butorphanol and morphine. *Clin Pharmacol Ther* 19:738, 1976.

56. Nunn JF, Chanarin I: Nitrous oxide and vitamin B_{12}. *Br J Anaesth* 50:1089, 1978.

57. Pantuck EJ, Pantuck CB: Cholinesterases and anticholinesterases. In Katz RL (ed): *Muscle Relaxants.* New York, Elsevier, 1975.

58. Parnass SM, Feld JM, Chamberlin WH, et al: Status asthmaticus treated with isoflurane and enflurane. *Anesth Analg* 66:193, 1987.

59. Pavlin EG: Respiratory pharmacology of inhaled anesthetic agents. In Miller RD (ed): *Anesthesia.* New York, Churchill Livingstone, 1981, vol 2.

60. Pierce EC, Lambertsen CJ, Deutsch S, et al. Cerebral circulation and metabolism during thiopental anesthesia and hyperventilation in man. *J Clin Invest* 41:1664, 1962.

61. Priebe HJ, Foex P: Isoflurane causes regional myocardial dysfunction in dogs with critical coronary artery stenoses. *Anesthesiology* 66:293, 1987.

62. Regan MJ, Eger EI II: Effect of hypothermia in dogs on anesthetizing and apneic doses of inhalational agents. *Anesthesiology* 28:689, 1967.

63. Reiz S, Balfors E, Sorensen MB, et al: Isoflurane: a powerful coronary vasodilator in patients with coronary artery disease. *Anesthesiology* 59:91, 1983.

64. Reynolds ES, Moslen ET: Halothane hepatotoxicity: enhancement by polychlorinated biphenyl pre-treatment. *Anesthesiology* 47:19, 1977.

65. Romagnoli A, Keats AS: Ceiling effect for respiratory depression by nalbuphine. *Clin Pharmacol Ther* 27:478, 1980.

66. Rosow CE, Moss J, Philbin DM, et al: Histamine release during morphine and fentanyl anesthesia. *Anesthesiology* 56:93, 1982.

67. Ross WT Jr, Daggy BP, Cardell RR Jr: Hepatic necrosis caused by halothane and hypoxia in phenobarbital-treated rats. *Anesthesiology* 51:327, 1979.

68. Saidman LJ, Eger EI II: The effect of thiopental metabolism on duration of anesthesia. *Anesthesiology* 27:118, 1966.

69. Sanford TJ, Smith NT, Dec-Silver H, et al: A comparison of morphine, fentanyl, and sufentanil anesthesia for cardiac surgery. Induction, emergence and extubation. *Anesth Analg* 65:259, 1986.

70. Savarese JJ: The autonomic margins of safety of metocurine and d-tubocurarine in the cat. *Anesthesiology* 50:40, 1979.

71. Savarese JJ: Clinical use of muscle relaxants. *Weekly Anesthesiol Update* 2(16):2, 1978.

72. Savarese JJ, Philbin DM: Cardiovascular effects of neuromuscular blocking agents. *Int Anesthesiol Clin* 17:13, 1979.

73. Schaner PJ, Brown RL, Kirksey TD, et al: Succinylcho-

line-induced hyperkalemia in burned patients. *Anesth Analg* 48:764, 1969.

74. Schwartz S: Treatment of status asthmaticus with halothane. *JAMA* 251:2688, 1984.

75. Shapiro HM: Intracranial hypertension: therapeutic and anesthetic considerations. *Anesthesiology* 43:445, 1975.

76. Sheffer L, Steffenson JL, Birch AA: Nitrous oxide induced diffusion hypoxia in patients breathing spontaneously. *Anesthesiology* 37:436, 1972.

77. Shnider SM, Papper EM: Anesthesia for the asthmatic patient. *Anesthesiology* 22:886, 1961.

78. Stanley TH: Nitrous oxide: new concepts about an old agent. *Anesthetic Update Series*, No. 16, 1978.

79. Stevens WC, Cromwell TH, Halsey MJ, et al: The cardiovascular effects of a new inhalation anesthetic, Forane, in human volunteers at constant arterial carbon dioxide tension. *Anesthesiology* 35:8, 1971.

80. Stevenson PH, Birch AA: Succinylcholine-induced hyperkalemia in a patient with closed head injury. *Anesthesiology* 51:89, 1979.

81. Stock JGL, Strunin L: Unexplained hepatitis following halothane. *Anesthesiology* 63:424, 1985.

82. Stoelting RK: The hemodynamic effects of pancuronium and d-tubocurarine in anesthetized patients. *Anesthesiology* 36:612, 1972.

83. Stoelting RK, Eger EI II: The effects of ventilation and anesthetic solubility on recovery from anesthesia: an in vivo and analog analysis before and after equilibration. *Anesthesiology* 30:290, 1969.

84. Stoelting RK, Peterson C: Heart rate slowing and junctional rhythm following intravenous succinylcholine with and without intramuscular atropine pre-anesthetic medication. *Anesth Analg* 54:705, 1975.

85. Strauer BE: Contractile responses to morphine, piritramide, meperidine and fentanyl: a comparative study of effects on the isolated ventricular myocardium. *Anesthesiology* 37:304, 1972.

86. Stulken EH, Milde JH, Michenfelder JD, et al: The nonlinear responses of cerebral metabolism to low concentrations of halothane, enflurane, isoflurane and thiopental. *Anesthesiology* 46:28, 1977.

87. Subcommittee on the National Halothane Study of the Committee on Anesthesia. National Academy of Sciences—National Research Council: Summary of the National Halothane Study. *JAMA* 197:775, 1966.

88. Waud BE, Waud DR: The relation between tetanic fade and receptor occlusion in the presence of competitive neuromuscular block. *Anesthesiology* 35:456, 1971.

89. Weil JV, McCullough RE, Kline JS, et al: Diminished ventilatory response to hypoxia and hypercapnia after morphine in normal man. *N Engl J Med* 292:1103, 1975.

90. Weintraub HD, Heisterkamp DV, Cooperman LH: Changes in plasma potassium concentration after depolarizing blockers in anesthetized man. *Br J Anaesth* 41:1048, 1969.

91. White PF, Way WL, Trevor AJ: Ketamine—its pharmacology and therapeutic uses. *Anesthesiology* 56:119, 1982.

92. Whittaker M: Genetic aspects of succinylcholine sensitivity. *Anesthesiology* 32:143, 1970.

93. Widger LA, Gandolfi AJ, Van Dyke RA: Hypoxia and halothane metabolism in vivo: release of inorganic fluoride and halothane metabolite binding to cellular constituents. *Anesthesiology* 44:197, 1976.

94. Wong KC, Martin WE, Hornbein TF, et al: The cardiovascular effects of morphine sulfate with oxygen and nitrous oxide in man. *Anesthesiology* 38:542, 1973.

95. Wood M, Berman ML, Harbison RD, et al: Halothane-induced hepatic necrosis in triiodothyronine-pretreated rats. *Anesthesiology* 52:470, 1980.

96. Zsigmond ED, Domino EF: Ketamine: clinical pharmacology, pharmacokinetics and current clinical uses. *Anesthesiol Rev* 7:13, 1980.

14

Use and Administration of Blood and Components

Patricia T. Pisciotto, M.D.
Edward L. Snyder, M.D., F.A.C.P.

Transfusion of the specific portion of whole blood required to treat a patient's disease is the main concept behind blood component therapy. This form of hemotherapy has evolved as a result of our ability to fractionate a single unit of whole blood into its component parts while maintaining a sterile "closed" system. The use of plastic collection containers with integrally attached satellite or transfer bags for separation of components has provided the means of avoiding an "open" collection system, which would limit the shelf-life of any blood component to a maximum of 24 hours (51). The appropriate elective and emergency use of blood and components is an area of increasing importance in critical care medicine. The various blood components available (Table 14.1) are reviewed here, in terms of their composition, indications and contraindications for use, potential adverse effects, and appropriate administration and dosage. In addition, we cover the varied nature of transfusion reactions and discuss general aspects of the administration of blood and components.

BLOOD COMPONENTS AND DERIVATIVES

Whole Blood

Product Description

A unit of whole blood has an approximate volume of 500 ml. It consists of red blood cells, a buffy coat of nonviable leukocytes and platelets, plasma, and an anticoagulant-preservative. Whole blood has a hematocrit of 35–40%. The amount of preservative solution added to the primary collection container is sufficient to anticoagulate 450 ± 50 ml of blood. Whole blood must be stored between 1° and 6°C in a monitored refrigerator; its shelf-life varies with the anticoagulant used. Blood collected in citrate-phosphate-dextrose (CPD) preservative can be stored up to 21 days. The 63 ml of CPD anticoagulant present in each collection bag contains 1.66 g of sodium citrate, 1.6 g of dextrose, 206 mg of citric acid, and 140 mg of sodium biphosphate. Dextrose supports glycolysis, bicarbonate maintains pH, and phosphate supports generation of adenosine triphosphate (ATP), which is necessary for red cell viability. The preservative CPD adenine-1 (CPDA-1), which allows storage of blood for 35 days, differs from CPD in that it contains 2 g of dextrose as well as 17.3 mg of adenine (66). The adenine present in CPDA-1 is an additional substrate used for the synthesis of greater levels of ATP, resulting in improved red cell viability (shelf-life) for CPDA-1–preserved blood (35 days) compared with CPD (21 days) (73). The amount of citrate present in both preservatives is sufficient to bind ionized calcium in the volume of donor blood collected, thus preventing activation of the coagulation system.

The concentration of 2,3-diphosphoglycerate (2,3-DPG) in stored red cells is important, since 2,3-DPG is required for hemoglobin to maintain its capacity to carry and release oxygen (60). The level of this compound is dependent on the arterial pH; as the pH falls, 2,3-DPG levels decline creating a high-oxygen-affinity hemoglobin. Blood collected and stored in CPD or CPDA-1 maintains a pH that preserves the level of 2,3-DPG (14).

Indications and Contraindications

Whole blood serves as a volume expander while simultaneously providing red cells to

Table 14.1
Blood Components[a,b]

Component/Product	Composition	Approx. Volume (ml)	Indications
Whole blood	RBC; plasma; WBC; platelets	500	Increase both red cell mass and plasma volume (WBC and platelets not functional; plasma deficient in labile clotting factors V, VIII)
Red blood cells	RBC; reduced plasma, WBC and platelets	250	Increase red cell mass in symptomatic anemia (WBC and platelets not functional)
Red blood cells, adenine-saline added	RBC; reduced plasma, WBC and platelets; 100 ml of additive solution	330	Increase red cell mass in symptomatic anemia (WBC and platelets not functional)
Leukocyte-poor RBC (prepared by filtration, centrifugation or saline washed)	RBC; few WBC and platelets; minimal plasma	200	Increase red cell mass; minimize febrile or allergic (if washed) reactions due to leukocyte antibodies or plasma proteins
Frozen-thawed-deglycerolized RBC	RBC; minimal WBC and platelets; no plasma	180	Increase red cell mass; minimize febrile or allergic transfusion reactions; used for rare blood storage
Granulocyte-platelet concentrate (centrifugation leukapheresis)	Granulocytes; lymphocytes; platelets ($>1.0 \times 10^{10}$ PMN/unit; $>2.0 \times 10^{11}$ platelets/unit); some RBC	220	Provide granulocytes for septic leukopenic patients; platelets present will treat thrombocytopenia (24-hour shelf-life)
Platelet concentrate (random donor)	Platelets; some WBC; plasma ($>5.5 \times 10^{10}$ platelets/unit); some RBC	50	Bleeding due to thrombocytopenia or thrombocytopathy (5-day shelf-life)
Platelet concentrate (single-donor platelet-pheresis)	Platelets; some WBC; plasma; ($>3 \times 10^{11}$ platelets/unit); some RBC	300	Bleeding due to thrombocytopenia in patients with HLA antiplatelet antibodies; product often HLA matched (24-hour or 5-day shelf-life; varies with storage bag)
Fresh frozen plasma	Plasma; all coagulation factors; complement (no platelets)	220	Treatment of some coagulation disorders
Liquid plasma	Plasma; stable clotting factors; no platelets	220	Treatment of stable clotting factor deficiencies (II, VII, IX, X, XI)
Cryoprecipitate-depleted plasma (modified plasma)	Plasma; stable clotting factors; no platelets	200	Treatment of stable clotting factor deficiencies (II, VII, IX, X, XI)
Cryoprecipitated AHF	Fibrinogen; factors VIII and XIII, von Willebrand factor; fibronectin	15	Deficiency of factor VIII (hemophilia A), factor XIII, fibrinogen; treatment of von Willebrand's disease
Lyophilized VIII	Factor VIII	25	Hemophilia A (VIII deficiency)
Lyophilized II, VII, IX, X	Factors II, VII, IX, X	25	Hereditary II, VII, IX, or X deficiency
Antiinhibitor coagulation complex	Factor VIII bypassing activity	30	Patients with antibody to factor VIII (note: indications for use not well established)
Albumin/plasma protein fraction	Albumin, some α, β globulins	(5%); (25%)	Volume expansion
Immune serum globulin	IgG antibodies	Varies	Treatment of hypo- or agammaglobulinemia; disease prophylaxis
Rh immune globulin	IgG anti-D	1	Prevention of hemolytic disease of the newborn due to D antigen

[a] From Snyder EL (ed): *Blood Transfusion Therapy.* Arlington, VA, American Association of Blood Banks, 1987, pp 4–5.
[b] RBC, red blood cells; WBC, white blood cells; PMN, polymorphonuclear leukocyte; AHF, antihemophilic factor.

carry oxygen to the tissues. It is indicated for patients suffering from a combined deficit of oxygen-carrying capacity (red cell mass) and hypovolemia, such as occurs in hemorrhagic shock when there is greater than 25% loss of blood volume. It may also be used for exchange transfusions in neonatal and pediatric patients.

The use of whole blood is contraindicated in patients with chronic anemia who are normovolemic, since fluid overload with subsequent congestive heart failure can occur. Neither is it indicated solely to replace blood volume; this can be better replenished using other volume expanders such as albumin or dextran, which do not transmit disease.

Whole blood is a source of stable coagulation proteins, but not the labile coagulation factors V and VIII. Accordingly, it should not be used to correct deficits of factors V and VIII, which occur in disseminated intravascular coagulation (DIC) (9). After 24 hours of storage, the platelets and granulocytes present in a unit of whole blood are no longer viable. Appropriate components, not whole blood, should be used to supply these cellular constituents when medically indicated. Fresh whole blood less than 24 hours old is not used in modern medicine. It is rarely available (because of the time required to process and test donated blood) and it is not indicated as the component of choice for any illness requiring blood transfusion. Appropriate use of specific blood components is the approach taken in contemporary critical care hemotherapy.

Adverse Reactions

There are several risks associated with transfusion of whole blood, as well as other blood components, which should be carefully considered when making the decision to transfuse any patient. These include hemolytic, allergic, and febrile reactions as well as circulatory overload and transmission of various infectious diseases. The hazards of transfusion are discussed in detail below.

Dosage and Administration

Transfused whole blood must be ABO identical with the recipient and must be administered through a blood filter (51). The volume and rate of the transfusion depend on the clinical status of the patient; infusion time, however, should not exceed 4 hours. Each unit of whole blood should raise the hemoglobin of a 70-kg adult by 1 g/dl or the hematocrit by 3%.

Red Blood Cells

Product Description

Red blood cells are separated from the plasma in whole blood by centrifugation or sedimentation. Plasma is transferred to an attached sterile bag, leaving the red cell component in the primary collection bag. A unit of red cells intended for transfusion consists of an approximate volume of 220 ml with a hematocrit (Hct) between 70 and 80% (4). The platelets and granulocytes remaining in the product are nonfunctional. Red blood cells must be stored between 1° and 6°C in a monitored refrigerator. The shelf-life depends on the anticoagulant present in the container used to collect the unit of whole blood: 21 days for CPD, 35 days for CPDA-1.

Indications and Contraindications

Transfusion of red blood cells is indicated for correction of symptomatic anemia such as may occur in bone marrow failure. This blood component supplies the same oxygen-carrying capacity (red cell mass) as the original whole blood unit. It is preferred to whole blood for treating patients with cardiac disease or renal failure in whom excess volume or sodium may be detrimental. A patient's clinical status and not a predetermined hemoglobin or hematocrit level should dictate when a transfusion is necessary. The amount of blood to be transfused also depends on the amelioration of symptoms. If a patient clinically improves after the infusion of a single unit of red cells, regardless of the hematocrit level achieved, the risks versus the benefits of further transfusion should be carefully considered. The concept of the single-unit red cell transfusion as an unnecessary transfusion is no longer valid; if it is used appropriately it can also be good medical practice.

Red blood cell transfusions are contraindicated in compensated anemias or when the patient is clinically stable and the red cell deficit can be corrected, over time, with specific hematinics such as iron, vitamin B_{12}, or folic acid. It is also generally considered inappropriate to transfuse chronically ill patients with the anemia of chronic disease (Hct, 32–36%). Nor is it acceptable to transfuse postoperative surgical patients with hematocrits of 28–34% merely to promote "wound healing."

Adverse Reactions

Reactions similar to those occurring with whole blood can also occur with the transfusion of red blood cells. The main benefit derived from removing the plasma is a decrease in the risk of fluid overload. The potential for disease transmission is similar to that of whole blood.

Administration and Dosage

Red blood cells, from which most of the original plasma and therefore most of the ABO alloantibodies have been removed, must be ABO compatible but not necessarily ABO identical with the recipient. The addition of approximately 50–100 ml of 0.9% sodium chloride (USP) to red blood cells prior to infusion is acceptable in order to reduce viscosity and increase the flow rate (51). The volume and rate of transfusion should be determined by the patient's clinical status. However, the infusion time for a unit of blood or components should not exceed 4 hours. A blood filter must be used. In a 70-kg adult, the transfusion of 1 unit of red blood cells should raise the hemoglobin concentration by 1 g/dl and the hematocrit by 3%. In a child, the transfusion of 10 ml of red cells per kilogram of body weight should raise the hemoglobin by 3 g/dl and the hematocrit 9–10% (70).

Additive Solutions

Additive solutions are used in conjunction with the anticoagulant present in the primary bag during the collection of whole blood. They increase red blood cell shelf-life and decrease the viscosity (Hct) of the transfused product. During the preparation of red blood cells from whole blood, a major portion of the plasma as well as the anticoagulant-preservative solution is removed as part of component processing. With an additive-solution system, the additive solution contained in one of the attached satellite containers is added to the separated red blood cells via the integrally attached closed system tubing. The solutions usually consist of additional dextrose and adenine in approximately 100 ml of isotonic saline. The extra adenine is required to maintain acceptable red

cell function for up to 42 days of storage. Additive-solution formula one (AS-1) (Adsol-Fenwal Corporation, Deerfield, IL), consists of 2.2 g of dextrose, 27 mg of adenine, and 0.75 g of mannitol in 100 ml of 0.9% sodium chloride. The mannitol serves to stabilize the red blood cell membrane (22). AS-3 (Nutricel-Cutter Biological, Emeryville, CA) contains in 100 ml of solution, 1100 mg of dextrose, 410 mg of sodium chloride, 42 mg of citric acid, 558 mg of sodium citrate, 276 mg of sodium phosphate, and 30 mg of adenine. The primary anticoagulant in AS-3 is CP2D, which contains citric acid, sodium phosphate, and 5110 mg of dextrose—twice that found in CPDA-1 and hence the designation CP2D (53). The hematocrit of red blood cells mixed with an additive solution is approximately 55–65%, thus allowing a rapid flow rate similar to that of whole blood. The final volume of these additive-solution red cell units is approximately 350 ml. Because of the presence of additional adenine these units can be stored for 42 days at 1–6°C. The posttransfusion in vivo survival of red cells stored for 42 days in these solutions is comparable with that of red cells stored for 35 days in CPDA-1 (23) or 21 days in CPD. Additive-solution red cells have the same indications and contraindications, adverse reactions, and administration and dosage requirements as does whole blood. Since most of the plasma with its ABO alloagglutinins has been removed, however, additive-solution units need only be ABO compatible with the recipient, not ABO identical as is necessary with whole blood. Most physicians consider additive-solution red cell units as suitable for pediatric patients even though the units contain additional adenine. If desired, the units can be centrifuged and the supernatant additive solution removed prior to transfusion. Rejuvenating solutions, which may be added near the end or shortly after the expiration date of a red blood cell unit, are available. These solutions, which are rarely used in blood banks because of the availability of indated blood, are intended to increase the levels of 2,3-DPG and ATP in order to restore red cell function and in vivo survival (18).

Leukocyte-Poor Red Blood Cells

Product Description

The leukocytes and platelets contained in units of whole blood or red blood cells can produce febrile transfusion reactions. Removal of the buffy coat can lessen or prevent these reactions, which are most likely to occur in multiply transfused patients or multiparous women. Several techniques are used to remove leukocytes from either whole blood or red blood cells, including inverted centrifugation, filtration, or cell washing (39). Regardless of the procedure used, it must ensure that at least 70% of the original leukocytes are removed and that 70% of the original red cell mass remains in the product (51). Units prepared by filtration or washing techniques have a 24-hour outdate since the primary collection bag must be entered, thus creating an "open" system. Washing of red cell units generally removes a greater percentage of leukocytes than does filtration or centrifugation. Cell washing also removes almost all of the original plasma.

Indications and Contraindications

Leukocyte-poor red cells are indicated for anemic patients with a history of recurrent febrile reactions. Since febrile reactions are usually related to transfusion rate and dose, inverted centrifugation or filtration of units to remove the buffy coat usually prevents further febrile reactions. If reactions continue with these products, presumably because of the small residual of buffy coat, it may be necessary to utilize washing techniques. Washing of red cell units may also be indicated for patients with paroxysmal nocturnal hemoglobinuria or those with serious allergic reactions to plasma, such as patients with IgA deficiency who have IgG, anti–Ig-A antibodies. Transfusion of any red cell component is generally contraindicated in well-compensated anemia.

Adverse Reactions

Adverse reactions relating to transfusion-transmitted diseases are similar to those occurring with red blood cells. Febrile reactions occur less frequently with leukocyte-poor units.

Administration and Dosage

Administration and dosage are the same as for red blood cells. Since washed red cells have a slightly decreased red cell mass compared with an unwashed unit of red blood cells, after an infusion of washed cells the rise in posttransfusion hematocrit may be reduced. Washed red cells must still be administered through a filter.

Deglycerolized Red Blood Cells

Product Description

Red blood cells can be preserved for an extended period of time by the addition of a cryoprotective agent, glycerol. The red cells are then frozen, usually at $-70°C$, and can be stored for up to 3 years; American Association of Blood Banks Standards permit storage for up to 7 years (51). The glycerol that enters the red cell protects the membrane from the hypertonic conditions occurring in the cell membrane as pure water freezes (38). Prior to transfusion, red cells that have been frozen must be thawed and washed with a graded series of saline and glucose solutions in order to remove the glycerol (deglycerolization). The deglycerolized-washed red cells, containing at least 80% of the original red cell mass (51), are suspended in isotonic saline to a volume of approximately 180 ml and a hematocrit of 50–70%. The washing process removes practically all of the original leukocytes, platelets, and plasma. Since the deglycerolization technique, with its multiple washing steps, creates an open system, the reconstituted red cell units have a shelf-life of 24 hours when stored at 1–6°C. The function and survival of these red cells are comparable with those of the unit when originally frozen.

Indications and Contraindications

The largest use of frozen blood today is for storage of rare blood types either for autologous use or for individuals who develop multiple antibodies. The indications for transfusion are basically similar to those for leukocyte-poor red cells, that is, the patient with a history of recurrent febrile or severe allergic transfusion reactions who shows symptoms of tissue oxygen deprivation (chest pain or ST segment depression on an electrocardiogram). Use of this blood product is contraindicated when the patient is clinically stable and the anemia can be corrected by other therapeutic modalities. Frozen-thawed-deglycerolized red blood cells are expensive and are not indicated for routine use or for use after one or two febrile transfusion reactions; washed or microaggregate filtered red cells are recommended for these situations.

Adverse Reactions

Adverse reactions associated with transfusion of red cells, such as immune hemolysis, transmission of hepatitis (B and non-A, non-B), and acquired immune deficiency syndrome (AIDS), can also occur with deglycerolized red cells. In addition, intravascular hemolysis can result from failure to remove residual glycerol (40).

Administration and Dosage

Because of the slightly reduced red cell mass remaining after washing, the posttransfusion increment in hematocrit may be lower than that achieved with a unit of red blood cells. Administration is similar to that for red blood cells; a blood filter must be used.

Platelet Concentrates

RANDOM-DONOR PLATELETS

Product Description

Platelet concentrates are prepared in a closed system from individual units of whole blood. A two-stage centrifugation technique is utilized in which platelet-rich plasma is first separated from donor red cells, followed by the removal of plasma from a platelet button formed by the second centrifugation. Platelet concentrates contain at least 5.5×10^{10} platelets suspended in a sufficient amount of the original plasma to maintain a pH of 6.0 or greater throughout its storage period (51). For platelets stored at 20–24°C, a plasma volume between 50 and 60 ml is usually required with the storage time restricted to a maximum of 5 days. Both constant gentle agitation and maintenance of a pH above 6.0 are essential to preserve platelet function during storage (55). Platelets can also be stored at 1–6°C suspended in 20–30 ml of plasma. However, to maintain optimal posttransfusion viability and function, since the microtubule apparatus is destroyed in the cold, the storage time is set at a maximum of 48 hours. Platelets are rarely stored at 1–6°C today.

Indications and Contraindications

Platelet transfusions are indicated for patients who are bleeding as a result of thrombocytopenia secondary to decreased platelet production, or in some cases, increased platelet destruction. However, in many of these latter cases, such as in DIC, platelet transfusion may fail to raise the platelet count. Platelet transfusions are also indicated for patients with abnormally functioning platelets. Platelet concentrates may be useful in massively transfused patients who are bleeding because of dilutional thrombocytopenia (platelet count less than 40,000/μl), or as a prophylactic measure to prevent serious hemorrhage in patients with low platelet counts (usually less than 15,000/μl) resulting from chemotherapy or malignancy.

Platelet transfusions are not indicated in patients with bleeding due to a deficiency or defect in a plasma factor or in patients with an anatomic vascular lesion. Platelet transfusions are not indicated, and usually not beneficial, in patients who are thrombocytopenic, because of rapid immune platelet destruction, such as in autoimmune thrombocytopenic purpura (AITP). In these cases, despite the thrombocytopenia, the patient's bone marrow usually shows megakaryocyte hyperplasia. Thus, the patient cannot keep up with platelet losses despite a substantial increase in endogenous production of platelets by the bone marrow. The relatively small number of transfused exogenous platelets are unlikely to be of value in such patients. However, their use could be considered for a limited clinical trial when bleeding is life-threatening and there is little else to offer. Efforts to correct the primary cause of the thrombocytopenia are usually more effective in raising the patient's platelet count. A National Institutes of Health Consensus Conference was held to review the indications for platelet transfusions (43).

Adverse Reactions

Many of the complications of transfusion, such as febrile and allergic reactions or circulatory overload, also occur with the transfusion of platelets. An order for platelet transfusion involves transfusing multiple, usually 4–8, individual units of platelets. Accordingly, the risk of adverse reactions, such as disease transmission, is directly proportional to the number of donor exposures (units).

Platelets possess not only ABO antigens but also HLA and platelet-specific antigens on their surface. Patients receiving repeated platelet transfusions may develop antibodies to antigens in the latter two systems, causing rapid destruction of transfused platelets. In some situations the patient may become refractory to all but HLA-matched platelets (32). Often even HLA-matched platelets lose their effectiveness, usually because of development of additional antiplatelet or HLA antibodies not identified.

Platelets do not possess Rh antigens. However, platelet concentrates contain a small amount of red blood cells that do possess Rh antigens. Rh-negative patients receiving platelets from an Rh-positive donor may become immunized by the contaminating Rh-positive red blood cells. For this reason, the administration of Rh immune globulin to prevent Rh immunization should be considered whenever the transfusion of Rh-positive concentrates to Rh-negative women of child-bearing potential is unavoidable. The transfusion of platelets that are ABO-incompatible with the patient's red blood cells may result in the development of a positive direct antiglobulin test and, rarely, hemolysis due to the presence of ABO isoagglutinins in the plasma contained in the platelets. This situation is particularly likely to occur in children, who have smaller blood volumes (44).

Administration and Dosage

Although it may be desirable to transfuse ABO type–specific platelets in order to maximize platelet recovery (3) and avoid potential hemolysis from incompatible plasma, if the patient's clinical status warrants an *immediate* transfusion, any platelets available, regardless of ABO type, should be used; pretransfusion testing is not required. There is no standard dose of platelets. Usually in an adult 6–8 units should be adequate, and in a child 0.1 unit/kg is a reasonable guideline. Platelet concentrates may be pooled prior to transfusion, but once pooled must be infused within 4–6 hours (51). The rate of infusion depends on the patient's clinical condition; but, platelets, like all blood components, must be infused within a 4-hour period. A blood filter is required for administration.

The effectiveness of a platelet transfusion can be monitored by assessing for cessation of bleeding, correction of the bleeding time, or presence of a posttransfusion platelet increment. In a 70-kg adult, 1 unit of random donor platelets usually results in a platelet increment of 5,000 to 10,000/μl (17). The expected response to platelets is not sustained if the patient's clinical condition results in either rapid platelet destruction (e.g., in patients with fever, sepsis, autoimmunization, or alloimmunization) or consumption (e.g., in those with DIC or hypersplenism). In order to evaluate whether a patient is truly refractory to random

donor platelets on the basis of alloimmunization, the platelet count must be monitored at approximately 1 hour after the transfusion, since counts obtained 12–24 hours later reflect platelet survival rather than an initial response to transfusion (13).

SINGLE-DONOR PLATELETS

Product Description

Therapeutic doses of platelets can be harvested from one individual by plateletpheresis. Platelet units obtained by an apheresis procedure usually contain more than 3×10^{11} platelets, which is the equivalent of six random donor platelet concentrates (51). The final product may have a plasma volume ranging from 200 to 300 ml. The number of contaminating red blood cells and lymphocytes present in the component varies depending on the cell separator utilized for the apheresis procedure and whether an additional centrifugation step was performed after the collection. Platelets prepared by apheresis using an open system have a 24-hour outdate. If a product is prepared in a closed system it may be stored at room temperature with continuous agitation for up to 5 days. As with random donor platelets, in order to maintain viability, the pH of the concentrate must be maintained at 6.0 or higher.

Indications and Contraindications

Single-donor platelet concentrates are indicated in patients who have been found to be refractory to random donor platelets as a result of alloimmunization, usually to HLA system antibodies (54). The donors who are chosen to provide this component are HLA-matched with the patient. The use of random (unmatched) single-donor platelets in this situation would likely be of no benefit. When patients have increased destruction of platelets for reasons other than alloimmunization (e.g., hypersplenism, fever, sepsis, DIC, AITP), the use of single-donor platelets (HLA-matched or unmatched) would be no more effective than random-donor platelets (50).

Adverse Reactions

The adverse reactions that occur with random-donor platelets can also be observed with the use of single-donor platelets.

Administration and Dosage

Since a substantial quantity of plasma from the single donor is used to resuspend platelets obtained by apheresis, the donor plasma should be ABO-compatible with the recipient's red blood cells. If the component is contaminated with red blood cells (5 ml or more), pretransfusion compatibility must be performed (51). Concerns about Rh antigens are the same for single-donor platelet products as for random-donor platelets.

In the absence of any clinical conditions known to be associated with a decreased platelet survival, 1 unit of single-donor platelets can be expected to raise the platelet count in a 70-kg adult by 30,000–60,000/μl. A blood filter must be used during administration.

Granulocyte Concentrates

Product Description

Granulocyte concentrates are prepared by centrifugation leukapheresis of a single donor. Each product contains a minimum of 1×10^{10} granulocytes with varying amounts of lymphocytes and red cells and is usually suspended in 200 ml of plasma. Hydroxyethyl starch, a sedimenting agent (also a volume expander), is often present in the concentrate as well.

Indications and Contraindications

Granulocytes are indicated for individuals with bone marrow hypoplasia, neutropenia of less than 500 granulocytes/μl and fever or sepsis unresponsive to appropriate antibiotic therapy. Prophylactic use of granulocytes is thought to be of little value (69). Indeed, use of granulocytes is declining generally as data have shown that appropriate antibiotic therapy may be more effective than granulocyte transfusion (61), probably because of the inability to transfuse sufficient granulocytes to be of value clinically. Granulocytes are rarely used today except in septic neonatal patients, when the number of granulocytes given may actually provide a significant amount in comparison to the infant's small size. Although still available, granulocyte concentrates are now of little use to the intensive care physician.

Adverse Reactions

Chills, fever, and allergic reactions often occur, as may hypotension. These reactions may be so severe as to require discontinuation of the concentrates.

Dose and Administration

Granulocytes must be administered through a blood filter. Depth microaggregate filters must be avoided. The product should be used as soon as it is available, and must be used within 24 hours of collection. Granulocyte concentrates should be stored when necessary at 20–24°C without agitation.

Fresh Frozen Plasma

Product Description

Fresh frozen plasma is prepared from whole blood by separating and freezing the plasma within 6 hours of phlebotomy. It may be stored for up to 1 year at −18°C or lower. The typical unit contains a volume of 200–230 ml. When frozen, factors V and VIII, the labile clotting factors, deteriorate to a minimal extent. Fresh frozen plasma is to be used only to provide replacement coagulation therapy. One milliliter of fresh frozen plasma contains approximately 1 unit of coagulation factor activity.

Indications and Contraindications

The indications for use of fresh frozen plasma are primarily in individuals with multiple coagulation factor problems often secondary to liver disease or DIC or due to massive transfusion and dilutional coagulopathy. All of these patients have documentable coagulopathies. It is also indicated for patients with congenital factor deficiencies, such as V or XI for which coagulation concentrates are not available. Fresh frozen plasma should *not* be used to provide volume expansion if this is the only indication for its use. Such an abuse of fresh frozen plasma exposes the recipient unnecessarily to the risks of hepatitis, AIDS, and other transfusion-transmitted diseases. Volume expanders without the same potential for infection, such as albumin, plasma protein fraction, crystalloid, or colloid, are preferred. Fresh frozen plasma is not to be used as a source of protein. A National Institutes of Health Consensus Conference outlined the appropriate indications for use of fresh frozen plasma (42).

Adverse Reactions

The problem with using fresh frozen plasma to treat patients with coagulopathies is the possibility of fluid overload. Treatment of severe coagulopathies with fresh frozen plasma, since it is not a concentrate, may require infusion of large amounts of plasma; fluid overload thus becomes a concern. Today, virus-inactivated heat and/or solvent/detergent-treated coagulation factor concentrates for hemophilia A and B (factor VIII and factor IX) are available, and their use may be preferred over fresh frozen plasma even in mild cases, as recommended by the National Hemophilia Society. Fresh frozen plasma has a risk of hepatitis and AIDS transmission equal to that of whole blood. Allergic reactions, febrile reactions, and noncardiogenic pulmonary edema may occur.

Dose and Administration

The dose of fresh frozen plasma depends on the clinical situation. Evaluation of coagulation status pre– and post–plasma infusion is important. This evaluation can be achieved by monitoring of a prothombin time, partial thromboplastin time, or specific factor assay. Fresh frozen plasma must be given through a filter; once thawed it should be used as soon as possible, and must be used within 24 hours of thawing. Compatibility testing is not required, but ABO-compatible fresh frozen plasma should be used.

Liquid Plasma

Liquid plasma is a blood component obtained by separating plasma from whole blood, any time up to 5 days after the expiration date of the unit of blood. It contains all the stable coagulation factors but has reduced levels of labile factors V and VIII. The indications for this plasma are for treatment of patients with deficiencies of stable coagulation factors and not for individuals with documented factor V or factor VIII deficiencies. The contraindications and precautions, dosage and administration are the same as for fresh frozen plasma.

Cryoprecipitated Antihemophilic Factor

Product Description

Cryoprecipitate is prepared by thawing fresh frozen plasma at 4°C. After thawing, a white precipitate forms that contains the cryoprecipitable proteins, factor VIII and fibrinogen. This material is concentrated by centrifugation and

stored in 10–15 ml at −18°C or lower. It has a shelf-life of 1 year.

Indications and Contraindications

Cryoprecipitate is primarily used to provide fibrinogen or factor VIII or as a source of factor VIII:von Willebrand factor (vWF) for individuals with von Willebrand's disease. Some factor XIII is also present because of the small amount of plasma contained in the cryoprecipitate. Each bag contains about 80–120 units of factor VIII:C and about 250 mg of fibrinogen. Fibrinogen concentrates, per se, are no longer available because of the risk of hepatitis associated with preparation of that blood fraction. Currently, the main source of fibrinogen is cryoprecipitate. Fibronectin, another cryoprecipitable protein, is also present. This opsonin may play a role in reticuloendothelial cell function to help clear foreign particles and bacteria from blood (49). However, the clinical value of fibronectin is as yet uncertain, and the risk of use of fibronectin from a pooled plasma source may outweigh any potential advantages of reticuloendothelial cell clearance (59).

Additional controlled clinical trials involving fibronectin are needed to determine its role in critical care medicine. Cryoprecipitate does not contain factor V. It should not be used to treat patients with deficiencies of clotting factors other than factor VIII:C, fibrinogen, von Willebrand's factor, or factor XIII. It should not be used as the sole source of coagulation factor replacement to treat DIC. ABO-compatible cryoprecipitate should be used whenever possible.

Adverse Reactions

Infusion of large amounts of ABO-incompatible cryoprecipitate can cause a positive direct antiglobulin test and rarely hemolysis. The risk of hepatitis and AIDS for each unit (bag) of cryoprecipitate is the same as that for a unit of whole blood. If large amounts are given, fibrinogen levels may become markedly increased and hyperfibrinogenemia can occur. Febrile and allergic reactions can occur as with any blood component.

Dose and Administration

Prior to infusion, cryoprecipitate is thawed, pooled, and administered through a standard blood filter. No compatibility testing is required. The dose of cryoprecipitate required is calculated by the following formulas:

40 ml/kg body weight × body weight in kg =
plasma volume (PV)

Factor VIII to be transfused =
PV × % increase in factor VIII level desired

To determine the number of bags of cryoprecipitate, the number of units of factor VIII needed is divided by 80, the minimum acceptable factor VIII activity in a unit of cryoprecipitate.

Coagulation Factor Concentrates

Product Description

Concentrates of factor VIII, IX, and antiinhibitor coagulation complex are available. They are prepared from pools of plasma collected from thousands of donors. Currently, these products are heat treated to decrease the risk of AIDS transmission. Some newer products are also treated with a solvent/detergent formula to render them less likely to transmit non-A, non-B hepatitis.

Indications and Contraindications

These products are indicated for individuals with factor VIII or factor IX deficiency or patients with high-titer antibodies to factor VIII who require factor VIII inhibitor–bypassing activity. The use of the antiinhibitor coagulation complex for this latter purpose should be undertaken only after consulting a qualified hematologist or physician familiar with its use. Patients with factor VIII inhibitor titers over 10 Bethesda units are considered candidates for treatment with antiinhibitor coagulation complex. A porcine factor VIII material for treatment of hemophiliacs with antibodies to factor VIII:C has also been licensed by the U.S. Food and Drug Administration. At present, the National Hemophilia Advisory Council advises that heat-treated or otherwise viral-attenuated factor VIII and factor IX may be the preferred products for treatment of patients in groups for which the use of cryoprecipitate or plasma was previously recommended. Whenever possible, 1-desamino-8-D-arginine vasopressin (dDAVP) is used to stimulate factor VIII production in patients with mild or moderate hemophilia and in patients with von Willebrand's disease. The dosage recom-

mended is 0.3 μg/kg body weight given as an intravenous drip over 15 minutes (35). The exact mechanism of action is unclear, but likely involves release of factor VIII and von Willebrand's factor from endothelial cells and other storage sites. dDAVP should not be used to treat patients with type IIB von Willebrand's disease, since platelet aggregation may be induced. Recent data suggest a role for dDAVP in acquired hemostatic disorders such as uremia (35).

Adverse Reactions

With use of large amounts of coagulation factor concentrates, anti-A and anti-B alloagglutinins present in the product can cause a positive direct antiglobulin test in non–group O recipients. Allergic and febrile reactions can occur, as noted for cryoprecipitate infusions.

Dose and Administration

All coagulation factor concentrates must be infused through a blood filter or through a filter needle supplied with the concentrate. The dose can be calculated using the units listed on the bottle label.

Albumin and Plasma Protein Fraction

Product Description

Albumin and plasma protein fraction (PPF) are initially obtained from donor plasma removed from whole blood or from plasmapheresis. The plasma is processed commercially by a cold alcohol-acid fractionation (Cohn) process in which it is separated from other blood proteins. Albumin contains 96% albumin and 4% globulins; PPF contains 83% albumin and 17% globulins. Both products are heated at 60°C for 10 hours to inactivate the hepatitis B virus as well as the HIV virus. Albumin for infusion is available as a 25% or 5% solution. Each has a sodium content of about 145 mEq/liter, and the 5% solution is osmotically and oncotically equivalent to plasma.

Indications and Contraindications

The indications for the administration of PPF or albumin to patients who are hypovolemic are described in Chapter 12. Neither albumin nor PPF should be used as a source of protein (56, 67). However, they are useful for supporting the intravascular volume in hypotensive individuals or in individuals undergoing procedures such as paracentesis or thoracentesis. In individuals with burns, albumin use is not indicated during the first 24 hours because of capillary leak. After the first 24 hours, in the presence of hypoproteinemia, albumin infusion is considered appropriate. Albumin or PPF transfusions are not effective in raising serum albumin levels in individuals with acute or chronic liver failure, and they are not effective in mobilizing ascites. They are, however, useful for treating hypotension in individuals with these conditions. For individuals in circulatory shock with serum albumin levels below 2.5 g/dl or total protein concentrations below 5.2 g/dl, albumin might be useful; it is probably of little value for treatment of patients with the adult respiratory distress syndrome, since albumin infusion does not effectively remove fluid from the pulmonary interstitial space.

Adverse Reactions

Complications associated with albumin administration relate to its use as a volume expander and the resulting potential for fluid overload. Other reported side effects include flushing, urticaria, chills, fever, and headache.

Administration and Dosage

As noted on the package insert, PPF is contraindicated for intraarterial administration or infusion during cardiopulmonary bypass when the lungs are removed from the perfusion circuit. Albumin is not intended to correct chronic hypoalbuminemia associated with a protein-losing enteropathy or nephropathy. It should not be used for long-term therapy, nor should it be used in total parenteral nutrition solutions. Administration of albumin and PPF does not require use of a blood filter since these derivatives are filtered at the manufacturing plant.

Blood bank physicians have removed fresh frozen plasma from the list of acceptable general volume expanders, because of the risk of transfusion-transmitted diseases, leaving albumin and PPF as the main therapeutic agents. Cost-conscious hospital administrators, however, may remove albumin and PPF from this list in an attempt to decrease inflated hospital budgets. This removal would leave synthetic colloids (such as hydroxyethyl starch or dextran) or crystalloid solutions for volume expansion. A combined approach involving the judicious and appropriate use of albumin, nonalbumin colloids, or crystalloid solutions is probably most acceptable to all parties and will likely be adopted as the optimal therapeutic approach as medicine enters the 1990s.

Acellular Oxygen-Carrying Compounds

PERFLUOROCARBON COMPOUNDS

Over the past decade much research has been undertaken to develop an "artificial blood." Perfluorocarbon emulsions have been developed that carry oxygen at high partial pressures of oxygen ($Fio_2, 1.0$) (20, 26, 30). Perfluorocarbons are derived from hydrocarbons, with fluorine substituted for hydrogen. These compounds have the ability to dissolve oxygen to a greater degree than does water. Perfluorocarbons carry oxygen in a physically dissolved form, not chemically combined, as is the case with hemoglobin. The perfluorocarbons, however, are immiscible with blood and form gaseous emboli, and therefore must be emulsified. Pluronic F-68, a nonionic detergent, is used as an emulsifier to maintain the emulsion in a stable form. In addition, yolk phospholipids and a variety of salts as well as hydroxyethyl starch are added, and the pH of the final product adjusted to 7.4. The final product is known as Fluosol-DA and patented by the Green Cross Corporation, Osaka, Japan. Perfluorocarbon emulsions have not been licensed by the FDA because the compounds have not been shown to be more effective than simple volume expansion for increasing tissue oxygenation. Pluronic present in Fluosol-DA activates complement and produces respiratory insufficiency. In addition, unless the patient is receiving an Fio_2 above 0.6, insufficient amounts of oxygen are carried to the tissues. Other problems associated with the perfluorocarbons include concern over long-term retention of the emulsion in the reticuloendothelial system and the rapid clearance of some perfluorocarbons from the vasculature because of a short half-life. Perfluorocarbon emulsions are not yet licensed for clinical transfusion. Other roles for perfluorocarbons being pursued include their use in increasing tissue oxygenation to ischemic brain tissue in patients with stroke, and in providing oxygen to ischemic myocardial tissue in patients with recent myocardial infarctions. It is also being evaluated for use in sickle cell anemia, as an ingredient in cardioplegia solutions, and for treatment of oxygen-sensitive neoplasms.

STROMA-FREE HEMOGLOBIN

Another acellular oxygen-carrying compound being developed is stroma-free hemoglobin (15, 26, 30). This material is prepared by osmotically lysing outdated red cells and preparing the stroma-free hemoglobin by various filtration and crystallization procedures. Major problems with stroma-free hemoglobin relate to the loss of 2,3-DPG after rupture of the cell membrane. This loss of 2,3-DPG shifts the P_{50} of the oxyhemoglobin dissociation curve to the left. In an attempt to shift the curve further to the right to provide a better oxygen-carrying compound, pyridoxal-5-phosphate has been added to the stroma-free hemoglobin. The pyridoxal-5-phosphate fits into the pocket in the hemoglobin molecule normally occupied by the 2,3-DPG. This alters the steric configuration of the hemoglobin molecule, permitting more efficient O_2 binding and shifting the curve more to the right, thus more toward normal (15). In an attempt to decrease the oncotic pressure of denatured stroma-free hemoglobin, the material has been polymerized with, for example, glutaraldehyde. This pyridoxylated, polymerized stroma-free hemoglobin may be clinically useful. Disadvantages of stroma-free hemoglobin solution include potential renal toxicity due to the inability to completely remove red cell stroma, a still existing left shift in the O_2-hemoglobin dissociation curve, a short intravascular half-life, and a high oncotic pressure. Development of a pyridoxylated, polymerized form of stroma-free hemoglobin, however, has reduced many of these effects. The possible transmission of infectious diseases including hepatitis and AIDS by stroma-free hemoglobin is being evaluated. Other concerns yet to be evaluated relate to the blockade of the reticuloendothelial system and the effect on the immune system of the infusion of multiple human hemoglobins. Thus far, neither perfluorocarbon emulsions nor stroma-free hemoglobin solutions have been licensed by the FDA or approved for human use. For general clinical use, stroma-free hemoglobin seems to be the most promising of the two acellular oxygen-carrying products. Its major use may be in cases of trauma and for military applications.

TRANSFUSION REACTIONS: ADVERSE EFFECTS OF BLOOD TRANSFUSION

Several risks are associated with the transfusion of whole blood and the various blood components (Table 14.2). These reactions are

Table 14.2
Risks Associated with Transfusion

Hazards	Cause	Prevention
Immediate		
Hemolysis		
Immunologic	Usually ABO incompatibility due to clerical error associated with patient misidentification	Appropriate patient identification prior to and during transfusion through the use of identification bracelets
Nonimmunologic	Mechanical lysis, overheating of blood, use of hypotonic i.v. fluids	Use of monitored blood warmers. Use of 0.9% sodium chloride only, when transfusing blood. Check with manufacturer to determine suitability of infusing packed cells with blood pump.
Febrile reaction	Antibody to leukocyte or platelet proteins	Washed or microaggregate filtered blood. For platelet or granulocyte infusions, premedicate with antipyretics and use a slow rate of infusion, 100 mg hydrocortisone i.v. for severe reactions.
Allergic reaction	Antibody to plasma proteins	Washed cells or premedication with diphenhydramine
Urticarial	Localized reaction in the skin involving transfused plasma proteins	Premedication with diphenhydramine

Table 14.2 (continued)

Hazards	Cause	Prevention
Allergic reaction (*continued*) Anaphylactoid	IgA deficiency with presence of IgG, anti-IgA antibody	Washed cells or use of IgA-deficient plasma or platelet concentrate collected from IgA-deficient donors
Bacterial contamination	Improper collection or storage of blood or components	Use of proper techniques of storage. Scrupulous attention to sterile technique during blood collection.
Fluid overload	Too much volume infused too quickly	Consider patient's volume, use of red blood cells in euvolemic patients, transfusion of smaller aliquots of blood. Judicious use of diuretics.
Noncardiogenic pulmonary edema	HLA or antileukocyte or platelet antibodies	Washed cells
Delayed Hemolysis	Usually non-ABO incompatibility due to Rh, Kell, or other non-ABO blood group systems	Use of antigen-negative blood. Avoid clerical errors involving patient identification.
Transmission of infectious diseases	Viruses causing hepatitis B, non-A, non-B hepatitis, AIDS, malaria, CMV	Decreased use of unnecessary blood components. Use of heat-treated products when available. Prevention through use of hepatitis B vaccine. Use of washed cells in individuals susceptible to CMV.
Alloimmunization	Transfusion of multiple units of blood or components	Decreased use of unnecessary blood components
Iron overload	Infusion of massive numbers of red cells over time	Desferrioxamine (iron chelation therapy)
Posttransfusion purpura	Anti-PL^{A1} antibody	Self-limited
Graft-versus-host disease	Transfusion of viable immunocompetent lymphocytes into an immunoincompetent host	In susceptible immuno-suppressed individuals, irradiation of blood or components with ≥1500 rads gamma irradiation

either immediate or acute, which could rapidly compromise patients in an already unstable condition, or may present as a delayed complication of transfusion. Physicians and paramedical personnel must correctly assess the potential risks of transfusion compared with its benefits in each individual patient, as well as recognize the many varied complications of transfusion therapy.

Immediate Adverse Reactions

IMMUNE HEMOLYSIS

An acute hemolytic transfusion reaction occurs when a patient receives a unit of blood containing antigens for which he or she already possesses a sufficient level of antibody to produce an immediate antigen-antibody reaction. If the reaction causes fixation of complement to C9, such as occurs with the ABO system, an acute intravascular reaction ensues with resulting hemoglobinemia and hemoglobinuria. If only IgG is fixed to the cell or if complement is fixed only to C3b, an acute extravascular reaction occurs. Immunologically mediated acute intravascular hemolytic transfusion reactions, although rare, are one of the most clinically severe complications of blood transfusion. Although an undetected or "missed" serologic incompatibility may occasionally account for a reaction, the most common cause of a hemolytic transfusion reaction is a clerical or patient identification error resulting in an ABO-incompatible transfusion (25). The A and B blood group antigens are the most highly reactive on the red cell membrane. Individuals lacking one or both of these antigens develop "naturally occurring" and potent anti-A and/or anti-B antibodies. When an ABO-incompatible unit is transfused, antigen-antibody complexes readily form and fix complement components C1q–C9 resulting in intravascular hemolysis. Anaphylatoxins I (C3a) and II (C5a) with their associated symptoms of shock, anaphylaxis, and bronchospasm are generated during the process. The immune complex stimulates the kinin and sympathetic nervous systems leading to vasomotor instability and activation of the coagulation system with the possible induction of DIC. The combination of renal vasoconstriction as well as intravascular thrombus formation may result in irreversible kidney damage (19).

Several factors are involved in determining the severity of an ABO-incompatible transfusion reaction, including the volume of incompatible red cells transfused, the patient's underlying clinical condition, and the delay from the time of recognition that a reaction has taken place to initiation of treatment. Depending on the rapidity of the antigen-antibody complex formation and complement activation, symptoms may occur within the first 15 minutes after the transfusion has been started or perhaps not at all, although this is rare. Fever, with or without chills, has been reported as the most common presenting symptom in the unanesthetized patient (45). If a transfusion reaction is suspected, the transfusion *must* be stopped immediately. The management of an immune intravascular hemolytic transfusion reaction includes hydration, induction of diuresis, and aggressive treatment of shock. In adults, fluid therapy to induce a urine output of at least 100 ml/hr should be maintained for 18 to 24 hours. A diuretic such as furosemide (up to 80–120 mg intravenously) should be used to improve blood flow to the kidneys and increase urine output (19). If DIC or renal failure occurs, appropriate therapy should be initiated. Acute extravascular reactions are clinically much more benign and rarely induce vasomotor instability or bronchospasm, largely because of the lack of generation of anaphylatoxins I and II. Severe acute extravascular reactions may produce hemoglobinemia, but this is a rare occurrence.

NONIMMUNE HEMOLYSIS

Hemolysis of transfused red cells can also occur secondary to nonimmunologic causes such as exposure to nonisotonic solutions (5% dextrose in water), improper storage of red cells, overheating or freezing red cells, mechanical destruction of red cells such as is seen with some blood pumps, or rarely, bacterial contamination of a unit of blood. In these cases, except for the infusion of bacterially contaminated blood or overheated blood, the patient's clinical response is usually associated with hemoglobinemia and hemoglobinuria, but not a full-blown intravascular hemolytic transfusion reaction with major vasomotor instability or bronchospasm. The major toxic mediators formed in an immune-generated ABO-incompatible transfusion reaction are C3a and C5a. The absence of these factors and of the powerful vasoconstrictive effects of antibody-coated red cell stroma is responsible for the comparatively benign clinical course seen in most patients presenting with nonimmune acute hemolytic transfusion reactions. For overheated blood, the clinical constellation can be attributed to lipoproteins released from the heat-damaged red cells. For bacterially contaminated units of blood, bacterial toxins (endotoxins or exotoxins) are the most likely cause of the acute clinical distress.

FEBRILE NONHEMOLYTIC REACTIONS

Fever is a common nonspecific sign of a transfusion reaction and may be associated with infusion of a bacterially contaminated unit of blood, immune-mediated hemolysis, or a leukoagglutination reaction. A febrile reaction is a diagnosis of exclusion, in which a core body temperature increase of 1–2°C or more occurs in association with a transfusion without any other cause for the fever being found. The temperature may rise shortly after starting the transfusion or up to 2 hours after completion. Febrile reactions occur in approximately 1% of transfusions and are usually attributed to antibodies directed against leukocytes or platelets (64). Recurrent febrile reactions are uncommon, and approximately 85% of patients experiencing a febrile reaction do not have a second episode. Therefore, the use of leukocyte-poor red cells is usually recommended only after two or more reactions (37). For patients with a history of febrile transfusion reactions who require platelet transfusion, premedication is also a consideration. Acetaminophen (600 mg orally) can be given, but is unlikely to prevent a severe febrile reaction. Aspirin should be avoided in patients with thrombocytopenia since this drug will increase the bleeding time. The acetyl group in aspirin (acetylsalicylic acid) acetylates the enzyme, cyclooxygenase, thus inhibiting or impairing synthesis of thromboxane which is required for the platelet release reaction and therefore for normal platelet function. Steroids such as hydrocortisone sodium succinate (100 mg intravenously) can be given in severe cases. Antihistamines do not decrease fever and are not indicated for treatment of patients with febrile transfusion reactions; they are more useful in allergic reactions. Premedication should not be considered a substitute for appropriate use of leukocyte-poor packed red blood cells, but may be required in patients who require platelet transfusions but in whom febrile reactions are a recurring problem.

ALLERGIC REACTIONS

Urticarial reactions consisting of "hives," itching, and erythema may occur in 1–2% of blood transfusion recipients. These reactions are usually mild and localized and respond to the administration of antihistamines such as diphenhydramine, 25–50 mg orally or parenterally. The exact cause is unknown, although antibodies against proteins in the donor's plasma is suspected.

Anaphylactic reactions, which may be characterized by bronchospasm, respiratory distress, and shock, often in the absence of fever, characteristically occur after transfusion of only a few milliliters of blood or plasma. These reactions are uncommon, usually occurring in individuals who have developed IgG, anti-IgA antibodies. Immediate treatment consists of the administration of epinephrine, 0.4 ml of a 1:1000 solution subcutaneously. Treatment with steroids, such as 100 mg of hydrocortisone intravenously, may also be useful. Anaphylactic reactions due to anti-IgA antibody, however, are rare and most IgA-deficient patients do not develop antibodies or symptoms. If, however, a patient with a history of severe allergic reactions to blood transfusion does have IgG, anti-IgA antibodies, this patient must be transfused with blood components that lack IgA, such as washed red cells (71). Plasma-containing components such as fresh frozen plasma or platelets must be collected from IgA-deficient donors.

BACTERIAL CONTAMINATION

Bacterial contamination of a unit of donor blood has become exceedingly rare as a result of the use of strict aseptic techniques for the collection of blood and adherence to protocols designed to maintain a closed system for the preparation of components. However, contamination of a unit of blood by psychrophilic Gram-negative bacteria, such as *Pseudomonas* species (62), can result in severe endotoxic shock, which must be recognized and treated immediately with appropriate antibiotics (e.g., aminoglycosides), combined with therapy to maintain blood pressure (e.g., dopamine) and urine output. Recent reports of contamination of random-donor platelets, which are stored at room temperature, has resulted in limiting the storage time of platelets to 5 days (8, 21). The most likely source of bacterial contamination in a unit of blood is an improperly cleaned donor arm. Phlebotomists should be ever mindful of the dangers inherent in passing a needle through an improperly cleaned skin surface.

CIRCULATORY OVERLOAD

Circulatory overload, which is characterized by respiratory distress, headache, vascular engorgement, pulmonary edema, and systolic hypertension, results from the transfusion of an excessive volume of blood or too rapid an infusion rate. The patients at highest risk for this complication are elderly patients who may already have preexisting cardiac or pulmonary compromise, patients with chronic anemia who are normovolemic, and pediatric patients with a smaller blood volume. This type of reaction can easily occur in infants, who require low-volume transfusions. Transfusion to such patients should be given over a 2- to 4-hour time period. When a hypervolemic reaction is suspected, the transfusion should be stopped, the patient placed in a sitting position, and oxygen and diuretics administered. If symptoms do not subside, phlebotomy should be considered.

NONCARDIOGENIC PULMONARY EDEMA

The acute onset of pulmonary edema unassociated with congestive heart failure or hypervolemia is a rare, but well-known, complication of transfusion. In such cases, cardiac pressures are normal, but copious amounts of pulmonary edema fluid can be suctioned from the patient's airway. The etiology of the edema is not clearly understood, although it is believed to be caused by either antibodies to leukocytes (63) or activation of complement (C5a) in the recipient, resulting in aggregation of leukocytes in the pulmonary vasculature with accompanying endothelial damage produced by the release of toxic oxygen radicals (27). Leukoagglutinins may be present either in the recipient, where they aggregate leukocytes present in any transfused blood or components, or in the donor plasma (16). The passive transfer of a potent donor leukoagglutinin with the resultant aggregation of recipient leukocytes is also known to occur (24, 31). The treatment of this type of reaction includes stopping the transfusion immediately and providing respiratory support. It has been proposed that corticosteroid therapy, when used in high concentrations, may be beneficial by inhibiting both C5a-induced granulocyte aggregation and superoxide production. Large intravenous doses, such as methylprednisolone, 30 mg/kg body weight every 6 hours for 48 hours, have been recommended (27). If future transfusions are necessary the use of washed cells should be considered. The potential risk versus benefit of future red cell, platelet, or granulocyte transfusions must be carefully evaluated, and if transfusion is necessary the patient must be monitored closely. Transfusion-related acute lung injury has been described by Popovsky and associates (47). This syndrome, caused by HLA or other leukoagglutinins, can cause severe pulmonary complications following blood transfusion.

Delayed Adverse Reactions

HEMOLYSIS

If the antigen-antibody reaction following transfusion occurs 3–10 days or longer after the transfusion, the reaction is classified as delayed. Depending on the degree of complement fixation, as was described for acute transfusion reactions, there may be delayed extravascular or delayed intravascular reactions. Delayed reactions usually occur in patients who have been previously sensitized to the foreign antigen through prior transfusions or pregnancy, but in whom antibody levels are too low to be detected in routine pretransfusion testing. After reexposure to the antigen, antibody production can occur rapidly (an an-

amnestic response), resulting in destruction of transfused red cells by macrophages in the reticuloendothelial system within 3–10 days. On rare occasions, primary exposure to a foreign red cell antigen may result in destruction of transfused and still circulating red cells; however, this event would likely occur several weeks after the transfusion. Delayed hemolytic reactions are characterized by an unexplained fall in the patient's hemoglobin, with or without fever or the development of icterus. A new positive direct antiglobulin (Coombs) test (posttransfusion) may be the first clue. Treatment is usually not required, although on rare occasions a delayed intravascular reaction may be severe enough to require support (as described for an acute reaction) (46).

TRANSMISSION OF INFECTIOUS DISEASE

Several infectious diseases can be transmitted through transfusion, non-A, non-B hepatitis being the most frequent (6). The exact incident of this infectious complication is unknown because of underreporting, although it has been stated that up to 10% of transfused recipients develop some degree of liver damage (1). Some blood products, because they are derived from pooled human plasma, carry a higher risk of transmitting hepatitis. Hepatitis A is rarely transmitted by a blood transfusion, although there are reported cases. The transmission of hepatitis B has been greatly reduced through specific HBsAg testing of donor blood and by the use of a volunteer donor system. Greater than 90% of the transfusion-associated hepatitis occurring today is due to a non-A, non-B agent for which there is no definitive test (52). Since there is no specific test, surrogate tests are used as markers for the presence of non-A, non-B hepatitis. The etiologic agent of non-A, non-B hepatitis is believed to be a virus—possibly several viruses. Blood-collecting facilities have recently instituted the screening of all donor blood for elevated alanine aminotransferase (ALT, formerly SGPT) activity as a marker for asymptomatic hepatitis. Testing for anti-HBc, the antibody to the hepatitis B core antigen, has also been adopted. Studies have shown that anti-HBc–positive individuals are more likely to also transmit non-A, non-B hepatitis because of their probable past exposure to multiple types of hepatitis. The clinical outcome of hepatitis is variable and may be fatal. Posttransfusion viral hepatitis must be suspected and investigated in any patient developing acute liver dysfunction 15–180 days after the transfusion of blood or blood components.

The acquired immune deficiency syndrome, which appears to be caused by a retrovirus called HIV (formerly HTLV-III or LAV), can be transmitted by blood transfusion (6, 10). The incidence of this transfusion-associated complication is not clear, but as of late 1987, 2% of cases of AIDS may be attributed to blood transfusion. Precautions taken to reduce the spread of AIDS through blood transfusion have included testing of all donor blood samples for HIV antibodies and the implementation of specific criteria to selectively exclude any donors who may be potential carriers of the virus, including homosexual men and intravenous drug users. Although the spread of AIDS by blood transfusion has captured most of the media attention, spread of non-A, non-B hepatitis by blood transfusion is clearly a more important public health risk.

Several other infectious diseases can be transmitted through blood transfusion, including malaria, Epstein-Barr virus, toxoplasmosis, and cytomegalovirus (CMV) (29). Transfusion-induced CMV infection has become a major concern in immunosuppressed patients, who may be at higher risk of developing severe complications. Neonates weighing less than 1200 g whose mothers are CMV antibody–negative are also believed to be at greater risk (72).

ALLOIMMUNIZATION

Every time an individual is transfused there is the chance of their becoming sensitized to red cell, white cell, platelet, or other foreign protein antigens. It has been estimated that for each unit of blood transfused there is a 1–1.6% risk of immunizing a recipient to a red cell antigen (34). Although this complication does not pose a problem at the time of the transfusion, it could present complications with subsequent transfusions in the form of a severe transfusion reaction or difficulty in finding compatible units of blood.

IRON OVERLOAD

Transfusion-induced hemosiderosis is a complication of chronic transfusion therapy. Since a milliliter of red blood cells contains about 1 mg of iron, each unit of red blood cells (about 250 ml) contains approximately 250 mg of iron. As a result of long-term transfusion

therapy, iron, which cannot be readily excreted by the body, deposits in parenchymal tissues resulting in organ dysfunction. Chelating agents such as desferrioxamine have been used in these patients to reduce body iron stores (28).

POSTTRANSFUSION PURPURA

Posttransfusion thrombocytopenic purpura is a rare complication of transfusion usually occurring in multiparous females. It may occur after a single transfusion of packed red cells (some platelets are still present in red cell units) and is manifest by a precipitous fall in the recipient's platelet count associated with the development of purpura approximately 1 week after transfusion. The development of a platelet-specific alloantibody, usually PL^{A1}, which destroys not only transfused platelets but also the patient's own PL^{A1}-negative platelets, has often been implicated in the etiology of this disorder. The thrombocytopenia tends to be severe but self-limiting, with no beneficial effects from transfused platelets (36); plasmapheresis has been suggested as a possible therapy.

GRAFT-VERSUS-HOST DISEASE

Posttransfusion graft-versus-host disease (GVHD) has been reported in severely immunosuppressed patients and results from the engraftment and proliferation of immunocompetent donor lymphocytes. Individuals who appear to be at greatest risk are children with severe combined immunodeficiency syndrome and bone marrow transplant patients (33).

Transfusion-induced GVHD is characterized by the development of fever, skin rash, diarrhea, liver dysfunction, and bone marrow suppression within 4–30 days after transfusion. The outcome is usually fatal, often secondary to infection (68). Irradiation (≥ 1500 rads) of blood components that contain viable lymphocytes (essentially all blood components except fresh frozen plasma and cryoprecipitate) has been recommended for patients who are highly susceptible to developing GVHD in order to reduce the risk of this complication.

TRANSFUSION PRACTICES

Emergency Transfusion

Emergency release of blood from the blood bank may be requested when a physician considers a patient's clinical condition so critical that the immediate transfusion of blood prior to completion of routine testing may be life-saving. Usually the goal of such therapy is to restore both intravascular volume and oxygen-carrying capacity. If the patient's blood type is unknown, group O, Rh-negative red cells may be issued immediately and used in conjunction with crystalloid or colloid solutions. This blood, although not risk-free, will eliminate the concern over life-threatening ABO incompatibility and avoid immunizing a possibly Rh-negative individual with the most immunogenic Rh antigen—the D antigen. The patient is still at risk, however, for reaction with one or more of the myriad of other blood group antigens if a preexisting antibody exists because of prior transfusion or pregnancy. If there is time to determine the patient's ABO and Rh type, then unmatched ABO-specific and Rh group–specific red blood cells or whole blood, if volume replacement is critical, may be released. When whole blood is requested, only ABO group–specific whole blood should be used to avoid any problems related to anti-A or anti-B incompatible isoagglutinins (51). Even though unmatched blood is being released, compatibility testing should be completed and the patient's physician notified if any incompatibility is detected. In the event that the patient's condition should stabilize prior to the infusion of the unmatched "emergency-release" units of blood, the blood should be returned to the blood bank *immediately* while the pretransfusion testing is being completed. The use of unmatched ABO-compatible and Rh-compatible red cells in a patient whose blood specimen has been tested and found to have no atypical antibodies, i.e., a negative antibody screen, has been reported to be 99.7% as safe as cross-matched blood (41). This fact is the basis of the type and screen procedure used for surgical procedures for which blood usage is extremely low (5).

Massive Transfusion

Massive transfusion can be defined as the transfusion of a quantity of blood equal to or greater than the individual's blood volume within a 24-hour period (e.g., transfusing 10 or more units of whole blood to a 70-kg patient). Although bleeding has been associated with transfusion of massive quantities of stored blood, this coagulopathy should not be attributed only to the use of stored blood, since often it is the tissue damage associated with the primary injury that contributes to abnormal hemostasis (11). The patient's clinical status as well as laboratory monitoring of platelet counts and coagulation profiles should guide the appropriate use of other blood components. The use of a predetermined formula stating that specific components such as platelets, fresh frozen plasma, or cryoprecipitate should be infused after transfusion of a fixed number of whole blood or red cell units frequently exposes the patient to unnecessary risks associated with transfusion of nonindicated blood products. These risks include febrile and allergic reactions, fluid overload, and transfusion-transmitted diseases. Massive transfusion, per se, is unlikely to produce an isolated deficiency of coagulation factors. Even labile factor VIII rarely falls below hemostatic levels after massive transfusion, unless accompanied by a disseminated intravascular coagulopathy (12). Dilutional thrombocytopenia leading to impaired hemostasis may occur, however (12). Administration of platelet concentrates in such situations would also serve as a source of stable coagulation factors, since 50–60 ml of plasma are present in each unit of platelets. Laboratory testing (PT, PTT, and platelet count) to evaluate the clinical coagulopathy followed by institution of appropriate component therapy based on these results is the most appropriate method of handling these cases. The days of "shotgun" therapy are all but gone. Such therapy can rarely be medically, economically, or legally justified. This fact does not mean that a "clinical trial" of a component is never warranted, but medical judgment must be used in such cases and the reasoning documented in the chart. When extensive bleeding continues postoperatively or posttransfusion in the absence of any detectable hemostatis defect, the possibility of an anatomic lesion necessitating surgical intervention should be carefully considered.

Blood Administration

A most critical but frequently overlooked area of transfusion practice is the actual administration of blood and components. The first and most important step is proper patient identification, which should be performed from a hospital identification bracelet, a bracelet that should not be removed from the patient's arm at any time during the stay in hospital. After a transfusion is started, the patient should remain under direct observation for 5 or 10 minutes. The time limit for administration of blood or blood components is currently recommended to be 4 hours because of the risk of bacterial growth in blood maintained at room temperature but not infused. If clinical conditions require the infusion to exceed 4 hours, the component can be divided into aliquots and portions stored in the blood bank until required. Changing the blood filter every 4 hours is also recommended. Blood that warms to above 10°C but is not transfused must be returned to the blood bank, where it will be discarded. Such blood cannot be put back on the shelf for long-term storage because of the potential for bacterial growth. Blood must not be stored in unmonitored refrigerators.

BLOOD FILTERS

All units of blood and components should be administered through a filter to remove protein, blood clots, and other debris (57). Blood filters with a pore size of 170 μm are the standard devices used. However, some individuals are concerned about the risk of respiratory distress syndrome (ARDS) due to the infusion of large amounts of blood containing microaggregates—degenerating platelets, fibrin strands, and granulocytes, which form during storage. Despite early reports from the Vietnam War that massive transfusion appeared to be associated with shock lung and ARDS, controlled studies in the civilian population have failed to show the benefit of microaggregate blood filtration for the prevention of respiratory distress. Today, we know that individuals more likely develop shock lung because of the initial trauma responsible for the need for infusion of massive amounts of blood. Microaggregate filters are currently not recommended for use except when the blood is being transfused into the arterial circuit, such as during cardiopulmonary bypass (57). If at least 3 or 4 units can be transfused, use of the filters is cost effective. Despite intensive research, microaggregate debris has not been proved to cause ARDS. Microaggregate filters may, however, be useful to prevent febrile transfusion reactions since these filters do remove white cells, which react with leukoagglutinins to cause febrile reactions.

BLOOD WARMERS

If blood is infused at such a rate that the sinoatrial node reaches temperatures below 30°C, ventricular fibrillation results (7). Accordingly, warming blood to 37°C prior to infusion has been recommended to prevent this complication. However, sinoatrial node hypothermia occurs very infrequently and usually is seen only in a truly massive transfusion setting, e.g., 1 unit every 5 minutes. There are several types of blood warmers: a simple coil of plastic tubing placed in a temperature-monitored (37°C) waterbath, or an electrical device in which blood flowing in a special large-surface-area plastic bag comes in contact with heated (37°C) plates. Blood warmers should have automatic warning devices such as visual and audible alarms to alert staff to the danger of overheating, since hemolysis occurs at temperatures over 40°C. Infusion of hemolyzed blood can cause anaphylaxis and shock and may possibly be fatal. Warming blood by use of a microwave oven or immersion of the blood bag in hot water is not acceptable because of the risk of hemolysis (2). Generally, blood warmer use is restricted to adult patients receiving rapid and multiple transfusions at rates over 50 ml/kg/hr, to exchange transfusion in infants, and to children receiving blood volumes in excess of 15 ml/kg/hr. Because blood infused through warmers must be given more slowly, a blood warmer should not be used in individuals for whom transfusion may be lifesaving, if it so impedes flow rates as to be detrimental to patient care.

INTRAVENOUS SOLUTIONS

Only normal saline (0.9% USP) should be administered with blood components. Other solutions are unacceptable since they are hypotonic (D5W) or contain calcium (lactated Ringer's solutions). Ringer's solution could initiate clotting in the citrated blood in vitro due to recalcification. Medication should never be added to a unit of blood for several reasons: (a) it may cause hemolysis due to excessive pH; (b) if medication is added and the unit is subsequently discontinued because of a transfusion reaction, the full dose of medication may not be given; and (c) if a drug is added to the blood and a reaction occurs, it would be difficult to determine whether the drug or the blood caused the reaction. Five percent albumin can be mixed with blood in special circumstances (48).

INFUSION DEVICES

A variety of electronic pumps are available for delivering blood. These may be syringe-type pumping systems, peristaltic devices, or electromechanical volume displacement pumps. Some systems require manufacturer-supplied cassettes; others use standard intravenous tubing. Most pump systems do not induce mechanical hemolysis when used with whole blood. However, with high-viscosity, high-hematocrit packed cells, hemolysis may occur. The package insert for each pump should be consulted. Infusion of granulocytes or platelet concentrates through some types of pumps is acceptable (58). Pumps should be used for special indications requiring slow metered infusion. If the device is set on "maximum" to pump blood in as quickly as possible, use of the pump should be questioned and probably omitted completely.

Autologous Transfusion

Currently, because of the concern over transfusion-transmissible diseases as well as the need to promote blood conservation, a variety of autologous transfusion techniques are used (65). These include preoperative donation, intraoperative salvage, intraoperative hemodilution, and postoperative salvage. Of most concern to the intensive care physician is the use of intraoperative salvage, in which blood can be salvaged from the operative field, eliminating the need for transfusing some units of allogeneic blood from the blood bank. Blood is usually recovered from the operative field by employing some type of suction device. The blood is then washed (in some systems) and filtered prior to reinfusion. Washing removes fibrin, cellular debris, free hemoglobin, potassium, and other metabolites. Blood collected by intraoperative salvage cannot be transfused into other patients. Critical to any type of intraoperative salvage involving collection into a container is appropriate labeling of that container to ensure proper identification of the blood. Postoperative salvage techniques are also available. In one type of technique, blood from the chest tube drainage is collected. This blood is processed by washing (in some systems) and filtration prior to reinfusion. Blood intended for retransfusion must not remain in a drainage device longer than 4 hours. These techniques should not be used when tumor or sepsis is present or suspected. Whatever risks are associated with transfusion of banked blood, they are outweighed by the risks inherent in infusion of improperly collected and stored autologous blood.

References

1. Aach RD, Kahn RA: Posttransfusion hepatatis: current perspectives. *Ann Intern Med* 92:539–546, 1980.
2. Arens JF, Leonard GL: Danger of overwarming blood by microwave. *JAMA* 218:1045–46, 1971.
3. Aster RH: Effect of anticoagulant and ABO incompatibility on recovery of transfused human platelets. *Blood* 26:732–734, 1965.
4. Beutler E, West C: The storage of hard-packed red blood cells in citrate-phosphate-dextrose (CPD) and CPD-adenine (CPDA-1). *Blood* 54:280–284, 1979.
5. Boral LI, Henry JB: The type and screen: a safe alternative and supplement in selected surgical procedures. *Transfusion* 17:163–168, 1977.
6. Bove JR: Transfusion-transmitted diseases: current problems and challenges. In Brown EB (ed): *Progress in Hematology.* Orlando, FL, Grune & Stratton, 1986, vol 14, pp 123–147.
7. Boyan CP, Howland WS: Cardiac arrest and temperature of bank blood. *JAMA* 183:58–60, 1963.
8. Braine HG, Kickler TS, Charache P, et al: Bacterial sepsis secondary to platelet transfusion: an adverse effect of extended storage at room temperature. *Transfusion* 26:391–393, 1986.
9. Caggiano V: Red blood cell transfusions. In Silver H (ed): *Blood, Blood Components and Derivatives in Transfusion Therapy.* Washington, DC, American Association of Blood Banks, 1980, pp 1–28.
10. Centers for Disease Control Update: Acquired immunodeficiency syndrome (AIDS)—United States. *MMWR CDC Surveill Summ* 33:661–664, 1984.
11. Collins JA: Massive blood transfusions. *Clin Haematol* 5:201–222, 1976.
12. Counts RB, Haish C, Simon TL, et al: Hemostasis in massively transfused trauma patients. *Ann Surg* 190:91–99, 1979.
13. Daly PA, Schiffer CA, Aisner J, et al: Platelet transfusion therapy—one hour post-transfusion increments are valuable in predicting the need for HLA-matched preparation. *JAMA* 243:435–438, 1980.
14. Dawson RB, Kocholaty WF, Gray JL: Hemoglobin function and 2,3-DPG levels in blood stored at 4°C in ACD and CPD: pH effect. *Transfusion* 10:299–304, 1970.
15. De Venuto F: Modified hemoglobin solution as a resuscitation fluid. *Vox Sang* 44:129–142, 1983.
16. Dubois M, Lotze MT, Diamond WJ, Kim YD, Flye MW, MacNamara TE: Pulmonary shunting during leukoagglutinin-induced noncardiac pulmonary edema. *JAMA* 244:2186–2189, 1980.
17. Freireich EJ, Kliman A, Gaydos LA, et al: Response to repeated platelet transfusion from the same donor. *Ann Intern Med* 59:277–287, 1963.
18. Gilbert R, Miripol J, Vaithianathan T, et al: Rejuvenation of outdated CPD-adenine red cells: in vitro and in vivo results (abstract). *Transfusion* 21:636, 1981.
19. Goldfinger D: Acute hemolytic transfusion reactions—a fresh look at pathogenesis and considerations regarding therapy. *Transfusion* 17:85–98, 1977.
20. Gould SA, Rosen AL, Sehgal LR: Fluosol-DA as a red cell substitute in acute anemia. *N Engl J Med* 314:1653–1656, 1986.
21. Heal JM, Singal S, Sardisco E, et al: Bacterial prolifer-

ation in platelet concentrates. *Transfusion* 26:388–390, 1986.

22. Heaton A, Miripol J, Aster R, et al: Use of Adsol preservation solution for prolonged storage of low viscosity AS-1 red blood cells. *Br J Haematol* 57:467–478, 1984.

23. Heaton A, Miripol J, Grapka B, et al: Improved storage of high hematocrit cell concentrates using a mannitol, adenine, saline, glucose solution (abstract). *Transfusion* 21:600, 1981.

24. Higby DJ, Burnett D: Granulocyte transfusions: current status. *Blood* 55:2–8, 1980.

25. Honig CL, Bove JR: Transfusion-associated fatalities: review of Bureau of Biologics reports 1976–1978. *Transfusion* 20:653–661, 1980.

26. International Forum on Oxygen Carrying Blood Substitutes. *Vox Sang* 42:97–109, 1982.

27. Jacob HS, Craddock PR, Hammerschmidt DE, et al: Complement-induced granulocyte aggregation. *N Engl J Med* 302:789–794, 1980.

28. Jacobs A: Iron chelation therapy for iron loaded patients. *Br J Haematol* 43:1–5, 1979.

29. Kahn RA: Diseases transmitted by blood transfusion. *Hum Pathol* 14:241–247, 1983.

30. Kahn RA, Allen RW, Baldassare J: Alternate sources and substitutes for therapeutic blood components. *Blood* 66:1–12, 1985.

31. Kernoff PBA, Durrant IJ, Rizza CR, et al: Severe allergic pulmonary edema after plasma transfusion. *Br J Haematol* 23:777–781, 1972.

32. Lee EJ, Schiffer CA: Management of platelet alloimmunization. In McCarthy LJ, Menitove JE (eds): *Immunologic Aspects of Platelet Transfusion.* Arlington, VA, American Association of Blood Banks, 1985, pp 1–19.

33. Leitman SF, Holland PV: Irradiation of blood products. Indications and guidelines. *Transfusion* 25:293–300, 1985.

34. Lostumbo MM, Holland PV, Schmidt PJ: Isoimmunization after multiple transfusions. *N Engl J Med* 275:141–144, 1966.

35. Mannucci PM: Desmopressin (dDAVP) for treatment of disorders of hemostasis. In Coller BS (ed): *Progress in Hemostasis and Thrombosis.* Orlando, FL, Grune & Stratton, vol 8, 1986, pp 19–45.

36. McFarland JG, Aster RH: Clinical significance of platelet-specific antigens. In McCarthy LJ, Menitove JE (eds): *Immunologic Aspects of Platelet Transfusion.* Arlington, VA, American Association of Blood Banks, 1985, pp 55–69.

37. Menitove JE, McElligott MC, Aster RH: Febrile transfusion reactions: what blood component should be given next. *Vox Sang* 42:318–321, 1982.

38. Meryman HT: Cryopreservation of blood and marrow cells: basic biological and biophysical considerations. In Petz LD, Swisher SN (eds): *Clinical Practice of Blood Transfusion.* New York, Churchill Livingstone, 1981, pp 313–331.

39. Meryman HT, Hornblower M: The preparation of red cells depleted of leukocytes. *Transfusion* 26:101–106, 1986.

40. Meryman HT, Hornblower M: Quality control for deglycerolizing red blood cells. *Transfusion* 21:235–240, 1982.

41. Oberman HA, Barnes BA, Friedman A: The risk of abbreviating the major crossmatch in urgent or massive transfusion. *Transfusion* 18:137–141, 1978.

42. Office of Medical Applications of Research, National Institutes of Health: Fresh frozen plasma: indications and risks. *JAMA* 253:551–553, 1985.

43. Office of Medical Applications of Research, National Institutes of Health: Platelet transfusion therapy. *JAMA*, 257:1777–1780, 1987.

44. Pierce RN, Reich LM, Mayer K: Hemolysis following platelet transfusions from ABO-incompatible donors. *Transfusion* 25:60–62, 1985.

45. Pineda AA, Brzica SM Jr, Taswell HF: Hemolytic trans-

fusion reaction: recent experience in a large blood bank. *Mayo Clin Proc* 53:378–390, 1978.

46. Pineda A, Taswell HF, Brzica SM Jr: Delayed hemolytic transfusion reaction, an immunologic hazard of blood transfusion. *Transfusion* 18:1–7, 1978.

47. Popovsky MA, Abel MD, Moore SG: Transfusion related acute lung injury associated with passive transfer of antileukocyte antibodies. *Am Rev Respir Dis* 128:185–189, 1983.

48. Ryden SE, Oberman HA: Compatibility of common intravenous solutions with CPD blood. *Transfusion* 15:250–255, 1975.

49. Saba TM, Jaffe E: Plasma fibronectin (opsonic glycoprotein): its synthesis by vascular endothelial cells and role in cardiopulmonary integrity after trauma as related to reticuloendothelial function. *Am J Med* 68:577–594, 1980.

50. Schiffer CA, Slichter ST: Platelet transfusions from single donors. *N Engl J Med* 307:245–247, 1982.

51. Schmidt PJ (ed): *Standards for Blood Banks and Transfusion Services,* ed 12. Washington, DC, American Association of Blood Banks, 1987.

52. Seeff LB, Wright EC, Zimmerman HJ, et al: VA cooperative study of post-transfusion hepatitis 1969–1974: incidence and characteristics of hepatitis and responsible risk factors. *Am J Med Sci* 270:355–362, 1975.

53. Simon TL, Marcus CS, Myhre BA, Nelson EJ: Effects of AS-3 nutrient additive solution on 42–49 day storage of red cells. *Transfusion,* 27:178–182, 1987.

54. Slichter SJ: Controversies in platelet transfusion therapy. *Ann Rev Med* 31:509–540, 1980.

55. Slichter SJ: Preservation of platelet viability and function during storage of concentrates. In Greenwalt TJ, Jamieson GA (eds): *The Blood Platelet in Transfusion Therapy.* New York, Alan R. Liss, 1978, pp 83–100.

56. Snyder EL: Clinical use of albumin, plasma protein fraction and isoimmune globulin products. In Silvergleid A, Britten A (eds): *Plasma Products: Use and Management.* Arlington, VA, American Association of Blood Banks, 1982, pp 87–107.

57. Snyder EL, Bookbinder M: Role of microaggregate blood filtration in clinical medicine. *Transfusion* 23:460–470, 1983.

58. Snyder EL, Ferri PM, Smith EO, Ezekowitz MD: Use of an electromechanical infusion pump for transfusion of platelet concentrates. *Transfusion* 24:524–527, 1984.

59. Snyder EL, Luban NLC: Fibronectin: applications to clinical medicine. *CRC Crit Rev Clin Lab Sci* 23:15–34, 1986.

60. Sohmer PR, Dawson RB: The significance of 2,3-DPG in red cell transfusion. *CRC Crit Rev Clin Lab Sci* 11:107, 1979.

61. Strauss RG, Connett JE, Gale RP, et al. A controlled trial of prophylactic granulocyte transfusions during initial induction chemotherapy for acute myelogenous leukemia. *N Engl J Med* 305:597–603, 1981.

62. Tabor E, Gerety RJ: Five cases of *Pseudomonas* sepsis transmitted by blood transfusions. *Lancet* 1:1403, 1984.

63. Thompson JS, Severson CD, Parmely MJ, et al: Pulmonary "hypersensitivity" reactions induced by transfusion of non-HLA leukoagglutinins. *N Engl J Med* 284:1120–1125, 1971.

64. Thulstrup H: The influence of leukocyte and thrombocyte incompatibility on nonhaemolytic transfusion reactions: a retrospective study. *Vox Sang* 21:233–250, 1971.

65. Thurer RL, Hauser JM: Autotransfusion and blood conservation. *Curr Probl Surg* 19:97–156, 1982.

66. Title 21. Food and Drug Administration. Chapter I, part 640. Code of Federal Regulations. Washington, DC, US Government Printing Office, 1985.

67. Tullis JL: Albumin 2. Guidelines for clinical use. *JAMA* 237:460–463, 1977.

68. von Fleidner V, Higby DJ, Kim U: Graft versus host

reaction following blood product transfusion. *Am J Med* 72:951–961, 1982.

69. Winston DJ, Ho WG, Gale RP: Prophylactic granulocyte transfusions during chemotherapy of acute nonlymphocytic leukemia. *Ann Intern Med* 94:616–622, 1981.

70. Wolfe L, Epstein M, Kevy SV: Blood transfusion for the neonatal patient. *Hum Pathol* 14:256–260, 1983.

71. Yap PL, Pryde EAD, McClelland DBL: IgA content of frozen-thawed-washed red blood cells and blood products measured by radioimmunoassay. *Transfusion* 22:36–38, 1982.

72. Yeager AS, Grumet FC, Hafleigh EB, et al: Prevention of transfusion-acquired cytomegalovirus infection in newborn infants. *J Pediatr* 98:281–287, 1981.

73. Zuck TF, Bensinger TA, Peck CC, et al: The in vivo survival of red blood cells stored in modified CPD with adenine: report of a multi-institutional cooperative effort. *Transfusion* 17:374–382, 1977.

15

Red Cell Substitutes: A Current Appraisal

Steven A. Gould, M.D.
Lakshman R. Sehgal, Ph.D.
Arthur L. Rosen, Ph.D.
Hansa L. Sehgal, B.S.
Gerald S. Moss, M.D.

The two acellular oxygen carriers currently being evaluated as red cell substitutes are hemoglobin solutions and fluorocarbon emulsions. The primary indication for such a product would be the unavailability of blood. The most important properties of a suitable red cell substitute should be the ability to effectively transport oxygen and carbon dioxide and to support circulatory dynamics. In addition, the preparation should be nontoxic and temperature stable, should have a long shelf storage time and a suitable intravascular persistence, should require no cross-match before administration, and should be effective when the recipient is on room air.

We have shown that both hemoglobin solutions and fluorocarbon emulsions can maintain normal levels of oxygen consumption, carbon dioxide production, and circulatory dynamics in primates in the virtual absence of red blood cells. Although each solution therefore satisfies the most important criteria for a red cell substitute, certain problems exist with both that must be resolved prior to their clinical application. This chapter will assess the current status of both products.

HEMOGLOBIN SOLUTIONS

For the last 15 years we have pursued the possibility that a hemoglobin solution prepared from outdated blood could serve as a temporary substitute for the red blood cell (17, 25, 26). This interest is based on several remarkable characteristics of the hemoglobin molecule. First, hemoglobin has the capacity to chemically bind oxygen: 1 g of hemoglobin binds 1.34 ml of oxygen. Second, the hemoglobin molecule has the ability to become fully

oxygen-saturated at ambient oxygen pressures. Few, if any, biologically acceptable substances have a greater oxygen capacity at physiologic pressures. Thus, hemoglobin is a fully effective oxygen carrier without the addition of supplemental oxygen to the inspired air. Third, oxygen is normally unloaded from hemoglobin in the capillary at oxygen pressures of approximately 40 torr. This unloading characteristic allows for oxygen molecules to flow from hemoglobin to the intracellular mitochondria without producing interstitial hypoxia. Despite these features, an acceptable hemoglobin solution has not yet been used in the clinical setting.

Unmodified Hemoglobin

The basic unmodified hemoglobin solution is currently prepared from outdated blood. The red cells are first washed and lysed with pyrogen-free water (Fig. 15.1). A series of filtration steps permits the complete separation of the red cell membrane debris ("stroma") from the hemoglobin molecules. The resultant hemoglobin solution is essentially free of these contaminants, and is commonly referred to as "stroma-free hemoglobin" or SFH. Since the blood type characteristics are located on the cell membrane, SFH is universally compatible and can be infused without regard to specific blood type. The properties of this unmodified tetrameric or "stripped" hemoglobin solution are shown in Table 15.1. The P_{50} of 12–14 torr compares with a normal value of 26 torr (25). Although SFH can be prepared with a [Hb] of 14 g/dl, the solution would have a colloid osmotic pressure (COP) of greater than 60 torr (17). This hyperoncotic solution would not be

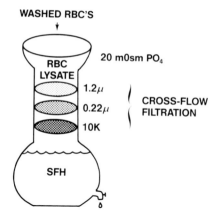

Figure 15.1. Schematic drawing of preparation process for stroma-free hemoglobin *(SFH)*. RBC, red blood cell.

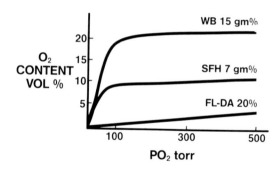

Figure 15.2. Oxygen content curves for 15 g/dl (gm%) of whole blood, *(WB)*, 7 g/dl (gm%) of stroma-free hemoglobin *(SFH)*, and 20% Fluosol-DA *(FL-DA)*.

acceptable for clinical use. The [Hb] of 7 g/dl is therefore required to maintain an isoncotic product. The low P_{50} is due to the loss of 2,3-diphosphoglycerate (2,3-DPG) during the preparation. The O_2 content curve of SFH is thus both anemic (↓ [Hb]) and leftward-shifted (↓ P_{50}). A comparison with a 15 g/dl whole blood product and Fluosol-DA, 20%, is shown in Figure 15.2.

Despite these limitations, SFH will support life in primates in the absence of red cells, documenting effective O_2 transport (25). Animals survive a total exchange transfusion with SFH to zero hematocrit with maintenance of normal O_2 consumption ($\dot{V}O_2$), cardiac output (CO), and arteriovenous O_2 content difference (AVDo$_2$). Although still normal, there is a decline in some of these parameters from the baseline values. In addition, a considerable decrease occurs in the mixed venous oxygen tension ($P_{mv}O_2$) from roughly 50 to 20 torr.

The $P_{mv}O_2$ is the tension at which oxygen unloads from the hemoglobin molecule, and is in equilibrium with the tissue P_{O_2}. This decline indicates a marked increase in O_2 extraction, and is the mechanism used to compensate for the fall in [Hb] and P_{50}. Such a low $P_{mv}O_2$ caused us concern, and led us to attempt to restore a more normal value.

Table 15.1
Properties of Stroma-free Hemoglobin (SFH)

Hemoglobin content	6–8 g/dl
P_{50}	12–14 torr
Colloid osmotic pressure	20–25 torr
Half-life	2–4 hr

Analysis of Mixed Venous Oxygen Tension

The factors that lower $P_{mv}O_2$ include a decrease in cardiac output, hemoglobin mass, P_{50} (↑ affinity state), and arterial saturation, and an increase in O_2 consumption (12). In reviewing the data we could eliminate changes in O_2 consumption, arterial saturation, and cardiac output as explanations for the decline in $P_{mv}O_2$. The major changes were the fall in [Hb] and P_{50} that occurred during the exchange transfusion. We believed that the low [Hb] and P_{50} of the infused SFH were responsible for these results (18). Our subsequent efforts have focused on normalizing these values, and obtaining a product with a normal O_2-carrying capacity.

Pyridoxylated Hemoglobin

Our initial efforts were focused on improving the oxygen affinity state of SFH. The increase in affinity state (↓ P_{50}) in SFH is related to the loss of the organic ligand, 2,3-DPG, normally found in the red blood cell. Figure 15.3 demonstrates how a leftward shift in the O_2 content curve with no change in $\dot{V}O_2$, CO, or AVDo$_2$ produces a decrease in the oxygen tension at which unloading occurs—the $P_{mv}O_2$ (15). Attempts to normalize P_{50} by the simple addition of 2,3-DPG to the hemoglobin solution were unsuccessful because the DPG disappears rapidly from the circulation after infusion (38). Benesch (1), Greenburgh (21), Sehgal (36) and their coworkers have described a modification of the hemoglobin molecule by the addition of pyridoxal phosphate. The resulting pyridoxylated hemoglobin (SFH-P) has

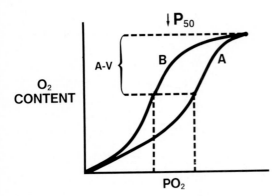

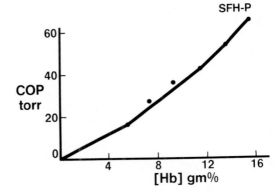

Figure 15.3. Oxygen content curves showing how a leftward shift (P_{50}) with a constant $AVDO_2$ leads to a lower $P_{mv}O_2$.

Figure 15.4. Relationship between [Hb] and colloid osmotic pressure *(COP)* for tetrameric SFH-P.

a P_{50} of 20–22 torr, considerably higher than the P_{50} of the unmodified SFH.

The SFH-P was evaluated in eight baboons (9). Four received SFH (P_{50}, 12 torr), and four received SFH-P (P_{50}, 22 torr). The hemoglobin concentration of both solutions was approximately 7 g/dl. The exchange transfusion again was carried out until zero hematocrit was achieved. The $P_{mv}O_2$ levels were significantly higher at the end of the exchange in the animals receiving SFH-P. Although the hemodynamics were maintained in a normal range, there was once again a decline from the baseline values in both groups.

These results illustrate three points. First, they confirm that rightward shifts in the dissociation curve ($\uparrow P_{50}$) result in an increased $P_{mv}O_2$ as long as the other determinants of $P_{mv}O_2$ remain constant (9). This fact is physiologically important because it allows O_2 unloading to occur at a higher tissue P_{O_2}. Second, although increased, the $P_{mv}O_2$ level (near 25 torr) in the animals treated with SFH-P still was substantially lower than the normal value of 40–50 torr found in control animals. Third, the hemodynamics still showed a reduction from the baseline values. Thus we began to search for other means to normalize the $P_{mv}O_2$ and the hemodynamics. The remaining option was to raise the hemoglobin concentration of the SFH (18).

Polymerized Hemoglobin

PREPARATION

It is possible to prepare a hemoglobin solution with a normal hemoglobin concentration.

However, the COP of such a product will be in excess of 60 torr (Fig. 15.4) (17, 26). Such a solution might produce large fluid shifts from the extravascular to the intravascular space following infusion, and therefore is not a suitable product. An alternative approach to developing a product with a normal O_2 capacity and a normal COP value is polymerization of the hemoglobin molecule. The COP of any solution is proportional to the number of colloidal particles in the solution. If a 15 g/dl solution of hemoglobin is polymerized, the number of molecules is reduced along with the COP, whereas no change occurs in hemoglobin concentration (Fig. 15.5). We have successfully prepared such a product in large volumes (33–35). The characteristics of such a polymerized, pyridoxylated hemoglobin solution (Poly SFH-P) are shown in Table 15.2.

PRELIMINARY STUDIES

Two kinds of preliminary studies have been completed. The first documented the efficacy of the polyhemoglobin in rats at otherwise

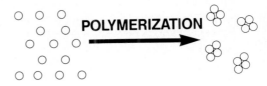

COP > 60 torr
[Hb] = 15 gm %

COP = 20 torr
[Hb] = 15 gm %

Figure 15.5. Schematic explanation of polymerization of 15 g/dl (gm%) tetrameric to 15 g/dl (gm%) polymerized hemoglobin. *COP*, colloid osmotic pressure.

Table 15.2
Properties of Polymerized, Pyridoxylated
Stroma-free Hemoglobin (Poly SFH-P)

Hemoglobin content	14–16 g/dl
P_{50}	16–20 torr
Colloid osmotic pressure	20–25 torr
Half-life	24–48 hr

lethal hematocrits (34), and the second investigated polyhemoglobin half-life in the baboon (33). Much of the tetramer is cleared by the kidneys following dissociation into dimers, with a resultant half-life of 2–4 hours. The polyhemoglobin shows a striking increase in half-life to 38 hours, compared with about 4 hours for pyridoxylated hemoglobin (33). Thus, at the same COP, the O_2 capacity is greater and the intravascular persistence is much longer for Poly SFH-P than for any unpolymerized product.

EFFICACY

We recently completed two studies to evaluate the efficacy of Poly SFH-P in baboons. The first examined the effects on P_{50} (11). Although the [Hb] of 14 g/dl of Poly SFH-P is a significant improvement over the [Hb] of the unpolymerized tetramer, the polymerization process results in a modest decrease in the P_{50}, from 22–24 torr for SFH-P to 16–20 torr for Poly SFH-P. Because O_2 unloading may decrease as P_{50} falls (18), there is concern about the ability of Poly SFH-P to transport O_2 effectively in the presence of red cells with their normal P_{50} of 26 torr. This issue is relevant because the clinical use of Poly SFH-P is likely to be in the presence of a reduced, but significant, red cell mass. In this setting, O_2 is carried in three separate compartments: the red cell (RBC), the plasma, and the Poly SFH-P, as shown:

$$[O_2]_{total} = [O_2]_{RBC} + [O_2]_{plasma} + [O_2]_{Poly\ SFH-P} \quad (1)$$

We previously reported that the efficacy of any O_2 carrier can be assessed quantitatively by determining its individual contribution to total O_2 delivery and O_2 consumption (11, 29). Using this methodology we evaluated the efficacy of Poly SFH-P as an O_2 carrier in a clinically relevant range of hematocrits, and have shown that SFH-P effectively transports O_2 in the presence of red cells.

Seven adult baboons underwent a total exchange transfusion with Poly SFH-P with a [Hb] of 14.3 ± 2 g/dl and a P_{50} of 19.6 ± 0.4 torr.

The data were compared with previously reported data using unpolymerized SFH-P with a [Hb] of 7.3 ± 0.2 g/dl and a P_{50} of 22.1 ± 1 torr. All animals receiving Poly SFH-P survived. The results show that Poly SFH-P supports life at zero hematocrit, and that it makes significant contributions to both total O_2 delivery and O_2 consumption in the presence of red cells. Poly SFH-P permits a higher plasma [Hb] (Fig. 15.6) and has a longer intravascular persistence than any unpolymerized hemoglobin solution. Poly SFH-P thus is an effective O_2 carrier (13).

The second study focused on the hemodynamics (19). As stated above, although animals survive exchange transfusion with SFH-P, there is a decrease from baseline values in $\dot{V}o_2$, mean arterial pressure (MAP), and CO, and an increase in heart rate (HR) at zero hematocrit. It is possible these changes are due to the low [Hb] of SFH-P, because the final plasma [Hb] in these animals is only 4 g/dl. Our hypothesis was that Poly SFH-P might normalize the final [Hb] and thus maintain baseline hemodynamics in the absence of red cells.

Six adult baboons were anesthetized, paralyzed, intubated, and mechanically ventilated on room air. Arterial, venous, and pulmonary artery catheters were inserted. A total exchange transfusion was performed with Poly SFH-P (Hb, 14.2 g/dl; P_{50}, 19.2 torr). The exchange volumes were adjusted to maintain the pulmonary capillary wedge pressure at baseline values. Cardiac output, O_2 consumption, MAP, and HR were measured. All baboons survived the exchange to a hematocrit (Hct) below 1%. The mean $\pm$ SEM for $\dot{V}o_2$, MAP, HR, and CO at baseline (before exchange) and Hct below 1% (after exchange) are shown in Table 15.3. The results are compared with our

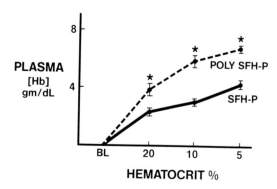

Figure 15.6. Plasma [Hb] (mean ± SEM) at intermediate hematocrits with Poly SFH-P or SFH-P. *BL*, baseline.

Table 15.3
Hemodynamics and Oxygen Consumption Before and After Exchange Transfusion

	Poly SFH-P		SFH-P	
	Baseline	Hct < 1%	Baseline	Hct < 1%
Oxygen consumption (ml/min)	60.1 ± 8.5	58.0 ± 4.8	85 ± 10	50 ± 10[a]
Mean arterial pressure (torr)	138 ± 8	140 ± 8	128 ± 7	95 ± 7[a]
Heart rate (beats/min)	114 ± 3	117 ± 10	108 ± 8	138 ± 11[a]
Cardiac output (liters/min)	1.63 ± 0.26	1.30 ± 0.2	2.72 ± 0.32	2.06 ± 0.46[a]

[a] Significant difference from baseline ($P < 0.05$).

prior data from six animals receiving the unpolymerized SFH-P ([Hb], 6.6 g/dl; P_{50}, 18.3 torr). The final plasma [Hb] at Hct below 1% was 9.7 g/dl for Poly SFH-P and 3.7 g/dl for the unpolymerized SFH-P. The hemodynamics and O_2 consumption were well maintained throughout with Poly SFH-P (19).

Poly SFH-P and SFH-P both support life in the absence of red cells. In contrast to SFH-P, Poly SFH-P achieves a near-normal plasma [Hb], and maintains baseline hemodynamics and O_2 consumption at zero hematocrit. Its intravascular persistence is prolonged significantly. These observations suggest that Poly SFH-P is an improved red cell substitute for use in the clinical setting.

SAFETY

The limiting factor prior to clinical testing is the concern about the safety of Poly SFH-P. The main uncertainty is the effect of this product on renal function. Nephrotoxicity was reported in early studies following the infusion of hemoglobin solution (22). Further investigations suggested that the stroma was the toxic factor, probably because of thrombosis of the small renal vasculature (27). In 1967 Rabiner and associates (28) reported that hemoglobin solution, relatively free of stroma, produced no deterioration in renal function following infusion in dogs. These findings were subsequently confirmed in monkeys, even in the stressful circumstances of dehydration and shock (2). The key observation was made in 1978 when Savitsky and coworkers (32) reported the results of a clinical safety trial in humans using stroma-free hemoglobin. Eight healthy male volunteers received a 250-ml infusion of stroma-free hemoglobin at a rate of 2–4 ml/min. The hemoglobin concentration of this solution was 6.4 gm/dl. The P_{50} was not reported. Two control patients received similar infusions at 5% albumin.

The most striking finding of this study was a decline in creatinine clearance in the hemoglobin solution recipients from a baseline value of 148 ml/min to 73 ml/min, 1 hour after infusion. This value returned to normal in the second hour following infusion. This alteration in kidney function was accompanied by a sharp decline in urine volume in these patients. In the albumin control patients, no changes were seen in urine volume or creatinine clearance. The authors stressed that this deterioration in kidney function was transient and not associated with permanent renal damage. Nevertheless, these results had a chilling effect on further clinical research.

As Savitsky and coworkers (32) pointed out, there are several possible explanations for the observed nephrotoxicity. The first is stromal toxicity—the authors did report a stroma lipid level of 1.6 mg/dl. However, since this represents only 1% of the original level of phospholipid, and since the infusion of hemoglobin solution did not produce detectable disseminated intravascular coagulation in the recipients, stromal toxicity is an unlikely explanation. A second possibility is that the changes in renal function were simply related to the filtration of free hemoglobin through the kidneys. Perhaps hemoglobin filtration in some way interferes with normal kidney function. Once the hemoglobinemia disappears, renal function returns to normal. This is an interesting argument, since the highest level of plasma hemoglobin in the human volunteers was only 57 mg/dl. In actual clinical practice, we expect plasma hemoglobin levels to rise to 6–8 g/dl, a 1000-fold increase over the levels seen in the clinical safety trials. Elevations of plasma hemoglobin of such a magnitude would probably produce even greater changes in renal function, especially in a setting of hemorrhagic shock.

A significant problem has been the absence of a reliable animal model to assess the safety of each product. We have recently developed a sensitive and reproducible animal model that virtually duplicates these findings (31). Infusion of tetrameric hemoglobin solution in the

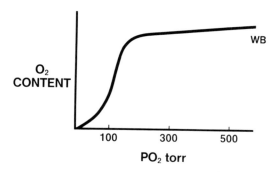

Figure 15.7. Oxygen content curve for whole blood *(WB)*.

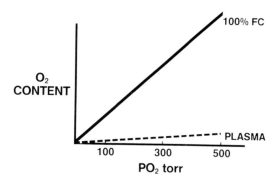

Figure 15.9. Oxygen content curves for 100% fluorocarbon *(FC)* and plasma.

unanesthetized primate produces the same changes in hemodynamics and renal function that were observed in the human volunteers. It is our hypothesis that since the large polymerized hemoglobin molecule will not traverse the renal tubules, it may not produce these same effects. We are currently completing the evaluation of Poly SFH-P in this same model. If no adverse effects are observed, a clinical trial with Poly SFH-P might be feasible.

PERFLUOROCHEMICAL EMULSIONS

Perfluorochemicals have potential as oxygen carriers because of their relatively high solubility for oxygen when compared with blood or plasma (3). However, this high solubility exists only for pure perfluorochemicals. Since perfluorochemicals are not miscible with water (i.e., plasma), current products are prepared as an emulsion, which lowers the concentration of fluorocarbon. The properties of the currently available perfluorochemical emulsions can best be understood by looking at several oxygen content curves. The oxygen content curve for whole blood is shown in Figure 15.7, and is

the composite of the oxygen content curves for red cell hemoglobin and plasma, as shown in Figure 15.8 (7). The curve illustrates that the majority of oxygen in whole blood is chemically bound to the hemoglobin molecule. The hemoglobin becomes fully saturated at a P_{O_2} of 150 torr. As the P_{O_2} increases beyond 150 torr, however, there is still an increase in the amount of oxygen in whole blood (Fig. 15.7), which reflects the dissolved O_2 in the aqueous phase of plasma (Fig. 15.8). Thus, as the oxygen tension in the blood is increased, the oxygen content will similarly increase despite the complete saturation of the hemoglobin molecule. Since the dissolved oxygen content of blood at the ambient P_{O_2} of 100 torr is only 0.3 ml/dl, it is generally ignored when discussing oxygen content.

The potential value of perfluorochemicals as oxygen carriers is shown in Figure 15.9 (20). The curve illustrates that pure fluorocarbons have a solubility coefficient approximately 10–20 times that of plasma. In a sense, the fluorocarbons are functioning as a "super water." Unfortunately, however, pure fluorocarbons cannot be administered. A major development in perfluorochemical research was the ability to make a stable emulsion using pluronic F-68 as the emulsifying agent. By creating this emulsion, the concentration of fluorocarbon is lowered dramatically. Figure 15.10 shows oxygen content curves for 20% and 40% fluorocarbon emulsions compared with plasma. Clearly, the lower the concentration of fluorocarbon, the lower the oxygen content. The oxygen content of the perfluorochemical depends on both the P_{O_2} and the volume concentration of fluorocarbon (fluorocrit). For any given fluorocrit, the higher the P_{O_2}, the higher the concentration of dissolved oxygen. Similarly, for any given P_{O_2}, the higher the amount of

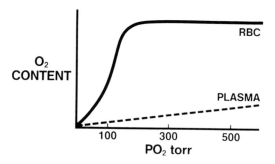

Figure 15.8. Oxygen content curves for red blood cells *(RBC)* and plasma.

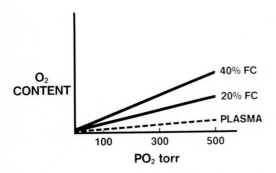

Figure 15.10. Oxygen content curves for plasma, and 20% and 40% fluorocarbons *(FC)*.

fluorocarbon, the higher the oxygen content (Fig. 15.10).

The commercially prepared perfluorochemical emulsion is Fluosol-DA, 20%. This product has been evaluated extensively in animals and humans in Japan, and in several series in the United States. A comparison of whole blood with a hemoglobin of 15 g/dl and Fluosol-DA, 20%, is shown in Figure 15.11 (20). Although the Fluosol-DA does offer some value as an oxygen carrier, there are several limiting factors. First, the patient must breathe a high concentration of inspired oxygen in order to maximize the O_2 content of the Fluosol-DA. Second, even at a P_{O_2} of 500 torr (Fractional inspired O_2 concentration (F_{IO_2}), 1.0), with the maximum achievable fluorocrit, the O_2 content is still less than 5 ml/dl compared with 20 ml/dl in whole blood. The infusion of Fluosol-DA would therefore add very little to the total O_2 content unless the [Hb] were considerably reduced from normal. The point of this observation is that although a potential benefit of

Fluosol-DA does exist, there are significant limitations. Furthermore, the restrictions on the amount of Fluosol-DA that can be administered to any patient (40 ml/kg) limits the achievable fluorocrit, which will further decrease the amount of oxygen that can be carried by the Fluosol-DA.

Laboratory Studies

Our initial effort was to answer the question: How good are fluorocarbon emulsions as oxygen carriers? Because the principal requirement of any O_2 carrier is the ability to load and unload oxygen, these functions must be accurately evaluated. We have shown that adult baboons can survive a total exchange transfusion with Fluosol-DA to zero hematocrit if they are ventilated at an F_{IO_2} of 1.0 (11). The animals maintain normal hemodynamics and oxygen transport in the virtual absence of red blood cells. Although these data suggest that Fluosol-DA is an effective oxygen carrier, we also demonstrated that control animals survive at zero hematocrit on an F_{IO_2} of 1.0 without Fluosol-DA (13). This remarkable observation leads to the conclusion that Fluosol-DA is not necessary at an F_{IO_2} of 1.0, at least in this acute setting.

These results can be explained by an understanding of the way in which the fluorocarbons carry oxygen. In the presence of red blood cells and fluorocarbon (FC), the total oxygen content in the blood can be considered as the sum of three separate oxygen carriers:

$$[O_2]_{total} = [O_2]_{RBC} + [O_2]_{plasma} + [O_2]_{FC} \quad (2)$$

Survival depends on total oxygen content, but does not distinguish between each of the oxygen carriers (14, 30). Thus, at a P_{O_2} of 500 torr the plasma becomes a very significant carrier of oxygen and is capable of supporting oxygen consumption even in the complete absence of both red cells and fluorocarbon. Because the plasma oxygen content will always be increased at an F_{IO_2} of 1.0, the actual need for the Fluosol-DA is unclear.

Although this study documents the efficacy of plasma as an oxygen carrier at an F_{IO_2} of 1.0, we are concerned about the potential risk of oxygen toxicity to the lungs in the clinical setting (5). A safe level of prolonged supplemental oxygen is thought to be an F_{IO_2} below 0.6. Our data suggest the Fluosol-DA might not be necessary at an F_{IO_2} of 1.0, but we cannot

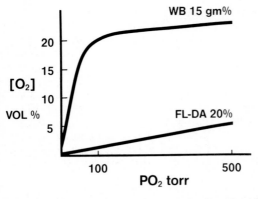

Figure 15.11. Oxygen content curves for 15 g/dl (gm%) of whole blood *(WB)* and 20% Fluosol-DA *(FL-DA)*.

assume the same to be true at lower levels of supplemental oxygen.

Clinical Trial

The results of the animal study led us to design a clinical trial to evaluate the safety and efficacy of Fluosol-DA as an oxygen carrier (7, 10). We sought to distinguish between the contribution of the dissolved oxygen in the plasma and the dissolved oxygen in the Fluosol-DA compartment, and to minimize the risk of toxicity from breathing 100% oxygen. The objective, therefore, was to provide sufficient O_2 delivery with Fluosol-DA at an Fio_2 below 0.6. Unlike most clinical trials, the protocol for Fluosol-DA was nonblinded, and had a crossover design, with each patient serving as his or her own control for each O_2 carrier. Such a design let us define the physiologic need for, and evaluate the efficacy of, Fluosol-DA in acute anemia.

Patients had to be at least 18 years old in order to be admitted into the study. Furthermore, the patient's arterial blood Po_2 (Pao_2) had to reach 300 torr or greater when receiving supplemental oxygen, and the patient had to be normovolemic. The physiologic criteria of need for supplementing oxygen content were derived from our control studies in baboons: [Hb] below 3.5 g/dl; $P_{mv}O_2$ below 25 torr, and O_2 extraction ratio above 50% (6, 14).

A patient who met one of the inclusion criteria was first treated with 100% oxygen. An attempt was made to stabilize the patient's condition at the clinically safe inspired oxygen level of 60% by a gradual tapering process. If successful, the patient was considered to have no physiologic need for an increased O_2 content, and did not receive Fluosol-DA. If unsuccessful, the patient was crossed over to the Fluosol-DA, and received up to a maximum permissible dose of 40 ml/kg of body weight. Once again, an attempt was made to stabilize the patient's condition at 60% oxygen with Fluosol-DA.

GOALS

The study had three goals: (a) to identify a physiologic need for an additional oxygen carrier when the red cell compartment became inadequate, as defined by the physiologic criteria; (b) to attempt an increase in the oxygen content using only the plasma as an oxygen carrier at a safe Fio_2; and (c) to evaluate Fluo-

sol-DA as an oxygen carrier if the physiologic criteria of need still existed at an unsafe Fio_2.

RESULTS

Twenty-three surgical patients with blood loss and having religious objections to receiving blood transfusions were evaluated. Fifteen moderately anemic patients with a mean hemoglobin level ($\pm$ SE) of 7.2 $\pm$ 0.5 g/dl had no evidence of a physiologic need for increased arterial oxygen content and did not receive Fluosol-DA. Eight severely anemic patients with a mean hemoglobin level of 3.0 $\pm$ 0.4 g/dl met the criteria of need, and received the drug until the physiologic need disappeared or a maximal dose of 40 ml/kg of body weight was reached. All patients breathed supplemental O_2. We observed no adverse reactions to Fluosol-DA.

The volume of Fluosol-DA infused ranged from 2 to 10 units. Six of the eight patients received the maximum allowable dose. One patient survived after receiving only 2 units. Another died before his total dosage had been infused.

The maximal arterial oxygen content added by Fluosol-DA in the eight patients ranged from 0.3 to 1.2 ml/dl, with a mean increment of 0.7 $\pm$ 0.1 ml/dl. The data for Fio_2, fluorocrit, and partial pressure of arterial oxygen at the time of this peak in arterial oxygen content are shown in Table 15.4. The simultaneous level of arterial oxygen carried by the plasma was 1.3 $\pm$ 0.1 ml/dl, and the level of oxygen carried by the red cells was 2.8 $\pm$ 0.6 ml/dl.

Table 15.5 shows the extent of oxygen unloading from the three phases. Eighty-two percent of the oxygen carried by the plasma and Fluosol-DA phases was unloaded. In contrast, only 19% was unloaded from the red cell phase. The relative contribution to total oxygen consumption for each of the three phases is also shown in Table 15.5. The plasma contributes

Table 15.4
Arterial Oxygen Content at Peak Effect of Fluosol-DA

	Mean $\pm$ SE
Partial pressure of arterial O_2 (torr)	430 $\pm$ 19
Fluorocrit (%)	5 $\pm$ 1
Fractional inspired O_2 concentration	1.0 $\pm$ 0.0
Arterial O_2 content (ml/dl)	
In Fluosol-DA phase	0.7 $\pm$ 0.1
In plasma phase	1.3 $\pm$ 0.1
Of red cells	2.8 $\pm$ 0.6

Table 15.5
Oxygen Dynamics of Three Phases at Peak Effect of Fluosol-DA

	Mean ± SE		
	Fluosol-DA	Plasma	Red Cells
Arterial O_2 content (ml/dl)	0.7 ± 0.1	1.3 ± 0.1	2.8 ± 0.6
Venous O_2 content (ml/dl)	0.2 ± 0.1	0.2 ± 0.1	2.2 ± 0.4
Oxygen unloaded (%)	82 ± 5	82 ± 5	19 ± 5
Contribution to O_2 consumption (%)	28 ± 5	50 ± 5	22 ± 7

the most (50%), whereas Fluosol-DA contributes 28% and the red cells only 22%.

The hemodynamic and oxygen transport values before and after Fluosol-DA are shown in Table 15.6. The only statistically significant differences were a minor reduction in heart rate and an increase in partial pressure of arterial oxygen (following an increased FiO_2 in one patient).

The intravascular persistence of the Fluosol-DA was determined in five patients. The mean half-life was 24.3 ± 4.3 hours, with a range of 12–37 hours.

SURVIVAL

Six of the eight patients receiving Fluosol-DA died. One of the surviving patients received red cell transfusions against his wishes, under a court order, after receiving his maximal allowable dose of Fluosol-DA (7). He prob-

ably would have died in the absence of red cell therapy. The minimal hemoglobin level observed in these eight patients was 1.8 ± 0.4 g/dl.

The 15 patients not receiving Fluosol-DA had a minimal hemoglobin level of 7.2 ± 0.5 g/dl during their hospital stay. Fourteen of these patients survived.

Implications of the Clinical Study

The principal requirement of any oxygen carrier is the ability to load and unload oxygen effectively. The product must remain in the intravascular space long enough to satisfy the need for which it was administered and it must be free from any undesirable side effects.

The data illustrate that Fluosol-DA provides poor arterial oxygen content supplementation. This study shows that the fluorocrit achieved clinically with the currently available product is only about 5%. As shown in Table 15.4, a 5% concentration of Fluosol-DA at a Po_2 of 430 torr has an oxygen content of 0.7 ml/dl or approximately half the oxygen carried by plasma (1.3 ml/dl). This is equivalent to an increase in hemoglobin concentration of only 0.5 g/dl. This relation between the amount of oxygen carried by Fluosol-DA at this fluorocrit and the amount carried by plasma is valid regardless of Po_2, since the oxygen content curves for both carriers are straight lines (Fig. 15.12). The potential benefit of the Fluosol-DA is that even this small amount of oxygen is additive to the amount carried by plasma (Equation 2). However, the observed increase in total oxygen content of 0.7 ml/dl was not clinically important in our eight patients, as evidenced by the absence of any discernible physiologic benefit after the Fluosol-DA infusion.

In contrast, Fluosol-DA unloads oxygen very effectively. The $AVDo_2$ of the Fluosol-DA phase is 0.5 ml/dl (Table 15.5). Most of the oxygen carried by the Fluosol-DA is thus unloaded. The data also confirm previous reports that

Table 15.6
Hemodynamics and Oxygen Transport Before and after Fluosol-DA Administration

	Mean ± SE	
	Before Fluosol-DA	After Fluosol-DA[a]
Heart rate beats/min	117 ± 5	106 ± 4[b]
Mean arterial pressure (torr)	74 ± 6	78 ± 5
Cardiac index (liters/min/m²)	4.5 ± 0.7	4.2 ± 0.7
Hemoglobin (g/dl)	3.0 ± 0.4	2.0 ± 0.4
Total arterial O_2 content (ml/dl)	5.3 ± 0.5	4.8 ± 0.6
O_2 delivery (ml/min/m²)	235 ± 27	197 ± 32
O_2 consumption (ml/min/m²)	109 ± 13	88 ± 11
Partial pressure of arterial O_2 (torr)	356 ± 24	430 ± 19[b]
Partial pressure of mixed venous O_2 (torr)	40.0 ± 3.9	78.2 ± 23.3
O_2 extraction ratio (%)	46.0 ± 2.5	47.6 ± 3.8

[a]Data were obtained at peak arterial oxygen content after Fluosol-DA.
[b]The difference between values before and after Fluosol-DA is statistically significant ($P < 0.05$).

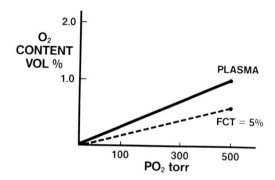

Figure 15.12. Oxygen content curves for plasma and Fluosol at a fluorocrit *(FCT)* of 5%.

Fluosol-DA makes an important contribution to total oxygen consumption (39–41). However, the lack of any apparent physiologic effect despite this efficient oxygen unloading again suggests that this contribution is inadequate.

The intravascular persistence of Fluosol-DA is also insufficient, at least when red cells cannot be subsequently used. The half-life of 24 hours and the maximal allowable dose of 40 ml/kg led to a loss of the Fluosol-DA from the circulation before the patients were able to regenerate an adequate red cell mass to recover from their severe anemia (8). The mean hemoglobin level in the eight patients fell from an initial level of 3.0 to a low of 1.8 g/dl. This hemoglobin level is not compatible with survival, and six of the eight patients died of progressive anemia. The combination of too small an increment in arterial oxygen content and an inadequate duration of Fluosol-DA probably contributed to this unsatisfactory outcome. One of the survivors did require and eventually received red cells (against his wishes) after his total Fluosol-DA dose. It is thus possible that an evaluation of Fluosol-DA in a setting of short-term unavailability of red cells might result in a better outcome.

The mortality results should be compared with those of previous studies (23, 24, 39, 41). In the four earlier reports, representing a total of 200 patients, only three patients had a hemoglobin level of less than 3 g/dl. Two of these three patients died. In contrast, the less severely anemic patients receiving Fluosol-DA had satisfactory outcomes. This is consistent with our experience. Fifteen of the 23 patients evaluated had no physiologic evidence of a need for increased arterial oxygen content, despite their minimal hemoglobin level of 7.2 g/ dl. They appeared to do as well as the comparable patients who received Fluosol-DA or those who would have received red cells if they were willing, because their hemoglobin level was below 10 g/dl. Fourteen of these moderately anemic patients not receiving Fluosol-DA survived. This good outcome justifies our physiologic assessment of when supplementation of oxygen content is needed, and raises some questions of the manner in which decisions about transfusions are made. The mortality rate is high among severely anemic patients refusing red cells, despite Fluosol-DA therapy. Patients with less extreme blood loss who refuse red cells do well, with or without Fluosol-DA.

In conclusion, the results suggest that in acute blood loss, Fluosol-DA is unnecessary when anemia is moderate and ineffective when it is severe. Fluosol-DA is therefore an inadequate red cell substitute. New formulations of perfluorochemicals that correct the observed shortcomings of Fluosol-DA may be more effective (4, 37), such as achieving higher fluorocarbon concentrations and a longer intravascular persistence. In the near future, however, there is no likely perfluorochemical that will be an effective red cell substitute.

SUMMARY

The possibilities for the use of these oxygen carriers in the future are rather exciting. Both products meet some of the criteria of an ideal red cell substitute; both have shortcomings that will influence their clinical utility. The fluorocarbons appear to be quite safe. Their major current deficiency is that they are not likely to be useful in the clinical setting because of the requirement for supplemental O_2. The fluorocarbons are ineffective O_2 carriers when patients are breathing room air. In contrast, Poly SFH-P has been shown to be highly effective, and has an O_2-carrying capacity equivalent to that of red blood cells. The unknown factor at this time is the safety of this hemoglobin solution. However, we are hopeful that Poly SFH-P will eliminate the undesirable effects of prior products. If the results are encouraging, it might be possible to design a clinical trial with Poly SFH-P. Other areas of use for these O_2 carriers are being explored, such as use in coronary angioplasty, myocardial and cerebral ischemia, and radiation and chemotherapy. In addition, both products may be useful in cardioplegia and organ preservation. Once the safety and efficacy issues are resolved, other innovative uses may be identified. The development of both products remains active.

References

1. Benesch RE, Benesch R, Renthal RD, et al: Affinity labeling of the polyphosphate binding site of hemoglobin. *Biochemistry* 11:3576, 1972.
2. Birndorf NI, Lopas H: Effects of red cell stroma-free hemoglobin solution on renal function in monkeys. *J Appl Physiol* 29:573, 1970.
3. Biro GP, Blais P: Perfluorocarbon blood substitutes. *CRC Crit Rev Oncol Hematol* 6(4):311, 1987.
4. Clark LC Jr, Clark EW, Moore RE, et al: Room temperature-stable biocompatible fluorocarbon emulsions. In Bolin RB, Geyer RP, Nemo GJ (eds): *Advances in Blood Substitute Research*. New York, Alan R Liss, 1983, p 169.
5. Davis WB, Rennard SI, Bitterman PB, Crystal RG: Pulmonary oxygen toxicity: early reversible changes in human alveolar structure induced by hyperoxia. *N Engl J Med* 309:878, 1983.
6. Gould SA, Rice CL, Moss GS: The physiologic basis of the use of blood and blood products. *Surg Annu* 16:13, 1984.
7. Gould SA, Rosen AL, Sehgal LR, et al: Clinical experience with Fluosol-DA. In Bolin RB, Geyer RP (eds): *Advances in Blood Substitute Research*. New York, Alan R Liss, 1983, p 331.
8. Gould SA, Rosen AL, Sehgal LR, et al: Depressed red cell recovery following acute blood loss. (abstract). *Fed Proc* 44:1265, 1985.
9. Gould SA, Rosen AL, Sehgal L, et al: The effect of altered hemoglobin-oxygen affinity on oxygen transport by hemoglobin solution. *J Surg Res* 28:246, 1980.
10. Gould SA, Rosen AL, Sehgal LR, et al: Fluosol-DA as a red cell substitute in acute anemia. *N Engl J Med* 315:1653, 1986.
11. Gould SA, Rosen AL, Sehgal LR, et al: How good are fluorocarbon emulsions as O_2 carriers? *Surg Forum* 32:299, 1981.
12. Gould SA, Rosen AL, Sehgal LR, et al: Is cardiac output the principal determinant of $P_{mv}O_2$? *Crit Care Med* 9:273, 1981.
13. Gould SA, Rosen AL, Sehgal LR, et al: Is polyhemoglobin an effective O_2 carrier? *J Trauma* 26:903, 1986.
14. Gould SA, Rosen AL, Sehgal LR, et al: O_2 extraction ratio: a physiologic indicator of transfusion need (abstract). *Transfusion* 23:416, 1983.
15. Gould SA, Rosen AL, Sehgal LR, et al: Plasma: an alternative oxygen carrier? (abstract 7864). *Fed Proc* 41:1615, 1982.
16. Gould SA, Rosen AL, Sehgal LR, et al: Red cell substitutes: hemoglobin solution or fluorocarbon? *J Trauma* 22:736, 1982.
17. Gould SA, Sehgal LR, Rosen AL, et al: The development of polymerized pyridoxylated hemoglobin solution as a red cell substitute. *Ann Emerg Med* 15:1416, 1986.
18. Gould SA, Sehgal LR, Rosen AL, et al: Hemoglobin solution: Is a normal [Hb] or P_{50} more important? *J Surg Res* 33:189, 1982.
19. Gould SA, Sehgal LR, Rosen AL, et al: Polyhemoglobin: an improved red cell substitute. *Surg Forum* 36:30, 1985.
20. Gould SA, Sehgal LR, Rosen AL, et al: Red cell substitutes: an update. *Ann Emerg Med* 14:798, 1985.
21. Greenburg AG, Hayashi R, Siefert I, et al: Intravascular persistence and oxygen delivery of pyridoxylated, stroma-free hemoglobin during gradations of hypotension. *Surgery* 86:13, 1979.
22. Hamilton PB, Hiller A, Van Slyke DD: Renal effects of hemoglobin infusions in dogs in hemorrhagic shock. *J Exp Med* 85:477, 1948.
23. Karn KE, Ogburn PL Jr, Julian T, et al: Use of a whole blood substitute, Fluosol-DA 20%, after massive postpartum hemorrhage. *Surg Obstet Gynecol* 65:127, 1985.
24. Mitsuno T, Ohyanagi H, Naito R: Clinical studies of a perfluorochemical whole blood substitute (Fluosol-DA): summary of 186 cases. *Ann Surg* 195:60, 1982.
25. Moss GS, DeWoskin R, Rosen AL, et al: Transport of oxygen and carbon dioxide by hemoglobin-saline solution in the red cell–free primate. *Surg Gynecol Obstet* 142:357, 1976.
26. Moss GS, Gould SA, Sehgal LR, et al: Hemoglobin solution—from tetramer to polymer. *Surgery* 95:249, 1984.
27. Rabiner SF, Friedman LH: The role of intravascular hemolysis and the reticuloendothelial system in the production of a hypercoagulable state. *Br J Haematol* 14:105, 1968.
28. Rabiner SF, Helbert JR, Lopas H, Friedman LH: Evaluation of a stroma-free hemoglobin solution for use as a plasma expander. *J Exp Med* 126:1127, 1967.
29. Rosen AL, Gould SA, Sehgal LR, et al: Evaluation of efficacy of stroma free hemoglobin solutions. In Bolin RB, Geyer RP (eds): *Advances in Blood Substitutes*. New York, Alan R Liss, 1983, p. 79.
30. Rosen AL, Sehgal LR, Gould SA, et al: Fluorocarbon emulsions: methodology to assess efficacy. *Crit Care Med* 10:149, 1982.
31. Rosen AL, Sehgal LR, Gould SA, et al: Renal response to hemoglobin solutions. *Physiologist* 29:4, 1986.
32. Savitsky JP, Doczi J, Black J, Arnold JD: A clinical safety trial of stroma-free hemoglobin. *Clin Pharmacol Ther* 23:73, 1978.
33. Sehgal LR, Gould SA, Rosen AL, et al: Polymerized pyridoxylated hemoglobin: a red cell substitute with normal O_2 capacity. *Surgery* 95:433, 1984.
34. Sehgal L, Rosen AL, Gould SA, et al: In vitro and in vivo characteristics of polymerized pyridoxylated hemoglobin solution (abstract 2383). *Fed Proc* 39:718, 1980.
35. Sehgal LR, Rosen AL, Gould SA, et al: Preparation and *in vitro* characteristics of polymerized pyridoxylated hemoglobin. *Transfusion* 23:148, 1983.
36. Sehgal LR, Rosen AL, Noud G, et al: Large volume preparation of pyridoxylated hemoglobin with high *in vivo* P_{50}. *J Surg Res* 30:14, 1981.
37. Sloviter HA, Mukherji B: Prolonged retention in the circulation of emulsified lipid-coated perfluorochemicals. In Bolin RB, Geyer RP (eds): *Advances in Blood Substitute Research*. New York, Alan R Liss, 1983, p 181.
38. Sunder-Plassman L, Dieterle R, Seifert J, et al: Stroma free haemoglobin solution as a blood replacement fluid: actual state and problems. *Eur J Intensive Care Med* 1:37, 1975.
39. Tremper KK, Friedman AE, Levine EM, et al: The preoperative treatment of severely anemic patients with a perfluorochemical oxygen-transport fluid, Fluosol-DA. *N Engl J Med* 307:277, 1982.
40. Tremper KK, Lapin R, Levine E, et al: Hemodynamic and oxygen transport effects of a perfluorochemical blood substitute. Fluosol-DA (20%). *Crit Care Med* 8:738, 1980.
41. Waxman K, Tremper KK, Cullen BF, Mason GR: Perfluorocarbon infusion in bleeding patients refusing blood transfusion. *Arch Surg* 119:721, 1984.

16

Thrombolytic Therapy

Paul R. Eisenberg, M.D., M.P.H.
Allan S. Jaffe, M.D.

Thrombolytic agents have been investigated extensively for the treatment of thrombotic disorders since the initial observations by Tillet and Garner in 1933 (126) that filtrates of β-hemolytic streptococci had fibrinolytic activity. However, because of the potential for bleeding and the lack of adequate documentation of benefit, the indications for the use of thrombolytic agents have been limited. Recently, enthusiasm for thrombolytic therapy has increased because of the development of agents with greater clot specificity, and the demonstration that prompt reperfusion of coronary arteries occluded by thrombi in patients with acute myocardial infarction leads to a reduction in mortality (49, 68, 114) and preservation of ventricular function (97, 112, 113). As a result, the optimum means for induction of fibrinolysis and indications for its use are now being extensively redefined.

OVERVIEW OF THE FIBRINOLYTIC SYSTEM

The fibrinolytic system is an enzymatic system present in blood that induces clot dissolution via the formation of the enzyme, plasmin. Plasmin is derived from the circulating zymogen, plasminogen, by the action of agents known as plasminogen activators. Once generated, plasmin degrades fibrin as well as fibrinogen, prothrombin, factor V, factor VIII, prekallikrein, several components of the complement system, and other circulating proteins (2). The proteolytic activity of plasmin is controlled by rapid interactions with several circulating inhibitors in blood (19).

Plasminogen is a single chain glycoprotein that exists in several forms. Native plasminogen has a glutamic acid at the amino terminus, and is referred to as "glu-plasminogen" (141). Limited plasmin digestion of plasminogen during activation results in a modified glycoprotein with lysine, alanine, or methionine at the amino terminus, referred to collectively as "lys-plasminogen." Within the plasminogen molecule are sites referred to as the lysine-binding sites, which serve as the points of interaction for the binding of plasminogen to fibrin or to its inhibitor, α-2-antiplasmin (19, 147). Lys-plasminogen has a higher affinity for fibrin than does glu-plasminogen and is also more rapidly converted to plasmin by the plasminogen activator, urokinase (18, 95).

MECHANISM OF ACTION OF PLASMINOGEN ACTIVATORS

Plasminogen can be activated by a number of mechanisms. It is activated by factor XII, prekallikrein, high molecular weight kininogen, and possibly other plasma constituents of the kallikrein system (66). The physiologic importance of this type of activation (intrinsic) is undetermined. The significance of activation due to the secretion of plasminogen activators from tissue or endothelium is better understood (extrinsic activation). Tissue-type plasminogen activator has been extensively studied and is probably identical to blood plasminogen activator and vascular plasminogen activator (101). It has very little plasminogen activator activity in isolation; however, in the presence of fibrin, activation of plasminogen increases markedly (58). Thus, in physiologic systems, tissue-type plasminogen activator converts only fibrin-bound plasminogen to plasmin, providing a localized mechanism for clot dissolution (21).

Urokinase is a two-chain serum protease that has been isolated from human urine and cultured kidney cells (91, 151). It exists in both a high and low molecular weight form (145). Two-chain urokinase activates plasminogen by lysis of a single arginine-valine bond (102). A single chain proenzyme form of urokinase (scu-PA) also has been isolated and has plasminogen activator activity even without conversion to the two-chain form (22, 50).

Streptokinase, in contrast, activates plasminogen indirectly. It first forms an equimolar complex with plasminogen, which exposes an active site on plasminogen and transforms it into an activator complex (16, 85). Streptokinase-plasminogen complexes have been modified by the synthesis of derivatives containing acyl groups at the active site (116). In the circulation, acylation prevents plasminogen activation. These derivatives are deacylated slowly, and active streptokinase-plasmin(ogen) activator complexes result. The less pronounced induction of systemic plasminogen activation and the potential for deacylation in the vicinity of clot allows for slightly greater clot specificity than with streptokinase alone.

Once generated, plasmin is rapidly inhibited by the formation of an equimolar complex with α-2-antiplasmin (146). Plasmin interacts with fibrin at the enzyme's lysine-binding site. Plasmin that is bound to fibrin is protected from rapid inhibition by α-2-antiplasmin since the lysine-binding site is occupied by fibrin. α-2-Macroglobulin also inhibits plasmin, though more slowly (19).

CLINICAL PHARMACOLOGY OF FIBRINOLYTIC AGENTS

Streptokinase

Because streptokinase (SK) is derived from a common bacterial species, antibodies to it are present in most patients. Although allergic reactions can occur, a well-documented case of anaphylaxis with currently available preparations has not been reported. When streptokinase is administered systemically, an initial large dose is used to overcome the inhibitory effect of high antibody titers. The administration of 250,000 units overcomes antibody resistance and induces a systemic lytic state in more than 90% of patients (55). The maintenance dose used subsequently varies, but in theory must be sufficient to generate enough plasmin to overcome circulating inhibitors. On the other hand, an excessive dose of streptokinase could consume or complex all of the available plasminogen, leaving none for further activation. Thus, both insufficient and/or excessive doses may result in failure to achieve a lytic state.

The half-life of streptokinase in vivo has not been precisely delineated. After an injection of radiolabeled streptokinase, an initial α-distributive half-life of 18 minutes has been observed, followed by a β-distributive half-life of 83 minutes (37). However, the clearance of functionally active SK-plasminogen complexes has been estimated to be only 23 minutes (86). Nonetheless, plasmin activity can be demonstrated for up to 4 hours after administration of streptokinase, documenting persistent fibrinolytic activity despite clearance of active complexes from plasma (35).

Since streptokinase activates both circulating plasminogen and plasminogen bound to fibrin, both local and systemic effects are observed after its administration. Degradation of circulating fibrinogen, plasminogen, and coagulation factors is the most significant hemostatic alteration (111). Formation of fibrinogen degradation products may exacerbate the tendency toward bleeding induced by the low levels of circulating fibrinogen and other coagulation factors by inhibiting thrombin and fibrin polymerization (76, 83). Low-dose local infusions of streptokinase have been used to limit these adverse systemic effects.

Urokinase

Urokinase (UK) has also been used extensively as a fibrinolytic agent. Since urokinase is not antigenic in humans and is a direct activator of plasminogen, the dose-response relationships of this activator are less complex. After administration, urokinase is cleared with a half-life of 14 ± 6 minutes. Since urokinase activates both circulating plasminogen and plasminogen bound to fibrin, intravenous administration results in systemic effects similar to those observed after streptokinase (38). Local infusions of urokinase have also been used to minimize these effects. In general, the effects of urokinase and those of streptokinase are similar but urokinase is considerably more expensive.

Tissue Plasminogen Activator

Human tissue-type plasminogen activator (t-PA) has recently become available for clinical use. Initial studies using a product isolated from a human melanoma cell line demonstrated successful thrombolysis in both dogs and humans (11, 134). More recently t-PA has become available in large quantities through the use of recombinant gene technology (25, 133). This product is functionally similar to that derived from cell culture. Tissue-type plasminogen activator exists as either a one-chain or two-chain form (140). Both forms have similar fibrinolytic activity in purified systems; however, in plasma, one-chain t-PA is converted to two-chain t-PA during fibrinolysis (100). After a bolus injection, t-PA is cleared from plasma with a half-life of approximately 6 minutes (88). However with larger infusions, a β half-life of 1.3 hours has been documented for one preparation of the recombinant product (138). More recent preparations have a slightly shorter half-life (43). Lytic activity after administration of t-PA persists for many hours after clearance of activator (35).

Unlike urokinase or streptokinase, t-PA has little systemic effect at low doses (24, 134). The markedly enhanced activation of plasminogen by t-PA in the presence of fibrin should result in clot lysis without significant systemic plasminogen activation. However, the selectivity for plasminogen bound to fibrin is only relative, and in the presence of very high concentrations of t-PA, circulating plasminogen is degraded as well (117, 125). Thus, in clinical trials in patients with acute myocardial infarction, higher doses (100–150 mg) of t-PA produce some systemic plasminogen activation and fibrinogen breakdown (20). Nonetheless, systemic effects are less with t-PA than with other activators.

Trials of recombinant t-PA (Genentech, Inc., San Francisco, CA) in patients with acute myocardial infarction have utilized intravenous administration in order to permit treatment at the earliest possible instance. However, infusions into the coronary artery and peripheral arteries have also been employed, and offer the advantage of a significantly lower dose with similar beneficial effects (25, 47) when the early administration of treatment is less critical. Heparin competes with t-PA for fibrin binding (5, 90); thus, the concomitant use of heparin may increase the plasminogenolytic activity of t-PA and reduce its fibrin specificity.

Acylated Streptokinase/Plasminogen Complex Derivatives

The acylated streptokinase-plasminogen complex chosen for clinical trials, BRL-26921 (ASPAC), in experimental models induces clot lysis, while inducing less systemic lytic activity than streptokinase (115). Deacylation occurs with a half-life of 40 minutes; subsequently, clearance is similar to that of unmodified streptokinase-plasminogen complexes. In humans there is little systemic fibrinogenolytic activity when 7–12 mg is administered as an intravenous bolus (93, 119). However, at higher doses, progressive systemic lytic activity has been observed (56, 67). In recent trials, bolus doses of 30 mg were required to induce rapid coronary thrombolysis (9, 82, 139). In this dose range, significant systemic lytic activity is observed.

Single Chain Urokinase Plasminogen Activator

Single chain urokinase plasminogen activator (scu-PA) directly activates plasminogen to plasmin. Circulating scu-PA is converted to the two-chain form of urokinase, resulting in still further plasminogen activation (26, 80). In plasma, activation of plasminogen by scu-PA is limited by competition with a specific inhibitor (80), which is thought to be inactivated in the presence of fibrin. The half-life of scu-PA in experimental models is similar to that of urokinase. Preliminary trials with scu-PA demonstrate greater clot selectivity in humans than with urokinase (135). Whether therapeutic doses will be as selective as those observed with t-PA is undetermined. Synergism with t-PA has been demonstrated (23).

MONITORING OF THE COAGULATION SYSTEM DURING FIBRINOLYSIS

Ideally, laboratory monitoring of coagulation during treatment with fibrinolytic agents should provide precise information regarding the effect of the activator on coagulation and hence the intensity of fibrinolytic activity, the extent of clot dissolution, and the potential for bleeding. Conventional assays of coagulation can only document the presence of a systemic lytic state when it is induced, and do not distinguish between the effects of the activators and those of heparin (111). With the newer, more clot-selective plasminogen activators, monitoring has focused primarily on detection of systemic lytic activity as an index of excessive dosage. Once the lytic state has waned, assays of coagulation are used to titrate heparin administration.

Conventional laboratory monitoring of thrombolytic therapy may include assays of thrombin time, activated partial thromboplastin time, prothrombin time, fibrinogen, fibrinogen degradation products, and euglobulin lysis time. An understanding of each test and how it is affected by plasminogen activation is essential to proper interpretation of assay results (111).

The *thrombin time* (TT) is critically dependent on the concentration of fibrinogen in plasma and is extremely sensitive to heparin and fibrinogen degradation products in the sample (61). The thrombin time is prolonged after administration of fibrinolytic agents if fibrinogen is depleted and/or fibrin(ogen) degradation products are formed. When heparin has been administered, the addition of protamine sulfate to the plasma sample reverses the effects of heparin, thus allowing for detection of the consequences of systemic lytic activity alone.

The *activated partial thromboplastin time* (aPTT) assesses the activity of the coagulation factors other than factors VII and XIII, and is used primarily to monitor the effects of heparin (92). It is affected by decreased fibrinogen and elevated fibrinogen degradation products, but to a lesser extent than the thrombin time. Once the systemic lytic state has resolved, the aPTT is the best presently available coagulation test for monitoring and titrating heparin.

The *prothrombin time* (PT) measures the activity of factors V, VII, and X, prothrombin, and fibrinogen. It is affected to an even lesser extent than the aPTT by low levels of fibrinogen and/or fibrin(ogen) degradation products.

Determination of *fibrinogen* degradation is one of the most common criteria for documenting systemic plasminogen activation. Several methods are available for measurement of fibrinogen. The Clauss procedure measures the kinetics of clot formation and hence clottable fibrinogen. This assay is sensitive to the presence of fibrin(ogen) degradation products that are not clottable or inhibit polymerization of fibrin, and is inaccurate when fibrinogen levels are extremely low (generally less than 55 mg/dl) as is frequently the case after intravenous administration of conventional activators (e.g., SK). The Ellis method of measuring fibrinogen is an endpoint assay that measures the total amount of fibrinogen clotted after prolonged incubation. This assay is less affected by fibrin(ogen) degradation products and generally yields higher values for fibrinogen than those obtained from the Clauss method,

particularly when the fibrinogen level is very low. Large amounts of heparin in the sample can lead to spuriously low values. Reversal of the effects of heparin with protamine sulfate corrects for this effect. Precipitation procedures and most immunologic methods generally do not differentiate fibrinogen from large nonclottable fibrinogen degradation products.

The most commonly used procedure for measurement of *fibrin(ogen) degradation products* utilizes antifibrinogen antibody–coated latex particles. This method and most others detect products of both fibrinogen and fibrinolysis (122).

The euglobulin fraction of plasma does not contain inhibitors of plasmin. Thus, the *euglobulin lysis time* measures the functional activity of plasminogen activators in plasma (75). Enhanced lytic activity in the euglobulin fraction on plasma clots or fibrin plates or on clots in other systems is evidence of the presence of functional plasmin activity in vivo.

With conventional activators such as streptokinase, monitoring generally should include baseline and posttreatment measurements of the aPTT, TT, fibrinogen, and/or fibrin(ogen) degradation products to document induction of the lytic state (111). Reduction of the fibrinogen to 50% of baseline values or less can be considered evidence of systemic lytic activity. When very low levels of fibrinogen are present, the Ellis assay is more likely to be accurate. Subsequently, a normal protamine-corrected TT can be used to document the absence of residual effects due to plasminogen activation. Once the systemic lytic state has resolved, the aPTT may be used to titrate heparin. With newer, more clot-specific activators such as t-PA that may not induce systemic plasminogen activation, a shortened euglobulin lysis time may be the only evidence of circulating plasminogen activator, since fibrinogen degradation and other alterations of coagulation may only be present after large doses.

Fibrinopeptide A (FPA) is a 16 amino acid polypeptide cleaved from fibrinogen by thrombin as part of the formation of fibrin. Elevated levels of FPA in plasma are common in patients with acute transmural myocardial infarction early after the onset of symptoms (34). Thus, this assay detects the thrombotic state associated with acute transmural myocardial infarction. When streptokinase is given, FPA decreases markedly when recanalization occurs (33). In patients in whom recanalization does not occur, FPA increases markedly, suggesting that continued thrombin activity is competing with thrombolysis and is an important determinant of the lack of recanalization (33). Increased levels of FPA are observed even 4 hours after the administration of streptokinase, but rapidly decrease in response to heparin. Thus, measurement of FPA may provide a useful index of the intensity of thrombin activity in vivo during therapy and may provide a criterion for the success or failure of treatment. In addition, since FPA directly measures thrombin activity, it may facilitate titration of heparin.

Several new assays have been developed recently to distinguish fibrin from fibrinogen degradation products (41, 107, 144). These assays have been used to show that fibrin dissolution (following tissue plasminogen activator and streptokinase) persists for many hours after these activators are cleared from the circulation (35). In the future these assays may permit both sensitive and specific quantitative detection of fibrin dissolution in vivo, allowing for more precise titration of thrombolysis.

CLINICAL APPLICATIONS OF THROMBOLYSIS

Deep Venous Thrombosis

The traditional objective of therapy for lower extremity venous thrombosis was to prevent pulmonary embolism and its often catastrophic complications (28, 63, 70). Treatment with heparin usually does not result in dissolution of the thrombus by itself. As a consequence of residual thrombosis, morbidity due to venous valvular insufficiency with lower extremity edema, aching, stasis dermatitis, and ulceration (postphlebitic syndrome) may occur, especially after extensive proximal venous thrombosis (13, 150). As many as 80% of patients treated with heparin for venous thrombosis ultimately develop signs and/or symptoms of the postphlebitic syndrome (89). Fibrinolytic agents have the potential to more thoroughly dissolve occlusive thrombi. If residual clot is the etiology of the "postphlebitic syndrome," this therapy should reduce its incidence.

RANDOMIZED TRIALS COMPARING STREPTOKINASE WITH HEPARIN

Nine randomized trials have compared the efficacy of clot lysis induced by streptokinase with that induced by heparin as assessed by

Table 16.1
Results of Trials Comparing Thrombolysis with Heparin Therapy for Deep Venous Thrombosis

Study	Venographic Improvement (% of patients)[a]	
	Streptokinase	Heparin
Anreson et al (6)	71 (15/21)	14 (3/21)
Beiger et al (10)	NA[b]	NA[b]
Elliot et al (36)	65 (17/26)	0 (0/25)
Kakkar et al (64)	78 (8/9)	22 (2/9)
Marder et al (84)	58 (7/12)	25 (3/12)
Robertson et al (103)	66 (6/9)	29 (2/7)
Rosch et al (105)	45 (10/22)	27 (7/26)
Tsapogas et al (130)	53 (10/19)	7 (1/15)
Watz and Savidge (142)	67 (12/18)	36 (6/17)
Average (totals)	62 (84/136)	20 (26/132)

[a]Number of patients in parentheses.
[b]Only late venograms were performed in this study.

venography (6, 10, 36, 64, 84, 103, 105, 130, 142). In six, long-term end-points also were assessed (7, 27, 36, 64, 65, 130). In response to streptokinase, generally administered as a bolus of 250,000 units followed by an intravenous infusion of 100,000 units/hr for 24–72 hours, improved venous patency was observed in 62% of patients (Table 16.1). Only 20% of patients treated with heparin demonstrated similar improvement. Bleeding complications after streptokinase occurred in up to 26% of patients. Despite the improved efficiency of clot lysis with streptokinase, the short-term clinical response was similar with either regimen in most series.

Long-term clinical benefit was also evident in those patients treated with streptokinase (Table 16.2). Approximately 60% of the patients who received streptokinase had normal or only minor abnormalities on follow-up venography at intervals from 2 to 6½ years; 74% were asymptomatic. In contrast, only 20% of the patients treated with heparin alone demonstrated similar findings by venography, and more than 70% had symptomatic postphlebitic syndrome. Thus, fibrinolytic therapy results in more rapid and more complete resolution of deep venous thrombosis acutely, and less morbidity chronically.

TRIALS WITH OTHER PLASMINOGEN ACTIVATORS

More recent trials have employed acylated plasminogen-streptokinase complex (BRL-26921) and t-PA activator to treat deep venous thrombosis in the hope that less systemic fi-

Table 16.2
Late Results of Trials Comparing Thrombolysis with Heparin Therapy for Deep Venous Thrombosis

| Study | Follow-up | Normal Venogram (% of patients)[a] | |
		Streptokinase	Heparin
Anreson et al (7)	6.5 yr	56 (9/16)	33 (6/18)
Beiger et al (10)	3–4 months	40 (2/5)	20 (1/5)
Elliot et al (36)	3 months	60 (12/20)	0
Kakkar et al (65)	6–12 months	57 (4/7)	12 (1/8)
Rosch et al and Common et al (27, 105)	7 months	40 (6/15)	8 (1/12)
Watz and Savidge (142)	1–2 months	92 (11/12)	13 (1/8)
Average (totals)		59 (44/75)	20 (10/51)

[a]Number of patients in parentheses.

brinogen degradation would be induced thus reducing bleeding. BRL-26921 is effective (116); however, at doses higher than 5 mg/day, significant fibrinogen degradation occurs (67). In two patients treated with a low dose of melanoma-derived t-PA, complete lysis of deep venous thrombi occurred without systemic plasminogen activation (143). Preliminary results from ongoing trials suggest that t-PA will be effective and may be safer. Thus, t-PA may become the therapy of choice for deep venous thrombosis once optimal regimens for its use are defined.

SUMMARY

Thrombolytic therapy of deep venous thrombosis is beneficial. The more complete dissolution of thrombi prevents venous valvular damage and venous hypertension, reducing the incidence of the postphlebitic syndrome. Thrombolytic therapy should be considered in well-selected younger patients with extensive proximal venous thrombosis, who are free of contraindications to treatment (Table 16.3). After treatment, patients should receive heparin titrated to maintain the aPTT at approximately twice normal, followed by long-term Coumadin. The availability of agents with greater clot selectivity such as t-PA may enhance the safety of therapy and ultimately make fibrinolytic agents the treatment of choice for deep venous thrombosis.

Pulmonary Embolism

The use of heparin for the treatment of pulmonary embolism has markedly reduced mortality from recurrent emboli (8). Once treatment has been initiated, mortality is ap-

proximately 8% and often is secondary to associated illness (30). Nonetheless, patients with severe reduction in the cross-sectional area of the pulmonary artery (greater than 50%) frequently have right ventricular failure and shock, and have a poor prognosis despite heparin treatment.

Several controlled trials have attempted to show that more rapid clot lysis induced by fibrinolytic agents improves prognosis. The largest trial, sponsored by the National Institutes of Health was performed in two phases. In the first phase, the effects of a 12-hour infusion of urokinase were compared with the effects of heparin alone (Urokinase Pulmonary Embolism Trial, (UPET) (131). In the second,

Table 16.3
Contraindications to Thrombolytic Therapy

Absolute contraindications
   Active bleeding
   Cerebrovascular accident within 2 months, or active intracerebral process
Major relative contraindications
   Major recent surgery, organ biopsy, or invasive vascular procedure within 10 days
   Active malignancy
   Recent serious trauma, including prolonged cardiopulmonary resuscitation
   Severe hypertension (systolic ≥ 170 mm Hg or diastolic ≥ 110 mm Hg)
Other relative contraindications
   Chronic or acute renal failure
   Endocarditis
   Pregnancy or immediate postpartum state
   Age > 75 yr
   Diabetic hemorrhagic retinopathy
   Chronic therapeutic anticoagulation
   Inflammatory bowel disease
   Cutaneous ulcerations
   Chronic liver disease
   Disorders of hemostasis
   History of cerebrovascular accident

Table 16.4
Resolution of Lung Scan Defects in the National Institutes of Health Trials with Thrombolytic Agents

Protocol	Lung Scan Resolution (%)				
	1 day	2 days	5 days	14 days	3 months
UPET					
Urokinase (12 hr)[a]	6.2	8.0	11.3	14.9	—
Heparin only	2.7	4.9	9.3	14.7	—
USPET					
Urokinase (12 hr)[a]	9.0	—	—	—	28.6
Urokinase (24 hr)[a]	11.6	—	—	—	26.0
Streptokinase (24 hr)[a]	7.0	—	—	—	21.6

[a]All patients received heparin after infusion of the fibrinolytic agent.

12- and 24-hour infusions of urokinase and a 24-hour infusion of streptokinase were compared (Urokinase-Streptokinase Pulmonary Embolism Trial, USPET) (132). In both studies, patients subsequently received heparin for 5 days, then Coumadin for 14 days (Table 16.4). Both of these trials, as well as several smaller series, demonstrated that fibrinolytic therapy accelerated the dissolution of pulmonary emboli.

In the 333 patients randomized in UPET and USPET, resolution of emboli, judged by perfusion scans and pulmonary angiography, was more complete during the first 24 hours after fibrinolytic agents (Table 16-4). This rapid resolution was associated with a more rapid decrease of mean pulmonary artery pressure and pulmonary vascular resistance, and modest improvements in cardiac index (Table 16.5). However, by 5 days or more after treatment, the degree of lung scan resolution was similar after urokinase or heparin (UPET). Mortality was similar in patients who presented in shock (5–6%), whether or not they received thrombolytic agents. Bleeding was more common following thrombolytic therapy, 45% of the patients given urokinase compared with 27% who received heparin.

In addition to the NIH trials, two smaller randomized controlled trials have compared the effects of streptokinase with those of heparin in patients with massive pulmonary emboli (81,124). In both, streptokinase was administered for 72 hours at a rate of 100,000 units/hr. Streptokinase resulted in more rapid and complete dissolution of emboli than heparin alone. Bleeding complications occurred in 30% of the patients who received streptokinase and 18% of those who received heparin alone. Thus, the more rapid dissolution of emboli appears to be associated with an improved clinical course in patients with massive insult; however, enthusiasm for fibrinolytic therapy has been blunted by the greater incidence of bleeding.

Recent studies suggest that use of t-PA for pulmonary embolism may be associated with fewer bleeding complications. In a case report, nearly complete dissolution of a massive pulmonary embolus occurred after a 90-minute

Table 16.5
Hemodynamic Response to Thrombolysis in the National Institutes of Health Trials[a]

Protocol	PA Mean (mm Hg)		Cardiac Index (liters/min/m²)		Total Pulmonary Resistance (dyne/sec/cm⁻⁵)	
	Pre	Post	Pre	Post	Pre	Post
UPET						
Urokinase (12 hr)	26.3	20.7	3.2	3.3	330.3	244.7
Heparin only	26.0	24.8	3.1	3.0	365.0	395.7
USPET						
Urokinase (12 hr)	27.4	20.1	2.9	3.0	403.4	298.9
Urokinase (24 hr)	27.5	20.0	2.6	2.9	365.0	244.7
Streptokinase (24 hr)	26.2	20.9	2.8	3.6	181.3	121.5

[a]Measurements made before (pre) and 24 hours after (post) start of infusion of the fibrinolytic agent. Urokinase 12-hour group had been on heparin for 12 hours at time of posttreatment measurements. PA, pulmonary artery pressure.

infusion of 30 mg of recombinant t-PA (12). A larger clinical trial (35 patients) demonstrated marked resolution of pulmonary emboli in 67% of patients and moderate to slight dissolution in an additional 23% after an intravenous dose of 50 mg of t-PA over 2 hours followed by an additional 40 mg over the next 4 hours (46). Heparin was given prior to and after treatment with t-PA. Major bleeding occurred in two patients and "minor bleeding" sufficient to halt administration of t-PA (usually at puncture sites) occurred in five. If the optimal doses of activator can be determined and the need for invasive procedures reduced, clot-selective activators may become the preferred treatment for patients with pulmonary emboli.

At present, thrombolytic therapy should be considered when pulmonary embolism is massive and complicated by right ventricular failure, hypotension, or obstruction of 50% or more of a major pulmonary artery. Therapy with streptokinase or urokinase (the only presently available activators) should be given for 24 hours or less. Streptokinase is generally given as an intravenous bolus of 250,000 units over 15–30 minutes, followed by infusion of 100,000 units/hr. For urokinase, a bolus of 300,000 units followed by infusion of 2,000 units/kg/hr is as efficacious as higher doses (4,400 units/kg/hr) (48). Prior to and during therapy, meticulous management to avoid bleeding due to vascular trauma is essential. Pulmonary artery catheters for monitoring or angiography should be placed through antecubital fossa venous cut down rather than percutaneously in noncompressible vessels (i.e., large central veins). Arterial blood gases should be obtained only if essential with a 23-gauge needle from the radial artery. The artery should then be compressed for a minimum of 15 minutes. Whenever possible, noninvasive monitoring of oxygen saturation is preferred.

Acute Myocardial Infarction

Much of the recent enthusiasm for thrombolytic therapy has been stimulated by the demonstration of improved outcome in acute myocardial infarction after treatment with fibrinolytic agents. When coronary reperfusion occurs within 2 hours after the onset of acute transmural myocardial infarction, regional left ventricular wall motion often improves and mortality is reduced, particularly in patients with anterior infarction. (49, 74, 97, 113, 114). When treatment is started later, benefit is of lesser magnitude and less consistent (3, 4, 68, 69, 71, 99, 104, 109). Thus, with acute myocardial infarction time is the most critical parameter.

The use of thrombolytic therapy for acute myocardial infarction was first reported in 1958 (39, 40). However, until recently the data demonstrating a benefit for such therapy were not sufficiently persuasive to justify its use in view of the potential for serious hemorrhage. In addition, during the 1970s, skepticism regarding the role of coronary thrombosis in acute myocardial infarction further discouraged the use of antithrombotic and fibrinolytic agents. The rediscovery of the importance of coronary thrombosis in transmural infarction can be attributed to DeWood and associates (31), who demonstrated total coronary occlusion in 87% of 126 patients studied within the first 4 hours of the onset of infarction, and nearly total obstruction in an additional 10%. In patients studied later (12–24 hours) the incidence of total occlusion decreased to 65%. These data, coupled with the retrieval of thrombus during subsequent emergent coronary revascularization in a large subset (51 patients), conclusively established the presence of coronary thrombosis early during the evolution of acute myocardial infarction. Although Chazov and coworkers (17) were the first to report pharmacologic coronary fibrinolysis, Rentrop and associates (98) popularized the concept that coronary reperfusion could be achieved by guide-wire fragmentation followed by intracoronary streptokinase. Subsequently it has been demonstrated that intracoronary administration of streptokinase elicits recanalization in approximately 70% of cases (Table 16.6).

Initially, intracoronary administration of fibrinolytic therapy was thought preferable since lower doses could be administered, systemic lytic effects were thought to be minimal, and the results of therapy could be immediately

Table 16.6
Recanalization Rates in Trials of Intracoronary Streptokinase for Coronary Thrombosis

Study	Recanalization Rate	
	No. of Patients	%
Anderson et al (4)	15/20	75
Khaja et al (71)	12/20	60
Kennedy et al (68)	73/108	83
Leibhoff et al (78)	15/22	68
Rentrop et al (98)	17/20	85
Rentrop et al (99)	32/43	74

appreciated. However, rapid mixing of the activator in the systemic circulation occurs after intracoronary administration and results in systemic activation of plasminogen and induction of a systemic lytic state (29, 106). In addition, the time needed to perform coronary angiography prior to the initiation of treatment results in a delay often as long as 90 minutes, during which the magnitude of potential benefit from reperfusion is diminishing. The relatively late initiation of therapy due to this obligatory time delay in most trials of intracoronary streptokinase may explain why consistent improvement in global left ventricular function has not been demonstrated in many randomized studies. However, when ventriculographic analysis of regional left ventricular wall motion (defined angiographically) is performed, improvement in regional performance can be documented in 82% of patients in whom recanalization is induced within 2 hours of the onset of symptoms (112, 113). Regional wall motion improvement is less consistent in those in whom recanalization occurs later.

Several studies also have documented reduced mortality in patients with acute myocardial infarction treated with intracoronary streptokinase. In the Western Washington trial, 134 patients who received intracoronary streptokinase were compared with 116 patients treated conventionally (68). Patients were eligible for randomization if they presented during the first 12 hours of acute infarction. The mean time to presentation was 4.7 ± 2.5 hours. Thirty-day mortality was dramatically reduced for those who received intracoronary streptokinase (3.7%) compared with controls (11.6%, $P < 0.02$). Patients with anterior infarction were more likely to benefit. However, mortality at 1 year was no longer significantly different between the two groups, in large part because of patients with no reperfusion, less than "complete reperfusion," or inferior infarction (68). In the Interuniversity Cardiology Institute Randomized Study, the mean time to reperfusion was 200 minutes after treatment with intracoronary streptokinase alone, in some instances preceded by intravenous streptokinase. The reduction in mortality in this trial was similar to that in the Western Washington study (114). At 28 days, 6% of the patients given streptokinase had died, compared with 12% of the control patients ($P = 0.03$). Improved survival was still evident at 12 months. Despite the encouraging results of these trials, not all of the studies employing intracoronary strepto-

kinase for treatment of acute myocardial infarction have shown benefit, likely because of the delays inherent in its initiation.

Intravenous administration of fibrinolytic agents has the advantage of permitting more prompt institution of therapy and simpler logistics. Although prior to 1980 several studies documented the benefits of treatment with intravenous streptokinase for evolving acute myocardial infarction, others did not and the reported benefits did not seem to justify the risk of bleeding, which was substantial (120). However, because of the delays inherent with intracoronary streptokinase, there was renewed interest in intravenous administration of fibrinolytic agents. In comparison with intracoronary streptokinase, intravenous streptokinase leads to recanalization less often (1, 42, 108, 118). In studies in which preinterventional coronary angiograms have been acquired, the success rate of intravenous streptokinase is approximately 45%, whereas it is approximately 70% with intracoronary administration (Table 16.7) (96). Studies in which preinterventional angiography was not performed suggested rates of recanalization of 70% or higher; however, this result reflected the inclusion of some patients without total thrombotic occlusion (5–21%). Nonetheless, early administration of intravenous streptokinase significantly decreases mortality in patients with acute myocardial infarction. In the largest study thus far (GISSI), 5,630 patients were treated with intravenous streptokinase at the time of admission to the emergency room and their course compared with 5,852 patients

Table 16.7
Recanalization Rate in Trials of Intravenous Streptokinase for Acute Myocardial Infarction

Study	Recanalization Rate	
	No. of Patients	%
Preinterventional angiogram performed		
Rogers et al (104)	7/16[a]	44
Schroeder et al (108)	11/21	52
Alderman et al (1)	8/13	62
Spann et al (118)	21/44[b]	48
Preinterventional angiogram not performed		
Ganz et al (42)	65/68	96
Schroeder et al (108)	42/52	84
Taylor et al (121)	99/121	82
Anderson et al (3)	16/22	73

[a] Patients given dose of 1,000,000 IU.
[b] Includes patients given 850,000 IU and those given 1,500,000 IU.

treated conventionally (49). No adjunctive therapy (including heparin) was given and the patients did not subsequently undergo coronary angiography. Nonetheless, mortality was less at 21 days in patients given streptokinase (10.7%) than in those treated conventionally (13%, P<0.002). The reduction in mortality was most marked in those patients treated within the first 3 hours of infarction (9.2% compared with 12% in controls). A modest but significant improvement in mortality was also observed for those patients treated 3–6 hours after onset of symptoms. On further analysis, it appeared that only those patients less than 65 years of age or those with anterior infarction were likely to benefit. In a smaller study, intravenous streptokinase was administered to 53 patients within 4 hours of the onset of symptoms, in some cases in a mobile care unit at the patient's home (74). Patients treated within 1.5 hours of the onset of infarction were found to have a significantly better left ventricular ejection fraction after infarction than those treated later.

When used for coronary thrombolysis, streptokinase is given in a dose of 750,000–1,500,000 units/hr intravenously. The intravenous dose for urokinase is 2,000,000 units/hr. Heparin is usually given prior to treatment or at the end of the infusion, and titrated to keep the aPTT at greater than 1.5–2 times normal.

OTHER PLASMINOGEN ACTIVATORS IN MYOCARDIAL INFARCTION

Tissue-type plasminogen activator has been the most extensively studied of the more recently developed activators for clinical use. Initial data demonstrated the ability of very low doses of intravenous t-PA to induce coronary thrombolysis in patients with acute myocardial infarction (25, 134). In a dose-finding study, t-PA given intravenously in a dose of 0.5 mg/kg produced reperfusion in 76% of patients by 90 minutes, results similar to those achievable with intracoronary streptokinase (25). Subsequently, the NIH-sponsored Thrombolysis in Myocardial Infarction Trial (TIMI) found that t-PA induced recanalization in 66% of patients given recombinant t-PA intravenously, compared with only 36% of those patients given intravenous streptokinase (123). These results have been confirmed by the European Cooperative Study, which reported a 70% rate of recanalization with t-PA, compared with 55% for streptokinase (137). Intravenous t-PA clearly has an efficacy similar to

that of intracoronary streptokinase, and by virtue of the greater degree of clot selectivity, intravenous t-PA is safer and can be administered without the delays inherent in a catheterization procedure. Recent studies suggest that prolonged low-dose infusion of t-PA may result in more complete thrombolysis and reduce the incidence of coronary reocclusion (44). Whether similar results might occur without adjunctive therapy with heparin is unknown but of potential importance, since bleeding has not been decreased in trials that have used t-PA, perhaps due to the effects of heparin (137).

Single chain urokinase (scu-PA) type plasminogen activator was also highly effective in inducing recanalization in acute myocardial infarction in two small clinical trials (135, 136). Coronary reperfusion was induced in patients with acute myocardial infarction at a rate similar to that observed for t-PA. However, complete thrombolysis requires a high dose (70 mg), which is associated with a fairly marked degree of systemic lytic activity in approximately half of the patients. Since the half-life of scu-PA is relatively short (approximately 8 minutes), a continuous infusion is required as for t-PA. At the present time, the therapeutic:toxic ratio seems to be less favorable than that demonstrated for t-PA. A recent preliminary report suggests that low doses of t-PA and scu-PA may by synergistic and both more potent and more selective than higher doses of either activator alone (23).

Acylated streptokinase plasminogen complexes (BRL-26921, ASPAC) have been used to induce coronary thrombolysis in a number of studies (9, 49, 50, 82, 119). Because deacylation to the active streptokinase plasminogen activator complex is relatively slow, the agent can be administered as an intravenous bolus. Optimal rates of recanalization appear to require a dose of at least 30 mg, which results in significant systemic lytic activity. In a recent large trial, recanalization after treatment with ASPAC did not appear to be as frequent as in most trials using t-PA (9). In addition, ASPAC resulted in far more systemic fibrinogen depletion. The primary advantage of ASPAC at the present time appears to be the ability to administer it as an intravenous bolus.

ADDITIONAL CONSIDERATIONS AFTER CORONARY THROMBOLYSIS

After successful coronary thrombolysis a high-grade residual stenosis generally persists.

Since this stenosis is a potential site for reocclusion and reinfarction, aggressive management of the residual stenosis is recommended by many. In most centers, if a high-grade residual stenosis is documented, coronary angioplasty (PTCA) is performed in order to improve flow to the injured region (32, 45, 57, 77, 110, 128, 129, 149). In the hands of experienced operators angioplasty can be safely performed even in the presence of a systemic lytic state. Urgent coronary artery bypass surgery has also been employed in selected patients; however, the presence of a systemic lytic state increases the potential for morbidity with this procedure.

Patients who have been given intravenous streptokinase should undergo coronary angiography if recanalization appears to have occurred. Clinical indicators of successful coronary recanalization include a rapid rise and early peaking of MB creatine kinase, evidence for reperfusion arrhythmias, rapid resolution of ST segment elevation, and rapid resolution of chest discomfort after administration of plasminogen activators. None of these findings is definitive; however, when they are used in concert, the clinician is often able to correctly predict the occurrence or failure of recanalization. Recurrent chest discomfort following the timely administration of plasminogen activators is often an indication of impending reocclusion after coronary recanalization.

The timing of coronary angiography and PTCA is controversial. In general, the bias has been that patients at high risk (i.e., those with extensive anterior infarction, previous infarction, recurrent pain or arrhythmia, congestive heart failure, or hypotension with or without shock) who cannot tolerate further loss of myocardium should have immediate or at least expeditious procedures, whereas those who are stable clinically and at lower risk can undergo angiography electively. If a high-grade residual stenosis is identified, angioplasty or coronary artery bypass surgery, depending on the overall coronary anatomy and the clinical condition of the patient, is recommended. Recent data have indicated that PTCA need not be done emergently unless the patient is unstable (127). In addition, prolonged infusions of t-PA may result in sufficient remodeling to reduce the need for PTCA in many patients (4).

β-Adrenergic blockers (54, 59) and to a lesser extent intravenous nitroglycerin (15, 60) have been reported to reduce infarct size and improve survival in patients with acute myocardial infarction. Recent data suggest that such agents may also be useful in conjunction with thrombolysis. Ongoing research suggests that calcium channel blockers (53, 72, 73), α-adrenergic blockers (148), β-adrenergic blockers (51), and oxygen free-radical scavengers (14, 62, 87, 94) may enhance the salvage of myocardium following thrombolysis. However, until the results of ongoing clinical trials are available these agents should not be used because of the potential for deleterious effects.

Heparin has been used almost universally following administration of fibrinolytic agents. Its use is predicated on the need to avoid recurrent coronary thrombosis. Reocclusion after coronary recanalization with streptokinase is common, occurring in 20–43% of patients despite use of heparin (52, 78). With t-PA, 20% of patients manifested reocclusion within 30 minutes of completion of the infusion despite use of heparin. However, reocclusion was prevented by a longer infusion of t-PA (44). It is prudent to administer heparin to patients following fibrinolytic therapy, at least for 72 hours. If bleeding develops, heparin may be discontinued, and subsequent angiography planned should recurrent symptoms develop. Although the logic for the use of heparin is compelling, little direct data support its use, and a substantial reduction in mortality was documented in the GISSI trial without it (49). In view of the possibility that heparin may exacerbate bleeding, more data are needed to define its importance.

SUMMARY

When coronary reperfusion is accomplished within 1–2 hours after the onset of symptoms, patients benefit, especially those with anterior wall myocardial infarction. When treatment is initiated later, benefit is less consistent. Thus, the decision to employ thrombolytic therapy more than 2 hours after the onset of infarction depends on consideration of both the risk and potential benefit for the individual patient. Since rapid initiation of therapy is essential, intravenous fibrinolytic agents appear to be the treatment of choice. Streptokinase is the most widely available fibrinolytic agent, but t-PA will likely become the preferred agent in the near future. The development of still newer types of plasminogen activators should ultimately make efficacious and safe therapy possible. (See Editor's note on p. 301.)

References

1. Alderman EL, Jutzky KR, Berte LE, et al: Randomized comparison of intravenous versus intracoronary streptokinase for myocardial infarction. *Am J Cardiol* 54:14, 1984.
2. Alkjaersig N, Fletcher AP, Sherry S: The mechanism of clot dissolution by plasmin. *J Clin Invest* 38:1086, 1959.
3. Anderson JL, Marshall HW, Askens JC, et al. A randomized trial of intravenous and intracoronary streptokinase in patients with acute myocardial infarction. *Circulation* 70:606, 1983.
4. Anderson JL, Marshall HW, Bray BE, et al: A randomized trial of intracoronary streptokinase in treatment of acute myocardial infarction. *N Engl J Med* 308:1312, 1983.
5. Andrade-Gordon P, Strickland S. Interaction of heparin with plasminogen activators and plasminogen: effects on the activation of plasminogen. *Biochemistry* 25:403, 1986.
6. Anreson H, Heilo A, Jakobsen E, et al. A prospective study of streptokinase and heparin in the treatment of deep vein thrombosis. *Acta Med Scand* 203:457, 1978.
7. Anreson H, Hoiseth A, Ly B. Streptokinase or heparin in the treatment of deep venous thrombosis. *Acta Med Scand* 211:65, 1982.
8. Barritt DW, Jordan SC. Anticoagulant drugs in the treatment of pulmonary embolism. A controlled trial. *Lancet* 1:1309, 1960.
9. Been M, de Bona DP, Muir AL, et al. Coronary thrombolysis with intravenous anisoylated plasminogen streptokinase complex BRL26921. *Br Heart J* 53:253, 1985.
10. Beiger R, Boehout-Mussert RJ, Hohmann F. Is streptokinase useful in the treatment of deep venous thrombosis? *Acta Med Scand* 199:81, 1976.
11. Bergmann SR, Fox KAA, Ter-Pogossian MM, et al. Clot selective coronary thrombolysis with tissue-type plasminogen activator. *Science* 220:1181, 1983.
12. Bounameaux HM, Vermylen J, Collen D. Thrombolytic treatment with recombinant tissue-type plasminogen activator in a patient with massive pulmonary embolism. *Ann Intern Med* 103:64, 1985.
13. Browse NL, Clemenson G, Lea Thomas ML. Is the postphlebitic leg always postphlebitic? Relationship between phlebographic appearances of deep-vein thrombosis and late sequelae. *Br Med J*. 281:1167, 1980.
14. Burton KP. Superoxide dismutase enhances recovery following myocardial ischemia. *Am J Physiol* 248:H637, 1985.
15. Bussman W, Passek D, Seidel E. Reduction of CK and CK-MB indices of infarct size by intravenous nitroglycerine. *Circulation* 63:615, 1981.
16. Castellino FJ. A unique enzyme-protein substrate modifier reaction: plasmin/streptokinase interaction. *Trends Biochem Sci* 4:1, 1979.
17. Chazov EL, Mateeva LS, Mazaev AV, et al. Intracoronary administration of fibrinolysis in acute myocardial infarction *Ter Arkh* 48:8–19, 1976.
18. Claeys H., Vermylen J. Physico-chemical and proenzyme properties of NH$_2$-terminal lysine human plasminogen. Influence of 6-aminohexanoic acid. *Biochim Biophys Acta* 342:351, 1974.
19. Collen D. On the regulation and control of fibrinolysis. *Thromb Haemost* 45:77, 1981.
20. Collen D, Bounameaux H, De Cock F, et al. Analysis of coagulation and fibrinolysis during intravenous infusion of recombinant human tissue-type plasminogen activator in patients with acute myocardial infarction. *Circulation* 73:511, 1986.
21. Collen D, Lijnen HR. The fibrinolytic system in man. An overview. In Collen D, Lijnen HR, Verstraete M. (eds): *Thrombolysis: Biological and Therapeutic Properties of New Thrombolytic Agents.* Edinburgh, Churchill Livingstone, 1985.
22. Collen D, Stassen JM, Blaber M, et al. Biological and thrombolytic properties of the proenzyme and active forms of human urokinase. III. Thrombolytic properties of natural and recombinant urokinase in rabbits with experimental jugular vein thrombosis. *Thromb Haemost* 52:26, 1984.
23. Collen D, Stassen J, Stump DC, et al. Synergism of thrombolytic agents in vivo. *Circulation* 74:838, 1986.
24. Collen D, Stassen JM, Verstraete M. Thrombolysis with human extrinsic (tissue-type) plasminogen activator in rabbits with experimental jugular vein thrombosis. Effect of molecular form and dose of activator, age of thrombus, and route of administration. *J Clin Invest* 71:1012, 1984.
25. Collen D, Topol EJ, Tiefenbrunn AJ, et al. Coronary thrombolysis with recombinant human tissue-type plasminogen activator: a prospective, randomized, placebo-controlled trial. *Circulation* 70:1012, 1984.
26. Collen D, Zamarron C, Lijnen HR, et al. Activation of plasminogen by pro-urokinase. 2. Kinetics. *J Biol Chem* 261:1259, 1986.
27. Common HH, Seaman AJ, Rosch J, et al. Deep vein thrombosis treated with streptokinase or heparin. *Angiology* 27:645, 1976.
28. Coon WW, Willis PW, Symons MJ. Assessment of anticoagulant treatment of venous thromboembolism. *Ann Surg* 170:559, 1969.
29. Cowley MJ, Hastillo A, Vetrovec GW. Effects of intracoronary streptokinase in acute myocardial infarction. *Am Heart J* 102:1149, 1981.
30. Dalen JE, Alpert JS. Natural history of pulmonary embolism. *Prog Cardiovasc Dis* 17:259, 1975.
31. DeWood MA, Spores J, Notske RN, et al. Prevalence of total coronary occlusion during the early hours of transmural myocardial infarction. *N Engl J Med* 303:897, 1980.
32. Dodge HT, Sheehan FH, Mathey DG, et al. Usefulness of coronary artery bypass graft surgery or percutaneous transluminal angioplasty after thrombolytic therapy. *Circulation* 72(part 2):39, 1984.
33. Eisenberg PR, Sherman LA, Rich M, et al. Importance of continued activation of thrombin reflected by fibrinopeptide A to the efficacy of thrombolysis. *J Am Coll Cardiol* 7:1255, 1986.
34. Eisenberg PR, Sherman LA, Schechtman K, et al. Fibrinopeptide A: a marker of acute coronary thrombosis. *Circulation* 71:912, 1985.
35. Eisenberg PR, Sherman LA, Tiefenbrunn AJ, et al. Sustained fibrinolysis after t-PA in man. *Thromb Haemost* 57:35, 1987.
36. Elliot MS, Immelman EJ, Jeffrey P, et al. A comparative randomized trial of heparin versus streptokinase in the treatment of acute proximal venous thrombosis: an interim report of a prospective trial. *Br J Surg* 66:838, 1979.
37. Fletcher AP, Alkjaersig N, Sherry S. The clearance of heterologous protein from the circulation of normal and immunized man. *J Clin Invest* 37:1306, 1959.
38. Fletcher AP, Alkjaersig N, Sherry S, et al. The development of urokinase as a thrombolytic agent. Maintenance of a sustained thrombolytic state in man by its intravenous infusion. *J Lab Clin Med* 65:713, 1965.
39. Fletcher AP, Alkjaersig N, Smyrniotis FE, et al. The treatment of patients suffering from early myocardial infarction with massive and prolonged streptokinase therapy. *Trans Assoc Am Physicians* 71:287, 1958.
40. Fletcher AP, Sherry S, Alkjaersig N, et al. The maintenance of a sustained thrombolytic state in man. II. Clinical observations on patients with myocardial infarction and other thromboembolic disorders. *J Clin Invest* 38:111, 1959.
41. Gaffney PJ, Perry MJ. Unreliability of current serum

fibrin degradation product (FDP) assays. *Thromb Hae-most* 53:310, 1984.

42. Ganz W, Geft I, Lew AS, et al. Intravenous streptoki-nase in evolving acute myocardial infarction. *Am J Cardiol* 53:1209, 1984.

43. Garabedian HD, Gold HK, Leinbach RC, et al. Com-parative properties of two clinical preparations of re-combinant human tissue-type plasminogen activator in patients with acute myocardial infarction. *J Am Coll Cardiol* 9:599, 1987.

44. Gold HK, Leinbach RC, Garabedian HD, et al. Acute coronary reocclusion after thrombolysis with recom-binant human tissue-type plasminogen activator: pre-vention by a maintenance infusion. *Circulation* 73:347, 1986.

45. Goldberg S, Urban PL, Greenspon A, et al. Combina-tion therapy for evolving myocardial infarction: intra-coronary thrombolysis and percutaneous transluminal angioplasty. *Am J Med* 72:994, 1982.

46. Goldhaber SZ, Vaughn DE, Markis JE, et al. Acute pulmonary embolism treated with tissue plasminogen activator. *Lancet* 2:886, 1986.

47. Graor RA, Risius B, Young JR, et al. Peripheral artery and bypass graft thrombolysis with recombinant hu-man tissue-type plasminogen activator. *J Vasc Surg* 3:115, 1985.

48. Groupe de Recherche Urokinase-Embolie Pulmonaire: Rapport prepare par B. Charbonnie, Tours. Etude Mu-liticentrique sur seux protocoles d'urokinase dans l'embolie pulmonaire grave. *Arch Mal Coeur* 7:773, 1984.

49. Gruppo Italiano per lo Studio della Sreptochinasi nell'Infarcto Miocardio (GISSI): Effectiveness of intra-venous thrombolytic treatment in acute myocardial infarction. *Lancet* 1:398, 1986.

50. Gurewich V, Pannell R, Louie S, et al. Effective and fibrin-specific clot lysis by a zymogen precursor form of urokinase (prourokinase). A study *in vitro* and in two animal species. *J Clin Invest* 73:1731, 1984.

51. Hammerman H, Kloner RA, Briggs LL, et al. Enhance-ment of salvage of reperfused myocardium by early beta-adrenergic blockade (timolol). *J Am Coll Cardiol* 3:1438, 1984.

52. Harrison DC, Ferguson DW, Collin SM, et al. Rethrom-bosis after reperfusion with streptokinase: importance of geometry of residual lesions. *Circulation* 69:991, 1984.

53. Henry PD, Schuchleib R, Davis J, et al. Myocardial contracture and accumulation of mitochondrial cal-cium in ischemic rabbit heart. *Am J Physiol* 233:H677, 1977.

54. Herltiz J, Elmfeldt D, Holmberg S, et al. Goteberg Metoprolol Trial: Mortality and causes of death. *Am J Cardiol* 53:9D, 1984.

55. Hirsch J, O'Sullivan EF, Martin M. Evaluation of a standard dosage schedule with streptokinase. *Blood* 35:341, 1970.

56. Hoffman JJML, van Rey FJW, Bonnier JJRM. Systemic effects of BRL 26921 during thrombolytic treatment of acute myocardial infarction. *Thromb Res* 37:567, 1985.

57. Holmes DR Jr, Smith HC, Vlietstra RE, et al. Percuta-neous transluminal coronary angioplasty, alone or in combination with streptokinase therapy, during acute myocardial infarction. *Mayo Clin Proc* 60:449, 1985.

58. Hoylaerts M, Rijken DC, Lijnen HR, et al. Kinetics of the activation of plasminogen by human tissue-type plasminogen activator. Role of fibrin. *J Biol Chem* 257:2912, 1982.

59. ISIS Group: Vascular Mortality after early IV beta blockade in acute myocardial infarction (MI). *Circu-lation* 72:III, 1985.

60. Jaffe AS, Geltman EM, Teifenbrunn AJ, et al. Reduc-tion of infarct size in patients with inferior infarction with intravenous glyceryl trinitrate. A randomized study. *Br Heart J* 49:452, 1982.

61. Jim RTS. A study of plasma prothrombin time. *J Lab Clin Med* 50:45, 1957.

62. Jolly SR, Kane WJ, Bailie MB, et al. Canine myocar-dium reperfusion injury, its reduction by the com-bined administration of superoxide dismutase and cat-alase. *Circ Res* 54:277, 1984.

63. Kakkar VV, Flank C, Howe CT, et al. Natural history of post-operative deep vein thrombosis. *Lancet* 2:230, 1969.

64. Kakkar VV, Flanc C, Howe CT, O'Shea M, Flute PT. Treatment of deep venous thrombosis. A trial of heparin, streptokinase, and Arvin. *Br Med J* 1:806, 1969.

65. Kakkar VV, Howe CT, Laws JW, et al. Late results of treatment of deep venous thrombosis. *Br Med J* 1:810, 1969.

66. Kaplan AP. Initiation of the intrinsic coagulation and fibrinolytic pathways of man: the role of surfaces, Hagemen factor, prekallekrein, HMW kininogen, and factor XI. *Prog Hemost Thromb* 4:127, 1978.

67. Kasper W, Erbel R, Meinertz T. Intracoronary throm-bolysis with an acylated streptokinase plasminogen activator (BRL 26921) in patients with acute myocar-dial infarction. *J Am Coll Cardiol* 4:357, 1984.

68. Kennedy JW, Ritchie RL, Davis KB, et al. Western Washington randomized trial of intracoronary strep-tokinase in acute myocardial infarction. *N Engl J Med* 309:1477, 1983.

69. Kennedy JW, Ritchie RL, Davis KB, et al. The Western Washington randomized trial of intracoronary strep-tokinase: a 12 month follow up. *N Engl J Med* 312:1073, 1985.

70. Kernogan RJ, Todd C. Heparin therapy in thromboem-bolic disease. *Lancet* 1:621, 1966.

71. Khaja F, Walton JA, Brymer JF, et al. Intracoronary fibrinolytic therapy in acute myocardial infarction: report of a prospective randomized trial. *N Engl J Med* 308:756, 1983.

72. Klein HH, Schobothe M, Nebendahl K, et al. The effects of two different diltiazem treatments on infarct size in ischemic reperfused porcine hearts. *Circulation* 69:1000, 1984.

73. Knabb RM, Rosamond TI, Fox KAA, et al. Enhanced salvage of reperfused ischemic myocardium by dilti-azem. *J Am Coll Cardiol* 8:861, 1986.

74. Koren G, Weiss AT, Hasin Y, et al. Prevention of myocardial damage in acute myocardial ischemia by early treatment with intravenous streptokinase. *N Engl J Med* 313:1384, 1985.

75. Kowalski E, Kopec M, Niewiarowski S. An evaluation of the euglobulin method for determination of fibri-nolysis. *J Clin Pathol* 12:215, 1959.

76. Larrieu MJ, Rigollot C, Marder VJ. Comparative effects of fibrinogen degradation products D and E on coag-ulation. *Br J Haematol* 72:719, 1973.

77. Lee G, Low RI, Takeda P, et al. Importance of follow-up medical and surgical approaches to prevent rein-farction, reocclusion, and recurrent angina following intracoronary thrombolysis with streptokinase in acute myocardial infarction. *Am Heart J* 104:921, 1982.

78. Leibhoff RH, Katz RJ, Wasserman AG, et al. A random-ized angiographically controlled trial of intracoronary streptokinase in acute myocardial infarction. *Am J Cardiol* 53:404, 1984.

79. Lew AS, Laramee P, Cercek B, et al. The hypotensive effect of intravenous streptokinase in patients without mycardial infarction. *Circulation* 72:1321, 1985.

80. Lijnen HR, Zamarron C, Blaber M, et al. Activation of plasminogen by pro-urokinase. I. Mechanism. *J Biol Chem* 261:1253, 1986.

81. Ly B, Anreson H, Eie H, et al. A controlled trial of streptokinase and heparin in the treatment of major pulmonary embolism. *Acta Med Scand* 1203:465, 1978.

82. Marder VJ, Rothbard RL, Fitzpatrick PG, et al. Rapid lysis of coronary artery thrombi with anisoylated plas-

minogen:streptokinase activator complexes. *Ann Intern Med* 104:304, 1986.

83. Marder VJ, Shulman NR. High molecular weight derivatives of human fibrinogen produced by plasmin. *J Biol Chem* 244:2120, 1969.

84. Marder VJ, Soulen BL, Atichartakarn V, et al. Quantitative venographic assessment of deep vein thrombosis in the evaluation of streptokinase and heparin therapy. *J Lab Clin Med* 89:1018, 1977.

85. McKlintock DK, Bell PH. the mechanism of activation of human plasminogen by streptokinase. *Biochem Biophys Res Commun* 43:694, 1971.

86. Mentzer RL, Budynski AZ, Sherry S. High-dose, brief duration intravenous infusion of streptokinase in acute myocardial infarction: description of effects on the circulation. *Am J Cardiol* 57:1220, 1986.

87. Myers ML, Bolli R, Lekich RF, et al. Enhancement of recovery of myocardial function by oxygen free-radical scavengers after reversible regional ischemia. *Circulation* 72:915, 1985.

88. Nilsson T, Wallen P, Mellbring G. Turnover of human extrinsic (tissue-type) plasminogen activator in man. *Haemostasis* 14:90, 1984.

89. O'Donnell TF, Browse NL, Burnand KG, et al.: The socioeconomic effects of an iliofemoral venous thrombosis. *J Surg Res* 22:483, 1977.

90. Paques EP, Stohr HA, Heimburger N. Study on the mechanism of action of heparin and related substances on the fibrinolytic systems: relationship between plasminogen activator and heparin. *Thromb Res* 42:797, 1986.

91. Ploug J, Kheldgaard NO. Urokinase: an activator of plasminogen from urine. I. Isolation and properties. *Biochim Biophys Acta* 24:282, 1957.

92. Proctor RR, Rapaport SI. The partial thomboplastin time with kaolin. *Am J Clin Pathol* 6:212, 1963.

93. Prowse CW, Davies J, Lane DA. Proteolysis of fibrinogen in healthy volunteers following major and minor *in vivo* plasminogen activation. *Thromb Res* 27:91, 1982.

94. Przyklenk K, Kloner RA. Superoxide dismutase plus catalase improve contractile function in the canine model of "stunned myocardium." *Circ Res* 58:148, 1986.

95. Rakoczi I, Wiman B, Collen D. On the biological significance of the specific interaction between fibrin, plasminogen, and antiplasmin. *Biochim Biophy Acta* 1540:295, 1978.

96. Rentrop KP. Thrombolytic therapy in patients with acute myocardial infarction. *Circulation* 71:627, 1985.

97. Rentrop P, Blanke H, Karsch KR, et al. Changes in left ventricular function after intracoronary streptokinase infusion in clinical evolving myocardial infarction. *Am Heart J* 102:1188, 1981.

98. Rentrop P, Blanke H, Karsch KR, et al. Selective intracoronary thrombolysis in acute myocardial infarction and unstable angina pectoris. *Circulation* 63:307, 1981.

99. Rentrop KP, Feit F, Blanke H, et al. Effects of intracoronary streptokinase and intracoronary nitroglycerine infusion on coronary angiographic patterns and mortality in patients with acute myocardial infarction. *N Engl J Med* 311:1457, 1984.

100. Rijken DC, Hoylaerts M, Collen D. Fibrinolytic properties of one-chain and two chain human extrinsic (tissue-type) plasminogen activator. *J Biol Chem* 257:2920, 1982.

101. Rijken DC, Wijngaards G, Collen D. Tissue-type plasminogen activator from human tissue and cell cultures and its occurrence in plasma. In Collen D, Lijnen HR, Verstraete M (eds:) *Thrombolysis: Biological and Therapeutic Properties of New Thrombolytic Agents.* Edinburgh, Churchill Livingstone, 1985.

102. Robbins KC. The human plasma fibrinolytic system: regulation and control. *Mol Cell Biochem* 20:149, 1978.

103. Robertson BR, Nilsson IM, Nylander G. Thrombolytic

effect of streptokinase as evaluated by phlebography of deep venos thrombi of the leg. *Acta Chir Scand* 136:173, 1970.

104. Rogers WJ, Mantle, JA, Hood WP: Prospective randomized trial of intravenous and intracoronary streptokinase in acute myocardial infarction. *Circulation* 68:1051, 1983.

105. Rosch J, Dotter CT, Seaman AJ, Porter JM, et al. Healing of deep venous thrombosis: Venographic findings in a randomized study comparing streptokinase and heparin. *AJR* 127:553, 1976.

106. Rothbard RL, Fitzpatrick PG, Francis CW, et al. Relationship of the lytic state to successful reperfusion with standard and low dose intracoronary streptokinase. *Circulation* 71:562, 1985.

107. Rylatt DB, Blake AS, Cottis LE, et al. An immunoassay for human D dimer using monoclonal antibodies. *Thromb Res* 31:767, 1983.

108. Schroeder R, Biamino G, Von Leitner ER, et al Intravenous short-term infusion of streptokinase in acute myocardial infarction. *Circulation* 67:536, 1983.

109. Schroeder R, Neuhaus KL, Leizorovicz A, et al. A prospective placebo-controlled double-blind multicenter trial of intravenous streptokinase in acute myocardial infarction (ISAM): long-term mortality and morbidity. *J Am Coll Cardiol* 9:197, 1987.

110. Serruys PW, Wijns W, van den Brand M, et al. Is transluminal coronary angioplasty mandatory after successful thrombolysis? Quantitative coronary angiographic study. *Br Heart J* 50:257, 1983.

111. Shafer KE, Santoro SA, Sobel BE, et al. Monitoring of fibrinolytic agents. A therapeutic challenge. *Am J Med* 76:879, 1984.

112. Sheehan FH, Detley GM, Schofer J, et al. Effect of interventions in salvaging left ventricular function in acute myocardial infarction: a study of intracoronary streptokinase. *Am J Cardiol* 52:431, 1983.

113. Sheehan FH, Mathey DS, Schofer J, et al. Factors that determine recovery of left ventricular function after thrombolysis in patients with acute myocardial infarction. *Circulation* 71:1121, 1985.

114. Simmons ML, Brand M, de Zwaan C, et al. Improved survival after early thrombolysis in acute myocardial infarction. *Lancet* 2:578, 1985.

115. Smith RAG, Dupe RJ, English PD, et al. Acyl-enzymes as thrombolytic agents in a rabbit model of venous thrombosis. *Thromb Haemost* 47:269, 1982.

116. Smith RAG, Dupe RJ, English PD, et al. Fibrinolysis with acyl-enzymes: a new approach to thrombolytic therapy. *Nature* 290:505, 1981.

117. Sobel BE, Gross RW, Robison AK. Thrombolysis, clot selectivity, and kinetics. *Circulation* 70:160, 1984.

118. Spann JF, Sherry S, Carabello BA, et al. Coronary thrombolysis by intravenous streptokinase in acute myocardial infarction: acute and follow-up studies. *Am J Cardiol* 53:655, 1984.

119. Stainforth DH, Smith RAG, Hibbs M. Streptokinase and anisoylated streptokinase plasminogen complex. Their action on haemostasis in human volunteers. *Eur J Pharmacol* 24:751, 1983.

120. Stampfer MJ, Goldhaber SZ, Yusef S, et al. Effect of intravenous streptokinase on acute myocardial infarction. Pooled results from randomized trials. *N Engl J Med* 307:1180, 1982.

121. Taylor GJ, Mikell SL, Moses HW, et al: Intravenous versus intracoronary streptokinase therapy for acute myocardial infarction in community hospitals. *Am J Cardiol* 54:256, 1984.

122. Thomas D, Niewiarowski S, Meyers AR, et al. A comparative study of four methods for detecting fibrinogen degradation products in patients with various diseases. *N Engl J Med* 283:663, 1970.

123. The Thrombolysis in Myocardial Infarction (TIMI) Trial: phase I findings. *N Engl J Med* 312:932, 1985.

124. Tibbutt DA, Davies JA, Anderson JA, et al. Comparison

by controlled clinical trial of streptokinase and heparin in treatment of life-threatening pulmonary embolism. *Br Med J* 1:343, 1974.

125. Tiefenbrunn AJ, Robison AK, Kurnik PB, et al. Clinical pharmacology in patients with evolving myocardial infarction of tissue-type plasminogen activator produced by recombinant DNA technology. *Circulation* 71:110, 1985.

126. Tillet WS, Garner RL. The fibrinolytic activity of hemolytic streptococci. *J Exp Med* 58:485, 1933.

127. Topol EJ, Califf RM, George BS, et al. A multicentered randomized trial of intravenous recombinant tissue plasminogen activator and emergency coronary angioplasty for acute myocardial infarction: preliminary report from the TAMI study. *Circulation* 74:II-74, 1986.

128. Topol EJ, O'Neill WW, Langburd AB, et al. A randomized, placebo-controlled trial of intravenous recombinant tissue-type plasminogen activator and emergency coronary angioplasty in patients with acute myocardial infarction. *Circulation* 75:420, 1987.

129. Topol EJ, Weiss JL, Brinker JA, et al. Regional wall motion improvement after coronary thrombolysis with recombinant tissue plasminogen activator: importance of coronary angioplasty. *J Am Coll Cardiol* 6:426, 1985.

130. Tsapogas MJ, Peabody RA, Wu KT, et al. Controlled trial of thrombolytic therapy in deep vein thrombosis. *Surgery* 74:973, 1973.

131. Urokinase Pulmonary Embolism Trial, phase 1 results. *JAMA* 214:2163, 1970.

132. Urokinase-Streptokinase Pulmonary Embolism Trial, phase 2 results. *JAMA* 229:1606, 1974.

133. Van de Werf F, Bergmann SR, Fox KAA, et al. Coronary thrombolysis with intravenously administered human tissue-type plasminogen activator produced by recombinant DNA technology. *Circulation* 69:605, 1984.

134. Van de Werf F, Ludbrook PA, Bergmann SR, et al. Coronary thrombolysis with intravenously administered human tissue-type plasminogen activator in patients with acute myocardial infarction. *N Engl J Med* 311:609, 1984.

135. Van de Werf F, Nobuhara M, Collen D. Coronary thrombolysis with human single-chain urokinase-type plasminogen activator (prourokinase) in patients with acute myocardial infarction. *Ann Intern Med* 104:345, 1984.

136. Van de Werf F, Vanhaecke J, de Geest H, et al. Coronary thrombolysis with recombinant single-chain urokinase type plasminogen activator in patients with acute MI. *Circulation* 74:1066, 1986.

137. Verstraete M, Bory M, Collen D, et al. Randomized trial of intravenous recombinant tissue-type plasminogen activator versus intravenous streptokinase in acute myocardial infarction, *Lancet* 1:842, 1985.

138. Verstraete M, Bounameoux H, De Cock F, et al. Pharmacokinetics and systemic fibrinogenolytic effects of recombinant human tissue-type plasminogen activator (rt-PA) in humans. *J Pharmacol Exp Ther* 235:506, 1985.

139. Walker ID, Davidson JR, Rae AP, et al. Acylated streptokinase-plasminogen complex in patients with acute myocardial infarction. *Thromb Haemost* 51:204, 1984.

140. Wallen P, Bergsdorf N, Ranby M. Purification and identification of two structural variants of porcine tissue plasminogen activator by affinity adsorption of fibrin. *Biochim Bioplys Acta* 719:318, 1982.

141. Wallen P, Wiman B. Characterization of human plasminogen. II. Separation and partial characterization of different molecular forms of human plasminogen. *Biochim Biophys Acta* 257:122.

142. Watz R, Savidge GF. Rapid thrombolysis and preservation of valvular function in high deep venous thrombosis. *Acta Med Scand* 205:293, 1979.

143. Weimar W, Stibbe AJ, van Seyen AJ, et al. Specific lysis of an iliofemoral thrombus by administration of extrinsic (tissue type) plasminogen activator. *Lancet* 2:1018, 1980.

144. Whitaker AN, Elms NJ, Masci PP. Measurement of crosslinked fibrin derivatives in plasma an immunoassay using monoclonal antibodies. *J Clin Pathol* 37:882, 1984.

145. White WF, Barlow GH, Mozen MN. The isolation and characterization of plasminogen activators (urokinase) from human urine. *Biochemistry* 5:2160, 1966.

146. Wiman B, Collen D. On the kinetics of the reaction between human antiplasmin and plasmin. *Eur J Biochem* 84:573, 1978.

147. Wiman B, Collen D. Purification and characterization of human antiplasmin, the fast-acting plasmin inhibitor in plasma. *Eur J Biochem* 78:19, 1977.

148. Yamada K, Saffitz JE, Sobel BE, et al. Enhanced salvage of reperfused ischemic myocardium by alpha-adrenergic blockade. *J Am Coll Cardiol* 7:54, 1986.

149. Yasuno M, Saito Y, Ishida M, et al. Effects of percutaneous transluminal coronary angioplasty: intracoronary thrombolysis with urokinase in acute myocardial infarction. *Am J Cardiol* 53:1217, 1984.

150. Young AE, Lea Thomas M, Browse NL. Comparison between sequelae of surgical and medical treatment of venous thromboembolism. *Br Med J* 4:127, 1974.

151. Zammarron C, Lijnen HR, Van Hoef B, et al. Biological and thrombolytic properties of proenzyme and active forms of human urokinase. 1. Fibrinolytic and fibrinogenolytic properties in human plasma *in vitro* of urokinases obtained from human urine or by recombinant DNA technology. *Thromb Haemost* 52:19, 1984.

Editor's note added in proof: After submission of this chapter, tissue plasminogen was approved by the FDA for the treatment of acute myocardial infarction.

Medication Groups

17

Diuretics and Other Medications Used in Renal Failure

Eric S. Marks, M.D.

When acute renal failure complicates the course of the critically ill patient, medical management becomes more difficult and the mortality rate often exceeds 50%. Therefore, an early attempt to identify the presence of known risk factors influencing morbidity and mortality and the preservation of existing renal function are of high priority (26). In some instances adverse effects of drugs cause the renal injury, whereas in others the hemodynamic abnormalities of the underlying disease induce renal dysfunction. Antecedent chronic renal failure also increases the hazards of therapy and the mortality rate of the critically ill patient. Because of the wide array of pharmacologic agents and of mechanical life-support systems available for such patients, the physician must be alert to a multitude of adverse, as well as beneficial, effects of therapeutic maneuvers. Such alertness requires an understanding of the organ-specific responses induced by the treatments employed.

The purpose of this chapter is to discuss the direct effects on the kidney of a number of pharmacologic agents and therapeutic interventions. In addition, brief reviews of renal physiology applicable to the class of drug under consideration are presented. Any manipulation that modifies systemic hemodynamics directly or through neurohumoral mechanisms can exert an influence on renal function. Thus, changes in blood pressure, cardiac output, ventilatory pattern, and peripheral resistance all affect the kidney.

In general, the maintenance of renal function depends on the intrinsic ability of the kidney to autoregulate both its blood flow and glomerular filtration rate (GFR) in response to changes in cardiac output and/or perfusion pressure. Autoregulation is accomplished by intrarenal adjustments in resistance and flow patterns, but these adjustments are finite and limited in scope. Any drug or process that interferes with this activity predisposes the kidney to injury. Regardless of etiology, increases or decreases in blood pressure outside the autoregulatory range or a fall in cardiac output can diminish renal function. In the critically ill patient the kidney is physiologically stressed with enhanced susceptibility to ischemic injury. An understanding of the pathogenesis of acute renal failure, particularly the effects of shock on the kidney, is essential in the care of these patients. The pathogenesis and management of acute renal failure and the kidney in shock is extensively covered elsewhere (21). In the critically ill patient, mul-

The opinions and assertions contained herein are those of the author and are not to be construed as official or as representing those of the Uniformed Services University of the Health Sciences or the Department of Defense.

tiple intrinsic compensatory mechanisms are operative at any given time. The major goal of therapy is management of the underlying disorder to avoid interference with these normal mechanisms and to restore stable systemic hemodynamics.

DIURETICS

Diuretics are used for a wide variety of conditions including congestive heart failure and hypertension. Critically ill patients who have been receiving these medications may have profound alterations in their body fluid volumes and electrolyte composition. Initial patient evaluation should consider antecedent diuretic-induced fluid and electrolyte changes, as well as the predicted acute effects of diuresis. Therapeutic approaches based on these considerations should decrease patient morbidity.

Diuretics can be classified in a number of ways based on chemical structure, potency, and site of action. Table 17.1 provides a concise summary of the major attributes of the commonly available agents. Detailed descriptions of the pharmacokinetics and mechanism

of action of each drug are available elsewhere (175).

General Guidelines for the Use of Diuretics

The following guidelines for use of diuretics take into account the effects on extracellular fluid volume, acid-base balance, and electrolyte composition.

1. Obtain a pretherapy body weight followed by daily weights on the same scale. Weights may be measured more frequently if acute alterations in volume status are expected. In addition, accurate records of fluid intake and output are essential. The detailed assessment of hemodynamics with invasive physiologic monitoring techniques provides important information that is useful in directing therapeutic interventions (161). Volume depletion leading to cardiac and renal decompensation may occur abruptly or gradually and may be subtle in presentation. In a prospective study of hospital-acquired renal insufficiency, decreased kidney perfusion was the most frequently identified cause (90).

2. Measure baseline serum urea nitrogen,

Table 17.1
Characteristics of Diuretics

Diuretic[a]	Site of Action	Onset of Action	Peak Action	Duration of Action (hr)
I. Potent: $Fe_{Na} > 15\%$				
Furosemide	Loop of Henle	1 hr (i.v.:5 min)	1–2 hr (i.v.:10 min)	6 (i.v.:2)
Ethacrynic acid	Loop of Henle	30 min (i.v.:5 min)	1–2 hr (i.v.:10 min)	6–8 (i.v.:3)
Bumetanide	Loop of Henle	30 min (i.v.:10 min)	1–2 hr (i.v.:15–30 min)	5–6 (i.v.:4)
II. Moderately potent: $Fe_{Na} = 5–10\%$				
Chlorothiazide	All act in	1 hr	4 hr	6–8
Hydrochlorothiazide	cortical	2 hr	4 hr	12–18
Indapamide	collecting	1–3 hr		12–36
Metolazone	tubule	1 hr	2 hr	12–24
Chlorthalidone		2 hr	8–10 hr	48–72
III. Potassium-sparing: $Fe_{Na} < 5\%$				
Triamterene	All act in	2 hr	4–6 hr	12–16
Amiloride	cortical	2 hr	6–10 hr	24
Spironolactone	collecting tubule	>24 hr		48–72
IV. Carbonic anhydrase inhibitor: $Fe_{Na} < 5\%$				
Acetazolamide	Proximal tubule	30–60 min (i.v.:1 min)	2 hr	6–8
V. Osmotic: $Fe_{Na} < 5\%$				
Mannitol	Proximal tubule; loop of Henle	i.v.: 1 min	5–10 min	2–4

[a]Fe_{Na}, maximal fractional excretion of sodium.

creatinine, and electrolyte concentrations, including magnesium, calcium, and phosphate. The frequency of follow-up blood and urine values is dictated by the clinical situation of the individual patient.

3. Use a single agent for initial diuretic therapy. The maximum safe dose should be employed before adding a second drug. If the desired diuretic response is not obtained, reevaluate volume status and fluid therapy, level of renal function, and presence of prostaglandin synthesis inhibitors. Combination therapy may be necessary in patients with resistant sodium retention in the setting of severe heart failure, renal failure, liver disease, or nephrotic syndrome. The very nature of these disease processes underscores the care that must be taken when diuretic therapy is used (143). The synergistic effect of two diuretics can produce a massive natriuresis, diuresis, and kaliuresis. The most common diuretic combination is one that blocks sodium chloride reabsorption in the ascending limb of Henle's loop and one that inhibits sodium-potassium exchange distally. A thiazide, usually metolazone, in a small dose is frequently effective. In addition, a supraadditive effect has been described with the combination of bumetanide and theophylline ethylenediamine (162).

Physiologic Side Effects of Diuretics

Hypovolemia may occur following diuretic use and poses a significant risk of hypotension for the elderly patient and for those with hepatic, cardiac, and renal disease. Hypotension due to a decrease in cardiac output may also occur in patients requiring high ventricular filling pressure, including those with severe cardiomyopathy, tricuspid insufficiency, and pericardial disease.

Disorders of acid-base status may occur as a result of specific actions of the diuretic on acidification or may be secondary to alterations in volume or potassium status. Development and perpetuation of a metabolic alkalosis can be due to extracellular fluid volume depletion, resultant enhancement of renal bicarbonate reabsorption, and release of aldosterone, a mediator of distal tubular hydrogen secretion. Furosemide enhances urinary acidification and potassium excretion. Hypokalemia can increase ammonia production, bicarbonate reabsorption, and chloride excretion; these factors tend to increase plasma bicarbonate concentration. Correction of the alkalosis

requires volume, potassium, and chloride replacement. At the other extreme, metabolic acidosis can develop with the use of the carbonic anhydrase inhibitor, acetazolamide. This drug reduces proximal tubular bicarbonate reabsorption and causes bicarbonaturia. The potassium-sparing agents also decrease hydrogen ion excretion.

Hypokalemia primarily results from an increased delivery of sodium to the distal nephron where it exchanges for potassium. Thiazides, "loop" agents, and acetazolamide are all capable of producing a moderate to marked kaliuresis. Some degree of total body potassium depletion should be expected in the patient on chronic diuretic therapy (180). Elderly patients or those with diabetes mellitus, chronic illness, malnutrition, or advanced heart or liver disease are at high risk for hypokalemia. The physiologic effects of hypokalemia relate not only to the absolute plasma level but also to the rate of decline. β_2-Adrenoceptor stimulation by circulating epinephrine can cause hypokalemia (25). This effect is potentiated in patients receiving concomitant diuretic therapy (173). The circulating levels of epinephrine produced by infusion in these studies were comparable with those noted in patients with acute myocardial infarction. The increase in ammonia production stimulated by hypokalemia may precipitate hepatic encephalopathy in patients with hepatic dysfunction. Severe hypokalemia has been implicated as a contributing cause in diuretic-induced hyponatremia (54). The relationship between diuretic-induced hypokalemia, hypomagnesemia, and cardiac arrhythmias is established (15). This relationship is particularly important in patients with acute myocardial infarction and/or those on digitalis. Magnesium plays an important role in the maintenance of potassium balance and is required for the activity of sodium-potassium ATPase. Urinary excretion of magnesium is markedly increased by loop-acting and to a lesser extent by thiazide diuretics. Amiloride decreases magnesium excretion. It is the coexistence of hypokalemia and hypomagnesemia that appears to place the patient at highest risk. In the critically ill patient, potassium should be replaced to maintain a plasma level greater than 3 mEq/liter. Correction of magnesium deficiency and continued careful monitoring of the serum magnesium concentration is mandatory for the adequate repletion of cellular potassium and the abolition of hypokalemic-induced cardiac problems.

Hyperkalemia can develop during use of the potassium-sparing diuretics. The concomitant use of potassium supplements, β-blockers, or the angiotensin II–converting enzyme inhibitors increases the probability of this occurrence (151).

Hyponatremia is a consequence of impaired water handling and the stimulated release of antidiuretic hormone by volume depletion. Thiazides and loop-acting agents all diminish free water formation (69). Hyponatremia is a frequent hospital-acquired electrolyte disorder, particularly in the postoperation period (2). Volume replacement with hypotonic solutions is a major contributing cause, as is the presence of hepatic, renal, or cardiac disease, and/or mechanical ventilation. As would be expected from the severity of the underlying clinical conditions, hyponatremia is a poor prognostic indicator. Serious attention to water balance is necessary if these complications are to be minimized. Of note, the hyponatremia associated with severe heart failure has been successfully treated with a combination of furosemide and converting enzyme inhibition (44).

Hypernatremia usually results from water loss in excess of sodium when an osmotic diuretic such as mannitol is used. This side effect is particularly hazardous in patients who have underlying volume contraction. (64).

Calciuresis is induced by furosemide and this effect has been used therapeutically in conjunction with volume replacement to treat hypercalcemia. Elevations of the serum calcium concentration have occurred in patients with hyperparathyroidism and in normal subjects receiving thiazides (23, 170, 178).

Role of Diuretics in Acute Renal Failure

The efficacy of diuretics in the prophylaxis and treatment of acute renal failure is controversial (114). A review of the studies suggests that the careful maintenance of an appropriate volume status is more important than the use of the diuretic. Interest has focused on the use of diuretics to convert oliguric renal failure to the nonoliguric type, which is associated with less morbidity and mortality. Patients with oliguric renal failure seem to have a greater reduction in filtration and tubular function than those with the nonoliguric form. Response to diuretics is related to the duration of oliguria and the level of renal tubular function as reflected by concentrating ability (urine-to-plasma osmolality) and sodium handling (absolute and fractional excretion) (39). Care must be exercised in the use of diuretics. High-dose furosemide can result in ototoxicity, and accumulation of mannitol can produce volume overload with pulmonary congestion. No definite statement concerning the impact of diuretic therapy on the ultimate outcome of acute renal failure can be made at this time. In a prospective study using furosemide to maintain urine output, no significant differences were observed in the number of dialyses, duration of renal failure, or mortality when compared with untreated controls (24).

ADRENERGIC INFLUENCE ON RENAL FUNCTION: AN OVERVIEW

The renal vasculature, tubular structures, cortex, and pelvis contain extensive neural innervation. Efferent renal nerve activity has the capability of altering renal function through a variety of mechanisms, including direct tubular effects on reabsorptive and secretory functions, effects on tubular gluconeogenesis, alterations in renal hemodynamics through direct vascular action, and effects on intrarenal renin and prostaglandin release (165). It has become apparent that in addition to the efferent renal nerves, there are renal afferents with central projections to the hypothalamic region in the brain. Animal studies have revealed intrarenal mechanoreceptors and chemoreceptors and have demonstrated a neural communication between the kidneys (renorenal reflex) that directly affects excretory function (71). The kidney contains adrenergic receptors of the α_1, α_2, β, and dopamine subtypes, which are defined pharmacologically through the use of specific agonists and antagonists. A number of these stimulatory and inhibitory ("blocking") agents (e.g., norepinephrine, dopamine, propranolol) are used frequently in clinical practice. Their observed renal effects are determined by both systemic and local actions.

The vast majority of the clinical studies evaluating the α- and β-receptor–specific drugs have been conducted in patients with underlying hypertension, usually of the essential type. Responses are determined in part by the age of the patient and the level and duration of hypertension. The natural course of the alterations in systemic hemodynamics in patients with essential hypertension has been evaluated in a longitudinal study of eight untreated subjects followed over 17 years. Cardiac index gradually decreased in these patients as mean arterial pressure and total peripheral resistance increased (122). Ljungman and associates (120) designed an age-controlled study to determine the effect of the level of mean arterial pressure on renal function. The 111 individuals evaluated in this study, all 49 years of age, were selected to represent the range of blood pressure seen in the general population. The data show that as the level of mean arterial pressure increases, renal vascular resistance increases, renal blood flow decreases, filtration fraction increases, and glomerular filtration is preserved. These changes appear as a continuum and do not start at a specific level of blood pressure. The preservation of GFR suggests that the increase in resistance at the efferent glomerular arteriole exceeds that at the afferent arteriole. This initial maintenance of GFR is not permanent; the natural rate of decline in creatinine clearance associated with aging is accelerated in patients with arterial pressures greater than 140/90 mm Hg (116).

SYMPATHOMIMETIC AMINES

The renal vascular bed is very sensitive to α-adrenergic receptor–mediated vasoconstriction, but is not as sensitive to β-receptor–induced vasodilation as are other vascular beds (100). Anticipating the result of pharmacologic intervention with sympathomimetic amines requires a general understanding of their specific renal actions. Use of these agents to restore a disruption in systemic hemodynamics should be balanced against their potential to affect renal function adversely. The underlying degree of stimulation of the sympathetic nervous system may modify the expected therapeutic response, especially when renal autoregulatory capacity is compromised. In a variety of hypoxic and hypoperfusion states, circulating catecholamine levels are high; in hemorrhagic shock, the levels correlate with total peripheral resistance (32, 93). Redistribution of intrarenal blood flow, particularly in the cortical region, frequently occurs in a number of these low-perfusion conditions. These abnormal flow patterns can be reproduced by exogenously administered catecholamines (30).

Norepinephrine

Norepinephrine is the neurotransmitter that, when released into the synapse, acts at both α_1- and α_2-adrenergic receptors. Levels of norepinephrine in renal venous effluent demonstrate intrarenal release, responsive to renal nerve stimulation (139). In the kidney, norepinephrine directly constricts both arterioles and venules, an action enhanced by salt restriction (70, 157). This constriction increases renal vascular resistance and may, depending on dose, induce a fall in glomerular filtration (157). Norepinephrine is a potent stimulator of renin release (100). The subsequent generation of angiotensin II, a vasoconstrictor, may contribute to the norepinephrine-induced vascular changes. Norepinephrine inhibits the action of antidiuretic hormone (ADH) on water excretion without altering osmolar clearance (106). The mechanism is most likely a norepinephrine-induced suppression of ADH release. Retention of sodium also occurs, probably because of the altered hemodynamics rather than a direct effect on tubular function (157). Patients with mild renal insufficiency have an enhanced pressor response to infused norepinephrine (12). In summary, infusion of norepinephrine can to varying degrees constrict the renal vasculature, influence salt and water excretion, and under most clinical conditions, diminish glomerular filtration.

Epinephrine

Epinephrine demonstrates affinity for α- and β-adrenergic receptors. The β-adrenergic effects predominate, especially at low doses, in all vascular beds except the kidney, where marked α-mediated vasoconstriction occurs (66). Salt restriction does not enhance this effect of epinephrine (70), unlike norepinephrine. The resultant decrease in blood flow and GFR is associated with sodium and water retention. Epinephrine stimulates renin release. Data from patients undergoing xenon washout and angiographic studies suggest an enhanced sensitivity of the cortical vasculature to epinephrine (49). Epinephrine administered therapeutically should enhance the vasoconstriction and potentiate the cortical ischemia and redistribution of blood flow that has been observed in patients with acute renal failure (84) and those with congestive heart failure (29). These adverse effects on renal function, coupled with the availability of other vasoactive agents, make the therapeutic use of epinephrine for hemodynamic abnormalities undesirable.

Isoproterenol

Isoproterenol, a synthetic β-adrenergic agonist, affects both β_1- and β_2-adrenergic receptors (66). Injection into the renal artery at low doses (0.125–0.32 μg) and high doses (50–100 μg) decreases renal vascular resistance and increases renal blood flow. At higher doses (50–100 μg) renal blood flow falls. The vasodilation is blocked by propranolol at both dosage levels. Following β blockade with propranolol, a vasoconstrictive response diminished by phentolamine is noted at the 50–100 μg dose, suggesting a degree of α stimulation. Systemic administration causes vasodilation in skeletal and mesenteric vascular beds with a redistribution of total blood flow. During infusion in normal subjects and in patients with heart disease, the percentage of cardiac output delivered to the kidney falls, probably because of systemic redistribution (156). Renal blood flow usually does not change, but may decrease when the circulating blood volume is low (66). Isoproterenol stimulates renin release and increases urinary osmolality with an associated fall in free water clearance. These changes are not associated with alterations in glomerular filtration or renal vascular resistance and are abolished by the destruction of the hypothalamo-neurohypophyseal system, most likely by a decrease in ADH (158). The clinical consequences of this impaired water handling may be the development of hyponatremia in the susceptible patient if water and salt intake are not well controlled.

Metaraminol

Metaraminol is a sympathomimetic amine, the pressor effect of which is decreased but not reversed by α-adrenergic antagonists. Its effects in humans resemble those of norepinephrine (46), although its duration of action is longer (82). In normal humans, the increase in mean arterial pressure is associated with a slight decrease in renal blood flow and an unchanged GFR (119). In hypotensive dogs, metaraminol increases renal blood flow and GFR (133). There appears to be some vascular specificity to metaraminol, with the renal vessels being less sensitive than the systemic circulation. Although renal vasoconstriction occurs, the more pronounced effect on systemic resistance makes this agent an attractive alternative to norepinephrine. However, this ben-

efit is relative and as with all vasopressor amines, the shorter the exposure the better.

Dopamine

Dopamine is a naturally occurring catecholamine and the immediate precursor of norepinephrine in the endogenous biosynthetic pathway of the catecholamines. It can interact at α_1, β_1, β_2, and specific neurotropic (DA$_2$) and postsynaptic (DA$_1$) dopaminergic receptors (47, 121). The specific receptors in the kidney appear to be DA$_1$ receptors and are coupled to the activation of the adenyl cyclase phosphodiesterase system (186). The observed physiologic responses elicited by these interactions are dose-dependent (67). Specific renal arterial dilation occurs at intravenous infusion rates of 0.5–2.0 μg/kg/min. At progressively higher doses, cardiac β-adrenergic effects occur (2–10 μg/kg/min), followed by mixed α- and β-adrenergic effects (10–20 μg/kg/min) and finally, α-adrenergic–mediated vasoconstriction predominates at high levels (>20 μg/kg/min) (32). This effect in the kidney causes a decrease in renal blood flow with sodium retention, mimicking the actions of norepinephrine. The dopamine augmentation of renal blood flow plateaus at doses of 10 μg/kg/min. Stimulation of renal dopamine receptors results in vasodilation with increases in blood flow, GFR, urine flow, and sodium excretion (1, 130, 181). In addition, urinary phosphate excretion is increased, an action that is important in the patient predisposed to hypophosphatemia (35). Haloperidol and chlorpromazine are dopaminergic antagonists that can alter the response to administered dopamine (68).

THERAPEUTIC APPLICATION OF DOPAMINE

The timing of pharmacologic intervention to prevent or modify the course of acute renal failure is highly pertinent, because most agents are not effective after failure is established. Use of dopamine to improve overall kidney function in acute renal failure has not received extensive study. Dopamine infusions are effective in increasing blood flow in patients with various types of underlying chronic renal insufficiency. The magnitude of the increase in blood flow and GFR is related to the pretreatment values. In addition, normal subjects have a greater increase in both blood flow and GFR than do patients with renal disease and a similar basal GFR. In chronic renal disease, no significant effect on GFR or renal blood flow is noted when the baseline GFR is less than 50 ml/min/1.73 m^2 of body surface area (181). The mechanism responsible for the natriuresis and diuresis has not been clearly defined. Although the alteration in renal hemodynamics could be responsible, a direct effect of dopamine on the tubules is considered likely. In a cross-over study conducted on patients following open heart surgery, individual infusions of dopamine or dobutamine were dose-adjusted to provide equivalent cardiac indices. Under these conditions, the resulting GFR, effective renal plasma flow, renal vascular resistance, and filtration fraction were essentially identical. However, dopamine caused a significantly greater urine flow, sodium excretion (both fractional and absolute), and potassium excretion and a less concentrated urine (83). In cases of acute oliguric renal failure, a continuous low-dose dopamine infusion (1.2–2.5 μg/kg/min) has been demonstrated to preserve and improve renal function (147). Dopamine alone increased creatinine clearance, osmolar clearance, and fractional excretion of sodium. In those patients who failed to increase urine flow with dopamine, the addition of a continuous infusion of furosemide (3–5 mg/kg/day) increased urine flow, and the effects of the two agents appeared to be additive (147). In two studies, patients with acute oliguric renal failure unresponsive to high-dose diuretic therapy (mannitol and furosemide) were treated with a combination of dopamine (1–3 μg/kg/min) and furosemide. The furosemide was delivered either as a continuous infusion of 10–15 mg/kg/hr or as bolus doses of 100–200 mg every 6–8 hours. The degree of response appeared to be related to both the severity of the renal insufficiency and the duration of the oliguria (73, 117). Early intervention is recommended after adequate volume status is confirmed. The significant increase in osmolar clearance has important therapeutic implications. Fluid overload is a common complication in the critically ill patient, particularly in those requiring mechanical ventilation. The enhanced solute and water excretion obtained with low-dose dopamine alone or in combination with furosemide may be of value in preventing and treating this problem.

Combination therapy with low-dose dopamine and other vasoactive agents allows the physician to take maximal advantage of the specific renal actions. Dobutamine, a β-adrenergic agonist with predominantly cardiac ef-

fects, has no affinity for the dopaminergic receptor (166). The simultaneous use of these two agents should improve salt and water excretion through an improvement in cardiac hemodynamics and a direct effect on the kidney. The combination allows for a lower effective dose of both drugs.

Summary

Sympathomimetic amines appreciably alter renal hemodynamics and may disrupt normal renal function. The essential factor in the treatment of low perfusion states is to maximize effective volume and improve cardiac function.

ANTAGONISTS OF SYMPATHETIC FUNCTION

α-Receptor Agents

The α_1 is the predominant receptor subtype in the human kidney and appears to be principally responsible for the vascular and tubular effects associated with efferent neural activity (38). The role of the α_2-receptor in renal function is currently under extensive study. α_2-Receptor stimulation decreases adenylate cyclase activity, and this may be the mechanism for its inhibitory effect on the tubular action of ADH (172, 177).

The α-receptor–specific agents are most commonly used for antihypertensive therapy (13). Agents of one type cross the blood-brain barrier and exert their agonist effects "centrally" by reducing sympathetic nervous system efferent activity. These include, in order of increasing specificity for the α_2-receptor, methyldopa, clonidine, and guanabenz. Although these agents do have activity in the periphery, it is their central antihypertensive action that is most prominent. Agents of the second type are active outside the central nervous system. These drugs include the α_1-specific antagonists, prazosin, indoramin, and the nonselective phentolamine.

α_2-ADRENORECEPTOR AGONISTS

α-Methyldopa is converted to an α_2-receptor agonist, α-methylnorepinephrine, in central adrenergic neurons. Acute oral administration is associated with a decrease in GFR, urine volume, and sodium. Renal blood flow is not affected and therefore the filtration fraction decreases (72). These effects persist with chronic use, and the development of edema is well documented. Patients with low plasma renin activity have the greatest weight gain and those with high renin have the least (61). A review of the reported cases suggests that the greatest decrement in renal function occurs in individuals with normal filtration rates.

Clonidine reduces renal vascular resistance and has a minimal effect on GFR and renal blood flow. Acute oral administration is associated with a decrease in cardiac output due to a fall in heart rate and stroke volume, with no change in renal hemodynamics but a decrease in urinary sodium excretion (142). The cardiac actions tend to diminish with chronic use. Intravenous administration can cause a fall in renal blood flow with a maintained GFR. This response is probably due to vasoconstriction caused by stimulation of extrajunctional α_2-receptors in the renal vasculature. Clonidine decreases the plasma level of norepinephrine, depresses renin secretion, and has been reported to promote renal prostaglandin release. Responsivity of the collecting duct to ADH appears blunted by clonidine, and although the mechanism is unclear, it may be related to the attenuating action of prostaglandins on ADH activity (92). Although chronic therapy tends to be associated with mild salt and water retention, the incidence and severity are significantly less than are observed with α-methyldopa (63).

Guanabenz has no significant effect on heart rate and cardiac output. Acute oral administration decreases GFR, renal blood flow, urine volume, sodium excretion, and free water clearance. These effects are transient, and with long-term use renal hemodynamics return essentially to baseline (18, 87). The state of hydration appears to be important in determining the acute renal effects of guanabenz. In patients who underwent volume expansion with normal saline (2% body weight) 24 hours prior to receiving 16 mg of the drug, there was no change in GFR or renal blood flow but a significant increase in urinary sodium, fractional excretion of sodium, and free water clearance (62). These data suggest that guanabenz possesses both diuretic and natriuretic properties. In addition, no evidence of weight gain, sodium retention, or alterations in body fluid volumes has been reported with chronic administration. Guanabenz decreases plasma levels of both norepinephrine and epinephrine during exercise(45).

α_1-ADRENORECEPTOR ANTAGONISTS

Prazosin does not appear to have any adverse effect on GFR or renal blood flow and has been reported to lower renal vascular resistance. As with other vasodilators, plasma and extracellular volume are noted to increase, and these actions may oppose the therapeutic response (9, 13, 107).

Indoramin lowers blood pressure by decreasing peripheral resistance without affecting cardiac output or causing a reflex tachycardia (88). In contrast to prazosin, indoramin decreases baroreceptor sensitivity (171). Few studies with a limited number of normal and hypertensive subjects have addressed the specific effects of indoramin on renal function. Acute and chronic oral administration have not been reported to decrease either GFR or renal blood flow (134). Vascular resistance has been noted to decrease. Acute intravenous infusion of 0.25 mg/kg is not accompanied by any significant changes in blood pressure, GFR, or effective renal plasma flow. One patient who received 0.5 mg/kg experienced a marked hypotensive response associated with transient anuria (81).

β-Adrenoreceptor Antagonists

β-Adrenergic antagonists are used in a variety of clinical situations, including postmyocardial infarction prophylaxis. Accordingly, there is an increasing likelihood that patients presenting for critical care will either have received these drugs or require their use during the course of their hospitalization. β-Blockers can be classified on the basis of their affinity for β-adrenergic receptors as either β_1-selective or β-nonselective. This selectivity is relative and can be overcome at high dosage levels.

Propranolol is β-nonselective, lacking in partial agonist activity, and well absorbed when given orally (90%). It undergoes appreciable postabsorption hepatic ("first pass") elimination, and plasma levels vary markedly after a given dose. Because of this initial hepatic clearance, the drug is much more potent per milligram when given intravenously compared with the oral route. Propranolol is highly lipid-soluble and has an elimination half-life of 3.5–6 hours (57, 191, 195). No adjustment in dosage is required during an acute decrease in renal function.

Nadolol is β-nonselective and has no intrinsic agonist activity. Oral absorption is approximately 30%, and it is excreted unchanged in the urine. Elimination half-life is the longest of all the β-blockers at 14–24 hours, and it is predominantly excreted in the urine. Decreases in renal function require adjustment of dosage, and the drug is dialyzable (56, 195).

Metoprolol is β_1-selective and without agonist activity. It is well absorbed orally and undergoes hepatic metabolism. Elimination half-life is 3–4 hours (57, 195). The drug requires no change in dose with renal insufficiency.

Atenolol is β_1-selective and is without intrinsic sympathomimetic activity. Protein binding is minimal and the drug is water-soluble. Elimination half-life is 6–7 hours but may be markedly prolonged with decreases in GFR below 35 ml/min/1.73 m² of body surface area. Gastrointestinal absorption is 60% following oral administration, with little variability in plasma levels (57, 136).

Labetalol is a nonselective β-antagonist with a minimal degree of β_1 and possible β_2 intrinsic agonist activity. In addition to its β activity, this agent is an α_1-selective competitive antagonist. In contrast to agents with only β-blocking activity, labetalol lowers blood pressure through a decrease in peripheral resistance with essentially no change in resting heart rate or cardiac output (126).

The effects of the β-receptor–blocking agents on renal function can be divided into those associated with acute oral or intravenous administration and with chronic oral therapy. The best characterized β-blocker is propranolol. Studies on the other agents are not numerous and allow a limited interpretation because of the small numbers of patients evaluated, the general use of patients with essential hypertension, and the heterogeneity of experimental designs (50).

Acute intravenous administration of propranolol decreases renal blood flow and increases renal vascular resistance in patients with essential hypertension. This decrement is unaffected by prior salt loading (176). In contrast, nadolol reportedly increases renal blood flow (55, 85). Infusion of metoprolol decreases GFR and renal blood flow while increasing renal vascular resistance (55). Intravenous labetalol decreases renal vascular resistance with no change in renal blood flow (41).

Patients receiving chronic treatment with oral propranolol demonstrate a fall in both renal blood flow and GFR. The decrease in filtration rate may not be associated with a rise

in serum creatinine concentration or a fall in endogenous creatinine clearance because of augmented tubular secretion, but inulin clearance decreases significantly. Changes in tubular secretion of creatinine in patients receiving propranolol make this an unsatisfactory marker of glomerular filtration (7). Oral therapy with nadolol or metoprolol does not appear to change GRF (77, 152, 187). Metoprolol does not appear to change plasma volume, GFR, or renal blood flow (174). The reported effects of atenolol are variable, with minor increases and decreases in GFR and renal blood flow. Atenolol reduces renal vascular resistance without changing creatinine clearance or renal plasma flow in patients with essential hypertension studied over a 4-week period (40).

Labetalol maintains both GFR and renal blood flow and decreases renal vascular resistance (188). The long-term use of labetalol has been associated with expansion of the plasma volume, a response that may be related to its unique vasodilating action. O'Malley and associates (141), evaluating the effects of β blockade in an "elderly population, reported that effective renal plasma flow was increased by atenolol, decreased by nadolol, and not changed by labetalol. GFR was not affected by any of the agents. It was suggested that age may be an important factor in determining the hemodynamic response to β-blockers.

These induced changes in renal function have not hampered the general use of β-blockers, although the degree of reversibility and long-term effects are not well defined. The situation in the critically ill patient may be different. The renal response to exercise provides a model for evaluating the relationship between neural activity and hemodynamics. The fall in GFR and renal blood flow that accompanies exercise in both normotensive and essential hypertensive patients is potentiated by propranolol but not labetalol (109, 148, 188). Adrenergic activity increases during exercise and stress, as evidenced by an elevated plasma norepinephrine level. Patients receiving propranolol have a greater rise in norepinephrine levels than do controls (59). This enhanced sympathetic activity may be a compensation for the decrease in β-receptor–dependent cardiac function. β Blockade in acutely ill patients with shock, hemorrhage, hypoxia, or cardiac decompensation may further compromise systemic hemodynamics. This, along with the potentiated elevation in circulating catecholamines (32) and unopposed α-adrenergic stimulation, may predispose the physiologically stressed kidney to ischemic injury.

VASODILATORS

Parenteral vasodilating agents are used in a variety of clinical situations. In experimental models of acute renal failure, response to their use is variable and no benefit is noted once renal failure is established (164). Most of the changes in renal function induced by these compounds, except for those caused by glucagon, are related to their effect on systemic hemodyanmics. In effect, a drug-induced fall in mean arterial pressure with resultant decrease in renal perfusion pressure outside the autoregulatory range overshadows any specific renal vasodilation.

Glyceryl trainitrate (nitroglycerin) acts directly on smooth muscle cells causing relaxation. Systemic effects on blood flow and resistances vary according to time, dose, and route of administration. Renal blood flow increases with both intravenous and sublingual administration. In both the mesenteric and iliac vascular beds, but not in the renal vasculature, a biphasic flow pattern is noted following termination of the drug. This response, which appears to be baroreceptor-mediated, is characterized by an initial increase in flow, followed by a rebound decrease in flow as a result of increased vascular resistances. The unique preservation of renal blood flow probably reflects renal autoregulatory activity (184). In patients with severe congestive heart failure, intravenous nitroglycerin failed to alter renal vascular resistance, and renal blood flow decreased along with a fall in mean arterial pressure (110).

Nitroprusside has a marked predilection for vascular smooth muscle (146). It is a weak renal vasodilator, and when administered into the renal artery increases renal blood flow and decreases vascular resistance, but has no major effect on GFR (6). Nitroprusside-induced systemic hypotension overrides the primary renal effects. As with nitroglycerin, a biphasic response in renal blood flow or resistance is not noted post infusion (145). In patients with class III congestive heart failure, intravenous nitroprusside increases renal blood flow and decreases vascular resistance and filtration fraction, with a minimal change in filtration rate. This fact suggests that the improvement in renal function is linked to the increase in

myocardial function rather than to a specific effect on the kidney (34).

In normal subjects, glucagon causes renal vasodilation and may increase urinary excretion of sodium, chloride, potassium, and inorganic phosphate (51). The natriuretic, kaliuretic, and diuretic effects of glucagon are diminished by indomethacin in a dose-related fashion and may in part be prostaglandin mediated (105). Glucagon can cause a transient increase in plasma potassium concentration followed by a prolonged decrease. The increase is probably due to a direct effect of glucagon. The decrease is most likely secondary to an insulin-induced increase in uptake of potassium by a variety of tissues. The hyperkalemic response may be a potential problem for those patients with absolute insulin deficiency (diabetes mellitus) or peripheral insulin resistance (uremia) (128, 132). In a variety of experimental models of renal ischemia, intravenous glucagon (5 mg/min) enhances renal blood flow and increases GFR and urine flow. These improvements in hemodynamics are more pronounced in the ischemic kidney (115). Unfortunately, glucagon is of no benefit once acute renal failure is established. This action of increasing both renal blood flow and glomerular filtration rate makes glucagon unique among the vasodilators (132).

INHIBITORS OF ANGIOTENSIN-CONVERTING ENZYME

The renin-angiotensin system is a major contributor to the control of renal function (113). Glomerular surface area and capillary pressure are major determinants of glomerular filtration affected by angiotensin II. Capillary hydraulic pressure is determined by the balance between afferent (preglomerular) and efferent (postglomerular) arteriolar resistance. Glomerular surface area is maintained by the supporting mesangium. Angiotensin II is the principal vasoconstrictor of the efferent arteriole and can cause mesangial contraction (43).

A detailed description of the mechanisms of renin release and angiotensin II formation is available in a number of comprehensive reviews (74, 101). In brief, renin enzymatically cleaves angiotensin I from renin substrate, an α_2-globulin. The converting enzyme, a dipeptidyl carboxy-peptidase, acts on angiotensin I to form angiotensin II. Angiotensin II is a potent vasoconstrictor and stimulates the adrenal release of aldosterone.

At present, captopril and enalapril maleate are the available orally active inhibitors of angiotensin-converting enzyme. These agents are used in the treatment of hypertension, both essential and renal, congestive heart failure, and scleroderma renal crisis (182). Additional clinical indications may be forthcoming since results from rodent studies suggest that the progressive loss of glomerular filtration observed in hypertension due to reduced renal mass or streptozotocin-induced diabetes can be prevented by converting-enzyme blockade. The mechanism responsible for these effects is believed to be a reduction in elevated glomerular capillary pressure (3, 198). Preliminary data from patients with diabetes mellitus show that captopril reduces the annual rate of decline in GFR (16).

Captopril is well absorbed orally, with peak blood levels appearing at approximately 1 hour and an elimination half-life of 2–3 hours. Following absorption, enalapril is hydrolyzed in the liver to its more active form, enalaprilat. Peak serum concentrations of enalaprilat appear 3–4 hours following ingestion, although delayed appearance has been noted in patients with hepatic dysfunction and congestive heart failure. Enalaprilat has a greater affinity for converting enzyme than does captopril, and has both a longer half-life (11 hours) and longer duration of action (183). Both drugs are principally cleared by the kidney, and appropriate dosage adjustments must be made based on renal function.

The majority of studies with both of these drugs have been conducted in patients with either hypertension or congestive heart failure. In normal subjects and hypertensives with normal renal function, captopril causes an acute increase in renal blood flow. The magnitude of the increase is related to sodium (volume) balance, with a greater increase noted in subjects on a low sodium intake. Essential hypertensives have a potentiated response greater than that of normal subjects at any level of intake. GFR fell slightly in normal subjects but was either unchanged or increased (based on baseline GFR) in hypertensives (86). Enalapril has been reported to produce similar effects, including the increase in filtration when baseline GFR is less than 80 ml/min (8). A natriuretic response has also been reported (137). An increase in plasma potassium concentration is common although usually minor. However, the presence of renal insufficiency or the concomitant use of potassium-sparing diuretic agents, potassium supplements, or β-blocking agents may cause clinically significant hyperkalemia.

Both agents appear relatively selective for the renal vascular bed and cause a reduction in vascular resistance. In the majority of congestive heart failure patients, converting-enzyme blockade increases renal blood flow and lowers vascular resistance without causing a significant effect on GFR (155). However, a recent study comparing enalapril with captopril in patients with congestive heart failure reported a decline in GFR and sustained hypotension with enalapril (144). The dose of enalapril employed was relatively large and was not titrated to effect. However, this fact emphasizes the importance of the careful monitoring necessary when using this class of drugs.

Deterioration in renal function has been reported with both of these agents in patients with renovascular occlusive disease. This problem is particularly true in patients with bilateral renal artery stenosis or stenosis in a single kidney (11, 91). When mean arterial pressure is reduced, perfusion pressure distal to the stenosis falls. As noted above, autoregulation of filtration requires the action of angiotensin II on the efferent glomerular arteriole. Use of these drugs should be undertaken with care in any patient with evidence of atherosclerotic vascular disease.

In summary, the renal hemodynamic and functional responses to angiotensin-converting enzyme blockade is determined by a number of factors including volume status, systemic hemodynamics, baseline level of renal function, and patency of the renal arterial vasculature.

CALCIUM ENTRY–BLOCKING DRUGS

Calcium plays a role in intrarenal hemodynamics, including autoregulation and volume regulation. The calcium entry–blocking agents inhibit channel-mediated calcium movement across the cell membrane (201).

Autoregulation requires normally responsive vascular smooth muscle to alter renal vascular resistance at various sites. This autoregulatory ability appears to be in part calcium-dependent. The potential for the calcium-blocking agents to blunt normal autoregulation is based on their ability to affect vascular smooth muscle directly, interfering with the "signal" that prompts the vascular response, and their ability to attenuate the intrarenal effects of angiotensin II. In vascular smooth muscle the influx of extracellular calcium, initiated by either electrical stimulation or receptor activation, releases stored intracellular calcium. The cytosolic free calcium binds to calmodulin and this complex activates a protein kinase that alters myosin, enabling an interaction with actin resulting in contraction (129).

In the majority of patients receiving these drugs, both GFR and renal blood flow remain stable or increase slightly as perfusion pressure decreases (10). This fact suggests that autoregulatory ability is maintained in most cases. The renal response to calcium antagonists in the critically ill patient has not yet been described. Of interest is a recent study in the mechanically ventilated, barbiturate-anesthetized dog, a preparation known to have high plasma renin activity and elevated renal vascular resistance. The renal response to graded doses of nitroprusside, diltiazem, and nifedipine were compared. When mean arterial pressure was decreased within the autoregulatory range, both effective renal plasma flow and GFR were maintained with nitroprusside. In contrast, nifedipine, and to a slightly lesser extent, diltiazem, decreased both renal plasma flow and GFR. All agents increased plasma renin activity, but the calcium-blocking drugs provoked a substantially larger increase. Plasma catecholamines were increased by all three drugs, with nifedipine causing the largest rise (17). These findings suggest that use of calcium-blocking agents, under certain clinical conditions, could provoke deterioration in renal function.

Alterations in GFR and renal blood flow can affect tubular handling of sodium and water. Both diltiazem and nifedipine have been clearly shown to cause a natriuresis and diuresis following acute administration, without an effect on potassium excretion. This action does not appear to be maintained with chronic administration. However, unlike other vasodilators, none of these agents has been reported to cause salt or volume retention (10, 197).

Verapamil, a derivative of papaverine, has been reported to produce no change in GFR, plasma renin activity, or the excretion of salt and water following acute and/or chronic oral administration (111, 112). Nifedipine, a dihydropyridine derivative, is a potent vasodilator. Its effect on renal blood flow in normotensive humans without renal disease appears to be minimal. In nifedipine-treated hypertensives and patients with congestive heart failure, renal blood flow has been reported to either increase or remain stable. GFR increases, decreases, or remains unchanged following acute nifedipine administration (167). The effect with chronic oral therapy appears minimal. Intravenous infusion of a nondepressor dose of nifedipine increased GFR in hypertensives with mild renal insufficiency, but not in normotensive controls or patients with severe renal disease. Renal blood flow increased only in the group with essential hypertension (111). Acute administration of nifedipine has both diuretic and natriuretic actions that are more pronounced in hypertensives (196). Increased uric acid excretion has also been reported (167). Plasma renin activity is increased with acute administration, but appears to return to baseline over time. Of interest is a recent report of four cases of acute renal insufficiency apparently induced by nifedipine in patients with underlying renal dysfunction of varying severity. The episodes were nonoliguric without any other apparent etiology. Renal function returned toward baseline relatively rapidly after nifedipine was discontinued (37).

Nitrendipine is another dihydropyridine presently under investigation. GFR and renal blood flow were unchanged in the presence of a reduced mean arterial pressure and total peripheral resistance following 2 weeks of oral drug therapy. Nitrendipine caused a significant increase in plasma renin activity without a concomitant rise in plasma aldosterone. No changes were noted in body weight, fractional sodium excretion, and osmolar or free water clearance (149).

Diltiazem, a benzothiazepine derivative, has not been shown to consistently affect either GFR or renal blood flow with acute administration. A preliminary report suggests that in hypertensives with an initial GFR of less than 80 ml/min/1.73 m^2, diltiazem significantly increased both GFR and renal blood flow (10). Diltiazem does not appear to increase plasma renin activity. Like nifedipine, diltiazem has been reported to increase urine flow rates and sodium excretion, without a change in potassium excretion. This effect has been noted in patients with hypertension, renal disease, and chronic congestive heart failure (31).

INHIBITORS OF PROSTAGLANDIN SYNTHESIS

Intrarenal production of prostaglandins and thromboxanes is well documented (42). These compounds have been the object of intense study and speculation, while the use of agents that inhibit prostaglandin synthesis has also proliferated.

Cyclooxygenase, the enzyme that converts arachidonic acid to prostaglandin G_2, can be inhibited by the nonsteroidal antiinflammatory drugs (NSAIDs) and aspirin. Cyclooxygenase is acetylated by aspirin and irreversibly inhibited. The rapid turnover of this enzyme by the kidney restricts the aspirin-mediated inhibition to 24–48 hours. Binding to the cyclooxygenase protein by the NSAIDs is reversible and their effects diminish over 8–24 hours (42).

Aspirin and the NSAIDs can compromise prostaglandin-dependent renal function (136). Although prostaglandins do not appear to play a significant role in the normal maintenance of GFR and renal blood flow, this finding is not the case during periods of hemodynamic stress (89). Under a variety of conditions, prostaglandins act as vasodepressors and attenuate the actions of a number of vasoconstricting systems.

Experiments with animal models of hypotensive hemorrhage (78), endotoxemia (79), hypoxemia (194), increased renal venous pressure (200), and diminished cardiac output (140) all demonstrate the importance of an intact renal prostaglandin production system. In addition, the renal vasodilatory response to mannitol during hypoperfusion appears to be prostaglandin-dependent (97). Decreases in renal blood flow and GFR and marked increases in renal vascular resistance occur when prostaglandin synthesis is inhibited under these conditions. The contribution of the sympathetic nervous system and circulating catecholamines as mediators of renal vascular tone is clearly observed when the vasodilator action of prostaglandins is lacking (80, 138).

A wide variety of clinical syndromes have been described with the use of NSAIDs (33). These include a decline in renal blood flow and GFR in patients with congestive heart failure or chronic liver disease, particularly those with ascites (19, 199). Drug-induced nephrotic syndrome with reversible renal failure has been reported (22). An increase in serum potassium is common, with a more severe degree of hyperkalemia associated with the concomitant use of other drugs that affect potassium homeostasis. Acute deterioration of renal function and marked hyperkalemia have been induced in patients with mild underlying renal dysfunction treated with indomethacin (60, 179, 190). Some patients with systemic lupus erythematosus have a decrease in both filtration rate and blood flow with therapeutic doses of aspirin, ibuprofen, napoxen, or fenoprofen (103, 104). The NSAIDs have been shown to attenuate the natriuretic actions of furosemide and spironolactone (52). A similar effect is suggested for the thiazides (192). Because the NSAIDs can induce sodium retention directly, this drug interaction has potentially serious clinical consequences. Of particular concern is the severe decline in renal function and the report of anuric renal failure induced by the combination of indomethacin and triamterene (53, 193). The action of the β-blocking drugs is also diminished by the NSAIDs (192).

All these data emphasize that when the kidney is under hemodynamic stress due to volume depletion, immunologic injury, hypoxia, or decreased perfusion of any cause, prostaglandins exert a potent and essential protective effect. Use of NSAIDs in critically ill patients must be undertaken with extreme caution.

If a NSAID is absolutely essential, of the agents presently available, the judicious use of sulindac appears to be the best choice. Although sulindac is claimed to be "renal sparing," the data are conflicting (20, 154).

PHARMACOLOGIC APPROACHES TO UREMIC BLEEDING

The bleeding diathesis of uremia is a major contributing factor to the continued high morbidity and mortality in patients with acute renal failure. Major disruptions of platelet function combined with coagulation defects and alterations in the production of prostaglandin I_2 by vascular endothelium contribute to the complex pathophysiology of the hemostatic abnormalities. A detailed description of this subject can be found in a number of recent excellent reviews (4, 36, 98).

The properly performed and interpreted simplate bleeding time appears to be the best discriminating test in predicting the occurrence of clinical bleeding in the uremic patient (168). The bleeding time is determined by a combination of factors including hematocrit, platelet function, vascular contractility, and VIII:von Willebrand's factor activity.

Both hemodialysis and peritoneal dialysis can shorten the bleeding time and improve platelet function, and may diminish clinical bleeding. Although the traditional therapy, they are not consistently efficacious. Based on observations from a number of other bleeding disorders, alternative treatments for uremic bleeding have been evaluated. These include the use of cryoprecipitate, desmopressin acetate (deamino-8-D-arginine vasopressin, dDAVP), and conjugated estrogen. At this time, the numbers of both studies and patients involved are small, and no definitive recommendations can be made. However, it appears that the judicious use of dDAVP may be beneficial under selected circumstances involving clinical bleeding unresponsive to dialysis, and prophylactically in patients at risk for bleeding because of a prolonged bleeding time prior to surgery.

Cryoprecipitate is the insoluble component remaining after plasma has been frozen and then thawed at 4°C. It has been used to shorten the bleeding time in storage disease, a type of platelet dysfunction. Janson and associates (94) reported the results of cryoprecipitate infusion in seven uremic patients. In one patient with a cecal mass, cryoprecipitate stopped a serious gastrointestinal hemorrhage, and it allowed surgically invasive procedures to be performed in five patients without the development of abnormal hemostasis. All patients were uremic and had prolonged bleeding times. The bleeding time was shortened in all subjects and the maximal effect was noted 1–12 (mean, 5.8) hours following infusion (94). Plasma preparations, however, carry the potential risk of infectious agent transmission.

dDAVP is a synthetic analogue of arginine vasopressin that is used to correct bleeding time in patients with either hemophilia A or mild to moderate von Willebrand's disease (type 1). In a randomized cross-over study involving 12 chronic dialysis patients, dDAVP effectively shortened the prolonged bleeding times. No abnormal bleeding was noted in an additional nine individuals either on dialysis or with acute renal failure who received dDAVP prior to elective surgery or kidney biopsy. The dose of dDAVP used was 0.3 μg/kg in 50 ml of normal saline infused over 30 minutes (125). The effect on bleeding time occurs within 1 hour and may persist for up to 8 hours. In two studies involving two patients, one with gastrointestinal bleeding and the other with surgical-induced bleeding, dDAVP given as a 0.4 μg/kg 10-minute infusion (189) or 3.0 μg/kg administered intranasally (159) was successful in shortening the bleeding time and decreasing clinical bleeding. The mechanism of action of dDAVP is not clearly defined but may involve a direct effect on the vessel wall that increases platelet adhesivity. No major side effects were reported in any of these studies. However,

dDAVP has potent antidiuretic activity as well as some vasoconstrictor activity, and its use requires careful monitoring of serum sodium concentration and blood pressure.

In a single report, the effectiveness of a conjugated estrogen preparation (Premarin) was studied in six chronic dialysis patients with persistently prolonged bleeding times and a history of clinical bleeding. The bleeding time normalized in four patients and decreased in two. The maximal effect was noted between 2 and 9 days and persisted for a variable period after the medication was stopped. Doses ranged from 10 to 50 mg/day (118). Further studies are required before any conclusions can be made about the role of this compound in the treatment of uremic bleeding.

RENAL RESPONSE TO MECHANICAL LIFE-SUPPORT SYSTEMS

Respiratory failure requiring mechanical ventilatory support occurs often in the critically ill patient. Management of these individuals requires an understanding of the renal response to this intervention and the effects of respiratory failure on renal function.

Changes in both arterial oxygen (Pa_{O_2}) and carbon dioxide (Pa_{CO_2}) tension can influence renal hemodynamics and sodium excretion. The response of the renal vasculature to changes in oxygen and carbon dioxide tensions appears to be a summation of the local direct and systemic effects of these gases (75). Autoregulation of renal blood flow operates effectively over a Pa_{O_2} range of 40–125 torr. Renal blood flow tends to decrease as Pa_{O_2} rises, and increases as Pa_{O_2} falls. Development of hypoxia or hyperoxia outside these levels is accompanied by decreases in renal blood flow, fractional excretion of sodium, urine output, and to a lesser degree, glomerular filtration rate (102). Severe hypoxia ($Pa_{O_2} < 40$ torr) enhances the baroreceptor-mediated, hypotension-induced vasoconstriction within the renal vasculature (150). Hypercapnea (Pa_{CO_2} levels > 65 torr) markedly decreases urine flow, sodium excretion, and renal blood flow (163). Both baseline GFR and blood flow tend to be reduced in the patient with acute respiratory failure, so changes in oxygen tension can have a marked effect on renal function. This fact may be particularly true in patients with underlying chronic obstructive pulmonary disease. These individuals as a group have a decreased GFR and effective renal plasma flow and an impaired ability to excrete a sodium load. The presence of hypoxia produces a further decline in GFR and sodium excretion (153).

The effect of positive pressure ventilation on the kidney is multifactorial. Initiation and maintenance of controlled mechanical ventilation alters both thoracic pressure and arterial concentrations of oxygen and carbon dioxide. Spontaneous breathing against positive pressure produces a fall in urine flow, free water clearance, osmolar clearance, and sodium excretion, and mild decreases in GFR and renal blood flow. The decline in urine volume is disproportionately greater than the fall in GFR (135).

In this discussion mechanical ventilation is subdivided into two major types: (a) intermittent positive pressure ventilation (IPPV) and (b) IPPV with positive end-expiratory pressure (PEEP) or continuous positive pressure ventilation (CPPV).

The long-term effects of IPPV include both sodium (65) and water retention (163). The effects of CPPV have been more extensively studied. The data from both human and animal experiments show a CPPV-induced decrease in urine flow, renal plasma flow, and sodium excretion. Filtration rate is maintained or decreases slightly (5, 96, 127). Both plasma renin and aldosterone increase. Changes in free water clearance are either absent or inconsistent, whereas plasma levels of ADH and norepinephrine are elevated (108). The increase in ADH has been considered the basis for the water retention found in patients requiring prolonged ventilatory support. These hormonal alterations are probably the result of the CPPV-induced changes in systemic hemodynamics. The primary change is a decrease in cardiac output that is due in part to changes in filling pressures and a decrease in left ventricular volume (95). It is the combination of the hemodynamic and humoral stimuli that produces the changes in renal function (5).

In order to modify these potential harmful alterations in renal function, careful attention must be paid to the patient's volume status. Expansion of circulating volume has been shown to attenuate the humoral, systemic hemodynamic, and renal function changes described above (14, 185). When acute or progressive fluid overload occurs, with the attendant problem of cardiopulmonary decompensation, careful use of loop-acting diuretics should be considered. Although a role for angiotensin II in the pressor response to acute hypoxemia and hypercapnic acidosis has been suggested, its participation in the maintenance of GFR during mechanical ventilation has not been clearly defined. Extreme caution is recommended in the use of the converting-enzyme inhibitors, captopril or enalapril, in patients on mechanical ventilatory support (see "Inhibitors of Angiotensin-Converting Enzyme").

Alternatives to volume expansion have been explored. Low-dose dopamine infusion (5 ± 0.05 μg/kg/min) in patients with acute respiratory failure on CPPV (PEEP = 20 cm H_2O) corrects the ventilator-induced decrease in mean arterial pressure and cardiac output, and in addition increases urine output, creatinine clearance, and urinary sodium excretion (77). Use of intermittent mandatory ventilation (IMV), both with and without PEEP, improves creatinine clearance, osmolar clearance, and urine volume compared with controlled mechanical ventilation (169).

Realistic considerations of the systemic and renal effects of mechanical ventilation and oxygenation in the total therapeutic approach to the critically ill patient should help to improve treatment-induced morbidity.

MEDICAL ANTISHOCK TROUSERS

Use of medical antishock trousers, the MAST garment, in the therapy of hypovolemic shock and to control intraabdominal hemorrhage is well established (160). In normal individuals placed in a 30° upright tilt, graduated increases in MAST suit pressure produce progressive increases in left ventricular end-diastolic dimension, cardiac output, stroke volume, mean arterial pressure, and forearm blood flow (124). The observed effects on systemic hemodynamics are attributed to volume redistribution with increased venous return to the heart (preload), and to a direct effect on peripheral vascular resistance (afterload) (58). The renal response to an increase in central blood volume, as caused by head-out water immersion in humans (48) or the application of lower body positive pressure in monkeys (99), is both a diuresis and natriuresis. Studies in normal humans wearing the MAST suit for 24 hours at a pressure of 20 cm H_2O show no effect on renal plasma flow (28). In patients with intraabdominal hemorrhage, use of the suit increases or sustains urine flow (11 of 15 cases, with a mild decrease in four cases) (27). The specific benefits derived from the appropriate application of the MAST suit are not counterbalanced by an adverse effect on renal function.

References

1. Adam WR: Aldosterone and dopamine receptors in the kidney: sites for pharmacologic manipulation of renal function. *Kidney Int* 18:623–635, 1980.
2. Anderson RJ: Hospital-associated hyponatremia. *Kidney Int* 29:1237–1247, 1986.
3. Anderson S, Rennke HG, Brenner, B: Therapeutic advantage of converting enzyme inhibitors in arresting progressive renal disease associated with systemic hypertension in the rat. *J Clin Invest* 77:1993–2000, 1986.
4. Andrassy K, Ritz E: Uremia as a cause of bleeding. *Am J Nephrol* 3:313–319, 1985.
5. Annat G, Viale JP, Xuan BB, Aissa OH, Benzoni D, Vincent M, Gharib C, Motin J: Effect of PEEP ventilation on renal function, plasma renin, aldosterone, neurophysins and urinary ADH, and prostaglandins. *Anesthesiology* 58:136–141, 1983.
6. Bastron RD, Kalozanides GJ: Effect of sodium nitroprusside on function in the isolated and intact dog kidney. *J Pharmacol Exp Ther* 181:244–249, 1972.
7. Bauer JH, Brooks CS: The long-term effect of propranolol on renal function. *Am J Med* 66:405–410, 1979.
8. Bauer JH, Gaddy P: Effects of enalapril alone and in combination with hydrochlorothiazide, on renin-angiotensin-aldosterone, renal function, salt and water excretion and body fluid composition. *Am J Kidney Dis* 6:222–232, 1985.
9. Bauer JH, Jones LB, Gaddy P: Effects of prazosin therapy on BP, renal function, and body fluid composition. *Arch Intern Med* 144:1196–1200, 1984.
10. Bauer JH, Sunderrajan S, Reams G: Effects of calcium entry blockers on renin-angiotensin-aldosterone system, renal function and hemodynamics, salt and water excretion and body fluid composition. *Am J Cardiol* 56:62H–67H, 1985.
11. Bender W, La France N, Walker WG: Mechanism of deterioration in renal function in patients with renovascular hypertension treated with enalapril. *Hypertension* 6(suppl 1):I193–I197, 1984.
12. Beretta-Piccoli C, Weidmann P, Schiffl H, Cottier C, Reubi FC: Enhanced cardiovascular pressor reactivity to norepinephrine in mild renal parenchymal disease. *Kidney Int* 22:297–303, 1982.
13. Bernstein KN, O'Connor DT: Antiadrenergic antihypertensive drugs: their effect on renal function. *Annu Rev Pharmacol Toxicol* 24:105–120, 1984.
14. Berry AJ: Respiratory support and renal function. *Anesthesiology* 55:655–667, 1981.
15. Birkenhager WH, Solomon RJ, Wills MR: Symposium on electrolyte disturbances and cardiac risks. *Drugs* 29(suppl 1):1–199, 1984.
16. Bjorck S, Nyberg G, Mulec H, Granerus G, Herlitz H, Aurell M: Beneficial effects of angiotensin enzyme inhibition on renal function in patients with diabetic nephropathy. *Br Med J* 293:471–475, 1986.
17. Blackshear JL, Orlandi C, Williams GH, Hollenberg NK: The renal response to diltiazem and nifedipine: comparison with nitroprusside. *J Cardiovasc Pharmacol* 8:37–43, 1986.
18. Bosanac P, Dubb J, Walker B, Goldberg M, Agus ZS: Renal effects of guanabenz: a new antihypertensive. *J Clin Pharmacol* 16:631–636, 1976.
19. Boyer TD, Zia P, Reynolds TB: Effect of indomethacin and prostaglandin A$_1$ on renal function and plasma renin activity in alcoholic liver disease. *Gastroenterology* 77:215–222, 1979.
20. Brater DC, Anderson S, Baird B, Campbell WB: Effects of ibuprofen, naproxen, and sulindac on prostaglandins in men. *Kidney Int* 27:66–73, 1985.
21. Brenner BM, Lazarus JM (eds): *Acute Renal Failure.* Philadelphia, WB Saunders, 1983.
22. Brezin JH, Katz SM, Schwartz AB, Chimitz JL: Reversible renal failure and nephrotic syndrome associated with nonsteroidal anti-inflammatory drugs. *N Engl J Med* 301:1271–1273, 1979.
23. Brickman AS, Massry SG, Coburn JW: Changes in serum and urinary calcium during treatment with hydrochlorothiazide: studies on mechanisms. *J Clin Invest* 51:945–954, 1972.
24. Brown CB, Ogg CS, Cameron JS: High dose furosemide in acute renal failure: a controlled trial. *Clin Nephrol* 15:90–96, 1981.
25. Brown MJ, Brown DC, Murphy MB: Hypokalemia from β$_2$-receptor stimulation by circulating epinephrine. *N Engl J Med* 309:1414–1419, 1983.
26. Bullock ML, Umen AJ, Finkelstein M, Keane WF: The assessment of risk factors in 462 patients with acute renal failure. *Am J Kidney Dis* 5:97–103, 1985.
27. Burdick JF, Warshaw AL, Abbott WM: External counterpressure to control postoperative intra-abdominal hemorrhage. *Am J Surg* 129:369–373, 1975.
28. Cangiano JL, Kest L: Use of a G-suit for uncontrollable bleeding after percutaneous renal biopsy. *J Urol* 107:360–361, 1972.
29. Cannon PJ: The kidney in heart failure. *N Engl J Med* 296(1):26–32, 1977.
30. Carriere S: Factors affecting renal cortical blood flow. A review. *Can J Physiol Pharmacol* 53:1–20, 1975.
31. Chaffman M, Brogden RN: Diltiazem: a review of its pharmacological properties and therapeutic efficacy. *Drugs* 29:387–454, 1985.
32. Chernow B, Rainey TG, Lake CR: Endogenous and exogenous catecholamines in critical care medicine. *Crit Care Med* 10:409–416, 1982.
33. Clive DM, Stoff JS: Renal syndromes associated with nonsteroidal anti-inflammatory drugs. *N Engl J Med* 310:563–572, 1984.
34. Cogan JJ, Humphreys MH, Carlson CJ, Rapaport E: Renal effects of nitroprusside and hydralazine in patients with congestive heart failure. *Circulation* 61(2):316–323, 1980.
35. Cuche JL, Marchand GR, Greger RF, Lang FC, Knox FG: Phosphaturic effect of dopamine in dogs: possible role of intrarenally produced dopamine in phosphate regulation. *J Clin Invest* 58:71–76, 1976.
36. Deykin D: Uremic bleeding. *Kidney Int* 24:698–705, 1983.
37. Diamond JR, Cheung JY, Fang LST: Nifedipine-induced renal dysfunction. *Am J Med* 77:905–909, 1984.
38. DiBona GF: Neural control of renal function: role of alpha adrenoceptors. *J Cardiovasc Pharmacol* 7(suppl 8):S18–S23, 1985.
39. Dixon BS, Anderson RJ: Nonoliguric acute renal failure. *Am J Kidney Dis* 6:71–80, 1985.
40. Dreslinski GR, Messerli FH, Dunn FG, Suarez DH, Reisen E, Frohlich ED: Hemodynamics, biochemical and reflexive changes produced by atenolol in hypertension. *Circulation* 65:1365–1368, 1982.
41. Dunn FG, Oigman W, Messerli FH, Dreslinski GR, Reisin E, Frohlich ED: Hemodynamic effects of intravenous labetalol in essential hypertension. *Clin Pharmacol Ther* 33:139–143, 1983.
42. Dunn MJ, Zambraski EF: Renal effects of drugs that inhibit prostaglandin synthesis. *Kidney Int* 18:609–622, 1980.
43. Dworkin LD, Ichikawa I, Brenner BM: Hormonal modulation of glomerular function. *Am J Physiol* 13:F95–F104, 1983.
44. Dzau VJ, Hollenberg NK: Renal response to captopril in severe heart failure: role of furosemide in natriuresis and reversal of hyponatremia. *Ann Intern Med* 100:777–782, 1984.

45. Dziedzic SW, Elijovich F, Felton K, Yeager K, Krakoff LR: Effect of guanabenz on blood pressure response to posture and exercise. *Clin Pharmacol Ther* 33:151–155, 1983.

46. Eckstein JW, Aboud FM: Circulatory effects of sympathomimetic amines. *Am Heart J* 63:119–135, 1962.

47. Elghozi JL, Earnhardt JT, Meyer P: Dopamine: vascular and renal effects and alterations in hypertension. *Adv Nephrol* 13:135–150, 1984.

48. Epstein M: Renal effects of headout water immersion in man: implications for an understanding of volume homeostasis. *Physiol Rev* 58(3):529–581, 1978.

49. Epstein M, Hollenberg NK, Merrill JP: The pattern of the renal vascular response to epinephrine in man. *Proc Soc Exp Biol Med* 134:720–724, 1970.

50. Epstein M, Oster JR: Beta-blockers and the kidney. *Miner Electrolyte Metab* 8:237–254, 1982.

51. Farah AE: Glucagon and the circulation. *Pharmacol Rev* 35:181–207, 1983.

52. Favre L, Glasson PH, Riondel A, Vallotton MB: Interaction of diuretics and nonsteroidal anti-inflammatory drugs in man. *Clin Sci* 64:407–415, 1983.

53. Favre L, Glasson P, Vallotton MB: Reversible acute renal failure from combined triamterene and indomethacin. *Ann Intern Med* 96:317–320, 1982.

54. Fichman MP, Vorhen H, Klaecman C, Telfer N: Diuretic induced hyponatremia. *Ann Intern Med* 75:853–863, 1971.

55. Foley J, Penner B, Fung H: Short-term renal hemodynamic effects of nadolol and metoprolol in normotensive and hypertensive subjects. *Clin Pharmacol Ther* 29:245, 1981.

56. Frishman W: Clinical pharmacology of the new beta-adrenergic blocking drugs. Part 9. Nadolol: a new long-acting beta-adrenoreceptor blocking drug. *Am Heart J* 99:124–128, 1980.

57. Frishman W: Part 1. Pharmacodynamic and pharmacokinetic properties. *Am Heart J* 97:663–670, 1979.

58. Gaffney FA, Thal ER, Taylor WF, Bastian BC, Weigelt JA, Atkins JM, Blomquist CG: Hemodynamic effects of medical anti-shock trousers (MAST garment). *J Trauma* 21(11):931–937, 1981.

59. Galbo H, Holst JJ, Christensen NJ, Hilsted J: Glucagon and plasma catecholamines during beta-receptor blockade in exercising man. *J Appl Physiol* 40:855–863, 1976.

60. Galler M, Folkert VW, Schlondorff D: Reversible acute renal insufficiency and hyperkalemia following indomethacin therapy. *JAMA* 246:154–155, 1981.

61. Gavras H, Gavras I, Brunner HR, Laragh JH: The antihypertensive action of methyldopa in relation to its effect on the renin-aldosterone system. *J Clin Pharmacol* 16:372–378, 1977.

62. Gehr M, MacCarthy EP, Goldberg M: Guanabenz: a centrally acting, natriuretic antihypertensive drug. *Kidney Int* 29:1203–1298, 1986.

63. Gehr M, MacCarthy EP, Goldberg M: Natriuretic and water diuretic effects of central alpha$_2$-adrenoreceptor agonists. *J Cardiovasc Pharmacol* 6:S781–S786, 1984.

64. Gennari FJ, Kassirer JP: Osmotic diuresis. *N Engl J Med* 291:714–720, 1974.

65. Gett PM, Jones S, Sheppard GF: Pulmonary edema associated with sodium retention during ventilator treatment. *Br J Anaesth* 43:460–470, 1970.

66. Goldberg LI: Recent advances in the pharmacology of catecholamines. *Intensive Care Med* 3:233–236, 1977.

67. Goldberg LI, Hsien YY, Resnekov L: Newer catecholamines for treatment of heart failure and shock: an update of dopamine and a first look at dobutamine. *Prog Cardiovasc Dis* 19:327–340, 1977.

68. Goldberg LI, Volkman PH, Kohli JD: A comparison of the vascular dopamine receptor with other dopamine receptors. *Annu Rev Pharmacol Toxicol* 18:57–79, 1978.

69. Goldberg M, Beck LH, Puschett JB, Schubert JJ: Sites of action of benzothiadiazines, furosemide and ethacrynic acid. In Tant AF, Wilson GM (Eds): *Modern Diuretic Therapy in the Treatment of Cardiovascular and Renal Disease.* London, Excerpta Medica, 1973, pp 135–147.

70. Gombos EA, Hulet WH, Bopp P, Goldring W, Baldwin DS, Chasis H: Reaction of renal and systemic circulations to vasoconstriction agents in normotensive and hypertensive subjects. *J Clin Invest* 41(2):203–217, 1962.

71. Gottschalk CW, Moss NG, Colindres RE: Neural control of renal function in health and disease. In Seldin DW, Giebish G (eds): *The Kidney: Physiology and Pathophysiology.* New York, Raven Press, 1985, pp 581–611.

72. Grabie M, Nussbaum P, Goldfarb S, Walker BR, Goldberg M, Agus ZS: Effects of methyldopa on renal hemodynamics and tubular function. *Clin Pharmacol Ther* 27:522–527, 1980.

73. Graziani G, Cantaluppi A, Casti S, Citterio A, Scalamogna A, Aroldi A, Silenzio R, Brancaccio D, Ponticelli C: Dopamine and furosemide in oliguric acute renal failure. *Nephron* 37:39–42, 1984.

74. Haber E, Carlson W: The biochemistry of the renin-angiotensin system. In Genest J, Kuchel O, Hamet P, Cantin M (eds): *Hypertension.* New York, McGraw Hill, 1983, pp 171–184.

75. Hall SV, Steinman TI: Alterations in renal function during acute respiratory failure. *Int Anesthesiol Clin* 14(1):179–213, 1976.

76. Heel RC, Brogden RN, Pakes GE, Speight TM, Avery GS: Nadolol: a review of its pharmacological properties and therapeutic efficacy in hypertension and angina pectoris. *Drugs* 20:1–23, 1980.

77. Hemmer M, Suter PM: Treatment of cardiac and renal effects of PEEP with dopamine in patients with acute renal failure. *Anesthesiology* 50:399–403, 1979.

78. Henrich WL, Anderson RJ, Berns AS, McDonald KM, Paulsen PJ, Berl T, Schrier RW: The role of renal nerves and prostaglandins in control of renal hemodynamics and plasma renin activity during hypotensive hemorrhage in the dog. *J Clin Invest* 61:744–750, 1978.

79. Henrich WL, Hamasaki Y, Said SI, Campbell WB, Cronin RE: Dissociation of systemic and renal effects in endotoxemia. *J Clin Invest* 69:691–699, 1982.

80. Henrich WL, Pettinger WA, Cronin RE: The influence of circulating catecholamines and prostaglandins on canine renal hemodynamics during hemorrhage. *Circ Res* 48:424–429, 1981.

81. Henry JA, Ohashi C, Britton CW, Britton KE: Acute effects of hydralazine and indoramin on renal function in man. *Br J Clin Pharmacol* 12:75S–77S, 1981.

82. Herbert P, Tinker J: Inotropic drugs in acute circulatory failure. *Intensive Care Med* 6:101–111, 1980.

83. Hilberman M, Maseda J, Stinson EB, Derby GC, Spencer RJ, Miller DC, Oyer PE, Myers BD: The diuretic properties of dopamine in patients after open-heart operation. *Anesthesiology* 61:489–494, 1984.

84. Hollenberg NK, Adams DF: Vascular factors in the pathogenesis of acute renal failure in man. In Friedman FA (ed): *Proceedings of the Acute Renal Failure Conference.* Washington, DC, Department of Health, Education and Welfare, DHEW Publication No. (NIH) 74-608, 1973, pp 209–229.

85. Hollenberg NK, Adams DF, McKinsty DN, Williams GH, Borucki LS, Sullivan JM: β-Adrenoceptor blocking agents and the kidney: effect of nadolol and propranolol on the renal circulation. *Br J Clin Pharmacol* 7(suppl 2):219S–225S, 1979.

86. Hollenberg NK, Meggs LG, Williams GH, Katz J, Garnic JD, Harrington DP: Sodium intake and renal responses to captopril in normal man and essential hypertension. *Kidney Int* 20:240–245, 1981.

87. Holmes B, Brogden RN, Heel RC, Speight TM, Avery GS: Guanabenz: a review of its pharmacodynamic

properties and therapeutic efficacy in hypertension. *Drugs* 26:212–229, 1983.

88. Holmes B, Sorkin EM: Indoramin: a review of its pharmacodynamic and pharmacokinetic properties, and therapeutic efficacy in hypertension and related vascular, cardiovascular and airway diseases. *Drugs* 31:467–499, 1986.

89. Horton R, Zipser R, Fichman M: Prostaglandins, renal function and vascular regulation. In Symposium on Prostaglandins. *Med Clin North Am* 65(4):891–914, 1981.

90. Hou SH, Bushinsky DA, Wish JB, Cohen JJ, Harrington JT: Hospital-acquired renal insufficiency: a prospective study. *Am J Med* 74:243–248, 1983.

91. Hricik DE, Browning PJ, Kopelman R, Goorno WE, Madias NE, Dzau VJ: Captopril-induced functional renal insufficiency in patients with bilateral renal-artery stenoses or renal-artery stenosis in a solitary kidney. *N Engl J Med* 308:373–376, 1983.

92. Itskovitz HD: Clonidine and the kidney. *J Cardiovasc Pharmacol* 2(suppl 1):S47–S60, 1980.

93. Jakschick BA, Marshall TR, Kourick JL, Needleman T: Profile of circulating vasoactive substances in haemorrhagic shock and their pharmacologic manipulation. *J Clin Invest* 54:842–852, 1974.

94. Janson PA, Jubeliere SJ, Weinstein MJ, Deykin D: Treatment of the bleeding tendency in uremia with cryoprecipitate. *N Engl J Med* 303:1318–1322, 1980.

95. Jardin F, Farcot JC, Boisante L, Curien N, Margairaz A, Bourdarias JP: Influence of positive end-expiratory pressure on left ventricular performance. *N Engl J Med* 304:387–392, 1981.

96. Jarnberg PO, Devillota D, Eklund J, Granberg PO: Effects of positive end-expiratory pressure on renal function. *Acta Anaesthesiol Scand* 22:508–514, 1978.

97. Johnston PA, Bernard DB, Perrin NS, Levinsky NG: Prostaglandins mediate the vasodilatory effect of mannitol in the hypoperfused rat kidney. *J Clin Invest* 68:127–133, 1981.

98. Jubeliere SJ: Hemostatic abnormalities in renal disease. *Am J Kidney Dis* 5:219–225, 1985.

99. Kass DA, Moore-Ede MC: Renal responses to prolonged central volume expansion in conscious primates. *Am J Physiol* 242:F649–F656, 1982.

100. Katz AI, Lindheimer MD: Actions of hormones on the kidney. *Annu Rev Physiol* 39:97–134, 1977.

101. Keeton TK, Campbell WB: The pharmacologic alteration of renin release. *Pharmacol Rev* 32:81–227, 1980.

102. Kilbern KH, Dowell AR: Renal function in respiratory failure: effects of hypoxia, hyperoxia and hypercapnea. *Arch Intern Med* 127:754–762, 1971.

103. Kimberly RP, Bowden RE, Keiser JR, Plotz PH: Reduction of renal function by new nonsteroidal anti-inflammatory drugs. *Am J Med* 64:804–807, 1978.

104. Kimberly RP, Gill JR Jr, Bowden RE, Keiser JR, Plotz PH: Elevated urinary prostaglandins and the effects of aspirin on renal function in lupus erythematosus. *Ann Intern Med* 89:336–341, 1978.

105. Kirschenbaum MA, Zawada ET: The role of prostaglandins in glucagon-induced natriuresis. *Clin Sci* 58:393–401, 1980.

106. Klein LA, Liberman B, Laks M, Kleeman CR: Interrelated effects of antidiuretic hormone and adrenergic drugs on water metabolism. *Am J Physiol* 221:1657–1665, 1971.

107. Koshy M, Mickley D, Bourgoignie J, Blaufox MD: Physiologic evaluation of a new antihypertensive agent: prazosin HCL. *Circulation* 55:533–537, 1977.

108. Kumar A, Pontoppidan H, Baratz RA, Laver MB: Inappropriate response to increased plasma ADH during mechanical ventilation in acute respiratory failure. *Anesthesiology* 40(3):215–221, 1974.

109. Larsen JS, Pedersen EB: Comparison of the effects of propranolol and labetalol on renal haemodynamics at rest and during exercise in essential hypertension. *Eur J Clin Pharmacol* 18:135–139, 1980.

110. Leier CV, Bambach D, Thompson MJ, Cattaneo SM, Goldberg RJ, Unverferth DV: Central and regional hemodynamic effects of intravenous isosorbide dinitrate, nitroglycerin and nitroprusside in patients with congestive heart failure. *Am J Cardiol* 48:1115–1123, 1981.

111. Leonetti G, Cuspidi C, Sampieri L, Terzoli L, Zanchetti A: Comparison of cardiovascular, renal, and humoral effects of acute administration of two calcium channel blockers in normotensive and hypertensive subjects. *J Cardiovasc Pharmacol* 4:S319–S324, 1982.

112. Leonetti G, Sala C, Bianchini C, Terzoli L, Zanchetti A: Antihypertensive and renal effects of orally administered verapamil. *Eur J Clin Pharmacol* 18:375–382, 1980.

113. Levans NR, Peach MJ, Carey RM: Role of the intrarenal renin-angiotensin system in the control of renal function. *Circ Res* 48:157–167, 1981.

114. Levinsky NG, Bernard DB, Johnston PA: Enhancement of recovery of acute renal failure: effects of mannitol and diuretics. In Brenner BM, Stein JH (eds): *Acute Renal Failure* (Contemporary Issues in Nephrology, vol. 6). New York, Churchill Livingstone, 1980, pp 163–179.

115. Levy M: The effect of glucagon on glomerular filtration rate in dogs during reduction of renal blood flow. *Can J Physiol Pharmacol* 53:660–668, 1978.

116. Lindeman RD, Tobin JD, Shock NW: Association between blood pressure and the rate of decline in renal function with age. *Kidney Int* 26:861–868, 1984.

117. Lindner A: Synergism of dopamine and furosemide in diuretic-resistant, oliguric acute renal failure. *Nephron* 33:121–126, 1983.

118. Liu YK, Kosfeld RE, Marcum SG: Treatment of uraemic bleeding with conjugated oestrogen. *Lancet* 2:887–889, 1984.

119. Livesay WR, Moyer JH, Chapman DW: The cardiovascular and renal hemodynamic effects of aramine. *Am Heart J* 47:745–756, 1954.

120. Ljungman S, Aurell M, Hartford M, Wikstrand J, Wilhelmsen L, Berglund G: Blood pressure and renal function. *Acta Med Scand* 208:17–25, 1980.

121. Lokhandwala MF, Barrett RJ: Cardiovascular dopamine receptors: physiological, pharmacological, and therapeutic implications. *J Auton Pharmacol* 2(3):189–215, 1982.

122. Lund-Johansen P: Short- and long-term (six-year) hemodynamic effects of labetalol in essential hypertension. *Am J Med* 75(4A):24–31, 1983.

123. MacCarthy EP, Bloomfield SS: Labetalol: a review of its pharmacology, pharmacokinetics, clinical uses and adverse effects. *Pharmacotherapy* 3:193–219, 1983.

124. Mannering D, Bennett ED, Mehta N, Davis AL: Application of the medical anti-shock trouser (MAST) increases cardiac output and tissue perfusion in simulated, mild hypovolaemia. *Intensive Care Med* 12:143–146, 1986.

125. Mannucci PM, Remuzzi G, Pusineri F, Lombardi R, Valsecchi C, Mecca G, Zimmerman TS: Deamino-8-D-arginine vasopressin shortens the bleeding time in uremia. *N Engl J Med* 308:8–12, 1983.

126. Mark AL, Eckstein JW, Abboud RM, Wendling MG: Renal vascular responses to isoproterenol. *Am J Physiol* 217:764–767, 1969.

127. Marquez JM, Douglas ME, Downs JB, Wu WH, Mantini EL, Kuck EJ, Calderwood HW: Renal function and cardiovascular responses during positive airway pressure. *Anesthesiology* 50:393–398, 1979.

128. Massara F, Martelli S, Cagliero E, Camanni F, Molinatti GM: Influence of glucagon on plasma levels of potassium in man. *Diabetologia* 19:414–417, 1980.

129. McCall D, Walsh RA, Frohlich ED, O'Rourke RA: Calcium entry blocking drugs: mechanisms of action, ex-

perimental studies and clinical uses. *Curr Prob Cardiol* 8:6–14, 1985.

130. McDonald RH, Goldberg LI, McNay JL, Tuhle EP: Effects of dopamine in man: augmentation of sodium excretion, glomerular filtration rate, and renal plasma flow. *J Clin Invest* 43:1116–1123, 1964.

131. McLeod AA, Shand DG: Atenolol: a long-acting beta$_1$ adrenoceptor antagonist. *Ann Intern Med* 96:244–245, 1982.

132. McNay JL: Pharmacology of the renal circulation. *Am J Med* 62:507–513, 1977.

133. Mills LC, Moyer JH: The effects of various catecholamines on specific vascular hemodynamics in hypotensive and normotensive subjects. *Am J Cardiol* 5:652–659, 1960.

134. Morrison G, Spar B, Walker BR, Goldfarb S: The acute and chronic effects of indoramin on renal function, hemodynamics, transport. *J Cardiovasc Pharmacol* 8(suppl 2):S25–S29, 1986.

135. Murdaugh HV, Sieker HO, Manfredi F: Effect of altered intrathoracic pressure on renal hemodynamic, electrolyte excretion and water clearance. *J Clin Invest* 38:834–842, 1959.

136. Muther RS, Potter DM, Bennet WM: Aspirin-induced depression of glomerular filtration rate in normal humans: role of sodium balance. *Ann Intern Med* 94:317–321, 1981.

137. Navis GJ, DeZeeuw D, de Jong PE: Enalapril and the kidney: renal vasodilation and natriuresis due to inhibition of angiotensin II formation. *J Cardiovasc Pharmacol* 8(suppl 1):S30–S34, 1986.

138. Needleman P, Marshal GR, Johnson EM: Determinants and modification of andrenergic and vascular resistance in the kidney. *Am J Physiol* 227:665–669, 1974.

139. Oliver JA, Pinto J, Sciacca RR, Cannon PJ: Basal norepinephrine overflow into the renal vein: effect of renal nerve stimulation. *Am J Physiol* 239:F371–F377, 1980.

140. Oliver JA, Sciacca RR, Pinto J, Cannon PJ: Participation of the prostaglandins in the control of renal blood flow during acute reduction of cardiac output in the dog. *J Clin Invest* 67:229–237, 1981.

141. O'Malley K, O'Callaghan WG, Laher MS, McGarry K, O'Brien E: Beta-adrenoreceptor blocking drugs and renal blood flow with special reference to the elderly. *Drugs* 25(suppl 2):103–107, 1983.

142. Onesti G, Schwartz AB, Kim KE, Swartz C, Brest AN: Pharmacodynamic effects of a new antihypertensive drug, catapres (ST-155). *Circulation* 39:219–228, 1969.

143. Oster JR, Epstein M, Smoller S: Combined therapy with thiazide-type and loop diuretic agents for resistant sodium retention. *Ann Intern Med* 99:405–406, 1983.

144. Packer M, Lee WH, Yushak M, Medicna N: Comparison of captopril and enalapril in patients with severe chronic heart failure. *N Engl J Med* 313:847–853, 1986.

145. Pagani M, Vatner SF, Braunwald E: Hemodynamic effects of intravenous sodium nitroprusside in the conscious dog. *Circulation* 57(1):144–151, 1978.

146. Palmer FR, Lasseter KC: Sodium nitroprusside. *N Engl J Med* 292:294–297, 1975.

147. Parker S, Carlon GC, Isaacs M, Howland WS, Kahn RS: Dopamine administration in oliguria and oliguric renal failure. *Crit Care Med* 9(9):630–632, 1981.

148. Pedersen EB: Abnormal renal haemodynamics during exercise in young patients with mild essential hypertension without treatment and during long-term propranolol therapy. *Scand J Clin Lab Invest* 38:567–571, 1978.

149. Pedrinelli R, Fouad FM, Tarazi RC, Bravo EL, Textor ES: Nitrendipine, a calcium-entry blocker. *Arch Intern Med* 146:62–65, 1986.

150. Pelletier CL, Shephard JT: Effect of hypoxia on vascular responses to the carotid baroreflex. *Am J Physiol* 228:331–336, 1975.

151. Ponce SP, Jennings AE, Madias NE, Harrington JT: Drug-induced hyperkalemia. *Medicine* 64:357–370, 1985.

152. Rasmussen S, Rasmussen K: Influence of metoprolol, alone and in combination with a thiazide diuretic, on blood pressure, plasma volume, extracellular volume and glomerular filtration rate in essential hypertension. *Eur J Clin Pharmacol* 15:305–310, 1979.

153. Reihman DH, Farber MO, Weinberger MH, Henry DP, Fineberg NS, Dowdeswell IG, Burt RW, Manfredi F: Effect of hypoxemia on sodium and water excretion in chronic obstructive lung disease. *Am J Med* 78:87–94, 1985.

154. Roberts DG, Gerber JG, Barnes JS, Zerbe GO, Nies AS: Sulindac is not renal sparing in man. *Clin Pharmacol Ther* 38:258–265, 1985.

155. Romankiewicz JA, Brogden RN, Heel RC, Speight TM, Avery GS: Captopril: an update review of its pharmacological properties and therapeutic efficacy in congestive heart failure. *Drugs* 25:6–40, 1983.

156. Rosenblum R, Berkowitz WD, Lawson D: Effect of acute intravenous administration of isoproterenol on cardiorenal haemodynamics in man. *Circulation* 38:158–168, 1968.

157. Schrier RW: Effects of adrenergic nervous system and catecholamines on systemic and renal hemodynamics, sodium and water excretion and renin secretion. *Kidney Int* 6:291–306, 1974.

158. Schrier RW, Lieberman R, Ufferman RC: Mechanism of antidiuretic effect of beta adrenergic stimulation. *J Clin Invest* 51:97–111, 1972.

159. Shapiro MD, Kelleher SP: Intranasal deamino-8-D-arginine vasopressin shortens the bleeding time in uremia. *Am J Nephrol* 4:260–261, 1984.

160. Shine KI, moderator: Aspects of the management of shock. *Ann Intern Med* 93:723–734, 1980.

161. Shoemaker WC, Bland RD, Appel PL: Therapy of critically ill postoperative patients based on outcome prediction and prospective clinical trials. *Surg Clin North Am* 65:811–833, 1985.

162. Sigurd B, Olesen KD: The supra-additive natriuretic effect of addition of theophylline ethylenediamine and bumetanide in congestive heart failure. *Am Heart J* 94:168–174, 1977.

163. Sladen A, Laver MG, Pontoppidan H: Pulmonary complications and water retention in prolonged mechanical ventilation. *N Engl J Med* 279(9):448–453, 1968.

164. Smolens P, Stein JH (eds): Hemodynamic factors in acute renal failure: pathophysiologic and therapeutic implications. In *Acute Renal Failure* (Contemporary Issues in Nephrology, vol 6). New York, Churchill Livingston, 1980, pp 180–201.

165. Snavely MD, Insel PA: Catecholamines and the kidney: receptors and renal function. *Annu Rev Physiol* 43:625–636, 1981.

166. Sonnenblick EH, Frishman WH, LeJemtel TH: Dobutamine: a new synthetic cardioactive sympathetic amine. *N Engl J Med* 300:17–22, 1979.

167. Sorkin EM, Clissold SP, Brogden RN: Nifedipine: a review of its pharmacodynamic and pharmacokinetic properties and therapeutic efficacy, in ischaemic heart disease, hypertension and related cardiovascular disorders. *Drugs* 30:182–274, 1985.

168. Steiner RW, Coggins C, Carvalho CA: Bleeding time in uremia: a useful test to assess clinical bleeding. *Am J Hematol* 7:107–117, 1979.

169. Steinhoff H, Falke K, Schwarzhoff W: Enhanced renal function associated with intermittent mandatory ventilation in acute respiratory failure. *Intensive Care Med* 8:69–74, 1982.

170. Stote RM, Smith L, Wilson D, Dube WJ, Goldsmith RS, Arnaud CD: Hydrochlorthiazide effects on sodium, calcium and immunoreactive parathyroid hormone concentrations. *Ann Intern Med* 77:587–591, 1972.

171. Strandhoy JW: Comparison of the renal effects of in-

doramin and prazosin. *J Cardiovasc Pharmacol* 8(suppl 2):S151–S155, 1986.

172. Strandhoy JW: Role of alpha-2 receptors in the regulation of renal function. *J Cardiovasc Pharmacol* 7(suppl 8):S28–S33, 1985.

173. Struthers AD, Whitesmith R, Reid JL: Prior thiazide diuretic treatment increases adrenaline-induced hypokalemia. *Lancet* 1:1358–1360, 1983.

174. Sugino G, Barg AP, O'Connor DT: Renal perfusion is preserved during cardioselective beta-blockade with metoprolol in hypertension. *Am J Kidney Dis* 3:357–361, 1984.

175. Suki WN, Steinbaugh BJ, Frommer JP, Eknoyan G: Physiology of diuretic action. In Seldin DW, Giebish G (eds): *The Kidney: Physiology and Pathophysiology.* New York, Raven Press, 1985, pp 2127–2162.

176. Sullivan JM, Adams DF, Hollenberg NK: Beta-adrenergic blockade in essential hypertension reduced renin release despite renal vasoconstriction. *Circ Res* 39:532–535, 1976.

177. Summers RJ: Renal alpha adrenoceptors. *Fed Proc* 43:2917–2922, 1984.

178. Sutton RA: Diuretics and calcium metabolism. *Am J Kidney Dis* 5:4–9, 1985.

179. Tan SY, Shapiro R, Franco R, Stockard H, Mulrow PJ: Indomethacin-induced prostaglandin inhibition with hyperkalemia: a reversible cause of hyporeninemic hypoaldosteronism. *Ann Intern Med* 90:783–785, 1979.

180. Tannen RL: Diuretic-induced hypokalemia. *Kidney Int* 28:988–1000, 1985.

181. ter Wee PM, Smit AJ, Rosman JB, Sluiter WJ, Donker AJM: Effect of intravenous infusion of low-dose dopamine on renal function in normal individuals and in patients with renal disease. *Am J Nephrol* 6:42–46, 1986.

182. Thurm RH, Alexander JC: Captopril in the treatment of scleroderma renal crisis. *Arch Intern Med* 144:733–735, 1984.

183. Todd PA, Heel RC: Enalapril: a review of its pharmacodynamic and pharmacokinetic properties, and therapeutic use in hypertension and congestive heart failure. *Drugs* 31:198–248, 1986.

184. Vatner SF, Pagani M, Rutherford JD, Millard RW, Manders WT: Effects of nitroglycerin on cardiac function and regional blood flow distribution in conscious dogs. *Am J Physiol* 234(3):H244–H252, 1978.

185. Venus B, Mathru M, Smith RA, Pham CG, Shirakawa Y, Sugiura A: Renal function during the application of positive end-expiratory pressure in swine: effects of hydration. *Anesthesiology:* 62:765–769, 1985.

186. Vlachozannis J, Weismuller G, Schoeppe W: Effects of dopamine on kidney function and on the adenyl cyclase phosphodiesterase system in man. *Eur J Clin Invest* 6:131–137, 1976.

187. Waal-Manney HJ, Hobson CH: Renal function in patients with essential hypertension receiving nadolol. *Br Med J* 3:423–424, 1980.

188. Wallin JD: Antihypertensives and their impact on renal function. *Am J Med* 75(4A):103–108, 1983.

189. Walshe JJ, Venuto RC: Acute oliguric renal failure induced by indomethacin: possible mechanism. *Ann Intern Med* 91:47–49, 1979.

190. Watson AJ, Keogh, JAB: 1-Deamino-8-D-arginine vasopressin as a therapy for the bleeding diathesis of renal failure. *Am J Nephrol* 4:49–51, 1984.

191. Weber MA, Drazer JIM: Renal effect of beta-adrenoceptor blockade. *Kidney Int* 18:686–699, 1980.

192. Webster J: Interactions of NSAIDS with diuretics and beta-blockers: mechanisms and clinical implications. *Drugs* 30:32–41, 1985.

193. Weinberg MS, Quigg RJ, Salant DJ, Bernard DB: Anuric renal failure precipitated by indomethacin and triamterene. *Nephron* 40:216–218, 1985.

194. Weismann DN: Altered renal hemodynamic and urinary prostaglandin response to acute hypoxemia after inhibition of prostaglandin synthesis in the anesthetized dog. *Circ Res* 48:632–640, 1981.

195. Wilkinson R: β-blockers and renal function. *Drugs* 23:195–206, 1982.

196. Yokoyama S, Kaburagi T: Clinical effects of intravenous nifedipine on renal function. *J Cardiovasc Pharmacol* 5:67–71, 1983.

197. Zanchetti A, Leonetti G: Natriuretic effects of calcium antagonists. *J Cardiovasc Pharmacol* 7(suppl 4):S33–S37, 1985.

198. Zatz R, Dunn R, Meyer TW, Reenke HG, Brenner BM: Prevention of diabetic glomerulopathy by pharmacological amelioration of glomerular capillary hypertension. *J Clin Invest* 77:1925–1930, 1986.

199. Zipser RD, Hoefs JC, Speckart PF, Zia PK, Horton R: Prostaglandins: modulators of renal function and pressor resistance in chronic liver disease. *J Clin Endocrinol Metab* 48:895–900, 1979.

200. Zipser R, Myers S, Needleman P: Exaggerated prostaglandin and thromboxane synthesis in the rabbit with renal vein constriction. *Circ Res* 47:231–237, 1980.

201. Zsoter TT, Church JG, Calcium antagonist: pharmacodynamic effects and mechanisms of action. *Drugs* 25:93–112, 1983.

18

Pharmacologic Approach to Gastrointestinal Disease in Critical Illness

David A. Johnson, M.D., F.A.C.P., F.A.C.G.
Edward L. Cattau, Jr., M.D., F.A.C.P., F.A.C.G.

A broad spectrum of gastrointestinal diseases may be manifested in an intensive care unit (ICU). A bleeding peptic or variceal lesion may be the primary reason for a patient's admission to the ICU, or a secondary complication, for example hepatic insufficiency, stress ulceration, or bowel ischemia, may develop during the course of an ICU stay. A working knowledge of the pharmacokinetic properties of drugs used to treat such conditions, as well as the indications and complications implicit with their use, is paramount in maximizing the care afforded to these patients during an ICU stay. The goal of this chapter is to discuss the gastrointestinal medications that may be used by the intensive care physician and to focus on special considerations that may be of importance in select patients.

ANTACIDS

The numerous antacids available differ in chemical composition, neutralizing capacity (39, 52), cost effectiveness (39, 52), potential side effects (171), and palatability. The major mechanisms of action of these agents, how-

Table 18.1
Neutralizing Capacity, Sodium Content, and Cost Effectiveness of Liquid Antacids

Antacid	Acid Neutralizing Capacity (mEq/ml)	Volume Containing 140 mEq (ml)[a]	Sodium Content (mg/5 ml)	Comparative Monthly Cost of Therapy ($)	Composition
Maalox TC	4.2	33	1.2	44	Aluminum hydroxide, magnesium hydroxide
Titralac	4.2	33	11.0	35	Calcium carbonate, glycine
Delcid	4.1	34	1.5	57	Aluminum hydroxide, magnesium hydroxide
Mylanta-II	3.6	39	1.1	63	Aluminum hydroxide, magnesium hydroxide, simethicone
Camalox	3.2	44	2.5	55	Aluminum hydroxide, magnesium hydroxide, calcium carbonate
Gelusil-II	3.0	47	1.3	74	Aluminum hydroxide, magnesium hydroxide, simethicone
Basaljel ES	2.9	48	23.0	101	Aluminum carbonate
ALternaGEL	2.5	56	2.0	71	Aluminum hydroxide
Digel	2.5	56	8.5	51	Aluminum hydroxide, magnesium hydroxide
Mylanta	2.4	58	0.7	67	Aluminum hydroxide, magnesium hydroxide, simethicone
Maalox Plus	2.3	61	2.5	68	Aluminum hydroxide, magnesium hydroxide, simethicone
Gelusil	2.2	64	0.7	80	Aluminum hydroxide, magnesium hydroxide, simethicone
Riopan Plus	1.8	78	0.3	78	Magaldrate, simethicone
Amphojel	1.4	100	7.0	114	Aluminum hydroxide

[a] 140 mEq, seven times per day.

ever, are similar, with the reduction of hydrogen ion concentration by neutralization and reduction of pepsin activity. Antacids range in the strength of acid neutralization (Table 18.1) from the oxyaluminum compounds, which raise the gastric pH to 3–4, to magnesium hydroxide, which can raise the pH to 9.

Antacids suppress pepsin activity when given in sufficient quantity to elevate the pH of gastric contents above 2.3, and irreversibly inactivate the enzyme at a pH above 6.9 (144). Antacids, however, do not appear to have direct antipepsin activity (92, 125).

The most commonly used antacids include calcium carbonate, aluminum hydroxide, and magnesium hydroxide, either alone or in combination. Each compound has some unique physical and chemical properties. A common feature of antacids is that they all contain sodium, although the content varies (Table 18.1). Antacids also cause alkalinization of the urine, which can alter renal excretion of several drugs. The tubular reabsorption of drugs that are weak bases such as quinidine, procainamide, or ephedrine may be increased, resulting in higher serum levels. In contrast, the reabsorption of drugs that are weak acids such as salicylates, phenobarbitone, and sulfonamides may be less, increasing their urinary excretion and lowering serum levels (171). Antacids also have a potential for influencing the gut absorption of various drugs (Table 18.2).

Calcium-Containing Antacids

Calcium carbonate has a relatively rapid onset and prolonged duration of action. The amount of calcium absorbed is dependent on the amount of gastric acid. After a single 2-g dose, 0–2% is absorbed in achlorhydric patients, 9–16% in normal subjects, and 11–34% in patients with peptic ulcers (74). Moreover, the fraction of calcium absorbed is the same during chronic therapy with daily doses of 20 g. A dose-absorption curve is not available; however, the amount absorbed probably reaches a plateau at a single dose of 40–50 g (63). Although there is a transient rise in serum calcium after a single oral 4-g dose of calcium carbonate, chronic hypercalcemia does not develop with daily doses as high as 20 g in patients with normal renal function. In patients with azotemia, hypercalcemia can develop with doses as low as 3.4 g/day. Calcium excretion varies directly with the creatinine clearance, and less than 1–9% of the amount absorbed is excreted in normal subjects, even after weeks of therapy (28).

Aluminum-Containing Antacids

Commercial preparations of aluminum hydroxide have varying low efficacy, partly because of nonreactive bulk (H_2O and fixed CO_2),

Table 18.2
Effect of Antacids on Drug Absorption and Excretion

Drugs *not affected* by concomitant antacid administration:	Drugs with *decreased absorption* during antacid administration:	Drugs with *increased absorption* during antacid administration:
Carbenoxolone[a]	Ampicillin	Aspirin[b]
Cimetidine	Carbenoxolone[a]	Bishydroxycoumarin
Chlordiazepoxide	Chlorpromazine	Levodopa
Ethionamide	Digitoxin	Nalidixic acid
Fenoprofen	Digoxin	Naproxen[a]
Glucocorticoids[a]	Glucocorticoids[a]	Pseudoephedrine hydroxide
Naproxen[a]	Iron	Sulfadiazine acid[a]
Theophylline	Isoniazid	
Quinidine sulfate	Naproxen[a]	
Warfarin sodium	Oral contraceptives	
	Pentobarbital	
	Phenytoin	
	Quinine sulfate	
	Sulfadiazine sodium[a]	
	Tetracyclines	
	Tolbutamide	
	Vitamin A	

[a] Presence in more than one group indicates conflicting data.
[b] Simultaneous alterations that may result in decreased serum levels.

but also because of the formation of polymers that dissolve very slowly. Moreover, proteins, peptides, amino acids, and certain dietary organic acids impair the neutralizing capacity of this antacid (58). A study of the ingestion of four aluminum-containing compounds (aluminum hydroxide, carbonate, aminoacetate, and phosphate) by normal volunteers revealed a significant increase in urinary aluminum levels with three of the four compounds (no rise with aluminum phosphate) (81). In renal failure, administration of aluminum hydroxide can elevate serum aluminum to potentially dangerous levels (8). Excessive aluminum intake in patients with renal failure may contribute to the development of dialysis encephalopathy (2), myopathy, and an osteomalacia provoked by undetected hypophosphatemia and compensating skeletal demineralization (4). High doses of aluminum hydroxide, even without renal failure, can lead to a phosphorus depletion syndrome (98), particularly if low phosphate intake or malabsorption is present. Aluminum hydroxide may also produce constipation and fecal impaction, especially in elderly patients (68).

Magnesium-Containing Antacids

Although magnesium hydroxide is classified as a nonabsorbed antacid, 5–33% of magnesium is absorbed (39, 101) and can lead to hypermagnesemia and death in patients with renal insufficiency (63). Supersaturation of the urine with magnesium may predispose patients to nephrolithiasis. Additionally, siliceous nephrolithiasis may be seen with use of magnesium trisalicylate.

The pathogenesis of the cathartic effect of magnesium may be multifactorial. The primary cause is the formation of magnesium salts, which are delivered as an osmotic load to the bowel and stimulate both secretion and motility (174). Another possible factor is that magnesium is a weak stimulant of gallbladder contraction and pancreatic secretion, although the clinical significance of this stimulation is not defined (102).

HISTAMINE H₂-ANTAGONISTS

With the synthesis of Burimamide in 1972, Black and coworkers (9) demonstrated the existence of two classes of histamine receptors: H_1 and H_2. In contrast to the H_1 type, H_2-receptors are not antagonized by conventional antihistamines and are involved in the action of histamine on the gastric parietal cell. Metiamide was the first H_2-blocker used clinically, but it caused agranulocytosis. Cimetidine was the first H_2-blocker to receive widespread use. The subsequent introduction of ranitidine and more recently famotidine has given the clinician several options directed at gastric acid suppression.

Cimetidine has an imidazole ring as does histamine, but has a much less basic and longer side chain. Cimetidine has a cyanoguanidine group whereas metiamide, its forerunner, had a thiourea group. This structural difference may explain why cimetidine has not been associated with the same incidence of severe agranulocytosis seen with metiamide.

The H_2-receptors have been identified in many sites including the atrium, stomach, uterus, ileum, mesenteric and cutaneous vascular beds, bronchial musculature, parathyroid cells, adipocytes, and T suppressor cells (55). The clinical importance of H_2-receptor blockade in organs other than the stomach is not clearly defined.

Cimetidine

MECHANISM OF ACTION

Cimetidine, acting as a reversible competitive antagonist of the action of histamine on H_2-receptors, predictably inhibits histamine-stimulated acid secretion on parietal cells. The mechanism by which cimetidine inhibits the acid secretion promoted by the other two endogenous secretagogues (acetylcholine and gastrin) is less well understood. The previously held view that histamine is the "final common mediator" of acid secretion has largely been replaced with the current concept that the parietal cell has separate receptors for each of the secretagogues. The interaction of histamine with its receptors increases the affinity of the parietal cell for gastrin and acetylcholine and thereby potentiates their effects (156). Since cimetidine and anticholinergics inhibit acid secretion by different mechanisms, their effects are synergistic (46).

Cimetidine is a potent inhibitor of all phases of gastric secretion. Both basal and nocturnal basal acid secretion are reduced 90–95% by a 300-mg dose (6). Pepsin output is reduced by cimetidine in humans, probably as a result of decreased secretion of gastric juice (6). Cimetidine-induced reduction in stimulated (but not basal) intrinsic factor secretion has been demonstrated and is related to decreased gastric volume (6, 149). The effects of H_2-antagonists on gastric mucus secretion in humans is less clear, although it seems unlikely that mucus secretion is mediated by H_2-receptors.

Fasting serum gastrin levels are unaffected by cimetidine; however, postprandial levels are raised because of the reduction in acid feedback and inhibition of gastrin release (97). There have been no reports of a "rebound" increase in peak acid output following therapy. Cimetidine has no apparent action on gastric emptying (97) or bile acid composition or secretion (97, 115).

PHARMACOKINETICS

Cimetidine can be administered orally, intravenously, and intramuscularly. Food delays absorption of the drug, so peak serum levels are lower but the duration of effect is prolonged when given with meals. Parenterally administered cimetidine achieves higher peak drug levels than those obtained by oral administration; however, the clinically effective drug level is maintained for approximately 4 hours, similar to the time achieved with the oral route. Measurement of blood cimetidine levels is not clinically useful (49).

Approximately 15% of cimetidine is metabolized in the liver and most of the drug is excreted unchanged in the urine. Use of cimetidine in patients with liver disease is not contraindicated, but reduced dosages may be necessary with severe liver impairment. In renal failure drug accumulation may occur, and

Table 18.3
Cimetidine Dosage in Patients with Impaired Renal Function

Estimated Creatinine Clearance[a] (ml/min/1.73 m^2)	Appropriate Dosing Regimen
>40 (mild)	300 mg/6 hr
20–40 (moderate)	300 mg/8 hr
0–20 (severe)	300 mg/12 hr

[a]Estimated creatinine clearance is calculated as follows:

Males:

$$Cl_{cr} = \frac{140 - age}{serum\ creatinine} \times \frac{weight\ (kg)}{72}$$

Females:

$$Cl_{cr} = \frac{140 - age}{serum\ creatinine} \times \frac{weight\ (kg)}{72} \times 0.85$$

therefore the lowest frequency of dosing compatible with an adequate patient response should be used (Table 18.3). Hemodialysis lowers the level of circulating drug by at least 50% and the dosage schedule should be adjusted so that the timing of a scheduled dose coincides with the end of hemodialysis (99, 168). A dosage of 400 mg/day on nondialysis days and 800 mg/day on dialysis days has been used effectively in acute duodenal ulceration, with 200 mg/day continued thereafter as maintenance therapy (37). Insufficient amounts of cimetidine are removed during peritoneal dialysis to warrant a postdialysis supplemental dose (71, 169). With advancing age, plasma cimetidine half-life and the volume of distribution tend to increase so that even in the absence of severe renal failure, reducing standard doses of oral cimetidine by one-third to one-half appears justified (139).

Experience with gross overdosage of cimetidine is limited. In the few cases that have been reported in humans, doses up to 10 g have not been associated with any untoward effects (110). The usual measures should be taken to remove unabsorbed material from the gastrointestinal tract, in addition to clinical monitoring and supportive therapy. Studies in animals indicate that toxic doses are associated with respiratory failure and tachycardia, which may be controlled by assisted respiration and administration of a β-blocker (142).

Small amounts of cimetidine are excreted in bile and, with unabsorbed drug, excreted in the feces. The drug crosses the placental barrier, is excreted in milk, and is widely distributed in almost all tissues except the brain (38). The blood-brain barrier may become more permeable to cimetidine, however, in patients with severe medical illnesses, especially uremia (114).

DOSAGE AND INDICATIONS

Cimetidine is approved for use in the short-term treatment of active duodenal or benign gastric ulcer as well as the long-term prevention thereof. Effective oral dosage regimens include 300 mg four times daily, 400 mg twice daily, or 800 mg at bedtime. For use in pathologic hypersecretory conditions, such as Zollinger-Ellison syndrome, dosage and dosing interval may need to be adjusted but should not exceed 2400 mg/day. For parenteral administration, cimetidine may be given as a 300-mg dose every 6–8 hours intramuscularly or intravenously. It may also be delivered by a continuous intravenous infusion starting at 40–50 mg/hr and adjusted to maintain a desired target gastric pH.

SPECIAL CONSIDERATIONS

The effect of H_2-blockers on hepatic function and hepatic drug metabolism needs consideration. Contrary to previous impressions, cimetidine does not cause a fall in hepatic blood flow. Cimetidine does, however, affect type I biotransformation and reduces microsomal mixed function oxidase activity, so there is a potential effect on other drugs that are metabolized by the microsomal cytochrome P-450 enzyme system. For example, it is generally accepted that blood levels of warfarin and theophylline rise when either is given simultaneously with cimetidine. Reduction of the doses of these agents by approximately one-third is advised, along with regular monitoring of serum theophylline concentrations and prothrombin

time. Other drugs that should be reduced when cimetidine is administered, particularly in the elderly, are benzodiazepines such as diazepam and chlordiazepoxide, since cimetidine inhibits the N-demethylation of these drugs. In contrast, lorazepam and oxazepam have limited hepatic biotransformation (glucuronide conjugation) that is not influenced by cimetidine, and doses need not be altered. A complete list of H_2-receptor drug interactions is shown in Table 18.4 (147).

Cimetidine inhibits gastric acid secretion and causes an increase in the pH of the stomach and proximal small bowel. An increased pH could lead to differences in the rate and extent of absorption of drugs that are destroyed at a low pH or require low pH for disintegration or dissolution. The known effects of H_2-antagonists on absorption of several orally administered drugs are shown in Table 18.5.

Cimetidine has decreased effectiveness in

Table 18.4
Drug Interactions with Cimetidine and Ranitidine

Drug	Comments	References
Antiarrhythmics	Inhibition of procainamide and quinidine metabolism have been reported.	62, 157
Anticoagulants (oral)	Cimetidine competitively inhibits metabolism, and a marked increase in prothrombin time has been demonstrated.	118, 148, 153
Anticonvulsants	Increased serum phenytoin and carbamazepine levels have been reported when used with cimetidine.	5, 66, 163, 176
Benzodiazepines	Potentiated sedation by inhibited metabolism of those agents metabolized by glucuronidation. Reduction in dose not required for oxazepam, lorazepam, temazepam.	87, 120, 140
β-Blockers	Clearance of propranolol is reduced by cimetidine by inhibition of drug-metabolizing enzymes and reduced hepatic blood flow.	45, 65
Carmustine (BCNU)	Increased bone marrow toxicity has been reported with concomitant use.	143
Chlormethiazole	Cimetidine alters the disposition of drug and results in increased pharmacologic effect.	150
Lidocaine HCl	Cimetidine increases serum levels by reducing systemic clearance; 50% reduction in maintenance infusion recommended following standard loading dose.	53, 88
Narcotic analgesics	Cimetidine may enhance activity of morphine, meperidine, methadone, and fentanyl citrate.	51, 95
Nifedipine	Both cimetidine and ranitidine increase the hypotensive activity of this drug.	85
Theophylline	Cimetidine inhibits clearance; 50% reduction in dose of theophylline should be considered when given together.	24, 75, 129

Table 18.5
Effects of H$_2$-Antagonists on Absorption of Orally Administered Drugs

	References
Increased absorption	
Aspirin	82
Decreased absorption	
Ketoconazole	167
Insignificant or inconsistent effects on absorption	
Penicillin	44, 136, 146
Furosemide	137
Digoxin	80
Cotrimoxazole	136
Tetracycline	146

burn patients and possibly other surgical patients (78). Increased clearance of cimetidine has been demonstrated, the total clearance correlating with the size of the burn. Trauma and surgical patients may be pharmacologically different from nonsurgical patients because of inflammation-induced alterations in hemodynamic and organ functions. Increased renal and hepatic blood flow occur as part of the response to tissue trauma and injury (78). Dosage schedules may need to be altered in this patient population to compensate for the enhanced clearance of cimetidine.

Cimetidine is stable in parenteral nutrition fluids. It is effective when administered via continuous intravenous infusion rather than intermittent intravenous injection, and continuous infusion is considerably less expensive overall (35). Incompatibility with certain drugs has been described (Table 18.6), and administration via separate intravenous lines is suggested when cimetidine is to be given simultaneously with these drugs (141, 180).

SIDE EFFECTS

Numerous adverse reactions have been attributed to cimetidine (Table 18.7), which is understandable in view of the attention and scrutiny the drug has received, its widespread use, and its systemic effects. The reported frequency of side effects has differed considera-

Table 18.6
Cimetidine Hydrochloride Incompatibilities

Aerosporin
Aminophylline
Amphotericin B
Barbiturates
Cephalosporins
Garamycin
Fat emulsions

Table 18.7
Comparison of Reported Adverse Effects for Cimetidine and Ranitidine

Adverse Effect, by System	Cimetidine	Ranitidine
Central nervous system		
Malaise	+	+
Confusion	+	+
Insomnia	+	+
Agitation	+	+
Hallucinations	+	+
Depression	+	+
Cardiovascular		
Bradycardia	+	
Tachycardia	+	+
Ectopy	+	+
Dermatologic		
Rash	+	+
Alopecia	+	+
Endocrine		
Gynecomastia	+	
Reversible impotence	+	
Prolactin elevation	+	
Chylomicronemia	+	
Gastrointestinal		
Diarrhea	+	+
Constipation	+	+
Hepatitis	+	+
Pancreatitis	+	
General		
Fever	+	+
Hematopoietic		
Leukopenia	+	+
Pancytopenia	+	+
Thrombocytopenia	+	
Musculoskeletal		
Arthralgias	+	+
Myalgias	+	
Renal		
Elevation in creatinine	+	+
Interstitial nephritis	+	

bly but is low in all studies (109, 178). A worldwide reporting system showed the incidence of adverse effects to be as follows: 7.3/100,000 patients treated (1.1/100,000 with mental confusion); gastrointestinal-hepatobiliary system abnormalities, 4.8/100,000; skin and musculoskeletal disturbances, 3.1/100,000; abnormal hematologic findings, 2.3/100,000; and interstitial nephritis, <0.1/100,000 (54).

Symptoms of central nervous system (CNS) toxicity are among the commonest of cimetidine's unwanted effects. Cimetidine crosses the blood-brain barrier, and the CNS symptoms tend to be more frequent in elderly and very young patients, those receiving high dosages, and those with renal or hepatic disease. The effects on the CNS may be due to blockage of the H$_2$-receptors and consequent partial inhibition of the neurotransmitter properties of histamine (181). Cimetidine may also interfere with the function of endogenous enkephalins (22). Physostigmine reverses cimetidine-induced confusion (114), but experience with use of this drug is limited and it is recommended only in the presence of life-threatening CNS toxicity.

Pharmacologic studies in humans show that both the myocardium and peripheral blood vessels possess H_2-receptors (162). Stimulation of cardiac H_2-receptors causes positive chronotropic and inotropic responses. Stimulation of H_2-receptors in peripheral vessels causes vasodilation. The physiologic role of these receptors has not been established. Bolus injection of cimetidine in critically ill patients is associated with a decrease in blood pressure, particularly in patients requiring vasoconstrictor support (84). This hypotension is probably induced by arterial vasodilation. Cardiac dysrhythmias may occur with cimetidine use, although such reactions have not been reported after oral or slow intravenous administration in normal subjects (14, 15).

Cimetidine has a weak antiandrogen effect. Gynecomastia may be caused by blockade of androgen receptors that mediate the normal suppression of breast tissue (160). Serum prolactin levels do not rise after oral administration of cimetidine, but bolus intravenous administration results in dose-dependent prolactin elevations (32). Chylomicronemia has been described with cimetidine use in a patient with hypertriglyceridemia (3). The clinical picture included musculoskeletal pain, abdominal pain, and splenomegaly on two separate occasions during cimetidine administration. This potentially treacherous complication should be considered, therefore, when prescribing cimetidine for patients with known hyperlipidemia.

Mild, self-limited elevations in liver transaminases may occur with cimetidine, and hepatitis of the idiosyncratic or hypersensitivity type has been described. Cholestasis is rare, and hepatotoxicity with cimetidine is uncommon and appears to be reversible (54).

Fever is an infrequent idiosyncratic effect of cimetidine use. The onset of fever varies from 5 to 13 days, persists the entire course of treatment, and is gone within 12–72 hours after stopping the drug (3). Rechallenges lead to new onset of fever within 12–24 hours. The range of temperature reported is 38.5–39.5°C. Associated findings include malaise, night sweats, epigastric pain, and leukopenia.

The hematologic effects of cimetidine have been scrutinized in view of the profound effects of metiamide. Several cases of granulo-cytopenia, thrombocytopenia, and pancytopenia have been reported, but are rare (56). Bone marrow suppression appears to occur by a dose-dependent idiosyncratic mechanism.

Cimetidine may have immunologic effects by influencing a subclass of human thymic-dependent suppressor T lymphocytes that have H_2-receptors. Histamine stimulates these suppressor cells and may thereby serve a local immunoinhibitory role. Blockage of these receptors conceivably could interfere with this inhibitory function and result in augmented cell-mediated immune responses. Skin reactivity to common antigens improves with cimetidine therapy in patients with chronic mucocutaneous candidiasis and Crohn's disease. Remission of symptoms also occurred in some patients with herpes virus infections. Cimetidine does not, however, appear to influence the function of grafts or increase the number or severity of rejection episodes (79, 138).

Small increases in serum creatinine occur commonly during cimetidine therapy. The values rarely exceed 2 mg/dl, are not associated with changes in blood urea or urinalysis, and return rapidly to baseline values on discontinuance of the drug. These mild elevations in creatinine are not regarded as an adverse reaction and do not require discontinuance of therapy. Acute interstitial nephritis has been described and appears to be an idiosyncratic or hypersensitivity reaction. Clinical features include fever, malaise, mild eosinophilia, and decreased renal function developing after several weeks of cimetidine therapy (108).

Ranitidine

Ranitidine is an H_2-receptor antagonist that was released 6 years after cimetidine was introduced. In contrast to cimetidine, which contains the same imidazole ring found in histamine, ranitidine includes a furan ring, which is not chemically related to histamine and does not occur naturally in the human body. Studies with ranitidine indicate that it is 5–12 times as potent as cimetidine (on a molar basis) in inhibiting stimulated gastric acid secretion in humans (18).

PHARMACOKINETICS

The pharmacokinetic profile of ranitidine is similar to that of cimetidine. Neither product is inherently long-acting and they have similar half-lives of 2.0–3.0 hours. If equipotent doses of cimetidine and ranitidine are administered, the duration of action is essentially the same. The bioavailability of oral ranitidine is about 50%, compared with 70% for cimetidine (182). The bioavailability of ranitidine is influenced by hepatic function. The drug is taken up and metabolized by the liver by "first pass" kinetics. Up to 30% of the drug is metabolized by the liver to nitrogen oxide, sulfuric oxide, and demethyl derivatives, and at least 50% is excreted by the kidney unchanged (18). When given orally, ranitidine is rapidly absorbed from the gastrointestinal tract, and absorption is not influenced by food ingestion.

DOSAGE AND INDICATIONS

Ranitidine has essentially the same indications as cimetidine. Oral dosage schedules for active peptic ulcer disease include 150 mg twice daily or 300 mg at bedtime. Ranitidine is very rapidly absorbed after intramuscular injection, with bioavailability of 90–100% compared with intravenous administration. The dosage for intramuscular or intravenous delivery is 50 mg every 8 hours, and the drug may also be given as a continuous infusion starting at 150 mg/day with dosage adjusted as required to attain the desired target gastric pH. When given as an intravenous bolus, the volume should be injected over a period of not less than 5 minutes.

OVERDOSAGE

There is no experience to date with deliberate overdosage. As with cimetidine, the usual measures to remove unabsorbed material from the gastrointestinal tract should be employed. Studies in dogs receiving ranitidine in excess of 225 mg/kg/day have shown muscular tremors, vomiting, and rapid respiration. Single oral doses of 1000 mg/kg in mice and rats were not lethal; intravenous LD_{50} values were 83 mg/kg and 77 mg/kg, respectively (124).

SPECIAL CONSIDERATIONS

The drug interaction potential for ranitidine was initially thought to be considerably less than for cimetidine, since ranitidine has a lesser effect on cytochrome P-450–mediated drug metabolism. As experience using ranitidine increases, more drug interactions have been defined. There are reports of interactions between ranitidine and warfarin (133), benzodi-

azepine (41), fentanyl (95), metoprolol (159), nifedipine (18), acetaminophen (133), and theophylline (48). Interaction with acetaminophen is particularly significant in view of hepatic dependence on glutathione for detoxification of acetaminophen, and suggests that ranitidine, like other furans, may have finite glutathione requirements for safe elimination and freedom from hepatotoxicity. Some drug interactions may also develop from the ability of ranitidine, like cimetidine, to reduce hepatic blood flow by 20–40%. As with cimetidine, strong antacids may reduce absorption of ranitidine.

In geriatric patients, the half-life of ranitidine is prolonged by about 50%, presumably as a result of a decrease in the glomerular filtration rate (68). The bioavailability of ranitidine in patients with liver disease is increased, and the serum half-life is slightly prolonged because of decreased hepatic metabolism and a slight reduction in glomerular filtration rate (179). It is probably not necessary to change the usual therapeutic dose in patients with mild hepatic disease, although caution should be observed in all patients with hepatic dysfunction. In patients with serious renal disease, therapeutic levels can be obtained with lower doses. The recommended dose in patients with a creatinine clearance below 50 ml/min is 50 mg every 18–24 hours. Should the patient's condition require, the frequency of dosing may be increased with caution. Hemodialysis reduces the level of circulating ranitidine. Ideally, the dosage schedule should be adjusted so that the timing of a scheduled dose coincides with the end of hemodialysis.

SIDE EFFECTS

Initially, ranitidine was thought to have fewer side effects than cimetidine; however, more reports are continually being generated as the experience with ranitidine increases. Unlike cimetidine, ranitidine binds minimally if at all to androgen receptors, the hepatic mixed function oxidase system, and peripheral lymphocytes (182). It once was believed that ranitidine, less lipophilic than cimetidine, would not enter the cerebrospinal fluid or cause the neurologic problems occasionally seen with cimetidine. However, ranitidine does enter the cerebrospinal fluid, and the lesser lipophilicity is offset by greater potency in the CNS. An overview of the side effects for both cimetidine and ranitidine is shown in Table 18.7.

Famotidine

Famotidine, another H_2-receptor antagonist drug, was released for clinical use in late 1986. As a result, the clinical data that come from widespread use are limited. Famotidine is a guanidinathiazole derivative containing neither the imidazole ring of cimetidine nor the furan ring of ranitidine. It acts as a reversible competitive H_2-receptor inhibitor, with an antisecretory potency in animal studies that is 30–100 times greater than that of cimetidine and 6–10 times greater than that of ranitidine (27).

PHARMACOKINETICS

Famotidine is incompletely absorbed, with bioavailability of 40–45% for orally administered dosages. There is a minimal first pass metabolism. Drug elimination is 65–70% renal and 30–35% metabolic (155).

DOSAGE AND INDICATIONS

Famotidine is likely to have the same indications as cimetidine and ranitidine, although at the time of its release, famotidine was indicated only for the short-term treatment of active duodenal ulcers, maintenance therapy for healed duodenal ulcers, and treatment of pathologic hypersecretory conditions, e.g., Zollinger-Ellison syndrome. The adult oral dosage is 40 mg at bedtime or 20 mg twice daily. The starting dose for hypersecretory conditions is 20 mg orally every 6 hours, with doses up to 160 mg every 6 hours having been administered to some patients with severe Zollinger-Ellison syndrome (69, 170).

OVERDOSAGE

There are no reported cases of deliberate overdosage, but the approach to treatment would be similar to that for cimetidine and ranitidine overdose. The oral LD_{50} of famotidine in rats and dogs is 3000 mg/kg and 2000 mg/kg, respectively (40).

SPECIAL CONSIDERATIONS

In patients with severe renal insufficiency (creatinine clearance <10 ml/min), the half-life of famotidine exceeds 20 hours and is approximately 24 hours if the patient is anuric. The dose should be reduced to 20 mg at bedtime or the dosing interval prolonged to 36–48 hours as indicated by the patient's clinical response (27). No drug interactions have yet been defined in controlled studies. Specific clinical interaction studies have shown no interference with compounds metabolized by hepatic microsomal enzyme processes, including diazepam, phenytoin, theophylline, and warfarin (155). In elderly patients, there are no clinically important age-related changes in pharmacokinetics.

SIDE EFFECTS

As was learned with ranitidine, the true incidence of side effects is not known until after several years of widespread clinical use. In the controlled trials to date, the reported side effects of famotidine include headache (4.7%), dizziness (1.3%), constipation (1.2%), and diarrhea (1.7%) (23, 40, 155). Other adverse reactions may be defined as drug exposure increases. Safety studies conducted in healthy volunteers have shown no famotidine-induced actions on the cardiovascular, endocrine, or renal systems (23).

OTHER DRUGS USED IN SUPPRESSION OF GASTRIC ACID SECRETION AND ULCER HEALING

Omeprazole

Omeprazole (5-methoxy-2-[4-methoxy-(3,5-dimethyl-2-pyridinyl)-methyl]-sulfinyl-1h-benzimidazole) is a substituted benzimidazole and a potent inhibitor of gastric acid secretion. This class of drugs is new and currently undergoing phase trials for clinical use in the United States. The agents act by selective noncompetitive inhibition of the hydrogen-potassium ATPase enzyme in the parietal cell. This action interferes with the hydrogen-potassium ATPase proton pump (the final common pathway of gastric acid secretion) and therefore abolishes all responses to all types of stimulation (172).

PHARMACOKINETICS

Omeprazole is a weak base ($pK_a = 4$) that is absorbed from the small bowel at an alkaline pH. In the parietal cell, the drug is trapped in the acid secretory canaliculus. The acid environment allows formation of a sulfoxide metabolite that binds to hydrogen-potassium

ATPase, irreversibly inactivating the enzyme and thereby inhibiting gastric acid secretion. Plasma concentrations of drug do not correlate with gastric acid inhibition because the drug irreversibly inactivates hydrogen-potassium ATPase with single-dose inhibition of secretion for up to 3 days (60 hours after the drug is cleared from the circulation) The bioavailability of oral omeprazole increases with repeated doses because absorption improves as gastric pH increases. After 7 days of treatment with 30 or 60 mg daily, there is almost 100% inhibition of basal and stimulated acid secretion (70).

DOSAGE AND INDICATIONS

Neither dosage nor indications for omeprazole have yet been established in the United States. With oral dosages in the range of 20–40 mg/day, omeprazole does appear to heal ulcers more rapidly than H_2-receptor antagonists. In addition, at 4 weeks following therapy more patients appear to have ulcer healing with omeprazole (94). For gastric ulcers, in limited trials omeprazole appears to be as effective as H_2-receptor blockers (29). Omeprazole is highly effective in treating patients with Zollinger-Ellison syndrome for prolonged periods (105).

SPECIAL CONSIDERATIONS

The dramatic effects of omeprazole in the suppression of gastric acid secretion have caused some concern about its long-term use. Of most concern is the possible relationship between omeprazole-induced achlorhydria, elevated serum gastrin concentrations, and gastric carcinoid tumors in rats (42). In humans, the treatment of duodenal and gastric ulcer patients for several weeks produces modest reversible elevations in serum gastrin concentrations. No changes in the number of gastric endocrine cells have been noted. Serum gastrin concentrations and endocrine cell numbers in the gastric mucosa of Zollinger-Ellison syndrome patients apparently do not change following treatment with omeprazole. Further concern has been raised about the long-term use of omeprazole and the development of bacterial overgrowth. To date, however, there have been no reports of illness related to bacterial overgrowth in patients treated with omeprazole for weeks or years. Omeprazole also inhibits drug metabolism by the hepatic microsomal P-450 monooxygenase system (61). Dosage adjustment of such drugs should be considered if omeprazole is used concomitantly.

Sucralfate

Sucralfate is a nonabsorbable salt of sucrose octasulfate and aluminum hydroxide that is effective in gastroduodenal ulcer healing (128). When the drug reaches the acidic environment (pH <3–4) of the stomach, some aluminum hydroxide dissociates from sucrose octasulfate molecules and the residual compound becomes negatively charged. Polymerization of the sucrose octasulfate molecule occurs and simultaneously, a paste-like substance is formed, which is the active form of sucralfate. This paste-like material binds to necrotic ulcer tissue in both the stomach and duodenum. The mechanism for this attachment is, in part, related to the binding of negatively charged sucralfate molecules to positively charged proteins such as albumin, fibrinogen, damaged mucosal cells, and dead leukocytes in the ulcer base (135).

There are two possible mechanisms to explain sucralfate's effectiveness in promoting ulcer healing. First, the adherent complex that sucralfate forms with protein at the ulcer site acts as an effective barrier against acid, pepsin, and bile (117). Second, since large doses of sucralfate increase prostaglandin release into gastric juice in rats, a cytoprotective effect may be due to prostaglandin release (67). It has also been suggested that the gastric protection afforded by sucralfate is related to a prostaglandin-independent increase in mucus production (151). Sucralfate has minimal acid-neutralizing capability and in vitro studies indicate that it absorbs bile acids (117).

PHARMACOKINETICS

Sucralfate is only minimally absorbed from the gastrointestinal tract. The small amounts of the sulfated disaccharide that are absorbed are excreted primarily in the urine.

DOSAGE AND INDICATIONS

The recommended adult oral dosage of sucralfate, when used for treatment of duodenal ulcer, is 1 g four times a day on an empty stomach. Alternatively, a dose of 2 g twice a day appears to be equally effective in the short-term treatment of duodenal ulcer (17). The tablet may be dissolved in 15–30 ml of water or 5–15 ml of glycerol, although the clinical efficacy of this dosing form has not been well studied. Although currently approved only for use in duodenal ulcer disease, this drug may also be effective in gastric ulcer, esophageal sclerotherapy–induced ulcers, and esophagitis, and for mucosal damage due to nonsteroidal antiinflammatory drugs (20).

SPECIAL CONSIDERATIONS

Although sucralfate appears to be most effective at low pH, prior administration of cimetidine had little effect on binding of sucralfate to ulcer tissue in rats. Despite this finding, if both drugs are to be used concomitantly, we recommend staggering the dosing intervals so that the sucralfate is given 60 minutes before the cimetidine. Animal studies have shown that simultaneous administration of sucralfate with tetracycline, phenytoin, digoxin, or cimetidine results in a statistically significant reduction in the bioavailability of these agents. This reduction may be prevented by separating the administration of these agents and sucralfate by 2 hours. The interaction appears to be nonsystemic and presumably results from sucralfate binding of these agents within the gastrointestinal tract. The clinical importance of these animal studies is unknown at present, but separate administration of sucralfate and these other agents is recommended when alterations in bioavailability are thought to be critical for the concomitantly administered drugs. Although sucralfate is only minimally absorbed from the gastrointestinal tract, it seems prudent to monitor for signs of aluminum toxicity when the drug is to be administered chronically to dialysis patients with end-stage renal disease. Concomitant dosing with antacids may be prescribed as needed for relief of pain, but should not be taken within one-half hour before or after sucralfate since it may impede sucralfate tissue binding.

SIDE EFFECTS

Because of minimal absorption, side effects are rare. Constipation is the most common (2.3%), followed by oral dryness (0.7%) and dizziness (0.4%) (73). There is no experience with overdosage in humans. Animal data with dosings of up to 12 mg/kg have not shown a lethal effect.

Prostaglandins

Prostaglandins (particularly those of the E and I series) exert pronounced effects on various functions of the digestive system. In the stomach, these agents stimulate bicarbonate secretion and also have antisecretory, antiulcer, and cytoprotective effects (90).

Several prostaglandins of the E type are being evaluated for the treatment of gastric and duodenal ulcer and gastroduodenal side effects of nonsteroidal antiinflammatory drugs, and for the management of upper gastrointestinal bleeding (16, 89). The release of these agents in the United States has been prevented because of concern over the uterotonic effects of certain prostaglandins and the possible abortive sequelae in child-bearing females. Diarrhea is another common side effect, but appears to be less if lower doses are used. The role of prostaglandins in the treatment of gastrointestinal disease may be limited in the United States if approval by the Food and Drug Administration is not granted.

PROKINETIC AGENTS

Metoclopramide

Metoclopramide is a methoxychlorinated derivative of procainamide and a dopamine antagonist. This drug has a prokinetic effect, most effective in the upper gastrointestinal tract. It has little, if any, effect on the gallbladder or colon. The esophagogastric effects of this drug include increases in acid clearance, esophageal peristaltic amplitude, lower esophageal sphincter pressure, gastric emptying, and gastric contraction rate and amplitude (1, 145). In the small bowel, metoclopramide induces the equivalent of a migrating motor complex, inasmuch as the increase in gastric motility that it induces extends into the duodenum and small bowel.

PHARMACOKINETICS

Metoclopramide is well absorbed when given orally, with an onset of action of 30–60 minutes and duration of pharmacologic effect of 1–2 hours. The onset of action following an intravenous dose is 1–3 minutes and following an intramuscular dose is 10–15 minutes (145). Approximately 85% of a radioactive dose appears in the urine within 72 hours, with approximately one-half present as free or unconjugated metoclopramide.

DOSAGE AND INDICATIONS

Metoclopramide may be administered in doses of 10–15 mg before meals and at bedtime. If symptoms occur intermittently or at specific times, the use of metoclopramide in doses of 20 mg may be preferred. Caution should be observed in using doses in excess of 40 mg/day, although larger doses have been used by oncologists in treating nausea and vomiting associated with emetogenic cancer chemotherapy.

The gastrointestinal uses of this drug include treatment of gastroesophageal reflux, diabetic gastroparesis, slowed gastric emptying after gastric resection, gastroparesis, and idiopathic gastric stasis (106). In patients with postoperative ileus, metoclopramide improves nausea and vomiting and abdominal pain, and facilitates return of bowel sounds and passage of flatus and stools. As mentioned above, the effects in the colon are less than those in the upper gastrointestinal system, and although metoclopramide may be helpful in some patients with colonic hypomotility, clinical evidence is lacking.

SPECIAL CONSIDERATIONS

The effects of metoclopramide on gastrointestinal motility are antagonized by anticholinergic drugs and narcotic analgesics. Additive sedative effects can occur when given with alcohol, sedatives, hypnotics, narcotics, or tranquilizers. Absorption of certain drugs from the stomach may be diminished (e.g., digoxin) by metoclopramide, whereas absorption of other drugs from the small bowel may be accelerated (e.g., acetaminophen, tetracycline, levodopa, ethanol). Diabetic gastroparesis may be responsible for poor glucose control in some patients, since administered insulin may begin to act before food has left the stomach, leading to hypoglycemia. Adjustment of insulin dosages may be necessary, therefore, if gastric stasis improves with the use of metoclopramide. Dosages in children, elderly patients, and those with renal failure must be carefully monitored. Metoclopramide elevates serum prolactin levels in all patients, some of whom may develop associated breast enlargement, nipple tenderness, galactorrhea, or menstrual irregularity. Metoclopramide is incompatible with the following intravenous admixtures: ce-

phalothin sodium, chloramphenicol sodium, and sodium bicarbonate (123). Contraindications to the use of metoclopramide include use whenever stimulation of gastrointestinal motility might be dangerous, as in the presence of mechanical obstruction or perforation. Metoclopramide is contraindicated in patients with pheochromocytoma because the drug may cause a hypertensive crisis, probably due to release of catecholamines from the tumor. Phentolamine may be used to control such crises if they occur (123). Metoclopramide should also not be used in epileptics or patients receiving other drugs that are likely to cause extrapyramidal reactions, since the frequency and severity of seizures or extrapyramidal reactions may be increased.

SIDE EFFECTS

The incidence of side effects due to metoclopramide is approximately 20% (145). The main problems are drowsiness, restlessness, and anxiety. Dry mouth, depression, lightheadedness, constipation, and diarrhea are less commonly reported. Extrapyramidal reactions such as oculogyric crises, opisthotonos, trismus, and torticollis occur in about 1% of patients. Rarely, dystonic reactions may present as stupor and dyspnea. These effects can be reversed with intramuscular administration of 50 mg of diphenhydramine hydrochloride and discontinuance of the drug.

Domperidone

Domperidone is another prokinetic agent currently in clinical trials in the United States. This drug is a specific dopamine antagonist that stimulates the gastrointestinal tract and has antiemetic properties, but does not cross the blood-brain barrier and rarely causes extrapyramidal side effects (57).

PHARMACOKINETICS

Peak plasma concentrations of domperidone are attained 10–30 minutes after intramuscular and oral administration, and 1–2 hours after rectal administration of suppositories. The bioavailability of intramuscular domperidone is 90%, whereas that of oral domperidone is 13–17% because of "first pass" hepatic and gut wall metabolism. The elimination half-life of domperidone is 7.5 hours in healthy subjects, but can be prolonged up to 20.8 hours in patients with severe hepatic insufficiency.

DOSAGE AND INDICATIONS

Dosage recommendations have not been established pending completion of clinical trials. Daily dosage regimens have ranged from 40 to 120 mg/day in divided doses. The drug has some promise for treatment of gastroesophageal reflux and gastric stasis. High concentrations of the drug are found in the esophagus, stomach, and small intestine. Domperidone probably has minimal effect on colonic motility.

SIDE EFFECTS

Domperidone is well tolerated and seldom causes important side effects. It has a potent effect in stimulating prolactin secretion. Other reported side effects include dry mouth, pruritus, headache, diarrhea, and nervousness. Extrapyramidal and true dystonic reactions are rare, and CNS effects have not been reported.

Cisapride

Cisapride is a new prokinetic agent currently under clinical investigation in both the United States and Europe. This agent is thought to facilitate acetylcholine release at the myenteric plexus without affecting the secretory gland level. In vitro, it stimulates ileal contractility, increases gastric tonic and phasic motility, and furthers antroduodenal coordination. In vivo, it stimulates digestive and interdigestive antroduodenal motility and improves gastric emptying. Animal data support a prokinetic effect on the esophagus, stomach, small bowel, and colon (106) Unlike metoclopramide and domperidone, cisapride has no dopamine antagonist properties.

PHARMACOKINETICS

In humans, the plasma level of cisapride decays triexponentially with a half-life of 19.4 hours after intravenous administration. The bioavailability after oral administration is in the range of 35–40%. Plasma levels after oral administration of a 10-mg tablet peak at 1.5–2.0 hours (106).

DOSAGE AND INDICATIONS

Dosage recommendations are not established pending completion of clinical trials. In humans, cisapride in doses of 2, 4, and 8 mg intravenously and 4, 10, and 16 mg orally increase gastric emptying, antral peristalsis, lower esophageal sphincter pressure, small bowel transit, and colonic transit (106, 107). Preliminary reports suggest that cisapride may be useful in patients with idiopathic gastric stasis, gastroparesis diabeticorum, and intestinal pseudoobstruction (47, 106). This agent appears to have the most pronounced colonic effect of the prokinetic agents studied to date and also holds special promise for use in patients with colonic ileus and idiopathic constipation.

ANTIDIARRHEAL AGENTS

Several agents may be used in the ICU for management of diarrhea. There are no absolute dosage recommendations for any one of these agents and dosages should be titrated to effect in each patient. Bismuth subsalicylate is commonly used as an over-the-counter treatment for diarrhea for adults; 2 tablespoons every ½–1 hours can be given (not to exceed eight doses a day). Signs of salicylism may be noted. Caution is advised when administering to patients taking medication for anticoagulation, diabetes, or gout. Opiates such as codeine (15–60 mg up to every 4 hours) or belladonna tincture (0.3–1.0 ml up to every 8 hours) are frequently used for treatment of diarrhea. The pharmacokinetics of opiates are altered with age, resulting in increased plasma levels in the older patient. Loperamide hydrochloride is a long-acting antidiarrheal agent given as a 4-mg dose initially, followed by a 2-mg dose after each unformed stool, not to exceed a maximum dose of 16 mg/day. It is relatively devoid of central effects and no specific side effects have been reported in the elderly. Diphenoxylate hydrochloride with a small amount of atropine is also commonly used for treatment of diarrhea. It is extensively metabolized before it is excreted, mostly in bile. The drug is chemically similar to meperidine and thus may potentiate the actions of barbiturates, tranquilizers, and alcohol. Respiratory depression can occur when excessive doses are administered, and concomitant administration of monoamine oxidase inhibitors are contraindicated. The adult dosage recommended is 2.5–5.0 mg, three to four times per day.

α-Adrenergic agonists stimulate sodium and chloride absorption in the intestine and the use of such agents may therefore have a potent antidiarrheal effect. Ion transport in the intestine is mediated by an α_2-adrenergic receptor.

Clonidine, a widely prescribed antihypertensive medication, is a specific α_2-adrenergic agonist. Both clonidine and lidamine, a structurally similar analogue, can stimulate water and electrolyte absorption and thereby inhibit diarrhea (104).These medications, however, have prominent cardiovascular and central nervous system effects. At present, they probably should be used to control diarrhea only in patients unresponsive to conventional treatment or unable to use opiate compounds.

Somatostatin is a 14-amino acid peptide found in the D cell, one of the endocrine cells of the gut. It stimulates water and electrolyte absorption in the intestine and inhibits diarrhea in patients with carcinoid tumors and short bowel syndrome. A synthetic analogue has been recently developed for use in controlling diarrhea in patients with carcinoid syndrome (93).

LAXATIVES

Successful management of constipation requires knowledge of normal bowel physiology, conditions with which constipation is associated, and potential complications. Table 18.8 shows some of the agents and conditions with which constipation is associated. Laxatives should be used in critically ill patients only after the differential diagnostic concerns have been fully considered.

Osmotic or Saline Laxatives

Osmotic or saline laxatives contain slowly absorbable or nonabsorbable salts, especially magnesium. These salts are hyperosmotic, drawing water into the lumen of the small intestine and causing a large quantity of fluid to enter the ascending colon producing a fluid overload with loose, easily passed stools. The most widely used saline laxative is magnesium hydroxide (milk of magnesia). Dosages of 1–2 tablespoons/day are usually effective. Magnesium citrate is useful, usually in doses of 5–10 oz/day. Care must be taken when giving magnesium salts to patients with renal insufficiency (hypermagnesemia may result) and when giving sodium salts to those with congestive heart failure.

Lactulose is an especially effective laxative. It is a carbohydrate that is not digested and therefore serves as an osmotic load, stimulating water secretion in the bowel. Lactulose

Table 18.8
Drugs and Abnormalities Associated with Constipation

Drugs
  Aluminum-containing antacids
  Anticholinergics
  Barium sulfate
  Calcium channel blockers (especially verapamil)
  Cholestyramine
  Chronic laxative abuse
  Chronic lead exposure
  Opiates
  Phenothiazines
  Tricyclic antidepressants
  Vincristine
Mechanical obstruction
Metabolic abnormalities
  Diabetes mellitus
  Hypercalcemia
  Hypothyroidism
  Porphyria
Muscular or connective tissue disorders
  Myotonic dystrophy
  Primary muscle abnormalities
  Scleroderma
Neurologic abnormalities
  Autonomic neuropathy
  Multiple sclerosis
  Parkinson's disease
  Spinal cord abnormalities
  Tabes dorsalis
Rectal disorders
  Anal fissures
  Hemorrhoids
  Ulcerative proctitis

syrup can be given in a dosage of 15–30 ml/day as needed, with increasing dosages of up to 60 ml/day.

Other Laxative Agents

Osmotic or stimulant laxatives include cascara sagrada, senna, bisacodyl, phenolphthalein, and castor oil. Suppositories, e.g. glycerol, act directly on the rectal mucosa to stimulate peristalsis. Small-dose (4-oz) phosphate solution enemas may be used, although serum phosphate may rise with repeated usage. Tap water enemas may be used with lukewarm water without soap. The volume should be less than 500 ml (16 oz). Several instances of soapsud-colitis have been reported (86). An electrolyte-polyethylene glycol solution (Colyte; GoLYTELY) used for preparation for colonoscopy or barium enema (43) can be used in constipated patients as long as there is no evidence of obstruction.

Table 18.9
Drugs Used for Pharmacologic Therapy of Portal Hypertension

Vasoconstrictors
  Vasopressin
  Somatostatin
  β-Adrenergic blockers
    Nonselective
    Selective
Vasodilators
  Nitroglycerin
  Isosorbide dinitrate
  Prazosin
  Sodium nitroprusside
  Clonidine
  Ketanserin
  Calcium channel blockers
Miscellaneous
  Pentagastrin
  Domperidone
  Metoclopramide

DRUGS FOR THE TREATMENT OF PORTAL HYPERTENSION

Pharmacologic efforts to treat portal hypertension are directed toward reducing the increased blood flow in the portal collateral system and reducing the increased intrahepatic resistance, thereby reducing variceal pressure (127, 134). Vasoconstrictors reduce splanchnic blood flow and therefore portal flow. Vasodilators dilate the intrahepatic vasculature, reducing vascular resistance to portal blood flow. Additionally, there are other drugs that reduce the blood flow or pressure in the gastroesophageal-variceal system by mechanisms other than active vasoconstriction or vasodilation (Table 18.9).

Vasoconstrictors

VASOPRESSIN

Vasopressin is a peptide produced by the posterior pituitary gland. When infused at pharmacologic doses, it causes splanchnic vasoconstriction with a consequent reduction in portal blood flow and portal pressure. Vasopressin may be given intraarterially as well as by intravenous infusion. Since the intraarterial administration requires special skills and facilities and superimposes complications related to catheterization and the maintenance of catheter position, continuous intravenous infusion is the route of choice with portal hypertensive bleeding.

Vasopressin infusion should be begun at a dose of 0.2–0.4 U/min intravenously. Dosages of up to 1.0 U/min are sometimes necessary to control bleeding, but this dose significantly increases the risk of toxicity. Tapering of the dose before discontinuation appears to be unnecessary because vasopressin does not prevent rebleed from varices.

The list of potential adverse effects of vasopressin is lengthy (127, 134). Vasopressin produces increased gut motility, presumably by stimulation of smooth muscle, with attendant abdominal cramps and occasionally diarrhea. The vasoconstrictive effects may result in bowel ischemia and necrosis. An increase in cardiac afterload, baroreceptor-mediated bradycardia, decreased coronary blood flow, and direct impairment of cardiac contractibility are responsible for the decreased cardiac output and myocardial performance observed with this agent (183). Severe arrhythmias and myocardial infarction may occur with the use of vasopressin in humans; therefore, close supervision and cardiac monitoring are advised during infusion. The drug is contraindicated in patients with known coronary artery disease and should be used cautiously in alcoholics who may have a subclinical cardiomyopathy. Vasopressin has also been associated with respiratory arrest and cerebral hemorrhage. Nonhemodynamic effects of vasopressin include antidiuresis and stimulation of endothelial release of plasminogen activator and factor VIII (25). Administration of vasopressin to nonbleeding patients with cirrhosis is not, however, associated with chemical evidence of fibrinolysis (132).

β-ADRENERGIC BLOCKADE

Propranolol, a universal β-blocker, reduces portal pressure both acutely and chronically when administered to patients with portal hypertension. The mechanism of effect seems to be via a reduction in splanchnic blood flow. This action is the result of both a reduction in cardiac output (β_1-blockade) and splanchnic vasoconstriction, the latter probably due to β_2-blockade with unopposed α-adrenergic–mediated constrictive effects on splanchnic blood flow in humans (e.g., 29% reduction) (130). The principal application of propranolol therapy has been in the prevention of variceal bleeding, although the results of clinical studies are mixed and further controlled studies are required to define the place of propranolol in prevention of variceal bleeding (30).

SOMATOSTATIN

The hormone somatostatin reduces splanchnic blood flow, although the mechanism is unclear. In cirrhotic patients, hepatic blood flow decreases progressively with somatostatin infusion rates of 2.5 and 7.5 μg/min, but there is no further decrease with larger doses. The effect on portal pressure in cirrhotic patients is controversial (158). In contrast to vasopressin, somatostatin has minimal systemic effects at the dose used.

Vasodilators

Nitrates by themselves are mild portal hypotensive agents. Portal blood flow actually rises rather than falls in response to these vasodilators. Portal pressure is presumably reduced because the fall in portal inflow pressure, secondary to systemic vasodilation, is greater than the fall in hepatic vein pressure. Direct dilation of the portal vein is another possible mechanism of action. Oral, transdermal, and intravenous administration of nitrates reduces portal pressure. The primary use of nitrates at present appears to be in conjunction with vasopressin. Nitroglycerin reverses the cardiotoxic effects of vasopressin. It enhances the portal hypotensive effects by reducing the increase in portal venous resistance induced by vasopressin. Hemodynamic studies supported the favorable results observed in clinical trials (60, 166).

The effects of several other vasodilators on portal pressure have been studied. Prazosin, an α-adrenergic blocker, at a dose of 5 mg twice a day produced a sustained decline of 17% in portal pressure without a mean change in arterial pressure or cardiac output (113). Clonidine, a centrally acting α-adrenergic agonist, has been evaluated in one report in which intravenously administered clonidine (2.5 mg/kg) lowered the hepatic venous pressure gradient by 25% (177). Ketanserin, a selective 5-hydroxytryptamine–blocking agent, reduces portal pressure in animals, suggesting a specific role for serotonin in the maintenance of portal hypertension (33). The effects of all of these agents require clinical confirmation, and their use in portal hypertension remains investigational.

Miscellaneous Agents

Several agents selectively increase lower esophageal sphincter pressure and contract the esophageal musculature and decrease blood flow through the esophageal vessels, supposedly by compression of collateral vessels feeding the varices. Agents such as pentagastrin, domperidone, and metoclopramide may have a future role in the medical therapy of portal hypertension (103).

Sclerosant Solutions

Injection sclerotherapy has become a first-line treatment modality for bleeding varices of the esophagus in many patients. A brief review of the pharmacology of the different sclerosing agents is included here. A common denominator among sclerosing agents is their ability to induce an inflammatory reaction within or outside the vascular endothelium, resulting in a fibrotic, varicopenic esophagus. The amount of sclerosant injected into each varix is approximately 1–2 ml with an average total of 15–25 ml used per session. The most commonly used variceal sclerosing agents in the United States are sodium morrhuate and sodium tetradecyl sulfate.

Sodium morrhuate is a mixture of sodium salts of cod liver oil. Preparation may be nonuniform, and allergic reactions ranging from rash to anaphylaxis may be seen. Fever, chest pain, pleural effusion, and deep postsclerosis ulceration are more common than with sodium tetradecyl sulfate. Acute respiratory distress syndrome has been reported in two patients within 24 hours of sclerotherapy with sodium morrhuate (116). A more recent study, however, has shown that only 20% of injected sodium morrhuate reaches the pulmonary circulation and as a result, pulmonary endothelium is exposed to only small amounts of this agent with no change in diffusing capacity (31).

Sodium tetradecyl sulfate is a synthetic anion detergent. The surface activity of the fatty acid anions of the soap is thought to be responsible for the physical properties leading to variceal thrombosis. The effect of long-term esophageal variceal sclerotherapy using this agent have recently been evaluated; no serious long-term or short-term impairment of lung function was noted (91). Sodium tetradecyl sulfate is commercially available in 1% and 3% solutions.

Ethanolamine oleate, although not commercially available in the United States, is a widely used effective sclerosing agent. It is derived from oleic acid and is similar in physical properties to sodium morrhuate—in fact, sodium oleate is one of the chief constituents of the fatty acids in sodium morrhuate. Ethanolamine produces rare allergic reactions and has resulted in one such death. Data at present do not appear to give this drug clear advantage in either safety or efficacy over other sclerosants available in the United States.

Polidocanol is a synthetic agent that has been used widely in Europe. A 1% solution is injected adjacent to the varices at several levels in the esophagus. Intravariceal injections are to be avoided because this agent has been associated with heart failure and death due to the action of the drug passing into the systemic circulation. The negative chronotropic effects may be ascribed to this agent's local anesthetic properties. Although, in general, use of poliodecanol is safe, it is not available in the United States.

In the United States sclerosing mixtures have been used primarily in an attempt to avoid the recognized toxicities of sodium morrhuate and sodium tetradecyl sulfate. Dilution of these agents with solutions such as 50% dextrose and 50–95% ethanol appears to be the most popular approach (116). Other mixtures including addition of cephalothin or thrombin have not been shown to be more efficacious (77).

DRUGS FOR ACUTE STRESS EROSIONS AND ULCERATIONS

Stress ulcer and acute erosive gastritis occur in patients with extensive burns, multiple injuries, or major operative procedures, especially when these conditions are accompanied by episodes of hypotension, sepsis, or renal, hepatic, and respiratory failure (26). The incidence of bleeding from these lesions is variable and has been estimated to occur in approximately 3–6% of patients who are seriously ill, and upwards of 54% of patients with intracranial disease. In the very sickest patients with sepsis, the mortality from this complication approaches 80% (154).

The pathogenesis of stress erosions and ulcers is not completely understood but may be examined in the light of the known mechanisms of mucosal integrity, which include maintenance of mucosal pH, intramural pH, integrity of the gastric mucosal barrier, gastric mucosal blood flow, the composition of gastric mucus, and the state of gastric epithelial renewal. Mucosal pH is the most clinically accessible of these factors and has been the most extensively studied. Although not a universal finding, hypersecretion of acid has been demonstrated to occur in some patients who subsequently develop stress ulceration and may be especially prominent in those with central nervous system injury (72).

Intramural gastric pH may also be associated with the development of stress ulceration by several different mechanisms. First, disruption of the mucosal barrier to back-diffusion of hydrogen ion may lead to accumulation of intramural hydrogen ions. Second, decreased gastric mucosal or subepithelial blood flow may cause localized anoxia with resultant anaerobiosis; lactic acid accumulates, with a consequent fall in tissue pH. Third, systemic acidosis that accompanies shock states may cause a local decrease in the pH of the blood perfusing the gastric mucosa. In one study, the presence of multiple clinical risk factors and a low intramural gastric pH correlated with the development of massive bleeding from stress ulceration (50). Furthermore, bleeding from stress ulceration was identified only in the presence of a markedly decreased intramural pH. All patients who developed bleeding had been treated with antacids, which suggested that intramural pH rather than luminal pH may be the more important factor in the development of stress ulceration.

Since most studies have shown that bleeding or evidence of gastric mucosal injury is associated with an increased overall mortality, a significant amount of attention has been directed toward prevention of stress ulcerations (131). Controlled randomized trials have shown that aggressive hourly intragastric antacid titration can reduce the incidence of acute upper gastrointestinal bleeding in critically ill patients. Hourly titration of gastric contents with antacids to maintain intragastric pH above 3.5 resulted in a significant reduction of bleeding in critically ill patients (64). Continuous infusion of antacids is effective, and given at a dose of 30–60 ml/hr may also facilitate nursing care by obviating the requirement for hourly dosage administration. Disadvantages of antacid prophylaxis include diarrhea, systemic alkalosis, hypophosphatemia, and hypomagnesemia or hypermagnesemia. In addition, the danger of pulmonary aspiration may be increased in patients receiving large volumes of antacids by nasogastric tube. The H_2-receptor antagonists are also effective in prophylaxis of stress-induced ulcerations and bleeding (122). Cimetidine (300 mg every 6 hours, intravenously) compares favorably but is not more effective than antacids in the prevention of stress erosions (126). Hourly antacid use, however, appears to be better for maintaining gastric pH above 4. The goal was accomplished in 97.9% of patients in one study (83) compared with 79.5% of patients receiving bolus cimetidine therapy. Ranitidine given as an intravenous bolus of 50 mg every 8 hours is another effective alternative. Intragastric pH can be much more effectively maintained above 4.0 if a continuous infusion of histamine H_2-antagonists is used instead of intermittent bolus dosing (119). In patients with normal renal function, cimetidine should be administered intravenously as a 300-mg bolus over 10–20 minutes, followed by a continuous infusion of 37.5 mg/hr. Gastric pH should be measured after 6 hours. In some patients, the infusion rate may need to be increased possibly to 50–100 mg/hr in order to maintain gastric pH above 4.0. Patients who have recently been treated with cimetidine may be resistant to its action and supplemental antacids may be required. The slow infusion of the cimetidine bolus is advised in the light of reports of serious cardiac dysrhythmias in critically ill patients who received rapid intravenous administration of cimetidine (100). Ranitidine given as a 50-mg initial bolus dose followed by an 8 mg/hr continuous infusion is an alternative, and at present is the preferred method in our intensive care units. Another advantage to continuous infusion of histamine H_2-antagonists is the time and material cost savings to the pharmacy and nursing services. These agents can be added to parenteral alimentation solutions, and in one study, costs for total parenteral nutrition–delivered cimetidine was $12,257 versus $34,769 for intermittently administered cimetidine (141).

The use of other agents in the prevention of stress bleeding awaits further studies. Sucralfate is effective, and unlike antacids and cimetidine, the efficacy of sucralfate is independent of intragastric pH (13, 165). One gram of sucralfate can be dissolved in 30 ml of water and administered every 6 hours orally or via a nasogastric tube. Preliminary experience with the use of famotidine (34) and omeprazole (173) in critically ill patients suggests that these agents will also be of therapeutic benefit in

controlling intragastric acidity in critically ill patients.

DRUG THERAPY FOR UPPER GASTROINTESTINAL BLEEDING

Bleeding from peptic ulcers usually ceases spontaneously, although rebleeding during hospitalization occurs in 25–30% of patients. Morbidity and mortality is increased if rebleeding occurs. As a consequence, attempts have been made to use endoscopic criteria of peptic ulcers to predict the likelihood of rebleeding and accordingly, better direct the care of the patient (161, 175). Endoscopic features of the ulcer that increase the likelihood of rebleeding are a central dark spot, adherent clot, visible vessel, or slow blood ooze from the ulcer crater. Studies have varied in defining rebleeding risk based on each of these parameters (Table 18.10).

Attempts to prevent recurrent bleeding from gastric or duodenal ulcers using cimetidine and/or antacids have not been successful (184). One possibility for these failures is that gastric pH may not be adequately elevated. In vitro data suggest that it may be necessary to raise gastric pH to 7.0 (achlorhydria) in order to prevent recurrent hemorrhage (59). In vitro experiments have confirmed that the process of normal blood coagulation is pH-dependent and requires a pH of 6.9–7.4 (Table 18.11). Pepsin acts in concert with acid to dissolve clots (7) and is not irreversibly inactivated until pH values of 7.0 or higher are achieved (59). If these in vitro pH data can be applied to intragastric pH levels in humans, poor clot formation or even clot dissolution might occur in the stomach of patients who have bled unless a pH of 7.0 or more is maintained.

The pharmacologic approach to sustaining medical achlorhydria is best directed by the

Table 18.10
Endoscopic Stigmata for Predicting Rebleeding

Endoscopic Finding	Prevalence (%)		Rebleeding (%)	
	Mean	Range	Mean	Range
Central dark spot	21	20–54	9	0–15
Adherent clot	19	5–32	20	0–24
Visible vessel	30	15–72	53	19–100
Ongoing ooze	22	18–72	45	32–100

Table 18.11
pH Effects on Intragastric Coagulation

pH	Comments
7.4	Reference pH
7.0	Pepsin irreversibly inactivated
6.8	$3\times$ decrease platelet aggregation
6.4	Clotting time $2\times$ increase; decreased availability of platelet phospholipid and platelet factor III
6.1	60% disaggregation of previously formed platelet aggregates
6.0	Clotting time $4\times$ increase; decreased availability of platelet phospholipid and platelet factor III
5.9	Platelet aggregation abolished; complete dissolution of previously formed platelet aggregates.
5.4	Clotting abolished

results of a recent comparison of different medical regimens (121). The effects of bolus doses of cimetidine (300 mg every 6 hours intravenously), antacid (30 ml/hr intragastrically), and a combination of these resulted in attaining intragastric pH values of 3.5, 4.6, and 6.8, respectively, but did not achieve achlorhydria. Constant infusion regimens of cimetidine (50 mg/hr intravenously), antacid (0.5 ml/min intragastrically), and the combination resulted in pH values of 4.3, 5.2, and 7.4, respectively. Sustained achlorhydria was still not produced in each patient until the infusion of cimetidine was increased to 100 mg/hr and administered with a constant infusion of antacid. Although the maintenance of gastric pH at 7.0 or higher should theoretically reduce bleeding and/or rebleeding, a clinical controlled patient trial has not yet been reported. The use of more potent acid inhibitors such as ranitidine, famotidine, and omeprazole may prove to be more effective in ensuring sustained achlorhydria. At present, we recommend coupling of a constant infusion of cimetidine or ranitidine with a continuous infusion of antacid in patients who present with nonvariceal upper gastrointestinal hemorrhage and who are at risk for rebleeding. Dosages of the medications should be carefully titrated to ensure a pH of 7.0 or higher. Endoscopic definition of the ulcer features may help in better identifying those patients with a higher likelihood of rebleeding. If a lesion with a high risk for rebleeding is identified, we would favor continuing the combination therapy for at least the first 24–48 hours of intensive support.

DRUGS USED FOR INTENSIVE TREATMENT OF INFLAMMATORY BOWEL DISEASE

Ulcerative Colitis

Before the corticosteroid era, severe or moderately severe attacks of ulcerative colitis (UC) had high mortality. Corticosteroids sharply reduced the fatality rate in moderately severe attacks of UC, but severe attacks continued to be dangerous until the policy of early colectomy was introduced. The dramatic decrease in mortality with surgery led some authors to abandon corticosteroid therapy. Successful medical treatment of a severe attack of UC may, however, be followed by a sustained remission (164). The aim, therefore, is to obtain the best possible timing between medical and surgical treatment.

Patients with severe UC are systematically ill with fever, leukocytosis, bloody diarrhea, abdominal pain, and tenderness. For such patients, treatment with parenteral steroids is mandatory. Oral steroids for such patients are a poor choice because of inferior response, and should not be used. Intravenous hydrocortisone, 300 mg daily, or prednisolone, 60 mg daily, in divided doses should be administered unless the intestine has already perforated. If the patient has not previously received adrenocortical steroids, some clinicians advise intravenous adrenocorticotropic hormone therapy, 120 U/day (112). Steroid therapy may lessen symptoms and signs expected with perforation, so careful physical examination for liver dullness at least twice daily and frequent flat plates of the abdomen should be done.

Intensive medical therapy improves or induces a remission in approximately 80% of patients with severe colitis (76, 111, 153). Continuation of medical therapy beyond 5–6 days without clear-cut objective evidence of improvement is very hazardous since colonic perforation with peritoneal soilage is a disaster that increases operative mortality and postoperative complications at least 10-fold (19). Antibiotics do not influence remission rates and should not be used routinely, but should be added when there is impending or definite colonic perforation or evidence of definite suppuration (111). When added, antibiotic coverage should be directed at both anaerobic and aerobic fecal flora. Sulfasalazine is not helpful in the severely ill patient with fulminant colitis. Total parenteral nutrition has no primary therapeutic effect in acute colitis, although it preserves body protein (36).

Medications that affect bowel activity have been associated with megacolon in patients with active ulcerative or Crohn's colitis. Drugs implicated include anticholinergics such as propantheline bromide and atropine; narcotics such as codeine, opium, paregoric, meperidine, and morphine; and narcotic derivative antidiarrheal agents such as diphenoxylate hydrochloride with atropine sulfate and loperamide.

Crohn's Disease

Patients with severely symptomatic Crohn's disease require hospitalization, bowel rest, and intravenous fluid therapy. Patients are usually febrile, and questions of extensive inflammation outside the lumen of the intestine and abscess formation frequently arise. Broad spectrum antibiotic coverage is frequently begun with aggressive attempts to identify an intraabdominal abscess. Metronidazole has received systematic investigation in patients with Crohn's disease. A powerful drug against intestinal anaerobics, metronidazole clearly is effective against mixed intestinal flora infections and suppurative foci in the acute case. It also is effective in treating perirectal disease and perirectal fistulae. If no definite abscess can be localized and no positive blood cultures are obtained, steroids, prednisolone or equivalent, should be given at a dose of 40–60 mg/day intravenously. With a regimen of bowel rest, high-dose steroids, and broad spectrum antibiotics if extraluminal extension is suspected, the disease remits in the majority of severely ill patients. The use of azothioprine, 1.0–2.0 mg/kg/day, or 6-mercaptopurine, 1.5–2.5 mg/kg/day, can be considered for patients who do not respond to this regimen. These agents, however, may not be of benefit in acute disease, in that there is often a protracted delay in attaining maximal therapeutic effect.

DRUGS FOR INTESTINAL ISCHEMIA

Acute mesenteric ischemia results from an abrupt diminution in the blood supply to the small bowel and is most commonly caused by an embolus or vasospasm (nonocclusive mesenteric ischemia). Less commonly, arterial thrombosis with insufficient collateralization and, rarely, a venous thrombosis is responsible. Patients at risk are usually older than 50 years of age, have valvular or arteriosclerotic heart disease and/or longstanding poorly controlled congestive heart failure, and are treated by rapid digitalization (a splanchnic vasoconstrictor) or with potent diuretics. Such patients frequently have a cardiac arrhythmia, an episode of hypotension (hypovolemia or shock), or a recent myocardial infarction. Also at risk are patients with inflammatory, degenerative, or structural diseases of the small mesenteric vessels. The clinical hallmark of early acute mesenteric ischemia is severe abdominal pain without significant abdominal findings. The disease can be diagnosed only by angiography, and selective intraarterial infusion of a number of potential dilators (including histamine, phenoxybenzamine, isoproterenol, dopamine, methylprednisolone, prescoline, gut peptides, prostaglandin E_1, and papaverine) has been tried (11, 12). Of these, papaverine appears to be the most effective (10).

The main actions of papaverine are exerted on cardiac and smooth muscle. It relaxes the smooth musculature of the larger blood vessels and reduces vasospasm. The antispasmodic effect is direct and unrelated to muscle innervation. In addition, this drug has direct cardiac effects with depression of conduction and prolongation of the refractory period. Systemic arterial pressure and cardiac rate must be monitored during the infusion because the amount of papaverine administered may cause cardiac arrhythmias, peripheral vasodilation, and increased myocardial oxygen demand. The duration of infusion depends both on the purpose for its use and the clinical and angiographic response of the patient.

References

1. Albibi R, McCallum RW: Metoclopramide—pharmacology and clinical application. *Ann Intern Med* 98:86–93, 1983.
2. Alfrey AC, Le Gendre GR, Kaehny WD: The dialysis encephalopathy syndrome: possible aluminum intoxication. *N Engl J Med* 294:184–188, 1976.
3. Averius PH, Brunzell JD: Chylomicronemia induced by cimetidine. *Gastroenterology* 89:664–666, 1985.
4. Baker LRI, Ackrell P, Catell WR, et al: Iatrogenic osteomalacia and myopathy due to phosphate depletion. *Br Med J* 3:150–152, 1974.
5. Bartle WR, Walter SE, Shapero T: Dose-dependent effect of cimetidine on phenytoin kinetics. *Clin Pharmacol Ther* 33:649–655, 1983.
6. Bender HJ, Donaldson RM Jr: Effect of cimetidine on

intrinsic factor and pepsin secretion in man. *Gastroenterology* 74:371–375, 1978.

7. Berstad A: Management of acute upper gastrointestinal bleeding. *Scand J Gastroenterol* 17:103–108, 1982.

8. Berylne GM, Ben-Ari J, Pest D, et al: Hyperaluminaemia from aluminum resins in renal failure. *Lancet* 2:494–496, 1970.

9. Black JW, Duncan WAM, Durant CJ, et al: Definition and antagonism of histamine H_2 receptors. *Nature* 236:385–390, 1972.

10. Boley SJ, Fernstein FR, Sammartano R, Brandt LJ, Sprayregen S: New concepts in the management of emboli of the superior mesenteric artery. *Surg Gynecol Obstet* 153:561–569, 1981.

11. Boley SJ, Sammartano R, Brandt LJ, Mitsudo S, Sheran M: Intra-arterial vasodilators and thrombolytic agents in experimental superior mesenteric artery embolus. *Gastroenterology* 82:1021, 1982.

12. Borden EB, Boley SJ: Acute mesenteric ischemia: Treat aggressively for best results. *J Crit Illness* 10:52–58, 1986.

13. Borrero E, Bank S, Margolis I, Schulman ND, Chardavoyne R: Comparison of antacid and sucralfate in the presentation of gastrointestinal bleeding in patients who are critically ill. *Am J Med* 79(suppl 2C):28–30, 1985.

14. Boyce MJ: Cimetidine and the cardiovascular system. In Baron JH (ed): *Cimetidine in the 80's*. Edinburgh, Churchill Livingstone, 1981, pp 227–237.

15. Boyce MJ, Wareham K: Histamine H_1, and H_2-receptors in the cardiovascular system of man. In Torsoli A, Zucchelli PE, Brimblecomb RW (eds): *H_2-Antagonists*. Amsterdam, Excerpta Medica, 1980, pp 280–293.

16. Brand DC, Roufail WM, Thomson ABR, Taper EJ: Misoprostil, a synthetic PGE_1 analog, in the treatment of duodenal ulcers: a multicenter double-blind study. *Dig Dis Sci* 30:1475–1585, 1985.

17. Brandstaetter G, Kratochvil P: Comparison of two sucralfate dosages (2 g twice a day versus 1 g four times a day) in duodenal ulcer healing. *Am J Med* 79(Suppl 2C):18–20, 1985.

18. Brogden RN, Carmine AA, Heel RC, Speight TM, Avery GS: Ranitidine: a review of its pharmacology and therapeutic use in peptic ulcer disease and other allied diseases. *Drugs* 24:267–303, 1982.

19. Brooke BN, Sampson PA: An indication for surgery in acute ulcerative colitis. *Lancet* 2:1272–1273, 1964.

20. Brooks WS: Sucralfate: non-ulcer uses. *Am J Gastroenterol* 80:206–209, 1985.

21. Brooks WS: *Variceal sclerosing agents. Am J Gastroenterol* 79:424–428, 1984.

22. Bulkard WP: Histamine H_2 receptor binding with ^3H-cimetidine in brain. *Eur J Pharmacol* 50:449–450, 1978.

23. Burck JD, Myka JA, Kokelman DK: Famotidine: summary of preclinical safety assessment. *Digestion* 32:7–14, 1985.

24. Campbell MA, Plachetka JR, Jackson JE, Moon FJ, Finley PR: Cimetidine decreases theophylline clearance. *Ann Intern Med* 95:68–69, 1981.

25. Cash JD, Gader AM, Da Costa J: The release of plasminogen activator and factor VIII to lysine vasopressin, arginine vasopressin, l-desamino-8-d-arginine vasopressin, angiotensin and oxytocin in man. *Br J Haematol* 27:363–364, 1974.

26. Cheung LY: Treatment of established stress ulcer disease. *World J Surg* 5:235–246, 1981.

27. Chremos AN: Pharmacodynamics of famotidine in humans. *Am J Med* 81(suppl 4B):3–12, 1986.

28. Clarkson EM, McDonald SJ, De Wardner HW: The effect of a high intake of calcium carbonate in normal subjects and patients with chronic renal failure. *Clin Sci* 30:425–438, 1966.

29. Classen M, Darnmann HD, Domshke W, Hutteman W, Londong W: Omeprazole heals duodenal but not gastric ulcers more rapidly than ranitidine. *Hepatogastroenterology* 32:243–245, 1985.

30. Conn HO: Propranolol in portal hypertension: problems in paradise? *Hepatology* 4:560–564, 1984.

31. Connors AF, Bacon BR, Miron SD: Sodium morruate delivery to the lung during endoscopic variceal sclerotherapy. *Ann Intern Med* 105:539–542, 1986.

32. Crossby RJ, Evers PW: Review of endocrine studies of cimetidine. In Baron JH (ed): *Cimetidine in the 80's*. Edinburgh, Churchill Livingstone, 1981, pp 247–252.

33. Cummings S, Daumann A, Groszmann RJ: Vascular reactivity to serotonin in a rat model of portal hypertension. *Hepatology* 5:1059, 1985.

34. Dammann HG, Burkhardt F, Kuhl U, Walter A, Muller P, Simon B: The effect of intravenous famotidine and ranitidine on intragastric pH and hormone levels in critical care patients. *Gastroenterology* 88:1359, 1985.

35. Davis TG, Picket DL, Schlosser JH: Evaluation of the worldwide spontaneous reporting system with cimetidine. *JAMA* 243:1912–1914, 1980.

36. Dickinson RJ, Ashton MG, Axon ATR, Smith RC, Yerind CK, Hill GL: Controlled trial of intravenous hyperalimentation and total bowel rest as an adjunct to the routine therapy of acute colitis. *Gastroenterology* 79:1199–1204, 1980.

37. Doherty CC, O'Connor FA, Buchanan KD, McGeown MG: Cimetidine for duodenal ulceration in patients undergoing haemodialysis. *Br Med J* 2:1506–1508, 1977.

38. Douglas WW: Histamine and 5-hydroxytryptamine (serotonin) and their antagonists. In Gilman AG, Goodman LS, Gilman A (eds): *The Pharmacological Basis of Therapeutics*, ed. 6. New York, Macmillan, 1980, pp 622–632.

39. Drake D, Hollander D: Neutralizing capacity and cost effectiveness of antacids. *Ann Intern Med* 94:215–217, 1981.

40. *Drug Information File*. West Point, PA, Merck Sharp & Dohme.

41. Dundee JW, McGowan WA, Elwood RJ, Hilderbran PJ: Plasma benzodiazepine concentrations following oral administration with and without H_2-receptor blockers. *Ir J Med Sci* 151:413–414, 1982.

42. Ekman L, Hansson E, Havu N, Carlson E, Lundberg C: Toxicological studies on omeprazole. *Scand J Gastroenterol* 108:53–69, 1985.

43. Ernstoff JJ, Howard DA, Marshall JB, Jumshyd A, McCullough JA: A randomized, blinded clinical trial of a rapid colonic lavage solution (GoLYTELY) compared with standard preparation for colonoscopy and barium enema. *Gastroenterology* 84:1512–1516, 1983.

44. Fairfax AJ, Adam J, Pagan FS: Effect of cimetidine on the absorption of oral benzylpenicillin. *Br Med J* 1:820, 1978.

45. Feely J, Wilkinson GR, Wood AJ: Reduction of liver blood flow and propranolol metabolism by cimetidine. *N Engl J Med* 304:692–695, 1981.

46. Feldman M, Richardson CT, Peterson WL, et al: Effect of low-dose propantheline on food-stimulated gastric acid secretion: comparison with an "optimal effective dose" and interaction with cimetidine. *N Engl J Med* 297:1427–1430, 1977.

47. Feldman M, Smith JH: Effect of cisapride on gastric emptying of indigestible solids in patients with gastroparesis diabeticorum. *Gastroenterology* 91:171–174, 1987.

48. Fernandes E, Melewicz FM: Ranitidine and theophylline. *Ann Intern Med* 100:459, 1984.

49. Festen HPM, Diemel J, Lamers CBH: Is the measurement of blood cimetidine levels useful? *Br J Clin Pharmacol* 12:417–421, 1981.

50. Fiddian-Green RG, McGough E, Pittenger G, et al: Predictive value of intramural pH and other risk factors for massive bleeding from stress ulceration. *Gastroenterology* 85:613–620, 1983.

51. Fine A, Churchill T: Potentially lethal interaction of cimetidine and morphine. *Can Med Assoc J* 124:1434–1436, 1981.
52. Fortran JS, Morawiki SG, Richardson CT: *In vivo* and *in vitro* evaluation of liquid antacids. *N Engl J Med* 288:923–928, 1973.
53. Freely J, Wilkinson GR, McAllister CB, Wood AJJ: Increased toxicity and reduced clearance of lidocaine by cimetidine. *Ann Intern Med* 96:592–594, 1982.
54. Freston JW: Cimetidine-adverse reactions and patterns of use. *Ann Intern Med* 97:728–734, 1982.
55. Freston JW: Cimetidine: developments, pharmacology, and efficacy. *Ann Intern Med* 97:573–580, 1982.
56. Fretwell MD, Pearlman RA, Vestal RE, Mease PJ, Hazzard WR: Fever and delirium in three elderly patients: a discussion of possible cimetidine toxicity, cimetidine pharmacology and application of decision analysis to cimetidine therapy. *Med Grand Rounds* 1:222–238, 1982.
57. Friedman G: The GI drug column: domperidone. *Am J Gastroenterol* 78:47–48, 1983.
58. Gibaldi M, Kanig JL, Amsel L: Critical *in vitro* factors in evaluation of gastric antacids. Inhibition of neutralization rate of dried aluminum hydroxide gel. *J Pharm Sci* 53:1375–1377, 1964.
59. Green FW, Kaplan MM, Curtis LE, Levine PH: Effect of acid and pepsin on blood coagulation and platelet aggregation. *Gastroenterology* 74:38–43, 1978.
60. Groszman RJ, Kravetz D, Bosch J, et al: Nitroglycerin improves the hemodynamic response to vasopressin in portal hypertension. *Hepatology* 2:757–762, 1982.
61. Gugler R, Jense JC: Omeprazole inhibits oxidative drug metabolism. *Gastroenterology* 89:1235–1241, 1985.
62. Hardy BG, Zador IT, Golden L, Lalka D, Schentag JJ: Effect of cimetidine on the pharmacokinetics and pharmacodynamics of quinidine. *Am J Cardiol* 52:172–174, 1982.
63. Harvey SC: Gastric antacids and digestants. In Gilman AG, Goodman LS, Gilman A (eds): *The Pharmacologic Basis of Therapeutics*, ed. 6. New York, Macmillan, 1980, pp 988–1001.
64. Hastings PL, Skillman JJ, Bushness LS, Silen W: Antacid titration in the prevention of acute gastrointestinal bleeding. A controlled, randomized trial in 100 critically ill patients. *N Engl J Med* 298:1041–1044, 1978.
65. Heagerty AM, Castleden CM, Patel L: Failure of ranitidine to interact with propranolol. *Br Med J* 284:1304, 1982.
66. Hetzel DJ, Bochner F, Hallpike JF, Shearman DJC, Hann CS: Cimetidine interaction with phenytoin. *Br Med J* 282:1512, 1981.
67. Hollander D, Tarnawski A, Gergely H, Zipser RD: Sucralfate protection of gastric mucosa against alcohol-induced necrosis: a prostaglandin mediated process. *Scand J Gastroenterol* 19:97–102, 1984.
68. Holt PR: Gastrointestinal drugs in the elderly. *Am J Gastroenterol* 81:403–411, 1986.
69. Howard JM: Famotidine: a new potent long acting histamine H2-receptor antagonist: comparison with cimetidine and ranitidine in the treatment of Zollinger-Ellison syndrome. *Gastroenterology* 88:1026–1033, 1985.
70. Howden CW, Meredith PA, Forrest JA, Reid JL: Oral pharmacokinetics of omeprazole. *Eur J Clin Pharmacol* 26:641–643, 1984.
71. Hyneck ML, Murphy JF, Lipschutz DE: Cimetidine clearance during intermittent and chronic peritoneal dialysis. *Am J Hosp Pharm* 38:1760–1762, 1981.
72. Idjadi F, Robbins R, Stahl WM, et al: Prospective study of gastric secretion in stressed patients with intracranial injury. *J Trauma* 11:681–686, 1971.
73. Ishimosi A: Safety experience with sucralfate in Japan. *J Clin Gastroenterol* 3:169–173, 1981.
74. Ivanovich P, Fellows H, Rich C: The absorption of calcium carbonate. *Ann Intern Med* 66:917–923, 1967.
75. Jackson JE, Powell JR, Wandell M, Bentley J, Dorr R: Cimetidine decreases theophylline clearance. *Am Rev Respir Dis* 123:615–617, 1981.
76. Janerot G, Rolny P, Sandberg-Gertzen H: Intensive intravenous treatment of ulcerative colitis. *Gastroenterology* 89:1005–1013, 1985.
77. Jansen DM: Sclerosants for injection sclerosis of esophageal varices. *Gastrointest Endosc* 29:315–317, 1983,
78. Jeevendra Martin JA, Greenblatt DJ, Abernethy DR: Increased cimetidine clearance of burn patients. *JAMA* 253:1288–1291, 1985.
79. Jones RH, Rudge CJ, Bewick M, Parsons V, Weston MJ: Cimetidine: prophylaxis against upper gastrointestinal haemorrhage after renal transplantation. *Br Med J* 1:398–400, 1978.
80. Jordaens L, Hoegaerts J, Belpaire F: Non-interaction of cimetidine with digoxin absorption. *Acta Clin Belg* 36:109–110, 1981.
81. Kaehny WD, Hegg AP, Alfrey AC: Gastrointestinal absorption of aluminum-containing antacids. *N Engl J Med* 296:1389–1390, 1977.
82. Khoury W, Geracik G, Askari A, et al: The effect of cimetidine on aspirin absorption (abstract). *Gastroenterology* 76:1169, 1979.
83. Kingsley AN: Prophylaxis for acute stress ulcers: antacids or cimetidine. *Am Surg* 51:545–547, 1985.
84. Kiowski W, Frei A: Bolus injection of cimetidine and hypotension in patients in the intensive care unit: incidence and mechanisms. *Arch Intern Med* 147:153–156, 1987.
85. Kirch W: Presentation at the Fourteenth Congress of the European Society of Pharmacology, Rome, Italy, March 1983.
86. Kirchner SG, Buckspan GS, O'Neill JA, et al: Detergent enema: a cause of caustic colitis. *Pediatr Radiol* 6:141–146, 1977.
87. Klotz V, Reimann I: Delayed clearance of diazepam due to cimetidine. *N Engl J Med* 302:1012–1014, 1980.
88. Knapp AB, Maguire W, Keren G, et al: The cimetidine-lidocaine interaction. *Ann Intern Med* 98:174–177, 1983.
89. Kollberg B, Slezak P: The effect of prostaglandin E2 on duodenal ulcer healing. *Prostaglandins* 24:527–536, 1982.
90. Konturek SJ: Prostaglandins in pathophysiology of peptic ulcer disease. *Dig Dis Sci* 30:105S–108S, 1985.
91. Korula J, Baydur A, Sassoon C, Sakimura I: Effect of esophageal variceal sclerotherapy (EVS) on lung function: a prospective controlled study. *Arch Intern Med* 14:1517–1520, 1986.
92. Kuruvilla JT: Antipeptic activity of antacids. *Gut* 12:897–898, 1971.
93. Kvols LK, Moertel GG, O'Connell MJ, Schutt AJ, Rubin J, Hahn RG: Treatment of the malignant carcinoid syndrome: evaluation of a long-acting somatostatin analogue. *N Engl J Med* 315:663–666, 1986.
94. Lauretsen K, Run SJ, Bytzer P, et al: Effect of omeprazole and cimetidine on duodenal ulcer: a double-blind comparative trial. *N Engl J Med* 312:958–961, 1985.
95. Lee HR: Cimetidine and narcotic analgesics. *Pharmacologist* 24:145–148, 1982.
96. Lee HR, Gandolfi AJ, Sipes IG, Bentley J: Effect of histamine H2-receptors on fentanyl metabolism. *Toxicologist* 2:145, 1981.
97. Longstreth AF, Go CLW, Malagelada JR: Postprandial gastric, pancreatic and biliary response to histamine H2 receptor antagonists in active duodenal ulcer. *Gastroenterology* 72:9–13, 1977.
98. Lotz M, Zisman E, Bartter FC: Evidence for a phosphorus depletion syndrome in man. *N Engl J Med* 278:400–415, 1968.

99. Ma KW, Brown D, Masler DS, et al: Effects of renal failure on blood levels of cimetidine. *Gastroenterology* 74(2):473–477, 1978.

100. MacMahon B, Bakshi J, Walsh MJ. Cardiac arrhythmias after intravenous cimetidine. *N Engl J Med* 305:832–833, 1981.

101. Malazelada JR, Carson GL: Antacid therapy. *Scand J Gastroenterol* 14 (suppl 55): 67–83, 1979.

102. Malazelada JR, Holtermuller KH, McCall JT, et al: Pancreatic, gallbladder, and intestinal responses to intraluminal magnesium salts in man. *Am J Dig Dis* 23:481–485, 1978.

103. Mastai R, Bosch J, Bruix J, et al: Effects of metoclopramide and domperidone on azygos blood flow in patients with cirrhosis and portal hypertension. *J Hepatology* 1:588, 1984.

104. McArthur KE, Anderson DS, Durbin TE, Orloff MJ, Dharmsathaporn K: Clonidine and lidamine to inhibit watery diarrhea in a patient with lung cancer. *Ann Intern Med* 96:323–325, 1982.

105. McArthur KE, Collen MJ, Maton PN, et al: Omeprazole: effect, convenient therapy for Zollinger-Ellison syndrome. *Gastroenterology* 28:939–944, 1985.

106. McCallum RW: Review of the current status of prokinetic agents in gastroenterology. *Am J Gastroenterol* 80:1008–1016, 1985.

107. McCallum RW, Petersen J, Caride V, Prokoff E: A scintigraphic evaluation of colonic transit in normal subjects: the prokinetic effects of cisapride. *Gastroenterology* 90:1540, 1986.

108. McGowan WR, Vermillion SE: Acute interstitial nephritis related to cimetidine therapy. *Gastroenterology* 79:746–749, 1980.

109. McGuigan JE: A consideration of the adverse effects of cimetidine. *Gastroenterology* 80:181–192, 1981.

110. Meredith TJ, Volans GN: Management of cimetidine overdose. *Lancet* 2:1367, 1979.

111. Meyers S, Janowitz HD: Systemic corticosteroid therapy of ulcerative colitis. *Gastroenterology* 89:1189–1891, 1985.

112. Meyers S, Sachar DB, Goldberg JD, Janowitz HD: Corticotropin versus hydrocortisone in the intravenous treatment of ulcerative colitis. *Gastroenterology* 85:351–357, 1983.

113. Mills PR, Rae AP, Farah DA, Russell RI, Lorimer AR, Carter DC: Comparison of three adrenoreceptor blocking agents in patients with cirrhosis and portal hypertension. *Gut* 25:73–78, 1984.

114. Mogelnicki SR, Waller JL, Finlayson DC: Physostigmine reversal of cimetidine-induced mental confusion. *JAMA* 241:826–827, 1979.

115. Mok HYI: Effects of cimetidine on biliary lipids in patients with reflux esophagitis. *Gastroenterology* 81:340–344, 1981.

116. Monroe P, Morrow CF, Millen JE, Fairman RP, Glauser FL: Acute respiratory failure after sodium morruate esophageal sclerotherapy. *Gastroenterology* 85:693–699, 1983.

117. Nagishuma R: Mechanisms of action of sucralfate. *J Clin Gastroenterol* 3(suppl 2):117–127, 1981.

118. O'Reilly RA: Comparative interaction of cimetidine and ranitidine with racemic warfarin in man. *Arch Intern Med* 144:989–991, 1984.

119. Ostro MJ, Russell JA, Solden SJ, Mahon WA, Jeyeeboy KN: Control of gastric pH with cimetidine: boluses versus primed infusion. *Gastroenterology* 89:532–536, 1985.

120. Patwardhan RV, Yarborough GW, Desmond GW, Johnson RF, Schenker S, Speeg KV: Cimetidine spares the glucuronidation of lorazepam and oxazepam. *Gastroenterology* 79:912–916, 1980.

121. Peterson WL, Richardson CT: Sustained fasting achlorhydria: a comparison of medical regimens. *Gastroenterology* 88:666–669, 1985.

122. Peura DA, Johnson LF: Cimetidine for prevention and treatment of gastroduodenal mucosal lesions in patients in an intensive care unit. *Ann Intern Med* 103:173–177, 1985.

123. *Physicians Desk Reference*. Oradell, NJ, Medical Economics Co, 1987, pp 1634–1636.

124. *Physicians Desk Reference*. Oradell, NJ, Medical Economics Co, 1986, p 922.

125. Piper DW, Fenton B: pH stability and activity curves of pepsin with special reference to their clinical importance. *Gut* 6:506–508, 1965.

126. Poleski MH, Spanier AH: Cimetidine versus antacids in the prevention of stress erosions in critically ill patients. *Am J Gastroenterol* 81:107, 1986.

127. Polio J, Groszmann RJ: Hemodynamic factors involved in the development and rupture of esophageal varices: a pathophysiologic approach to treatment. *Semin Liver Dis* 6:318–331, 1986.

128. Pop P, Nikkels RE, Thys O, Dorrestein GCM: Comparison of sucralfate and cimetidine in the treatment of duodenal and gastric ulcers. A multicenter study. *Scand J Gastroenterol* 18:43–47, 1983.

129. Powell JR, Rogers JF, Wargen WA, Cross RE, Eshelman FN: Inhibition of theophylline clearance by cimetidine but not ranitidine. *Arch Intern Med* 144:484–486, 1984.

130. Price HL, Cooperman LH, Warden JC: Control of the splanchnic circulation in man: role of beta-adrenergic receptors. *Circ Res* 21:333–340, 1967.

131. Priebe J, Skillman JJ: Methods of prophylaxis in stress ulcer disease. *World J Surg* 5:223–233, 1981.

132. Prowse CV, Douglas JG, Forest JA, Forsling ML: Haemostatic effects of lysine vasopressin and triglycyl lysine vasopressin infusion in patients with cirrhosis. *Eur J Clin Invest* 10:49–54, 1980.

133. Ranitidine. *Med Lett Drugs Ther* 24:111–113, 1982.

134. Rector WG: Drug therapy for portal hypertension. *Ann Intern Med* 105:96–107, 1986.

135. Richardson CT: Sucralfate. *Ann Intern Med* 97:269–271, 1982.

136. Rogers HJ, James CA, Morrison PJ, Bradbrook ID: Effect of cimetidine on oral absorption of ampicillin and cotrianoxazole. *J Antimicrob Chemother* 6:297–300, 1980.

137. Rogers HJ, Morrison P, House FR, et al: Effect of cimetidine on the absorption and efficacy of orally administered furosemide. *Int J Clin Pharmacol Ther Toxicol* 20:8–11, 1982.

138. Rowley-Jones D, Flind AC: Continuing evaluation of the safety of cimetidine in the 80's. In Baron JH (ed): *Cimetidine in the 80's*. Edinburgh, Churchill Livingstone, 1981, pp 261–269.

139. Rudolfi A: Bleed level of cimetidine in relation to age. *Eur J Clin Pharmacol* 15:257–261, 1982.

140. Ruffalo RL, Thompson JF: Effect of cimetidine on the clearance of benzodiazepines. *N Engl J Med* 303:753–754, 1980.

141. Russell JA: Pharmacokinetics and pharmacodynamics of cimetidine in critically ill patients. *Clin Pharmacol Ther* 33:260, 1983.

142. Sawyer D, Conner CS, Scalley R: Cimetidine: adverse reactions and acute toxicity. *Am J Hosp Pharm* 38:188–197, 1981.

143. Sazie E, Jaffe JP: Severe granulocytopenia with cimetidine and phenytoin. *Ann Intern Med* 93:151–153, 1980.

144. Schneider RP, Roach AC: An antacid tasting: the relative palatability of 19 liquid antacids. *South Med J* 69:1312–1313, 1976.

145. Schulze-Delview K: Metoclopramide. *Gastroenterology* 77:768–779, 1979.

146. Schwinghammer TL: Drug interactions with cimetidine. *Am J Hosp Pharm* 38:1976–1978, 1981.

147. Sedman AJ: Cimetidine-drug interactions. *Am Intern Med* 76:109–114, 1984.

148. Serlin MJ, Sibeon RG, Mossman S, et al: Cimetidine: interaction with oral anticoagulants in man. *Lancet* 2:317–319, 1979.
149. Sharpe PC, Mills JG, Horton L, et al: Histamine H₂ receptors and intrinsic factor secretion. *Scand J Gastroenterol* 15:377–384, 1980.
150. Shaw G, Bury RW, Mashford ML, Breen KJ, Desmond PV: Cimetidine impairs the elimination of chlormethiazole. *Eur J Clin Pharmacol* 21:83–85, 1981.
151. Shea-Donohue T, Steel L, Montcalm E, Dubois A: Gastric protection by sucralfate: role of mucus and prostaglandins. *Gastroenterology* 91:660–666, 1986.
152. Silver BA, Bell WR: Cimetidine potentiation of the hypoprothrombinemic effect of warfarin. *Ann Intern Med* 90:348–349, 1979.
153. Singleton JW: Medical therapy of inflammatory bowel disease. *Med Clin North Am* 64:1117–1133, 1980.
154. Skillman JJ, Bushness LS, Godlman H, Silen W: Respiratory failure, hypotension, sepsis and jaundice: a clinical syndrome associated with lethal hemorrhage from acute stress ulceration of the stomach. *Am J Surg* 117:523–526, 1969.
155. Smith J, Torey C: Clinical pharmacology of famotidine. *Digestion* 32:15–23, 1985.
156. Soll AH: Three-way interactions between histamine, carbacol, and gastrin on aminopyrine uptake by isolated canine parietal cells (abstract). *Gastroenterology* 74:1146, 1978.
157. Somogyi A, Heinzow B: Cimetidine reduces procainamide. *N Engl J Med* 307:1080–1081, 1982.
158. Sonnenberg GE, Keller J, Pernichoud A, et al: Effects of somatostatin on splanchnic hemodynamics in patients with cirrhosis of the liver and in normal subjects. *Gastroenterology* 80:526–532, 1981.
159. Spahn H, Mutschler E, Kirch W, Ohnhaus EE, Janisch HD: Influence of ranitidine on plasma metoprolol and atenolol concentrations. *Br Med J* 286:1546–1547, 1983.
160. Spence RW, Celestin LR. Gynaecomastia associated with cimetidine. *Gut* 20:154–157, 1979.
161. Storey DW, Brown SG, Swain CP, et al: Endoscopic prediction of recurrent bleeding in peptic ulcers. *N Engl J Med* 305:915–916, 1981.
162. Takayanagi I, Iwayama Y, Kasuya Y: Narcotic antagonistic action of cimetidine on the guinea-pig ileum. *J Pharm Pharmacol* 30:519–520, 1978.
163. Tellerman-Toppet N, Duret ME, Coers C: Cimetidine interaction with carbamazepine [letter]. *Ann Intern Med* 94:544, 1981.
164. Truelove SC, Jewell DP: Intensive intravenous regimen for severe attacks of ulcerative colitis. *Lancet* 1:1067–1070, 1974.
165. Tryba M, Zevounow F, Torok M, Zenz M: Prevention of acute stress bleeding with sucralfate, antacids or cimetidine. *Am J Med* 79(supple 2C):21–27, 1985.
166. Tsai YT, Lay CS, Lai KH, et al: A controlled trial of vasopressin plus nitroglycerin vs. vasopressin alone in the treatment of bleeding esophageal varices. *Hepatology* 6:406–409, 1986.
167. Van Der Meer JWM, Kevning JJ, Scheijgrond AW, Heykants J, Van Cutsem J, Brugmans J: The influence of gastric acidity on the bioavailability of ketoconazole. *J Antimicrob Chemother* 6:552–554, 1980.
168. Vaziri ND, Ness RL, Barton CH: Hemodialysis clearance of cimetidine. *Arch Intern Med* 138:1685–1686, 1978.
169. Vaziri ND, Ness RL, Barton CH: Peritoneal dialysis clearance of cimetidine. *Am J Gastroenterol* 71(6):572–576, 1979.
170. Vinayek R, Howard JM, Maton PN, et al: Famotidine in the therapy of gastric hypersecretory states. *Am J Med* 81(suppl 4B):49–59, 1986.
171. Walan A: Antacids, metabolic side effects, and interactions. *Scand J Gastroenterol* [Suppl]25:63–68, 1982.
172. Wallmark B, Brandstrom A, Larsson H: Evidence for acid-induced transformation of omeprazole into an active inhibitor of (H⁺ + K⁺)-ATPase within the parietal cell. *Biochim Biophys Acta* 718:549–558, 1981.
173. Walt RR, Reynolds JR, Langman MJS, et al: Intravenous omeprazole rapidly raises intragastric pH. *Gut* 26:902–906, 1985.
174. Wanetschke R, Ammon HV: Effects of magnesium sulfate on transit time and water transport in the human jejunum (abstract). *Gastroenterology* 70:949, 1976.
175. Wara P: Endoscopic prediction of major rebleeding: a prospective study of stigmata of hemorrhage in bleeding ulcer. *Gastroenterology* 88:1209–1214, 1985.
176. Watts RW, Hetzel DJ, Bochner F, et al: Lack of interaction between ranitidine and phenytoin. *Br J Clin Pharmacol* 75:499–500, 1983.
177. Willet I, Esler M, Jennings F, Dudley F: Effect of clonidine on systemic and portal hemodynamics in alcoholic cirrhosis (abstract). *Gastroenterology* 86:1705, 1985.
178. Wilmore DW, Goodwin CW, Aulock LH, et al: Effect of injury and infection on visceral metabolism and circulation. *Ann Surg* 192:491–504, 1980.
179. Young CJ, Daneschmend TK, Roberts CJC: Effects of cirrhosis and aging on the elimination and bioavailability of ranitidine. *Gut* 23:819–832, 1980.
180. Yuhas EM, Lofton, FT, Baldinus JG, et al: Cimetidine hydrochloride compatibility with preoperative medications. *Am J Hosp Pharm* 38:1173–1174, 1981.
181. Yuhas EM, Lofton FT, Rosenberg HA, et al: Cimetidine hydrochloride compatibility III: Room temperature stability in drug admixtures. *Am J Hosp Pharm* 38:1919–1922, 1981.
182. Zeldis JB, Friedman LS, Isselbacher KJ. Ranitidine: a new H₂-receptor antagonist. *N Engl J Med* 309:1368–1373, 1983.
183. Zito RA, Diez A, Groszmann RJ: Comparative effects of nitroglycerin and nitroprusside on vasopressin-induced cardiac dysfunction in the dog. *J Cardiovasc Pharmacol* 5:586–591, 1983.
184. Zuckerman G, Welch R, Douglas A, et al: Controlled trial of medical therapy for active upper gastrointestinal bleeding and prevention of rebleeding. *Am J Med* 76:361–366, 1984.

19

Vasodilator Therapy

Joseph E. Parrillo, M.D.

Although the principles of afterload reduction with vasodilator therapy were enumerated more than 40 years ago (104), it is only in the past 15 years that clinical applications of vasodilator therapy in the treatment of moderate to severe cardiac failure have gained relatively widespread acceptance (16, 29). As early as 1944, spinal anesthesia–induced vasodilation was employed successfully to reverse cardiogenic pulmonary edema (100). In the early 1960s, the principles of afterload reduction as a method to improve cardiac performance were confirmed and extended (12, 103). However, frequent clinical use of vasodilators required the ability to document a salutary hemodynamic response and the capability of closely monitoring adverse consequences of this therapy. In the 1970s, the development of the Swan-Ganz balloon flotation catheter (108) allowed hemodynamic monitoring at the bedside, which was previously only available in the cardiac catheterization laboratory. Today, the physician can serially measure cardiac outputs and calculate systemic vascular resistance to document a salutary or adverse response to therapy. Further, routine use of arterial pressure catheters allows a beat-to-beat measure of the major adverse consequence of vasodilators, namely, hypotension.

In 1971, phentolamine, an α-adrenergic receptor antagonist, was reported to be effective in relieving symptoms and improving the hemodynamics of patients with severe heart failure secondary to ischemic heart disease (75). One year later, nitroprusside-induced vasodilation was shown to increase cardiac output, reduce ventricular filling pressures, and relieve symptoms in post–myocardial infarction patients with severe heart failure, or even cardiogenic shock (46). Subsequent studies have documented the usefulness of vasodilation therapy in subsets of patients with severe intractable heart failure (58), cardiogenic shock

(32), and severe mitral (20) or aortic (9) regurgitation.

The purpose of this chapter is to review the physiologic mechanisms underlying vasodilator therapy, the appropriate indications for use of vasodilators, and the usefulness of specific vasodilator agents. The practical considerations of vasodilator therapy in the management of critically ill patients are reviewed. Emphasis is placed on the physiology and pathogenic mechanisms that provide a foundation for proper patient care. Reviews of more specific aspects of vasodilator therapy are available (6, 7, 24, 40, 41, 50, 76, 80, 86, 88, 98, 113, 114, 119).

PHYSIOLOGIC MECHANISMS OF ACTION OF VASODILATORS

Factors Determining Ventricular Function

The heart's major function is to supply blood flow to the tissues to satisfy the metabolic requirements of the body. There are four major determinants of cardiac function: preload, afterload, contractility, and heart rate (12, 25). These factors can be manipulated clinically to produce optimal ventricular function in any given patient. Depending on the patient's physiology, pathology, and clinical status, the physician can choose from a wide variety of methods to augment cardiovascular function.

PRELOAD

Preload is defined as the amount the myocardium is stretched prior to the onset of contraction. Isolated papillary muscle experiments originally demonstrated an increase in myocardial tension development with an increase in the resting length of the cardiac mus-

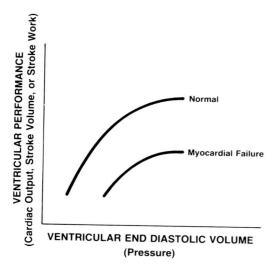

Figure 19.1. Frank-Starling ventricular performance curves. In the normal ventricle, as ventricular end-diastolic volume is increased, there is a concomitant increase in ventricular performance until a plateau is reached. Patients with myocardial dysfunction and heart failure demonstrate a shift of this curve downward and to the right. In heart failure, an increase in end-diastolic volume produces less of an increase in ventricular performance and a "plateau" is reached at a much lower level of ventricular performance.

cles (13), with maximal tension development occurring when there was the most overlap of action and myosin filaments. In the intact ventricle, this Frank-Starling relationship is manifested by enhanced ventricular performance as the end-diastolic volume of the left or right ventricle is increased (13) (Fig. 19.1). In the normal heart, at low end-diastolic volumes, small increases in preload cause a substantial increase in stroke volume and cardiac output; as one increases end-diastolic volume further, similar increases in end-diastolic volume produce progressively less of an increase in stroke volume, finally reaching a plateau beyond which increases in diastolic volume do not increase stroke volume (or other measures of ventricular performance) (107).

Clinically, measuring end-diastolic ventricular volumes is difficult, whereas end-diastolic pressure can be relatively easily obtained from intracardiac catheter readings. When plotting the relationship between end-diastolic pressure and ventricular performance, one sees a relationship similar to that shown in Figure 19.1, i.e., on increasing end-diastolic pressure, ventricular performance increases substan-

tially, then more modestly, finally plateauing. It is clinically useful to recognize that the relationship between end-diastolic pressure and volume is not linear (Fig. 19.2). Thus, at low volumes, a substantial increase in end-diastolic volume (producing an increase in stroke volume) can cause little or no change in end-diastolic pressure. At higher volumes, the relationship between volume and pressure becomes more linear, and changes in volume will be associated with increases in the end-diastolic ventricular pressure. Therefore, when dealing with low end-diastolic volumes, increasing the end-diastolic volume with fluid administration can produce considerable increases in stroke volume with little or no change in ventricular filling pressures.

The ventricle's intrinsic ability to increase its volume and pressure in response to an increase (or decrease) in intravascular volume is termed compliance, a measure of the ventricle's distensibility. Ischemia, fibrosis, hypertrophy, and certain pharmacologic agents such as vasodilators (see below) can profoundly influence ventricular compliance (11). Several studies suggest that left ventricular compliance is altered by high right ventricular diastolic pressures (8), which presumably alter left ventricular geometry with a displaced septum. Other studies suggest that an intact pericardium is important in right ventricular in-

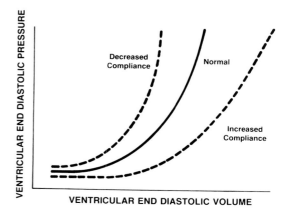

Figure 19.2. Diastolic pressure-volume relationship of the left ventricle. At low ventricular volumes, substantial changes in volume produce little change in ventricular pressure. At higher ventricular volumes, small changes produce exponentially greater increases in pressure. Increasing ventricular compliance with vasodilator therapy shifts the curve to the right, allowing a greater end-diastolic volume at a lower pressure. See text for details.

duced decreases in left ventricular compliances (92), arguing that changes in the right side of the heart affect the left side because of the pericardial "closed space."

In a more compliant ventricle, for any ventricular end-diastolic volume the ventricular pressure will be lower. This is a practical clinical concern since pulmonary edema occurs when left ventricular end-diastolic pressure rises above approximately 20 mm Hg. Thus, a more compliant ventricle allows for a greater increase in end-diastolic volume (enhancing systolic ventricular performance) than a noncompliant ventricle, which will develop a high pressure at a lower ventricular volume.

AFTERLOAD

Afterload is defined as the sum of the factors that oppose the shortening of muscle fibers—a definition derived from isolated papillary muscle experiments (83). In the intact cardiovascular system, afterload refers to the impedance against which the ventricle must eject during systole. Precise determination of aortic impedance to ventricular ejection requires sophisticated analysis of a series of harmonics, each of which depends on amplitude, phase angle, and frequency. These harmonics describe a spectrum of instantaneous relationships between pressure and flow (83, 99). Because of its complexity and the difficulty of its determination, afterload is usually clinically defined as vascular resistance, a value that defines the steady state (frequency-independent) characteristics of impedance to aortic flow.

Systemic vascular resistance (SVR) is defined by the following equation:

$$SVR = \frac{MAP - mean\ right\ atrial\ pressure}{CO}$$

where MAP is mean arterial blood pressure and CO is cardiac output. This equation demonstrates why afterload cannot be derived from blood pressure measurements alone: an arterial dilator can reduce SVR and cause an increase in CO resulting in no change in blood pressure, though the afterload confronting the ventricle is substantially reduced. Thus, SVR has become the most commonly used clinical parameter to reflect afterload or outflow impedance.

The nature of the relationship between afterload and stroke volume is important to an understanding of changes in cardiac function

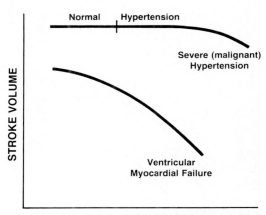

**SYSTEMIC VASCULAR RESISTANCE
(Afterload)**

Figure 19.3.   Relationship of systemic vascular resistance to stroke volume in a normal and dysfunctional ventricle. Increases in afterload do not cause a decrease in stroke volume in a normal ventricle *(upper curve)* except at very high levels of afterload when severe hypertension causes ventricular decompensation. In a failing ventricle *(lower curve),* however, an increase in afterload causes a progressive depression of stroke volume and cardiac output. Thus, vasodilator-induced reductions in afterload enhance stroke volume in patients with severe ventricular dysfunction.

when SVR varies. Stroke volume varies as the function of increasing SVR (Fig. 19.3). In the normally functioning ventricle *(upper curve),* mild to moderate increases in SVR do not decrease stroke volume, although the blood pressure rises modestly. Severe increases in SVR, e.g., malignant hypertension, may depress stroke volume (16, 29, 103). One of the major reasons that the normal ventricle's stroke volume does not become depressed with increasing afterload is the ventricle's ability to increase preload by rising on the steep portion of the Starling curve (Fig. 19.1) (23, 31, 103). Thus, in an experimental setting in which preload and contractility are kept constant, an increase in afterload decreases stroke volume secondary to a reduction in the extent and velocity of myocardial wall shortening (15, 115). Analogously, a ventricle with myocardial dysfunction operates on the plateau of the Starling function (Fig. 19.1) and is unable to increase stroke volume by increasing end-diastolic volume. Therefore, in a dysfunctional ventricle increases in SVR depress stroke volume. These physiologic principles provide the basis for effective vasodilator therapy: in a moderately or severely dysfunctional ventricle, a decrease in SVR commonly causes an increase in stroke volume, therefore augmenting CO (Fig. 19.3, *lower curve*).

CONTRACTILITY

Contractility refers to the inherent ability of the ventricle to increase the velocity and/or extent of contraction. Studies have defined contractility as changes in ventricular performance that cannot be ascribed to preload or afterload. Another useful operational definition is that an increase in contractility (holding afterload constant) produces a shift in the Starling preload curve upward and to the left (Fig. 19.4). A negative inotropic effect shifts the Starling curve downward and to the right. Positive inotropic agents that augment the contractility of the ventricle include the catecholamines, digitalis, glucagon, and thyroxine. Negative inotropic agents include phenobarbital, most general anesthetics, and propranolol.

The relationship of intrinsic myocardial contractility to afterload is also important in optimal vasodilator therapy. In the normal ventricle, increases in afterload are well tolerated with no decrease in stroke volume; however, in a depressed, poorly contractile ventricle, increases in afterload result in decreased stroke volume and CO (Fig. 19.3, *lower*

curve). Thus, in many patients with heart failure and an elevated SVR, reducing SVR results in an augmented stroke volume and CO (Fig. 19.3).

HEART RATE

If stroke volume is held constant, CO increases linearly with increases in heart rate, since CO is equal to the product of heart rate and stroke volume. However, faster heart rates allow less time for diastolic filling and may decrease preload; the ultimate CO depends on the extent of the increase in heart rate versus the decrease in preload. In addition, increases in heart rate cause an increase in ventricular contractility; this augmented contractility with increased heart rate occurs in ventricles with myocardial dysfunction and in normal ventricles (63, 70).

Many pharmacologic interventions have important effects on several of the above parameters affecting CO. The ultimate pharmacologic effect on cardiac performance depends on the magnitude and direction of the changes produced in each individual parameter, and also on the baseline hemodynamics of the treated patient. Further, one must consider reflex responses (autonomic or renin-angiotensin system) activated by the pharmacologic intervention; these reflexes tend to counteract many of the therapeutic effects. Thus, in order to predict the ultimate outcome of any particular pharmacologic intervention on cardiac performance, one must know the pharmacologic effect on each individual parameter (preload, afterload, contractility, and heart rate) and the patient's hemodynamic status (70, 103). Even with the above knowledge, one cannot always accurately predict the ultimate outcome of certain interventions; in such cases, a therapeutic trial following objective hemodynamic parameters is required.

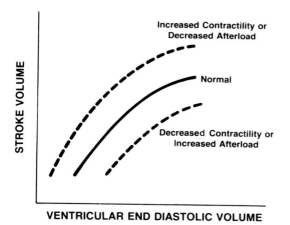

VENTRICULAR END DIASTOLIC VOLUME
(Pressure)

Figure 19.4. Ventricular function curves demonstrating the effects of changes in contractility or afterload. If afterload is held constant, an increase in contractility of the ventricle will shift the functional curve upward and to the left, demonstrating improved ventricular performance at any given level of end-diastolic volume. If ventricular contractility is left unchanged, a decrease in afterload will produce a similar shift in the ventricular function curve.

Pathophysiologic Abnormalities in Congestive Heart Failure

When myocardial function is depressed, the body activates a number of compensatory mechanisms designed to maintain CO and systemic blood pressure (11–13, 16, 29). The possible etiologies of the cardiac dysfunction and failure include ischemic heart disease, primary cardiomyopathy, infiltrative cardiomyopathies, chronic pressure overload (e.g., aortic stenosis), and chronic volume overload (e.g., mitral regurgitation, aortic regurgitation, ventricular septal defect). Regardless of the underlying causes of heart failure, the compensatory mechanisms are similar and include the following. First, dilation of the left ventricle, i.e., increasing the left ventricular end-diastolic volume optimizes preload. Patients with heart failure are operating on the plateau portion of a depressed left ventricular function curve (Fig. 19.1). Once the end-diastolic volume reaches the plateau, further elevations of preload do not improve stroke volume or ventricular performance and have an undesirable effect, namely, elevation of left ventricular end-diastolic pressure, elevated pulmonary capillary wedge pressure, and pulmonary edema (11, 13, 15). Further increases in end-diastolic volume increase left ventricular wall stress (La Place relationship) and in turn increase myocardial oxygen consumption, potentially precipitating acute ischemic events in patients with coronary artery disease (16). In some patients with heart failure, left ventricular dilation causes mitral regurgitation, adding a regurgitant volume load to an already compromised ventricle (103). Although elevation of end-diastolic volume is a useful mechanism in increasing cardiac performance, it can have deleterious effects on cardiac function once preload increases past the plateau of the Starling curve. In some patients, reduction of this inappropriately elevated preload (especially the pressure component) to prevent pulmonary congestion becomes important. This reduction can be performed clinically with diuretics, but vasodilators, with the ability to venodilate and increase the capacitance of the venous system, are also highly effective in reducing even severe elevations of ventricular end-diastolic pressure and volume (16, 29, 76).

A secondary compensatory mechanism in many patients with congestive heart failure is an increase in adrenergic stimulation of the heart, enhancing cardiac contractility and increasing heart rate and subsequently CO (121).

A third mechanism that serves to maintain blood pressure, presumably a response to depressed stroke volume, is elevated SVR (29, 117). This mechanism is at least partially mediated via baroreceptor activation of the sympathetic nervous system, increased activation of the renin-angiotensin system, accumulation of salt and water in blood vessel walls, and some other mechanisms (47, 117–120). Importantly, in many patients with heart failure, the SVR becomes inappropriately elevated, i.e., the resistance is higher than that

needed to maintain an adequate blood pressure, and is high enough to actually depress stroke volume because of the effect of an increased afterload on a dysfunctional ventricle (29). If this inappropriately high SVR is lowered with a vasodilator agent, stroke volume and CO may improve with little change in blood pressure. It is important to realize that this reflex increase in afterload does not depress stroke volume in a normal ventricle (Fig. 19.3) (107), but does reduce stroke volume in a dysfunctional and failing ventricle. Thus, paradoxically, one of the compensatory mechanisms (increased afterload) in the clinical syndrome of heart failure, in which a depression of stroke volume is likely to occur, may actually worsen overall cardiac performance.

Mechanism of Vasodilator Action

The major mechanism by which vasodilators increase CO and reduce ventricular filling pressures is by decreasing arterial and venous vasoconstriction. Vasodilators that cause predominantly arterial dilation reduce afterload or outflow impedance, and those that produce predominantly venodilation decrease preload (ventricular end-diastolic volume and/or pressure). Most vasodilators produce their effect by relaxing vascular smooth muscle in resistance and capacitance vessels. Some agents produce this relaxation by a direct smooth muscle effect, other agents stimulate or inhibit mechanisms that regulate smooth muscle tone.

The relationship of vascular resistance to the size of the vascular bed is expressed in Poiseuille's law:

$$\frac{\text{Resistance}}{\text{to flow}} = \frac{\text{viscosity} \times \text{vessel length} \times 8}{(\text{vessel radius})^4}$$

Resistance varies inversely with the vessel radius to the fourth power. The arterial vascular radius (or cross-sectional area) is determined largely by the smooth muscle tone in the arterioles, and this smooth muscle tone is the direct or indirect site of vasodilator action. Changes in smooth muscle tone have a different effect on the arterial and venous circulations. Increases in arteriolar vessel tone increase resistance to blood flow in the arterial circuit (i.e., increased afterload). Increases in venular and venous vessel tone decrease the amount of blood stored in the venous system. Since the venous system and venules have approximately 70–80% of the body's blood volume, venous vasoconstriction decreases the amount of blood returned to the heart (57, 80). When conceptualizing the circulatory system and comparing it to electrical systems, the arterial circuit is best considered as a resistor and the venous system as a capacitor circuit.

Different vasodilator agents may have effects on arteriolar vessel tone, venous vessel tone, or on a combination of arteriolar and venous tone. Further, vasodilators can have different effects on the systemic versus the pulmonary circulation (57). Depending on these effects and the baseline clinical hemodynamics, the ultimate effect or the general direction of hemodynamic change of a vasodilator agent can be predicted (Fig. 19.5). Although specific vasodilators are classified as venous or arterial in their action, none has "pure" effects on one circuit; nonetheless, the major effect is commonly regarded as predominantly arterial or venous.

In general, the goal of vasodilator therapy in heart failure is to improve CO by reducing unnecessary increases in afterload and to improve elevated ventricular filling pressures by

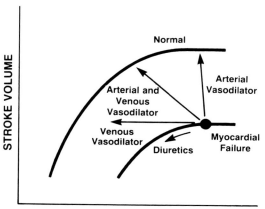

LEFT VENTRICULAR END DIASTOLIC VOLUME (Pressure)

Figure 19.5. Ability of different types of vasodilators to shift depressed ventricular function curve toward normal. Arterial vasodilators produce an increase in stroke volume with little or no changes in preload. Venous vasodilators produce a reduction in end-diastolic volume with little or no change in stroke volume. Vasodilators with both arterial and venous effects improve stroke volume and reduce filling pressures. An inotropic agent, along with a vasodilator, would shift the depressed curve even closer toward normal. At low levels of end-diastolic volume (on the slope rather than the plateau of the ventricular function curve), vasodilators may cause decreases in stroke volume and/or end-diastolic volume, resulting in decreased cardiac performance and hypotension. See text for details.

reducing preload. On the arterial side, a decrease in outflow impedance increases stroke volume and thus CO. In most patients with heart failure treated with vasodilators, the heart rate does not increase and the blood pressure decreases slightly or not at all. The lack of change in blood pressure is due to a proportional increase in stroke volume enhancing CO in response to the vasodilator-induced decrease in SVR (16, 29).

Thus, the vasodilator reverses an inappropriate elevated vascular resistance and induces a rise in CO. When this occurs, most patients report symptomatic improvement with decreased dyspnea and fatigue. Patients commonly demonstrate reversal of signs of poor organ perfusion such as mental obtundation, cool, clammy skin, and elevations of blood urea nitrogen secondary to depressed renal perfusion. Better renal perfusion increases the excretion of salt and water, which tends to decrease vascular filling pressures (16, 29, 57, 103). Decreased sodium concentrations in vessel walls further decrease vessel tone. If mitral or aortic regurgitation is a part of the cardiovascular pathophysiology, the regurgitant fraction is reduced with an increase in forward stroke volume.

Vasodilators become more effective as ventricular function worsens, and these agents can dramatically improve severe heart failure. Several studies have found a correlation between baseline CO and the vasodilator-induced increase in CO, i.e., the patients with the lowest resting CO have the best response to vasodilators (18, 42, 43, 45, 46, 73, 74, 82, 84). One study shows a strong positive correlation between the initial SVR and the ability of the vasodilators to reduce SVR, i.e., the highest impedance has the greatest chance of response (49). Most patients with severe myocardial dysfunction and failure have a steep impedance to stroke volume relationship (Fig. 19.3, *lower curve*) and decreasing impedance raises stroke volume. In contrast, patients with normal or near-normal cardiac function have no change in stroke volume with decreased impedance (Fig. 19.3, *upper curve*); the preload reduction depresses stroke volume because these patients are operating on the steep portion of the Starling curve, and the depressed stroke volume and CO may result in substantial decreases in blood pressure. The hypotensive effect is desirable in hypertensive patients, and vasodilator therapy is an effective antihypertensive regimen (90); however, in patients with severe heart failure, blood pressure usually changes minimally for the reasons enumerated above.

With venodilation, ventricular filling pressures decrease. Since most patients with heart failure are operating on the plateau portion of a depressed Starling curve (Fig. 19.1), reductions in preload generally do not reduce ventricular performance. However, reductions of filling pressures below a certain level reduce the stroke volume and can result in serious hypotension and/or a low output syndrome. The pulmonary capillary wedge pressure or left ventricular end-diastolic pressures can be reduced to approximately 15 mm Hg without affecting stroke volume in most patients; reductions below this level should be avoided because they depress stroke volume and CO (16, 29).

Despite many studies suggesting that vasodilator therapy in moderate to severe heart failure is not associated with an important blood pressure reduction, an occasional patient does develop symptomatic hypotension with vasodilator administration. If this occurs, one should suspect that the filling pressures are not elevated and preload has been reduced too low, or that ventricle function is only mildly impaired. Patients with obstructive cardiac lesions in whom forward output cannot be increased (e.g., aortic stenosis, mitral stenosis, or obstructive hypertrophic cardiomyopathy) also may have a hypotensive response to vasodilators. Patients with restrictive cardiomyopathy from amyloidosis or endomyocardial fibrosis are also prone to hypotensive responses to vasodilators in the author's experience. After the above possible causes of a hypotensive reaction to vasodilators are considered, an occasional patient with proven high filling pressures and poor CO, in severe heart failure, does not tolerate vasodilator therapy because of hypotension. It is assumed that this patient has not developed the usual inappropriate elevation of SVR seen in most patients with severe heart failure, though the reasons for this fact remain obscure.

Cellular and Biochemical Mechanisms Involved in Vasodilator Actions

The final common pathway of vasodilator effect is to relax vascular smooth muscle tone. At the cellular and biochemical level, three major classes of vasodilators are presently recognized to produce this vasodilation: (a) direct smooth muscle relaxers, as exemplified by nitroprusside, nitrates, hydralazine, and minoxidil; (b) sympathetic nervous system blocking agents that negate α-adrenergic stimulation, e.g., phentolamine, prazosin, and trimethaphan; and (c) inhibitors of the renin-angiotensin system, e.g., saralasin and captopril. Much of the clinical experience with vasodilators has been gained with the direct-acting smooth muscle relaxers such as nitroprusside in the acute setting and hydralazine and/or nitrates in chronic heart failure; however, more experience is accumulating with sympathetic and renin-angiotensin blockers. The specific mechanisms of action of the individual vasodilator agents are considered below ("Specific Vasodilator Agents").

Effects of Vasodilators on Myocardial Ischemia

An area of myocardial ischemia represents an imbalance between myocardial oxygen demand and supply. In patients with coronary artery disease, blood supply is limited by coronary artery narrowing and, in some patients, by coronary spasm (10, 62, 105). When myocardial oxygen demand increases, blood cannot reach certain areas of myocardium, which then become segmentally ischemic and dysfunctional. The major determinants of myocardial oxygen consumption are arterial (or ventricular) systolic pressure, heart rate, heart size, and the ventricular contractile state. Arterial systolic pressure and heart size are the major determinants of wall stress, according to the La Place relationship (11–13). Vasodilators have a number of mechanisms for favorably altering the balance between myocardial oxygen demand by decreasing preload and reducing ventricular size, and the ventricular pressure also reduces myocardial oxygen needs.

Vasodilators can increase blood flow to an ischemic area by reducing vasoconstrictor influences in the collateral flow to ischemic zones. Vasodilators reduce end-diastolic pressures, favoring subendocardial flow. Several studies have shown that segmental wall motion abnormalities are improved following nitroglycerin administration (61), providing evidence that certain vasodilators can influence the myocardial oxygen supply/demand balance favorably. The ultimate effect of a vasodilator on ischemic myocardium in a particular patient depends on a number of factors: the baseline hemodynamic state of the ventricle, the coronary anatomy and collateral flow, and the type of vasodilator employed. Conflicting and contradictory results are common in this field. Some have reported that nitroglycerin decreases, whereas nitroprusside increases, evidence of myocardial ischemia (22). Others have reported that nitroprusside can decrease the ST segment, evidence of ischemia (5). Two large, controlled studies investigated the effects of nitroprusside infusion in patients with acute myocardial infarction (30, 38). One study found a statistically significant reduction in mortality in the nitroprusside group, along with a nitroprusside-induced reduction in the incidence of cardiogenic shock, clinical signs of heart failure, and levels of creatine kinase isoenzymes (38). In a second multicenter trial, nitroprusside was not associated with any change in overall mortality when given to patients with myocardial infarction and a pulmonary capillary wedge pressure greater than 12 mm Hg (30). In this latter study, patients whose nitroprusside infusions were begun within 9 hours of chest pain had an increased mortality, whereas infusions begun later were associated with a decreased mortality. These two studies do not lend themselves to a simple interpretation of the effect of this vasodilator agent on myocardial ischemia in the postinfarction phase of acute myocardial infarction. Nonetheless, the two studies were well controlled and properly performed, and the contradictory results argue for the complexity of predicting the response of vasodilators in patients with myocardial ischemia. Further, large trials are necessary to determine which subsets of patients with acute myocardial infarction benefit from vasodilator therapy.

Effect of Vasodilators on Ventricular Compliance

Another possible mechanism by which vasodilators improve ventricular function is induction of an increase in ventricular compliance (17, 96). The volume-pressure relationship of the ventricle is curvilinear (Fig. 19.2). At small end-diastolic volumes, ventricular size can change with little change in pressure; at higher ventricular volumes, a small change in volume produces a much greater pressure rise. If a pharmacologic agent shifts the volume-pressure curve to the right, there is a greater increase in end-diastolic volume without

reaching a ventricular pressure that induces pulmonary edema. Assuming one has not reached the plateau portion of the Starling curve (Fig. 19.1), this increased volume at lower pressure produces better ventricular performance.

Studies suggest that vasodilators improve ventricular compliance (11, 71, 72, 97, 100), though further investigation is necessary to decide if this is an important mechanism of vasodilator-induced improvement in ventricular performance. The mechanism of this improvement in compliance is not clear. Some investigators postulate a reduction in ischemia, others argue for an intrinsic increase in ventricular relaxation (14, 17), or right ventricular relaxation causing increased left ventricular compliance within a confined pericardial space (32, 72). Further studies are needed to determine the true mechanism of vasodilator-induced increases in compliance.

Vasodilator-Induced Redistribution Effects

Most of the literature on vasodilators focuses on their ability to reduce afterload and/or preload and improve ventricular performance. Another potentially important capability of vasodilators in critical care medicine is reduction or redistribution of blood flow away from certain nonessential vascular beds and toward vital areas. For example, patients with septic shock commonly have a high CO, low filling pressures, and a low overall peripheral vascular resistance; however, many organs in the body are not receiving appropriate blood supply as evidenced by lactic acidosis and progressive organ system dysfunction, e.g., rising blood urea nitrogen with renal dysfunction. In this setting, the appropriate vasodilator could potentially redirect blood flow toward the vital organs. Many forms of shock are postulated to have inappropriate sympathetic outflow causing arteriolar vasoconstriction; some investigators advocate vasodilators in the treatment of shock (100). However, in shock, where one is faced with hypotension that is commonly difficult to control, vasodilators may further decrease blood pressure. In the absence of clear efficacy and with the potential of worsening already existing hypotension, vasodilators are not widely accepted in the treatment of noncardiogenic shock.

In cardiogenic shock and severe intractable

heart failure (32, 58), vasodilator therapy increases stroke volume and CO, and in some cases reverses cardiogenic shock. Commonly, vasodilator therapy in cardiogenic shock is used in conjunction with an inotropic agent such as dopamine (79, 87) or with intraaortic balloon counterpulsation (59). In severe heart failure, the body's compensatory mechanisms (sympathetic outflow, the renin-angiotensin system, and the organ's autoregulatory capacity) redistribute blood flow to preferentially maintain cerebral and coronary perfusion. In this setting, renal perfusion does not change or fall, and flow to the mesenteric and limb circulations is considerably diminished (122). If vasodilator therapy increases CO, flow to these vascular beds increases. In cardiogenic shock, the body's compensatory mechanisms are redistributing a very reduced CO to those organs of vital importance to survival. In other forms of shock (e.g., septic shock), there is an adequate or increased CO, but the distribution of flow is commonly inappropriate, resulting in lactic acidosis and vital organ dysfunction. The cause of this inappropriate redistribution of flow in septic shock, and whether vasodilators can redirect the flow, are questions that are unanswered and will require further study.

Vasodilator Therapy in Mechanical Defects

Patients with mitral regurgitation, aortic regurgitation, or a ventricular septal defect frequently respond to vasodilator therapy with an improvement in their hemodynamics and clinical symptoms of heart failure (9, 20). Although the definitive treatment for these mechanical lesions is corrective cardiac surgery, vasodilator therapy can be employed when surgery is not possible or when it is wise to defer surgery.

In mitral regurgitation, the severity of the regurgitation is dependent on the degree of anatomic derangement of the mitral apparatus as well as aortic outflow impedance (20, 96). Increasing afterload increases the regurgitant fraction (11, 12); vasodilator-induced reduction of aortic impedance should decrease regurgitation through the mitral valve. A number of clinical studies have documented that vasodilator-induced reductions in SVR produce marked hemodynamic improvements in patients with mitral regurgitations (20, 52, 56, 60, 116). Nitroprusside increases forward stroke volume and CO (mean increase, approximately

50%), decreases regurgitant volumes, decreases pulmonary artery and capillary wedge pressures, and causes large V waves in the pulmonary capillary wedge tracing to decrease markedly or disappear. These effects are a result of vasodilator-induced redistribution of the left ventricular stroke volume, causing more blood to be ejected into the aorta than into the left atrium. The major mechanism for this effect is a reduction of aortic impedance; however, a reduction in ventricular size with closer approximation of mitral leaflets and, in some cases, a reduction of papillary muscle ischemia may also contribute to the vasodilator-induced improvement in regurgitation.

In severe aortic regurgitation, the body may reflexly increase SVR to maintain blood pressure and thereby initiate a vicious cycle that increases regurgitation further. Nitroprusside is capable of reducing the aortic regurgitant fraction and increasing the forward stroke volume in chronic aortic regurgitation (9, 14, 81, 112). Vasodilators also produce increases in forward CO in acute aortic regurgitation (96).

In a large ventricular septal defect, the magnitude of the left-to-right shunt is largely determined by the ratio of the vascular resistances in the pulmonary versus systemic circuits. A reduction in SVR decreases the left-to-right shunt and favors flow from the left ventricle to the aorta, i.e., it increases systemic CO. Nitroprusside induces a favorable hemodynamic response in patients with acute ventricular septal defects complicating myocardial infarction (110). It should be recognized that if vasodilator therapy reduces pulmonary more than systemic resistance, the left-to-right shunt increases and systemic flow decreases. One must repeatedly measure flows and shunts to be sure that a sustained beneficial effect is resulting from such therapy.

Effect of Vasodilator Therapy on Mortality in Patients with Moderate to Severe Congestive Heart Failure

Vasodilators have been shown to produce profound changes in cardiovascular physiology, especially in patients with moderate to severe congestive heart failure. There is no question that vasodilator therapy can decrease elevated filling pressures and increase cardiac output and stroke volume in many patients with significant heart failure. Concomitant with these improved hemodynamics, many patients note a decrease in symptomatology and improvement in signs of heart failure: decreased dyspnea, improved energy, and improved organ blood flow and function. However, one of the most important but unanswered questions regarding vasodilator therapy is its effect on survival of patients with such severe heart failure.

Although retrospective studies have suggested that vasodilator-treated patients fare better, only in the past year have two excellent studies appeared that directly address this question. A Veterans Administration Cooperative Study at multiple centers assigned 642 men with heart failure already receiving digitalis and diuretics to receive additional double-blind treatment with (a) placebo, (b) prazosin (20 mg/day), or (c) a combination of hydralazine (300 mg/day) and isosorbide dinitrate (160 mg/day) (26, 27). The mortality in the hydralazine/isosorbide dinitrate group was lower than that in the placebo group throughout the entire follow-up period (average, 2.3 years). The mortality risk reduction in the group treated with hydralazine/isosorbide dinitrate was 36% by 3 years. The mortality in the prazosin group was similar to that in the placebo group. Further, the serially determined left ventricular ejection fraction increased in the hydralazine/isosorbide dinitrate group but not in the placebo or prazosin groups. Thus, this study demonstrates that addition of hydralazine/isosorbide dinitrate to digitalis/diuretic therapy can result in improved left ventricular function and decreased mortality.

An even more recent prospective, double-blind analysis evaluated the effect of an angiotensin-converting enzyme inhibitor, enalapril, in 253 patients under treatment for severe heart failure (33). The enalapril group had a highly significant 27% increase in mortality compared with the placebo group. Interestingly, the entire reduction in total mortality was found to be among patients with progressive heart failure, and no reduction was seen in the incidence of sudden cardiac death.

These two studies demonstrate that some vasodilators have the ability to decrease mortality as well as improve the hemodynamics and symptoms of chronic severe heart failure. If these results are confirmed, vasodilator therapy will be indicated in all moderate to severe chronic heart failure patients to induce the improvement in mortality. The inability of prazosin to produce an improvement in survival suggests that this agent lacks the pharmacologic action or consistency (tachyphylaxis occurs with this agent; see the section

"Prazosin" below) to produce a favorable response.

The studies were performed on patients with chronic severe heart failure. Whether vasodilators would also demonstrate an improvement in survival when used in critically ill patients with acute heart failure has not been evaluated. It will require further clinical investigation. However, the ability of vasodilators to improve mortality in chronic heart failure suggests that these agents can produce a favorable response in cardiovascular performance, and may have a positive role in other clinical settings. Which specific vasodilator agent will prove to be best in specific settings will require further clinical investigation.

SPECIFIC VASODILATOR AGENTS

Clinically, the most useful method of classifying vasodilator agents is based on their major peripheral vascular actions (Fig. 19.5, Table 19.1) (121). One group of vasodilators is considered to have its major effect by dilating arterioles, a second group dilates predominantly veins and venules, and a third group has relatively equal effects dilating arterioles and veins ("balanced" vasodilation). In general, vasodilators that affect arterioles increase CO through an enhanced stroke volume but have little or no effect on pulmonary or systemic venous pressures. Agents that dilate veins and venules reduce pulmonary and systemic venous pressures with little or no change in CO. Vasodilators with effects on both the arterial and venous circuits reduce pulmonary and systemic venous hypertension and increase CO (Fig. 19.5).

Although this classification is clinically useful, it has several limitations. Of the presently available vasodilator agents, none has pure

Table 19.1
Vasodilators Classified by Their Principal Site of Action

Arterial and venous vasodilators—"balanced vasodilators"
Nitroprusside
Phentolamine
Prazosin
Captopril
Nifedipine
Arterial vasodilators
Hydralazine
Minoxidil
Venous vasodilators
Nitrates (nitroglycerin, isosorbide dinitrate)

arteriolar or venodilator properties; all have some effect on both circuits, though certain agents have such a predominant effect on the arteriolar or venous side that they are best regarded as arteriolar or venous vasodilators. Perhaps the most accurate representation of these vasodilator properties would be as a spectrum of effects ranging from pure venodilation to balanced venous and arteriolar effects to pure arteriolar dilation. A second limitation is that the hemodynamic response to any vasodilator depends on the baseline hemodynamic status of the patient (see "Mechanism of Vasodilator Action"). Patients' responses to the same vasodilator agent are usually variable and one must consider this fact when instituting therapy. Despite these limitations, the classification proposed (Table 19.1) is highly useful both conceptually and clinically and allows prediction of a vasodilator's probable site of action and probable hemodynamic outcome.

In the critical care setting, use of rapidly acting parenteral vasodilator agents predominates, and therefore the emphasis is on parenteral (usually intravenous) vasodilator agents. However, some mention is also made of nonparenteral agents that are of use in the intensive care unit.

Arterial and Venous Vasodilators

NITROPRUSSIDE

Because of its rapid onset of action, rapid reversibility when discontinued, relatively specific effect on vascular smooth muscle, balanced effect on the arteriolar and venous systems, and lack of tachyphylaxis, nitroprusside is the vasodilator of choice for many situations in the critical care unit.

Nitroprusside has both an interesting history and chemistry. It was originally used in the 1850s as a chemical color indicator. Its hypotensive properties were not described until 1929 (64). The chemical structure of nitroprusside contains five cyanide groups per molecule (28, 95), and concern about cyanide toxicity delayed development of the agent as a pharmaceutical until 1955 when its safety and potent hypotensive effects were demonstrated in a group of hypertensive patients (94). In 1972, nitroprusside was shown to improve left ventricular function in patients with acute myocardial infarction (46), and subsequent studies have shown the drug's ability to improve left ventricular function in severe heart failure due to ischemic heart disease, cardio-

myopathy, or cardiac regurgitant lesions (9, 14, 20, 32, 58).

Nitroprusside causes direct relaxation of arterial and venous smooth muscle. At therapeutic doses, it has no effect on uterine or duodenal smooth muscle or on myocardial contractility (28). Nitroprusside relaxes the lower esophageal sphincter (36); however, in general the drug affects vascular smooth muscle in a relatively specific manner. Nitroprusside-induced vascular smooth muscle relaxation is not dependent on the sympathetic nervous system or adrenergic receptors. Its cellular mechanism of action is unknown, though possible mechanisms include interaction with intracellular sulfhydryl groups, inhibition of calcium transport, or changes in intracellular cyclic nucleotides (103).

Nitroprusside is useful for all of the clinical indications outlined below ("Clinical Indications for Vasodilator Therapy"). It is the classical example of a balanced vasodilator with capability to reduce both pulmonary venous and systemic venous pressures as well as to increase stroke volume and CO in patients with severe heart failure. Heart rate usually decreases slightly or remains unchanged, and blood pressure may fall slightly or remain unchanged. Concomitant with this salutary hemodynamic effect, most patients have symptomatic improvement with relief of dyspnea, lessened fatigue, warming of the skin, and diuresis (16, 29, 46, 58).

In patients with severe heart failure requiring intensive care, nitroprusside therapy should be initiated and continued using constant arterial pressure monitoring and employing a Swan-Ganz pulmonary artery catheter to determine serial pulmonary artery pressures, pulmonary capillary wedge pressures, and thermodilution COs. Nitroprusside has an onset of action within seconds of initiating the drug, and its duration of effect is only 1–3 minutes, allowing slow increase of the dose every few minutes while watching the arterial pressure carefully. Serial determinations of hemodynamic values allow correlation of clinical with hemodynamic improvement. Once an optimal pulmonary capillary wedge pressure (usually 14–18 mm Hg) and maximal CO are achieved, oral vasodilator agents can be started and nitroprusside tapered. Serial hemodynamics can again help determine the optimal dose and combination of vasodilator agents for a particular patient.

The major complication of nitroprusside therapy is hypotension. Most patients with severe heart failure respond to relatively low doses of nitroprusside with an increase in CO and only minimal decreases in pressure; however, patients with low filling pressures commonly respond to nitroprusside with a reduced CO and hypotension due to inadequate preload (Fig. 19.1). Some authors recommend that vasodilators not be used with a diastolic pressure of less than 60 mm Hg (16, 96), but others state that nitroprusside therapy can be used in most patients with systolic pressures between 90 and 105 mm Hg without precipitating hypotension (28). Most patients whose blood pressure decreases with nitroprusside respond to discontinuation of the drug, and the nitroprusside can usually then be restarted at a lower dosage. A hypotensive response to nitroprusside should always cause the physician to consider whether the filling pressures are lower than suspected. Profound hypotension with nitroprusside that does not respond to discontinuation of infusion and fluid administration within a few minutes should be treated with an inotropic agent such as dopamine; this therapy usually restores blood pressure promptly.

For patients with severe heart failure, a nitroprusside infusion is started at 10 μg/min and may be increased by 10 μg/min increments every 5–15 minutes. There is great variability in individual responses to nitroprusside, but most patients with heart failure show a positive response by 1–2 μg/kg/min (approximately 70–140 μg/min) with a drop in the pulmonary capillary wedge pressure and/or an increase in CO. Although hemodynamic responses are highly variable, a decrease of 20–50% in wedge pressure and an increase of 20–40% in CO are considered positive responses to nitroprusside. In patients with pulmonary edema with hypertension, nitroprusside is started at 10 μg/min but is increased by 20 μg/min increments every 3–5 minutes in order to rapidly reduce filling pressures and relieve symptoms. When nitroprusside is used for hypertension, usually the doses required to decrease blood pressure are considerably higher than those to treat heart failure.

Other than hypotension, the other major side effects of nitroprusside are thiocyanate/cyanide toxicity and mild reductions in arterial oxygen tension due to nitroprusside-induced inhibition of the pulmonary vasoconstrictor response (85, 101). Thiocyanate toxicity is manifest by confusion, hyperreflexia, and convulsions; cyanide toxicity is first manifest by a metabolic acidosis due to cyanide combining with cytochromes and inhibiting aerobic cellular metabolism. Thiocyanate or cyanide toxicity occurs almost exclusively in patients receiving high doses of nitroprusside for a prolonged period. Infusion rates of less than 3 μg/kg/min for less than 72 hours are not associated with toxicity.

Deaths during long infusions of high doses of nitroprusside have been ascribed to cyanide toxicity. Cyanide conversion to thiocyanate is facilitated by thiosulfate, sodium nitrate, or hydroxycobalamin (25, 34), and these three agents should be considered as therapy in patients demonstrating toxicity from nitroprusside with metabolic acidosis and confusion when discontinuation of the nitroprusside does not reverse the toxicity. Monitoring blood thiocyanate levels is useful to follow toxicity in patients requiring infusions for longer than 2–3 days. Levels of thiocyanate below 10 mg/dl are considered safe.

On rapid discontinuation of a nitroprusside infusion, a rebound beyond the prenitroprusside baseline occurs, with an increase in SVR, increase in pulmonary capillary wedge pressure, and decrease in CO (92). This phenomenon probably results from vasodilator-induced activation of the sympathetic and renin-angiotensin systems. A slow nitroprusside taper while instituting oral vasodilator therapy usually avoids this rebound depression of cardiac performance.

PHENTOLAMINE

Phentolamine was the first vasodilator used clinically to improve cardiovascular performance in heart failure (75). It is considered one of the classical α-adrenergic blocking agents and causes blockade at both the postsynaptic (α_1) and presynaptic (α_2) receptors. Its potent vasodilator capabilities are secondary to both α blockade (53, 103) and a direct vasodilator effect on vascular smooth muscle (109). Norepinephrine release may actually increase reflexly because of baroreceptor activation caused by the fall in blood pressure and the blockade of the presynaptic α_2-receptors, the inhibition promoting further release. This circulating norepinephrine frequently results in a tachycardia and positive cardiac inotropic stimulation.

Phentolamine can relax arteriolar as well as venous vascular smooth muscle and thus can increase CO and reduce pulmonary and systemic venous pressures in patients with moderate to severe heart failure of all etiologies.

The ability of phentolamine to increase CO is comparable with that of nitroprusside; however, it produces less of a decrease in filling pressures. The ability of phentolamine to increase CO and its less than expected decreases in venous tone may be caused by the enhanced release of norepinephrine, which increases cardiac contractility and heightens venous vasoconstriction. Although phentolamine is generally well tolerated in ischemic cardiac failure, the tachycardia and norepinephrine release can worsen ischemia in patients with coronary artery disease.

Phentolamine is given as an intravenous infusion starting at 0.1 mg/min and increasing slowly up to 2 mg/min in increments of 0.2–0.4 mg/min every 10–30 minutes. Hemodynamic effects occur at 15 minutes, usually peak by 30 minutes, and persist up to 60 minutes after the drug is stopped. The drug can be given orally in doses of 50–150 mg every 4–6 hours.

In addition to the tachycardia, the major side effects of phentolamine are gastrointestinal: vomiting, abdominal pain, diarrhea, and hypermotility. Because tolerance to the drug develops rapidly, phentolamine is only used on an acute basis.

PRAZOSIN

Prazosin is a selective α_1 (postsynaptic) adrenergic receptor antagonist that causes arteriolar and venous vasodilation exclusively by its receptor-blocking effects (54, 106). Since it is only available in oral form, its use in the intensive care environment is as a subacute or chronic agent after therapy is initiated with a parenteral vasodilator. In patients with heart failure, prazosin has balanced hemodynamic actions similar to those of nitroprusside, with elevation in CO and reductions in systemic and pulmonary venous pressures (55).

Prazosin is well absorbed from the gastrointestinal tract and is given in doses of 1–10 mg every 6–8 hours. Its onset of action is 30–60 minutes, with maximal hemodynamic effect at 2–6 hours post dose. In many patients, the first dose of drug will produce orthostatic syncope, so patients should be warned to rise slowly from the supine position.

A subset of patients develop tachyphylaxis to the beneficial hemodynamic effect of this drug after several days of therapy (4, 37, 89). The mechanism is unknown, but increasing the drug dose or adding diuretics does not help. If tachyphylaxis occurs, prazosin should be discontinued and another vasodilator used.

CAPTOPRIL

With the onset of moderate to severe heart failure, the renin-angiotensin-aldosterone system is activated and serves as an important compensatory mechanism to maintain blood pressure and cause volume retention. In advanced heart failure, some of the "inappropriate" increase in afterload may be maintained by the vasoconstrictor substance, angiotensin II. Inhibition of the renin-angiotensin system reduces afterload or impedance and enhances cardiac performance. A number of inhibitors of the renin-angiotensin system are being tested and presently captopril, an inhibitor of angiotensin-converting enzyme, is one of the pharmaceutical agents commercially available.

In patients with heart failure, captopril produces a hemodynamic pattern similar to that seen with nitroprusside (69) or prazosin (65). From what is known of angiotensin II physiology, one would predict that a pure inhibitor of angiotensin II production would cause a reduction in afterload with little effect on preload. Yet captopril does reduce preload, prompting some to argue that captopril has an additional mechanism of action causing vasodilation. The mechanism of captopril-induced vasodilation is unknown, but it is postulated to be due to inhibition of the enzyme that degrades bradykinin leading to an increase in the circulating level of this potent vasodilator (39).

Captopril is only available in an oral preparation, and therapy is started with 25 mg every 6 hours and increased to a maximum daily dosage of 450 mg. Onset of a hemodynamic change is within 30 minutes, with peak effect at 1–3 hours and disappearance by 4–8 hours. The duration of the hemodynamic effect is dose-dependent, but the magnitude is not. Tolerance to the drug does not develop in patients treated for as long as 6–12 months.

NIFEDIPINE

Calcium channel blockers inhibit the contraction of vascular smooth muscle and therefore have vasodilator properties; however, few studies are available to evaluate the efficacy of these agents in heart failure. In one study, patients in cardiogenic pulmonary edema were treated with nifedipine (10 mg sublingually), causing reduction in symptoms of dyspnea, decreases in systemic and pulmonary venous pressures, and a rise in CO (102). Nifedipine also produces a sustained hemodynamic improvement in patients with chronic heart failure (7). Many clinicians are reluctant to use calcium channel blockers in heart failure because these agents have a direct depressant effect on the myocardium. With nifedipine, the decrease in afterload is more profound than the myocardial depressant effect, resulting in overall enhanced hemodynamics.

Verapamil, another calcium channel blocker, has vasodilator properties but its direct myocardial depressant effect is more profound, and this may seriously aggravate heart failure in patients with severe myocardial dysfunction.

Arterial Vasodilators

HYDRALAZINE

Hydralazine has been used in the treatment of hypertension for 30 years. It is a potent direct dilator of vascular smooth muscle and mostly affects arterioles. In patients with heart failure, hydralazine produces impressive increases in stroke volume by reducing arteriolar resistance and has no effect or only a modest lowering effect on systemic or pulmonary venous pressures (9, 21). For a given change in blood pressure, hydralazine increases CO more than nitroprusside or nitrates. There is conflicting evidence whether hydralazine has a reflex or direct cardiac inotropic effect as an explanation for its potent ability to increase CO (91, 103). Hydralazine can also increase limb and renal blood flow, thus promoting diuresis.

When using hydralazine in a critical care setting, intravenous administration is the most reliable route, but it must be given slowly and with constant hemodynamic monitoring to avoid hypotension. Administration should begin with 5–10 mg given as a slow intravenous drip over 20 minutes. Maximal effect occurs 15–45 minutes after injection and the effect can last 4–24 hours. One can administer up to 20 mg intravenously every 6 hours. Given orally, the dosage is usually 25–100 mg every 6 hours, with onset of action at 60 minutes and peak effect at 2–3 hours. Some studies suggest that high doses of hydralazine (150–200 mg)

are necessary in some patients to produce a beneficial effect on cardiac performance (19, 90); the need for this high oral dose in some patients may be due to mesenteric venous hypertension causing malabsorption of the drug.

A small number of patients with heart failure develop tachycardia with hydralazine administration. Exacerbation of angina pectoris can occur with hydralazine, especially (but not exclusively) in patients with ischemic heart disease who develop a tachycardia during therapy (66). Prolonged administration of hydralazine is associated with a lupus-like syndrome in 10–20% of patients, especially in those taking more than 400 mg daily (2).

MINOXIDIL

Minoxidil is a potent, direct-acting, vascular smooth muscle relaxant that acts largely on the arterial bed (48). In doses of 5–20 mg orally, the drug produces hemodynamic effects similar to those of hydralazine in patients with heart failure, i.e., a rise in CO, decrease in SVR, and no change in pulmonary venous (or arterial) pressure (44). Side effects include hirsutism and pericardial effusion. Minoxidil is presently being tested on large populations and, if it has fewer side effects than hydralazine, it may become the arterial vasodilator of choice.

Venous Vasodilators

Organic esters of nitric acid have been established therapy for angina pectoris for more than 100 years. Only in the past 10 years have they been used to treat congestive heart failure. Nitrates have a direct smooth muscle–relaxing capability, especially on vascular smooth muscle. Recent evidence suggests that nitrates may act on smooth muscle by releasing prostacyclin (a potent vasodilator) from vessel endothelial cells (68).

In patients with heart failure, the most prominent action of nitrates is to lower ventricular filling pressures by dilation of pulmonary and systemic veins (51). The volume of the left and right ventricles decreases and the compliance of the left ventricle increases (35, 71). The mechanism of this improved compliance is unclear; however, it may result from altered constraints on the left ventricle due to a decrease in right ventricle size.

Nitrates also decrease arterial vascular resistance, but CO may increase, remain unchanged, or decrease in response to nitrates (103). In some patients treated with nitrates, the CO does not increase because a concomitant fall in preload causes a depression in stroke volume (17, 96). Other patients not showing an increase in CO in response to nitrates have received a dose that is insufficient to produce a significant fall in impedance. At lower doses of nitrate, the vasodilatory effect is largely on the venous system with decreases in filling pressures. At higher nitrate doses, impedance falls and CO rises. As with nitroprusside, the increase in CO with nitrates is proportional to the reduction in SVR (42, 93) and is inversely correlated with the patient's baseline CO (42, 74, 93). Some authors note a positive correlation between baseline SVR and the nitrate-induced rise in CO (49), although others do not support this finding (3, 93).

The effects of nitrates and nitroprussides on ischemic heart disease were considered above ("Effects of Vasodilators on Myocardial Ischemia").

In an intensive care environment, the optimal nitrate preparation is intravenous nitroglycerin because it allows exact titration of dose and the ability to quickly terminate drug infusion. It is important to be certain that the left ventricular filling pressures are high or optimal because even low doses of nitroglycerin can precipitously decrease filling pressures. Intravenous infusions should begin at 10 μg/min, and one can increase the dosage in increments of 10 μg/min every 5–10 minutes to a dose of 50–100 μg/min. Most patients demonstrate a vasodilator effect at this dose, but up to 400 μg/min can be given if clinically indicated. High doses of nitroglycerin are well tolerated for several days. Treatment can then be changed to oral isosorbide dinitrate, 20–100 mg every 4 hours, nitroglycerin ointment, $\frac{1}{2}$–$1\frac{1}{2}$ inches every 4 hours, or a transdermal delivery system for nitroglycerin (1, 111).

Side effects of nitrate therapy include headache, which usually abates after several days, if therapy is continued. A nitrate withdrawal syndrome occurs in nitroglycerin factory workers and consists of coronary-like chest pain and acute myocardial infarction. Because of the sustained high doses of nitrates presently being employed, patients on high sustained nitrate regimens must be told not to discontinue therapy abruptly.

Nitrates and hydralazine are used together to combine nitrate-induced reductions in filling pressures with hydralazine's ability to increase CO, producing an oral regimen comparable with that of nitroprusside (66, 77, 78). The hemodynamic changes seen with the combination are roughly additive (67, 77, 78), and are similar to those produced by nitroprusside. As with all vasodilator regimens, hypotension can complicate this therapy and necessitate alteration in dosage or discontinuation of one of the drugs.

CLINICAL INDICATIONS FOR VASODILATOR THERAPY

The following are the clinical situations in which vasodilator therapy is beneficial:

1. Severe heart failure unresponsive to diuretics and digitalis. Vasodilators are most efficacious in patients with low CO, high left ventricular filling pressures, and elevated SVR.

2. Acute cardiogenic pulmonary edema. Vasodilator therapy with acute vasodilation can rapidly reduce high filling pressures and reverse symptoms. Vasodilators can be used in conjunction with supplemental oxygen, rotating tourniquets, morphine, and intravenous diuretics.

3. Acute or chronic mitral regurgitation, aortic regurgitation, or ventricular septal defect. Vasodilator-induced decreases in SVR increase forward (systemic) CO. Vasodilators are usually employed in these situations as a temporizing measure to allow time to prepare the patient for cardiac surgery.

4. Based on present data, vasodilators are not recommended for the routine therapy of patients with acute myocardial infarction. Nitrate therapy is useful in treating stable and unstable angina. Vasodilators such as nitroprusside can reduce myocardial oxygen consumption in patients with persistent chest pain who are hypertensive. In normotensive patients with myocardial infarction and no or only mild to moderate heart failure, the effectiveness of vasodilator therapy is not proven. As noted above, vasodilators are useful in severe heart failure.

5. In patients with cardiogenic shock, vasodilator therapy combined with inotropic drugs (e.g., dopamine) or intraaortic balloon counterpulsation can produce substantial hemodynamic improvement.

6. As reviewed in other chapters of this book, vasodilators are highly useful to treat hypertension, malignant hypertension, and dissecting aortic aneurysms (in conjunction

with β-blockade), and are possibly useful in primary pulmonary hypertension.

Acknowledgments

The author thanks Ms. Kathy Kiefer for her excellent secretarial assistance and Ms. Sandy Montgomery for her superb administrative and editorial assistance.

References

1. Abrams JA: Nitroglycerin and long-acting nitrates. *N Engl J Med* 302:1234–1237, 1980.
2. Alarcon-Segovia D: Drug-induced antinuclear antibodies and lupus syndromes. *Drugs* 12:69–77, 1976.
3. Armstrong PW, Armstrong JA, Markes CS: Pharmacokinetic hemodynamic studies of intravenous nitroglycerin in congestive heart failure. *Circulation* 62:160–166, 1980.
4. Arnold SB, Williams RL, Ports TA, Baughman RA, Benet LZ, Parmley WW, Chatterjee K: Attenuation of prazosin effect on cardiac output in chronic heart failure. *Ann Intern Med* 91:345–349, 1979.
5. Awan NA, Miller RR, Zakanddin V, DeMaria AN, Amsterdam EA, Mason DT: Reduction of ST segment elevation with infusion of nitroprusside in patients with acute myocardial infarction. *Am J Cardiol* 38:425–439, 1976.
6. Bache RJ, Dymek DJ: Local and regional regulation of coronary vascular tone. *Prog Cardiovasc Dis* 24:191–212, 1981.
7. Bellocuui F, Ansalone G, Scabia E, Viencenzo A, Peitro S, Laperfido F, Paolo Z: Sustained beneficial effect of nifedipine in chronic refractory heart failure. *Am J Cardiol* 47:407, 1981.
8. Bemis CF, Serue JR, Borkenhagen D, Sonnenblick EH, Urschel CW: Influence of right ventricular filling pressure on left ventricular pressure and dimension. *Circ Res* 34:498–504, 1974.
9. Bolen JL, Alderman EL: Hemodynamic consequence of afterload reduction in patients with chronic aortic regurgitation. *Circulation* 53:879–883, 1976.
10. Braunwald E: Control of myocardial oxygen consumption. *Am J Cardiol* 27:416–432, 1971.
11. Braunwald E: Pathophysiology of heart failure. In Braunwald E (ed): *Heart Disease: A Textbook of Cardiovascular Medicine*, ed 3. Philadelphia, WB Saunders, 1988, pp 426–448.
12. Braunwald E, Ross J, Sonneblick EH: *Mechanisms of Contraction of the Normal and Failing Heart*. Boston, Little, Brown & Co, 1976.
13. Braunwald E, Sonnenblick EH, Ross J: Contraction of the normal heart. In Braunwald E (ed): *Heart Disease: A Textbook of Cardiovascular Medicine*. Philadelphia, WB Saunders, 1980.
14. Brodie BR, Grossman W, Mann T, McLaurin LP: Effects of sodium nitroprusside on left ventricular diastolic pressure/volume relations. *J Clin Invest* 59:59–68, 1977.
15. Burns JW, Covell JW, Ross J: Mechanics of isotonic left ventricular contractions. *Am J Physiol* 224:725–732, 1973.
16. Chatterjee K, Parmley WW: The role of vasodilator therapy in heart failure. *Prog Cardiovasc Dis* 19:301–325, 1977.
17. Chatterjee K, Parmley WW: Vasodilator therapy for chronic heart failure. *Annu Rev Pharmacol Toxicol* 20:475–512, 1980.
18. Chatterjee K, Parmley WW, Ganz W, Forrester J, Walinsky P, Crexells C: Hemodynamic and metabolic responses to vasodilator therapy in the acute myocardial infarction. *Circulation* 48:1183–1193, 1973.
19. Chatterjee K, Parmley WW, Massie B: Oral hydralazine therapy for chronic refractory heart failure. *Circulation* 54:879–883, 1976.
20. Chatterjee K, Parmley WW, Swan HJ, Berman G, Forrester J: Beneficial effects of vasodilator agents in severe mitral regurgitation due to dysfunction of subvalvular apparatus. *Circulation* 48:684–690, 1973.
21. Chatterjee K, Ports TA, Brundage BH, Massie B, Holly AN, Parmley WW: Oral hydralazine in chronic heart failure: sustained beneficial hemodynamic effects. *Ann Intern Med* 92:600–604, 1980.
22. Chiariello M, Gold HK, Leinbach RC, Davis MA, Maroko PR: Comparison between the effects of nitroprusside and nitroglycerin on ischemic injury during acute myocardial infarction. *Circulation* 54:766–773, 1976.
23. Clancy RI, Graham TP, Ross J, Sonnenblick EH, Braunwald E: Influence of aortic pressure induced homeometric autoregulation on myocardial performance. *Am J Physiol* 214:1186–1192, 1968.
24. Cohn JN: Marriage of the heart and the peripheral circulation. *Prog Cardiovasc Dis* 24:189–190, 1981.
25. Cohn JN: Vasodilator therapy for heart failure. *Circulation* 48:5–8, 1973.
26. Cohn JN, Archibald DG, Ziesche S, Franciosa JA, Harston WE, Trostamo FE, Dunkman WB, Jacobs W, Francis GS, Flohr KH, Goldman S, Cobb FR, Shah PM, Saunders R, Fletcher RD, Loeb HS, Hughes VC, Baker B: Effects of vasodilator therapy on mortality in chronic congestive heart failure. Results of a Veterans Administration Cooperative Study. *N Engl J Med* 314:1547–1552, 1986.
27. Cohn JN, Archibald DG, Francis GS, Ziesche S, Franciosa JA, Harston WE, Tristani FE, Dunkman WB, Jacobs W, Flohr KH, Goldman S, Cobb FR, Shah PM, Saunders R, Fletcher RD, Loeb HS, Hughes VC, Baker B: Veterans Administration Cooperative Study on vasodilator therapy of heart failure: influence of prerandomization variables on the reduction of mortality by treatment with hydralazine and isosorbide dinitrate. *Circulation* 75(suppl IV):IV-49, 1987.
28. Cohn JN, Burke LP: Nitroprusside. *Ann Intern Med* 91:752–757, 1979.
29. Cohn JN, Franciosa JA: Vasodilator therapy of cardiac failure. *N Engl J Med* 297:254–258, 1977.
30. Cohn J, Franciosa JA, Francis GS, Archibald D, Tristani F, Fletcher R, Montero A, Cintron G, Clarke J, Hager D, Saunders R, Cobb F, Smith R, Loeb H, Settle H: Effect of short term infusion of sodium nitroprusside on mortality rate in acute myocardial infarction complicated by left ventricular failure. Results of a Veterans Administration Cooperative Study. *N Engl J Med* 306:1129–1135, 1982.
31. Cohn JN, Masniro I, Levine TB, Mehta J: Role of vasoconstrictor mechanisms in the control of left ventricular performance of the normal and damaged heart. *Am J Cardiol* 44:1019–1022, 1979.
32. Cohn JN, Mathew KJ, Franciosa JA, Snow JA: Chronic vasodilator therapy in the management of cardiogenic shock and intractable left vasodilator failure. *Ann Intern Med* 81:777–790, 1974.
33. CONSENSUS Trial Study Group: Effects of enalapril on mortality in severe congestive heart failure. Results of the Cooperative North Scandinavian Enalapril Survival Study (CONSENSUS). *N Engl J Med* 316:1429–1435, 1987.
34. Cottrell JE, Casthely P, Brodie JO, Patel K, Klein A, Turndorf H: Prevention of nitroprusside-induced cyanide toxicity and hydroxycobalamin. *N Engl J Med* 298:808–811, 1978.
35. DeMaria AN, Vismara LA, Auditore K, Amsterdam EA, Aelis R, Mason DT: Effects of nitroglycerine on left ventricular cavity size and cardiac performance determined by ultrasound in man. *Am J Med* 57:754–760, 1974.

36. Dent J, Dodds WJ, Arndorfer RC: Effect of nitroprusside and verapamil on esophageal smooth muscle contractility in the opposum. *Gastroenterology* 74:1119, 1978.

37. Desch CE, Magorien RD, Triffon DW, Blanford MF, Unverferth DV, Leier CV: Development of pharmacodynamic tolerance to prazosin in congestive heart failure. *Am J Cardiol* 44:1178–1182, 1979.

38. Durrer JD, Lie KI, Van Capelle FJL, Durrer D: Effect of sodium nitroprusside on mortality in acute myocardial infarction. *N Engl J Med* 306:1121–1128, 1982.

39. Dzau VJ, Colucci WS, Williams GH, Curfoman G, Meggs L, Hollenberg NK: Sustained effectiveness of converting-enzyme inhibition in patients with severe congestive heart failure. *N Engl J Med* 302:1373–1379, 1980.

40. Finkelstein SM, Collins VR: Vascular hemodynamic impedance measurement. *Prog Cardiovasc Dis* 24:401–418, 1982.

41. Franciosa JA, Effectiveness of long-term vasodilator administration in the treatment of chronic left ventricular failure. *Prog Cardiovasc Dis* 24:319–330, 1982.

42. Franciosa JA, Blank RC, Cohn JN, Miculec E: Hemodynamic effects of topical, oral and sublingual nitroglycerin in left ventricular failure. *Curr Ther Res* 22:231–245, 1977.

43. Franciosa JA, Blank RC, Cohn JN: Nitrate effects on cardiac output and left ventricular outflow resistance in chronic congestive heart failure. *Am J Med* 64:207–213, 1978.

44. Franciosa JA, Cohn JN: Effects of minoxidil on hemodynamics in patients with congestive heart failure. *Circulation* 63:652–657, 1981.

45. Franciosa JA, Cohn JN: Sustained hemodynamic effects without tolerance during long-term isosorbide dinitrate treatment of chronic left ventricular failure. *Am J Cardiol* 45:648–654, 1980.

46. Franciosa JA, Cuiha NH, Limas CJ, Rodriguera E, Cohn JN: Improved left ventricular function during nitroprusside infusion in acute myocardial infarction. *Lancet* 1:650–654, 1972.

47. Gaffney TF, Braunwald E: Importance of the adrenergic nervous system in the support of circulatory function in patients with congestive heart failure. *Am J Med* 34:320–324, 1963.

48. Gilmore E, Weil J, Chidsey C: Treatment of essential hypertension with a new vasodilator in combination with beta-adrenergic blockade. *N Engl J Med* 282:521–531, 1970.

49. Goldberg S, Mann T, Grossman W: Nitrate therapy of heart failure in valvular heart disease. Importance of resting level of peripheral vascular resistance in determining cardiac output response. *Am J Med* 65:161–166, 1978.

50. Goldstein RE: Coronary vascular responses to vasodilator drugs. *Prog Cardiovasc Dis* 24:419–436, 1982.

51. Gomes JAC, Carambas CR, Moran HE: The effect of isosorbide dinitrate on left ventricular size, wall stress and left ventricular function in the chronic refractory heart failure. *Am J Med* 65:794–801, 1978.

52. Goodman DJ, Rossen RM, Holloway FL, Alderman EF, Harrison DC: Effect of nitroprusside on left ventricular dynamics in mitral regurgitation. *Circulation* 50:1025–1032, 1974.

53. Gould L, Zahir M, Ettinger S: Phentolamine and cardiovascular performance. *Br Heart J* 31:154–162, 1969.

54. Graham RM, Oats HF, Stoker LM, Stokes GS: Alpha blocking action of the antihypertensive agent, prazosin. *J Pharmacol Exp Ther* 201:747–762, 1977.

55. Graham RM, Pettinger WA: Prazosin. *N Engl J Med* 300:232–236, 1979.

56. Grossman W, Harshaw CW, Munro AB, Becker L, McLaurin LP: Lowered aortic impedance as therapy for severe mitral regurgitation. *JAMA* 230:1011–1013, 1974.

57. Grossman W, McLaurin LP: Clinical measurement of vascular resistance and assessment of vasodilator drugs. In Grossman W (ed): *Cardiac Catheterization and Angiography*, ed 2. Philadelphia, Lea & Febiger, 1980.

58. Guiha NH, Cohn JN, Mikulic E: Treatment of refractory heart failure with infusion of nitroprusside. *N Engl J Med* 291:587–592, 1974.

59. Harper RW, Gold HK, Leinbach RC: Acute myocardial infarction. In Harper E, Austen WC (eds): *The Practice of Cardiology*. Boston, Little, Brown & Co, 1980.

60. Harshaw CW, Grossman W, Munro AB, McLaurin LP: Reduced systemic vascular resistance as therapy for severe mitral regurgitation of valvular origin. *Ann Intern Med* 83:312–316, 1975.

61. Helfant RH, Banka VS, Bodenheimer MM: Left ventricular dysfunction in coronary heart disease: a dynamic problem. *Cardiovasc Med* 2:557–571, 1977.

62. Herman MV, Heinle RA, Klein MD, Gorlin R: Localized disorders in myocardial contraction. *N Engl J Med* 277:222–232, 1967.

63. Higgins CB, Vatner SF, Franklin D, Braunwald E: Extent of regulation of the heart's contractile state in the conscious dog by alteration in the frequency of contraction. *J Clin Invest* 52:1187–1194, 1973.

64. Johnson CC: The actions and toxicity of sodium nitroprusside. *Arch Int Pharmacodyn Ther* 35:481–482, 1929.

65. Kluger J, Cody RF, Smith V, Laragh JH: Comparative hemodynamic effects and humoral correlations of prazosin and captopril in heart failure. *Clin Res* 29:215A, 1981.

66. Koch-Weser J: Hydralazine. *N Engl J Med* 295:320–323, 1976.

67. Leier CV, Magorien RD, Desch CE, Thompson MJ, Unverferth DV: Hydralazine and isosorbide dinitrate: comparative central and regional hemodynamic effects when administered alone or in combination. *Circulation* 63:102–107, 1981.

68. Levin RI, Weksler BB, Jaffe EA: Nitroglycerin induces production of prostacyclin by human endothelial cells. *Clin Res* 28:471A, 1980.

69. Levine TB, Franciosa JA, Cohn JN: Acute and long-term response to an oral converting-enzyme inhibitor, captopril, in congestive heart failure. *Circulation* 62:35–41, 1980.

70. Liedtke AJ, Buoncristiani JF, Kirk ES, Sonnenblick EH, Urschel CW: Regulation of cardiac output after administration of isoproterenol and ouabain: interactions of systolic impedance and contractility. *Cardiovasc Res* 56:325–332, 1972.

71. Ludbrook PA, Byrne JD, Kurnik PB, McKnight RC: Influence of reduction of preload and afterload by nitroglycerin on left ventricular diastolic pressure-volume relations and relaxation in man. *Circulation* 56:937–943, 1977.

72. Ludbrook PA, Byrne JD, McKnight RC: Influence of right ventricular diastolic pressure-volume relations in man. *Circulation* 59:21–31, 1979.

73. Lukes SA, Romero CA, Resnekov L: Hemodynamic effects of sodium nitroprusside in 21 subjects with congestive heart failure. *Br Heart J* 41:187–191, 1979.

74. Magrini F, Niarchos AP: Ineffectiveness of sublingual nitroglycerin in acute left ventricular failure in the presence of massive peripheral edema. *Am J Cardiol* 45:841–847, 1980.

75. Majid PA, Sharma B, Taylor SH: Phentolamine for vasodilator treatment of severe heart-failure. *Lancet* 22:719–726, 1971.

76. Mason DT: Afterload reduction and cardiac performance. *Am J Med* 65:106–107, 1978.

77. Massie B, Chatterjee K, Werner J, Greenberg B, Hart R, Parmley WW: Hemodynamic advantage of combined administration of hydralazine orally and nitrates non-

parenterally in the vasodilator therapy of chronic heart failure. *Am J Cardiol* 40:794–801, 1977.

78. Massie BM, Kramer B, Shen E, Haughloom F: Vasodilator treatment with isosorbide dinitrate and hydralazine in chronic heart failure. *Br Heart J* 45:376, 1981.
79. Miller RR, Awan NA, Joyce JA: Combined dopamine and nitroprusside, therapy in congestive heart failure. Greater augmentation of cardiac performance by addition of inotropic stimulation to afterload reduction. *Circulation* 55:881–884, 1977.
80. Miller RR, Fennell, WH, Young, JB, Palomo AR, Quinones MA: Differential systemic arterial and venous actions and consequent cardiac effects of vasodilator drugs. *Prog Cardiovasc Dis* 24:353–374, 1982.
81. Miller RR, Vismara LA, DeMaria AN, Salel AF, Mason DT: Afterload reduction therapy with nitroprusside in severe aortic regurgitation: improved cardiac performance and reduced regurgitant volume. *Am J Cardiol* 38:564–567, 1976.
82. Miller RR, Vismara LA, Zelis R, Amsterdam EA, Mason DT: Clinical use of sodium nitroprusside in chronic ischemic heart disease. *Circulation* 51:328–336, 1975.
83. Milnor WR: Arterial impedance as ventricular afterload. *Circ Res* 36:565–570, 1975.
84. Mookherjee S, Henion W, Warner R, Erch RH, Smulyan H, Obeid AI: Sodium nitroprusside therapy in congestive cardiomyopathy: variability in hemodynamic response. *J Clin Pharmacol* 18:67–75, 1978.
85. Mookherjee S, Keighley JFH, Warner RA, Bowser MA, Obeid AI: Hemodynamic, ventriculatory and blood gas changes during infusion of sodium nitroferricyanide (nitroprusside). *Chest* 72:273–278, 1977.
86. Nichols WW, Pepine CJ: Left ventricular afterload and aortic input impedance: implications of pulsatile blood flow. *Prog Cardiovasc Dis* 24:293–306, 1982.
87. Packer M, Leier CV: Survival in congestive heart failure during treatment with drugs with positive inotropic actions. *Circulation* 75(suppl IV):IV-55, 1987.
88. Packer M, LeJemtel TH: Physiologic and pharmacologic determinants of vasodilator response: a conceptual framework for rational drug therapy for chronic heart failure. *Prog Cardiovasc Dis* 24:275–292, 1982.
89. Packer M, Meller J, Gorlin R, Herman MV: Hemodynamic and clinical tachyphylaxis to prazosin mediated afterload reduction in severe chronic congestive heart failure. *Circulation* 59:531–539, 1979.
90. Packer M, Meller J, Medine N, Gorlin R, Herman MV: Dose requirements of hydralazine in patients with severe chronic congestive heart failure. *Am J Cardiol* 45:655–660, 1980.
91. Packer M, Meller J, Medina N, Gorlin R, Herman MV: Hemodynamic evaluation of hydralazine dosage in refractory heart failure. *Clin Pharmacol Ther* 27:337–346, 1980.
92. Packer M, Meller J, Medina N, Gorlin R, Herman MV: Rebound hemodynamic events after the abrupt withdrawal of nitroprusside in patients with severe chronic heart failure. *N Engl J Med* 301:1193–1197, 1979.
93. Packer M, Meller J, Medine N, Yushak M, Gorlin R: Determinants of drug response in severe chronic heart failure. I. Activation of vasoconstrictor forces during vasodilator therapy. *Circulation* 64:506–514, 1981.
94. Page IH, Corcoran AC, Dustan HP, Kuppanyi T: Cardiovascular actions of sodium nitroprusside in animals and hypertensive patients. *Circulation* 11:188–198, 1955.
95. Palmer RF, Lasseter KC: Sodium nitroprusside. *N Engl J Med* 292:294–497, 1975.
96. Parmley WW, Chatterjee K: Vasodilator therapy. In Harvey P (ed): *Current Problems in Cardiology.* Chicago, Year Book, 1978.
97. Parmley WW, Chuck L, Chatterjee K, Swan HJC, Klausner SC, Glantz SA, Ratshin RA: Acute changes in the

98. diastolic pressure volume relationship of the left ventricle. *Eur J Cardiol* 4:105–120, 1976.
98. Pepine CJ, Nichols WW: Aortic input impedance in cardiovascular disease. *Prog Cardiovasc Dis* 24:307–318, 1982.
99. Pepine CJ, Nichols WW, Conti CR: Aortic input impedance in heart failure. *Circulation* 58:460–465, 1978.
100. Petersdorf RG, Dale DC: Gram negative bacteremia and septic shock. In Petersdorf RG, Wilson (eds): *Harrison's Textbook of Medicine.* New York, McGraw-Hill, 1980.
101. Pierpont G, Hale KA, Franciosa JA, Cohen JN: Effects of vasodilators on pulmonary hemodynamics in gas exchange in left ventricular failure. *Am Heart J* 99:208–216, 1980.
102. Polese A, Fiorentine C, Olivari MT, Guazzi MD: Clinical use of a calcium antagonistic agent (nifedipine) in acute pulmonary edema. *Am J Med* 66:825–830, 1979.
103. Ribner HS, Breshnan D, Hsieh A, Silverman R, Tommaso C, Coath A, Askenazi J: Acute hemodynamic responses to vasodilator therapy in congestive heart failure. *Prog Cardiovasc Dis* 25:1–45, 1982.
104. Sarnoff SJ, Farr HW: Spinal anesthesia in the therapy of pulmonary edema: a preliminary report. *Anesthesiology* 5:69–76, 1944.
105. Schlant RC: Altered cardiovascular physiology of coronary atherosclerotic disease. In Hurst JW, Logue RB, Schlant RC (eds): *The Heart.* New York, McGraw-Hill, 1978.
106. Scivolett R, Toledo AJO, Gomes Da Silva AC, Nigro D: Mechanism of the hypotensive effect of prazosin. *Arch Int Pharmacodyn Ther* 223:333–338, 1976.
107. Sonnenblick EH: Force velocity relations in mammalian heart muscle. *Am J Physiol* 202:931–936, 1962.
108. Swan HJ, Ganz W, Forrester JS, Marcus H, Doamond G, Chonette D: Catheterization of the heart in man with the use of a flow-directed balloon tip catheter. *N Engl J Med* 283:444–451, 1970.
109. Taylor SH, Sutherland GR, MacKenzie CJ, Staunton HP, Donald KW: The circulatory effects of intravenous phentolamine in man. *Circulation* 31:741–754, 1965.
110. Teckleberg PL, Fitzgerald J, Allaire BI, Alderman EL, Harrison DC: Afterload reduction in the management of post-infarction ventricular septal defect. *Am J Cardiol* 38:956–958, 1976.
111. Transdermal delivery systems for nitroglycerin. *Med Lett Drugs Ther* 24:35, 1982.
112. Warner RA, Bowser M, Zuehlke A, Mookherjee S, Obeid AI: Treatment of acute aortic insufficiency with sodium nitroferricyanide. *Chest* 72:375–379, 1977.
113. Webb RC, Bohr DF: Regulation of vascular tone, molecular mechanisms. *Prog Cardiovasc Dis* 24:213–242, 1981.
114. Weber KT, Janicki JS, Hunter WC, Shroff S, Perlman ES, Fishman AP: The contractile behavior of the heart and its functional coupling of the circulation. *Prog Cardiovasc Dis* 24:375–400, 1982.
115. Weber KT, Janicki JS, Reeves RC: Determinants of stroke volume in the isolated canine heart. *J Appl Physiol* 37:742–746, 1974.
116. Yoran C, Yellin EL, Becker RM, Gabbay S, Frater R, Sonnenblick EH: Mechanism of reduction of mitral regurgitation with vasodilator therapy. *Am J Cardiol* 43:773–777, 1979.
117. Zelis R: The contribution of local factors to the elevated venous tone of congestive heart failure. *J Clin Invest* 54:219–224, 1974.
118. Zelis R, Delea CS, Coleman HN, Mason DT: Arterial sodium content in experimental congestive heart failure. *Circulation* 41:213–224, 1970.
119. Zelis R, Flaim SF: Alterations in vasomotor tone in congestive heart failure. *Prog Cardiovasc Dis* 24:437–459, 1982.

120. Zelis R, Lee G, Mason DT: Influence of experimental edema on metabolically determined blood flow. *Circ Res* 34:482–490, 1974.

121. Zelis R, Mason DT, Braunwald E: A comparison of the effects of vasodilator stimuli on peripheral resistance vessels in normal subjects and in patients with congestive heart failure. *J Clin Invest* 47:960–970, 1968.

122. Zelis R, Nellis SH, Longhurst J: Abnormalities in the regional circulations accompanying congestive heart failure. *Prog Cardiovasc Dis* 18:181–197, 1975.

20

Antihypertensive Therapy

Michael G. Ziegler, M.D.

Hypertension is the most common chronic illness of industrialized societies. Hypertensives develop critical cardiovascular disease at a much higher rate than normal subjects, thus patients arriving at intensive care units frequently have received antihypertensive drugs.

Table 20.1
Antihypertensive Therapies

Nutritional
    Weight loss
    Sodium restriction
    Ethanol restriction
    Potassium
Diuretics
    Thiazides
    Loop diuretics
Sympatholytics
    α-Blockers
        Phenoxybenzamine
        Phentolamine
        Prazosin
    β-Blockers
        Atenolol
        Metoprolol
        Nadolol
        Propranolol
        Timolol
        Acebutolol
        Labetalol
    α_2-Agonists
        Clonidine
        Guanabenz
        Methyldopa
        Guanfacine
    Ganglionic blockers
Vasodilators
    Diazoxide
    Hydralazine
    Minoxidil
    Nitroprusside
Calcium channel blockers
    Nifedipine
    Diltiazem
    Verapamil
Converting-enzyme inhibitors
    Captopril
    Enalapril
    Lisinopril

These drugs alter cardiovascular responses to severe illness and may diminish the ability to maintain the circulation during shock. Many other common drugs such as caffeine, ethanol, nicotine, and over-the-counter decongestants and diet pills alter blood pressure and are considered in this chapter. Food is also an important determinant of blood pressure, especially in patients dependent on intravenous nutrition. The interaction of all these chemicals is a complex but important facet of the regulation of the cardiovascular system. This chapter deals with each aspect of antihypertensive therapy under a separate subheading for quick reference. The sections are arranged in a logical sequence to describe the cardiovascular system of hypertensive subjects and how the hypertension can be controlled by medication.

High blood pressure was once considered "essential" to adequate tissue perfusion and thus acquired the name, "essential hypertension." The name remains, but we now know that the higher the pressure, the worse the prognosis for development of cardiovascular disease. Fifteen to 25% of the inhabitants of industrialized countries have high blood pressure; therefore, hypertension is one of the most common diagnoses among patients in a critical care unit. Some patients are there for therapy of malignant hypertension, but most have other illnesses, often of cardiovascular origin. All need care of their hypertension with attention to diet, intravenous fluids, and drugs (Table 20.1).

NUTRITIONAL PHARMACOLOGY OF HYPERTENSION

Diet is not an alternative usually considered in the drug therapy of hypertension, but dietary factors have potent effects on blood pressure and interact with antihypertensive drugs.

Dietary manipulations alone can often provide effective therapy of hypertension and may be prescribed in place of antihypertensive medication. The most important dietary factors are caloric intake, ethanol, sodium, potassium, and tyrosine.

Caloric Intake

Carbohydrate ingestion increases sympathetic nervous system activity, whereas consumption of protein or fat has little acute effect (34). When obese adults are switched from a 2600-kcal/day diet to a 600-kcal/day diet, they have a 40% decrease in the urinary excretion of 3-methoxy-4-hydroxymandelic acid, a metabolite of norepinephrine (95). The acute effects of carbohydrate ingestion on sympathetic nervous activity may be mediated by insulin, since maintenance of a constant serum insulin level prevents the carbohydrate-associated increase in circulating norepinephrine levels (45). All antihypertensive drugs have direct or indirect influences on the sympathetic nervous system, and carbohydrate ingestion can alter the effect of these drugs.

Obesity has chronic effects on the sympathetic and cardiovascular systems (48). Obesity augments cardiac output, stroke volume, left ventricular filling pressure, and intravascular volume, and lowers total peripheral resistance. Obesity is strongly associated with hypertension. Sixty-two percent of hypertensive subjects are more than 20% overweight. Weight loss can decrease or cure hypertension (18). The hyperinsulinemia of obesity promotes sodium retention (76) and sympathetic neuronal overactivity.

Fasting lowers blood pressure by decreasing sympathetic nervous activity and by activating an opiate-mediated vasodepressor response (21). After 8–12 weeks of a low calorie diet, plasma renin activity and aldosterone levels both decrease, irrespective of sodium intake (81). Weight loss thus reduces plasma insulin, norepinephrine, renin, and aldosterone levels, and cardiac output, all of which lower blood pressure.

The average hypertensive can expect to decrease systolic blood pressure by 1 mm Hg and diastolic pressure by ¾ mm Hg for every pound lost. As long as the weight is not gained back, there is no evidence of any rebound in blood pressure, thus the cure of a patient's obesity may simultaneously cure hypertension.

Diet has short-term effects on blood pressure as well. If dietary intake is less than 600 kcal/day, starvation ketosis causes natriuresis and hypotension. Carbohydrate consumption increases sympathetic nervous activity, but foods rich in the amino acid tyrosine may increase central norepinephrine release and thereby act to decrease peripheral sympathetic tone (1).

Ethanol

The consumption of more than three alcoholic drinks daily is associated with an increase in mean blood pressure and in the incidence of hypertension. Approximately 5% of the hypertension in the United States may be attributed to alcohol consumption. Surprisingly, the incidence of myocardial infarction decreases with increasing alcohol ingestion, even in the face of elevated blood pressure; however, stroke is more common in alcoholics. Moderate doses of ethanol increase plasma renin activity, plasma aldosterone, and cortisol (33). The cardioprotective effects of ethanol may be due to a direct effect on the heart or an interaction with norepinephrine release. Extremely high doses of ethanol may acutely activate central enkephalin neurons and lower blood pressure (32). The acutely ill patient in alcoholic coma is usually hypotensive while intoxicated. As time progresses, blood pressure in this intoxicated patient can be expected to increase, frequently into the hypertensive range, as the patient undergoes alcohol withdrawal.

Sodium

Patients with malignant hypertension reduce their blood pressure dramatically by eating a 10-mEq/day sodium diet (36). However, an increase in sodium from 10 to 35 mEq/day increases the blood pressure almost to pretreatment levels (88). The value of moderate sodium restriction has been contested, but controlled studies of moderate sodium restriction in hypertension show a fall in mean blood pressure of about 7 mm Hg (50) and a marked decrease in the requirement for antihypertensive medications (4). A similar decrement in blood pressure occurs in hospitalized patients who receive a 35-mEq/day sodium diet (87). Moderate sodium restriction can control mild hypertension, but severe hypertension requires severe sodium restriction for blood pressure control. The change in blood pressure that occurs with sodium restriction is acutely related to a change in plasma volume (87).

DIURETICS

Thiazides

Thiazide diuretics and closely related phthalimidine derivatives are customarily the first drugs used for hypertension. They cause sodium loss and vasodilation. Initially, thiazide therapy decreases blood volume and cardiac output. During chronic treatment these parameters return to normal, however, and blood pressure falls as peripheral resistance decreases (19). The antihypertensive effects of thiazide diuretics can be negated by a large salt intake or infusion of saline, although a similar increase in blood volume by a dextran infusion fails to increase blood pressure (93). The thiazides have a variety of biochemical effects early in treatment, particularly hypokalemia, hyperglycemia, hyperuricemia, decrease in plasma volume, and increase in renin, aldosterone, and sympathetic nervous activity (44). With chronic therapy, the hypokalemia, hyperglycemia, and hyperuricemia persist and a hypochloremic alkalosis may develop. A thiazide-induced decrease in blood pressure is accompanied by a decrease in peripheral resistance. Several homeostatic mechanisms, such as a stimulation of renin or aldosterone, may prevent a decrease in blood pressure. These reactions follow the increased sympathetic activity (44) that is particularly prominent in those who fail to respond to thiazides (43). Patients who fail to respond to thiazides because of compensatory homeostatic mechanisms are especially prone to the antihypertensive effect of sympatholytic drugs (43). Other patients do not respond to thiazides because they eat too much salt.

Current doses of thiazide diuretics used to treat hypertension are excessive. Treatment with 12½ mg of hydrochlorothiazide (5) and 25 mg of chlorthalidone (55) lowers blood pressure maximally in patients with normal renal function. It is best to use the lowest effective dose to treat hypertension because deleterious side effects multiply with increasing dose. Thiazides raise serum cholesterol by increasing low density lipoprotein levels without causing a similar increase in high density lipoproteins. These effects are most prominent in men and postmenopausal women, and these

changes might underlie an increased mortality in patients receiving thiazides (39).

Since the antihypertensive actions of thiazide diuretics take up to 3 weeks to fully manifest, thiazides are not useful as single agents in the acute care of hypertension. The lack of initial antihypertensive efficacy is due to homeostatic mechanisms, such as an increase in norepinephrine and renin release. These mechanisms can be blocked by sympatholytic drugs, thus acute therapy with a diuretic and sympatholytic drugs can rapidly lower blood pressure.

Loop Diuretics

Loop diuretics such as furosemide are more effective natriuretic agents than the thiazides. Furosemide decreases blood volume but not peripheral resistance. Rather, it elicits a reflex increase in sympathetic nervous activity and in renin release (42, 80), which may increase peripheral resistance. If a vasodilator or sympatholytic is given to diminish peripheral resistance, the combined effects may adequately decrease blood pressure. Furosemide is useful for patients with renal insufficiency or for those who have fluid retention. Patients with malignant hypertension are often volume-depleted, and loop diuretics may impair tissue perfusion and worsen vasospasm. Potent diuretics may be essential to combat the fluid-retaining effects of other potent antihypertensive medications. Many patients develop a photosensitivity dermatitis in response to furosemide and the thiazides. Ethacrynic acid and bumetanide are useful alternatives for these patients.

β-BLOCKING DRUGS

β-Blocking drugs lower blood pressure by several mechanisms. Cardiac output is promptly reduced, but increased peripheral resistance compensates for this. Days to weeks later, peripheral resistance diminishes, almost reaching pretreatment values, and blood pressure decreases. The β-blocking drugs inhibit renin secretion and lower blood pressure more in high-renin patients than in those with low renin (11), but these agents still have some hypotensive effect in low-renin patients. The β-blockers may alter prostaglandin levels in vascular tissue, and indomethacin can diminish some of their hypotensive effects (31). In animals, the β-blocking drugs enhance the central release of norepinephrine, which diminishes peripheral sympathetic tone. They also increase baroreflex sensitivity (66). β-Blocking drugs diminish cardiac output and renin release; they may alter blood pressure through interactions with prostaglandins and by central nervous system effects, but it is unclear how important these latter mechanisms are.

The effectiveness of β-blocker therapy depends on the patient's age, race, and renin status, and how recent the onset of hypertension. Patients with high plasma renin levels have the greatest hypotensive response to β-blocker therapy. Although this effect is statistically significant, it is not sufficiently striking to justify the use of renin-sodium classification in individual hypertensives (94). Both cardiac chronotropic and inotropic responsiveness to β stimulation diminishes with age (90), and β blockade has less of a cardiac effect in the elderly than in the young. The net effect is that β-blocking drugs work less well to lower blood pressure in the elderly than in the young, but can be more dangerous in the elderly since they may accentuate heart block and lung disease. In contrast, young patients with the recent onset of hypertension tend to have a hyperdynamic cardiac output and have hypertension based more on increased cardiac output than on increased peripheral resistance. These young hypertensives respond very well to β blockade (23).

Black hypertensives respond poorly to β blockade. A group of black patients who had

a decrease in mean blood pressure of 14 mm Hg with diuretic therapy had only a 5 mm Hg blood pressure decrease in response to β blockade (27). Hollifield and associates (28) reported that when low-dose propranolol fails to work, doses in the range of 320–960 mg/day diminish blood pressure. However, other investigators found that 80 mg of propranolol per day was as effective as 480 mg/day. It is not clear whether extremely high doses of β-blockers provide any additional hypotensive effect, but they do increase side effects and cost. β-Blocking drugs differ in their receptor affinity and pharmacokinetic properties (Table 20.2). Propranolol has a half-life of only 3–6 hours, but its effect persists with one daily dosing (83), with fewer nighttime side effects.

Propranolol blocks both β_1- and β_2-adrenergic receptors. The β_1-receptors mediate cardiac effects and β_2-receptors mediate bronchodilation and arteriolar dilation. A variety of other effects, including renin release, are influenced by both types of receptors (Table 20.3). Atenolol and acebutolol are β_1-selective and thus are less likely to block β-adrenergic bronchodilation or vasodilation. Their cardioselectivity is not absolute, however, and in the higher dose range these agents can cause bronchoconstriction. When a β-blocking agent is necessary in the treatment of a patient with bronchospasm or a diabetic receiving insulin (17), β_1-selective agents are safer than nonselective agents. However, β-blocking drugs should not be used at all in these patients unless absolutely necessary. Atenolol and me-

Table 20.2
Properties of β-Blocking Drugs

Generic name	Propranolol	Atenolol	Metoprolol	Nadolol	Pindolol	Timolol	Acebutolol	Labetalol
Brand name	Inderal	Tenormin	Lopressor	Corgard	Visken	Blocadren	Sectral	Trandate
Oral bioavailability (%)	30	40	50	30	90	75	40	25
Dose in hypertension (mg)	80–640	50–100	100–450	80–320	15–60	20–60	200–1200	200–2400
Variation in plasma levels between patients	20×	4×	10×	7×	4×	7×	7×	7×
Protein bound (%)	93	<5	12	30	60	10	25	50
Half-life (hr)	3–6	6–9	3–4	14–24	3–4	3–4	3–13	6–8
Fat solubility	+	0	±	0	±	0	0	+
Route of elimination	Liver	Kidney	Liver	Kidney	Kidney and liver	Liver	Kidney and liver	Kidney and liver
Membrane-stabilizing effect	+ +	0	±	0	+	0	+	+
Cardioselectivity	0	+	+	0	0	0	+	0
Intrinsic sympathomimetic activity	0	0	0	0	+ +	±	+	0
Active metabolites	+	0	0	0	0	0	+	0
Potency (relative)	10	10	10	10	60	60	5	2

Table 20.3
α-Adrenergic and β-Adrenergic Responses

Organ	Effect[a]	α	β_1	β_1 and β_2	β_2
Blood vessels	Constricts arterioles and venules	+	0		0
	Dilates arterioles (especially in skeletal muscle)	0	0		+
Heart	↑ Rate of S-A node discharge	0	+		0
	↑ Contractility	0	+		0
	↑ Conduction velocity	0	+		0
Lungs	Dilates bronchial muscles	0	0		+
Gastrointestinal tract	↓ Peristalsis	+		+	
Metabolic effects	Lipolysis	0		+	
	↓ Insulin release	+		0	
	↑ Insulin release	0		+	
	↑ Formation of cAMP	0		+	
	↑ Fasting blood sugar	±		+	
	↑ Renin secretion			+	

[a] S-A, sinoatrial; cAMP, cyclic AMP.

toprolol can be successfully used with β_2-agonist agents.

β-Blocking drugs also differ in their fat solubility and rate of elimination (Table 20.2). Atenolol and nadolol are not soluble in fat and are not extensively metabolized by the liver. They do not undergo a "first pass" metabolism by the liver as rapidly as more lipophilic agents. Their longer half-lives allow once daily dosing, but the dose needs to be adjusted in renal failure because these drugs are excreted by the kidneys. Nonlipophilic agents do not penetrate the brain very effectively. Although several β-blocking drugs impair renal perfusion during treatment of hypertension, nadolol lowers blood pressure without impairing glomerular filtration rate or renal blood flow (65). The decrease in renal blood flow with most β-blocking agents is too small to elevate serum creatinine or urea and is usually neglected in clinical practice. Most side effects of the different β-blocking agents are similar. In a study of 10,000 patients, propranolol worsened exercise tolerance dyspnea. It tended to cause nausea and rhinorrhea early in therapy and cold hands later in therapy (58). Rhinorrhea and Raynaud's phenomenon may be less of a problem with cardioselective β-blocking drugs, and central nervous system side effects may be less frequent with nonlipophilic agents.

People metabolize β-blockers at very different rates, and dosage must be adjusted by clinical response. If heart rate slows and the increment in heart rate decreases when the patient is standing, β blockade is effective. As shown in Table 20.2, the variation in plasma levels with the same dose of drug is greatest with propranolol and tends to be less with agents that are excreted by the kidney than those that are metabolized by the liver.

The first β-blocker synthesized was dichloroisoproterenol. It was a partial β-agonist and was not used in humans because of its β-receptor stimulant activity. Pindolol and acebutolol have sympathomimetic activity since they are partial agonists as well. They do not decrease resting heart rate but antagonize the increase in heart rate with exercise. Pindolol has the most intrinsic sympathomimetic activity and is unlikely to cause heart block or bradycardia. It may cause angina in a patient abruptly changed from another β-blocker to pindolol, because of its stimulant activity. Acebutolol has less intrinsic sympathomimetic activity and usually does not change heart rate (84).

The available β-blocking agents differ in their pharmacokinetic profile and in their β_1 selectivity. There is no convincing evidence that any of these agents is either more effective or associated with fewer side effects in the average hypertensive patient. However, in particular patients there is some clear advantage to specific agents—cardioselectivity is an advantage for patients with bronchospasm or those who tend to develop cold hands or Raynaud's phenomenon. These drugs can also be used with β_2-agonist bronchodilators, and are the drugs of choice when a β-blocker must be used in a patient with impaired respiratory function. The longer half-life of nadolol and atenolol may be important when these agents are used in the treatment of angina pectoris, but shorter acting drugs, such as propranolol, seem equally effective for the treatment of hypertension when given once daily.

β-Blocking drugs should not be withdrawn abruptly in patients with angina pectoris. Patients treated with β-blockers for hypertension can develop a reproducible hyperadrenergic withdrawal syndrome when β-blockers are stopped abruptly (70). Twenty-four hours after drug withdrawal, blood pressure and heart rate may rise. These symptoms increase to a maximum at 48 hours and disappear by 7 days. This syndrome is mediated by an increased sensitivity of β-receptors. Longer-lasting agents, such as atenolol and nadolol, or agents with intrinsic sympathomimetic activity, such as pindolol and acebutolol, may be less likely to cause the syndrome.

Labetalol is a nonspecific β-blocking drug that also possesses some α-blocking activity. Other β-blocking drugs initially increase peripheral vascular resistance, but this increased resistance is prevented by the α-blocking activity of labetalol. This quality makes labetalol useful for the acute therapy of severe hypertension. The drug may be given by slow intravenous injection in initial doses of 2.5–5 mg. The intravenous dose may be increased to 20 mg, 40 mg, then 80 mg, or by infusion at 2 mg/min up to a total dose of 300 mg or until blood pressure is controlled. The patient can then be maintained on 100–1200 mg of labetalol twice daily.

After intravenous injection of labetalol, symptomatic postural hypotension is common. In chronic use the drug possesses the side effects of β- and α-blockers and may cause nausea. However, labetalol is more effective than other β-blockers in lowering blood pressure, and its effects are potentiated by diuretics (60).

α-ADRENERGIC CONTROL OF BLOOD PRESSURE

The antihypertensive drugs methyldopa, clonidine, guanabenz, prazosin, phenoxybenzamine, and phentolamine all act on α-adrenergic receptors. Their hypotensive effect is most easily understood in terms of their effects on various types of α-receptors with differing anatomic distribution. The α_1- and α_2-receptors (commonly referred to as postsynaptic and presynaptic receptors) can be distinguished by their affinity for various drugs (Table 20.4). Epinephrine and norepinephrine stimulate, whereas phentolamine and phenoxybenzamine block, both types of receptors. However, newer drugs, such as prazosin or clonidine, can selectively block α_1-receptors or stimulate α_2-receptors. Because of their specificity, these agents cause fewer side effects than nonspecific drugs. The drugs can be classified by receptor binding affinities or physiologic effect, and these classifications are in agreement.

In the vasculature, α-receptors near noradrenergic nerve terminals are usually of the α_1 type, whereas receptors distant from these terminals, but accessible to circulating catecholamines, are of the α_2 type. α-Receptors in the brain are predominantly of the α_2 type, although all adrenergically innervated organs have both types of receptor.

Presynaptic α_2-adrenergic receptors on sympathetic nerve terminals inhibit the release of norepinephrine (46). When α_2-receptors on the nerves are stimulated, they antagonize calcium influx and enhance calcium efflux, thereby inhibiting further release of norepinephrine. These presynaptic α_2-receptors inhibit norepinephrine release from nerves in the periphery and in the brain. α_2-Receptors in the brain are also located postsynaptically, and postsynap-

Table 20.4
Relative Binding Affinity of Drugs for α_1- and α_2-Receptors

	Agonists	Antagonists	
α_2 ↓	Guanfacine Guanabenz Clonidine α-Methylnorepinephrine Epinephrine	Yohimbine	α_2 ↓
α_1 and α_2 ↓	Norepinephrine	Phentolamine Phenoxybenzamine	α_1 and α_2 ↓
α_1	Phenylephrine Methoxamine	Labetalol Prazosin	α_1

tic α-receptors mediate the central antihypertensive actions of clonidine and methyldopa (37).

There are two possible ways that α_2-receptors might lower blood pressure in humans. The stimulation of peripheral α-receptors inhibits norepinephrine release from sympathetic nerves (46), and stimulation of central α_2-receptors diminishes peripheral sympathetic nervous electrical activity. The central action is by far the more important and because of this central mode of action, clonidine-like drugs have central side effects such as sedation.

In general, peripheral α_1-receptors mediate vasoconstriction and peripheral α_2-receptors inhibit norepinephrine release. Central α_2-receptors depress sympathetic nervous activity and enhance vagal activity. Drugs that stimulate α_2-receptors or block α_1-receptors lower blood pressure and can do so with fewer side effects than nonspecific agents.

Prazosin

Because prazosin is structurally related to papaverine and to cyclic nucleotides, it was first thought to act as a vasodilator. However, it fails to vasodilate vasculature that is not stimulated by α-agonists, such as norepinephrine. Prazosin preferentially blocks α_1-receptors, and this blockade is responsible for its antihypertensive efficacy. The α-blocking agents, phenoxybenzamine and phentolamine, are of little use in treating hypertension because they nonselectively block both α_1- and α_2-receptors. The nonselective blockade of α_2-receptors enhances norepinephrine release, which causes tachycardia and increases renin release. In contrast, prazosin causes little or no heart rate increase in humans and may lower plasma renin activity. Prazosin does not affect presynaptic α_2-receptors, and allows them to inhibit norepinephrine release normally. Prazosin does not decrease cardiac output, but lowers blood pressure by reducing systemic vascular resistance. Prazosin and clonidine are no more effective in combination than clonidine alone (64).

Prazosin is readily absorbed from the gastrointestinal tract, and peak plasma levels occur between 1 and 3 hours after oral administration. The drug is metabolized primarily in the liver, and hepatic inactivation of the compound is so effective that there is a "first pass" clearance of almost 60% of the drug. This first pass clearance of prazosin is markedly diminished in uremic patients (25), thus very small doses of prazosin (approximately one-third the usual dose) are effective in renal failure.

In treating hypertension, prazosin may be used by itself, with a diuretic, or with multiple antihypertensive agents. When used alone, the antihypertensive efficacy of chronically administered prazosin may diminish because fluid retention leads to an increased plasma volume. However, some observers have noted a 6- to 8-week delay before prazosin affects diastolic pressure demonstrably (62). Alone, it is less effective than methyldopa (6), but prazosin's effect is almost doubled when used in conjunction with thiazide diuretics. The combination of prazosin with methyldopa, clonidine, or propranolol may not be particularly effective, however (41).

As might be expected from its α-blocking activities, prazosin is extremely effective in the treatment of hypertension due to pheochromocytoma (86). Prazosin rapidly lowers blood pressure when given to patients with untreated severe hypertension, although the hypotensive effect in this setting may be extreme and unpredictable. The "first dose effect" is the major side effect of prazosin. When first taken, there may be a massive pooling of blood in the venous system as a consequence of abrupt α blockade, and an abrupt lowering of blood pressure with severe postural hypotension (13). This complication is dose-related, and in a group of 74 hypertensive patients initially treated with a 2-mg dose of prazosin, two patients experienced syncope and 10 others had significant symptoms of postural hypotension (75). First dose syncope can be avoided by withholding diuretics the day before the first dose and administering a 1-mg capsule at bed time (79). The dose of prazosin may then be gradually increased to a maximum of 10 mg twice daily; doses beyond this range do not worsen side effects, but also do not increase antihypertensive efficacy. The postural hypotension from prazosin during chronic therapy is more severe than that seen with methyldopa or propranolol, but usually does not cause symptoms. Other side effects are mild and uncommon. Prazosin is devoid of CNS side effects.

Prazosin preserves renal blood flow and glomerular filtration (67) and is effective at low doses in patients with renal disease. The drug may cause bronchodilation, decrease serum cholesterol and triglyceride levels, and increase the ratio of high density lipoprotein cholesterol to low density lipoprotein cholesterol. These effects contrast with those of propranolol, which diminishes renal blood flow and causes bronchoconstriction and hyperlipidemia. The combination of prazosin and propranolol results in a partial amelioration of propranolol's effects on cholesterol and triglyceride levels.

In summary, prazosin is an antihypertensive agent with a unique mode of action. It is not as effective when used by itself as the thiazide diuretics or methyldopa, but is effective in combination with thiazides. Its unique mode of action makes it an effective drug in patients who may not tolerate other antihypertensive agents, since it may improve bronchospasm and lower cholesterol. Prazosin is nearly devoid of CNS side effects and appears to have no effect on sexual potency. The drug is particularly effective in patients with pheochromocytoma, and a prolonged response to prazosin should make one suspicious of the presence of this tumor.

Phenoxybenzamine

Phenoxybenzamine is an α-blocking drug that differs from phentolamine in being more specific for α-receptors and blocking them noncompetitively. Phenoxybenzamine is also a potent antihistamine and has a fairly weak effect on serotonin and acetylcholine receptors, but its important clinical effects are almost all related to its α-blocking activity. It is chemically related to the nitrogen mustards and has a tertiary amine that cyclizes to form a reactive intermediate molecule. This reactive intermediate is the active form of the drug and must be made to bind with α-adrenergic receptors. Phenoxybenzamine has a relatively slow onset of action, and peak effect is not attained until 1 hour after intravenous administration because of the time required for the formation of the reactive intermediate. The α-adrenergic blockade has a half-life of about 1 day, and the effects may be observable for 1 week after the drug is discontinued. This prolonged duration of action is most likely due to the requirement for synthesis of new α-receptors to replace those covalently bound to the drug. Phenoxybenzamine also inhibits the uptake of catecholamines into nerves and extraneuronal tissue.

Phenoxybenzamine blocks feedback mechanisms, increases the rate of turnover of nor-

epinephrine, and increases the amount of norepinephrine released by each nerve impulse by blocking presynaptic α_2-receptors (77). The most striking physiologic effect is a reflex tachycardia, the result of lower blood pressure, enhanced release of norepinephrine, and decreased inactivation of norepinephrine. Impaired venoconstriction causes postural hypotension, which becomes more pronounced during exercise or other vasodilating activities. Although phenoxybenzamine effectively lowers blood pressure, reflex reponses to hypotension limit its clinical usefulness. The drug can reverse the pressor effects of epinephrine by blocking its α-adrenergic effects and leaving β effects unopposed. Because of this, phenoxybenzamine can cause hypotension during stress. The drug exaggerates the vasodepressor effects of opiates and vasodilators by preventing compensatory vasoconstriction. The α blockade also leads to miosis, nasal stuffiness, and inhibition of ejaculation. It has CNS effects that include a characteristic loss of time perception, and in high doses causes nausea, vomiting, hyperventilation, and even convulsions. Lower doses cause sedation and fatigue, but it is not clear if α-blocking activity induces these CNS effects since they develop and terminate more rapidly than does the peripheral α blockade.

The major use of phenoxybenzamine is for treating hypertension caused by pheochromocytoma. Prazosin may be an equally useful α-blocker in this setting, but there is less clinical experience with prazosin. Phenoxybenzamine is available for oral use in 10-mg capsules; the intravenous form is available only by special arrangement with the manufacturer.

Phentolamine and Tolazoline

Phentolamine competitively blocks both α_1- and α_2-receptors. Its effects are most dramatic in patients with a pheochromocytoma. However, adequate doses of the drug have hemodynamic effects in almost all individuals. The blockade of vascular receptors causes vasodilation of arterioles and veins, with a prompt decrease in peripheral resistance and a fall in blood pressure. The blockade of α_2-receptors on adrenergic nerve terminals disinhibits norepinephrine release, which stimulates β-adrenergic receptors. This β stimulation can cause tachycardia, arrhythmias, and angina. The drug probably also has nonspecific effects on serotonin, histamine, and acetylcholine receptors, which frequently lead to gastrointestinal stimulation and occasionally stimulate salivary, lachrymal, respiratory tract, and pancreatic secretions.

Phentolamine is available in 50-mg oral tablets but is most frequently used in parenteral form, supplied in 5-mg ampules. An injected 5-mg dose dramatically decreases blood pressure in patients with pheochromocytoma or clonidine withdrawal.

Tolazoline is chemically and pharmacologically related to phentolamine. It is used in the treatment of clonidine overdose, since it blocks the α-receptors that are stimulated by clonidine and penetrates the central nervous system more easily than does phentolamine. The side effects of tolazoline are similar to those of phentolamine, but tend to be more severe since it is less specific for α-receptors than is phentolamine.

Clonidine, Guanfacine, and Guanabenz

Clonidine stimulates α_2-receptors, and its presynaptic action inhibits norepinephrine release in both the brain and peripheral sympathetic nervous systems. Its main hypotensive action is through stimulation of α_2-receptors in the vasomotor centers of the medulla oblongata, particularly at the nucleus tractus solitarius. This α_2 stimulation decreases sympathetic activity, increases vagal stimulation, and lowers plasma norepinephrine, epinephrine, and renin release (61). Even in the presence of β-blocking drugs, clonidine further lowers heart rate by enhancing vagal activity.

Since the primary mode of action of clonidine is through the central nervous system, the drug must penetrate the CNS in order to have its hypotensive effects. Intravenously administered clonidine transiently increases blood pressure, with a subsequent fall in blood pressure that is maximal at 20 minutes but persists for many hours. The pressor phase is not seen when clonidine is given orally since peak blood levels are not reached until 90 minutes after ingestion. Glomerular filtration rate is usually decreased and sodium excretion is considerably and acutely reduced. Over longer-term therapy, sodium retention tends to occur only at the higher dose ranges.

Clonidine increases cerebral vascular resistance and decreases cerebral blood flow (47). These physiologic changes are associated with a fall in resting blood pressure, but reflex control of capacitance vessels is intact, which helps maintain cardiac output during exercise.

Cardiac index, heart rate, and blood pressure increase normally with the drug during exercise. Renal blood flow is maintained because of a reduction in renal vascular resistance, but glomerular filtration rate may decrease. Clonidine has a small direct effect on the kidney, but decreases renin by its central actions.

After acute oral administration of clonidine, peak blood levels occur in 90 minutes. The drug is about 75% bioavailable, with a half-life of 8 hours. Sixty percent of the drug is cleared unchanged by the kidney. The hypotensive effect of clonidine and its side effects of sedation and dry mouth follow plasma levels very closely during acute therapy (16). With longer-term treatment, rate of absorption and half-life are unchanged and clonidine blood levels are still closely related to the decline in blood pressure. Clonidine's depressant effect on sympathetic nervous activity persists, and plasma norepinephrine levels and plasma renin activity remain low with chronic therapy. Some of clonidine's central effects may occur via release of β-endorphin (40). Naloxone reverses the antihypertensive effect of clonidine in laboratory animals and in some, but not all, human subjects. Although clonidine is used clinically in conjuction with β-blocking drugs, there is evidence that β-blockers that penetrate the CNS, such as propranolol, may interfere with the antihypertensive effects of clonidine (24). β-Blockers may also be dangerous in clonidine withdrawal. Sedation and dry mouth are inevitable side effects of clonidine and are a direct result of central α_2 stimulation. Although many people find the sedative effects of a nighttime dose of clonidine pleasant, it produces a dose-dependent inhibition of paradoxical sleep, which may be related to nighttime hallucinations and dementia when clonidine is given to the elderly (9). Sympathetic nervous activity and blood pressure decrease during sleep, and clonidine further lowers sympathetic activity and blood pressure at night (52).

Clonidine progressively lowers blood pressure with increasing dose up to 0.8 mg daily, but beyond this dose range it has a U-shaped dose-response curve. In the range of 1.2–1.6 mg daily, clonidine begins to increase blood pressure as its peripheral vasoconstrictor effects override its central hypotensive effects (72). Although the hypotensive effect diminishes with increasing dosage, sedation and dry mouth become more troublesome. When patients receiving high doses of clonidine abruptly discontinue their medication, a withdrawal syndrome begins about 18 hours later. They suffer insomnia, headache, flushing, sweating, apprehension, and tremulousness. Sympathetic nervous activity increases, and plasma norepinephrine levels and blood pressure are elevated above pretreatment levels. Symptoms are most marked 24–72 hours after clonidine is withdrawn, but then subside spontaneously (72). The withdrawal syndrome is most severe in patients taking more than 1.2 mg clonidine daily (8) and seems particularly likely to occur postoperatively (7, 8). The patient with tremulousness, tachycardia, and hypertension, may be treated with a β-blocker, but this approach may only exaggerate the hypertension by providing unopposed α-adrenergic vasoconstriction from the increased norepinephrine release. A patient receiving both clonidine and a β-blocker who stops taking just the clonidine becomes susceptible to severe hypertension during the withdrawal syndrome. The clonidine withdrawal syndrome only rarely occurs at doses of less than 0.3 mg daily, but patients receiving doses higher than this should be cautioned not to stop the drug abruptly.

Oral clonidine has been recommended for treating severe hypertension (2) in a dose of 0.2 mg initially followed by 0.1 mg hourly. Since clonidine acutely decreases cardiac output and cerebral blood flow, there are some theoretical objections to the safety of this procedure, but the clinical experience has been favorable.

Guanabenz, like clonidine, stimulates α_2-receptors and has blood pressure–lowering effects and similar side effects. Guanabenz's half-life of 6 hours is short, and it can cause a withdrawal syndrome similar to that of clonidine. Clinical reports suggest that guanabenz withdrawal is not as severe as clonidine withdrawal. Guanabenz is given in a dose of 4–32 mg twice daily, but the highest doses may cause a pressor response and severe side effects, similar to the action of high doses of clonidine.

Guanfacine was recently released in the United States. It has a relatively long half-life of 16 hours, which permits once daily dosing of 1–3 mg with effective control of blood pressure. The longer half-life should also diminish the severity of withdrawal from the drug.

α-Methyldopa

α-Methyldopa is metabolized to an α_2-agonist with actions similar to those of clonidine.

Only about one-fourth of methyldopa is absorbed unchanged since it is metabolized in the gut wall and in the liver before gaining access to the systemic circulation. The drug is enzymatically converted to active metabolities (Fig. 20.1), and inhibitors of the enzymes dopa-decarboxylase and dopamine-β-hydroxylase prevent its hypotensive effects. Methyldopa is converted to α-methyldopamine, then to α-methylnorepinephrine, a potent agonist at α_2-receptors (Fig. 20.1). α-methylnorepinephrine is stored in nerve endings and released by nerve stimulation. When formation of α-methylnorepinephrine is blocked, α-methyldopa fails to lower blood pressure. Several hours may elapse after methyldopa is given before enough metabolite is formed to lower blood pressure. Since the body stores this active metabolite, the effect of an oral dose persists for as long as 24 hours, even though the half-time of elimination for plasma α-methyldopa is about 2 hours. The O-methylated metabolites of methyldopa may also contribute to its hypotensive action (Fig. 20.1).

Methyldopa metabolites stimulate α_2-receptors, causing side effects similar to those of clonidine. Acute doses of methyldopa impair

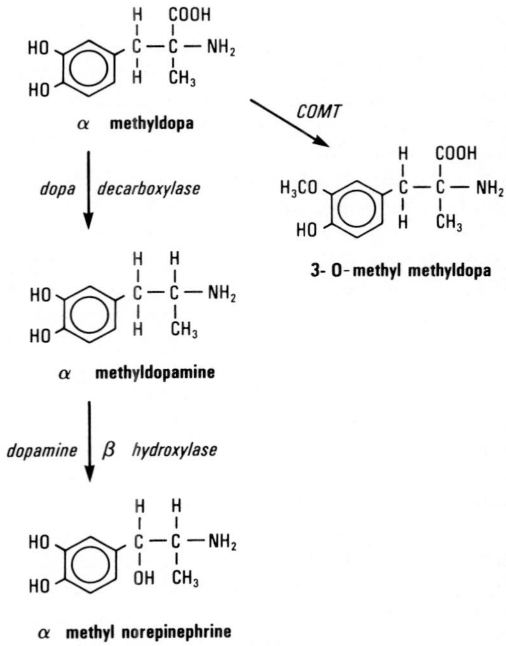

Figure 20.1. The metabolic conversion of methyldopa to its active metabolites. The metabolic enzymes are those normally involved in the production and degradation of norepinephrine. *COMT*, catechol-O-methyltransferase.

judgment (3) and depress behavior. The drug causes hypothermia and prolactin secretion. In contrast to clonidine, it increases rapid eye movement sleep in humans and causes less dry mouth and bradycardia than clonidine. Methyldopa also has important immunologic side effects. Twenty-five percent of patients taking 1 g of methyldopa daily for 6 months develop a positive direct Coombs' test. The drug stimulates production of an IgG antibody directed at the red cell membrane and not reacting with methyldopa itself. The positive Coombs' test is not a contraindication to continuation of therapy; however, in somewhat under 25% of individuals with a positive Coombs' test, a hemolytic anemia occurs. It sometimes causes drug fever or hepatic dysfunction. Rebound hypertension can occur after abrupt withdrawal of methyldopa (12), but this rebound is much rarer than with clonidine.

Both methyldopa and clonidine lower blood pressure by stimulating central α_2-receptors. This central action diminishes sympathetic nervous activity and increases vagal activity and sedation. The agents differ in that the effective half-life of methyldopa is much longer than that of clonidine, and there is less danger of hypertension on rapid withdrawal of the drug. However, methyldopa has occasional severe immunologic side effects that are not seen with clonidine. Guanfacine combines the long duration of action of methyldopa with the lack of immunologic side effects of clonidine.

The α_2-agonists can increase blood pressure when given in doses high enough to stimulate peripheral vasoconstriction. They should not be given in higher than recommended doses. Methyldopa, clonidine, guanabenz, and guanfacine should not be given in combination since their α_2-stimulating activities may be additive.

VASODILATORS

Vasodilators increase blood flow to vital organs, such as the brain and kidney; their peripheral mode of action avoids CNS side effects. When used properly, vasodilators are potent hypotensive agents. Some of these drugs can lower blood pressure to normal even in patients with hypertension that is resistant to all other modes of therapy.

The vasodilating activity of these drugs leads to predictable side effects. Hydralazine, minoxidil, and diazoxide dilate the precapillary arterioles with little effect on postcapillary circulation or capacitance vessels. Nitroprusside

has a balanced effect, dilating both arterioles and veins; the nitrates, such as nitroglycerin, are primarily venodilators. The arterial vasodilators lower blood pressure by allowing a relatively unimpeded flow of blood through the arterial circulation. Since capacitance vessels are not dilated, this blood returns promptly to the heart. The lower blood pressure reflexly increases sympathetic tone to the heart. Increased blood return to the heart and increased sympathetic stimulation cause a tachycardia and a greater cardiac output. The patient may experience these combined effects as a racing heart beat with palpitations, a pounding headache, and rushing vascular noises in the head. All of these cardiac manifestations of unopposed arterial vasodilation can be blocked by the β-blocking drugs or methyldopa or clonidine.

Although the vasodilators tend to increase renal blood flow, they cause sodium retention. This problem is particularly prominent with diazoxide, which has an intrinsic antinatriuretic effect, and with minoxidil. These agents cause a redistribution in renal blood flow, a decrease in perfusion pressure to the kidney, and an increase in renal renin output. Diuretics and sympatholytic agents that lower renin output can counteract these effects.

Blood pressure lowering with vasodilators has several major advantages. These agents counteract hypertensive vasoconstriction, preserve renal and cerebral blood flow, and are effective antihypertensives. However, the side effects of the arterial vasodilators prevent them from being used alone and they should be combined with a sympatholytic and a diuretic.

Hydralazine

Hydralazine is available for both parenteral and oral administration. The drug is extensively metabolized by the liver. After oral administration, bioavailability may be low because of first pass metabolism in the liver. Hepatic acetylation is a major route of metabolism and rapid acetylators have about 30% bioavailability of the drug, compared with 50% bioavailability in slow acetylators. The plasma elimination half-time of hydralazine is about 4 hours, but plasma hydralazine levels correlate poorly with antihypertensive efficacy, probably because the agent is directly bound to arterioles at its site of action. Although the drug's circulating half-life is about 3 hours, the half-time of its effect on blood pressure is about 100 hours (68). As a result, the drug is as effective when given twice a day as when given four times a day (68).

Hydralazine acts by vasodilation, which is most marked in the splanchnic, coronary, cerebral, and renal vasculature. Blood flow does not increase in skin or muscle, however. The antihypertensive potency of hydralazine is severely limited by a reflex increase in cardiac output and fluid retention. β-Blocking drugs that diminish the reflex increase in plasma renin activity are synergistic with hydralazine, and it is possible to devise a careful regimen of diuretic, β-blocker, and hydralazine that can markedly lower blood pressure with minimal side effects (96).

Although symptomatic side effects elicited by use of hydralazine can be combated with a diuretic and β-blocker, other side effects idiosyncratic to the drug cannot be blocked. A drug-induced lupus-like syndrome occurs in 10–20% of patients who receive prolonged therapy in doses exceeding 400 mg daily. This syndrome occurs more rarely at doses in the range of 200 mg/day and manifests primarily in caucasians who eliminate the drug slowly because of their acetylation phenotype. This lupus-like syndrome is reversible when the drug is withdrawn and is characterized by joint pain with skin rash; renal toxicity is infrequent. It can also cause drug fever. A peripheral neuropathy may occur, which can be corrected with pyridoxine, probably because the drug binds with this vitamin (38).

Hydralazine is available for intravenous or intramuscular injection. The usual parenteral dose is 10–40 mg, but response is quite variable and its effects develop gradually over 15–20 minutes after intravenous administration. Hydralazine is available for oral use in tablets of 10, 25, 50 and 100 mg. It is usually started in low doses so that the side effects of tachycardia and fluid retention can be combated with sympatholytics and diuretics before they become severe.

Minoxidil

Minoxidil is an extremely effective vasodilator with actions similar to those of hydralazine. However, the agent is more efficacious and more potent than hydralazine and causes different side effects.

Ninety percent of an orally administered dose of minoxidil is absorbed; 85% of the drug is metabolized by the liver and 15% is excreted unchanged in the kidney. The plasma half-life of minoxidil is approximately 4 hours, but it is effective for over 24 hours, probably because it is retained by vascular smooth muscle (49). The maximum effect of the drug is apparent 6 hours after an oral dose.

The ultimate dose of minoxidil required to control hypertension is extremely varied, and therapy should be begun with a small dose, such as 2½ or 5 mg. This dose may then be doubled every 6 hours as the maximum effect of the prior dose becomes apparent, until blood pressure control is obtained. The effective dose can then be administered every 12–24 hours. As with hydralazine, minoxidil must always be administered with a diuretic and a sympatholytic agent, such as a β-blocker or clonidine. The drug is presently approved only for therapy of hypertension resistant to other avenues of treatment. Minoxidil is effective in renal failure, and has successfully controlled blood pressure in patients with severe hypertension and end-stage renal disease.

Minoxidil's potent vasodilating effects can elicit marked hemodynamic responses. The sympathetic nervous system is activated to such a degree that plasma catecholamine levels may mimic those seen in patients with a pheochromocytoma (59). This sympathetic nervous activation stimulates renin secretion, and the vasoconstrictor effects of norepinephrine and angiotensin II diminish the hypotensive effects of minoxidil unless blocked with a sympatholytic. The renal tubules avidly retain sodium in the patient treated with minoxidil although glomerular filtration is not changed. Early in the course of therapy, even patients given large doses of furosemide may retain sodium. This fluid retention may be overcome by combining furosemide with a thiazide diuretic or metolazone, and with subsequent therapy fluid retention is less avid. It is sometimes necessary to lower the dose of minoxidil to effect a diuresis in patients who have some degree of renal insufficiency.

Minoxidil causes hypertrichosis (excessive hair growth involving the face, arms, and legs), which occurs in most patients several weeks to months after the drug is instituted and sometimes takes up to 6 months to disappear after the drug is stopped. Many women find this side effect intolerable. Pathologic lesions of the heart have been reported in two animal studies using minoxidil, but no such lesions have been reported in humans. Pulmonary hypertension has been reported during treatment with minoxidil, but there have also been reports of decreased pulmonary vascular resistance during therapy. Pericardial effusion occasionally progressing to pericardial tamponade has been described in patients receiving minoxidil, but these effects usually occur in those who have congestive heart failure or renal failure. Approximately 2% of patients treated with this drug show no response, even to a large dose (91). In 98% of hypertensives, minoxidil is one of the most effective drugs available.

Diazoxide

Diazoxide is chemically related to the thiazide diuretics, but it causes fluid retention rather than a natriuresis. Thiazide diuretics have a minor vasodilating effect, but diazoxide is a very effective vasodilator. Diazoxide directly dilates arterioles but has little effect on large veins, although it can dilate the small postcapillary resistance vessels. Diazoxide is usually given by rapid intravenous injection for the treatment of hypertension, and when given by this route, 90% of the drug is eventually bound to albumin and about one-third of the drug is cleared through the kidneys. The serum half-life of diazoxide is about 30 hours because it binds to albumin, and in patients with impaired renal function, the half-life increases proportionately. Diazoxide tends to accumulate with repeated administration, but there is no correlation between the total serum concentration and the intensity of its hypotensive action, because the hypotensive effects depend on the concentration of drug in the arterioles. Since the drug binds to both albumin and the arterioles, competition occurs between these sites and only the drug in the arterioles has a hypotensive effect. As a result, if a bolus of the drug is injected rapidly, it can reach arteriolar sites more effectively than when given slowly and its hypotensive usefulness is more beneficial and dramatic. When given this way, maximum hypotensive effect is attained in 3–5 minutes. Fifty to 150 mg of the drug can be given as a bolus, injected over 30 seconds or less. If the patient has already received a diuretic and a β-blocker, the drug may be given by slow intravenous infusion.

Diazoxide increases cardiac output and causes sympathetic stimulation and fluid retention. Its effects can be greatly potentiated by sympatholytic agents or diuresis. If the patient is volume-depleted or receiving a sympatholytic agent, the dose of diazoxide must be reduced to avoid hypotension. There are other side

effects characteristic of this agent. Cerebral blood flow is diminished (69) and the drug may cause extrapyramidal symptoms with prolonged use (63). It inhibits release of insulin from the pancreas, thereby raising blood glucose levels. In patients with diabetes mellitus or renal failure, treatment of the hyperglycemia may become necessary in a few days. Diazoxide suppresses tubular transport of uric acid and leads to hyperuricemia, as do the other thiazides. Since the drug binds strongly to albumin, it displaces warfarin anticoagulants.

In clinical practice, the side effects of diazoxide are usually relatively minor and its ease of use is one of its major advantages. In contrast to nitroprusside, diazoxide can be given in hypertensive emergencies to a patient who is not on continuous blood pressure monitoring, because its maximum effect is reached at 5 minutes and blood pressure gradually returns to pretreatment level within 5–12 hours. This allows time to introduce other antihypertensive therapies that can be maintained over a longer period. The drug should not be used alone when cardiac stimulation may be deleterious, such as in patients with severe coronary artery disease or aortic dissection. In most patients with severe hypertension, diazoxide can successfully lower blood pressure without the need for continuous monitoring.

Sodium Nitroprusside

Sodium nitroprusside's hypotensive capability has been recognized for 50 years, but it was little used until it was commercially marketed and promoted as Nipride. Its hypotensive effect is probably due to the iron-nitroso (Fe-NO) grouping in the intact nitroprusside molecule; the drug causes both venous and arterial vasodilation, as do the nitrates. This balanced vascular dilation, which includes venous capacitance vessels, gives nitroprusside a spectrum of effect slightly different from that of the other vasodilators. The venodilation results in a decreased cardiac preload instead of the increased preload seen with the "pure" arterial vasodilators. In the absence of heart failure, cardiac output either falls or does not change in response to nitroprusside. However, if myocardial disease has diminished cardiac output, nitroprusside may increase output as a result of diminished afterload. Nitroprusside usually causes a 20–30% increase in heart rate, but if there is a preexisting tachycardia due to heart failure, heart rate may actually decrease slightly. The decreased preload may diminish cardiac work, and angina often improves when nitroprusside is given; this finding is in contrast to the "pure" arterial vasodilators, which may cause myocardial ischemia.

Since nitroprusside causes venous pooling, it can induce a profound postural hypotension, unlike the pure arterial vasodilators. A critically ill patient who is receiving nitroprusside and becomes acutely hypotensive is usually intravascularly depleted and requires fluid replacement. With the patient in the upright posture, nitroprusside causes a fall in cardiac output, which may have a major effect on the drug's hypotensive impact. In supine patients, the fall in cardiac output is responsible for about one-fourth of its hypotensive activity. Nitroprusside-induced hypotension activates the sympathetic nervous system, which increases renin output and heart rate. Renal blood flow, glomerular filtration rate, and cerebral circulation do not change. Since nitroprusside does not increase cardiac preload, it is a good drug for treating patients with congestive heart failure, myocardial insufficiency, or aortic dissection in which hyperkinetic cardiac output would be harmful. It is also useful in treating hypertension associated with myocardical infarction and an unstable blood pressure since its effects can be rapidly terminated by stopping infusion.

Sodium nitroprusside given by intravenous infusion (0.25–2.5 μg/kg/min, advancing to a maximum of 10 μg/kg/min) lowers blood pressure within seconds, and the hypotensive effect dissipates within 1–2 minutes after stopping the infusion. The drug is extremely effective and can lower blood pressure markedly in any person. Because of its rapid action and potency, nitroprusside should be administered with an infusion pump while blood pressure is continuously monitored. After the first 2 hours of administration, the rate of drug infusion frequently needs to be increased to maintain an equivalent hypotensive effect because nitroprusside causes a rise in cardiac index without inducing tachycardia (73). The increased cardiac index is due to fluid accumulation and sympathetic nervous stimulation and can be effectively counteracted with a diuretic or β-blocking agent. The drug can increase or maintain cerebral blood flow, and this response can lead to increased intracranial pressure, which might be deleterious in patients with head injury.

Nitroprusside is broken down to cyanide, which is rapidly coverted in the body to thiocyanate. Cyanide toxicity from the drug is uncommon, but thiocyanate is handled by the body in essentially the same manner as are chloride and bromide. The thiocyanate may thus be retained by patients with renal failure or by those receiving low sodium diets; its half-life is normally 4 days. If the concentration of thiocyanate exceeds 10 mg/dl, weakness, hypoxia, nausea, tinnitus, muscle spasm, disorientation, and psychosis may occur. Thiocyanate interferes with transport of iodide by the thyroid gland and may cause hypothyroidism. If nitroprusside is infused for a long time and in high doses, blood levels of thiocyanate must be monitored. When standing, nitroprusside-treated patients may experience postural hypotension, and some may encounter nasal stuffiness and increased body warmth, dizziness, weakness, muscle twitching, and nausea.

Sodium nitroprusside (Nipride) is supplied as a powder (50-mg vials) for reconstitution in 250 ml of 5% dextrose (yielding a concentration of 200 μg/ml). This solution may be used for 24 hours after reconstitution, but should be protected from light. Deeply colored solutions should be discarded because development of color indicates loss of potency.

Patients given sodium nitroprusside must have their blood pressure continuously measured, therefore the drug can only be used where monitoring is available. Although nitroprusside is not necessary for treating most cases of severe hypertension, it is one of the better agents available for treating hypertensive emergencies. Since the drug becomes less effective and leads to accumulation of thiocyanate with prolonged infusion, patients should be given antihypertensive drugs soon after the initiation of therapy. Diuretics and sympatholytics markedly potentiate the effects of this vasodilator and decrease the dose of drug required.

Calcium Antagonists

The myocardium and smooth muscle cells have slow calcium channels in their cell walls that regulate the influx of calcium into the cytoplasm. Elevated free intracellular calcium increases smooth muscle contractility, peripheral resistance, and blood pressure. Calcium-blocking drugs lower intracellular calcium levels and thus cause vasodilation. The calcium channel blockers, nifedipine, diltiazem, and verapamil, are licensed for therapy of arrhythmias in the United States, but are also effective antihypertensives (71). Nifedipine decreases blood pressure in hypertensives but not in normal subjects (14). It can rapidly lower blood pressure when given sublingually (15) or orally (30), and the effect of a single dose lasts about 7 hours (30). The drug's vasodilating effect reflexly increases sympathetic nervous stimulation to the heart. However, nifedipine's direct cardiodepressant activity counteracts its reflex stimulant effects so that heart rate and contractility do not change much (78). After several months, the hypotensive effect of nifedipine tends to diminish when the drug is given alone, but the hypotensive effect is maintained when the drug is administered with propranolol or clonidine (30). About one-fourth of the patients receiving nifedipine accumulate fluid and require a diuretic.

Calcium channel blockers can cause ankle swelling in some people, but overall they have a mild diuretic effect. Their hypotensive effect is potentiated by β-blocking drugs. Calcium antagonists thus are useful in both emergency and chronic treatment of hypertension (22). There is not yet enough experience with these drugs to suggest that they be used as initial therapy in the treatment of hypertension. However, many hypertensive patients develop cardiac arrhythmias or congestive failure that is amenable to treatment with nifedipine, and in these patients, it is reasonable to increase the dose to obtain an antihypertensive effect. The choice of calcium channel blocker depends on the desired effect. Verapamil is the most strongly cardiodepressant; nifedipine is the most effective vasodilator, with relatively little effect on the heart. Diltiazem has effects intermediate between the other two drugs. A 240-mg timed release formulation of verapamil was recently approved for therapy of hypertension in the United States.

ANGIOTENSIN-CONVERTING ENZYME INHIBITORS (ACE INHIBITORS)

Renin is released from the kidney and enzymatically converts circulating angiotensinogen to angiotensin I. Angiotensin I is then rapidly converted to angiotensin II by angiotensin-converting enzyme, which is present in blood vessel walls and in the lung (Fig. 20.2). Angiotensin II is a very potent vasoconstrictor that also stimulates aldosterone release. Renin levels are markedly elevated in renovascular hypertension and malignant hy-

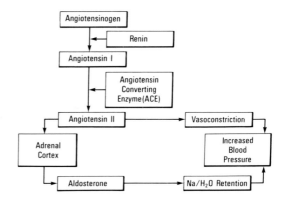

Figure 20.2.   The renin-angiotensin-aldosterone system.

pertension, and are above normal in about one-fourth of patients with essential hypertension. The pressor effects of renin can be blocked by inhibition of angiotensin-converting enzyme. The first inhibitor of this enzyme, teprotide, was derived from snake venom. Captopril was specifically designed to interfere with the active site of angiotensin-converting enzyme, and enalapril has a similar mode of action. ACE inhibitors are potent antihypertensive agents that act primarily by preventing the production of angiotensin II. Angiotensin-converting enzyme also causes the breakdown of circulating bradykinin, a potent vasodilator (20). Bradykinin acts in tissues to release vasodilatory prostaglandins; treatment with indomethacin diminishes the hypotensive activity of infused bradykinin and the hypotensive activity of captopril. ACE inhibitors also inhibit the pressor responses to sympathetic nerve stimulation, which may be mediated by inhibition of local angiotensin II formation in the blood vessel wall. Angiotensin II potentiates both the release and the pressor responses to norepinephrine. ACE inhibitors lower blood pressure by lowering levels of angiotensin II, and possibly by enhancing bradykinin levels and by inhibiting the effects of angiotensin II on sympathetic nerves (35).

The hemodynamic effects of ACE inhibitors differ from those of other antihypertensive agents and may be beneficial in patients with hypertensive damage to the kidneys and heart (26). After an acute dose of captopril, blood pressure reduction is related to the initial plasma renin activity (10). Patients with high renin levels have a triphasic blood pressure response to captopril. Their blood pressure falls abruptly, sometimes to dangerous levels in the first few hours, and then rebounds nearly to pretreatment levels. Over subsequent days, blood pressure slowly decreases, but not to the level encountered during the initiation of therapy. Patients with normal or low renin levels have a more prolonged and gentler decrease in blood pressure. The initial hypotensive response is exaggerated in patients who are volume-depleted, and this excessive hypotension can be treated with saline intravenous infusions.

Enalapril is a prodrug that is converted in the liver to the active metabolite, enalaprilat. Captopril can have hypotensive effects 15 minutes after a sublingual dose, but enalapril takes several hours to reach peak effects.

ACE inhibitors lower total peripheral resistance and cause little change in cardiac output, heart rate, or pulmonary wedge pressure in most hypertensives. However, in patients with congestive heart failure, they can increase cardiac output by diminishing afterload (82). ACE inhibitors decrease renal vascular resistance enough so that renal plasma flow increases even when blood pressure is low. In patients with renal artery stenosis, glomerular filtration rate may decrease. Serum creatinine may increase during the early stages of therapy, particularly if there is bilateral renal artery stenosis. ACE inhibitors do not cause postural hypotension and they lower blood pressure without a reflex increase in sympathetic nervous activity. Norepinephrine levels thus remain unchanged during therapy, but during exercise norepinephrine and epinephrine levels respond normally (54).

ACE inhibitors are particularly useful in the treatment of severe renovascular hypertension not amenable to surgery and in patients with congestive heart failure. They correct both the hypertension and electrolyte imbalances caused by markedly elevated renin levels. Angiotensin II stimulates the release of aldosterone, which causes renal potassium wasting. Serum potassium usually does not increase to dangerous levels with ACE inhibitors, but potassium supplementation should be discontinued. In patients who do not respond initially to ACE inhibition alone, the addition of a diuretic such as hydrochlorothiazide, which normally stimulates the release of renin by the kidney, enhances hypotensive effects. The addition of a vasodilator such as minoxidil to this drug regimen greatly increases the antihypertensive effect, even in patients resistant to the individual components of therapy (56). Captopril (25 mg) can be successfully em-

ployed in hypertensive emergencies (74). It is usually a very potent agent in malignant hypertension, but its effects are difficult to control in this setting.

Captopril contains a sulfhydryl grouping that can cause many immunologic side effects. A rash, occasionally accompanied by pruritus, fever, and eosinophilia, can occur. The symptoms usually arise in the first several weeks of therapy and may be dose-related. A reduction of the dose or continued therapy with the same dose often results in diminution of the rash, although the skin lesions may progress. Temporary loss of taste has been reported in about 6% of patients. This symptom is usually transient and does not respond to zinc therapy. Proteinuria of greater than 1 g/day occurs in just over 1% of the patients on captopril, and the nephrotic syndrome may develop in some of these individuals. The drug causes a glomerulopathy and electron-dense deposits similar to those caused by penicillamine and other sulfhydryl-containing drugs.

Neutropenia is the most severe side effect of captopril and occurs in about 0.3% of patients (85). It develops in the first 3–12 weeks of treatment, and blood counts should be obtained frequently during the first 3 months of therapy and periodically thereafter.

Captopril is provided in tablets of 12.5, 25, 50, and 100 mg. After oral administration, blood levels peak in 30–90 minutes and approximately 70% of the drug is absorbed, although food in the gastrointestinal tract may reduce absorption. After absorption, the drug is distributed to most tissues except the nervous system. Fifty percent of the drug is excreted by the kidneys within the first 4 hours of administration, and elimination of captopril and its metabolites correlates closely with creatinine clearance. Patients with renal insufficiency reach much higher peak plasma levels, and the dose may be considerably reduced in patients with impaired renal function. The hypotensive effect of captopril depends on 95% inhibition of angiotensin-converting enzyme, since this enzyme is present in great excess in the body. Once angiotensin-converting enzyme is inhibited, only negligible amounts of angiotensin II are generated and captopril's maximal hypotensive effect is obtained. Increasing the dose of captopril given at a single time thus does not lower blood pressure further. Larger doses maintain adequate captopril blood levels for a longer time, however.

Enalapril is the first of many nonsulfhydryl-containing ACE inhibitors that have been developed. It is converted to enalaprilat in the liver, which is the active form of the drug. This conversion step provides a slow onset of action and diminishes the possibility of an initial severe hypotensive response. Enalaprilat has a long half-life, thus enalapril is effective when given once daily. The drug does not cause sulfhydryl-related immune side effects.

Enalapril is available in tablets of 5, 10, and 20 mg, with a maximum recommended dose of 40 mg daily. Enalaprilat is under investigation as an intravenous ACE inhibitor for use in emergencies.

All of the ACE inhibitors impair the breakdown of bradykinin. This action may manifest as a chronic cough or as life-threatening angioedema requiring tracheostomy.

COMBINED DRUG THERAPY OF HYPERTENSION

The critically ill patient with severe hypertension can only rarely attain normal blood pressure in response to a single drug. Large doses of an individual drug are likely to cause a number of side effects, and many antihypertensive drugs potentiate the effects of others. It is often possible to take advantage of this potentiation to attain an adequate hypotensive effect with minimal side effects by using more than one drug. However, some drug combinations are ineffective or toxic. Many drugs lower blood pressure as a side effect of their primary use (Table 20.5), and some are potent antihypertensive agents when used with a diuretic.

Diuretics

The thiazide diuretics are the most useful agents in the treatment of hypertension and can be successfully employed in very low doses. Daily doses of 25 mg of chlorthalidone or 12.5 mg of hydrochlorothiazide provide the maximum hypotensive effect; larger doses are more toxic but not more effective in patients with normal renal function. The thiazide diuretics increase blood cholesterol, triglycerides, uric acid, and blood sugar, and cause hypokalemia. All of these undesirable side effects are dose-dependent and are slight at low doses. It is not necessary to routinely supplement low doses of thiazides with potassium-sparing diuretic agents, such as triamterene, amiloride, or spironolactone. Low doses of these thiazides should not cause hypokalemia, and if hypokalemia occurs, it suggests an aldosterone-secreting adrenal adenoma, adrenal hyperplasia, Cushing's syndrome, or renovascular hypertension.

Sympatholytic Drugs

The sympatholytic drugs include the β-blockers; the α-agonist drugs, clonidine, guanabenz, guanfacine, and α-methyldopa; and the α-blocking drug, prazosin. The α-blockers, phenoxybenzamine and phentolamine, are not very useful in the treatment of essential hypertension, and guanethidine and reserpine are rarely used now that less toxic drugs are available. The effects of sympatholytic drugs

Table 20.5
Drugs That Lower Blood Pressure[a]

Drug	Action	Drug Interactions
Neuroleptics, especially chlorpromazine	α Blockade	Potentiated by diuretics

Dopamine agonists
  L-Dopa
  Bromocriptine
  Dopamine
  Pimozide
	Stimulate dopamine receptors, inhibit NE release	

Fenfluramine	Inhibits NE release	Potentiated by diuretics
Tricyclic antidepressants	?	Inhibits clonidine effect
MAO inhibitors	?	Hypertension with tyramine, reserpine
Marijuana	Inhibits NE effects	
Opiates	Vasodilation, inhibits NE release	

Antiarrhythmics
  Nifedipine
  Verapamil
  Disopyramide
	Myocardial depression, vasodilation	

[a] NE, norepinephrine; MAO, monoamine oxidase.

are often potentiated by combination with a diuretic. Diuretics activate the sympathetic nervous system in response to volume depletion and hypotension. The body is then dependent on sympathetic nervous activity for maintenance of blood pressure, and the sympatholytic drugs become more effective in this setting.

The β-blocking drugs are all quite similar in their antihypertensive efficacy and in no instance is the use of more than one β-blocker at a time worthwhile. Clonidine acts to diminish the sympathetic nervous system release of norepinephrine, and the β-blockers antagonize the effects of norepinephrine. In experimental animals, β-blockers such as propranolol that penetrate the central nervous system inhibit the antihypertensive efficacy of clonidine. In humans, the combination of clonidine and propranolol has been reported as both effective and ineffective (89, 92). It appears unwise to combine these drugs because of potential toxicity. Although the combination of methyldopa with β-blockers has not been as extensively studied, methyldopa has actions very similar to those of clonidine.

The combination of the α-blocking agent, prazosin, with a β-blocking drug seems to be a reasonable approach to the control of hypertension. Labetalol, a drug with both peripheral α- and β-blocking activity, is an effective antihypertensive agent. However, according to some reports the antihypertensive efficacy of prazosin combined with propranolol is not more effective than either agent used alone (41, 57). Prazosin also does not enhance the antihypertensive efficacy of clonidine (29).

There is no clear evidence that the combination of β-blockers, clonidine, methyldopa, or prazosin is effective. In fact, these combinations may be dangerous. For example, the addition of clonidine to the regimen of a patient treated with a β-blocker caused dramatic pressor responses; and in a more complex situation with the patient on multiple sympatholytic drugs, just an increase in the dose of clonidine caused a pressor response (41).

In no cases has it proved clearly beneficial to combine sympatholytic drugs in the treatment of hypertension, except for the combination of α- and β-blocking agents in a patient with pheochromocytoma. On the other hand, there are numerous reports of unexpected pressor responses, and a predictable increase in the number of side effects occurs as more drugs are added. In general, patients should be treated with a single sympatholytic agent.

If they are treated with a β-blocker or prazosin, some do not respond, in which case it is reasonable to change to an α₂-agonist or to add an agent from another class of antihypertensive drugs, such as the vasodilators.

Drug Combinations with Vasodilators

The arterial vasodilators, hydralazine, minoxidil, and diazoxide, lower blood pressure by decreasing arteriolar tone, but they do not dilate venous capacitance vessels. They thus permit a relatively unimpeded flow of blood back to the heart and reflexly increase sympathetic nervous activity because of their effect on blood pressure. The increased blood supply and sympathetic stimulation can greatly increase cardiac output. The vasodilators also cause fluid retention by increasing renin and aldosterone production. Consequently, vasodilators are not very effective in lowering blood pressure by themselves; they need to be combined with a diuretic and a sympatholytic for maximal hypotensive effect and to avoid the side effects of edema and palpitations. A thiazide diuretic can sometimes control fluid accumulation, but minoxidil and diazoxide cause such avid fluid retention that a powerful diuretic such as furosemide is often necessary.

A variety of sympatholytic drugs potentiate the antihypertensive effects of the vasodilators, including β-blockers, α₂-agonists, reserpine, and guanethidine. β-Blocking drugs can block the increased cardiac output and renin secretion engendered by the vasodilators and do so with a minimum number of side effects. In fact, when β-blockers are used in appropriate doses, they can eliminate the palpitations, headache, and vascular noises that may be caused by the vasodilators. β-Blockers diminish β-adrenergic effects engendered by vasodilators, but they do not block α-adrenergic effects. If β-blockers do not lower blood pressure adequately, it is reasonable to change to an α₂-agonist such as clonidine. Clonidine should be substituted for the β-blocker, not added to the previous drug regimen, since clonidine can raise blood pressure in a patient treated with diuretic, hydralazine, and β-blocker (41).

Many hypertensives develop coronary insufficiency and angina pectoris. A vasodilator used alone can worsen the angina, but a vasodilator can safely be used if the patient is already on adequate doses of diuretic and β-blocker. Moreover, in some of these patients, vasodilators decrease cardiac work and diminish angina symptoms.

Drug Combinations with Angiotensin-Converting Enzyme Inhibitors

The ACE inhibitors can be used as single agents in many hypertensives. The drugs work well in patients with high renin levels or high circulating catecholamines and are sometimes beneficial in those with heart failure. An ACE inhibitor plus thiazide diuretic controls blood pressure in 90% of hypertensives (51). The addition of a vasodilator to this regimen lowers blood pressure even more.

PRACTICAL APPLICATIONS FOR THE CRITICAL CARE PRACTITIONER'S EVALUATION OF THE SEVERELY HYPERTENSIVE PATIENT

Essential hypertension is a lifelong disease and therapy ideally should be initiated slowly with the drugs least likely to cause side effects. However, patients presenting with severe hypertension may have a poor prognosis unless they receive prompt, effective treatment. The most common cause of a markedly elevated blood pressure is a stress reaction (53). Some patients who are only slightly hypertensive in their normal environment respond to the stress of a medical examination with severe hypertension, which promptly subsides when they return to their usual surroundings. This type of patient is always anxious and may conceal this anxiety at the expense of increased internal stress. A hypertensive stress reaction is particularly likely in patients receiving β-blocking drugs. They secrete epinephrine in response to stress and then have an "epinephrine reversal." The marked elevation in blood pressure is mediated by epinephrine's α-adrenergic effects without any compensatory β-adrenergic vasodilation. Ganglionic-blocking drugs such as guanethidine can block this stress-induced hypertension but clonidine or methyldopa do not. The effects of clonidine or methyldopa can be overridden during severe stress, allowing normal discharge from the sympathetic nervous system. There are several clues to the stress reaction, including pupillary dilation, sweaty palms, and a nervous and sometimes overly helpful behavior. On physical examination, the patient lacks the stigmata of hypertensive disease and funduscopic ex-

amination shows a relatively undamaged retinal vasculature. Administering potent antihypertensive agents to these patients leaves them hypotensive when they return to a less stressful environment.

A patient with persistent severe hypertension needs to have blood pressure lowered rapidly. The drug used depends on the cause of the hypertension and the presence of coexisting illnesses.

Patients with hypertension are prone to develop cerebrovascular occlusion, intracerebral bleeding, or subarachnoid hemorrhage. These customarily produce an increase in hypertension, ECG abnormalities, and focal neurologic signs. Blood pressure should be lowered very carefully in these patients to prevent extension of the damage; vasodilators that tend to increase intracranial pressure should be avoided.

Pheochromocytoma

Pheochromocytoma can produce episodic severe hypertension in response to circulating norepinephrine. Patients with pheochromocytoma are usually volume-depleted from the pressor effects of norepinephrine, thus treatment with diuretics may cause circulatory compromise to vital organs. β-Blocking drugs should not be given to the patient with a pheochromocytoma until adequate α blockade has been achieved, since blockade of β-adrenergic–mediated vasodilation allows unopposed α vasoconstriction and may worsen the hypertension. On the other hand, treatment with α-blocking drugs such as prazosin may be strikingly effective in lowering blood pressure, and a prolonged hypotensive response to a low dose of prazosin should make one suspicious of the presence of a pheochromocytoma. Calcium channel blocking drugs are also very effective in pheochromocytoma because they impair catecholamine release from the tumor.

Drug Reactions

Several drugs can cause reactions that mimic the pressor response to a pheochromocytoma (Table 20.6). Phenylpropanolamine is a popular over-the-counter anorectic agent, frequently combined with ephedrine or caffeine and marketed for the treatment of obesity, drowsiness, and nasal congestion. These drugs cause α-adrenergic–mediated vasoconstriction and raise blood pressure even when given in

Table 20.6
Drugs That Increase Blood Pressure

Drug	Action	Drug Interactions
Ethanol	↓ Aldosterone metabolism	Enhances diuretic K$^+$ loss; enhances sedation with methyldopa, clonidine
Nicotine	Vasoconstriction	
Caffeine	Sympathetic stimulation	Synergistic with nicotine, mild diuresis
Stimulants		
Amphetamine		
Methylphenidate		
Methamphetamine	Norepinephrine release, blockage of reuptake	Paradoxical hypertension with β-blockers
Phenmetrazine		
Cocaine		
Ephedrine		
Isoproterenol		
Isoetharine	β Stimulation	Inhibited by β-blockers
Terbutaline		
Phenylephrine	α Stimulation	Inhibited by prazosin
Phenylpropanolamine		
MAO inhibitor and tyramine[a]	Enhanced tyramine effect	
Mineralocorticoids	Na$^+$ retention	Enhance K$^+$ loss with diuretics
Glucocorticoids	?	
Estrogens, oral contraceptives	↑ Angiotensinogen	
Indomethacin	Blocks prostaglandin vasodilation	↓ Diuretic effects
Atropine	Tachycardia	
Antihistamines		

[a] MAO, monoamine oxidase.

normal doses and can cause marked hypertension when taken in excessive doses.

Monoamine oxidase inhibitors have had a resurgence in popularity for treatment of depression. They ordinarily lower blood pressure, but when taken with a food containing tyramine, such as cheese or wine, they can cause severe hypertension. They can also worsen the hypertension caused by drugs such as ephedine or phenylpropanolamine, which are degraded by monoamine oxidase. Other drugs that can increase blood pressure are listed in Table 20.6.

Abrupt withdrawal of clonidine in doses over 0.3 mg/day can cause a rebound increase in sympathetic nervous release of norepinephrine and an overshoot of hypertension. All of the above-mentioned drug reactions increase blood pressure through α-adrenergic stimulation and they are best treated acutely with α-blocking drugs. Although patients with a pheochromocytoma or one of these drug reactions are usually tachycardic and tremulous, they should not receive β-blocking drugs, which worsen their hypertension.

Malignant Hypertension

As opposed to the mislabeled "benign essential hypertension," which is neither benign nor essential, malignant hypertension is often fatal if not treated. Malignant hypertension usually develops slowly over a period of a few weeks and should be brought under control within days of its diagnosis. Diastolic blood pressure is characteristically above 130 mm Hg and the patient often presents because of symptoms caused by the hypertension, unlike the asymptomatic patient with lesser degrees of hypertension. Patients usually complain of headache, dizziness, and occasional blurred vision, and on questioning admit to some cardiorespiratory decompensation. Physical examination reveals signs of congestive heart failure and pulmonary edema, and the optic fundi have hemorrhages, exudates, and papilledema. Untreated malignant hypertension has a 50% fatality in 6 months, and prior to effective treatment it was generally fatal in 2 years. Because of their poor prognosis, these patients need to be treated quickly, usually in the hospital. A variety of drugs can bring the blood pressure down gradually and safely, without the need for continuous intensive monitoring (Table 20.7). These patients always have some renal damage due to their hypertension, and their fluid status needs to be evaluated on an individual basis. Serum creatinine and blood urea nitrogen levels are elevated, and proteinuria and hematuria are always present. The patient who has oliguria may be volume-over-

Table 20.7
Parenteral Antihypertensive Drugs

Drug	Administration	Dose	Time of Onset	Use in [a]	Avoid in [a]
Diazoxide	i.v. push	50–300 mg	1–2 min	Encephalopathy, glomerulonephritis	Acute MI, aortic aneurysm, pulmonary edema
Nitroprusside	i.v. drip	0.5–8 μg/kg/min	<1 min	Acute MI, aortic aneurysm, encephalopathy, intracranial bleeding	
Trimethaphan camsylate	i.v. drip	1–15 mg/min	<1 min	Intracranial bleeding, aortic aneurysm	Glomerulonephritis
Hydralazine	i.v. or i.m.	10–25 mg	20 min	Glomerulonephritis	Aortic aneurysm, acute MI
Methyldopa	i.v.	250–500 mg	3 hr		Encephalopathy, intracranial bleeding
Labetalol	i.v.	20–300 mg	2 min	Angina pectoris	Congestive heart failure, asthma

[a] MI, myocardial infarction.

loaded, but many of these patients have a low blood volume and should not receive diuretics. Circulating renin and catecholamines are uniformly extremely high, so that excess volume depletion may allow these vasopressors to compromise the circulation of vital organs. These elevated circulating pressor agents make these patients very susceptible to the hypotensive effects of certain drugs. Captopril may lower blood pressure with dangerous rapidity, whereas the sympatholytic drugs such as clonidine, methyldopa, reserpine, and the ganglionic blockers are usually very effective. Vasodilators sufficiently potent to counteract the intense vasospasm encountered in malignant hypertension are quite effective, but the diuretics usually do not lower blood pressure. β-Blockers are often ineffective acutely, and they may worsen the congestive heart failure that these patients experience. Malignant hypertension is also aptly called "acute vasospastic hypertension," and treatment aimed at the vasospasm is usually successful. Diuretics and β-blockers may worsen the vasospasm and thus are not very effective in the treatment of the hypertension, but they may be used to treat fluid retention or excess cardiac stimulation.

These basic principles allow for a wide variety of antihypertensive drugs that can be used in this situation, and the drug should be selected for the individual patient's symptoms and physical status. The vasodilators, hydralazine and diazoxide, can be given intravenously (Table 20.7). Diazoxide works very

quickly and hydralazine takes effect in about 15 minutes. If the patient has a long history of resistance to other hypertensive drugs, it may be appropriate to start treatment with minoxidil; the peak of an oral dose is seen 6 hours after administration. The sympatholytic agent, methyldopa, may be given intravenously but often takes hours before it has a hypotensive effect. An oral dose of 0.2 mg of clonidine is convenient and usually quite effective in lowering blood pressure. Its effect may be titrated by adding 0.1 mg hourly up to a total dose of 0.5 mg to lower blood pressure. Both methyldopa and clonidine are sedating. This action may be beneficial in the hospitalized patient, but may be dangerous in outpatients. An oral dose of prazosin has an acute effect to lower blood pressure; however, experience with this agent in the setting of malignant hypertension is very limited. Intravenous labetalol can be slowly titrated, but it often causes postural hypotension.

There is no one best drug for this disease because the choice of agents should depend on the patient being treated. The vasodilators may worsen coronary insufficiency or an aortic aneurysm, but they reduce afterload in congestive heart failure and usually preserve renal blood flow. The sympatholytic agents are often convenient to use in a patient without severe signs of cardiac or renal dysfunction. However, in a patient suspected of having a myocardial infarction or intracerebral hemorrhage, nitroprusside may be one of the safest agents to use because it causes a balanced arterial and venous dilation, and can be rapidly withdrawn during hypotensive episodes. Often, the best guide to a choice of drugs is the record of a patient's prior response to antihypertensive drugs.

Hypertensive Encephalopathy

The patient with hypertensive encephalopathy has a severe headache and frequently has visual disturbances, paralysis, convulsions, vomiting, stupor, and coma. The onset of encephalopathy occurs over a few hours, and diastolic blood pressure is usually above 140 mm Hg. Because of the abrupt onset, patients may not have developed papilledema, but arteriolar spasm and a retinal sheen are always present. There may be evidence of pulmonary edema and renal failure, and if untreated, the patient will die in several hours or days. This condition needs to be treated immediately, and intravenous nitroprusside or ganglionic blockers are the agents of choice. Intravenous diazoxide can be used in hypertensive encephalopathy if the patient cannot be continuously monitored in an intensive care unit. Rapid institution of therapy in hypertensive encephalopathy is life-saving. However, hypertensive encephalopathy is now a far less frequent occurrence than several years ago since most patients with severe hypertension can now have their blood pressure adequately controlled.

References

1. Agharanya JC, Alonso R, Wurtman RJ: Changes in catecholamine excretion after short-term tyrosine ingestion in normally fed human subjects. Am J Clin Nutr 34:82–87, 1981.
2. Anderson RJ, Hat GR, Crumpler CP, Reed WG, Matthews CA: Oral clonidine loading in hypertensive emergencies. JAMA 246:848–850, 1981.
3. Beal D, Dujovne C, Gillis JS: The effect of methyldopa on human judgment in hypertensive patients and normal volunteers. Res Commun Psychol Psychiatry Behav 5:205–217, 1980.
4. Beard TC, Gray WR, Cooke HM, Barge R: Randomised controlled trial of a no-added sodium diet for mild hypertension. Lancet 2:455–458, 1982
5. Berglund G, Andersson O: Low doses of hydrochlorothiazide in hypertension: antihypertensive and metabolic effects. Eur J Clin Pharmacol 10:177–182, 1976.
6. Bradley WF, Hoffman GF, Hutchison JC, Kalams Z, Waldron SL: Comparison of prazosin and methyldopa in mild to moderate hypertension: a multicenter cooperative study. Curr Ther Res 21:28–35, 1977.
7. Brenner WI, Lieberman AN: Acute clonidine withdrawal syndrome following open-heart operation. Ann Thorac Surg 24:80–82, 1977.
8. Brodsky JB, Bravo JJ: Acute postoperativve clonidine withdrawal syndrome. Anesthesiology 44:519–521, 1976.
9. Brown MJ, Salmon D, Rendell M: Clonidine hallucinations. Ann Intern Med 93:456–457, 1980.
10. Brunner HR, Gavras H, Waeber B, Kershaw GR, Turini GA, Vukovich RA, McKinstry DN, Gavras I: Oral angiotensin-converting enzyme inhibitor in long-term treatment of hypertensive patients. Ann Intern Med 90:19–23, 1979.
11. Buhler FR, Laragh JH, Baer L, Vaughan ED, Brunner HR: Propranolol inhibition of renin secretion. N Engl J Med 287:1209–1214, 1972.
12. Burden AC, Alexander CPT: Rebound hypertension after acute methyldopa withdrawal. Br Med J, 1:1056–1057, 1976.
13. Cavero I, Roach AG: The pharmacology of prazosin, a novel antihypertensive agent. Life Sci 27:1525–1540, 1980.
14. Corea L, Bentivoglio M, Cosmi F, Alunni G: Catecholamines, plasma levels and haemodynamic changes induced by nifedipine in chronic severe heart failure. Curr Ther Res 30:698–707, 1981.
15. Corea L, Miele N, Bentivoglio M, Boschetti E, Agabiti-Rosei E, Muiesan G: Acute and chronic effects of nifedipine on plasma renin activity and plasma adrenaline and noradrenaline in controls and hypertensive patients. Clin Sci 57:115s–117s, 1979.
16. Dollery CT, Davies DS, Draffan GH, Dargie HJ, Dean CR, Reid JL, Clare RA, Murray S: Clinical pharmacology and pharmacokinetics of clonidine. Clin Pharmacol Ther 19:11–17, 1975.
17. Dornhorst A, Powell SH, Pensky J: Aggravation by propranolol of hyperglycaemic effect of hydrochlorothiazide in type II diabetics without alteration of insulin secretion. Lancet 1:123–126, 1985.
18. Dustan HP: Obesity and hypertension. Ann Intern Med 103:1047–1049, 1985.
19. Dustan HP, Bravo EL, Tarazi RC: Volume dependent, essential and steroid hypertension. Am J Cardiol 32:606, 1973.
20. Edwards CR, Padfield PL: Angiotensin-converting enzyme inhibitors: past, present, and bright future. Lancet 1:30–34, 1985.
21. Einhorne D, Young JB, Landsberg L: Hypotensive effect of fasting: possible involvement of the sympathetic nervous system and endogenous opiates. Science 217:727–729, 1982.
22. Frishman W, Klein N, Beer N: Nifedipine in hypertension: expanding applications of a new drug. Arch Intern Med 141:843, 1981.
23. Frolich ED, Dustan HP, Page IH: Hyperdynamic beta-adrenergic circulatory state. Arch Intern Med 117:614–619, 1966.
24. Garvey HL, Ram N: Centrally induced hypotensive effects of beta adrenergic blocking drugs. Eur J Pharmacol 33:283–294, 1975.
25. Graham RM, Thornell G, Gain IR: Prazosin: the first dose phenomenon. Br Med J 2:1293, 1976.
26. Helgeland A, Strommen R, Hagelund CH, Tretli S: Enalapril, atenolol and hydrochlorothiazide in mild to moderate hypertension. Lancet 1:872–875, 1986.
27. Holland OB, Fairchild C: Renin classification for diuretic and beta blocker treatment of black hypertensive patients. J Chronic Dis 35:179–182, 1982.
28. Hollifield JW, Sherman K, Zwagg RV, Shand DG: Proposed mechanisms of propranolol's antihypertensive effect in essential hypertension. N Engl J Med 295:68–73, 1976.
29. Hubbell FA, Weber MA, Drayer JM, Rose DE: Central alpha-adrenergic stimulation by clonidine overrides the antihypertensive effect of peripheral alpha adrenergic blockadge induced by prazosin. Presented at the 8th Meeting of the International Society of Hypertension, Milan, Italy, 1981.
30. Imai Y, Abe K, Otsuke Y, Iorkawa N, Yasumina M, Saito

K, et al: Management of severe hypertension with ni-fedipine in combination with clonidine or propranolol. *Arzneimittelforschung* 30:674–678, 1980.

31. Jackson EK, Campbell WB: A possible antihypertensive mechanism of propranolol: antagonism of angiotensin II enhancement of sympathetic nerve transmission through prostaglandins. *Hypertension* 3:23–33, 1981.
32. Jeffreys DB, Flanagan RJ, Volans GN: Reversal of ethanol-induced coma with naloxone. *Lancet* 1:308–309, 1980.
33. Jenkins JS, Conolly J: Adrenocortical response to ethanol in man. *Br Med J* 2:804–805, 1968.
34. Joossens JV, Geboers J: Nutrition and essential hypertension. *Bibl Nutr Dieta* 37:104–118, 1986.
35. Katzman PL, Hulthen UL, Hokfelt B: The effect of 8 weeks treatment with the calcium antagonist felodipine on blood pressure, heart rate, working capacity, plasma renin activity, plasma angiotensin II, urinary catecholamines and aldosterone in patients with essential hypertension. *Br J Clin Pharmacol* 21:633–640, 1986.
36. Kempner W: Treatment of hypertensive vascular disease with rice diet. *Am J Med* 4:545–577, 1948.
37. Kobinger W: Alpha-adrenocepters in cardiovascular regulation. In Ziegler MG, Lake CR (eds): *Norepinephrine* (Frontiers of Clinical Neuroscience, vol 4). Baltimore, Williams & Wilkins, 1984.
38. Koch-Weser J: Vasodilator drugs in the treatment of hypertension. *Arch Intern Med* 133:1017–1025, 1974.
39. Kolata G: Heart study produces a surprise result. *Science* 218:31, 1982.
40. Kunos G, Farsang C: Beta endorphin: possible involvement in the antihypertensive effect of central alpha-receptor activation. *Science* 211:82–84, 1981.
41. Kuokkanen K, Mattila MJ: Antihypertensive effect of prazosin in combination with methyldopa, clonidine or propranolol. *Ann Clin Res* 11:18–24, 1979.
42. Lake CR, Ziegler MG: Effect of acute volume alterations on norepinephrine and dopamine-beta hydroxylase in normotensive and hypertensive subjects. *Circulation* 57:774–778, 1978.
43. Lake CR, Ziegler MG, Coleman MD, Kopin IJ: Fenfluramine potentiation of antihypertensive effects of thiazides. *Clin Pharmacol Ther* 28:22–27, 1980.
44. Lake CR, Ziegler MG, Coleman MD, Kopin IJ: Hydrocholorthiazide-induced sympathetic hyperactivity in hypertensive patients. *Clin Pharmacol Ther* 26:428–432, 1979.
45. Landsberg L, Young JB: Fasting, feeding and regulation of the sympathetic nervous system. *N Engl J Med* 298:1295–1302, 1978.
46. Langer SZ: The role of alpha and beta-presynaptic receptors in the regulation of noradrenaline release elicited by nerve stimulation. *Clin Sci Mol Med* 51:423s–426s, 1976.
47. Larbi JI, Zaimise E: Effect of acute intravenous administration of clonidine on cerebral blood flow in man. *Br J Pharmacol* 39:198P-199P, 1970.
48. Lavie CJ, Messerli FH: Cardiovascular adaptation to obesity and hypertension. *Chest* 90:275–279, 1986.
49. Linas SL, Nies AS: Minoxidil. *Ann Intern Med* 94:61–65, 1981.
50. MacGregor GA, Best FA, Cam JM, Markandu ND, Elder DM, Sagnella GA, Squires M: Double-blind randomised crossover trial of moderate sodium restriction in essential hypertension. *Lancet* 1:351–354, 1982.
51. MacGregor GA, Markandu ND, Smith SJ, Sagnella GA: Captopril: contrasting effects of adding hydrochlorothiazide, propranolol, or nifedipine. *J Cardiovasc Pharmacol* 7:S82–S87, 1985.
52. Maling TJB, Dollery CT, Hamilton CA: Clonidine and sympathetic activity during sleep. *Clin Sci* 57:509–514, 1979.
53. Mancia G, Grassi G, Pomdiossi G, Gregorini L, Bertinieri G, Parati G, Ferrari A, Zanchetti A: Effects of blood-pressure measurements by the doctor on patient's blood pressure and heart rate. *Lancet* 2:695–697, 1983.

54. Manhem P, Bramnert M, Hulthen UL, Hokfelt B: The effect of captopril on catecholamines, renin activity, angiotensin II and aldosterone in plasma during physical exercise in hypertensive patients. *Eur J Clin Invest* 11:389–395, 1981.
55. Materson BJ, Oster JR, Michael UF, Bolton SM, Burton ZC, Stambaugh JE, Morlege J: Dose responses to chlorthalidone in patients with mild hypertension. *Clin Pharmacol Ther* 24:192–198, 1978.
56. Matson JR, Norby LH, Robillard JE: Interaction of minoxidil and captopril in the treatment of refractory hypertension. *Am J Dis Child* 135:256–258, 1981.
57. Mattila MG: Antihypertensive effect of prazosin in combination with methyldopa. Clonidine or propranolol? *Ann Clin Res* 11:18, 1979.
58. Medical Research Council: Adverse reactions to bendroflumethazide and propranolol for the treatment of mild hypertension. *Lancet* 2:539–542, 1981.
59. Meier A, Weidmann P, Ziegler WH: Catecholamines, renin, aldosterone, and blood volume during chronic minoxidil therapy. *Klin Wochenschr* 59:1231–1236, 1981.
60. Michelson E, Frishman WH, Lewis JE, Edwards WT, Flanigan WJ, Bloomfield SS, Johnson BF, Lucas C, Freis ED, Finnerty FA, Sawin HS, Sabol SA, Long C, Poland MP: Multicenter clinical evaluation of long-term efficacy and safety of labetalol in treatment of hypertension. *Am J Med* 75:68–80, 1983.
61. Mitchell HC, Pettinger WA: Dose-response of clonidine on plasma catecholamines in the hypernoradrenergic state associated with vasodilator beta-blocker therapy. *J Cardiovasc Pharmacol* 3:647–654, 1981.
62. Mrozzek WJ, Finnerty FA: A double-blind evaluation of a new antihypertensive agent. In Cotton (ed): *Prazosin*. Amsterdam, Excerpta Medica, 1974.
63. Neary D, Thurston H, Pohl JEF: Development of extra-pyramidal symptoms in hypertensive patients treated with diazoxide. *Br Med J*, Sept 1, 1973, pp 474–475.
64. Oates HF, Stoker LM, Stokes GS: Interactions between prazosin, clonidine and direct vasodilators in the anaesthetized rat. *Clin Exp Pharmacol Physiol* 5:85–89, 1978.
65. O'Connor DT, Barg AP, Duchin KL: Preserved renal perfusion during treatment of essential hypertension with the beta blocker nadolol. *J Clin Pharmacol* 22:187–195, 1982.
66. O'Connor DT, Preston RA: Propranolol effects on autonomic function in hypertensive men. *Clin Cardiol* 5:340–346, 1982.
67. O'Connor DT, Preston RA, Sasso EH: Renal perfusion changes during treatment of essential hypertension: prazosin versus propranolol. *J Cardiovasc Pharmacol* 1(suppl 1):S38–S42, 1979.
68. O'Malley K, Segal JL, Israili ZH, Boles M, McNay JL, Dayton PG: Duration of hydralazine action in hypertension. *Clin Pharmacol Ther* 18:581–586, 1975.
69. Pearson RM, Griffith DNW, Woollard M, James IM: Comparison of effects on cerebral blood flow of rapid reduction in systemic arterial pressure by diazoxide and labetalol in hypertensive patients: preliminary findings. *Br J Clin Pharmacol* 8:195S–198S, 1979.
70. Pederson OL, Mikkelsen E, Nielsen JL, Christensen NJ: Abrupt withdrawal of beta-blocking agents in patients with arterial hypertension. Effect on blood pressure, heart rate and plasma catecholamines and prolactin. *Eur J Clin Pharmacol* 15:215–217, 1979.
71. Pool PE, Massie BM, Venkataraman K, Hirsch AT, Samant DR, Seagren SC, Gaw J, Salel AF, Tubau JF: Diltiazem as monotherapy for systemic hypertension: a multicenter, randomized, placebo-controlled trial. *Am J Cardiol* 57:212–217, 1986.
72. Reid JL, Dargie HJ, Davies DS, Wing LMH, Hamilton CA, Dollery CT: Clonidine withdrawal in hypertension. *Lancet* 1:1171–1174, 1977.
73. Rouby JJ, Gory G, Bourrelli B, Glaser P, Viars P: Resis-

tance to sodium nitroprusside in hypertensive patients. *Crit Care Med* 10:301–304, 1982.

74. Sakano T, Okuda N, Sakura N, Yahata H, Tabe Y, Eno S, Kurogane H, Usui T: Captopril in hypertensive emergencies. *Hiroshima J Med Sci* 30:30–45, 1981.

75. Semplicini A, Pessina AC, Pallatini P, et al: Orthostatic hypotension after the first administration of prazosin in hypertensive patients. *Clin Exp Pharmacol Physiol* 8:1–10, 1981.

76. Sims EAH, Berchtold P: Obesity and hypertension. Mechanisms and implications for management. *JAMA* 247:49–52, 1982.

77. Starke K: Regulation of noradrenaline released by presynaptic receptor systems. *Rev Physiol Biochem Pharmacol* 77:1–124, 1977.

78. Stern HC, Matthews JH, Belz GG.: Intrinsic and reflex actions of verapamil and nifedipine: assessment in normal subjects by noninvasive techniques and autonomic blockade. *Eur J Clin Pharmacol* 29:541–547, 1986.

79. Stokes GS, Braham RM, Gain JM, Davis PR: Influence of dosage and dietary sodium on the first-dose effects of prazosin. *Br Med J* 1:1507, 1977.

80. Taylor AA, Pool JL, Lake CR, Ziegler MG, Rosen RA, Rollins DE, Mitchell JR: Plasma norepinephrine concentrations: no differences among normal volunteers and low, high or normal renin hypertensive patients. *Life Sci* 22:1499–1510, 1978.

81. Tuck ML, Sowers J, Dornfeld L, Kledzik G, Maxwell M: The effect of weight reduction on blood pressure, plasma renin activity, and plasma aldosterone levels in obese patients. *N Engl J Med* 304:930–933, 1981.

82. Turini GA, Bribic M, Brunner HR, Waeber B, Gavras H: Improvement of chronic congestive heart-failure by oral captopril. *Lancet* 1:1213–1215, 1979.

83. van den Brink G, Boer P, van Asten P, Mees EJD, Geyskes GG: One and three doses of propranolol a day in hypertension. *Clin Pharmacol Ther* 27:9–15, 1980.

84. Vandongen R, Margetts B, Deklerk N, Beilin LJ, Rogers P: Plasma catecholamines following exercise in hyper-

tensives treated with pindolol: comparison with placebo and metoprolol. *Br J Clin Pharmacol* 21:627–632, 1986.

85. Vidt DG, Bravo EL, Fouad FM: Captopril. *N Engl J Med* 306:214–219, 1982.

86. Wallace JM, Gill DP: Prazosin in the diagnosis and treatment of pheochromocytoma. *JAMA* 240:2752–2753, 1978.

87. Warren SE, O'Connor DT: The antihypertensive mechanism of sodium restriction. *J Cardiovasc Pharmacol* 3:781–790, 1981.

88. Watkin DM, Frobe HF, Hatch TF, Gutman AB: Effects of diet in essential hypertension II. Results with unmodified Kempner rice diet in 50 hospitalized patients. *Am J Med* 9:441–493, 1950.

89. Weber MA, Drayer JIM, Laragh JH: The effects of clonidine and propranolol separately and in combination on blood pressure and plasma renin activity in essential hypertension. *J Clin Pharmacol* 18:233, 1978.

90. Weisfeldt ML: Aging of the cardiovascular system. *N Engl J Med* 303:1172–1173, 1980.

91. Wells JD. Unusual cases of resistance to minoxidil therapy. *J Cardiovasc Pharmacol* 2(suppl 1)):S228–S235, 1980.

92. Wilja M, Jonnela AJ, Juustila H, Mattila MJ: Interaction of clonidine and beta blockers. *Acta Med Scand* 207:173, 1980.

93. Winer BM: The antihypertensive actions of benzothiadiazenes. *Circulation* 23:211–218, 1961.

94. Woods JW, Pittman AW, Pulliam CC, Werk EE, Waider W, Allen CA: Renin profiling in hypertension and its use in treatment with propranolol and chlorthalidone. *N Engl J Med* 294:1137–1143, 1976.

95. Young JR, Landsberg L: Suppression of sympathetic nervous system during fasting. *Science* 190:1473–1475, 1977.

96. Zacest R, Gilmore E, Koch-Weser J: Treatment of essential hypertension with combined vasodilation and beta-adrenergic blockade. *N Engl J Med* 286:617–622, 1972.

21

Antiarrhythmics

John P. DiMarco, M.D., Ph.D.

The introduction of cardiac defibrillation and the development of pharmacologic agents with potent antiarrhythmic activity have made possible the successful reversal and prevention of many forms of cardiac arrhythmia. Optimal antiarrhythmic therapy requires a knowledge of the basic pathophysiology for a patient's arrhythmia. Frequently, if the etiology of the arrhythmia can be identified and reversed, the use of agents with specific electrophysiologic effects may be avoided. Particularly in the setting of the critical care unit where such factors are common, the first step in evaluation of the patient with an arrhythmia should be a search for reversible causes of the arrhythmia such as hypoxia, myocardial ischemia, abnormal intracardiac pressures, acid-base imbalance, or electrolyte abnormalities. However, in many situations antiarrhythmic drugs will be required either as temporary measures to permit stabilization of a patient's rhythm until reversible factors may be normalized, or continuously in those patients whose underlying cardiac disease makes them chronically susceptible to paroxysmal arrhythmias.

During the last several decades progress in both clinical and basic investigation has greatly enhanced our understanding of the mechanisms responsible for cardiac arrhythmias and for the actions of antiarrhythmic drugs. In the basic research laboratory, investigators have described the effects of antiarrhythmic agents on the various ionic currents that determine the electrical activities of cardiac cells. The parallel development of techniques for intracardiac stimulation and recording has allowed many clinical arrhythmias to be studied under controlled laboratory conditions. It has become apparent from these studies that therapy for each patient's arrhythmia must be individualized since electrocardiographically similar arrhythmias in different patients may require totally different forms of therapy.

CELLULAR ELECTROPHYSIOLOGY

The electrical properties of cardiac cells have been extensively studied and excellent reviews are available (8, 13, 69, 80, 124, 135, 153). Only a brief review of current concepts is presented in this section.

Electrically active myocardial cells at rest maintain a potential difference between their cytoplasm and the surrounding extracellular fluid. When excited, these cells manifest a characteristic sequence of transmembrane potential changes called the action potential, which has traditionally been divided into five phases (Fig. 21.1). When the diastolic potential spontaneously reaches or is brought to a certain level, termed the threshold potential, a rapid depolarization occurs with a transient reversal of polarity (phase 0). Repolarization is then accomplished in three stages: a brief but rapid repolarization (phase 1), a plateau period during which there is little change in the transmembrane potential (phase 2), and a final period of repolarization back to the maximal diastolic potential (phase 3). Cells of the specialized conduction system, but not normal working atrial or ventricular myocytes, possess an intrinsic capacity for spontaneous depolarization during diastole (phase 4) that will continue until either the threshold potential is reached or the cell is brought to threshold by a conducted or exogenous stimulus. The action potential differs in various tissues within the heart depending on the relative activities of the currents discussed below in each tissue.

The action potential is produced by a complex interplay of a number of ionic currents (Table 21.1), which are, in turn, regulated by changes in the selected permeabilities of the cellular membrane. At rest, the cell membrane is permeable to potassium and highly impermeable to sodium, chloride, and calcium. Thus, the resting transmembrane potential ap-

389

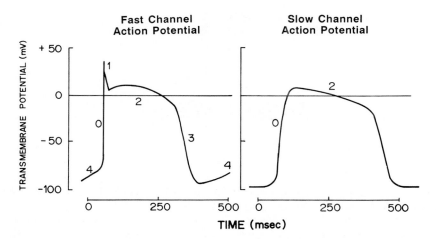

Figure 21.1. Representative cardiac action potentials from tissues dependent on either fast response (Na$^+$ channels) or slow response (Ca^{2+} channels) for action potential generation.

proximates the equilibrium potential for K$^+$ predicted by the Nernst equation for the transmembrane K$^+$ concentration gradient (K$^+$ concentration is approximately 4 mM in the extracellular space and 150 mM intracellularly). As a result, at the maximal point of repolarization in diastole, the transmembrane potential of a myocardial Purkinje fiber will be between -75 and -95 mV. If the threshold potential is reached, a dramatic change in membrane permeability and ionic currents take place. Sodium ion permeability increases and an inward Na$^+$ current (i_{Na}) is rapidly activated, pushing the transmembrane potential toward the equilibrium potential for Na$^+$ (approximately $+70$ mV). This change in membrane Na$^+$ conductance is probably due to the activation of molecular gates or channels that control the flow of specific ions through the membrane. Current theory describes a model in which each ionic channel is a protein that spans the lipid bilayer membrane (Fig. 21.2)

(68–70). In this model, an activation gate, called the "m gate," opens during phase 0 permitting an influx of Na$^+$ into the cell, which results in depolarization. An inactivation gate, termed the "h gate," then closes the Na$^+$ channel in a voltage-dependent manner before the full Na$^+$ equilibrium potential is reached. The kinetics of activation and inactivation of the channel are rapid, and the duration of the Purkinje fiber action potential upstroke is only 1 or 2 msec. For the remainder of the cardiac cycle the Na$^+$ channel remains in a resting state, closed but available for activation. Presumably by similar molecular mechanisms, the other ionic channels described below contribute to the full cardiac action potential.

During phase 1 of the action potential, inactivation of i_{Na} is completed and a Cl$^-$ current (i_{qr}) is activated leading to a transient period of rapid repolarization.

Phase 2 of the action potential, the plateau phase, involves the interactions of several fac-

Table 21.1
Ionic Currents Responsible for the Action Potential

Symbol[a]	Ion(s) Responsible	Activity
i_{Na}	Na$^+$	Activation produces phase 0 rapid depolarization
i_{qr}	Cl$^-$	Contributes to rapid repolarization (phase 1)
i_{si}	Ca^{2+}	Produces plateau phase and action potential in sinus and atrioventricular nodes
i_{x1}	K$^+$	Repolarizes fiber in phase 3
i_{bi}	Na$^+$	Contributes to phase 4 depolarization
i_{K1}	K$^+$	Background K$^+$ current
i_f	Na$^+$(K$^+$)	Pacemaker current in sinoatrial node
i_{K2}	K$^+$(Na$^+$)	Pacemaker current in Purkinje fiber

[a]The symbols used to denote specific currents have not been standardized and vary widely in discussions by different authors.

OUTSIDE

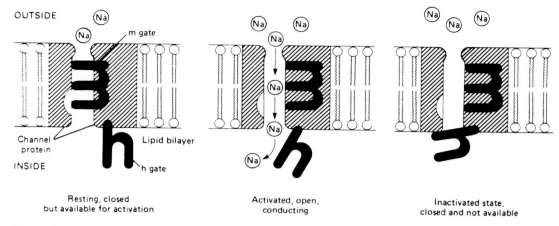

Resting, closed
but available for activation

Activated, open,
conducting

Inactivated state,
closed and not available

Figure 21.2. Schematic representation of the cardiac sodium channel. Shown is a protein *(shaded area)* spanning the bilayered lipid membrane with m and h gates. At rest, the m gate is closed but the h gate is open. With activation, the m gate opens and current flow is possible. Sodium current flow ceases with the rapid closing of the h gate ending phase 0. (From Hondeghem LM, Mason JW: Agents used in cardiac arrhythmias. In Katzung BG (ed): *Basic and Clinical Pharmacology.* Norwalk, CT, Appleton & Lange, 1987, pp. 151–167.)

tors. An outward background K^+ current, i_{K1}, is present throughout the action potential and it is balanced by an inward current (i_{si}) carried by Ca^{2+}, and to a lesser extent by Na^+, that is slowly activated by membrane depolarization in phase 0 and then slowly decays during the plateau period.

As i_{si} decays, more rapid repolarization occurs as a transient outward K^+ current (i_{x1}) is activated and the combined actions of i_{x1} and i_{K1} drive the transmembrane potential toward full diastolic depolarization.

The electrophysiologic characteristics of the action potential in sinus and atrioventricular (AV) nodal cells are quite different from those observed in Purkinje fibers. In the former, maximum negative diastolic potential is only -40 to -60 mV, and phase 0 of the action potential is not generated by the fast Na^+ channel but rather by a slow channel dependent on Ca^{2+} (Fig. 21.1). During phase 0, these cells exhibit a much slower rate of depolarization and a lower action potential amplitude and lack the overshoot seen in Purkinje fibers. Since conduction velocity is proportional to the rate of phase 0 depolarization, conduction in cells dependent on slow channel action potentials is also markedly slower.

The ionic mechanisms responsible for spontaneous diastolic depolarization remain incompletely understood. Early experiments in Purkinje fibers suggested that decay of an outward K^+ current in association with the constant effects of two time-independent back-

ground currents, i_{bi} and i_{K1}, led to diastolic depolarization. More recent experiments have suggested that a time-dependent inward current (i_f) carried by K^+ and Na^+ may be the primary mechanism for phase 4 depolarization. However, in sinus node cells, K^+ background currents, i_{si}, and electrogenic sodium pumping also may play a role in determining spontaneous activity.

DEFINITIONS: AUTOMATICITY, EXCITABILITY, REFRACTORINESS, RESPONSIVENESS, AND CONDUCTION

Effects of pharmacologic agents on the electrophysiologic characteristics of cardiac cells are often described in terms of several basic properties. Automaticity refers to the frequency of spontaneous impulse formation. Normally, it depends on three factors: the level of maximum diastolic depolarization, the rate of depolarization, and the level of the threshold potential. Excitability describes the strength of a stimulus required to initiate a new action potential at any given point during the action potential cycle. Refractoriness is the period during which the cell remains unexcitable after an action potential. Its most commonly used measure is the effective refractory period (ERP), the minimal interval between two propagated action potentials using an exciting stimulus of fixed intensity. In Purkinje fibers and working atrial and ventricular myocytes, the ERP is a function chiefly of the duration of the action potential. In cells located in the sinus and AV node, however, refractorineses is prolonged well after recovery of full diastolic depolarization. Membrane responsiveness describes the characteristics of a transmembrane potential response produced by an exciting stimulus. It has been demonstrated that the maximum rate of rise of the transmembrane potential ($\dot{V}_{max}$) during phase 0 may be used an an appropriate measure of the state of activation of the fast sodium channel and thus of sodium conductance. $\dot{V}_{max}$ in turn is related to the degree of membrane depolarization, and the relationship of the two has been termed the membrane responsiveness. Conduction occurs when an exciting stimulus brings a section of tissue to its threshold and the action potential generated serves as source of depolarizing current enabling adjacent sections to also reach threshold. The speed of conduction will depend on the passive electrical properties (cable properties) of the fiber and the membrane responsiveness.

MECHANISMS OF ARRHYTHMIAS

In broad terms, arrhythmias may be thought of as secondary to disorders of impulse formation (automaticity), impulse conduction, or a combination of the two (Table 21.2).

Arrhythmias Due to Abnormal Automaticity

In the normal heart, the cells of the sinoatrial (SA) node exhibit the most rapid rate of depolarization during diastole and reach threshold first. Cells in the distal AV junction and the His-Purkinje system also possess intrinsic automaticity, but because they manifest a slower rate of phase 4 depolarization, they normally are only latent or subsidiary pacemakers. The primary role of the SA node, the pacemaker for the rest of the heart, is reinforced by the phenomenon known as "overdrive suppression." Repetitive depolarization of a pacemaker cell by a stimulus from another source results in increased activity of the Na^+-K^+ exchange pump, thus generating a hyperpolarizing current. As a result, should a transient alteration in frequency of impulses from the SA node occur, a period of recovery is required before subsidiary pacemaker activity becomes manifest. Overdrive suppression enables the SA node to change rate modestly without competition from lower pacemakers and forms the basis for several clinical tests used to assess sinus node function.

The normal sinus node is highly responsive to alterations in autonomic nervous system output and in its biochemical surroundings. Increased adrenergic innervation produces major changes in ionic current activity in SA nodal cells. Catecholamine stimulation increases i_{si}, i_{x1}, and i_f, leading to a shorter action potential duration and an increase in the spontaneous rate of diastolic depolarization. Vagal stimulation and endogenous purines such as adenosine increase outward K^+ currents, thus hyperpolarizing the cells and inhibiting depolarization. In some cases, latent pacemakers may be more subject to the increase in adrenergic tone, and increased AV nodal or His-Purkinje automaticity induced by catecholamines may be responsible for the clinical occurrence of arrhythmias such as nonparoxysmal junctional tachycardia. In other situations, capacity for spontaneous depolarization may be induced by disease in working atrial or ventricular myocytes that would normally manifest a stable diastolic potential.

Other mechanisms for arrhythmias due to abnormal impulse formation are also possible. Under certain conditions, most notably intracellular calcium overload, oscillations, termed afterdepolarizations, in the transmembrane potential may be recorded either during phase 3 (early afterdepolarizations) or during the early part of phase 4 (late afterdepolarizations). Should these afterdepolarizations reach threshold, a new action potential will be generated and under appropriate conditions, propagated to adjacent cells (Fig. 21.3). Early and late afterdepolarizations may be observed

Table 21.2
Mechanisms for Arrhythmias

I. Disorders of automaticity
  A. Normal mechanisms—abnormal rate
    1. Sinus bradycardia or tachycardia
    2. Irregular sinus rhythm
  B. Abnormal mechanisms
    1. Enhanced spontaneous depolarization
    2. Early afterdepolarizations
    3. Late afterdepolarizations
    4. Triggered activity
II. Disorders of conduction
  A. Blocked normal impulse (sinoatrial exit block, AV block, etc.)
  B. Unidirectional block and reentry
    1. Random over multiple pathways (fibrillation)
    2. Organized over single pathway

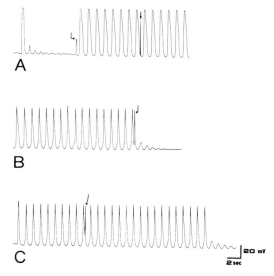

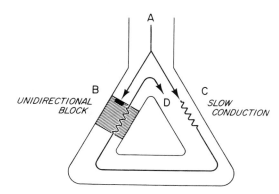

Figure 21.4.   Diagram of the requirements for reentry. A premature impulse from some proximal point arrives at a branch point *(A)* with unequal conduction in the two branches. On side *B,* the tissue is still refractory and antegrade conduction block occurs. On side *C,* the impulse is slowed but traverses the area. It can then conduct around to point *B,* which has sufficiently recovered to permit retrograde conduction. If the tissue at *D* has recovered excitability, the reentry loop is completed and may continue.

Figure 21.3.   Triggered automaticity in an isolated superfused guinea pig myocyte. **A, B,** and **C** depict action potential recordings obtained from an impaled myocyte in the presence of isoproterenol, 10 μM. **A,** The first action potential is followed by several delayed afterdepolarizations that fail to achieve threshold. At the *arrow,* an applied stimulus initiates sustained rhythmic activity. **B,** A single extrastimulus terminates the arrhythmia. Subthreshold delayed afterdepolarizations are again observed. As shown in **C,** triggered activity may also terminate spontaneously. (Courtesy of Dr. L. Belardinelli, University of Virginia.)

in response to hypothermia, electrolyte imbalance, catecholamine excess, or stretch. Late afterdepolarizations may also be of particular importance in some of the arrhythmias due to digitalis intoxication.

Disorders of Impulse Conduction

Many cardiac arrhythmias are probably due to a recirculation or reentry of impulses within circuits of conducting cells. This concept may be described as follows. An impulse reaches a branch point in the cardiac conduction system and is conducted unequally down the two limbs available for conduction (Fig. 21.4). On one side, antegrade conduction is blocked and the area distal to the site of block remains inactivated. On the opposite side, impulse conduction is delayed but the impulse still traverses the region of delay. The impulse can now complete the loop and under appropriate conditions traverse the area of the original antegrade block in the retrograde direction. If

the conduction velocity through the pathway has been slow enough so that the tissue encountered by the reentrant impulse distal to the region of block has recovered excitability, reactivation may occur and the process repeated. Thus, in this model, for reentry to occur, there must be an inhomogeneity of electrical properties within the circuit such that delayed conduction, unidirectional block, and the recovery of excitability simultaneously coexist during one or multiple cycles.

Conduction velocity in normal atrial or ventricular myocardium is so rapid relative to the duration of refractoriness that reentry could not occur unless very long pathways were involved. Conduction in the sinus and AV nodes and in fibers that have been damaged by disease, and are therefore partially depolarized, is quite slow, however, and reentry over anatomically feasible circuits becomes possible. The classic example of a reentrant arrhythmia is paroxysmal supraventricular tachycardia in patients with extranodal accessory pathways. In these patients an exact sequence of activation of various parts of the heart by the reentrant impulse can be measured. In other cases in which reentry pathways are thought to occur either within atrial or ventricular muscle or within the AV node, such clear-cut evidence for the presence of reentry is, however, lacking; nonetheless, the reentry model has still provided an adequate explanation for many types of clinically important arrhythmias.

MECHANISM OF ANTIARRHYTHMIC DRUG ACTION

Antiarrhythmic drugs exert their effects by means of interactions with ion channels. As shown in Figure 21.5, these drugs usually have a high affinity for open channels and inactive channels, but low affinity for channels in the resting state. When channels are in the drug-bound state, conductance of the ion regulated by that channel is inhibited.

Several phenomena observed to be associated with antiarrhythmic drugs may be explained using this modulated receptor hypothesis. Since at faster rates cells will spend less time in the resting or drug-insensitive state, antiarrhythmic drugs will typically produce greater effects at faster rates (68, 111). This phenomenon is called use or frequency dependence. Also, the increased activity of many drugs on damaged cells is explained by the fact that loss of resting potential results in many inactivated channels that will show an increased sensitivity to drugs. Finally, the relative kinetics of association and dissociation of the channel in each state may be used to explain the differences between the various drugs' effects on the action potential. Although the modulated receptor hypothesis has been most extensively tested for the interaction of drugs with sodium channels, it is likely that other ionic channels behave similarly.

DRUG CLASSIFICATION

Over the years, various schemes have been proposed for the classification of antiarrhythmic drugs. These classifications are all limited in their ability to predict the efficacy of an individual antiarrhythmic drug in a given clinical situation, but they do allow a grouping of agents into classes with similar mechanisms of action and potential clinical spectrum (Table 21.3). The most widely used classification groups antiarrhythmic drugs into four major classes based on their predominant effects on the electrophysiologic properties of isolated normal cells (141).

Class I agents are local anesthetic agents that have as their predominant effect a depression of sodium conductance during phase 0 of the action potential. These drugs produce depression of $\dot{V}_{max}$, slow conduction velocity, and decrease excitability. Most of the drugs in class I also affect potassium repolarization currents and suppress automaticity in ectopic pacemakers. Recently it has been proposed that class I agents should be further divided into several subclasses (141). Class Ia agents, such as quinidine, procainamide, and disopyramide, produce a moderate depression of sodium conductance during phase 0 of the action potential, thereby depressing $\dot{V}_{max}$, slowing conduction velocity, and decreasing excitability. These drugs also depress K^+ cur-

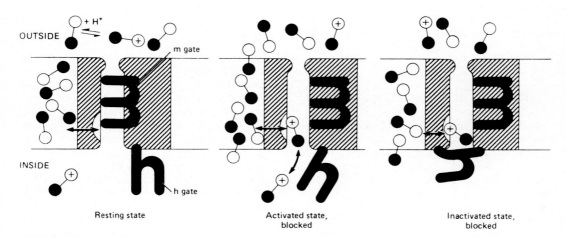

Figure 21.5. Interactions between antiarrhythmic drugs and the sodium channel. The *unshaded semicircular area* on the channel represents a hypothetical binding for the antiarrhythmic agent. In the resting state, closure of the m gate interferes with drug access and binding. In the activated and inactivated states, access is possible and the drug can bind to the receptor, blocking the channels. The kinetics of drug association and dissociation and the frequency of use of the channel all influence drug activity. (From Hondeghem LM, Mason JW: Agents used in cardiac arrhythmias. In Katzung BG (ed): *Basic and Clinical Pharmacology.* Norwalk, CT, Appleton & Lange, 1987, pp 151–167.)

Table 21.3
Classification of Antiarrhythmic Drugs

Class	Major Action	ECG Effects	Examples
I	Na$^+$ channel blockade	Ia: moderate ↓ conduction; moderate ↑ repolarization	Quinidine, procainamide, disopyramide
		Ib: mild ↑ conduction; little effect on repolarization	Lidocaine, mexiletine, tocainide, phenytoin
		Ic: marked ↓ conduction; little effect on repolarization	Encainide, flecainide, propranolol
II	β-Adrenergic blockade	Antagonizes endogenous catecholamines	Propranolol, metoprolol, many others
III	Variable and mixed	Prolongs action potential duration	Bretylium, amiodarone, sotalol
IV	Ca^{2+} channel blockade	Slows conduction in AV node; inhibits triggered activity	Verapamil, diltiazem

rents and prolong repolarization. Class Ib agents have minimal effects on sodium conductance and may actually shorten repolarization in normal fibers, but have more typical class I actions in partially depolarized fibers. Class Ic agents produce marked effects on sodium conductance and conduction velocity in normal and depolarized cells but have relatively little effect on repolarization.

Class II agents act by blocking β-adrenergic receptor stimulation. Some of these agents may produce class I–type effects at high concentrations, but their principal actions are to depress phase 4 depolarization in the sinus node, slow AV nodal conduction, and block catecholamine-induced changes in other electrophysiologic properties of cardiac tissues.

Class III agents are so grouped because they produce in vitro a marked prolongation of the action potential duration. Bretylium, sotalol, and amiodarone are placed in class III, but these drugs differ markedly in their clinical utility, and the mechanisms by which they exert their antiarrhythmic effects remain poorly understood.

Class IV agents depress the activity of the calcium-dependent slow channel and as a result are often referred to as "calcium blockers." These agents have been most useful clinically in the management of supraventricular arrhythmias that utilize the AV node for antegrade conduction, but may also prove to be of value in arrhythmias due to triggered automaticity.

There are numerous limitations to this classification scheme. The groupings are made on the basis of the single major effect of a drug on the action potential. Effects on other ionic channels or on the autonomic nervous system that may provide important contributions to a drug's overall antiarrhythmic effects are ignored. The classification is often based on ex-

perimental data obtained using normal tissues in vitro, but these observations may not accurately describe a drug's effect in a diseased tissue. Metabolites of a drug may be effective and may produce different electrophysiologic actions than the parent compound. Finally, since the mechanisms responsible for a given arrhythmia may differ from patient to patient, it is frequently not possible to predict accurately a drug's effectiveness based solely on this classification. Despite these limitations, however, this classification schema is widely used and does provide a rough guide on which to base therapy.

INDIVIDUAL ANTIARRHYTHMIC AGENTS

The pharmacokinetic properties of the antiarrhythmic drugs discussed in this text are listed in Table 21.4. Table 21.5 provides a brief index of the major side effects that may be expected to occur during therapy.

Quinidine

Quinidine, one of the cinchona alkaloids, has been used to treat cardiac arrhythmias for almost 200 years. Early in this century, Frey (41) reported on its efficacy in the management of atrial fibrillation, and it has subsequently been used to treat other atrial and ventricular arrhythmias.

ELECTROPHYSIOLOGIC AND ECG EFFECTS (61, 64, 77)

In clinically relevant concentrations, quinidine depresses fast channel sodium conductance, thus decreasing $\dot{V}_{max}$ and the amplitude

Table 21.4
Pharmacokinetic Properties of Antiarrhythmic Drugs

Drug	Class	Oral Absorption	Systemic Bioavailability (%)	Estimated Volume of Distribution (Steady State) (liters/kg)	Amount Protein-Bound (%)	Mode of Elimination	Estimated Elimination Half-life (hr)	Effective Serum Concentration	Comments
Quinidine	Ia	Good	60–90	2.0–3.0	90	Hepatic, renal	4.0–8.0	1.5–4.0 µg/ml	Concentration ranges vary with different assays currently in use; range quoted here is for quinidine-specific assays only
Procainamide	Ia	Good	70–90	2.5–3.5	15	Renal	2.0–4.0	4.0–16.0 µg/ml	Active metabolite may accumulate, especially with renal failure
Disopyramide	Ia	Good	80–90	1.0–1.5	5–65 (see text)	Renal	6.0–8.0	2.0–4.0 µg/ml	Protein binding decreases at high serum levels
Lidocaine	Ib	Good	<30	1.5 (see text)	50	Hepatic	1.5–2.5	1.0–5.0 µg/ml	Elimination dependent on hepatic blood flow
Phenytoin	Ib	Good	90	0.6	90	Hepatic	18.0–30.0	10.0–20.0 µg/ml	
Mexiletine[a]	Ib	Good	80–90	6.0–8.0	30–50	Hepatic	10.0–24.0	0.5–2.0 µg/ml	Elimination half-life highly variable
Tocainide[a]	Ib	Good	90–100	1.5–3.0	50	Hepatic, renal	10.0–15.0	6.0–12.0 µg/ml	
Encainide[a]	Ic	Variable	Variable	1.0	70	Hepatic	<2.0	See comment	Major metabolites with longer half-lives accumulate during therapy and may account for therapeutic effects
Flecainide[a]	Ic	Good	90–100	1.0–2.0	40	Hepatic, renal	14.0–20.0	400.0–800.0 ng/ml	
Propafenone	Ic	Good	Nonlinear	2–3	95	Hepatic	6–13	See comment	Active metabolites contribute to effects
Bretylium	III	Poor	10–30	3.0–5.0	Low	Renal	8.0–13.0	Unknown	
Amiodarone[a]	III	Poor	10–30	>20	>95	Unknown	Weeks	0.5–2.0 µg/ml	
Verapamil	IV	Good	10–30	4.0	90	Hepatic	3.0–6.0	70.0–200.0 ng/ml	
Diltiazem	IV	Good	30–40	NA	80	Hepatic	3.0–4.0	50.0–200.0 ng/ml	

[a] Experience with new or investigational agents is limited and additional side effects may be noted in the future.

Table 21.5
Major Extracardiac Side Effects of Antiarrhythmic Drugs

Drug	Gastrointestinal	Hematologic	Ocular	CNS	Dermatologic	Other
Quinidine	Nausea, vomiting, diarrhea, hepatitis	Thrombocytopenia, anemia			Rash	Fever, cinchonism, anaphylaxis, increased serum digoxin levels
Procainamide	Anorexia, nausea	Agranulocytosis, leukopenia			Rash	Fever, lupus-like syndrome
Disopyramide	Constipation, nausea		Blurred vision, glaucoma			Dry mouth, urinary retention
Lidocaine				Dizziness, dysarthria, convulsions		
Phenytoin		Lymphadenopathy, neutropenia		Drowsiness, ataxia, nystagmus	Rash	Gingival hyperplasia, disorders of calcium metabolism
Mexiletine	Nausea, vomiting			Tremor, dizziness, paresthesias, ataxia		
Tocainide	Nausea	Agranulocytosis		Headache, tremor, paresthesias	Rash	Pulmonary fibrosis
Encainide[a]	Nausea, vomiting			Dizziness, ataxia, tremor	Rash	
Flecainide[a]	Dysgeusia	N/A	Blurred vision	Dizziness, vertigo	N/A	N/A
Propafenone[a]	Gastrointestinal upset	N/A	Blurred vision	Dizziness	N/A	N/A
Bretylium	Nausea, vomiting, parotitis (late)	N/A	N/A	N/A	N/A	Hypotension, often severe
Sotalol[a]				Fatigue		
Amiodarone[a]	Nausea, vomiting, constipation, and elevated hepatic enzymes	N/A	Corneal deposits	Peripheral neuropathy, myopathy	Bluish discoloration, photosensitivity	Pulmonary infiltrates and thyroid dysfunction
Verapamil	Constipation			Vertigo		

[a] Experience with new or investigational agents is limited and additional side effects may be noted in the future.

of phase 0 of the action potential. Conduction in Purkinje fibers is thereby slowed. Quinidine also slows the rate of phase 4 depolarization in isolated Purkinje fibers and makes the threshold potential less negative, thus decreasing normal automaticity. There is little effect on early or late afterpotentials or on the slow channel-mediated automaticity of depolarized fibers. The duration of the action potential is mildly increased and the ERP is prolonged as a function of increasing quinidine concentration. The normal sinus node shows little direct influence from quinidine, but in patients with intrinsic sinus node dysfunction, marked sinus slowing is occasionally noted.

Quinidine has mixed effects on AV nodal conduction. The direct depressant effect seen in isolated preparations is often overcome clinically by a vagolytic acceleration of AV nodal conduction. Accessory pathways, which resemble atrial or ventricular muscle in their response to quinidine, display slowed conduction and prolonged refractoriness. When studied in patients undergoing clinical electrophysiologic studies, quinidine increases the HV interval and the ERP of atrial and ventricular muscle, while minimally decreasing the AH interval and the antegrade refractory period of the AV node. The PR interval usually remains unchanged, whereas small dose-related increases in the QRS duration and larger increases in the QT$_c$ interval are noted. At toxic concentrations, a widened QRS, AV block, and marked prolongation of the QT interval may occur. When quinidine is given to patients with atrial flutter or atrial fibrillation, its vagolytic effects on AV nodal conduction may produce dangerous increases in ventricular rate. This is a particular problem in atrial flutter in which the vagolytic effect in conjunction with a quinidine-induced increase in atrial cycle length may allow 1:1 AV conduction. Ventricular arrhythmias may also be aggravated by quinidine and this aggravation may occur even at usual plasma concentrations. The emergence of these arrhythmias is often but not always preceded by a marked prolongation of the QT interval.

PHARMACOKINETICS (49)

Quinidine is most commonly used orally, although intravenous infusions may be used safely in appropriate settings. The drug is well absorbed after oral administration but does undergo some first pass hepatic metabolism. This results in a systemic bioavailability of between 60% and 90%, depending on the preparation used. After intravenous administration, quinidine distributes rapidly (distribution half-life < 5 minutes) into a volume of distribution of approximately 2–3 liters/kg. The drug is highly bound (85–95%) to plasma proteins.

Hepatic metabolism is the principal method of elimination of quinidine. The major metabolites are (3S)-3-hydroxyquinidine and quinidine-N-oxide, and smaller quantities of 2'-oxoquinidine and O-desmethylquinidine may also be detected. The elimination half-life is between 6 and 8 hours. Quinidine metabolism is accelerated if the drug is administered in conjunction with a compound known to induce oxidative enzymes in hepatic microsomes. The clinical significance of this effect has been demonstrated during coadministration with either phenytoin or phenobarbital. The rate of quinidine metabolism is decreased in patients with congestive heart failure and in the elderly.

Renal excretion of unchanged quinidine accounts for only about 10–20% of drug elimination. However, azotemic patients on hemodialysis manifest decreased hepatic clearance and a decreased volume of distribution, and the dosage should be titrated in renal failure based on serum quinidine concentrations.

A variety of analytic techniques have been used in reports correlating plasma concentrations of quinidine and clinical efficacy. The older protein precipitation methods measured inactive or weakly active metabolites, and a therapeutic range of 4–8 µg/ml was usually reported. Plasma levels, measured either fluorometrically after extraction of metabolites or with more specific chromatographic assays, are considerably lower. When serum levels are measured by these latter techniques, serum concentrations in effectively treated patients will usually be between 1.5 and 4 µg/ml.

DIGOXIN-QUINIDINE INTERACTIONS (12, 89)

An interaction between quinidine and digoxin was first reported in 1978 (89) and the initial observations have been subsequently confirmed and extended in many studies. Initiation of quinidine therapy in a patient receiving a stable dose of digoxin decreases the volume of distribution of digoxin and decreases renal and possibly nonrenal clearance of digoxin. As a result, the serum digoxin concentration will gradually rise over 4–8 days, and with therapeutic doses of quinidine, a 1.5- to 3-fold increase in serum digoxin level is produced. A smaller rise in serum digitoxin level also occurs after initiation of quinidine therapy.

HEMODYNAMIC EFFECTS

During oral therapy, adverse hemodynamic effects from quinidine are rarely seen. When given intravenously, however, quinidine produces an α-sympatholytic effect that commonly causes hypotension and reflex tachycardia. This effect has limited the use of intravenous quinidine to special situations.

SIDE EFFECTS

In addition to the hemodynamic and ECG toxicity that may be associated with the drug, other side effects are commonly observed in patients treated with quinidine. Gastrointestinal intolerance is the most common side effect associated with quinidine therapy. Nausea, vomiting, and diarrhea are frequently seen and may preclude further therapy. Such reactions are common, occurring in up to one-third of those treated even if plasma concentrations are monitored within the "therapeutic range" (114).

Cinchonism is a syndrome that includes tinnitus, hearing loss, visual problems, and gastrointestinal upset caused by dose-related toxicity to quinidine or other cinchona alkaloids.

Immunologic reactions to quinidine include fever, thrombocytopenia, and anaphylaxis. Quinidine occasionally produces hemolytic anemia mediated either by a red cell antigen or by glucose-6-phosphate dehydrogenase deficiency. Blood cell counts should be monitored for several weeks after quinidine therapy has been initiated.

CLINICAL USE

Quinidine is useful in a variety of atrial arrhythmias. It may suppress ectopic atrial contractions that precipitate reentrant arrhythmias, convert established atrial flutter or atrial fibrillation to normal sinus rhythm, and by slowing conduction in accessory AV nodal pathways and in the "fast pathway" of patients with dual AV nodal pathways, can prevent or terminate some paroxysmal supraventricular tachycardias.

Ventricular arrhythmias may also be treated successfully with quinidine. Premature ventricular beats in the setting of acute myocardial infarction and in patients with chronic ventricular ectopy may be suppressed by quinidine. During electrophysiologic testing, quinidine suppresses the initiation of ventricular tachycardia with programmed ventricular stimulation in about one-third of patients studied (27). If ventricular tachycardia is not suppressed, the effect on tachycardia cycle length is somewhat variable, but the tachycardia in most patients shows cycle length prolongation. gation.

DOSAGE AND ADMINISTRATION

Quinidine is available for oral administration in several forms. A 200-mg tablet of quinidine sulfate contains 165 mg of quinidine base, and a 324-mg tablet of quinidine gluconate contains 206 mg of quinidine base. A 275-mg tablet of quinidine polygalacturonate is equivalent to 200 mg of quinidine sulfate. The gluconate and polygalacturonate are more slowly, but also more variably, absorbed than is the sulfate salt. The useful dose range is usually 800–2000 mg of quinidine sulfate daily in three or four divided doses, but plasma concentration monitoring should be used to guide therapy. Intramuscular administration of quinidine causes local irritation and should be discouraged. Quinidine gluconate may be given by a slow intravenous infusion if arterial pressure is carefully monitored. The usual initial intravenous loading dose is between 600 and 1000 mg (approximately 10 mg/kg) administered over 30–60 minutes.

Procainamide

First introduced in 1951, procainamide remains an important antiarrhythmic agent.

ELECTROPHYSIOLOGIC AND ECG EFFECTS (64, 75)

The electrophysiologic and ECG effects of procainamide are essentially the same as those produced by quinidine. In contrast to quinidine, however, procainamide has little anticholinergic activity. Procainamide, therefore, will widen the QRS, lengthen the QT interval, and prolong the HV interval while having little effect on AV nodal conduction. Sinus node function is usually not affected except in patients with sinus node disease. The ERPs of atrial and ventricular muscle and of many extranodal bypass tracts are prolonged by procainamide, thus procainamide given during a tachycardia often produces a dose-related prolongation of tachycardia cycle length and may eventually terminate the arrhythmia and block its reinitiation.

PHARMACOKINETICS (43, 44)

Procainamide may be used orally or parenterally. When administered orally, the drug is readily absorbed from the small intestine with a systemic bioavailability of 70–90%. Peak serum concentrations are achieved within 30–120 minutes of ingestion. The volume of distribution is approximately 1.5–2.5 liters/kg. Only about 15% of circulating procainamide is bound to plasma proteins.

The major mode of elimination of procainamide is renal tubular excretion of the unchanged compound. Procainamide also undergoes acetylation in the liver to N-acetylprocainamide. The rate of acetylation is variable, with patients separable into slow and fast acetylator subgroups (150). N-Acetylprocainamide has some antiarrhythmic activity and may contribute to the overall antiarrhythmic effect of procainamide. The elimination half-life for procainamide in normal subjects is approximately 3 hours. In patients with renal failure, renal elimination of procainamide and its metabolite are markedly prolonged and high levels of N-acetylprocainamide may accumulate.

The therapeutic range for procainamide plasma concentrations is broad. Little effect is seen below 4 μg/ml. Recent studies have shown that increased efficacy may be achieved with plasma concentrations up to 20 μg/ml (53), but this may often not be of clinical value (104). Different conditions may require different serum concentrations. However, toxicity is more frequent as plasma levels increase and may limit aggressive therapy in many patients.

HEMODYNAMIC EFFECTS

In high concentrations, procainamide may depress myocardial performance. Rapid intravenous infusion may lower peripheral resistance and blood pressure, but the latter effect is less commonly seen and is usually less marked than the hypotension associated with an electrophysiologically equivalent intravenous dose of quinidine.

SIDE EFFECTS

Side effects are uncommon during the first few days of procainamide therapy if low serum concentrations (≤ 10 μg/ml) are maintained. With increasing doses, nausea, vomiting, and anorexia become increasingly prominent and may limit therapy. These gastrointestinal side effects may be seen even after parenteral administration.

Procainamide produces a variety of immunologically mediated reactions that limit its clinical use. Fever, leukopenia, and agranulocytosis may occur during the first days to weeks of therapy. The most common immunologic side effect, however, is development of a clinical syndrome resembling systemic lupus erythematosus (150). During chronic therapy about 60–70% of patients develop positive antinuclear antibodies. With continued therapy, some of these patients will develop a clinical syndrome characterized by arthralgia, fever, and serositis. Lupus erythematosus cell preparations may be positive. The syndrome is reversible if procainamide is discontinued, but recovery may be prolonged and persistent symptoms may require treatment with salicylates or corticosteroids.

The development of this syndrome is more common in slow acetylators, and a plasma concentration–related exposure to procainamide itself seems to be required for its development. Procainamide-induced lupus has not been observed during treatment with only N-acetylprocainamide. Since N-acetylprocainamide (NAPA) has electrophysiologic activity, trials with this compound have been performed. However, although ventricular premature beat suppression in some patients treated with NAPA has been shown, results in patients with chronic ventricular tachycardia have been disappointing.

CLINICAL USE

The ease of its oral or parenteral administration and its relative freedom from early side effects at moderate serum concentrations have made procainamide a popular choice in the treatment of many atrial and ventricular arrhythmias. Its clinical spectrum is similar to that of quinidine, although the latter has been more commonly used for termination of, or prophylaxis against, atrial flutter or fibrillation. The recent introduction of sustained-release preparations (44) has obviated the need for short dosing intervals, and patients who reliably absorb these preparations may often be managed on only three or four daily doses. The development of hypersensitivity reactions during chronic therapy remains a major problem.

DOSAGE AND ADMINISTRATION

Procainamide may be given either intravenously, orally, or intramuscularly. Intravenous infusion should be given cautiously and slowly to avoid marked hypotension. A loading dose of 10–20 mg/kg should be given by intermittent bolus injection of 100 mg every 1–3 minutes or as an infusion over 30–45 minutes. Careful blood pressure and rhythm monitoring are mandatory during intravenous loading. Intramuscular injections of procainamide may be used since the drug is well absorbed from intramuscular injection sites and does not cause tissue necrosis. Oral therapy with procainamide requires multiple daily doses because of the drug's short elimination half-life. The introduction of sustained-release preparations has improved this situation, but oral absorption of these preparations is more variable and monitoring of plasma concentrations is essential. The usual dose of procainamide needed to achieve adequate serum concentrations is 3–6 g/day. Occasionally, patients may respond to still larger doses but the risk of toxicity becomes substantial.

Disopyramide

Disopyramide was approved for clinical use in the United States in 1977. Its antiarrhythmic activity was first reported in 1963 and it became available in some European countries in 1969 (84). Since it has electrophysiologic effects similar to those of quinidine and procainamide, it was initially hoped that it might effectively substitute for these drugs, with a decreased incidence of side effects. With several years clinical experience, however, an increased incidence of toxicity has been noted and chronic therapy with disopyramide is not feasible in many patients.

ELECTROPHYSIOLOGIC AND ECG EFFECTS (58, 84)

The direct electrophysiologic effects of disopyramide are similar to those of quinidine and procainamide. It depresses the rate of phase 0 depolarization, prolongs the duration of the action potential, and increases the ERP of atrial and ventricular muscle. In Purkinje fibers, conduction velocity is delayed and the slope of spontaneous diastolic depolarization is decreased. Disopyramide has significant anticholinergic properties and these tend to cancel out a direct depressant effect on atrioventricular conduction. Although sinus node testing in normal subjects shows few effects from disopyramide, the drug may produce marked depression of the sinus node in patients with a clinical history of sinus node dysfunction. Disopyramide prolongs the HV interval and in rare patients may precipitate AV block. During routine clinical usage, disopyramide at usual concentrations produces little change in sinus cycle length and PR interval, a minor prolongation of QRS duration, and a moderately prolonged QT_c interval.

PHARMACOKINETICS (58)

Disopyramide may be administered either orally or intravenously, but only the oral preparation is currently available for use in the United States. The drug is well absorbed orally and reaches a peak serum concentration approximately 1–2 hours after ingestion. The drug's volume of distribution after an intravenous bolus is about 1.0–1.5 liters/kg and is decreased in patients with acute myocardial infarction, congestive heart failure, or renal failure.

Renal excretion of unchanged drug is the major mode of elimination for disopyramide. The compound also undergoes N-dealkylation to a mono-N-dealkylated inactive metabolite. In normal volunteers, the elimination half-life is approximately 6–8 hours. Elimination is prolonged in renal failure and doses must be adjusted according to serum concentration. The effects of hemodialysis on disopyramide metabolism are variable, but resin or charcoal hemoperfusion has been used in the emergency treatment of poisoning with the drug.

Protein binding of most antiarrhythmic drugs remains constant within the therapeutic range. In contrast, the degree of protein binding for disopyramide decreases markedly with increasing total concentrations within the usually observed range of plasma concentrations of 2–4 mg/ml (102). This fact has potential clinical significance since most clinical laboratories report only total drug concentrations, and a small increase in total concentration may represent a large increase in active drug.

HEMODYNAMIC EFFECTS

Disopyramide has markedly negative inotropic effects that complicate its use in patients with congestive heart failure. Disopyramide has been reported to lower cardiac output, raise systemic vascular resistance, and depress left ventricular function. In one clinical series, symptomatic congestive heart failure was exacerbated or precipitated by disopyramide in 16 of 100 patients (119). This event occurred in 50% of the treated patients with a prior history of congestive heart failure. As a result of these observations, disopyramide therapy should be initiated in patients with congestive heart failure with great caution and only if no suitable alternative is available.

SIDE EFFECTS

Disopyramide has potent anticholinergic activity in many organ systems and produces dry mouth, urinary hesitancy, and constipation. Acute urinary retention may occur in patients with prostate enlargement or diabetes mellitus. The drug may also precipitate acute glaucoma. Rare cases of hepatitis have been reported.

DOSAGE AND ADMINISTRATION

At the present time, disopyramide is available for administration in the United States only as capsules containing 100 or 150 mg of the drug and as sustained-release capsules of the same size. The usual loading dose is 300 mg, with subsequent doses of 100–200 mg every 6 or 8 hours for the regular capsules. The interval between doses should be decreased in the presence of renal failure.

Lidocaine

Lidocaine is readily administered intravenously and has few side effects at therapeutic serum concentrations; its effects dissipate rapidly after an infusion is terminated. For these and other reasons, it has gained acceptance as the drug of choice for the short-term treatment of many acute ventricular arrhythmias (128).

ELECTROPHYSIOLOGIC AND ECG EFFECTS

Although lidocaine is grouped with quinidine and procainamide as a class I antiarrhythmic drug, there are marked differences in its electrophysiologic effects. Lidocaine depresses fast channel sodium conductance, but its effects are more prominent in partially depolarized fibers (3, 131). In normal fibers, lidocaine shortens the action potential duration, shortens the ERP, and decreases spontaneous automaticity. Conduction velocity shows little change. In depolarized fibers or in fibers damaged by ischemia, however, lidocaine prolongs the action potential and slows conduction. When given to normal subjects, lidocaine has little effect on sinus cycle length, PR interval, QRS duration, or QT interval. The AH and HV intervals usually remain normal. Lidocaine may rarely produce AV block in patients with severe preexisting intraventricular conduction disorders.

PHARMACOKINETICS (129, 151)

Lidocaine is well absorbed orally, but extensive first pass hepatic metabolism makes oral administration unreliable and the drug is used only parenterally. After intravenous administration, lidocaine distributes rapidly into a central compartment with a volume of distribution of approximately 0.5 liter/kg. The size of the central compartment is decreased in patients with heart failure or shock. With prolonged infusion of lidocaine, peripheral tissues become saturated and the steady state volume of distribution is approximately 1.5 liters/kg. In the blood, about 50% of the total lidocaine is bound to plasma proteins, principally albumin. Intramuscular lidocaine is also well tolerated and has been used in an emergency setting before hospital admission.

Lidocaine is eliminated chiefly via hepatic metabolism with the metabolic rate proportional to hepatic blood flow. A variety of metabolites have been detected. The major pathway is oxidative N-deacylation to monoethylglycinexylidide, an active metabolite, with subsequent hydrolysis to 2,6-xylidine. A number of other hydroxylated metabolites may also be found. In congestive heart failure, the volume of distribution in the central compartment is decreased and hepatic blood flow may be decreased if cardiac output is depressed. Hepatic failure slows clearance rate but does not affect the volume of distribution. Since less than 10% of lidocaine is excreted unchanged in the urine, little adjustment is required in renal failure. The elimination half-life after short-term infusion averages 1.5–2.5 hours, but is often prolonged in critically ill patients or in patients who have had prolonged courses of therapy.

The desired serum concentration of lidocaine should be 1–5 μg/ml. Toxicity begins to appear at a serum concentration between 5 and 10 μg/ml and a severe toxicity is common at higher levels.

HEMODYNAMIC EFFECTS

At the concentrations normally employed clinically, lidocaine produces few adverse hemodynamic changes.

SIDE EFFECTS

The principal side effects associated with lidocaine therapy are concentration-related and are manifest clinically as disturbances of central nervous system function. These effects may be quite subtle and are commonly overlooked in the critical care setting. The side effects are more frequent in elderly patients and those with compromised cardiac output in whom the volume of distribution is usually decreased. In such patients, lidocaine toxicity may be mistakenly thought to be due to the patient's overall condition and drug toxicity not suspected. Dysarthria is often the first warning of lidocaine toxicity, with paresthesias, disorientation, and agitation also frequent complaints. At higher concentrations, seizures and respiratory arrest may occur. These latter side effects are most commonly seen in patients with reduced central volumes of distribution due to age or heart failure in whom bolus injection may transiently produce marked elevations in serum concentrations.

CLINICAL USE

Lidocaine has been used chiefly for treating ventricular arrhythmias. Its ease of parenteral administration has made it the most common drug chosen for the initial therapy of acute arrhythmias in the critical care setting. Controlled data concerning lidocaine efficacy in most clinical situations are unfortunately lacking. In the absence of such data, however, the relative safety of lidocaine and its ease of use justify its traditional role.

The use of prophylactic lidocaine in cases of acute myocardial infarction remains controversial since conflicting data have been reported from equally well-designed studies (Table 21.6) (33, 87, 91, 115, 140). A decision as to whether lidocaine should be administered to patients with known or suspected myocardial infarction must continue to be made on an individualized basis.

DOSAGE AND ADMINISTRATION

Lidocaine may be used intramuscularly or intravenously, but the intravenous route is most commonly used. The initial loading dose of 1.5–2.5 mg/kg should be given in two injections separated by 20–30 minutes or as a continuous infusion over 30 minutes. Maintenance therapy may require infusion rates of 1–4 mg/min, but plasma level monitoring should be used if long-duration, high-dose infusions are used. The decreased central volume of distribution seen in congestive heart failure and shock requires that both loading and maintenance doses be lowered. In particular, caution is required when bolus injections of lidocaine are given to severely ill patients already on a maintenance infusion. In such situations it is often safer to switch to a second agent rather than risk major toxicity while attempting to achieve a maximal lidocaine effect.

Mexiletine

Mexiletine was first developed as an anticonvulsant, but subsequent studies indicated significant antiarrhythmic activity. It has been

Table 21.6
Prophylactic Lidocaine in Suspected Acute Myocardial Infarction

Authors	Lidocaine Dose	Period of Evaluation (hr)	No. of Patients[a]				
				Sustained VT or VF		Asystole or CHB	
			Total	Lidocaine	Placebo	Lidocaine	Placebo
Lie et al (91)	100 mg i.v. +3 mg/min	48	212	2	15	NR	NR
O'Brien et al (115)	75 mg i.v. +2.5 mg/min	48	300	18	18	7	2
Valentine et al (140)	300 mg i.m.	2	269	3	7	NR	NR
Koster and Dunning (87)	400 mg i.m.	1	6024	8	17	26	13
Dunn et al (33)	300 mg i.m. +100 mg i.v.	1	402	3	3	3	1

[a]CHB, complete heart block; NR, not reported; VT, ventricular tachycardia; VF, ventricular fibrillation.

widely used for a number of years in Europe and Great Britain and was released in the United States in 1986. It is usually classified as a class Ib agent.

ELECTROPHYSIOLOGIC AND ECG EFFECTS (127)

Mexiletine is structurally similar to lidocaine and its electrophysiologic effects are similar. In usual clinical concentrations, mexiletine produces no change in AH or HV intervals or in sinus or AV nodal function. The effect on the ERP in ventricular muscle is somewhat variable but most patients will manifest no change in sinus rate, PR, QRS, or QT_c intervals.

PHARMACOKINETICS (17)

Mexiletine is well absorbed orally, with peak concentrations achieved 30–90 minutes after a dose. After intravenous administration, the volume of distribution is large (6–8 liters/kg) reflecting extensive tissue binding. Thirty to 50% of the drug in plasma is protein bound. The major mode of elimination is hepatic transformation via oxidation or reduction to a variety of metabolites. The antiarrhythmic activities of these metabolites are unknown. Only a small fraction of the dose is excreted as unchanged drug in the urine. Although the urinary excretion is increased at lower urinary pH, this fact is of limited clinical significance. The elimination half-life of mexiletine is about 10 hours in normal volunteers, but is increased to 10–24 hours in patients with cardiac disease. The useful plasma therapeutic range for mexiletine appears to be about 0.5–2.0 μg/ml.

HEMODYNAMIC EFFECTS

Mexiletine has few or no clinically important hemodynamic effects during chronic oral therapy (136). Mild or moderate depression of left ventricular function has been reported after intravenous infusion. These effects have been similar to those observed with therapeutic doses of lidocaine.

SIDE EFFECTS (17)

The clinical use of mexiletine is limited by a high incidence of gastrointestinal and central nervous system reactions. Nausea, vomiting, and gastrointestinal upset are frequently seen. In some patients, these toxic effects may be prevented by administering small doses in association with meals. Neurologic toxicity is also prominent. Tremor, dizziness, confusion, and ataxia are often seen and may require discontinuation of therapy. These side effects may occur with plasma levels well within the useful range described above. Hypotension and increased AV block are not usually seen.

CLINICAL USE

Although mexiletine has been evaluated in a variety of clinical settings, no consensus about its current role in antiarrhythmic therapy exists. It does provide symptomatic relief in some patients with palpitations due to ventricular premature beats and nonsustained ventricular tachycardia. Mexiletine, however, has not proven to be consistently effective as single therapy in patients with a history of sustained ventricular tachycardia (26, 144), or in postinfarct patients (19, 73). The use of mexiletine in combination with a second antiarrhythmic drug or with a β-adrenergic blocker has seemed more promising, however, in patients with sustained arrhythmias (31).

DOSAGE AND ADMINISTRATION

The normal dosage range of mexiletine is 300–900 mg daily in three or four divided doses. Occasional patients may tolerate a twice-a-day dosage schedule.

Tocainide

Tocainide is another compound structurally related to lidocaine that has similar electrophysiologic properties. Its chief advantage over lidocaine is its long elimination half-life and its ability to be taken orally.

ELECTROPHYSIOLOGIC AND ECG EFFECTS (95)

The effects of tocainide on electrophysiologic parameters parallel those of lidocaine and mexiletine. After intravenous infusion, the drug produces only minor changes in sinus rate or in the PR, QRS or QT_c intervals. The AH and HV intervals and the ERPs of the His-Purkinje system and right ventricular muscle show no change. When given to some patients with ventricular tachycardia, tocainide may paradoxically shorten the tachycardia cycle length and cause degeneration to ventricular fibrillation (34).

PHARMACOKINETICS (95)

Tocainide is rapidly absorbed orally with almost 100% bioavailability. Peak serum levels are seen 1–2 hours are oral ingestion. About 50% of the drug is bound to plasma proteins at clinically relevant plasma concentrations. The volume of distribution is about 1–2 liters/kg. The drug is eliminated both by hepatic metabolism and by renal filtration. The principal metabolites detected in urine are the glucuronide conjugate of N-carboxytocainide and lactylxylide. The elimination half-life is between 10 and 15 hours. Antiarrhythmic effects are noted at plasma concentrations of 5–12 μg/ml.

HEMODYNAMIC EFFECTS

Only limited information is available on the hemodynamic actions of tocainide. Tocainide probably produces only minor changes in systolic function even in patients with heart failure.

SIDE EFFECTS

Central nervous system toxicity is a frequent complication of tocainide therapy, with tremors, headache, visual disturbances, dizziness, and paresthesia observed frequently with plasma levels below 10 μg/ml. Nausea, vomiting, dyspepsia, and anorexia are seen in approximately 10–25% of patients. Other rare adverse reactions include an allergic rash, leukopenia, and pulmonary fibrosis.

CLINICAL USE

Tocainide has been shown to suppress ventricular premature beats in 40–70% of patients with stable, asymptomatic arrhythmias (95). The response rate to tocainide for patients with sustained ventricular tachycardia or ventricular fibrillation is much lower, however, and like mexiletine, it should probably not be used as a single agent in therapy of sustained ventricular tachyarrhythmias. Tocainide has not been shown to be of significant benefit during acute myocardial infarction (18).

Encainide

Encainide is a benzanilide derivative that has recently been released for use in the United States. It is considered to be a class Ic antiarrhythmic agent.

ELECTROPHYSIOLOGIC AND ECG EFFECTS (126, 148)

In Purkinje fibers, encainide depresses $\dot{V}_{max}$ during phase 0 of the action potential, shortens action potential duration, prolongs the ERP relative to the action potential duration, and decreases the rate of spontaneous phase 4 depolarization. Conduction velocity in Purkinje fibers is markedly reduced. Normal sinus node function and AV nodal conduction are only slightly affected by intravenous encainide, but the HV interval is markedly prolonged. During chronic therapy, however, accumulation of active metabolites may cause prolongation of the AH interval. The ECG of patients during chronic therapy will usually show a prolonged PR interval and a widened QRS, but the JT_c interval will only rarely be lengthened.

PHARMACOKINETICS (143, 149)

Encainide is rapidly and well absorbed after oral administration, but in approximately 90% of the North American population, extensive first pass hepatic extraction and metabolism occur before the drug reaches the systemic circulation. Two major metabolites, O-desmethylencainide (ODE) and 3-methoxy-O-desmethylencainide (MODE), and a third, minor metabolite, N-desmethylencainide, have been identified. The former two compounds are both pharmacologically active, producing electrophysiologic effects similar to those of encainide itself (125). In patients who possess the capacity to metabolize encainide rapidly, the parent compound itself has an elimination half-life of only 1–2 hours, but ODE and MODE have elimination half-lives of approximately 11 and 24 hours, respectively, with final elimination occurring via conjugation and renal excretion. Thus, in these patients most of the clinically apparent effects are produced by the metabolites.

Approximately 6–10% of the North American population genetically lacks the ability to metabolize encainide readily (143). In these patients much higher plasma concentrations of encainide are seen; the parent compound itself has an elimination half-life of about 12 hours and is responsible for any antiarrhythmic activity.

Since the effects of encainide are due to the combined actions of several compounds, no firm guidelines for using plasma concentrations to guide therapy have been described.

HEMODYNAMIC EFFECTS (139)

Encainide has not produced significant acute changes in left ventricular function even in patients with moderate congestive heart failure, but long-term data concerning this question are not available.

SIDE EFFECTS

Encainide causes dose-related side effects that limit therapy in about 25% of patients treated with the drug. The most common adverse reactions reported are dizziness, blurred vision, ataxia, tremor, headache, and gastrointestinal upset. The nature of the relationships between these side effects and the individual plasma concentrations of encainide and its major metabolites is unknown.

Encainide, like flecainide and other similarly acting drugs, has a potential for producing proarrhythmic effects without warning. In the most severe form, these arrhythmias are sustained ventricular tachycardia with unusually wide QRS complexes that may be resistant to cardioversion attempts (147).

CLINICAL USE

Encainide is a generally safe and effective agent for suppressing ventricular premature beats and nonsustained ventricular tachycardia in patients without important structural heart disease. Results in patients with a history of sustained arrhythmias are less predictable (99). In addition, since antiarrhythmic effects in each patient are the sum of effects of the parent compound and the active metabolites, a standardized range of plasma concentrations to guide therapy is not available. In patients with sustained ventricular tachycardia, encainide at lower doses usually results in a slower tachycardia if the arrhythmia recurs.

Encainide may be useful in patients with supraventricular arrhythmias. If relatively high doses (150–200 mg/day) are used, encainide can markedly prolong the ERP of, or even block conduction in, accessory pathways (1, 121). The role of encainide in patients with paroxysmal atrial flutter or fibrillation has not been thoroughly investigated.

DOSAGE AND ADMINISTRATION

Encainide therapy is usually initiated at a dose of 25 mg three times daily, and this dose may be cautiously increased every 3–4 days up to a maximum dose of 200 mg daily. Rapid loading should be avoided because of the risk of overshooting the desired effects and either adversely affecting AV conduction or producing proarrhythmic effects. Although the population may be divided into two genetically determined groups based on their ability to metabolize encainide, phenotyping is unnecessary since the clinical results of therapy are similar in both groups.

Flecainide

Flecainide acetate was first synthesized in 1975 and was recognized to have significant antiarrhythmic activity in early preclinical and clinical trials. It was released for general use in the United States in 1986. Flecainide is classified as a type Ic antiarrhythmic agent.

ELECTROPHYSIOLOGIC AND ECG EFFECTS (66, 108)

Flecainide is a potent inhibitor of fast sodium channel activity and thus markedly depresses the upstroke of the action potential during phase 0. Conduction velocity in Purkinje fibers and both atrial and ventricular muscle is slowed. Normal sinus node automaticity is usually not changed, but Purkinje fiber automaticity is inhibited. Conduction velocity in the AV node is also decreased. During electrophysiologic studies, flecainide prolongs both the AH and HV intervals, prolongs or blocks conduction times in accessory pathways, and produces minor increases in atrial and ventricular refractoriness.

During chronic flecainide therapy, increases in the PR interval and QRS duration may be seen. Increases in QRS duration of more than 25% are related to elevated plasma concentrations and indicate toxicity.

PHARMACOKINETICS (23)

Oral flecainide is well absorbed, with 90–95% of an oral dose bioavailable. There is no alteration of bioavailability by food or antacids. Little first pass hepatic extraction occurs. The degree of plasma protein binding is approximately 40%. The steady state volume of distribution is 7–9 liters/kg. There are two major hepatic metabolites: *meta-O*-dealkylated flecainide and the *meta-O*-dealkylated lactan. These compounds do not have clinically relevant antiarrhythmic activity. During chronic therapy, about 40–60% of flecainide is excreted in the urine as unchanged drug. The average elimination half-life is between 12 and 24 hours, but this time may be prolonged in patients with congestive heart failure or renal insufficiency. Careful monitoring is required to maintain plasma concentrations within the desired range. For the reasons discussed below, this desired range requires adjustment from patient to patient to avoid toxicity. Therapeutic effects begin to be seen at concentrations over 200 ng/ml. Plasma concentrations should be maintained below 600 ng/ml in patients with congestive heart failure. Concentrations up to 1000 ng/ml may be tolerated by patients with normal ventricular function and may yield increased antiarrhythmic activity.

HEMODYNAMIC EFFECTS (76)

Flecainide has important negative inotropic effects in both animal and clinical studies. After intravenous administration, flecainide decreases left ventricular ejection fraction, cardiac index, and stroke work index and increases left and right ventricular filling pressures. During chronic oral therapy, 5–15% of patients treated with flecainide will either develop new congestive heart failure or a worsening of preexisting failure. This is a particularly difficult problem, since as heart failure develops, flecainide elimination is prolonged leading to further depression of ventricular function or to drug-induced arrhythmias if the dose is not reduced.

SIDE EFFECTS

The prevalence of adverse reactions during flecainide therapy is highly dependent on the patient population studied. In stable patients with normal ventricular function, minor extracardiac side effects including dizziness, dysgeusia, blurred vision, nausea, and headache may be seen. These adverse reactions are usually associated with plasma concentrations above 800 ng/ml and are manageable with dosage adjustments (39).

In contrast, patients with more serious cardiac disease are susceptible to several life-threatening forms of cardiac toxicity. Flecain-ide has been associated with a 10–15% incidence of worsened arrhythmias when given to patients with a history of sustained ventricular tachycardia or cardiac arrest (110, 118). This proarrhythmic effect often presents as sustained ventricular tachycardia with a very wide, poorly defined QRS complex that despite a relatively long cycle length may not support a blood pressure. This rhythm may be resistant to attempts at DC cardioversion and may prove fatal despite immediate and appropriate resuscitation attempts. In most but not all cases, this phenomenon has been associated with elevated plasma concentrations (>600 ng/ml) that occurred either during the first few days of therapy or after a change in dosage or metabolism.

Complete AV block may also be seen if flecainide is used in patients with preexisting AV conduction system disease. Worsened congestive heart failure is also common, as discussed above.

CLINICAL USE

In a large number of clinical trials, flecainide has been shown to suppress frequent and complex ventricular ectopy in over 80% of clinically stable patients (6, 37, 63). Results in patients with a history of sustained ventricular tachycardia and structural heart disease have not been as promising and further data are required (4, 38, 146). In these patients, response rates of 20–30% may be expected in previously untreated subjects. A history of prior failure of one or more agents may be expected to lower this rate of response.

Flecainide has also been reported to be effective in patients with several types of supraventricular arrhythmias (60, 79). Since the drug affects the AV node as well as atrial and ventricular muscle, it has shown promise in the treatment of both paroxysmal atrial fibrillation and paroxysmal supraventricular tachycardia. Patients with the Wolff-Parkinson-White syndrome and antegrade preexcitation may manifest greater increases in bypass tract refractoriness with well-tolerated doses of flecainide than may be achievable with quinidine or procainamide therapy.

At present, flecainide seems a reasonable first choice drug in patients with normal ventricular function and symptomatic sustained or nonsustained atrial and ventricular arrhythmias. Although it may be used in patients with compromised ventricular function, this approach requires caution and careful monitoring to prevent the appearance of adverse cardiac reactions.

DOSAGE AND ADMINISTRATION

Since cardiac toxicity to flecainide has been commonly seen during the first few days of therapy, rapid loading with flecainide is not recommended. In stable patients without congestive heart failure, the initial dose should be 100 mg twice daily, with increases up to 200 mg twice daily possible after steady state plasma concentrations have been measured. In patients with heart failure, 50 mg twice daily is a more appropriate initial dose, and upward increments should be made with caution. During chronic therapy, plasma concentrations should be monitored at frequent intervals since flecainide elimination may vary over time. Because of its potential for producing life-threatening adverse reactions, it is usually unwise to increase dosage aggressively in hopes of maximizing antiarrhythmic effects.

Propafenone

Propafenone is an antiarrhythmic agent that has been readily available in Europe for a number of years.

ELECTROPHYSIOLOGIC AND ECG EFFECTS (21, 22)

Propafenone depresses sodium conductance and results in a depression in $\dot{V}_{max}$ during phase 0 of the action potential. Conduction velocity in the His-Purkinje system in atrial and ventricular muscle is slowed. In cardiac tissues that display spontaneous automaticity, the rate of phase 4 depolarization is also decreased. In electrophysiologic studies, propafenone has variable effects on the sinus node recovery time; lengthens the refractorial periods of the atrium, AV node, and ventricle; and slows intraatrial, AV nodal, His-Purkinje, and intraventricular conduction. The PA, AH, and HV intervals are all prolonged. The surface ECG shows a modest increase in the PR interval and QRS duration but little change in the JT_c interval.

Propafenone also produces a mild degree of β-adrenergic blockage with a potency of about $\frac{1}{40}$ that of propranolol. The clinical significance of this latter effect remains undefined.

PHARMACOKINETICS (22, 132)

Propafenone is well absorbed (>95%) after oral ingestion, but undergoes extensive first pass hepatic metabolism before reaching the systemic circulation. This extraction system is partially saturable, thus first pass clearance decreases with larger single doses and during chronic therapy. Peak plasma concentrations are seen 2–3 hours after oral dosing. The steady state volume of distribution is between 0.7 and 1.1 liters/kg. Propafenone is highly (>95%) protein bound in the circulation.

Propafenone is extensively metabolized in most subjects, unchanged propafenone excretion accounting for less than 1% of total elimination. The rate of metabolism is at least partially genetically determined, with patients known to be slow metabolizers of debrisoquine having a correspondingly slow metabolism. During propafenone therapy, several metabolites including 4-hydroxypropafenone, hydroxymethoxypropafenone, and various glucuronide and sulfate conjugates have been identified. It is known that at least the 4-hydroxy metabolite has significant antiarrhythmic activity and contributes to propafenone's activity during clinical usage. Since oxidative metabolism of propafenone is genetically determined, the measured elimination half-life may vary greatly from patient to patient, with a range of 1.8–32 hours reported. Thus, the antiarrhythmic effects seen during propafenone therapy are due to the combined actions of the parent compound and its metabolites, and a practical "therapeutic range" for all patients is difficult to define. In rapid metabolizers, however, plasma propafenone concentrations are usually between 0.5 and 1.5 μg/ml.

HEMODYNAMIC EFFECTS (9)

Propafenone has been demonstrated to produce negative inotropic effects in both preclinical and clinical trials. As with other agents, these effects are most pronounced in subjects with preexisting congestive heart failure.

SIDE EFFECTS

Propafenone is usually well tolerated. Minor extracardiac side effects including dysgeusia, xerostomia, nausea and vomiting, constipation, dizziness, and blurred vision may be seen in up to 20% of patients. These problems are usually dose-related and can often be managed by dosage adjustment. Cardiac toxicity in the form of congestive heart failure, bradycardia due to sinus node suppression or AV block, and aggravation of tachyarrhythmias may occur at any dose and usually require discontinuation of therapy. Like other drugs with similar electrophysiologic effects, propafenone has been associated with a hemodynamically unstable, ventricular tachycardia that is resistant to attempts at cardioversion (109).

CLINICAL USE

Propafenone has been shown to produce antiarrhythmic effects in both ventricular and supraventricular arrhythmias. In studies on patients with chronic, stable ventricular premature beats, between 60% and 75% of patients manifest suppression of the arrhythmias (117, 130); however, when used in patients with sustained ventricular tachycardia, response rates have been much lower (10–40%) (21, 22, 29, 59). Propafenone usually lengthens the tachycardia cycle length in the latter patients, but despite this fact, hypotension during tachycardia may be more profound.

Propafenone appears to be useful for managing a variety of supraventricular arrhythmias (16, 56). In patients with preexcitation, propafenone prolongs the ERP and may cause block even in patients with a short ERP. Successful therapy of paroxysmal atrial flutter or atrial fibrillation and AV nodal reentry has also been reported.

DOSAGE AND ADMINISTRATION

Propafenone therapy is usually initiated at a dosage of 150 mg or 200 mg three times daily. Few patients have been treated with daily doses of over 1200 mg. The appearance of extracardiac side effects, worsened congestive heart failure, or QRS widening is an indication to decrease dosage since plasma level monitoring is unreliable.

Amiodarone

Amiodarone is a heavily iodinated benzofuran derivative that was initially developed as an antianginal agent. During early clinical use in Europe, it was observed to produce powerful antiarrhythmic effects in patients with both supraventricular and ventricular arrhythmias. However, its unusual pharmacokinetic profile and its potential for producing toxicity in many organ systems have limited the drug's overall utility.

ELECTROPHYSIOLOGIC AND ECG EFFECTS (97, 98)

Since amiodarone is virtually insoluble in aqueous media, few reports on its acute, in vitro electrophysiologic effects are available. In preparations taken from animals treated chronically with the drug, action potential duration is prolonged with the major effect apparent during phases 2 and 3. Phase 0 depolarization under baseline conditions is little affected, but a use-dependent depression of sodium channel conductance may be demonstrated. Amiodarone also produces a mild noncompetitive β-blockade and inhibits peripheral conversion of thyroxine (T_4) to triiodothyronine (T_3), thus producing indirect effects as well.

During chronic amiodarone therapy in humans, a number of electrophysiologic changes have been reported. Sinus node automaticity is decreased. AV nodal conduction velocity and refractoriness are both depressed. His-Purkinje conduction intervals are increased, as are the effective and functional refractory periods of atrium and ventricle. In patients with accessory pathways, both antegrade and retrograde refractory periods are increased.

The surface ECG during chronic amiodarone therapy usually shows a moderate sinus bradycardia, a slight prolongation of the PR interval, a marked prolongation in the QT_c, and the appearance of prominent U-waves, particularly in the midprecordial leads.

PHARMACOKINETICS (2, 54, 67)

Amiodarone has variable and unusual pharmacokinetic parameters. Bioavailability after a single oral dose has been reported to range from 22% to 86%, with peak plasma concentrations seen between 2 and 10 hours after ingestion. The volume of distribution is greater than 20 liters/kg, reflecting extensive tissue binding particularly in liver, lung, muscle, and adipose tissue. Elimination kinetics are complex. Plasma levels decline very slowly after discontinuation of chronic therapy, with detectable plasma concentrations present as long as 6–12 months after the last dose.

During chronic amiodarone therapy, an active metabolite, desethylamiodarone, accumulates and eventually achieves plasma concentrations of 60–80% of those of the parent drug. The mechanisms of final elimination of amiodarone and desethylamiodarone from the body are still uncertain.

The value of plasma concentration monitoring to guide therapy with amiodarone has remained controversial (36, 48). During chronic therapy (200–400 mg/day), plasma concentrations of amiodarone usually range between 0.5 and 3.5 μg/ml. Although weak correlations between dose and plasma concentrations and between electrophysiologic effects and plasma concentrations can be demonstrated, there is wide interindividual variability and the correlations are not of clinical value. In addition, significant toxicity from amiodarone may occur at all clinically useful doses and over a wide range of plasma concentrations.

HEMODYNAMIC EFFECTS (86)

Since steady state amiodarone effects cannot be practically achieved with short courses of administration, the direct hemodynamic effects of amiodarone remain uncertain. There seems to be little change in left ventricular ejection fraction or cardiac output during chronic oral therapy, but some patients may not tolerate the sinus bradycardia usually seen during therapy. Acute intravenous infusion of amiodarone has been reported to lower vas-

cular smooth muscle tone and to produce a modest negative inotropic effect.

SIDE EFFECTS

Chronic amiodarone therapy commonly produces at least minor toxicity, the majority of patients treated for several years experiencing one or more adverse reactions (48, 97). Adverse reactions may be seen at all clinically useful dosage levels, but are more common with higher doses and with increased durations of exposure.

The most dangerous side effect associated with amiodarone therapy is pulmonary infiltrates (134). This reaction has been reported in up to 10–20% of patients treated with amiodarone for several years. It may appear at any point during therapy. Patients with amiodarone pulmonary toxicity usually present with dyspnea and a nonproductive cough. Pyrexia may also occur. The chest x-ray shows diffuse interstitial infiltration (Fig. 21.6). Arterial blood gases show marked hypoxemia with a low or normal P_{CO_2}. Pulmonary function tests show restrictive lung volumes but no new obstruc-

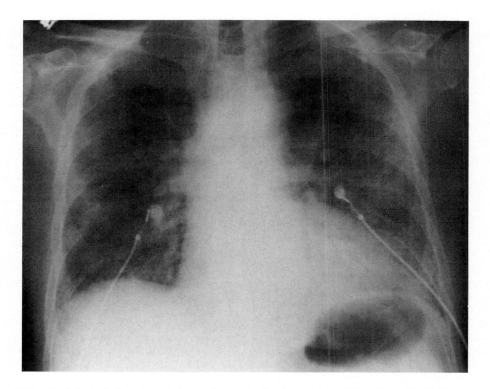

Figure 21.6. Radiologic findings in amiodarone-induced pulmonary toxicity. Diffuse interstitial infiltrates that may be difficult to distinguish from those seen with infection or heart failure characterize this syndrome.

tive defect. Diffusion capacity is usually markedly reduced.

Amiodarone pulmonary toxicity may develop gradually, but more commonly presents after a short course of rapid deterioration. The differential diagnosis at presentation often includes aggravated congestive heart failure and pulmonary infection. Catheterization of the right side of the heart and gallium scanning may be used to distinguish drug toxicity from these conditions. In equivocal cases, lung biopsy may be helpful. Biopsies show thickened alveolar septa and fibrosis with macrophages and other inflammatory cells in the alveoli. The macrophages contain lipid-containing lysosomal inclusion bodies.

Therapy of amiodarone pulmonary toxicity requires discontinuation of the drug, support of respiratory function, and control of arrhythmias. Although steroid therapy is frequently recommended, no conclusive evidence of its benefit has been shown. Amiodarone pulmonary toxicity, once clinically evident, usually takes weeks to resolve, and infection, respiratory failure, and recurrent arrhythmias often intervene to produce an overall mortality that may reach 20–40%.

Almost all patients receiving amiodarone chronically develop corneal microdeposits. Although these are readily visible during a slit lamp examination, they only rarely affect visual activity (74). However, approximately 10% of patients report visual blurring or halo vision.

Amiodarone has several interactions with thyroid hormone metabolism (15, 96). Each 200-mg tablet contains 75 mg of organic iodine. Iodine-induced hypothyroidism or hyperthyroidism may be seen, with the relative prevalence dependent on the dietary iodine content of the population studied. Amiodarone also inhibits conversion of T_4 to T_3. In patients who remain euthyroid, plasma concentrations of T_4 and reverse T_3 are elevated, whereas T_3 and thyroid-stimulating hormone concentrations should remain normal. Supplementation with thyroxine will prevent clinical symptoms of hypothyroidism without affecting antiarrhythmic activity; the development of hyperthyroidism is frequently signalled by arrhythmia recurrence.

Dermatologic toxicity is common after therapy with amiodarone and may present in two forms (152). Up to 50% of patients develop increased photosensitivity to UVA waveband light sources. In a smaller percentage of patients, bluish-gray skin discoloration on sun-exposed areas may develop because of an accumulation of lipofuscin granules in dermal macrophages. All patients treated with amiodarone should be instructed to use photoprotective topical therapy and clothing during periods of sun exposure.

Neuromuscular toxicity is commonly seen during amiodarone therapy, particularly in older patients treated with doses over 200 mg/day (20). Proximal muscle weakness, tremor, and peripheral neuropathy are the most frequent presentations. Other symptoms include distal paresthesias and numbness, muscle weakness and wasting, and areflexia. Other forms of neurologic reactions, including ataxia and sleep disturbance, are also common, particularly during the first weeks of treatment. All of these neurologic reactions appear to respond, albeit slowly, to reduction in dosage.

Liver function abnormalities may be detected in approximately one-third of patients receiving amiodarone. The usual finding is a minor ($<$ 2-fold) elevation of serum glutamic-oxaloacetic transaminase (SGOT), glutamic-pyruvic transaminase (SGPT), and lactic dehydrogenase (LDH) that may be either persistent or transient. A few cases of hepatitis or hepatic failure have been reported. Nausea, vomiting, and constipation have also been re-

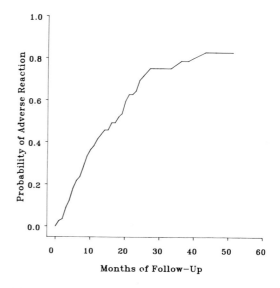

Figure 21.7. Expected incidence of adverse reactions during amiodarone therapy. (From Greenberg ML, Lerman BB, Shipe JR, et al: Relation between amiodarone and desethylamiodarone plasma concentrations and electrophysiologic effects, efficacy and toxicity. *J Am Coll Cardiol* 9:1148–1155, 1987.)

ported, but rarely limit therapy except during high-dose oral loading (50).

Bradycardias due to either sinus node suppression or drug-induced AV block are frequently encountered during long-term amiodarone therapy. Because of the long period that would be required for drug elimination, permanent pacing is often required.

Because of the frequent and serious adverse reactions produced by amiodarone, careful surveillance during long-term treatment is required. Blood tests for liver function and thyroid function abnormalities should be obtained, and periodic chest x-rays are also recommended. Such routine testing, along with a careful interim history and physical examination, is necessary to minimize the risk to any individual patient.

Amiodarone has a number of important drug interactions. It raises serum digoxin concentrations and interferes unpredictably with warfarin therapy (97, 105). The plasma levels of many other drugs also rise during amiodarone therapy.

CLINICAL USE

Although it has not been subjected to rigorous, placebo-controlled trials, amiodarone is undoubtedly an extremely potent antiarrhythmic agent. Most studies have dealt almost exclusively with patients who had previously failed one or more antiarrhythmic drug trials (40, 50, 72, 97, 101, 145). Nevertheless, long-term efficacy rates of 75–90% in patients with supraventricular arrhythmias and 45–75% in patients with ventricular arrhythmias have commonly been achieved. Amiodarone is highly effective in patients with recurrent atrial flutter and with paroxysmal supraventricular tachycardia due to either AV nodal reentry or reentry involving an accessory AV pathway. Paroxysmal atrial fibrillation also responds in many cases to amiodarone.

In patients with sustained ventricular tachycardia, amiodarone will often either eliminate or decrease the frequency of episodes. The rate of the tachycardia, should it recur, is usually significantly slowed (78). Although early reports suggested that programmed electrical stimulation was of little value for guiding amiodarone therapy (55, 107, 145), more recent reports have shown that ventricular stimulation can be used to define those at low risk of recurrence and to predict the characteristics of a potentially recurrent arrhythmia (72, 101).

DOSAGE AND ADMINISTRATION

Because of its great potential for producing toxicity and its unusual pharmacokinetics, amiodarone must be administered cautiously. In stable patients with supraventricular arrhythmias, an initial dose of 600 mg/day for 2–3 weeks followed by a maintenance dose of 200 mg/day is usually employed. In patients with serious ventricular arrhythmias, the usual starting dose of 1200–1800 mg/day is continued for 7–14 days and then decreased to 200–400 mg/day. There is no agreement on whether a gradual tapering of dosage after the early load is necessary, and clinical judgment is required. Chronic doses of over 400 mg/day are associated with significant morbidity and should only be used if no alternatives exist.

Amiodarone has also been used with success intravenously in unstable patients. The usual reported dose has been 600–1800 mg/day for 2–3 days (83). Intravenous amiodarone, however, causes severe phlebitis and only infusion into a central vein should be used.

β-Adrenergic Blockers

A large number of β-adrenergic blocking agents are now available for clinical use for a variety of cardiac indications. Used alone as antiarrhythmic drugs, they are useful in arrhythmias that depend on increased sympathetic tone and for their depressant effect on AV nodal conduction. However, β-adrenergic blockers are frequently helpful during antiarrhythmic therapy either to potentiate the effects of other antiarrhythmic agents or to indirectly affect the etiologic factors (e.g., ischemia, catecholamine excess) responsible for the arrhythmia.

Although significant differences have been described between β-adrenergic blocking drugs in terms of β_1 selectivity, membrane-stabilizing activity, and intrinsic sympathomimetic activity, the practical value of these variables for selecting the optimal β-blocking drug for treating arrhythmias in most situations has not been defined (42). Sotalol is an unusual drug with β-blocking and antiarrhythmic properties.

ELECTROPHYSIOLOGIC AND ECG EFFECTS

β-Adrenergic blockers decrease the slope of phase 4 depolarization in the sinus node and in Purkinje fibers. Phase 0 of the action potential is unchanged. At moderate concentrations, the effects of isoproterenol to shorten the refractory period of atrial and ventricular muscle and to lower the threshold for ventricular fibrillation are blocked. The other major effects of clinical relevance are increases in conduction time and refractoriness in AV nodal tissue.

Patients on β-adrenergic blocking agents without intrinsic sympathomimetic activity usually have a modest sinus bradycardia with normal PR, QRS, and QT_c intervals. Exercise-related or stress-related sinus tachycardia is usually blunted. Significant bradycardias may be precipitated in patients with sinus node dysfunction, autonomic dysfunction, or AV conduction system disease.

PHARMACOKINETICS (42)

β-Adrenergic blocking agents with a wide range of pharmacokinetic properties are currently available. Agents such as propranolol and metoprolol that are highly lipid soluble tend to be well absorbed, undergo extensive first pass hepatic extraction, and have a relatively short elimination half-life. Agents such as nadolol and atenolol are relatively water soluble, are incompletely absorbed, are cleared by renal excretion, and have longer elimination half-lives. Other agents exhibit properties between these extremes. The properties of some of these agents are summarized in Table 21.7.

HEMODYNAMIC EFFECTS

The hemodynamic effects of β-adrenergic blocking drugs are dependent on the level of intrinsic adrenergic activity and on the functional reserve of the heart. In general, β-adrenergic blockers lower heart rate and arterial blood pressure, decrease indices of myocardial contractility, and lower cardiac output.

SIDE EFFECTS

The side effects of β-adrenergic blocking agents are related to their effects on adrenergic receptors in various organs. Bronchospasm may be seen in patients with asthma and chronic obstructive pulmonary disease, and this risk is not totally eliminated by the use of relatively selective β_1-antagonists. Heart failure, hypotension, and bradycardia may be produced in susceptible patients. Some patients on β-blockers complain of fatigue, sleep disturbance, or impotence.

CLINICAL USE

β-Adrenergic drugs share several common uses. They may be used to increase AV nodal refractoriness and therefore control ventricular rate in atrial fibrillation and prevent episodes of paroxysmal supraventricular tachycardia. They also may act synergistically with other antiarrhythmic drugs whose actions to prolong conduction and increase refractoriness in atrial

Table 21.7
Selected Properties of β-Adrenergic Blocking Drugs[a]

Drug	Relative β_1 Selectivity	ISA	MSA	Absorption (%)	Bio-availability (%)	Elimination Half-life	Major Route of Elimination	Usual Intravenous Dose	Usual Oral Dose (mg)
Acebutolol	+	+	+	70	50	3–4 hr	Renal	—	200–600 b.i.d.
Atenolol	+	−	−	50	40	6–9 hr	Renal	—	50–100 q.d.
Esmolol	+	−	−	—	—	9–10 min	Hepatic	500 μg/kg load, then 100–300 μg/kg/min	—
Metoprolol	+	−	−	90	50	3–4 hr	Hepatic	5 mg × 3 over 10 min	25–100 b.i.d. or t.i.d.
Nadolol	−	−	−	30	30	14–24 hr	Renal	—	20–80 q.d.
Pindolol	−	+ +	+	90	90	3–4 hr	Renal, hepatic	—	5–20 b.i.d.
Propranolol	−	−	+ +	90	30	3–4 hr	Hepatic	5–10 mg at 1 mg/2–3 min	40–80 q.i.d.
Sotalol	−	−	−	70	60	8–10 hr	Renal	—	80–320 b.i.d.
Timolol	−	−	−	90	75	4–5 hr	Renal, hepatic	—	2.5–10 b.i.d.

[a] ISA, intrinsic sympathomimetic activity; MSA, membrane stabilizing activity.

or ventricular muscle are antagonized by adrenergic stimulation.

A number of studies have described a beneficial effect when β-blocking drugs are administered prophylactically to patients recovering from myocardial infarction (11, 62, 113). The precise mechanism by which this effect is achieved remains controversial.

Esmolol is a β-adrenergic blocking agent with an extremely brief elimination half-life (<10 minutes) and is available only for intravenous use. Because of this fact it is of particular value in the intensive care unit since it permits rapid intravenous titration of dosage and thus rapid control of ventricular rate in atrial arrhythmias. It appears to be of particular value in patients with postoperative atrial flutter and fibrillation (35, 45).

Sotalol is a β-adrenergic drug with mixed antiarrhythmic properties (90, 106). In addition to possessing about one-third the β-blocking potency per milligram of propranolol, it also has direct effects on the action potential similar to those produced by amiodarone. It has been successfully used to treat both supraventricular and ventricular arrhythmias. Sotalol produces QT prolongation, and when used in the setting of hypokalemia has been associated with the induction of polymorphic ventricular tachycardias.

Bretylium

Bretylium tosylate is a benzyl quaternary ammonium compound that was first introduced as an antihypertensive during the 1950s. The development of more effective and less toxic agents for blood pressure control prevented its widespread use for this purpose. It was subsequently reintroduced as an antiarrhythmic drug for parenteral use in 1974.

ELECTROPHYSIOLOGIC AND ECG EFFECTS (85, 93)

The majority of bretylium's electrophysiologic effects are due to its complex interactions at sympathetic nerve terminals. Early after acute administration of this drug, norepinephrine is released from the presynaptic nerve endings of postganglionic adrenergic neurons. Subsequently, bretylium accumulates in the nerve ending, produces depletion of norepinephrine stores, inhibits norepinephrine release, and blocks reuptake of catecholamines. These lat-

ter effects require 3–6 hours to become apparent.

After initial administration, bretylium causes a transient increase in sinus rate, AV conduction, and ventricular automaticity, effects presumably due to intramyocardial catecholamine release. Chronically, bretylium prolongs the ventricular action potential duration and ERPs without changing V_{max} and conduction velocity. In animal models, bretylium increases ventricular fibrillation threshold, particularly during myocardial ischemia (65).

PHARMACOKINETICS (5, 32)

Bretylium is poorly absorbed after oral administration and is usually administered intravenously or more rarely, intramuscularly. The apparent volume of distribution is 3–5 liters/kg and the drug is not bound to plasma proteins. Bretylium is not metabolized in the body and is excreted in unchanged form by the kidney. Bretylium is highly bound in tissues, and plasma concentrations are not accurate indicators of antiarrhythmic activity. The half-life of elimination is 8–13 hours, but elimination kinetics are not linear and are not accurately described using a two-compartment model. Since bretylium has two phases of activity, initial responses are not predictive of more chronic efficacy. No useful "therapeutic range" of effective plasma concentrations has been described.

HEMODYNAMIC EFFECTS

The initial positive chronotropic and inotropic effects of bretylium are related to the sympathetic discharge seen immediately after administration. Hypertension may be seen initially after bretylium administration is started, but with continued therapy, severe hypotension is commonly observed. The hypotension is aggravated by postural changes, but may persist even if the patient remains supine. Cardiac index is usually maintained unless adverse effects are produced by the hypotension.

SIDE EFFECTS

The immediate toxicity associated with bretylium is mediated via its effects on the sympathetic nervous system. Transient hypertension, increased automaticity in either the sinus node or in ectopic foci, and an increase in myocardial oxygen demand may all produce deleterious effects. With prolonged intravenous treatment, severe hypotension is the major side effect. Pretreatment with tricyclic antidepressants may block uptake of bretylium into adrenergic nerve terminals, but this has not been of practical clinical value. An analogue, bethanidine, which is well absorbed orally, has undergone testing for the chronic suppression of ventricular arrhythmias. In these studies, bethanidine has been administered along with the tricyclic antidepressant, protriptyline. Unfortunately, bethanidine has not been shown to be a particularly effective antiarrhythmic agent, and hypotension associated with its use has been particularly severe.

Rapid intravenous infusion of bretylium frequently produces nausea and vomiting. This may be ameliorated if the drug is given by slow injection over 8–10 minutes. Chronic oral therapy with bretylium has also been associated with parotitis.

CLINICAL USE (57, 116)

The role of bretylium in the treatment of ventricular arrhythmias requires continued assessment. The immediate and delayed antiarrhythmic effects of bretylium are presumably mediated by different mechanisms and data from clinical trials are difficult to analyze. Since it has electrophysiologic properties that are strikingly different from those of other conventionally available antiarrhythmic agents, bretylium may well prove useful in a different spectrum of arrhythmias and data obtained in traditional models may not be relevant. At present, it seems to be of sufficient potential efficacy to warrant consideration for the short-term control of ventricular fibrillation only. Antiarrhythmic effects may be delayed, and a trial of at least 6–8 hours of therapy seems indicated before bretylium can be considered a failure. Unfortunately, since the chief clinical experience with bretylium has been in cases of cardiac arrest or in the management of patients with multiple factors contributing to their arrhythmias, an objective analysis of bretylium's clinical efficacy even in cardiac arrest patients is not possible based on the current data (57, 116). There are no convincing data that bretylium is effective for hemodynamically stable ventricular tachycardia outside the setting of acute myocardial infarction, and considerable experience shows that the hypotension it causes can be harmful (10, 51).

DOSAGE AND ADMINISTRATION

Bretylium is available in 10-ml ampules containing 500 mg of bretylium tosylate. Ex-

cept in cardiopulmonary resuscitation, when it is usually injected as a bolus of 5 mg/kg, the drug should be diluted with either 5% dextrose or saline to a concentration of 10 mg/ml and infused slowly over 8–10 minutes. The initial loading dose should be 5 mg/kg. A second dose of 5 mg/kg may be administered if the first is ineffective. Maintenance therapy, for those rare cases in which it is indicated, usually requires 5–10 mg/kg every 6–8 hours or 1–2 mg/min by continuous infusion. Intramuscular therapy is possible and requires no dosage adjustment if peripheral circulation is intact. Careful monitoring of arterial blood pressure is mandatory and intraarterial monitoring is often necessary. Dosage should be reduced in patients with reduced renal function.

Verapamil

Verapamil is the prototype for a class of agents that selectively affect calcium transport. These "calcium blockers" have potential clinical utility in a variety of clinical situations: hypertension, variant and typical angina, and hypertrophic myopathies as well as for the treatment of various arrhythmias.

ELECTROPHYSIOLOGIC AND ECG EFFECTS (7, 94, 133)

Verapamil produces its electrophysiologic effects by altering the kinetics of activation, inactivation, and recovery of the calcium-dependent slow channel. At high concentrations, verapamil has local anesthetic activity, but this activity is absent at clinically relevant drug concentrations. Verapamil depresses action potentials dependent on slow channel activity in normal cells of the sinus and AV nodes and those slow action potentials seen in partially depolarized fibers. Conduction velocity in these cells is selectively depressed, whereas fibers in which the action potential is mediated by fast channel currents are relatively unaffected. Verapamil also suppresses triggered activity via its influence on intracellular calcium concentrations.

During electrophysiologic studies, verapamil may produce depression of sinus node function, particularly in patients with sinus node disease. Verapamil prolongs the AH interval and the refractory period of the AV node, but has no effect on the ERPs of atrial or ventricular muscle. The refractory period for antegrade conduction over accessory bypass tracts may either show no effect or actually shorten, but the latter effect may be reflex mediated. The ECG may show slight prolongation of the PR interval whereas the QRS and QT$_c$ usually remain unchanged.

PHARMACOKINETICS (81, 100)

Verapamil may be administered either orally or intravenously. After intravenous administration, the drug initially distributes into a central compartment with a volume of distribution of approximately 2 liters/kg. At steady state, the volume of distribution is about 4 liters/kg. When administered orally, the drug is well absorbed but undergoes substantial first pass hepatic degradation. The system for hepatic extraction and metabolism is saturable so that initial doses and lower doses are more completely cleared. The systemic bioavailability of the drug is only 10–30%. Ninety percent of the drug in plasma is protein-bound. Verapamil elimination is via hepatic metabolism. The principal metabolite, norverapamil, accumulates in plasma to a concentration greater than that of the parent compound during chronic therapy. Norverapamil has measurable antiarrhythmic activity, but is much less potent than verapamil. The elimination half-life for verapamil is about 3–6 hours. Elimination is prolonged in cirrhosis and in conditions of decreased hepatic blood flow. If hepatic blood flow is decreased, however, the fractional transhepatic extraction increases, partly compensating for the decreased flow. Effective serum concentrations during chronic oral therapy for arrhythmias have not been reported, but serum concentrations observed during verapamil therapy for hypertrophic cardiomyopathy are 30–150 ng/ml. In patients who receive 0.075 mg/kg intravenously for the termination of reentrant supraventricular tachycardias, concentrations ranging from 72 to 195 ng/ml have been seen (138).

HEMODYNAMIC EFFECTS (138)

Verapamil has marked negative inotropic effects and produces relaxation of vascular smooth muscle. In most patients, the decrease in blood pressure after intravenous verapamil is principally due to peripheral vasodilation, but left ventricular end-diastolic pressure increases and the drug may precipitate congestive heart failure. In many patients with mild or moderate heart failure, however, the improvement in afterload and attenuation of ischemia may al-

low the negative inotropic effects to be well compensated. Verapamil and other calcium channel blockers are also useful in angina, hypertension, and other disorders.

SIDE EFFECTS

The principal extracardiac side effect reported with oral verapamil is constipation. Nausea, vomiting, vertigo, headache, and nervousness have also been reported. After intravenous administration, hypotension and bradycardia may be seen. Ventricular asystole has been reported in patients who previously received intravenous β-adrenergic blocker. Verapamil causes a rise in serum digoxin concentrations in patients previously taking digoxin. The magnitude of the increase is less than that seen with quinidine.

CLINICAL USE (137, 138)

Verapamil administered intravenously at a dose of 0.075 or 0.15 mg/kg (5–10 mg total) terminates most episodes of reentrant supraventricular tachycardia in which the AV node is involved in the reentry loop. In atrial flutter or fibrillation, conduction through the AV node is delayed and a stable ventricular rate may be achieved. Reflex adrenergic stimulation in response to hypotension seen after verapamil injection may blunt these effects in unstable patients. Verapamil has no predictable effect on ventricular arrhythmias except in rare cases, and the hypotension it causes may prove dangerous. When given to patients with Wolff-Parkinson-White syndrome conducting antegradely over an accessory pathway, verapamil may actually speed antegrade conduction and increase ventricular rates. As a general rule, verapamil should never be given to a patient with a wide complex tachycardia of unknown mechanism.

Chronic oral verapamil is useful in the chronic prophylaxis of recurrent paroxysmal supraventricular tachycardia. It also can provide a stable ventricular rate in selected patients with chronic atrial fibrillation. The optimal dose ranges for these purposes are not firmly established, but therapy is usually initiated with 80–120 mg three or four times daily.

Other Calcium Antagonists

Several other calcium channel antagonists are now available in the United States. Nifedipine and nitrendepine have no electrophysiologic effects and therefore no potential as antiarrhythmic agents. Diltiazem has electrophysiologic actions similar to those of verapamil and may be of potential use as an antiarrhythmic drug. Further studies to characterize the antiarrhythmic actions and dose requirements of diltiazem are necessary, however, before it can be recommended as a substitute for verapamil in treating arrhythmias.

Other Antiarrhythmic Drugs

There has been an explosive growth in the number of pharmacologic agents that may be used for treating cardiac arrhythmias. The role of many of the more recently developed agents has not as yet been fully defined and these agents are not discussed in detail in this chapter. However, some relevant properties of selected new agents are listed in Table 21.8.

PACING AND CARDIOVERSION

Electrical pacing of the heart may be useful in the prevention or termination of many arrhythmias. The earliest uses of pacing were for treating bradycardia-dependent arrhythmias. Some arrhythmias are triggered by late diastolic premature beats. In bigeminal rhythms, the long pause after the premature beat can prolong repolarization after the subsequent normal beat and lead to an "R-on-T" phenomenon. In these two instances, overdrive pacing at faster rates may prove effective in preventing arrhythmias. In patients having a relative bradycardia associated with hemodynamic compromise that causes a secondary arrhythmia, either atrial, ventricular, or dual chamber pacing may help prevent further episodes. Unfortunately, for the long-term management of most arrhythmias, overdrive pacing by itself is only occasionally successful.

Pacing techniques, however, may be extremely valuable for the termination of an acute arrhythmia. This fact has been particularly true in patients after cardiac surgery in whom temporary epicardial pacing wires are often implanted, thus facilitating the procedure. As new technologies become available, implantable pacing units with antitachycardia capabilities may become more common.

The arrhythmia most commonly treated with pacing is atrial flutter (47). The delivery of bursts of atrial stimuli at cycle lengths shorter than the atrial cycle lengths results in atrial capture and a change in the flutter wave on the ECG, and in most cases will either terminate flutter or accelerate it to atrial fibrillation. If atrial capture can be reliably achieved, most episodes of atrial flutter can be terminated in this fashion. Even if atrial fibrillation is produced, it is often easier to control the ventricular rate with medications with resultant hemodynamic improvement. Reentrant supraventricular tachycardias may also be terminated in this manner. Atrial fibrillation, multifocal atrial tachycardia, and automatic atrial or junctional tachycardias do not respond.

Ventricular tachycardia may also be terminated with pacing. Single or double extrastimuli or bursts of rapid pacing terminate a

Table 21.8
Investigational Antiarrhythmic Drugs—Preliminary Data

Agent	Action	Elimination Half-life	Major Side Effects	Possible Future Use
Adenosine (28)	Slows AV nodal conduction	1–3 sec	Dyspnea	Termination of paroxysmal supraventricular tachycardia
Cibenzoline (88)	Ic and III	4 hr	Nausea, vomiting, headache	Ventricular arrhythmia
Clofilium (52)	III	?	Flushing	Ventricular arrhythmia
Indecainide (112)	Ic	6–12 hr	Dizziness, blurred vision	Ventricular arrhythmia
Lorcainide (82)	Ic	7–9 hr	Sleep disturbance, tremor	Ventricular arrhythmia
Meobentine (30)	Ic and III	11–27 hr	Hypotension, dyspnea	Ventricular arrhythmia
Moricizine (120)	Ib ?	6–14	Nausea, vomiting, rash	Ventricular arrhythmia
Pirmenol (123)	Ia	4–15 hr	Flushing, dysgeusia, constipation	Ventricular arrhythmia
Recainam (24)	Ic	7–12 hr	Nausea	Ventricular arrhythmia

majority of relatively slow, recurrent ventricular tachycardias and may decrease the need for frequent cardioversions. There is a substantial risk of producing acceleration of the tachycardia or inducing ventricular fibrillation, however, and the operator should be prepared for emergency resuscitation. This potential for arrhythmia acceleration has limited the introduction of automatic antitachycardia pacemakers for recurrent sustained ventricular tachycardia.

Direct current countershock is the treatment of choice for any arrhythmia that is associated with hemodynamic collapse or with severe angina in a patient with coronary artery disease, or one that is resistant to other forms of treatment. When used to treat supraventricular arrhythmias or a well-tolerated ventricular tachycardia, the DC countershock delivery should be synchronized with the peak of the QRS complex to avoid precipitating ventricular fibrillation by delivering the shock during the T wave. Digitalis toxicity should be excluded, if possible, prior to elective cardioversion since digitalis toxicity may lead to irreversible ventricular fibrillation after countershock.

The automatic internal cardioverter defibrillator was approved for general use in the United States in 1986 (103). This fully implantable device continually senses the heart's rhythm and is set to deliver shocks from internal electrodes in response to rapid or disorganized ventricular rhythms. As this technology develops, further modifications can be expected to improve arrhythmia detection, add antitachycardia pacing capability, eliminate the need for thoracotomy, and miniaturize the components. When such advances are realized, devices, probably in conjunction with drugs, may become the standard treatment for the more life-threatening forms of ventricular arrhythmias.

ASSESSMENT OF ANTIARRHYTHMIC THERAPY

When choosing to initiate therapy with an antiarrhythmic drug, the physician must balance the indication for treatment against the potential for toxicity associated with each agent. The goals of antiarrhythmic therapy may include termination of an acute arrhythmia, modification of an acute or chronic arrhythmia so that adverse hemodynamic effects are eliminated, or prophylaxis against the future oc-

Table 21.9
Goals of Antiarrhythmic Therapy

I. Short-term therapy
  A. Termination of an acute arrhythmia
  B. Modification of an arrhythmia to minimize hemodynamic effects
  C. Prevention of a life-threatening arrhythmia
II. Chronic Therapy
  A. Prevention of sudden cardiac death
  B. Elimination of symptomatic arrhythmia

currence of a life-threatening or symptomatic arrhythmia (Table 21.9). The likelihood of achieving these goals must be weighed against the potential adverse reactions and the cost of therapy. Arrhythmias that are not associated with symptoms and do not indicate a substantial risk for a life-threatening arrhythmia seldom require therapy.

The optimal methods for assessing antiarrhythmic therapy remain controversial. Except when arrhythmia termination provides an easily assessed therapeutic objective, the physician is often forced to use intermediate endpoints for assessing the efficacy of antiarrhythmic therapy. The endpoint selected, however, may vary depending on the clinical circumstances in which therapy is considered. Whatever the endpoint used to evaluate therapy, it should correlate with the ultimate goal of treatment.

It is essential to determine the optimal method for evaluating intermediate endpoints beginning chronic therapy when a treatment failure would result in an arrhythmia with life-threatening potential. Ventricular arrhythmias not associated with transmural myocardial infarction are responsible for the majority of sudden cardiac deaths, and prevention of these arrhythmias has become an important therapeutic challenge. The optimal method for the selection of chronic therapy for preventing sporadic sustained ventricular arrhythmias has not been determined, but several approaches are currently in use.

When coronary care units were first introduced, it was observed that some patients who later developed an episode of ventricular fibrillation would develop so-called "warning arrhythmias" before the event. Lown and Wolf (92) proposed a grading system for ventricular premature beats (VPBs) that ranked them in five grades of severity (Table 21.10). Although the maximum grade achieved is strongly related to the frequency of total VPBs and the concept of warning arrhythmias has been

Table 21.10
Lown-Wolf Grading System for Ventricular Premature Beats (VPBs)

Grade 0	No VPBs
Grade 1	Occasional VPBs (<20/hr, <1/min)
Grade 2	Frequent VPBs (≥30/hour)
Grade 3	More than one ECG morphology
Grade 4	Repetitive VPBs
4A	Paired VPBs
4B	Three or more consecutive VPBs
Grade 5	R-on-T VPBs

questioned, the basic Lown-Wolf grading system has been widely used to assess the prognostic significance of asymptomatic arrhythmias in certain populations and to evaluate responses to antiarrhythmic therapy. The various criteria for VPB suppression used in clinical studies have not been subjected to rigorous validation, but are based either on reduction of total VPB count or on both a reduction in VPB total and elimination of higher grade VPBs during ambulatory or, in some studies, exercise ECG. Such an approach has recently been reported to predict accurately the chronic efficacy of antiarrhythmic therapy in patients with a prior history of malignant ventricular arrhythmias (46). This method is limited, however, in that as many as 30–40% of patients with a history of sustained ventricular tachycardia or fibrillation will not have enough spontaneous VPBs to guide therapy, and is also limited by the extreme variability of VPB frequency and grade over time. In addition, some of the newer antiarrhythmic drugs are extremely potent suppressors of VPBs but do not prevent sustained ventricular tachycardia or fibrillation over the long term.

A second approach for the selection of chronic antiarrhythmic therapy has also been advocated. Electrode catheters are placed within the heart and the response to premature extrastimuli determined. In many patients, arrhythmias that have been observed clinically may be reproduced by these techniques, and if the ability to initiate the arrhythmia with stimulation is abolished by medical or surgical therapy, long-term efficacy of that therapy is accurately predicted. Therapy based on this electrophysiologic approach is useful in many patients with both ventricular and supraventricular arrhythmias (25, 122). Since electrophysiologic testing was first used in patients with ventricular arrhythmias, many questions about its value have been answered but some problems still remain. The technique works best in patients with coronary artery disease and prior myocardial infarction. In these patients, electrophysiologic testing is essential for guiding surgical or device-based therapy, and drugs likely to prove highly effective are readily identified. Unfortunately, 40–50% of patients may not achieve "control" by electrophysiologic criteria yet may remain arrhythmia-free. In patients with cardiac diagnoses other than coronary artery disease, the results of electrophysiologic testing are less reliable and further studies are required for reproducing arrhythmias and defining drug therapy.

PROARRHYTHMIC EFFECTS OF ANTIARRHYTHMIC DRUGS

The ability of antiarrhythmic drugs to induce or exacerbate arrhythmias has been appreciated for many years. A number of different mechanisms may be responsible. Most antiarrhythmic drugs produce changes in conduction and under appropriate conditions, might facilitate rather than abolish reentrant arrhythmias. This phenomenon may be seen with subthreshold doses of a drug that may be effective if higher concentrations are maintained. Many agents prolong repolarization and may result in a drug-induced long QT syndrome in which the prolonged and nonuniform recovery of excitability makes the tissue susceptible to the initiation of fibrillation by a critically timed premature beat. Some drugs may produce deleterious hemodynamic effects or conduction abnormalities that secondarily precipitate arrhythmias. Aggravation of arrhythmia has been reported during therapy with almost every antiarrhythmic agent, but the exact frequency of the reaction has only recently been appreciated. Current estimates based on data from both invasive and noninvasive studies suggest that proarrhythmic effects occur during approximately 10% of drug trials in patients with sustained ventricular arrhythmias (14, 71, 142). Therefore, it is important to suspect a proarrhythmic effect whenever an arrhythmia is seen in a patient receiving an "antiarrhythmic" drug.

MANAGEMENT OF SPECIFIC ARRHYTHMIAS

The usual therapies of some common arrhythmias are listed in Table 21.11.

Table 21.11
Therapy of Specific Arrhythmias

Arrhythmia	Maneuvers or Agents	
	Acute Termination	Chronic Prophylaxis
Paroxysmal supraventricular tachycardia (AV node or AV reentry)	Vagal maneuvers, verapamil, adenosine	Digoxin, β-blockers, Ca^{2+} blockers, Ia, Ic
Atrial flutter	Rapid atrial pacing, cardioversion, procainamide	Ia, Ic(?), amiodarone, sotalol
Atrial fibrillation	Cardioversion, rate control, Ia antiarrhythmics	Ia, Ic(?), amiodarone, sotalol
Nonparoxysmal junctional tachycardia	Reverse etiology	Atrial pacing (?)
Multifocal atrial tachycardia	Reverse etiology	Verapamil (?)
Sustained ventricular tachycardia	Cardioversion, lidocaine, procainamide	See text
Ventricular fibrillation	DC shock	See text

Sinus Tachycardia

Sinus tachycardia is characterized by normal P waves with 1:1 AV conduction usually at rates between 100 and 220 beats/min. In most cases, sinus tachycardia is an appropriate physiologic response to an acute stress and does not require specific therapy. Therefore, therapy should be directed at improving the underlying condition. However, if sinus tachycardia causes symptoms or contributes to an increased myocardial oxygen demand with resultant ischemia, it may require treatment. β-Adrenergic blockers are the usual drugs of choice.

Paroxysmal Supraventricular Tachycardia

Paroxysmal supraventricular tachycardia (PSVT) may be due to several mechanisms. Atrioventricular reentry, either with manifest preexcitation or in patients with concealed bypass tracts that function in retrograde fash-

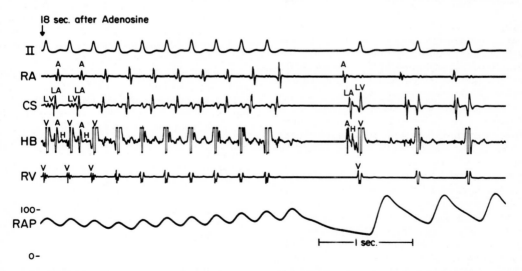

Figure 21.8. Termination of supraventricular tachycardia by adenosine. The tracings represent surface ECG leads II and intracardiac recordings from the right atrium *(RA),* coronary sinus *(CS),* bundle of His *(HB),* and right ventricle *(RV),* and a radial artery pressure *(RAP).* With arrival of the adenosine bolus at the heart 21 seconds after injection, AV nodal conduction is blocked and sinus rhythm and a normal blood pressure are restored. (From DiMarco JP, Sellers TD, Lerman BB, et al: Diagnostic and therapeutic use of adenosine in patients with supraventricular tachyarrhythmias. *J Am Coll Cardiol* 6:417–425, 1985.)

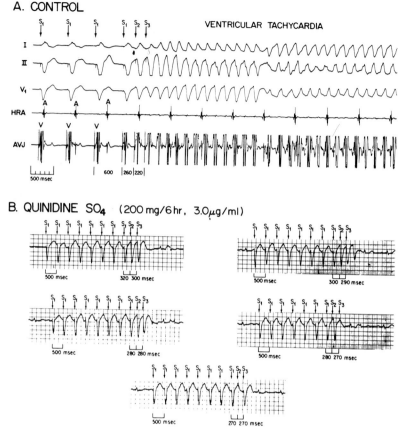

Figure 21.9. Electrophysiologic testing in a patient with cardiac arrest. **A,** Surface ECG leads I, II, and V₁ and intracardiac recordings from the high right atrium *(HRA)* and the AV junction *(AVJ)*. Two extrastimuli with coupling intervals of 260 and 220 msec initiated a rapid ventricular tachycardia that required countershock for termination. **B,** Repeat testing on quinidine shows that no arrhythmia is inducible. (From DiMarco JP, Garan H, Ruskin JN: Quinidine for ventricular arrhythmias: value of electrophysiologic testing. *Am J Cardiol* 51:90–95, 1983.)

ion only, or AV nodal reentry are the most common mechanisms. Intraatrial and sinus node reentry may also be seen. Automatic atrial tachycardia is a relatively rare chronic arrhythmia in adults, but may be more common in critically ill patients in whom increased adrenergic influences may unmask ectopic automatic atrial foci.

Since the majority of episodes of PSVT involve the AV node as part of the reentry pathway, initial attempts to terminate the arrhythmia usually involve maneuvers or agents that slow AV nodal conduction. Vagal maneuvers (e.g., Valsalva, carotid sinus massage) are often effective and some patients with repeated episodes are able to use them to self-terminate their arrhythmias. If drug therapy is required, the most effective agent for acute termination

is intravenous verapamil; the usual dose is 5 or 10 mg.

Recently, the electrophysiologic properties of the endogenous nucleoside adenosine have been described (28). Adenosine depresses AV nodal conduction and is cleared from the circulation within seconds after a bolus injection. When administered to patients with PSVT due to AV nodal or AV reentry, adenosine terminates the tachycardia by producing block within the AV node within 30 seconds after injection (Fig. 21.9). Individual dosage titration is usually required, the average dose being approximately 100 μg/kg.

Intravenous digoxin, propranolol, and edrophonium (Tensilon) were traditionally used in attempts to terminate PSVT prior to the availability of verapamil and adenosine. At the present time, however, they should be considered as second choice agents for acute therapy. The use of pressor agents is not recommended.

The chronic prophylaxis of PSVT must be individualized for each patient. Some patients respond best to agents that slow antegrade AV nodal conduction (digoxin, verapamil, and β-blocking drugs), whereas others respond better to agents that either suppress the premature beats that trigger the arrhythmias or depress retrograde atrioventricular conduction (class Ia or Ic agents, β-blockers, or amiodarone). Electrophysiologic studies are often helpful in drug selection in patients with severe symptoms during PSVT who have not responded to digoxin, propranolol, or verapamil.

Atrial Flutter and Atrial Fibrillation

Atrial flutter is characterized by repetitive atrial activity at an atrial rate of 250–350 beats/min. The QRS is normal. A second form of atrial flutter ("type II") has been described, but this latter arrhythmia is managed more like atrial fibrillation. In atrial flutter, the discrete atrial impulses bombard the AV conduction system at regular intervals and in most patients, 2:1 conduction due to alternating conduction and block is seen. Since the alternate impulse arrives during the absolute refractory period of the AV node, no part of the node is depolarized and it therefore can fully recover by the arrival of the next impulse 200 msec later. Smooth control of ventricular rate in atrial flutter is therefore difficult since major changes in AV nodal refractoriness would have to be produced and changes in rate would occur suddenly with fixed increments.

Atrial flutter is thought to involve intraatrial reentry and therefore is unlikely to terminate following administration of agents selective for the AV node. Quinidine has traditionally been used as the drug of choice if chemical cardioversion is to be attempted, but procainamide is probably equally effective. Unfortunately, only about 20–30% of patients with stable atrial flutter undergo successful cardioversion within 48 hours after starting one of these agents. During the start of therapy the patient's ventricular rate should be monitored since both quinidine and procainamide may slow the atrial rate, and quinidine by its vagolytic action may facilitate AV nodal conduction, thus resulting in 1:1 AV conduction at rates in excess of 200

beats/min. Quinidine raises serum digoxin concentrations, and since digoxin is the usual drug chosen to block this vagolytic effect, careful monitoring of the patient's condition is required. In the majority of patients either atrial pacing or cardioversion must be employed to terminate atrial flutter, since chemical conversion is usually unsuccessful and ventricular rates may be difficult to control.

In atrial fibrillation there is chaotic or very rapid atrial electrical activity and an irregularly irregular ventricular rate. Multiple impulses reach the AV node and either conduct, partially penetrate the node, or are totally blocked. Those that partially penetrate the node reset the refractory period of the penetrated nodal tissue and thereby affect the conduction of subsequent impulses. Agents that prolong AV nodal refractoriness cause a higher degree of partial penetration, and thus a relatively weak drug effect can produce major changes in ventricular rate in atrial fibrillation.

The usual initial approach to the patient with new onset atrial fibrillation is control of ventricular rate. Digoxin, verapamil, or β-adrenergic blockers are all effective and each may have advantages in certain patients. Patients with grossly enlarged atria or those who cannot be maintained in sinus rhythm on chronic drug therapy, may be successfully managed long-term with these drugs to control ventricular rates.

Conversion of the first episode of atrial fibrillation should always be attempted if the rhythm persists after treatment of reversible causes and if the atria are normal or only moderately enlarged. Twenty to 30% of patients undergo successful cardioversion with type Ia or Ic antiarrhythmic agents, and new agents such as sotalol or amiodarone may be more effective. Patients who do not respond to medications alone should undergo transthoracic cardioversion after a 2- to 3-week period of anticoagulation to reduce the small risk of thromboembolism. In patients with new and highly symptomatic atrial fibrillation, cardioversion may be performed emergently without chronic anticoagulation.

Nonparoxysmal Junctional Tachycardia

Nonparoxysmal junctional tachycardia (NPJT) is an automatic tachycardia arising from AV junctional tissue above the bifurcation of the bundle of His. The ECG shows a tachycardia with normal QRS at rates between 60 and 150 beats/min. Either AV dissociation or 1:1 AV conduction may be seen. NPJT usually arises in the setting of simultaneous sinus node depression and catecholamine stimulation. Drug toxicity (lithium, lidocaine, digoxin, etc.) and cardiac surgery are the most common precipitating factors.

Like other automatic arrhythmias, NPJT is difficult to manage. Efforts should be directed to reverse the causes for sympathetic overactivity and to stop drugs that may have depressed the sinus node. Atrial pacing at a faster rate may provide hemodynamic improvement. No specific drug therapy is likely to be effective.

Multifocal Atrial Tachycardia

Multifocal atrial tachycardia (MAT) is produced by enhanced automaticity in multiple atrial foci. The ECG will show three or more discrete P wave morphologies with an average rate of between 120 and 190 beats/min. There is usually 1:1 AV conduction. This arrhythmia is most commonly seen in patients with severe acute illness, especially in those with chronic obstructive pulmonary disease. Excess catecholamine stimulation or methylxanthine toxicity are frequent causes. MAT cannot be terminated acutely either with antiarrhythmic drugs or with electrical countershock. Treatment of the underlying etiology of the arrhythmia is the only effective means of therapy.

The ECG of the patient in MAT may superficially resemble atrial fibrillation and may lead to therapy with digoxin or another cardiac glycoside. In MAT, however, toxic concentrations of digoxin are required before a reduction in ventricular rate is observed, and digitalis-induced arrhythmias may occur. Propranolol is usually contraindicated when MAT is seen. Verapamil may slow the atrial rate in milder forms of MAT, but its use might aggravate the more critically ill patient's hemodynamic status. In most cases, MAT must be tolerated until the factors that precipitated it can be reversed.

Ventricular Tachycardia and Ventricular Fibrillation

The acute management of the patient with cardiac arrest is discussed elsewhere in this text. The elective treatment of ventricular tachycardia that is hemodynamically well tolerated remains largely empiric. Episodes in a small number of patients may be terminated rapidly by intravenous administration of a class I antiarrhythmic agent, usually either lidocaine or procainamide. In tachycardias with long cycle lengths, increasing intravenous doses of procainamide can produce gradual prolongation of the cycle length and may eventually terminate the arrhythmia. Acute drug therapy is often ineffective and either ventricular pacing or cardioversion is usually the treatment of choice for terminating ventricular tachycardia. If the patient is already on an antiarrhythmic drug at the time of the arrhythmia, knowledge of the plasma concentration of that agent is helpful when future prophylactic therapy is designed.

The best approach for selecting prophylactic therapy against ventricular arrhythmias remains controversial. However, clinical experience has shown that there is substantial variability among patients in response to the different antiarrhythmic agents and therapy must be individualized. At the present time, no single agent possesses such obvious clinical advantages that it should be recommended over all the other drugs currently in use. Each drug should be selected for trial and its results evaluated in systematic fashion. A better understanding of the mechanisms responsible for ventricular arrhythmias will allow a more rational approach to therapy in the future.

References

1. Abdollah H, Brugada P, Green M, et al: Clinical efficacy and electrophysiologic effects of intravenous and oral encainide in patients with accessory atrioventricular pathways and supraventricular arrhythmias. *Am J Cardiol* 54:544–549, 1984.
2. Adams PC, Holt DW, Storey GCA, et al: Amiodarone and its desethyl metabolite: tissue distribution and morphologic changes during long-term therapy. *Circulation* 72:1064–1075, 1985.
3. Allen JD, Brennan FJ, Wit AL: Actions of lidocaine on transmembrane potentials of subendocardial Purkinje fibers surviving in infarcted canine hearts. *Circ Res* 43:470–481, 1978.
4. Anderson JL, Lutz JR, Allison SB: Electrophysiologic and antiarrhythmic effects of oral flecainide in patients with inducible ventricular tachycardia. *J Am Coll Cardiol* 2:105–14, 1983.
5. Anderson JL, Patterson E, Wagner JG, et al: Clinical pharmacokinetics of intravenous and oral bretylium tosylate in survivors of ventricular tachycardia or fibrillation: clinical application of a new assay for bretylium. *J Cardiovasc Pharmacol* 3:485–499, 1981.
6. Anderson JL, Stewart JR, Perry BA, et al: Oral flecainide acetate for the treatment of ventricular arrhythmias. *N Engl J Med* 305:473–477, 1981.
7. Antman EM, Stone PH, Muller JE, et al: Calcium channel blocking agents in the treatment of cardiovascular

disorders. Part I: Basic and clinical electrophysiologic effects. *Ann Intern Med* 93:875–885, 1980.

8. Arnsdorf MF: Basic understanding of the electrophysiologic actions of arrhythmic drugs. Sources, sinks, and matrices of information. *Med Clin Am* 68:1247–1280, 1984.

9. Baker BJ, Dihn H, Kroskey D, et al: Effect of propafenone on left ventricular ejection fraction. *Am J Cardiol* 54:20D–22D, 1984.

10. Baurenfeind RA, Hoff JV, Swiryn S, et al: Electrophysiologic testing of bretylium tosylate in sustained ventricular tachycardia. *Am Heart J* 105:973–980, 1983.

11. β-Blocker Heart Attack Trial Research Group: A randomized trial of propranolol in patients with acute myocardial infarction. I. Mortality results. *JAMA* 247:1707–1714, 1982.

12. Bigger JT Jr: The quinidine-digoxin interaction. *Mod Concepts Cardiovasc Dis* 51:73–78, 1982.

13. Bigger JT Jr, Hoffman BF: Antiarrhythmic drugs. In Goodman, Gilman (eds): *The Pharmacological Basis of Therapeutics*, ed 5. New York, Macmillan, 1985, pp 748–791.

14. Bigger JT Jr, Sahar DI: Clinical types of proarrhythmic response to antiarrhythmic drugs. *Am J Cardiol* 59:2E–9E, 1987.

15. Borowski GD, Garofano CD, Rose LI: Effect of longterm amiodarone therapy on thyroid hormone levels and thyroid function. *Am J Med* 78:443–450, 1985.

16. Breithardt G, Borggrefe M, Wiebringhaus E, et al: Effect of propafenone in the Wolff-Parkinson-White syndrome: electrophysiologic findings and long-term follow-up. *Am J Cardiol* 54:29D–39D, 1984.

17. Campbell RWF: Drug therapy: mexiletine. *N Engl J Med* 36:29–34, 1987.

18. Campbell RWF, Hutton I, Elton RA, et al: Prophylaxis of primary ventricular fibrillation with tocainide in acute myocardial infarction. *Br Heart J* 49:557–563, 1983.

19. Chamberlain DA, Jewiit DE, Julian DG, et al: Oral mexiletine in high-risk patients after myocardial infarction. *Lancet* 2:1227, 1980.

20. Charness ME, Morady F, Scheinman MM: Frequent neurologic toxicity associated with amiodarone therapy. *Neurology* 34:669–671, 1984.

21. Chilson DA, Heger JJ, Zipes DP, et al: Electrophysiologic effects and clinical efficacy of oral propafenone therapy in patients with ventricular tachycardia. *J Am Coll Cardiol* 5:1407–1413, 1985.

22. Connolly SJ, Kates RE, Lebsack CS, et al: Clinical efficacy and electrophysiology of oral propafenone for ventricular tachycardia. *Am J Cardiol* 52:1208–1213, 1983.

23. Conrad GJ, Ober RE: Metabolism of flecainide. *Am J Cardiol* 53:41B–51B, 1984.

24. Davies RF, Lineberry MD, Echt DS, et al: Dose titration and pharmacokinetics of recainam, a new antiarrhythmic drug (abstract). *Circulation* 74:II-103, 1987.

25. DiMarco JP: Intracardiac electrophysiology in cardiac catheterization and angiography. In Grossman W (ed): ed 3. Philadelphia, Lea & Febiger, 1986, pp 339–358.

26. DiMarco JP, Garan H, Ruskin JN: Mexiletine for refractory ventricular arrhythmias: results using serial electrophysiologic testing. *Am J Cardiol* 47:13–38, 1981.

27. DiMarco JP, Garan H, Ruskin JN: Quinidine for ventricular arrhythmias: value of electrophysiologic testing. *Am J Cardiol* 51:90–95, 1983.

28. DiMarco JP, Sellers TD, Lerman BB, et al: Diagnostic and therapeutic use of adenosine in patients with supraventricular tachyarrhythmias. *J Am Coll Cardiol* 6:417–425, 1985.

29. Doherty JU, Waxman HL, Kienzle MG, et al: Limited role of intravenous propafenone hydrochloride in the treatment of sustained ventricular tachycardia: electrophysiologic effects and results of programmed ventricular stimulation. *J Am Coll Cardiol* 4:378–381, 1984.

30. Duff HJ, Oates JA, Roden DM, et al: The antiarrhythmic activity of meobentine sulfate in man. *J Cardiovasc Pharmacol* 6:650–656, 1984.

31. Duff HJ, Roden D, Primm RK, et al: Mexiletine in the treatment of resistant ventricular arrhythmias. Enhancement of efficacy and reduction of dose-related side effects by combination with quinidine. *Circulation* 67:1124–1128, 1983.

32. Duff HJ, Roden DM, Yacobi A, et al: Bretylium: relations between plasma concentrations and pharmacologic actions in high-frequency ventricular arrhythmias. *Am J Cardiol* 55:395–401, 1985.

33. Dunn HM, McComb JM, Kinney CD, et al: Prophylactic lidocaine in the early phase of suspected myocardial infarction. *Am Heart J* 110:353–362, 1985.

34. Engler RL, LeWinter M: Tocainide-induced ventricular fibrillation. *Am Heart J* 101:494–496, 1981.

35. The Esmolol vs Placebo Multicenter Study Group: Comparison of the efficacy and safety of esmolol, a short-acting beta blocker, with placebo in the treatment of supraventricular tachyarrhythmias. *Am Heart J* 111:42–48, 1986.

36. Falik R, Flores BT, Shaw L, et al: Relationship of steady-state serum concentrations of amiodarone and desethylamiodarone to therapeutic efficacy and adverse effects. *Am J Med* 82:1102–1108, 1987.

37. The Flecainide-Quinidine Research Group: Flecainide versus quinidine for treatment of chronic ventricular arrhythmias. A multicenter clinical trial. *Circulation* 67:1117–1123, 1983.

38. Flecainide Ventricular Tachycardia Study Group: Treatment of resistant ventricular tachycardia with flecainide acetate. *Am J Cardiol* 57:1299–1304, 1986.

39. Flowers D, O'Gallagher D, Torres V, et al: Long-term treatment using a reduced dosing schedule. *Am J Cardiol* 55:79–83, 1985.

40. Fogoros RN, Anderson KP, Winkle RA, et al: Amiodarone: clinical efficacy and toxicity in 95 patients with recurrent, drug-refractory arrhythmias. *Circulation* 68:88–94, 1983.

41. Frey W: Weitere erfahrunger mit clinidin bei absoluter nezunregelin assigkeit. *Wien Klin Wochenschr* 55:849–853, 1918.

42. Frishman WH, Teicher M: Beta-adrenergic blockade. An update. *Cardiology* 72:280–296, 1985.

43. Giardina E-GV, Dreyfuss J, Bigger JT Jr, et al: Metabolism of procainamide in normal and cardiac subjects. *Clin Pharmacol Ther* 19:339–351, 1975.

44. Graffner C, Johnson G, Sjigren J: Pharmacokinetics of procainamide intravenously and orally as conventional and slow release tablets. *Clin Pharmacol Ther* 17:414–423, 1974.

45. Gray RJ, Bateman TM, Czer LSC, et al: Esmolol: a new ultrashort-acting beta-adrenergic blocking agent for rapid control of heart rate in postoperative supraventricular tachyarrhythmias. *J Am Coll Cardiol* 5:141–56, 1985.

46. Grayboys TB, Lown B, Podrid PJ, et al: Long-term survival of patients with malignant ventricular arrhythmias treated with antiarrhythmic drugs. *Am J Cardiol* 50:437–443, 1982.

47. Greenberg ML, Kelly TA, Lerman BB, et al: Atrial pacing for conversion of atrial flutter. *Am J Cardiol* 58:95–99, 1986.

48. Greenberg ML, Lerman BB, Shipe JR, et al: Relation between amiodarone and desethylamiodarone plasma concentrations and electrophysiologic effects, efficacy and toxicity. *J Am Coll Cardiol* 9:1148–1155, 1987.

49. Greenblatt DJ, Pfeifer HJ, Ochs JR, et al: Pharmacokinetics of quinidine in humans after intravenous, intramuscular and oral administration. *J Pharmacol Exp Ther* 202:365–377, 1977.

50. Greene HL, Graham EL, Werner JA, et al: Toxic and therapeutic effects of amiodarone in the treatment of cardiac arrhythmias. *J Am Coll Cardiol* 2:1114–1128, 1983.

51. Greene HL, Werner JA, Gross BW, et al: Failure of bretylium to suppress inducible ventricular tachycardia. Am Heart J 105:717–721, 1983.

52. Greene HL, Werner JA, Gross BW, et al: Prolongation of cardiac refractory times in man by clofilium phosphate, a new antiarrhythmic agent. Am Heart J 106:492–501, 1983.

53. Greenspan AM, Horowitz LN, Spielman SR, et al: Large dose procainamide therapy for ventricular tachyarrhythmias. Am J Cardiol 46:453–463, 1980.

54. Haffajee CI, Love JC, Canada AT, et al: Clinical pharmacokinetics and efficacy of amiodarone for refractory tachyarrhythmias. Circulation 67:1347–1355, 1983.

55. Hamer AW, Finerman WB, Peter T, Mandel WJ: Disparity between the clinical and electrophysiologic effects of amiodarone in the treatment of recurrent ventricular tachyarrhythmias. Am Heart J 103:992–1000, 1981.

56. Hammill SC, McLaran CJ, Wood DL, et al: Double-blind study of intravenous propafenone for paroxysmal supraventricular reentrant tachycardia. J Am Coll Cardiol 9:1364–1368, 1987.

57. Haynes RE, Chinn TL, Copass MK, et al: Comparison of bretylium tosylate and lidocaine in management of out-of-hospital ventricular fibrillation: a randomized clinical trial. Am J Cardiol 48:353–356, 1981.

58. Heel RC, Brogden RN, Speight TM, et al: Disopyramide: a review of its pharmacological properties and therapeutic use in treating cardiac arrhythmias. Drugs 15:331–368, 1978.

59. Heger JJ, Hubbard J, Zipes DP, et al: Propafenone treatment of recurrent ventricular tachycardia: comparison of continuous electrocardiographic recording and electrophysiologic study in predicting drug efficacy. Am J Cardiol 54:40D–44D, 1984.

60. Hellestrand KJ, Nathan AW, Bexton RS, et al: Cardiac electrophysiologic effects of flecainide acetate for paroxysmal reentrant junctional tachycardias. Am J Cardiol 51:770–776, 1983.

61. Hirschfeld DS, Veda CT, Rowland M, et al: Clinical and electrophysiological effects of quinidine in man. Br Heart J 39:309–316, 1977.

62. Hjalmarson A, Elmfeldt D, Herlitz J, et al: Effect on mortality of metoprolol in acute myocardial infarction: a double-blind randomised trial. Lancet 2:823–827, 1981.

63. Hodges M, Haugland M, Granrud G, et al: Suppression of ventricular ectopic depolarizations by flecainide acetate, a new antiarrhythmic agent. Circulation 65:879–885, 1982.

64. Hoffman BF, Rosen MR, Wit AL: Electrophysiology and pharmacology of cardiac arrhythmias. VII. Cardiac effects of quinidine and procainamide. Am Heart J 89:804–808, 1975.

65. Holland K, Patterson E, Lucchesi BR: Prevention of ventricular fibrillation by bretylium in a conscious canine model of sudden coronary death. Am Heart J 105:711–717, 1983.

66. Holmes B, Heel RC: Flecainide: a preliminary review of its pharmacodynamic properties and therapeutic efficacy. Drugs 29:1–33, 1985.

67. Holt DW, Tucker GT, Jackson PR, et al: Amiodarone pharmacokinetics. Br J Clin Pract 40(suppl 4):109–14, 1986.

68. Hondeghem LM: Antiarrhythmic agents: modulated receptor applications. Circulation 75:514–520, 1987.

69. Hondeghem LM, Katzung BG: Antiarrhythmic agents: the modulated receptor mechanism of action of sodium and calcium channel–blocking drugs. Annu Rev Pharmacol Toxicol 24:387–423, 1984.

70. Hondeghem LM, Mason JW: Agents used in cardiac arrhythmias. In Katzung BG (ed): Basic and Clinical Pharmacology, ed 3. Norwalk, CT, Appleton & Lange, 1987, pp 151–167.

71. Horowitz LN, Greenspan AM, Rae AP, et al: Proar-

72. Horowitz LN, Greenspan AM, Spielman SR, et al: Usefulness of electrophysiologic testing in evaluation of amiodarone therapy for sustained ventricular tachyarrhythmias associated with coronary heart disease. Am J Cardiol 55:367–371, 1985.

73. Impact Research Group: International mexiletine and placebo antiarrhythmic coronary trial: I. Report on arrhythmia and other findings. J Am Coll Cardiol 4:1148–1163, 1984.

74. Ingram DV: Ocular effects in long-term amiodarone therapy. Am Heart J 106:902–904, 1983.

75. Josephson ME, Caracta AR, Ricciotti MA, et al: Electrophysiologic properties of procainamide in man. Am J Cardiol 33:596–603, 1974.

76. Josephson ME, Kaul S, Hopkins J, et al: Hemodynamic effects of intravenous flecainide relative to the level of ventricular function in patients with coronary artery disease. Am Heart J 109:41–45, 1985.

77. Josephson ME, Seides SF, Batsford WP, et al: The electrophysiologic effects of quinidine on the atrioventricular conducting system in man. Am Heart J 87:55–64, 1974.

78. Kadish AH, Buxton AE, Waxman HL, et al: Usefulness of electrophysiologic study to determine the clinical tolerance of arrhythmia recurrences during amiodarone therapy. J Am Coll Cardiol 10:90–96, 1987.

79. Kappenberger LJ, Fromer MA, Shenasa M, et al: Evaluation of flecainide acetate in rapid atrial fibrillation complicating Wolff-Parkinson-White syndrome. Clin Cardiol 8:321–326, 1985.

80. Kass RS: The ionic basis of electrical activity in the heart. In Sperelakis N (ed): Physiology and Pathology of the Heart. Boston, Martinus Nijhoff, 1984, pp 63–92.

81. Kates RE: Calcium antagonists. Pharmacokinetic properties. Drugs 25:113–24, 1983.

82. Keefe DL, Peters F, Winkle RA: Randomized double-blind placebo controlled crossover trial documenting oral lorcainide efficacy in suppression of symptomatic ventricular tachyarrhythmias. Am Heart J 103:511–518, 1982.

83. Kerin NZ, Blevins RD, Frumin H, et al: Intravenous and oral loading versus oral loading alone with amiodarone for chronic refractory ventricular arrhythmias. Am J Cardiol 55:90–91, 1985.

84. Koch-Weser J: Disopyramide. N Engl J Med 300:957–962, 1979.

85. Koch-Weser J: Drug therapy—bretylium. N Engl J Med 300:473–477, 1979.

86. Kosinski EJ, Albin JB, Young E, et al: Hemodynamic effects of intravenous amiodarone. J Am Coll Cardiol 4:565–570, 1984.

87. Koster RW, Dunning AJ: Intramuscular lidocaine for prevention of lethal arrhythmias in the prehospitalization phase of acute myocardial infarction. N Engl J Med 313:105–110, 1985.

88. Kostis JB, Krieger S, Moreyra A, et al: Cibenzoline for treatment of ventricular arrhythmias: a double-blind placebo-controlled study. J Am Coll Cardiol 4:372–377, 1984.

89. Leahey EB Jr, Reiffel JA, Drusin RE, et al: Interaction between digoxin and quinidine. JAMA 240:533–534, 1978.

90. Lidell C, Rehnqvist N, Sjogren A, et al: Comparative efficacy of oral sotalol and procainamide in patients with chronic ventricular arrhythmias: a multicenter study. Am Heart J 109:970–975, 1985.

91. Lie KI, Wellens HJ, van Capelle FJ, et al: Lidocaine in the prevention of primary ventricular fibrillation. N Engl J Med 291:1324–1326, 1974.

92. Lown B, Wolf M: Approaches to sudden death from coronary heart disease. Circulation 4:130–142, 1972.

93. Lucchesi BR, Patterson E: Therapeutic advances in the

management of cardiac arrhythmias: Part II—brety-lium. *Pract Cardiol* 8:101–112, 1982.

94. Lucchesi BR, Patterson E: Therapeutic advances in the management of cardiac arrhythmias: Part III—verapamil. *Pract Cardiol* 8:43–59, 1982.

95. Lynch JJ, Lucchesi BR: New antiarrhythmic agents: Part IV—the pharmacology and clinical use of tocainide. *Pract Cardiol* 11:108–137, 1985.

96. Martino E, Safran M, Aghini-Lombardi F, et al: Environmental iodine intake and thyroid dysfunction during chronic amiodarone therapy. *Ann Intern Med* 101:28–34, 1984.

97. Mason JW: Amiodarone. *N Engl J Med* 316:455–458, 1987.

98. Mason JW, Hondeghem LM, Katzung BG: Block of inactivated sodium channels and of depolarization-induced automaticity in guinea pig papillary muscle by amiodarone. *Circ Res* 55:277–285, 1984.

99. Mason JW, Peters FA: Antiarrhythmic efficacy of encainide in patients with refractory recurrent ventricular tachycardia. *Circulation* 63:670–675, 1981.

100. McAlister RG: Clinical pharmacology of slow channel blocking agents. *Prog Cardiovasc Dis* 25:83–102, 1982.

101. McGovern B, Garan H, Malacoff RF, et al: Long-term clinical outcome of ventricular tachycardia or fibrillation treated with amiodarone. *Am J Cardiol* 53:1558–1563, 1984.

102. Meffin PJ, Roberts EW, Winkle RA, et al: Role of concentration dependent plasma protein binding on disopyramide disposition. *J Pharmacol Kinet Bio Pharm* 7:29–46, 1979.

103. Mirowski, M: The automatic implantable cardioverter-defibrillator: an overview. *J Am Coll Cardiol* 6:461–466, 1985.

104. Morady F, DiCarlo LA Jr, deBuitleir MD, et al: Effects of incremental doses of procainamide on ventricular refractoriness, intraventricular conduction and induction of ventricular tachycardia. *Circulation* 74:135–164, 1986.

105. Moysey JO, Jaggarao NSV, Grundy EN, et al: Amiodarone increases plasma digoxin concentrations. *Br Med J* 282:272–274, 1981.

106. Nademanee K, Feld G, Hendrickson J, et al: Electrophysiologic and antiarrhythmic effects of sotalol in patients with life-threatening ventricular tachyarrhythmias. *Circulation* 72:555–564, 1985.

107. Nademanee K, Hendrickson J, Kannan R, Singh BN: Antiarrhythmic efficacy and electrophysiologic actions of amiodarone in patients with life-threatening ventricular arrhythmias: potent suppression of spontaneously occurring tachyarrhythmias versus inconsistent abolition of induced ventricular tachycardia. *Am Heart J* 103:950–959, 1982.

108. Nathan AW, Hellestrand KJ: Flecainide acetate: a review. *Clin Prog Pacing Electrophysiol* 2:43–53, 1984.

109. Nathan AW, Hellestrand KJ, Bexton RS, et al: Fatal ventricular tachycardia in association with propafenone, a new class IC antiarrhythmic agent. *Postgrad Med J* 60:155–156, 1984.

110. Nathan AW, Hellestrand KJ, Beston RS, et al: Proarrhythmic effects of the new antiarrhythmic agent flecainide acetate. *Am Heart J* 107:222–228, 1984.

111. Nattel S, Zeng F-D: Frequency-dependent effects of antiarrhythmic drugs on action potential duration and refractoriness of canine cardiac Purkinje fibers. *J Pharmacol Exp Ther* 229:283–291, 1984.

112. Nestico PF, Morganroth J, Horowitz LN, et al: Efficacy of oral and intravenous indecainide in ventricular arrhythmias. *Am J Cardiol* 59:1332–1336, 1987.

113. The Norwegian Multicenter Study Group: Timolol-induced reduction in mortality and reinfarction in patients surviving acute myocardial infarction. *N Engl J Med* 304:801–807, 1981.

114. Nygaard TW, Sellers TD, Cook TS, et al: Adverse reactions to antiarrhythmic drugs during therapy for ventricular arrhythmias. *JAMA* 256:55–58, 1986.

115. O'Brien KP, Taylor PM, Croxson RS: Prophylactic lidocaine in hospitalized patients with acute myocardial infarction. *Med J Aust* 2:536–537, 1973.

116. Olson DW, Thompson BM, Darin JC, et al: A randomized comparison study of bretylium tosylate and lidocaine in resuscitation of patients from out-of-hospital ventricular fibrillation in a paramedic system. *Ann Emerg Med* 13:807–810, 1984.

117. Podrid P, Lown B: Propafenone: a new agent for ventricular arrhythmia. *J Am Coll Cardiol* 4:117–125, 1984.

118. Podrid PJ, Morganroth J: Aggravation of arrhythmia during drug therapy: experience with flecainide acetate. *Pract Cardiol* 11:55–70, 1985.

119. Podrid PJ, Schoeneberger A, Lown B: Congestive heart failure caused by oral disopyramide. *N Engl J Med* 302:614–617, 1980.

120. Pratt CM, Yepsen SC, Taylor AA, et al: Ethmozine suppression of single and repetitive ventricular premature depolarizations during therapy: documentation of efficacy and long-term safety. *Am Heart J* 106:85–90, 1983.

121. Prystowsky EN, Klein GJ, Rinkenberger RL, et al: Clinical efficacy and electrophysiologic effects of encainide in patients with Wolff-Parkinson-White syndrome. *Circulation* 69:278–287, 1984.

122. Rae AP, Greenspan AM, Spielman SR, et al: Antiarrhythmic drug efficacy for ventricular tachyarrhythmias associated with coronary artery disease as assessed by electrophysiologic studies. *Am J Cardiol* 55:1494–1499, 1985.

123. Reiter MJ, Mann DE, Easley AR: New antiarrhythmic agents: Part VIII—antiarrhythmic properties of pirmenol. *Pract Cardiol* 11:129–147, 1985.

124. Reuter H: Ion channels in cardiac cell membranes. *Annu Rev Physiol* 46:473–484, 1984.

125. Roden DM, Dawson AK, Duff HJ, et al: Electrophysiology of O-demethyl encainide in a canine model of sustained ventricular tachycardia. *J Cardiovasc Pharmacol* 6:588–595, 1984.

126. Roden DM, Reele SB, Higgins SB, et al: Total suppression of ventricular arrhythmias by encainide: pharmacokinetic and electrocardiographic characteristics. *N Engl J Med* 302:877–882, 1980.

127. Roos JC, Paalman ACA, Duxning AJ: Electrophysiological effects of mexiletine in man. *Br Heart J* 38:1262–1271, 1976.

128. Rosen MR, Hoffman BF, Wit AL: Electrophysiology and pharmacology of cardiac arrhythmias. V. Cardiac antiarrhythmic effects of lidocaine. *Am Heart J* 89:52–56, 1975.

129. Routledge PA, Stargel WW, Barchowsky A, et al: Control of lidocaine therapy: new perspectives. *Ther Drug Monit* 4:265–270, 1980.

130. Salerno DM, Granrud G, Sharkey P, et al: A controlled trial of propafenone for treatment of frequent and repetitive ventricular premature complexes. *Am J Cardiol* 53:77–83, 1984.

131. Sanchez-Chapula J, Tsuda Y, Josephson IR: Voltage- and use-dependent effects of lidocaine on sodium current in rat single ventricular cells. *Circ Res* 52:557–565, 1983.

132. Siddoway LA, Roden DM, Woosley RL: Clinical pharmacology of propafenone: pharmacokinetics, metabolism and concentration-response relations. *Am J Cardiol* 54:9D–12D, 1984.

133. Singh BN, Nademanee K, Baky SH: Calcium antagonists. Clinical use in the treatment of arrhythmias. *Drugs* 25:125–153, 1983.

134. Sobol SM, Rakita L: Pneumonitis and pulmonary fibrosis associated with amiodarone treatment: a possible complication of a new antiarrhythmic drug. *Circulation* 65::819–824, 1982.

135. Sperelakis N: Electrical properties of cells at rest and maintenance of the ion distributions. In Sperelakis N (ed): *Physiology and Pathology of the Heart.* Boston, Martinus Nijhoff, 1984, pp 59–82.

136. Stein J, Podrid P, Lown B: Effects of oral mexiletine on left and right ventricular function. *Am J Cardiol* 54:575–578, 1984.

137. Stone PH, Antman EM, Muller JE, et al: Calcium channel blocking agents in the treatment of cardiovascular disorders. Part II: Hemodynamic effects and clinical applications. *Ann Intern Med* 93:886–904, 1980.

138. Sung RJ, Elser B, McAlister RG: Intravenous verapamil for termination of re-entrant supraventricular tachycardias. *Ann Intern Med* 93:682–689, 1980.

139. Tucker CR, Winkle RA, Peters FA, et al: Acute hemodynamic effects of intravenous encainide in patients with heart disease. *Am Heart J* 104:209–215, 1982.

140. Valentine PA, Frew JL, Mashford MC, et al: Lidocaine in the prevention of sudden death in the pre-hospital phase of acute infarctions. *N Engl J Med* 291:1327–1331, 1974.

141. Vaughn-Williams EM: A classification of antiarrhythmic actions reassessed after a decade of new drugs. *J Clin Pharmacol* 24:129–147, 1984.

142. Velebit V, Podrid P, Lown L, et al: Aggravation and provocation of ventricular arrhythmias by antiarrhythmic drugs. *Circulation* 65:886–894, 1982.

143. Wang T, Roden DM, Wolfenden HT, et al: Influence of genetic polymorphism on the metabolism and disposition of encainide in man. *J Pharmacol Exp Ther* 228:605–611, 1984.

144. Waspe LE, Waxman HL, Buxton AE, et al: Mexiletine for control of drug-resistant ventricular tachycardia: clinical and electrophysiologic results in 44 patients. *Am J Cardiol* 51:1175–1181, 1983.

145. Waxman HL, Groh WC, Marchlinski FE, et al: Amiodarone for control of sustained ventricular tachyarrhythmia: clinical and electrophysiologic effects in 51 patients. *Am J Cardiol* 50:1066–1074, 1982.

146. Webb CR, Morganroth J, Senior S, et al: Flecainide: steady state electrophysiologic effects in patients with remote myocardial infarction and inducible sustained ventricular arrhythmia. *J Am Coll Cardiol* 8:214–220, 1986.

147. Winkle RA, Mason JW, Griffin JC, et al: Malignant ventricular tachyarrhythmias associated with the use of encainide. *Am Heart J* 102:857–864, 1981.

148. Winkle RA, Peters F, Kates RE, et al: Clinical pharmacology and antiarrhythmic efficacy of encainide in patients with chronic ventricular arrhythmias. *Circulation* 64:290–296, 1981.

149. Winkle RA, Peters F, Kates RE, Harrison DC: Possible contribution of encainide to the long-term antiarrhythmic efficacy of encainide. *Am J Cardiol* 51:1182–1188, 1985.

150. Woosley RL, Drayer DE, Reidenberg MM, et al: Effect of acetylator phenotype on the rate at which procainamide induces antinuclear antibodies and the lupus syndrome. *N Engl J Med* 298:1157–1159, 1978.

151. Woosley RL, Echt DS, Roden DM: Effects of congestive heart failure on the pharmacokinetics and pharmacodynamics of antiarrhythmic agents. *Am J Cardiol* 56:25B–33B, 1986.

152. Zachary CB, Slater DN, Holt DW: The pathogenesis of amiodarone-induced pigmentation and photosensitivity. *Br J Dermatol* 110:451–456, 1984.

153. Zipes DP: Genesis of cardiac arrhythmias: electrophysiologic considerations. In Braunwald E (ed): *Heart Disease: A Textbook of Cardiovascular Medicine*, ed 2. Philadelphia, WB Saunders, pp 605–647.

22

Digitalis Pharmacodynamics: Considerations in Critical Illness

Paul M. Heerdt, M.D., Ph.D.

Although relatively toxic, the sugar-steroid complexes extracted from such plants as *Digitalis purpurea, Digitalis lanata,* and *Strophanthus gratus* (known generically as "digitalis") remain widely used to slow transmission of cardiac impulses through the atrioventricular (AV) node when atrial contractions are aberrant or abnormally rapid, and to enhance the contractility of failing myocardium (10). Since the time of ancient Egyptians, however, plant extracts containing cardiac glycosides have been used as everything from emetics and diuretics to rat poison (27).

Structurally, the cardiac glycosides are composed of a steroid moiety (a cyclopentanoperhydrophenanthrene nucleus with an unsaturated lactone ring attached to the C-17 position), with one to four sugar molecules bound to the C-3 position. In general, the sugar moiety dictates kinetic properties and potency of the drug, and the steroid (or aglycone) component contributes pharmacologic activity, with a double bond at the C-14 position of the lactone ring an essential feature.

By far the most commonly used digitalis compound is digoxin. Derived from the leaves of *Digitalis lanata,* digoxin may be given orally or intravenously, has a relatively long duration of action (plasma half-life of 36–48 hours), and can be readily assayed in the serum.

Until recently, the long history of digitalis therapeutics provided little insight into the precise mode or site of action. In 1785 William Withering published his book "An Account of The Foxglove and Some of its Medicinal Uses: with Practical Remarks on Dropsy and Other Diseases" (58), and although he noted that the heart was influenced by the drug, he did not regard it as the primary site of action. In 1799 John Ferriar (12) suggested that therapeutic effects of digitalis resulted from the drug's action on the heart. It was not until Wiggers

and Stimson (57) found an effect on ventricular contractile force in 1927, however, that digitalis was suggested to have a beneficial property other than slowing heart rate.

The cardiovascular response to digitalis reflects both direct and indirect actions and is profoundly influenced by cardiac disease and basal sympathetic nervous tone. There is substantial evidence to suggest that *direct* cellular actions of digitalis result from inhibition of sodium, potassium–activated adenosine triphosphatase (Na K-ATPase) (2, 49). In contrast, the ability of digitalis to stimulate autonomic nervous activity accounts for the vast majority of *indirect* actions.

INOTROPIC AND VASCULAR EFFECTS

Cardiac glycosides are employed in the treatment of congestive heart failure because of their ability to shift the ventricular function curve upward and to the left. The intact heart, therefore, is capable of producing more stroke work at any given filling pressure. Studies on isolated cardiac muscle under isometric conditions have demonstrated that at any given muscle length, digitalis increases the rate of force development as well as the peak force achieved and also accelerates muscle relaxation. The inotropic response to digitalis is influenced greatly by the initial state of the myocardium. In isolated tissue preparations under isometric and isotonic conditions, as well as in intact animals, depressed myocardium responds more vigorously than normal muscle to digitalis (27).

In all probability, digitalis-positive inotropism results from inhibition of Na K-ATPase, biochemical correlate of the "sodium pump" (30, 49). This magnesium-dependent sarcolemmal enzyme supplies energy for the exchange of three intracellular sodium ions for two extracellular potassium ions. Since the ion exchange is not stoichiometrically balanced, the interior of the cell becomes negatively charged with respect to the extracellular environment and the pump is said to be "electrogenic" (23). The moderate degree of sodium pump inhibition produced by therapeutic levels of digitalis leads to an accumulation of intracellular sodium. There is general agreement that increased intracellular sodium leads to accumulation of intracellular calcium, which is responsible for enhanced myocardial contractility (23, 30). However, whether increased intracellular calcium results from augmented exchange of intracellular sodium for extracellular calcium or from reduced calcium egress from the cell remains controversial (4).

Digitalis administration to healthy subjects increases systemic vascular resistance, which acts to oppose the positive inotropism of the drug (6, 46, 56). As a consequence, cardiac output tends to fall or remain unchanged. Conversely, when cardiac glycosides are administered during congestive heart failure, vasodilation results, which tends to augment direct inotropy. Clearly these findings exemplify the contribution of basal sympathetic tone to the therapeutic actions of digitalis. When "tone" is high (as during heart failure) increased cardiac output brought about by digitalis leads to a withdrawal of vascular tone, which counterbalances direct vasoconstriction by the drug and vasodilation occurs (27).

Digitalis causes constriction of isolated arteries (42), and studies in humans and animals have demonstrated a rise in arterial pressure following digitalis administration (40, 48). Specific investigations on regional systemic and pulmonary circulations have further demonstrated the vasoconstrictor actions of digitalis (26, 41). In critically ill patients, vascular actions of digitalis are worthy of consideration. Vasoconstriction of coronary, mesenteric, and renal circulations in response to digoxin infusion has been reported (26, 56), as has potentiation of the pressor actions of norepinephrine and angiotensin (20).

Early investigation suggested that digitalis causes vasoconstriction via a direct action on vascular smooth muscle. More recent findings, however, have indicated that activation of the sympathetic nervous system is responsible for digitalis-induced constriction of some vascular beds (17).

Three mechanisms have been proposed to explain *direct vasoconstriction* and all involve inhibition of vascular Na K-ATPase (34):

1. Release of catecholamines from sites within the vasculature secondary to sodium pump inhibition.
2. Partial depolarization of vascular smooth muscle cells secondary to sodium pump inhibition.
3. An increase in intracellular sodium, which leads to an accelerated rate of exchange of intracellular sodium for extracellular calcium and an accentuation of vascular tone.

Many data have accumulated to demonstrate that stimulation and/or facilitation of the sympathetic nervous system contributes to *indirect* digitalis-induced vasoconstriction. The sympathetic contribution to constriction seems to vary with the circulation studied. In normal, conscious dogs, digitalis causes vasoconstriction via a direct action in the renal, mesenteric, external iliac, and carotid beds (25, 26, 55). In contrast, other studies have demonstrated a sympathetically mediated vasoconstriction in skeletal muscle and the pulmonary circulation (14, 40). Early reports suggested that coronary vasoconstriction in response to digitalis was locally mediated (56). More recent studies, however, have showed an antagonism of the event by α-adrenergic and ganglionic blockade in both normal and ischemic hearts, and neurogenic coronary vasoconstriction in response to intracerebroventricular digitalis (15, 22, 47).

The specific manner in which cardiac glycosides influence sympathetic tone remains unclear. The subject has been recently reviewed (17). A number of investigators have observed that electrical stimulation of discrete areas within the brain causes cardiovascular alterations similar to those seen during digitalis toxicity. Intravenous injection of digitalis increases preganglionic nerve transmission, and administration directly into the cerebral ventricles or hypothalamus produces systemic hypertension and arrhythmias, which can be prevented by α-adrenergic blockade or spinal transection. Somberg and Smith (51) employed discrete brain lesions to localize the site of digitalis arrhythmogenesis to a small area of the medulla outside the blood-brain barrier, probably in the area postrema.

At a molecular level, digitalis has been suggested to influence central catecholaminergic, cholinergic, dopaminergic, and serotoninergic systems. None of the studies has provided definite conclusions, and in all probability a variety of neurotransmitter systems are involved (17).

In peripheral nervous tissue, digitalis sensitizes ganglia to chemical and electrical stimulation, and there are indications that glycosides may stimulate ganglia directly, thus initiating postganglionic events. Additional data demonstrate a facilitation of postganglionic nervous transmission by recruitment of nerve fibers and enhancement of nerve excitability.

At the sympathetic nerve terminal, digitalis-induced alterations in catecholamine synthesis, degradation, release, and uptake have been described (17). Digitalis has been theorized to increase the tissue concentration of norepinephrine, although clear evidence for this theory is lacking. It logically follows that an elevation in catecholamine content could arise from increased synthesis or reduced degradation. Goldstein and associates (18) applied digitalis directly to areas of the brain and found an initial increase followed by a decrease in norepinephrine synthesis. This response was independent of any alteration in tyrosine hydroxylase activity. Other studies have indicated that the cardiac glycosides may increase norepinephrine content in nerve terminals by inhibiting monoamine oxidase (38). Digitalis also influences catecholamine release via facilitation or direct stimulation of terminals in the heart, spleen, adrenal glands, and blood vessels.

A number of investigators have observed a potentiation of norepinephrine-induced vasoconstriction by digitalis, and this effect has been attributed to an inhibition of catecholamine reuptake (53). Further studies examining the uptake of [^{3}H]norepinephrine into slices of heart and spleen have suggested that digitalis inhibition of uptake may be a consequence of Na K-ATPase inhibition (53).

CARDIAC ELECTRICAL ACTIVITY

In the critical care setting, digitalis is frequently used to slow conduction of atrial impulses to the ventricles through the AV node (10). During atrial tachydysrhythmias, slowed AV conduction can prevent ventricular tachycardia. At therapeutic concentrations, the predominant electrical effects of digitalis are due to increased parasympathetic input to the heart as well as enhanced sensitivity of sinoatrial (SA) and AV node tissue to acetylcholine and reduced sensitivity to norepinephrine (44).

Cardiac glycosides stimulate or facilitate vagal activity at central nuclei and the nodose ganglion, at peripheral autonomic ganglia, and in vagal efferents (17). Additionally, there is evidence to suggest that digitalis sensitizes baroreceptors to produce a greater increase in vagal tone for a given elevation in pressure (11, 54) and is capable of directly stimulating cardiac receptors involved with the bradycardic Bezold-Jarisch reflex.

Arrhythmogenicity

Although nausea is the most common side effect of digitalis treatment, the most serious is the development of cardiac arrhythmias. Digitalis cardiotoxicity has been widely investigated and the literature well reviewed (1, 50). The diagnosis of digitalis toxicity is a clinical one and should not be based entirely on elevated digoxin levels or ECG alterations (3). Factors frequently encountered in the critical care setting, such as old age, myocardial ischemia or acute infarction, hypokalemia, hypomagnesemia, renal insufficiency, hepatic dysfunction, carotid sinus massage, electrical cardioversion, hypothyroidism, and concomitant quinidine therapy, all have been shown to influence digitalis kinetics or dynamics in such a way as to enhance cardiotoxicity. Mechanistically, digitalis arrhythmogenesis can also be regarded as having two components: (a) a direct effect on cardiac tissue secondary, perhaps, to excessive inhibition of the sodium pump and overaccumulation of intracellular calcium, and (b) an indirect component due to activation of the sympathetic nervous system. Both components serve to enhance the automaticity and excitability of cardiac tissue.

DIRECT CARDIOTOXICITY

As discussed above, beneficial electrophysiologic effects of digitalis at therapeutic levels stem primarily from increased vagal activity. When toxic concentrations of cardiac glycoside are achieved, however, the predominant electrophysiologic effects are secondary to direct cellular actions. Hypokalemia enhances the effect of digitalis on the sodium pump and thus serves to potentiate the direct component of cardiotoxicity.

In the SA and AV nodes, toxic digitalis concentrations directly magnify the indirect vagotonic properties of the drug. Hypopolarization of SA nodal tissue can eventually lead to cessation of impulse generation. AV nodal tissue displays a decrease in the maximal diastolic potential and the rate of rise and amplitude of action potentials. These alterations translate into a decrease in nodal conduction velocity (already depressed by increased vagal tone) and an increase in effective refractory period. Digitalis toxicity at the AV node, therefore, is manifest as varying degrees of conduction blockade.

In Purkinje fibers, digitalis is capable of directly producing arrhythmias by two mechanisms: an increase in the slope of phase 4 depolarization (and thus increased automaticity) and the development of delayed afterdepolarizations. In contrast to nodal tissue, Purkinje fibers have scant parasympathetic innervation and increased vagal tone has little influence to accentuate or ameliorate arrhythmia development. Purkinje fibers are, however, extremely responsive to norepinephrine, and enhanced sympathetic activity secondary to neural stimulation by digitalis may serve to accentuate ventricular ectopy (17).

Ventricular muscle fibers are less sensitive to direct digitalis toxicity than Purkinje fibers. Although the muscle fibers may develop afterdepolarizations at high drug concentrations (from overaccumulation of calcium), they are not subject to alterations in the slope of phase 4 (13). Since ventricular muscle comprises the major portion of cardiac mass, changes in ventricular electrical activity account for many of the ECG alterations produced by digitalis (27).

In contrast to other cardiac tissues, atrial fibers (both specialized and nonspecialized) are influenced oppositely by the therapeutic, indirect response to digitalis and the toxic, direct effects. Enhanced vagal tone to the atria increases membrane resting potential, reduces phase 4 of specialized fibers, shortens action potential duration, and reduces the effective refractory period. In contrast, digitalis acts directly to decrease resting membrane potential (hypopolarize the cell) and increase action potential duration (28). Toxic levels of digitalis also facilitate the development of afterdepolarizations in the specialized atrial fibers, thus contributing to the genesis of premature atrial contractions.

INDIRECT CARDIOTOXICITY

As noted above, digitalis stimulates the sympathetic nervous system at central, preganglionic, ganglionic, and postganglionic sites.

Considerable evidence demonstrates that this stimulation is a major contributor to arrhythmogenesis. Both surgical and chemical interruption of sympathetic influences on the heart increase cardiac resistance to the arrhythmogenic actions of intravenous cardiac glycosides, and arrhythmias can be produced when digitalis is injected directly into the cerebral ventricles, thus suggesting that sympathetic stimulation at central sites is an important feature.

Investigation has also revealed that activation of the sympathetic nervous system either chemically or behaviorally lowers the arrhythmogenic dose of ouabain (7, 43). These findings serve to underscore the sympathetic component of digitalis arrhythmogenesis and have clinical implications for the prevention of cardiac glycoside cardiotoxicity in critically ill patients with increased sympathetic "tone."

At a cellular level, enhanced adrenergic input to the heart serves to increase the slope of phase 4 depolarization and enhance automaticity in nodal, atrial, and ventricular tissue. At toxic doses, digitalis has a similar direct effect on Purkinje fibers and thus the two components may work in concert (1).

Electrocardiographic Changes

The multiple influences of digitalis on cardiac muscle and conducting system electrophysiology are manifest, in part, as alterations in the ECG. At nontoxic doses, relatively consistent changes include lengthening of the P-R interval, ST segment depression and shortening (often described as "sagging"), and reduction of T wave amplitude. In the His-Purkinje system at least, these changes appear to reflect changes in the duration and slope of phases 2 and 3 of the action potential (1). Less frequently, U waves appear, and symmetric T wave inversion similar to that seen during ischemia or pericarditis may occasionally occur. Electrocardiographic alterations, particularly ST segment changes, may become magnified by underlying myocardial disease, concomitant tachycardia, and high-amplitude QRS complexes.

CLINICAL USE OF DIGITALIS

Indications for digitalis therapy are outlined in Table 22.1. The drug is of established benefit

Table 22.1
Clinical Use of Digitalis

A. Indications
   1. Congestive heart failure from primary myocardial dysfunction or chronic hypertensive, coronary vascular, or valvular disease
   2. Supraventricular dysrhythmias: atrial flutter or fibrillation, paroxysmal atrial tachycardia
B. Little or no usefulness
   1. Mitral stenosis with sinus rhythm
   2. Obstructive cardiac tumors
   3. Cor pulmonale
   4. Myocardial hyperkinesis
   5. Acute myocarditis
   6. Constrictive pericarditis
C. Contraindications
   1. Suspected digitalis intoxication
   2. Idiopathic hypertrophic subaortic stenosis
   3. Heart block
   4. Severe hypokalemia

in the treatment of (a) congestive heart failure secondary to a variety of chronic processes, (b) atrial flutter or fibrillation with rapid ventricular response, and (c) recurrent paroxysmal atrial tachycardia. Digitalis therapy is of little or no benefit in the treatment of many other forms of cardiac disease (Table 22.1). The only absolute contraindication to digitalis administration is digitalis toxicity. Relative contraindications include idiopathic hypertrophic subaortic stenosis, heart block, and severe hypokalemia.

Dosing of digitalis compounds should be "titrated" to the patient's cardiovascular pathology, concomitant noncardiac disease, and age. In general, larger initial doses are required to slow ventricular response in supraventricular tachydysrhythmias than are needed in the treatment of congestive heart failure. Additionally, renal failure lowers the maintenance dose, and elderly patients tend to re-

quire less drug. Specific digitalis preparations and considerations for their use are outlined in Table 22.2. Digoxin is by far the most widely used preparation in the critical care setting.

The benefit of serum digoxin levels as a guide to therapeutic response is limited. There is a wide variability among patients in the serum concentration of drug required to achieve a desired response. Also, a number of other frequently used drugs raise serum digoxin levels. Quinidine, amiodarone, verapamil, diltiazem, spironolactone, triamterene, and indomethacin (preterm infants) have all been shown to increase serum digoxin levels (37). Furthermore, falsely elevated serum digoxin levels (either from an endogenous digitalis-like factor or altered biotransformation) have been reported in neonates and in the setting of hypertension, renal and hepatic disease, and pregnancy (16). Serum digoxin levels are of most benefit in assuring that the dose given is sufficient to achieve measurable blood concentrations and in confirming the clinical suspicion of overdose or toxicity.

When toxic drug levels are achieved, digitalis compounds are capable of producing virtually every ECG abnormality known. Relatively frequent disturbances include (a) atrial tachycardia with or without block, (b) AV conduction delay more pronounced than simple lengthening of the P-R interval, (c) AV dissociation, (d) junctional escape rhythms, and (e) ventricular dysrhythmias, particularly premature ventricular contractions.

Digitalis-induced arrhythmias may be life-threatening, particularly in critically ill patients with underlying multisystem disease. Initial intervention should include discontinuation of the drug; ECG monitoring, since arrhythmias may be intermittent or progressively malignant; and assessment of the patient for predisposing factors (e.g., hypokalemia, renal

Table 22.2
Digitalis Preparations, Dosages, and Pharmacokinetic Considerations

Compound	Average Digitalizing Dose (mg)		Onset of Action (min)	Peak Effect (hr)	Average Half-life (hr)	Major Metabolic Route
	Oral[a]	Intravenous[b]				
Ouabain	—	0.30–0.50	5–10	0.5–2	21	Renal; minor gastrointestinal
Digoxin	1.25–1.50	0.75–1.00	15–30	1.5–5	36–48	Renal; minor gastrointestinal
Digitoxin	0.70–1.20	1.00	25–120	4–12	96–144	Hepatic metabolism, renal excretion

[a]Three divided doses over 12–24 hours
[b]One-quarter to one-half maximal dose followed by small supplemental doses until desired response is achieved.

compromise). Administration of potassium chloride is often beneficial in the treatment of ventricular or supraventricular ectopy even if the patient is normokalemic. A solution of 60 mEq of potassium per liter in normal or half-normal saline infused through a large vein at the rate of 0.5 mEq/min may be used. Potassium may not be advantageous when the primary toxicity is a conduction disturbance since potassium has been shown to further depress conductivity. Diuretics should not be administered, nor glucose solutions without potassium. High-degree AV block and bradydysrhythmia may require temporary pacing. Supraventricular and ventricular tachydysrhythmias are frequently responsive to diphenylhydantoin or lidocaine, although additional therapy with propranolol, procainamide, or verapamil may be required. Direct current countershock should be avoided because of the potential for worsening arrhythmias. Hemodialysis is of no benefit for drug removal because of extensive tissue binding. Severe digoxin toxicity with malignant arrhythmias refractory to antiarrhythmic agents and producing hemodynamic compromise may require administration of digoxin-specific F_{ab} fragments (Digibind, Burroughs Wellcome). This fragment of antidigoxin antibody binds serum digoxin, rendering it pharmacologically inactive. The fragment-digoxin complex is then renally excreted.

CONSIDERATIONS FOR THE INTENSIVE CARE SPECIALIST

Potassium, Calcium, and Magnesium Homeostasis

Hypokalemia predisposes to digitalis cardiotoxicity under both clinical and experimental conditions. Mechanistically, low potassium augments inhibition of Na K-ATPase and the development of afterdepolarizations (1). Administration of potassium chloride can effectively oppose early manifestations of digitalis cardiotoxicity, but should be done carefully since hyperkalemia may augment cardiac glycoside–induced slowing of AV nodal conduction velocity (32). Particular diligence should be paid to assessing potassium homeostatsis during the initiation of digitalis therapy in patients dependent on parenteral nutrition, as well as those who are receiving diuretic therapy or carbohydrate and insulin infusion (21).

Calcium influences both the therapeutic and direct toxic effects of digitalis and thus should be considered during both the initiation and maintenance of therapy. Inhibition of Na K-ATPase by the cardiac glycosides leads to an accumulation of intracellular calcium and enhanced inotropy. Not surprisingly, insensitivity to digitalis has been reported in the setting of hypocalcemia (8). Alternatively, overaccumulation of calcium predisposes to afterdepolarization development and cardiac ectopy. Hypercalcemia has been demonstrated to exacerbate virtually all forms of cardiotoxicity, a phenomenon that is opposed by calcium channel blockade (29).

Magnesium is required for the appropriate functioning of Na K-ATPase. The amount required, however, is miniscule and thus magnesium infusion will not readily overcome inhibition of the sodium pump (52). Clinical hypomagnesemia probably has minimal influence on the inotropic response to cardiac glycosides, but there is evidence that it nearly doubles the amount of digoxin required to acutely control ventricular rate in patients with atrial fibrillation (9). Animal studies have shown a reduction in the arrhythmogenic dose of digitalis during concomitant hypomagnesemia (33), and magnesium sulfate infusion has been effective in the treatment of various digitalis-induced arrhythmias including some resistant to lidocaine (32). As with replacement of potassium or calcium, magnesium should be administered judiciously since hypermagnesemia can produce AV block and slowing of intraventricular conduction.

Nontherapeutic Effects

A major limitation to digitalis use is an exceptionally low therapeutic index. Many side effects of digitalis are well appreciated and relatively common in outpatients, but particular diligence should be paid to assessing possible adverse effects in debilitated patients with multisystem disease.

Digoxin administration may potentially exacerbate myocardial ischemia by causing both increased oxygen demand and coronary vasoconstriction. Since digitalis compounds are expected to produce ST segment changes on the ECG, alterations due to ischemia may well be missed. There is also good evidence that ischemic myocardium is much more susceptible to cardiotoxicity (24, 31).

Although the effects of cardiac glycosides on pulmonary function are widely variant and difficult to interpret (17), cardiotoxicity is apparently increased in patients with pulmonary disease (19). Additionally, digoxin causes pulmonary vasoconstriction (41), which may worsen underlying pulmonary hypertension or shunting; and ouabain alters ion transport in respiratory surface epithelial cells and macromolecular glandular secretion from submucosal cells (39).

In the kidney, cardiac glycosides produce a diuresis by inhibition of intrarenal Na K-ATPase, and a natriuresis most probably by inhibition of sodium reabsorption in the distal nephron (5). As noted above, digitalis compounds can produce relatively intense renal vasoconstriction, an action that may be detrimental in patients with compromised renal perfusion.

Inhibition of Na K-ATPase increases smooth muscle tone in a variety of organ systems, the most evident of which is the gastrointestinal tract, with resultant diarrhea. Nausea is a common side effect of digitalis treatment, most probably a consequence of stimulation of the medullary vomiting center. Mesenteric vasoconstriction in response to digitalis has been well documented, appears to be potentiated by nonsteroidal antiinflammatory agents (45), and has been implicated in bowel ischemia (35).

Central nervous system manifestations of digitalis treatment are common and should be considered in debilitated patients who may be confused or disoriented. Nightmares, hallucinations, mania, and depression have also been reported. Visual symptoms are frequent, especially halos and yellow discoloration (xanthopsia), and appear to reflect stimulation of visual pathways by the glycoside (36).

Summary

Digitalis compounds have a limited but relatively well-defined place in critical care. Practioners caring for critically ill patients with multisystem disease should be aware of digitalis's low therapeutic index, ability to produce virtually any arrhythmia in the setting of cardiotoxicity, noncardiac effects, and pharmacologic interactions. These considerations will enhance the safety and efficacy of digitalis use.

References

1. Akera T, Brown BS: Cardiovascular toxicity of cardiotonic drugs and chemicals. In Van Stee EW (ed): *Cardiovascular Toxicology.* New York, Raven Press, 1982 pp 109–134.
2. Allen JC, Entman ML, Schwartz A: The nature of the transport ATPase-digitalis complex. VIII. The relationship between *in vivo* bound ^{3}H-ouabain-Na$^+$,K$^+$-ATPase complex and ouabain-induced positive inotropism. *J Pharmacol Exp Ther* 192:105–112, 1975.
3. Atlee JL: Drugs used for the treatment of cardiac dysrhythmias. In *Perioperative Cardiac Dysrhythmias: Mechanisms, Recognition, Management.* Chicago, Year Book, 1985, pp 272–322.
4. Barry WH, Hasin Y, Smith TW: Sodium pump inhibition, enhanced calcium influx via sodium-calcium exchange, and positive inotropic response in cultured heart cells. *Circ Res* 56(2):231–241, 1985.
5. Brady JM, Nechay BR: Maximal effects of ouabain on renal sodium reabsorption and ouabain-sensitive adenosine triphosphatase activity in the dog. *J Pharmacol Exp Ther* 190:346–357, 1974.
6. Braunwald E, Bloodwell RD, Goldberg LI, Morrow AG: Studies on digitalis. IV. Observations in man on the effects of digitalis preparations on the contractility of the non-failing heart and on total vascular resistance. *J Clin Invest* 40:52–59, 1961.
7. Cagin NA, Natelson BA: Cholinergic activation produces psychomatic digitalis toxicity. *J Pharmacol Exp Ther* 218:709–711, 1981
8. Chopra D, Janson R, Sawin CT: Insensitivity to digoxin associated with hypocalcemia. *N Engl J Med* 296:917, 1977.
9. DiCarli C, Sprouse G, LaRosa JC: Arrhythmias and conduction disturbances: serum magnesium levels in symptomatic atrial fibrillation and their relation to rhythm control by intravenous digoxin. *Am J Cardiol* 57:956–959, 1986.
10. Duca P, Brest AW: Indications, contraindications, and nonindications for digitalis therapy. *Cardiovasc Clin* 4:131–139, 1974.
11. Ferrari A, Gregorini L, Ferrari MC, Prete L, Mancia G: Digitalis and baroreceptor reflexes in man. *Circulation* 63:279–285, 1981.
12. Ferriar J: An Essay on the Medical Properties of the Digitalis Purpurea of Foxglove. London, Souler and Russel, 1799.
13. Ferrier, GR, Moe, GK: Effect of calcium on acetylstrophanthidin-induced depolarization in canine Purkinje tissue. *Circ Res* 33:508, 1973.
14. Garan H, Powers ER, Powell WJ Jr: Dependence of the neurogenic vascular resistance effect of digitalis on the background level of sympathetic activity in skeletal muscle. *Fed Proc* 33:584, 1974.
15. Garan H, Smith TW, Powell WJ Jr: The central nervous system as a site of action for coronary vasoconstrictor effect of digoxin. *J Clin Invest* 54:1365–1372, 1974.
16. Gault H, Vusdev S, Vlusses P, et al: Interpretation of serum digoxin levels in renal failure. *Clin Pharmacol Ther* 39:530–536, 1986.
17. Gillis RA, Quest JA: The role of the nervous system in the cardiovascular effects of digitalis. *Pharmacol Rev* 31:19–97, 1980.
18. Goldstein M, Ohi Y, Backstrom T: The effect of ouabain on catecholamine biosynthesis in rat brain cortex slices. *J Pharmacol Exp Ther* 174(1):77–82, 1970.
19. Green LH, Smith TW: The use of digitalis in patients with pulmonary disease. *Ann Intern Med* 87:459–465, 1977.
20. Guthrie GP: Effects of digoxin on responsiveness to the pressor actions of angiotensin and norepinephrine in man. *J Clin Endocrinol Metab* 58:76–80, 1984.
21. Hall RJ, Gellbart A, Silverman M, Goldman RH: Studies on digitalis-induced arrhythmias in glucose and insulin-induced hypokalemia. *J Pharmacol Exp Ther* 201:711, 1977.
22. Hamlin NP, Willerson JT, Garan H, Powell WJ Jr: The neurogenic vasoconstriction effect of digitalis on coro-

nary vascular resistance. *J Clin Invest* 53:288–296, 1974.

23. Hanson O: Interaction of cardiac glycosides with $(Na^+ + K^+)$-activated ATPase: a biochemical link to digitalis-induced inotropy. *Pharmacol Rev* 36:143–162, 1984.

24. Harriman RJ, Zeiler RH, Gough WB, El-Sherif N: Enhancement of triggered activity in ischemic Purkinje fibers by ouabain: a mechanism of increased susceptibility to digitalis toxicity in myocardial infarction. *J Am Coll Cardiol* 5:672–679, 1985.

25. Harrison LA, Blasche J, Phillips RS, Price WE, Cotten M De V, Jacobson ED: Effects of ouabain on the splanchnic circulation. *J Pharmacol Exp Ther* 169:321–327, 1969.

26. Higgins CB, Vatner SF, Braunwald E: Regional hemodynamic effects of a digitalis glycoside in the conscious dog with and without experimental heart failure. *Circ Res* 30:406–417, 1972.

27. Hoffman BF, Bigger T Jr: Digitalis and allied cardiac glycosides. In Gilman AG, Goodman LS, Rall TW, Murad F (eds): *The Pharmacological Basis of Therapeutics.* ed 7. New York, Macmillan, 1985, pp 716–747.

28. Hordorf AJ, Spotnitz A, Mary-Labuse L, Edu RN, Rosen MR: The cellular electrophysiologic effects of digitalis on human atrial fibers. *Circulation* 57:223–229, 1978.

29. Jonkman FAM, Boddeke HWGM, van Zweiten PA: Protective activity of calcium entry blockers against ouabain intoxication in anesthetized guinea pigs. *J Cardiovasc Pharmacol* 8:1009–1013, 1986.

30. Kazazoglou, T, Renaud J, Rossi B, Lazdunski M: Two classes of ouabain receptors in chick ventricular cardiac cells and their relation to (Na^+,K^+)-ATPase inhibition, intracellular Na^+ accumulation, Ca^{2+} influx, and cardiotonic effect. *J Biol Chem* 258:12163–12170, 1983.

31. Kim DH, Akera T, Kennedy RH: Ischemia-induced enhancement of digitalis sensitivity in isolated guinea pig heart. *J Pharmacol Exp Ther* 226:335–342, 1983.

32. Kleeman K, Singh BN: Serum electrolytes and the heart. In Maxwell, MH, Kleeman CR (eds): *Clinical Disorders of Fluid and Electrolyte Metabolism.* New York, McGraw-Hill, 1980, pp 169–173.

33. Kleiger RE, Katsutaka S: Effects of chronic depletion of potassium and magnesium on the action of acetylstrophanthidin. *Am J Cardiol* 17:520, 1966.

34. Lang S, Blaustein MP: The role of the sodium pump in the control of vascular tone in the rat. *Circ Res* 46:463–470, 1980.

35. Levinsky RA, Lewis RM, Bynum TE, Hanley HG: Digoxin induced intestinal vasoconstriction. *Circulation* 52:130–136, 1975.

36. Longhurst JC: Extracardiac and coronary vascular effects of digitalis. *J Am Coll Cardiol* 5:99A–105A, 1985.

37. Lorenz RR, Powers DA, Vanhoutte PM, Shepard JT: The effects of acetylstrophanthidin and ouabain on the sympathetic adrenergic neuroeffector junction in canine vascular smooth muscle. *Circ Res* 47(6):845–854, 1980.

38. Marcus FI: Pharmacokinetic interaction between digoxin and other drugs. *J Am Coll Cardiol* 5:82A–90A, 1985.

39. Marin M: Pharmacology of airway secretion. *Pharmacol Rev* 38:273–289, 1984.

40. Mason DT, Braunwald E: Studies on digitalis. X. Effects of ouabain on forearm vascular resistance and venous tone in normal subjects and patients in heart failure. *J Clin Invest* 43:532–543, 1964.

41. Mecca TE, Elam JT, Caldwell RW: Mechanism of the pulmonary vasoconstrictor action of digoxin in the dog. *J Cardiovasc Pharmacol* 7:833–840, 1985.

42. Mikkelson E: Effects of digoxin on isolated human pulmonary vessels. *Acta Pharmacol Toxicol* 45:139–144, 1979.

43. Morrow DH: Anesthesia and digitalis toxicity. IV. Relationship of digitalis tolerance to catecholamines during cyclopropane or halothane anesthesia. *Anesth Analg* 46:675–681, 1967.

44. Nadeau RA, Amir-Jahad AK, Gauther P, Porlier GA: Effects of cardiac glycosides injected into the atrioventricular node artery of the dog. *Can J Physiol Pharmacol* 49:113–126, 1971.

45. Nies AS, Gerber JG: Non-steroidal anti-inflammatory drugs potentiate the vasoconstrictor effects of ouabain in the dog. *Circ Res* 48(6):844–849, 1981.

46. Ross J Jr, Braunwald E, Waldhausen JA: Studies on digitalis. II. Extracardiac effects on venous return and on capacity of the peripheral vascular bed. *J Clin Invest* 39:937–942, 1960.

47. Sagar KB, Horson EC, Powell WJ Jr: Neurogenic coronary vasoconstrictor effects of digitalis during acute global ischemia. *Am J Cardiol* 39:261, 1977.

48. Schinz A, Schnelle K, Klein G, Blomer H: Time sequence of direct vascular and inotropic effects following intravenous administration of digoxin in normal man. *Int J Clin Pharmacol* 15(4): 189–193, 1977.

49. Schwartz A, Lindenmayer GE, Allen JC: The sodium-potassium adenosine triphosphatase: pharmacological, physiological and biochemical aspects. *Pharmacol Rev* 27:1–134, 1975.

50. Smith TW, Autman EM, Freidman PL, et al: Digitalis glycosides: mechanisms and manifestations of toxicity. Parts I, II, and III. *Prog Cardiovasc Dis* 26:413, 495; 27:21, 1984.

51. Somberg JC, Smith TW: Localization of the neurally mediated arrhythmogenic properties of digitalis. *Science* 204:321–323, 1979.

52. Specter MJ, Schweizer E, Goldman RH: Studies on magnesium's mechanism of action in digitalis-induced arrhythmias. *Circulation* 52:1001, 1975.

53. Stickney JL: Differential species sensitivity to the inhibitory effect of cardiac glycosides on ^3H-noradrenalin accumulation by tissue slices. *Arch Int Pharmacodyn* 224:215–229, 1976.

54. Thames MD: Acetylstrophanthidin-induced reflex inhibition of canine renal sympathetic nerve activity mediated by cardiac receptors with vagal afferents. *Circ Res* 44:8–15, 1979.

55. Treat E, Ulano HB, Jacobson ED: Effects of intra-arterial ouabain on mesenteric and carotid hemodynamics. *J Pharmacol Exp Ther* 179:144–148, 1971.

56. Vatner SF, Higgins CB, Franklin D, Braunwald E: Effects of a digitalis glycoside on coronary and systemic hemodynamics in conscious dogs. *Circ Res* 28:470–479, 1971.

57. Wiggers CJ, Stimson B: Studies on cardiodynamic action of drugs. III. The mechanism of cardiac stimulation by digitalis and g-strophanthidin. *J Pharmacol Exp Ther* 30:251–269, 1927.

58. Withering W: *An Account of the Foxglove and Some of Its Medicinal Uses: with Practical Remarks on Dropsy and Other Diseases.* London, CGJ and J Robinson, 1785. Reprinted in *Medical Classics* 2:305–443, 1937.

23

Bronchodilators

Marissa Seligman, Pharm.D.

The use of drugs with potent bronchodilator action has proven to be highly effective therapy for the treatment of reversible airway obstruction. In bronchospastic patients, bronchodilator therapy may reverse hypoxia and normalize acid-base abnormalities, thereby helping to improve tissue perfusion and oxygenation. Additionally, these drugs may be used prophylactically to prevent the development of bronchospasm.

Effective use of bronchodilators requires a knowledge of the basic pathophysiology responsible for airway obstruction and the effect of drugs on airway caliber. Clinicians should also employ a systematic approach to the use of the various bronchodilators in patients with reversible airway obstruction.

AIRWAY OBSTRUCTION

Airway caliber and tone are regulated by the parasympathetic and sympathetic divisions of the autonomic nervous system (4, 44). The vagally mediated mechanisms of the parasympathetic nervous system are the primary determinants of bronchomotor tone and bronchial submucosal gland secretion (4, 12, 44). On stimulation of vagal efferent nerves, the neurotransmitter acetylcholine is released from the presynaptic nerve terminal. The acetylcholine then diffuses through the synaptic cleft and binds to muscarinic cholinergic receptors found on postsynaptic tissue cell membranes throughout the respiratory tree. Stimulation of the cholinergic receptors results in an increase in intracellular levels of cyclic guanosine monophosphate (cGMP) in the cytoplasm, thereby increasing the activity of the effector mechanism (44). Acetylcholine receptors are located in or adjacent to the respiratory epithelium, submucosal glands, mast cells, and airway smooth muscle (4, 12, 44). The highest number of receptors is found within the trachea and large bronchi (52). Stimulation of the acetylcholine receptors in the lung causes bronchoconstriction, decreased airway caliber, mast cell degranulation, and increased glandular secretion.

Direct sympathetic nervous system innervation of the respiratory tree is sparse (52). Nevertheless, bronchial smooth muscle cells, especially those located in the smaller airways (52), are well-populated with β_2-adrenergic receptors. β_1-Adrenergic receptors are also found in the lung, but have only a minimal role in lung physiology (27). β_2-adrenergic receptors are stimulated by adrenergic agonists, either endogenous (the presynaptic neurotransmitter norepinephrine, or epinephrine released by the adrenal medulla) or exogenous (drugs). This stimulation results in activation of membrane-bound adenylate cyclase to catalyze the conversion of adenosine triphosphate to cyclic adenosine monophosphate (cAMP) (26). A cascade of enzymatic reactions then progresses, resulting in bronchodilation and possibly increased secretion of mucus (55).

α-Adrenergic receptors are also found in the lung (44). Postsynaptic α_1-receptors are located predominantly in the bronchial and vascular smooth muscle and submucosal glands. Stimulation of these receptors by α-adrenergic agonists such as norepinephrine activates phosphatidylinositol turnover in the cytoplasm (47). The resulting bronchial smooth muscle and submucosal gland tissue responses are bronchoconstriction and increased mucus secretion. In the lung, α_2-receptors are located on the postsynaptic nerve terminal, although they are also located presynaptically elsewhere in the body. Presynaptic α_2-receptors regulate the release of norepinephrine from the presynaptic nerve terminal (47).

To summarize, the primary autonomic innervation of bronchial smooth muscle and the respiratory epithelium is via the parasympathetic (cholinergic) nervous system. This system is excitatory to the lungs; its activation causes bronchial smooth muscle contraction and bronchial gland secretion. This tonic activity is opposed, albeit minimally, by the sympathetic (adrenergic) nervous system. Bronchodilation results from activation of the β_2-receptors of the sympathetic nervous system.

In addition to autonomic nervous system control of airway tone, respiratory tree caliber may be altered by a third neural innervation pathway, the so-called "purinergic" or "nonadrenergic noncholinergic (NANC) nervous system" (1, 4, 12, 52). Stimulation of this pathway produces bronchial smooth muscle contraction. The exact role of the NANC nervous system remains to be defined, but further investigation of this system might eventually lead to novel forms of treatment of airway diseases (45).

Various endogenous substances, e.g., histamine, prostaglandins, and the leukotrienes (the slow-reacting substance of anaphylaxis) also have documented effects on smooth muscle tone (1).

Nonneurogenic factors may alter airway caliber by affecting either airway anatomy or physiology. The most common causes of increased airway resistance are asthma (acute or chronic), emphysema, chronic bronchitis, and cystic fibrosis. Mechanical factors, e.g., tumors, mucous plugging, and foreign bodies, are also frequent causes of airway obstruction (1). Less commonly, airway obstruction develops from inhalation of toxic materials and resultant airway injury, drug-induced bronchoconstriction, infectious bronchitis, or bronchiolitis (1). Acute left ventricular failure may infrequently present as airway obstruction, as can pulmonary emboli. When airway obstruction occurs as a result of immunologic disorders (e.g., collagen-vascular disorders, dust sensitivity) or aspiration, bronchoconstriction is often not involved (1). Accordingly, drug-induced bronchodilation may not reverse the resistance to airflow associated with these conditions.

Clinically, patients with airflow obstruction usually manifest tachypnea, labored respiration with accessory muscle use, pulsus paradoxus, thoracic overinflation, and ventilation-perfusion mismatching (1). Auscultation of the airways commonly demonstrates rales and prolongation of the expiratory phase. Wheezing is a prominent sign but may be absent if airway obstruction is so severe that a wheeze cannot be generated (1). Most patients with airway obstruction demonstrate abnormalities in peak expiratory flow measurements and spirometry. For example, if presenting with an forced expiratory volume in 1 second (FEV-1) of less than 800 ml or a peak expiratory flow rate of less than 100 ml/min, the patient should usually receive aggressive pharmacotherapy (1).

Critically ill patients who are mechanically ventilated may experience airflow obstruction due to abnormalities in lung compliance, thoracic deflation, laryngeal spasm, laryngeal edema, epiglottitis, blunt laryngeal trauma, and tracheal avulsion (1). Thus, when assessing these patients, care should be taken in evaluating artificial airway position and upper airway function.

CLASSIFICATION OF BRONCHODILATOR DRUGS

The classification system used to group bronchodilator drugs is based on their mechanism of action:

a. Direct respiratory smooth muscle relaxants: theophylline and related salts
b. β-Adrenergic agonists: isoetharine, isoproterenol, epinephrine, metaproterenol, albuterol, terbutaline, bitolterol
c. Anticholinergics: atropine, glycopyrrolate, ipratropium

Their sites of action are depicted in Figure 23.1 (48).

Theophylline

Theophylline, a naturally occurring methylxanthine closely related to caffeine and found in tea, has been used to treat bronchospasm for more than 100 years (46). An enormous number of pharmacokinetic and pharmacodynamic data relative to this drug have been generated over the past 20 years. These findings have contributed to renewed interest in theophylline and the introduction of a wide variety of theophylline products into clinical use. Accordingly, theophylline has become one of the most extensively prescribed drugs for the treatment of reversible airway obstruction. In addition, the development of methods to monitor serum theophylline concentrations in patients has contributed to the safe and efficacious clinical use of this drug.

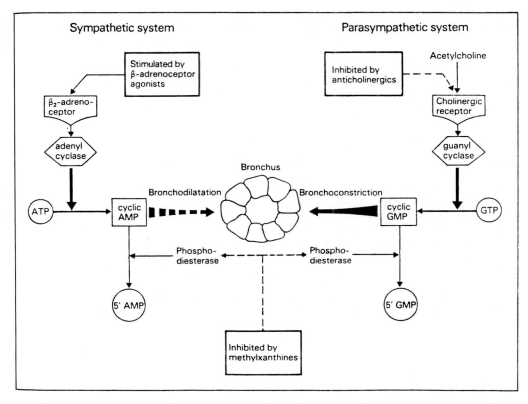

Figure 23.1. Mechanism of action of bronchodilator drugs (Originally published in Kelly HW: Controversies in asthma therapy with theophylline and the beta-2-adrenergic agents. *Clin Pharm* 3:386–395, 1984. Copyright © 1984, American Society of Hospital Pharmacists, Inc. All rights reserved. Reprinted with permission.)

PHARMACOLOGY

The exact mechanism by which theophylline exerts its pharmacologic effects is unclear (21). It is well established that theophylline competitively inhibits the activity of cytoplasmic phosphodiesterase, the enzyme that catalyzes the degradation of cAMP to 5′-AMP (56). This inhibition increases intracellular levels of cAMP, resulting in smooth muscle relaxation. However, this effect can only be demonstrated in vitro using very high concentrations of theophylline (5, 21). Additionally, unlike theophylline, other more potent phosphodiesterase inhibitors do not produce bronchodilation (21). Other postulated mechanisms of action include inhibition of intracellular calcium activity (18), prostaglandin inhibition (17), and increased binding of cAMP to cAMP-binding protein (6, 36). Recently, adenosine receptor antagonism has been proposed as the primary mediator of the pharmacologic and therapeutic actions of methylxanthines (16, 58).

Theophylline is a direct bronchial smooth muscle relaxant (13). If bronchospasm is not present, its effects on air flow and respiratory mechanics are minimal. The drug may also act by decreasing mucosal edema and reducing the production of excessive secretions (13). Other effects of theophylline include direct augmentation of myocardial inotropy and chronotropy (39); stimulation of diaphragmatic contractility (3, 38); dilation of the coronary, pulmonary, renal, and systemic arterioles and veins (2); diuresis (21, 32); stimulation of epinephrine and norepinephrine synthesis and release by the adrenal medulla (46); stimulation of the medullary respiratory center; relaxation of the smooth muscle of the gall bladder and gastrointestinal tract (32); stimulation of gastric acid secretion (18); and decreased cerebral blood flow (58).

SIDE EFFECTS

The most common side effects of theophylline include gastrointestinal effects that are both locally and centrally mediated (32). Frequently reported side effects include nausea, vomiting, and anorexia. Central nervous system effects include headache, irritability, restlessness, nervousness, dizziness, and seizures (5, 14). The incidence and severity of all of these adverse reactions usually decrease with reduction in the daily theophylline dosage (32). Unfortunately, mild side effects such as nausea and vomiting do not necessarily become manifest before serious life-threatening problems such as seizures develop (14, 15, 60). Additionally, theophylline-induced seizures are often unresponsive to standard anticonvulsive therapy, and the mortality rate associated with this problem has been estimated to be as high as 50% (5, 60). Theophylline may cause a number of cardiovascular side effects that are often poorly tolerated by critically ill patients. These effects include palpitations, sinus tachycardia, extrasystoles, and multifocal atrial tachycardia (5). Flushing, hypotension, circulatory collapse, and ventricular arrhythmias have also been reported.

Prior to 1983, the only parenteral form of theophylline was aminophylline. Aminophylline is theophylline compounded with ethylenediamine, which confers water solubility to the insoluble theophylline molecule. By weight, aminophylline is 80% theophylline (e.g., 100 mg of aminophylline is equivalent to 80 mg of theophylline). Interestingly, ethylenediamine contributes to both the efficacy and toxicity of theophylline. Ethylenediamine may augment the respiratory and cardiac stimulant effects of theophylline, but the significance of these effects is questionable (32). More importantly, it is well established that ethylenediamine can induce hypersensitivity reactions characterized by urticaria, generalized pruritus, angioedema, and bronchospasm (32). Recently, a premixed intravenous solution of theophylline in 5% dextrose in water was introduced into clinical use. Although adverse reactions to ethylenediamine occur rarely, theophylline therapy in critically ill patients can be simplified by use of these premixed theophylline solutions.

Because the rapid intravenous injection of aminophylline or theophylline may cause dizziness, palpitations, flushing, hypotension, and profound bradycardia, these drugs must be administered by slow intravenous injection or, preferably, by use of an infusion pump (13, 18). Cardiac arrest may also occur with the rapid administration of aminophylline. Intramuscular injections of theophylline salts are painful and the free drug is slowly and erratically absorbed from the site of administration. Therefore, this route of administration is not recommended (14, 32).

PHARMACOKINETICS

Theophylline is manufactured as a variety of salts for oral, rectal, and parenteral administration (in excess of 150 different products in the United States alone!) (14, 15, 18, 32, 60). Although rectal preparations of theophylline and its related salts are available, their absorption, especially from suppositories, into the systemic circulation is very erratic and unreliable. Use of the suppositories should be avoided in all patients (57). Fixed-dose combinations of theophylline with other drugs such as ephedrine should be avoided (9). The intravenous forms of theophylline are primarily limited to hospitalized patients, particularly those who are critically ill and unable to take oral medications.

The pharmacokinetics of theophylline have been well described (13, 18, 32, 35). Following oral administration, gastric acidity prompts the release of free theophylline from the theophylline salt or compound preparation. The rate of this release and the subsequent absorption of theophylline into the systemic circulation depends on the theophylline product used. For example, theophylline is rapidly absorbed from any of the many available oral solutions and uncoated tablet formulations. Peak serum levels are obtained 1–2 hours after administration. In contrast, extended-release and slow-release tablets are designed to release theophylline over a longer period of time (thereby decreasing the number of required drug doses per day); peak serum levels are usually reached 4 hours after administration. The actual rate of theophylline absorption from slow-release or extended-release formulations varies among formulations and routes of administration (e.g., oral route with or without food).

Theophylline distributes into a volume of distribution of 0.3–0.7 liters/kg in children and adults (14, 16, 32). In premature infants, the volume of distribution increases almost 2-fold. The drug is 56% bound to plasma proteins in children and adults and 36% in premature infants (18, 32, 35).

Hepatic metabolism of theophylline is the principal method of elimination. Eighty-eight to 92% of a theophylline dose is metabolized to three inactive metabolites; 1,3-dimethyluric acid, 1-methyluric acid, and 3-methylxanthine (32). In premature infants, a high percentage of theophylline is metabolized to caffeine. Theophylline and its metabolites are excreted from the body by the kidneys. Small amounts of unchanged theophylline may be excreted in the feces.

The metabolism of theophylline varies widely owing to differing rates of metabolism in different patient populations (18, 19, 32). In otherwise healthy, nonsmoking asthmatic adults, the elimination half-life averages between 7 and 9 hours; in children, between 1.5 and 9.5 hours; and in premature infants, between 15 and 58 hours (18, 32). Patients who are cigarette or marijuana smokers have a much shorter average elimination half-life of 4–5 hours (13). In contrast, patients with congestive heart failure, cor pulmonale, chronic obstructive pulmonary disease, or liver disease may have a markedly prolonged elimination half-life (14, 32).

Because theophylline has a low therapeutic ratio, the drug must be administered by careful dosage titration. Dosages should be calculated by use of lean body weight and consideration of underlying disease states and smoking history (Table 23.1) (14, 18). In addition, a variety of analytic techniques have been used to assess plasma or serum levels of theophylline and assist in reducing clinical toxicity (Table 23.2).

In isolated tracheal and bronchial smooth muscle preparations, theophylline induces bronchodilation in proportion to the log of the serum or plasma concentration over the range of 5–25 μg/ml (21, 37). Based on this relationship, a clinical "therapeutic range" for theophylline has been generated; the most frequently cited range is 10–20 μg/ml (14). Within this range, serious side effects of theophylline, including seizures, are reduced in incidence and severity, while efficacy is maintained. Most patients do not require levels in excess of 25 μg/ml to obtain adequate bronchodilation (35). This therapeutic range only represents the serum levels at which the majority of patients respond to theophylline; some patients respond outside this range. For example, bronchodilation can be produced at the lower end of the therapeutic range, i.e., serum concentrations of 2–10 μg/ml, in chronic asthmatic children (21). However, some patients may require levels in excess of 20 μg/ml (35). Marked interpatient and intrapatient variability exists for the dose-response curves for theophylline (5). Consequently, the ideal use of serum theophylline determinations is as an adjunct for titrating patient response and in determining

Table 23.1
Initial Intravenous Theophylline Maintenance Dosages[a]

Patient Population	Age	Theophylline Infusion Rate[b] (mg/kg/hr)
Neonates	Postnatal age up to 24 days	1 mg/kg q. 12 hours[c]
	Postnatal age above 24 days	1.5 mg/kg q. 12 hours[c]
Infants	6–52 weeks	0.008 × (age in weeks) + 0.21
Young children	1–9 yr	0.8
Older children	9–12 yr	0.7
Adolescents (smokers)	12–16 yr	0.7
Adolescents (nonsmokers)	12–16 yr	0.5[d]
Adults (healthy, smokers)	16–50 yr	0.7[d]
Adults (healthy, nonsmokers)	Above 16 years (including the elderly)	0.4[d]
Adults with cardiac decompensation, cor pulmonale, or liver dysfunction	Above 16 years	0.2[e]

[a]Originally published in Iafrate RP, Massey KL, Hendeles L: Current concepts in clinical therapeutics: asthma. *Clin Pharm* 5:206–227, 1986. Copyright © 1986, American Society of Hospital Pharmacists, Inc. All rights reserved. Reprinted with permission.
[b]Assumes an appropriate loading dose has been given. To achieve a target concentration of 10 μg/ml. Use lean body weight for obese patients. Although these doses are generally safe, many patients will require higher infusion rates as determined by serial serum measurements. These dosages differ from the current FDA recommendations, which include a higher infusion rate for the first 12 hours. Further dosage reductions may be required for patients receiving other drugs that decrease theophylline clearance.
[c]For a target concentration of 7.5 μg/ml (for neonatal apnea).
[d]Not to exceed 900 mg/day unless clinical symptoms and/or serum levels indicate the need for a larger dose.
[e]Not to exceed 400 mg/day unless clinical symptoms and/or serum levels indicate the need for a larger dose.

Table 23.2
Adverse Effects of Theophylline[a]

Serum Concentration	Symptoms	Frequency	Duration	Comments
5–20 μg/ml	Nausea, cramps, insomnia headache	Rare—if dose is slowly titrated over 1–2 weeks	Transient	
		Common—if therapeutic serum concentrations are rapidly attained	Transient	Avoided by dose titration
	Tremor	Rare—with concurrent administration of oral β_2-adrenergic	Unknown	Avoided if β_2-agonist is administered by inhalation
	Excessive gastric acid secretion	Rare		
15–35 μg/ml	Nausea, vomiting, diarrhea, stomach ache, headache, irritability, nervousness, insomnia, sinus tachycardia	Common—at serum concentrations >20 μg/ml	Persistent	Decrease dose
	Hyperglycemia	Rare—may occur in neonates	Persistent	
>35 μg/ml	Seizures, cerebral hypoxia, arrhythmias, cardiorespiratory arrest, death	Common	Persistent	Minor adverse effects often do not precede life-threatening toxicity

[a] Adapted from Hendeles L, Weinberger M: Theophylline: therapeutic use of serum concentration monitoring. In Taylor WJ, Finn AL (eds): *Individual Drug Therapy: Practical Applications of Drug Monitoring*. New York, Gross, Townsend, Frank, Hoffman, 1981, vol 1, pp 32–65. Used with permission of the publishers.

the optimal drug level and drug dosage that are necessary to achieve maximal bronchodilation.

DRUG INTERACTIONS

Theophylline clearance may be altered by a number of disease states and drugs (Table 23.3). Theophylline is reported to augment myocardial sensitivity to digitalis glycosides (32). In addition, theophylline may act synergistically with the β-adrenergic agonists to induce cardiac arrhythmias (21, 32).

CLINICAL USE

The primary role of theophylline is the prevention of bronchospasm in patients with either hyperactive airway disease or chronic obstructive pulmonary disorders (13, 18). For treatment of chronic bronchospasm in patients over 1 year of age, theophylline may be given initially at 16 mg/kg/day or 400 mg/day, whichever is less (14, 15). Depending on patient

response, the dose may be increased up to the following maximum daily doses (14, 15):

Age (yr)	Dosage (mg/kg/day)
1–9	24
9–12	20
12–16	18
>16	13, or 900 mg/day (whichever is less)

Note that in the prophylaxis of chronic bronchospasm, measurement of serum theophylline levels is usually necessary only (a) when these daily dosage recommendations are exceeded, (b) when drug toxicity is suspected, (c) when poor patient compliance to the prescribed regimen is suspected, or (d) to assess why a patient may not be responding to theophylline (e.g., rapid metabolism of the drug) (32, 35). Treatment should be started with an oral preparation of theophylline. The products that should be used are those with consistent 100% bioavailability: uncoated tablets, micro-

Table 23.3
Factors Affecting Theophylline Clearance[a]

Increase theophylline clearance	Decrease theophylline clearance
Smoking (cigarettes or marijuana)	Hepatic cirrhosis
Phenobarbital	Cor pulmonale
High protein/low carbohydrate diet	Congestive heart failure
Charcoal broiled diet	Propranolol
Phenytoin	Allopurinol ($>$600 mg/day)
Carbamazepine	Erythromycin
Rifampin	Cimetidine
	Troleandomycin
	Oral contraceptives

[a]Originally published in Iafrate RP, Massey KL, Hendeles: Current concepts in clinical therapeutics: asthma. *Clin Pharm* 5:206–227, 1986. Copyright © 1986, American Society of Hospital Pharmacists Inc. All rights reserved. Reprinted with permission.

crystalline dosage forms, or oral solutions. Once the patient's response has been demonstrated and dosages titrated, the daily drug dosage may then be converted to an equivalent amount of an extended-release theophylline product (56). For example, if a patient is taking theophylline oral tablets, 100 mg/4 hr, the total daily dose of 600 mg may be given as two 300-mg tablets of an extended-release product and manufacturer's recommendations followed as to the method of administration. Theophylline products should be chosen in accord with patient age and underlying disease state (37). At present a number of extended-release or slow-release theophylline products are available, each with different absorption profiles (18); not all clinicians consider these products to be interchangeable (18).

No theophylline product, oral or intravenous, should be used for the initial treatment of acute bronchospasm. Rather, only if repeated administration of inhaled β-adrenergic agonists, e.g., isoetharine or albuterol, produces a suboptimal effect should theophylline be administered (13, 18). Either intravenous or oral liquid theophylline can be used to treat acute bronchospasm; the former is more commonly used in critically ill patients (13, 14, 18).

Theophylline therapy in an acutely bronchospastic patient (assuming normal volume of distribution) can be initiated as follows (18). If the patient has not received any theophylline during the previous 24 hours, 5 mg/kg of theophylline should be administered as a loading dose over 30 minutes. If the patient has received theophylline within the past 24 hours, the loading dose should be reduced to 2.5 mg/kg. Subsequent intravenous infusion rates should be titrated based on patient response, using the dosing recommendations in Table 23.1. Theophylline levels can be used to maximize therapy, in that each additional 1 mg/kg of theophylline will produce a 2 μg/ml rise in the serum concentration. For example, if a 70-kg bronchospastic patient has a serum concentration of 8 μg/ml, the administration of an additional 210 mg of theophylline will, in the majority of patients, elevate the serum drug concentration to 14 μg/ml, well within the "therapeutic range" for theophylline.

β-Adrenergic Receptor Agonists

The value of β-adrenergic agonist therapy in the treatment of reversible airway obstruction was documented at the turn of the century when Solis-Cohen (51) reported the use of desiccated adrenal glands for the treatment of asthma. This discovery was followed by the isolation of ephedrine and the synthesis of isoproterenol. Subsequently, a variety of β-adrenergic agonists have been introduced into clinical use, which vary in affinity for the β_1- and β_2-adrenergic receptors and duration of action. These drugs have become well established as effective medications in the treatment of both acute and chronic reversible airway obstruction.

PHARMACOLOGY

All β-adrenergic receptor agonists act by binding to β_1 and β_2 cell membrane receptors (Fig. 23.1), which results in activation of adenyl cyclase; accordingly, intracellular levels of cAMP are increased (47). This action induces a relaxation of bronchial and vascular smooth muscle. β-Adrenergic agonists may also induce increased mucociliary transport of respiratory secretions (55, 56). Stimulation of β_2-receptors on mast cells inhibits the release of

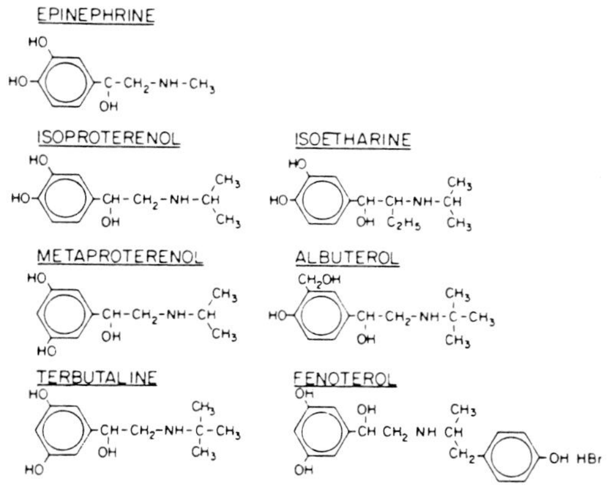

Figure 23.2. Structures of β-adrenergic agonists. (Originally published in Kelly HW: New beta-2-adrenergic agonist aerosols. *Clin Pharm* 4:393–403, 1985. Copyright © 1985, American Society of Hospital Pharmacists, Inc. All rights reserved. Reprinted with permission.)

mediators of bronchospasm, i.e., histamine and slow-reacting substance of anaphylaxis (27).

Distinctions between the β-adrenergic agonists are based on differences in chemistry and selectivity for the β_2-receptor over the β_1-receptor. Chemically, all β-adrenergic agonists are structural derivatives of phenylethylamine (Fig. 23.2). Structural modifications of the phenylethylamine nucleus result in compounds with differing durations of action and receptor activity (Table 23.4).

The catecholamine agents possess adjacent hydroxyl groups on positions 3 and 4 of the benzene ring of the catechol molecule (47). All catecholamines are capable of acting on both β_1- and β_2-adrenergic receptors. Whereas epinephrine and isoproterenol have equal β_1- and β_2-adrenergic receptor activity, isoetharine and bitolterol are reported to have greater affinity for the β_2-receptor than for the β_1-receptor (33). All catecholamines are readily inactivated by the enzymes catechol-O-methyltransferase, found in high concentrations in the liver and kidney, and monoamine oxidase, located in the presynaptic neurons (47). The duration of action of the catecholamines is short because of their rapid metabolism. The exception to this rule among β-agonists is bitolterol (53). Bitolterol is actually a prodrug; hydrolysis by plasma esterases results in the generation of the active drug colterol, which is a catecholamine (18). Because colterol must be generated in the systemic circulation, the duration of action of bitolterol is longer than that of other catecholamines. Catecholamines are usually not administered orally because they are rapidly conjugated and inactivated in the mucosa of the gastrointestinal tract (33).

The substitution of the catecholamine nucleus with resorcinol or saligenin has resulted in the development of drugs with longer durations of action than the catecholamines because they are resistant to the actions of both catechol-O-methyltransferase and monoamine oxidase (18). In addition, they are effective after oral administration and have relatively greater affinity for the β_2-receptor than for the β_1-receptor. The resorcinols include metaproterenol, terbutaline, and the investigational agent fenoterol; the only currently available saligenin is albuterol.

Table 23.4
β-Adrenergic Agents[a]

Drug	Route of Administration			Duration of Action (hr)	Receptor		
	Injection	Inhaled	Oral		β_2	β_1	α
Catecholamines							
Epinephrine	Yes	Yes	No	1–2	+	+	+
Isoproterenol	Yes	Yes	No	2–3	+	+	−
Isoetharine	No	Yes	No	2–3	+ +	+	−
Bitolterol	No	Yes	No	4–6	+ +	+	−
Resorcinols							
Metaproterenol	No	Yes	Yes	3–5	+ +	+	−
Terbutaline	Yes	No	Yes	4–6	+ +	+	−
Fenoterol	No	Yes	No	4–6	+ +	+	−
Saligen							
Albuterol	No	Yes	Yes	4–6	+ +	±	−

[a] Adapted from Iafrate RP, Massey KL, Hendeles L: Current concepts in clinical therapeutics: asthma. *Clin Pharm* 5:206–227, 1986. Copyright © 1986, American Society of Hospital Pharmacists, Inc. All rights reserved. Used with permission.

PHARMACOKINETICS

As previously discussed, the catecholamines are ineffective following oral administration. Accordingly, their only route of enteral administration is oral inhalation, either as a powder in a metered-dose inhaler or as a solution for nebulization. However, the noncatecholamine β-adrenergic agonists, metaproterenol, terbutaline, and albuterol, are also available as oral tablets, and metaproterenol and albuterol are also manufacturered as oral liquids.

Epinephrine, isotharine, isoproterenol, metaproterenol, albuterol, and bitolterol are the only β-adrenergic agents available for administration by nebulization. The only parenteral β-adrenergic agonists are epinephrine, isoproterenol, and terbutaline; the latter is available for subcutaneous administration only. Not all dosage forms of each drug are marketed in the United States. For example, terbutaline is not approved for use as an aerosol, despite its documented efficacy and the availability in Europe and Canada of an oral solution for nebulization.

Increasingly, the inhaled route of administration is becoming a preferred method of administration for β-adrenergic agonists (18, 22, 33, 40 ,48); nebulization is one of the most common methods of administration used in intensive care units. The reason for this strong interest in oral inhalation of these drugs is 3-fold (22, 40). First, inhalation delivers the drug directly to the site of activity, the airways. Second, administration by inhalation requires a smaller dose of drug to achieve a desired therapeutic response, and the drug is distributed over the large tissue surface area of the lungs, up to 70 m². Third, onset of action is very rapid following oral inhalation and side effects are minimal (40). There are disadvantages to this route of administration, however. In non–mechanically ventilated patients, a great deal of patient cooperation is required to deliver the drug adequately (40). However, spacer devices may improve drug delivery in patients who may have difficulty coordinating the discharge of medication from the inhaler with inhalation (9). Additionally, a high percentage of each drug dose commonly gets trapped in the upper airways or is swallowed; only 13% of a dose from a metered-dose inhaler and 1–5% of a dose administered by nebulization reach the lower respiratory tract (40). Administration by inhalation can result in mouth irritation and dryness. One particular disadvantage occurs in patients with severe bronchospasm: the drug may not be administered to the lower airways where it is needed. In this circumstance, much larger doses of drug are required to achieve a satisfactory response (40).

Few pharmacokinetic data are available on β-adrenergic agonists owing to the very low serum levels of drugs that are achieved after dosing, particularly following inhalation. However, it is well established that most of these drugs have short plasma half-lives and important first pass metabolism (18). For all inhaled catecholamine β-adrenergic agonists (except bitolterol), peak effects occur 5–15 minutes after administration and persist for 1–3 hours. Bitolterol's actions are maximal at 0.5–2 hours after administration and continue for up to 6 hours (22). Metaproterenol has a slow onset of action, up to 30 minutes after administration, and peak effects occur within 1 hour. The duration of action of metaproterenol is usually 3–5 hours. Terbutaline and fenoterol have similar pharmacokinetic profiles (onset of action 5–15 minutes, peak effects in 1–2 hours), and their effects may persist for as long as 6 hours. Like most of the inhaled β-adrenergic drugs, albuterol has a rapid onset of 5–15 minutes after administration, with peak effects in 0.5–2 hours and a persistence of 3–6 hours.

SIDE EFFECTS

The side effects of the β-adrenergic agonists are similar; the majority are transient (22, 28, 40, 43). The most common adverse effects are skeletal muscle tremor, nervousness, insomnia, tachycardia, and palpitations (49). The cardiac effects are primarily due to direct β_1-receptor stimulation. Reflex tachycardia may also result owing to β_2-mediated peripheral vasodilation (18, 22).

Less commonly reported side effects of these drugs include paradoxical bronchoconstriction, skin flushing, headache, and dizziness (43).

Although the incidence of all side effects is very low following inhalation, the oral and parenteral routes commonly induce side effects. The side effects may be so severe that the drugs may have to be discontinued (49). For example, muscle tremor is believed to result primarily from β_2 stimulation and appears to be dose-related (18, 22). In some patients, the tremor can be so serious as to be disabling. Use of oral β-adrenergics should be reserved for patients who are unable or unwilling to use the inhalation dosage forms. Some patients

Table 23.5
β_2-Adrenergic Aerosol Preparations and Dosages[a]

Drug	Preparations	Pediatric Dosages	Adult Dosages
Isoproterenol hydrochloride and sulfate			
Various manufacturers	0.25% (1:400) 2.5 mg/ml 0.50% (1:200) 5 mg/ml 1.0% (1:100) 10 mg/ml	0.05–0.1 mg/kg q. 2–4 hr	One to two inhalations of 0.25% solution by hand-bulb nebulizer; via nebulizer q. 2–4 hr

Isuprel Mistometer
  Norisodrine Aerotrol
  Medihaler-Iso
  Norisodrine Sulfate
	131 µg/spray
	120 µg/spray
	80 µg/spray
	110 µg/spray
		One to two inhalations q. 4–6 hr	One to two sprays q. 2–4 hr

Isoetharine			
Isoetharine hydrochloride for inhalation	0.1%, 0.125%, 0.2%	0.1–0.2 mg/kg q. 2–4 hr	3–5 mg undiluted via nebulizer with oxygen at 4–6 liters/min over 15–20 min q. 2–4 hr
Bronkosol	0.25%, 0.5%, 1%		0.5% and 1% solutions diluted 1:3 with 0.9% sodium chloride q. 2–4 hr
Bronkometer	340 µg/spray	One to two sprays q. 4–6 hr	One to two sprays q. 4–6 hr
Metaproterenol			
Alupent	5% (50 mg/ml) solution for nebulization	0.25–0.5 mg/kg q. 2–4 hr (15 mg maximum single dose)	0.3 ml (15 mg) diluted with 2.5 ml of 0.9% sodium chloride nebulized q. 2–4 hr
Metaprel	0.6% (15 mg/2.5 ml)		
Alupent MDI, Metaprel MDI	0.65 mg/puff, powder suspension	One to two puffs q. 4–6 hr and before exercise	Two to three puffs q. 4–6 hr and before exercise
Albuterol			
Ventolin Proventil	90 µg/puff, powder suspension	One to two puffs q. 4–6 hr and before exercise	One to two puffs q. 4–6 hr and before exercise
	0.5% (2.5 mg/ml)	0.05–0.15 mg diluted with 1–2 ml 0.9% normal saline q. 4–6 hr	2.5–5 mg diluted with 0.9% normal saline q. 4–6 hr
Terbutaline			
Brethaire	0.2 mg/puff, powder suspension	One to two puffs q. 4–6 hr and before exercise	One to two puffs q. 4–6 hr and before exercise
Brethine	0.1% (1 mg/ml) (not FDA approved for this use)	0.1–0.3 mg/kg q. 2–6 hr	5–7 mg undiluted q. 4–6 hr
Bitolterol			
Tornalate	0.37 mg/spray	One to three sprays q. 4–6 hr	One to three sprays q. 4–6 hr
Fenoterol hydrobromide[b]			
Berotec	0.16 mg/puff, powder solution	One to two puffs q. 4–6 hr	One to two puffs q. 4–6 hr

[a]Originally published in Kelly HW: New beta-2-adrenergic agonist aerosols. *Clin Pharm* 4:393–403, 1985. Copyright © 1985, American Society of Hospital Pharmacists, Inc. All rights reserved. Used with permission.
[b]Pending FDA approval.

who achieve only suboptimal effects with the inhalant products may benefit from supplementation with an oral β-adrenergic (18).

Because intravenous epinephrine and isoproterenol are associated with myocardial ischemia, infarction, and death (25, 30), their use is generally limited to patients with drug-unresponsive bronchospasm, i.e., status asthmaticus.

Following chronic use of β-adrenergic agonists, decreased responsiveness may develop. Commonly referred to as tolerance or tachyphylaxis, this effect has been documented to occur in both animals and humans (34). Interestingly, although tolerance has been demonstrated to develop to the nonbronchial β-adrenergic responses (e.g., heart rate, tremor), conflicting information exists regarding the bronchial response. Most data indicate that prolonged use of β-adrenergic agonists, either oral or inhaled, can result in a decrease in the duration of drug effect (18, 34).

DRUG INTERACTIONS

β-Adrenergic agonists may act synergistically when administered concurrently either with other β-adrenergic agonists or with theophylline (21, 41). The most important risk of these combinations would be in patients with underlying cardiac disease, with a limited capacity to tolerate high heart rate or arrhythmias (49).

CLINICAL USE

As previously discussed, inhaled β-adrenergic agonists are increasingly considered as the drug therapy of choice for the treatment of acute bronchospasm, particularly in critically ill patients (18). Other indications for their usage include prophylaxis of chronic asthma and exercise-induced asthma (18).

Practically, all of the inhaled β-adrenergics can be considered to be equally effective in treating bronchospasm. However, it has been suggested that metaproterenol and the catecholamines are less effective than albuterol, terbutaline, and isoproterenol (33). Choice of an individual agent reflects both clinician and patient preference, as well as economic factors. In hospitalized patients, isoetharine and metaproterenol are the most commonly used inhaled agents for administration by nebulization (18); an oral solution for nebulization of albuterol has recently been marketed.

DOSING

The dosages of the various β-adrenergic agents are listed in Table 23.5.

Anticholinergic Agents

In the early 1800s, the practice of inhaling burning powders of the anticholinergic alkaloids stramonium and belladonna for the treatment of asthma was introduced to Great Britain by travelers from India (59). Although effective, this practice was accompanied by a high number of adverse effects such as tachycardia, urinary retention, inspissation of secretions, and delirium. Following the development of inhaled bronchodilators, the use of anticholinergic agents for treatment of asthma was abandoned.

Over the last 20 years, interest in the use of anticholinergic drugs for treatment of bronchospasm has been renewed. This interest derives from documentation of the effective use of atropine by inhalation in the treatment of asthma. Additionally, two synthetic anticholinergics have been developed that are much safer and easier to use than atropine: glycopyrrolate and ipratropium.

PHARMACOLOGY

Atropine is a naturally occuring tertiary ammonium alkaloid obtained from plants of the Solanaceae family, including *Atropa belladonna* (deadly nightshade) and *Datura stramonium* (jimson weed) (40, 49). Also known as dl-hyoscyamine, atropine is the prototypic anticholinergic (antimuscarinic) agent. Other antimuscarinic drugs used in the treatment of bronchospasm—glycopyrrolate and the newly marketed compound, ipratropium—are synthetic quaternary ammonium derivatives of atropine (12, 59). Atropine methylnitrate is a quaternary ammonium compound that is available only for investigational use in the United States, but is commercially available in Europe as methylatropine nitrate (59).

All of the antimuscarinic drugs produce their effects by competitively inhibiting the effects of acetylcholine on muscarinic receptors. Specifically, these drugs act by inhibiting the generation of intracellular cGMP (Fig. 23.1) (48). This action results in bronchodilation, especially in the large airways and decreased tracheobronchial secretions. Of these available antimuscarinic agents, only ipratropium is approved by the Food and Drug Administra-

Atropine
Atropine sulfate

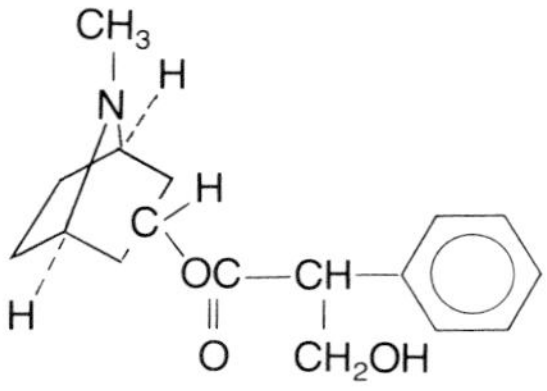

Glycopyrrolate

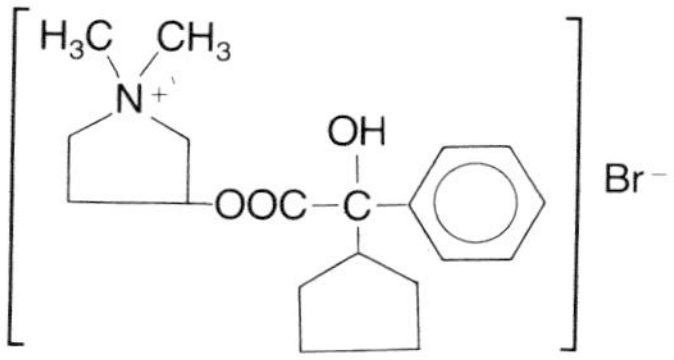

Ipratropium

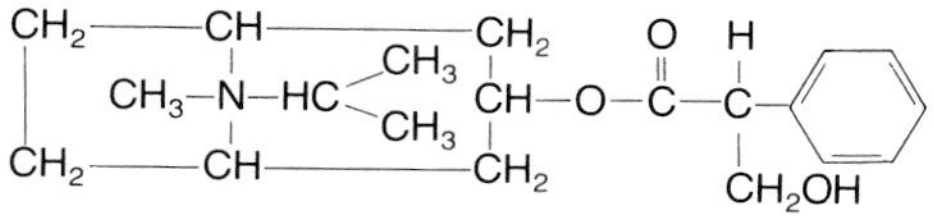

Figure 23.3. Structure of anticholinergic agents.

tion for inhalation in the treatment of bronchospasm.

PHARMACOKINETICS

Atropine is a tertiary ammonium alkaloid (Fig. 23.3), most commonly used as the sulfate salt. Inasmuch as atropine readily crosses epithelial mucosa, it may be administered via the gastrointestinal tract, by inhalation, and parenterally (24, 59). In contrast, atropine methylnitrate, glycopyrrolate, and ipratropium are quaternary ammonium antimuscarinics. The quaternary structure confers an electrical charge on these drugs, resulting in their poor absorption into the systemic circulation following administration by mouth or inhalation (12, 59).

The comparative pharmacokinetics of the inhaled anticholinergic agents are shown in Table 23.6. Following an aerosol dose, onset of action of atropine sulfate is 15–30 minutes; peak effects occur 30–170 minutes after administration. The duration of action of atropine sulfate is 3–5 hours (12, 59). Atropine is widely distributed in the body, including the central nervous system. The plasma half-life is 2–3 hours and the drug is eliminated by hepatic metabolism. About 30–50% of a given dose is metabolized to a variety of inactive metabolites, with the remainder of the dose being eliminated unchanged in the urine. Atropine methylnitrate exhibits a pharmacokinetic profile similar to that of atropine, but has a slightly longer duration of action, 4–6

Table 23.6
Bronchodilator Properties of Anticholinergic Drugs[a]

Drug	Dosages	Route of Administration	Time of Onset (min)	Peak Effect (min)	Duration (hr)
Atropine sulfate	0.025–0.075 mg/kg	Inhalation	15–30	30–170	3–5
	0.4–1 mg	Oral	NA	NA	NA
Atropine methonitrate	1–1.5 mg	Inhalation	15–30	40–60	4–6
Glycopyrrolate	0.0044 mg/kg	Inhalation	15–30	30–45	2–8
		Intramuscular Subcutaneous	15–30	30–45	2–7
	0.2 mg	Intravenous	1	NA	NA
Ipratropium	20–40 μg	Inhalation	3–30	90–120	3–8

[a]Adapted from Ziment I, Au JP: Anticholinergic agents. *Clin Chest Med* 7:355–366, 1986.

hours. In addition, this drug does not diffuse through the pulmonary epithelium nor does it cross the blood-brain barrier (12, 59).

Glycopyrrolate is a quaternary ammonium antimuscarinic, but it is also a complex aminoalcohol ester. Following inhalation, glycopyrrolate, like atropine, has an onset of action of 15–30 minutes; peak effects occur between 30 and 45 minutes after administration (12, 59). The drug has a longer duration of action than atropine, up to 8 hours (59). Like all quaternary ammonium salts, glycopyrrolate does not cross the blood-brain barrier or the pulmonary mucosa.

Ipratropium, also known as N-isopropylnortropine tropic acid ester, is a quaternary methyl derivative of atropine. As with other inhaled antimuscarinic drugs, the onset of action of ipratropium is rapid, 15–30 minutes. Peak effects are noted 90–120 minutes after administration and last for at least 4 hours and up to 6 hours in some patients (59). Systemic absorption is minimal after inhalation, and owing to the drug's quaternary structure, tissue distribution is limited. Ipratropium does not cross the blood-brain barrier (12, 59).

SIDE EFFECTS

As previously discussed, the side effect profile of the antimuscarinics is largely determined by their chemical structure and route of administration. Atropine, being a tertiary ammonium compound, readily crosses the mucosal epithelium into the systemic circulation (24). Accordingly, systemic side effects are common following oral and systemic administration; these effects tend to be dose-related. Because low doses of the drug are used for inhalation, however, side effects are greatly reduced in number and severity with this route of administration (24). Following inhalation of atropine most patients develop mouth dryness. Other possible side effects include flushing, lightheadedness, and slight tachycardia (24, 59). Urinary retention and blurred vision are rare, as are tremors, arrhythmias, and blood pressure changes (59).

For all of the quaternary ammonium compounds, the incidence of systemic side effects is extremely low following inhalation. As previously mentioned, these compounds poorly diffuse across the pulmonary epithelium and therefore have minimal systemic absorption. They do not cross the blood-brain barrier and are therefore devoid of central nervous system effects (12, 59).

Theoretically, the inhaled anticholinergics should alter mucociliary clearance and increase the viscosity of secretions. In practice, these side effects occur most commonly with atropine and not at all with ipratropium (54).

CLINICAL USE

Data are available on the efficacy of atropine (7, 8, 23, 29, 50), but there is only limited information regarding the use of glycopyrrolate as bronchodilator (10, 20, 24). The most information generated concerns the efficacy and safety of ipratropium in the treatment of bronchospasm (42).

Based on controlled and noncontrolled clinical trials, the use of inhaled anticholinergic drugs appears to be primarily as an alternative therapy in the treatment of bronchospastic diseases (12, 34). In contrast to inhaled β-adrenergic drugs, the anticholinergic bronchodilators have been demonstrated to be most effective in decreasing bronchial smooth muscle tone in patients with chronic bronchitis and emphysema. Their efficacy in asthma is inferior to that of β-adrenergic agonists (18). Because the onset of action of inhaled anticholinergics is slower than that of the inhaled β-adrenergics, they should not be used in the treatment of acute bronchospasm. In addition, although they have a longer duration of action than most inhaled β-adrenergics, the anticholinergics produce less bronchodilation and relief of symptoms in asthma (18, 42, 59).

Based on efficacy studies, the use of inhaled anticholinergic drugs should generally be limited to those patients who do not adequately respond to maximal β-adrenergic therapy (18). These patients usually are afflicted with chronic obstructive pulmonary disease, including emphysema and chronic bronchitis. In addition, because of the longer duration of action of these agents, anticholinergics may be found to be useful in special circumstances such as the prevention of nocturnal asthma, but such potential roles remain to be defined.

DOSING

The dosages of anticholinergics by inhalation are listed in Table 23.5

Acknowledgment

The author thanks Dr. Kenneth Shepherd for his critical review of this chapter.

References

1. Adair NE: Airflow obstruction. In *Current Therapy In Critical Care Medicine.* Philadelphia, BC Decker, 1987, pp 164–169.
2. Andersson KE, Persson CG: Extra-pulmonary effects of theophylline. *Eur J Respir Dis* 61(S109):17–28, 1980.
3. Aubier M, DeTroyer A, Sampson M, et al: Aminophylline improves diaphragmatic contractility. *N Engl J Med* 305:249–252, 1981.
4. Barnes PJ: State of the art: neural control of human airways in health and disease. *Am Rev Respir Dis* 134:1289–1314, 1986.
5. Bergstrand H: Phosphodiesterase inhibition and theophylline. *Eur J Respir Dis* 61(S109):37–44, 1980.
6. Brisson GR, Malaisse-Lagal F, Malaisse-Lagal WJ: The stimulus-secretion coupling of glucose-induced insulin release. 7. A proposed site of action for adenosine 3'5'-cyclic monophosphate. *J Clin Invest* 51:232–241, 1972.
7. Cavanaugh MJ, Cooper DM: Inhaled atropine sulfate: dose-response characteristics. *Am Rev Respir Dis* 114:517–524, 1976.
8. Chick TW, Jenne JW: Comparative bronchodilator response to atropine and terbutaline in asthma and chronic bronchitis. *Chest* 72:719–723, 1977.
9. Drugs used in treatment of asthma. *Med Lett Drugs Ther* 29:11–16, 1987.
10. Gal TJ, Suratt PM, Lu JY: Glycopyrrolate and atropine inhalation: comparative effects on normal airway function. *Am Rev Respir Dis* 129:871–873, 1984.
11. Ginchansky E, Weinberger M: Relationship of theophylline clearance to oral dosage in children with chronic asthma. *J Pediatr* 91:655–660, 1977.
12. Gross NJ, Skorodin MS: The place of anticholinergic agents in the treatment of airways obstruction. *Immunol Allergy Pract* 7:224–231, 1986.
13. Hendeles L, Weinberger M: Theophylline: a state of the art review. *Pharmacotherapy* 3:2–44, 1983.
14. Hendeles L, Weinberger M: Theophylline: therapeutic use of serum concentration monitoring. In Taylor WJ, Finn AL (eds): *Individualizing Drug Therapy: Practical Application of Drug Monitoring.* New York, Gross, Townsend, Frank, Hoffman. 1981, vol 1, pp 32–65.
15. Hendeles L, Weinberger M, Wyatt R: A guide to oral theophylline therapy for treatment of chronic asthma. *Am J Dis Child* 132:876–880, 1978.
16. Holgate ST, Mann JS, Cushey MJ: Adenosine as a bronchoconstriction mediator in asthma and its antagonism by methylxanthines. *J Allergy Clin Immunol* 74:302–306, 1984.
17. Horrobin DF, Manku MS, Franks DJ, et al: Methylxanthine phosphodiesterase inhibitors behave as prostaglandin antagonists in a perfused rat mesenteric artery preparation. *Prostaglandins* 13:33–40, 1977.
18. Iafrate RP, Massey KL, Hendeles L: Current concepts in clinical therapeutics: asthma. *Clin Pharm* 5:206–227, 1986.
19. Jenne JW, Wyze E, Rood FS, MacDonald IM: Pharmacokinetics of theophylline: application to adjustment of clinical dose of aminophylline. *Clin Pharmacol Ther* 13:349–368, 1972.
20. Johnson BE, Suratt PM, Gal TJ, Wilhort SL: Effects of inhaled glycopyrrolate and atropine in asthma precipitated by exercise and cold air inhalation. *Chest* 85:325–328, 1984.
21. Kelly HW: Controversies in asthma therapy with theophylline and the beta-2-adrenergic agonists. *Clin Pharm* 3:386–395, 1984.
22. Kelly HW: New beta-2-adrenergic agonist aerosols. *Clin Pharm* 4:393–403, 1985.
23. Klock LE, Miller TD, Morris AH, et al: A comparative study of atropine sulfate and isoproterenol hydrochloride in chronic bronchitis. *Am Rev Respir Dis* 112:371–376, 1975.
24. Kradjan WA, Lakshminarayan S, Hayden PW, et al: Serum atropine concentration after inhalation of atropine sulfate. *Am Rev Respir Dis* 123:471–472, 1981.
25. Kurland G, Williams J, Lewiston N: Fatal myocardial toxicity during continuous infusion of intravenous isoproterenol therapy for asthma. *J Allergy Clin Immunol* 63:407–411, 1979.
26. Lefkowitz RJ: Clinical physics of adrenoreceptor regulation. *Am J Physiol* 243:E43–E47, 1982.
27. Lofdahl CG, Svedmyr N: Selectivity of beta-adrenergic stimulant and blocking agents. *Eur J Respir Dis* 65(S136):101–113, 1984.
28. Lourenco RV, Eotromanes E: Clinical aerosols II. Therapeutic aerosols. *Arch Intern Med* 142:2299–2308, 1982.
29. Marini JJ, Lakshminarayan S: Inhaled atropine improves airflow in irreversible chronic bronchitis. *Am Rev Respir Dis* 119:148, 1979.
30. Matson JR, Coughlin G, Strunk R: Myocardial ischemia complicating the use of isoproterenol in asthmatic children. *J Pediatr* 92:776–778, 1978.
31. Matthay RA, Berger JH, Loke J, et al: Effects of aminophylline on right and left ventricular performance in chronic obstructive pulmonary disease—noninvasive assessment by radionuclide angiography. *Am J Med* 65:903–910, 1978.
32. McEvoy GK: Theophylline. In McEvoy GK (ed): *AHFS Drug Information 1987.* Bethesda, American Society of Hospital Pharmacists, 1987, pp 1952–1959.
33. McFadden ER Jr: Beta-2 receptor agonist: metabolism and pharmacology. *J Allergy Clin Immunol* 68:91–97, 1981.
34. McFadden ER: Clinical use of beta-adrenergic agonists. *J Allergy Clin Immunol* 76:352–356, 1985.
35. McFadden ER: Introduction: methylxanthine therapy and reversible airway obstruction. *Am J Med* 79(S6A):1–4, 1985.
36. Miech RP, Niedzwick JG, Smith TR: Effect of theophylline on the binding of c-AMP to soluble protein from tracheal smooth muscle. *Biochem Pharmacol* 28:3687–3688, 1979.
37. Mitenko PA, Ogilvie RI: Rational intravenous doses of theophylline. *N Engl J Med* 289:600–603, 1973.
38. Murciano D, Aubier M, Lecocguic Y, Pariente R: Effects of theophylline on diaphragmatic strength and fatigue in patients with chronic obstructive pulmonary disease. *N Engl J Med* 311:349–353, 1984.
39. Nassif EG, Weinberger M, Thompson R, et al: The value of maintenance theophylline in steroid-dependent asthma. *N Engl J Med* 304:71–75, 1981.
40. Newhouse MT, Dolovich MB: Control of asthma by aerosols. *N Engl J Med* 315:870–874, 1986.
41. Nicklas RA, Whitehurst VE, Donohue RF, et al: Concomitant use of beta adrenergic agonists and methylxanthines. *J Allergy Clin Immunol* 73:20–24, 1984.
42. Pakes GE, Brogden RN, Heel TM, et al: Ipratropium bromide: a review of its pharmacologic properties and therapy efficacy in asthma and chronic bronchitis. *Drugs* 20:237–266, 1980.
43. Paterson JW, Woolcock AJ, Shenfield GM: State of the art: bronchodilator drugs. *Am Rev Respir Dis* 120:1149–1188, 1979.
44. Richardson JB, Farguson CC: Neuromuscular structure and function in the airways. *Fed Proc* 38:202–208, 1979.
45. Sackner MA: Effect of respiratory drugs on mucociliary clearance. *Chest* 73:958–966, 1978.
46. Salter H: On some points in the treatment and clinical history of asthma. *Edinburgh Med J* 4:1109–1115, 1858.
47. Seligman M, Chernow B: Use of adrenergic agents in the critically ill patient. *Hosp Formul* 223:348–360, 1987.
48. Shenfield GM: Combination bronchodilator therapy. *Drugs* 24:414–439, 1982.
49. Sly RM, Anderson JA, Bierman CW, et al: Adverse effects and complications of treatment of beta-adrener-

gic agonist drugs. *J Allergy Clin Immunol:* 75:443–449, 1985.

50. Snow RM, Miller WC, Blair HT, et al: Inhaled atropine in asthma. *Ann Allergy* 42:286–289, 1979.
51. Solis-Cohen S: The use of adrenal substance in the treatment of asthma. *JAMA* 34:1164–1168, 1900.
52. Theodore AC, Beer DJ: Pharmacotherapy of chronic obstructive pulmonary disease. *Clin Chest Med* 7:657–671, 1986.
53. Walker SB, Kradgan MA, Bierman CW: Bitolterol mesylate: a beta-adrenergic agent. *Pharmacotherapy* 5:127–137, 1985.
54. Wanner A: Clinical aspects of mucociliary transport. *Am Rev Respir Dis* 116:73–125, 1977.
55. Wanner A: Effects of methylxanthines on airway mucociliary function. *Am J Med* 79(S6A):16–21, 1985.
56. Weinberger M, Hendeles L: Slow-release theophylline: rationale and basis for product selection. *N Engl J Med* 308:760–764, 1983.
57. Weinberger MM, Hendeles L: Theophylline use: an overview. *J Allergy Clin Immunol* 76:277–284, 1985.
58. Winn HR: Methylxanthines, adenosine, and the pulmonary system. *Chest* 91:800–801, 1987.
59. Ziment I, Au JP: Anticholinergic agents. *Clin Chest Med* 7:355–366, 1986.
60. Zwillich CW, Sutton TD, Neft TA, et al: Theophylline-induced seizures in adults: correlations with serum concentration. *Ann Intern Med* 82:784–787, 1975.

24

Oxygen/Respiratory Stimulants

John W. Hoyt, M.D.

The minute-to-minute delivery of oxygen to the cell for its metabolic needs is an essential part of sustaining life. Oxygen is an irreplaceable and consumable element in cellular function, because of its role in the Krebs cycle for the production of high energy phosphates by the mitochondria. Oxygen can also be viewed as a therapeutic agent, used in the management of various cardiopulmonary disease processes when atmospheric concentrations of oxygen are inadequate.

Measurement of oxygen consumption ($\dot{V}o_2$) has been done for many years in the laboratory setting, and now in the ICU, by determining the difference between inspired and expired oxygen concentrations (37). A second technique measures disappearance of oxygen from a closed system that contains a carbon dioxide absorber (4). The adaption of these techniques to the critical care environment for $\dot{V}o_2$ monitoring has been slow to evolve (40). Recent interest in predicting caloric needs during hyperalimentation by indirect calorimetry and use of the Weir equation has fostered the development of numerous instruments to directly monitor $\dot{V}o_2$ and carbon dioxide production ($\dot{V}co_2$) in the ICU (11).

Indirectly, $\dot{V}o_2$ can be determined by calculating arterial (Cao_2) and mixed venous (Cvo_2) oxygen contents (Table 24.1) and measuring thermodilution cardiac output solving the Fick equation for $\dot{V}o_2$:

$$\text{Cardiac output} = \frac{\dot{V}o_2}{(Cao_2 - Cvo_2)10} \quad (1)$$

This technique for monitoring $\dot{V}o_2$ is readily available to clinicians in the ICU whenever a pulmonary artery catheter is utilized, and is significantly less complicated than the new metabolic carts for directly measuring $\dot{V}o_2$.

Experience with assessing $\dot{V}o_2$ has shown that normally, 3 ml of oxygen per kilogram of body weight is consumed each minute. Other

authors have expressed normal $\dot{V}o_2$ as 110–130 ml/m^2/min (4). The proverbial 70-kg man with a body surface area of about 1.8 m^2 consumes about 200–250 ml of oxygen per minute. When critical illness intervenes, $\dot{V}o_2$ can easily double.

OXYGEN DELIVERY

Oxygen delivery refers to a physiologic journey that begins with the uptake of oxygen from the atmosphere and ends with the distribution of oxygen to the mitochondria of the cell for oxidative phosphorylation. This process starts with inspiring air which is 20.9% oxygen.

The partial pressure of inspired oxygen, (Pio_2) at sea level and 760 mm Hg barometric pressure (Pb) is 159 mm Hg. The progressive decrease in this partial pressure as oxygen traverses the lungs, blood, and tissues is known as the oxygen cascade (29). The first decrease occurs when inspired air is humidified in the airway and diluted by water vapor. Water vapor, at a temperature of 37°C, has a partial pressure (Ph_2o) of 47 mm Hg. Fully humidified, inspired air has a Pio_2 of 149 mm Hg. As inspired gas passes into the alveolus, it is

Table 24.1
Oxygen Contents[a]

Arterial content	= bound oxygen + dissolved oxygen
Cao_2	= (Hb × Sao_2 × 1.34) + (0.0031 × Pao_2)
Cao_2	= 20 ml O_2/100 ml blood
Venous content	= bound oxygen + dissolved oxygen
Cvo_2	= (Hb × Svo_2 × 1.34) + (0.0031 × Pvo_2)
Cvo_2	= 16 ml O_2/100 ml blood

[a]Sao_2, arterial oxygen saturation; Svo_2, venous oxygen saturation; Hb, hemoglobin. Other symbols explained in text.

further diluted by carbon dioxide. Solving the alveolar air equation, alveolar oxygen tension (P_{AO_2}) is 99 mm Hg:

$$P_{AO_2} = (Pb - P_{H_2O}) \, Fio_2 - (Paco_2/R) \qquad (2)$$
$$= (760 - 47)0.209 - (40/0.8)$$
$$= 99 \text{ mm Hg}$$

where Fio_2 is fractional inspired oxygen and $Paco_2$ is arterial carbon dioxide tension.

From the alveolus, oxygen moves across the gas exchange membrane composed of the epithelial lining of the alveolus and endothelial lining of the pulmonary capillary. Oxygen enters the blood stream, where it is carried bound to hemoglobin (Hb) or dissolved in blood. Because some deoxygenated blood enters the left side of the heart from bronchial and thebesian veins, there is a further reduction in the partial pressure of oxygen as the blood enters the aorta ($Pao_2 = 90-95$ mm Hg). A major decrease in oxygen partial pressure occurs as blood flow completes tissue perfusion in the systemic capillaries ($Pvo_2 = 40$ mm Hg). Oxygen molecules pass across cell membranes to the mitochondria, where oxygen participates in intracellular respiration. Oxygen partial pressure at the mitochondrial level varies from 4 to 25 mm Hg depending on the organ system.

If normal $\dot{V}o_2$ is 3 ml/kg/min, the cardiovascular system must transport about 250 ml of oxygen per minute from the lungs to the tissues. Hemoglobin makes this possible without excessive demands on the cardiovascular system. Without Hb, oxygen transport would be dependent on oxygen dissolved in plasma. One liter of cardiac output with a Pao_2 of 100 mm Hg would, without Hb, transport 3.1 ml of oxygen. A cardiac output of 65 liter/min would be required to meet cellular $\dot{V}o_2$ needs if one assumed total extraction of oxygen from plasma at the capillary level.

Hemoglobin carries 1.34 ml of oxygen per gram of Hb. One liter of cardiac output with 15 g of Hb transports 200 ml of oxygen. A normal cardiac output (CO) of 5 liters/min and normal Hb of 15 g results in an oxygen transport (Do_2) of 1000 ml/min:

$$Do_2 = CO \times Cao_2 \times 10 \qquad (3)$$

Each Hb molecule binds four oxygen molecules to the heme part of the structure. The relationship describing this binding is known as the oxygen-Hb dissociation curve. The curve is sigmoid with the flat portion in the area of high Po_2, greater than 100 mm Hg, and the steep portion of the curve in the physiologic

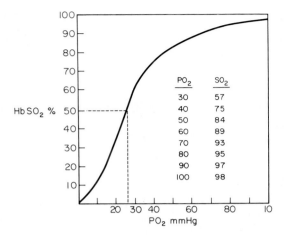

PO_2	SO_2
30	57
40	75
50	84
60	89
70	93
80	95
90	97
100	98

Figure 24.1. Oxyhemoglobin dissociation curve.

range of Po_2, 20–100 mm Hg (Fig. 24.1). This relationship facilitates oxygen unloading at the tissues when there are large changes in Po_2 and small changes in Hb saturation (So_2).

The position of this curve is best described by examining the 50% saturation point, which has a partial pressure of 27 mm Hg ($P_{50} = 27$) in normal adult Hb. This value expresses the affinity of Hb for oxygen. This affinity can be decreased by acidemia, hypercarbia, or hyperthermia, which increase P_{50}. Increased 2,3-diphosphoglycerate (2,3-DPG) in the red cell also shifts the curve to the right and increases P_{50}. Alkalosis, hypocarbia, hypothermia, and decreased 2,3-DPG shift the curve to the left when affinity increases and P_{50} decreases (1).

The adequacy of Do_2 can be assessed by looking at oxygen in the blood returning to the right side of the heart after perfusion of peripheral tissues and oxygen extraction. Normal Pvo_2 is 40 mm of Hg, which is 75% saturated. The Cvo_2 is about 16 ml/dl. These measurements must be made on blood obtained from the pulmonary artery because of discrepancies between superior and inferior vena caval oxygen contents. When Do_2 becomes inadequate, for whatever reason, to meet the $\dot{V}o_2$ needs of the peripheral tissues, mixed venous oxygen partial pressure and saturation fall, and the difference between arterial and mixed venous oxygen contents ($AVDo_2$) widens (28):

$$AVDo_2 = Cao_2 - Cvo_2 \qquad (4)$$

The oxygen utilization coefficient, $AVDo_2/Cao_2$, has been recommended as another technique for evaluating the delivery of oxygen.

CAUSES OF HYPOXIA

Hypoxia is the inadequate delivery of oxygen to tissues, leading to a failure of oxidative phosphorylation. There are four types of hypoxia as described by Barcroft in 1920 (3): anoxic hypoxia, referring to inadequate delivery of oxygen from the lungs to the blood; anemic hypoxia, which results from low, abnormal, or damaged Hb; stagnant hypoxia secondary to low cardiac output; and histotoxic hypoxia which is a failure of oxygen utilization by the cells. Only hypoxic anoxia responds to therapeutic oxygen administration.

Cyanosis is frequently thought to be a useful sign of *anoxic hypoxia*. There must be 5 g of unsaturated Hb for cyanosis to be clinically recognizable. For a normal patient with 15 g of Hb, this results in an SaO_2 of 66%, which is a PaO_2 of 35 mm Hg. A patient who is anemic and has only 10 g of Hb will be 50% desaturated with a PaO_2 of 27 mm Hg before cyanosis is apparent. Patients with 5 or 6 g of Hb never appear cyanotic. Thus, cyanosis is both a late and inadequate sign of anoxic hypoxia (8).

Tachycardia and mild increases in blood pressure occur with early hypoxia. If anoxic hypoxia worsens and persists, bradycardia and hypotension occur, eventually leading to cardiac arrest.

Anoxic hypoxia increases respiratory drive. The carotid and aortic bodies respond to PaO_2 values of less than 50 mm Hg, promoting large increases in minute ventilation. Acute reduction in PaO_2 below 50 mm Hg causes progressive neurologic dysfunction, with loss of consciousness below a PaO_2 of 32 mm Hg. Metabolic changes of anoxic hypoxia include a shift from

Table 24.2
Barometric pressure (Pb) and Partial Pressure of Inspired Oxygen (PIO_2) at Various Altitudes

Altitude (feet)	Pb	PIO_2
Sea level	760	159
5,000	632	132
10,000	523	109
20,000	349	73
30,000	225	47

$$PIO_2 = Pb \times 20.9$$

aerobic to anaerobic metabolism with the production of lactic acidosis.

There are essentially only five causes of anoxic hypoxia; low PIO_2, ventilation/perfusion ($\dot{V}_A/\dot{Q}$) abnormalities, right-to-left shunt ($\dot{Q}_s/\dot{Q}_t$), diffusion defect, and alveolar hypoventilation.

A low PIO_2 is most commonly seen at high altitudes (Table 24.2) and is also associated with mining or industrial accidents. In the hospital environment, a low PIO_2 can occur in the operating room if nitrous oxide is delivered to a patient from an anesthesia machine without an appropriate blend of oxygen or safety system. Other accidents can occur with hospital oxygen–nitrous oxide piping systems.

$\dot{V}_A/\dot{Q}$ abnormalities are the major clinical cause of hypoxia (41). Under normal physiologic circumstances there is a balancing of ventilation and perfusion. Normal alveolar ventilation and cardiac output are each about 70 ml/kg/min. Proper matching of $\dot{V}_A/\dot{Q}$ optimizes the uptake and distribution of oxygen from the lungs to the tissues. When ventilation predominates over perfusion, a high $\dot{V}_A/\dot{Q}$ ratio

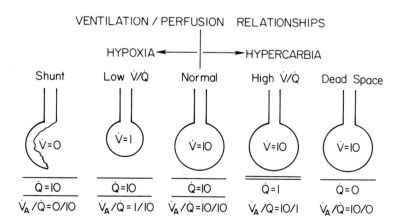

Figure 24.2 Ventilation-perfusion ($\dot{V}/\dot{Q}$) abnormalities as an etiology of hypoxia or carbon dioxide retention.

and wasted ventilation occurs. The highest $\dot{V}_A/\dot{Q}$ ratio occurs in ventilation in the absence of perfusion, which is known as dead space. When perfusion predominates over ventilation, hypoxia results since there is an inadequate oxygen delivery to the alveolus to be picked up by unsaturated Hb in the pulmonary capillary blood flow. The lowest $\dot{V}_A/\dot{Q}$ ratio occurs in perfusion in the absence of ventilation. This situation is known as right-to-left intrapulmonary shunt $(\dot{Q}_s/\dot{Q}_t)$ (Fig. 24.2).

Anoxic hypoxia due to a diffusion defect is uncommon except in the exercising patient. In chronic interstitial lung disease, diffusion represents as much as 20% of the source of hypoxia when the patient is exercising (9).

In alveolar hypoventilation, carbon dioxide rises in the poorly ventilated alveolus and displaces oxygen, resulting in hypoxia. This effect is most prominent when the patient is breathing room air and has the lowest initial Pao_2.

Of the clinically important causes of anoxic hypoxia seen in critically ill patients, therapeutic oxygen primarily benefits those patients with low $\dot{V}_A/\dot{Q}$ alveolar units. Enriching the alveolar oxygen content makes more oxygen available for the unsaturated Hb. Oxygen administration does not benefit $\dot{Q}_s/\dot{Q}_t$, because oxygen cannot reach the collapsed alveolus. In this situation, positive end-expiratory pressure (PEEP) is needed to open the alveolus, splint it open in a position of function, and recruit it to the family of both ventilated and perfused alveoli. Oxygen therapy may temporarily benefit a patient with alveolar hypoventilation, but mechanical ventilation is eventually needed as carbon dioxide continues to accumulate and respiratory acidosis occurs. The patient with a diffusion gradient during exercise is also benefited by oxygen therapy.

The second type of hypoxia in Barcroft's classification is *anemic hypoxia*, referring to an inadequate quantity of Hb to transport oxygen for the consumption needs of the tissues. When Hb is inadequate, various compensatory mechanisms are employed such as increasing cardiac output or decreasing hemoglobin's affinity for oxygen. The latter is accomplished by increasing intracellular 2,3-DPG, which raises P_{50} and facilitates unloading at the tissues.

For 15 years an arbitrary minimum Hb level of 10 g has been used in the critical care environment, below which level transfusion is indicated. Little scientific evidence supports this arbitrary level of Hb, and individual patient variation in ability to adjust to changing Hb levels is certainly more important than a hard-and-fast rule about minimal Hb levels in the ICU (36). Work with Jehovah's Witness patients who refuse blood transfusion has indicated that survival following critical illness is possible with Hb levels well below 10 g.

A form of anemic hypoxia may occur when Hb is present in adequate quantities, but is rendered nonfunctional by some change in the Hb molecule or by blocking of access to the heme component where oxygen must temporarily and reversibly bind. An example of nonfunctional hemoglobin is methemoglobin in which the iron in the ferrous state is oxidized to the ferric state and is no longer capable of binding oxygen. Chemicals and drugs that are nitrites or aniline derivatives can cause acquired methemoglobinemia (10). The most common drug used in the ICU that is known to cause methemoglobinemia is nitroglycerin (42). Some local anesthetics such as benzocaine and prilocaine can cause methemoglobinemia (22).

There are two forms of hereditary methemoglobinemia. In one form an abnormal Hb, hemoglobin M, has a crucial amino acid substitution (25). A second hereditary cause is NADH-MetHb reductase deficiency (20 This enzyme is responsible for reducing naturally oxidized hemoglobin that occurs in normal humans at a low frequency, which is correctable if there is adequate enzyme activity.

Access to the iron component of the Hb molecule can be blocked by both carbon monoxide and sulfur. Carbon monoxide binds 218 times more tightly to Hb than does oxygen and as a result effectively competes with oxygen for attachment to the iron molecule, forming carboxyhemoglobin. Sulfur from such compounds as sulfonamides and sulfur-containing ointments can also bind to the Hb molecule and prevent oxygen from forming oxyhemoglobin (30). Sulfhemoglobin is an irreversibly blocked Hb, whereas carboxyhemoglobin can be treated by using high oxygen concentrations or hyperbaric oxygen, the high concentration allowing oxygen to be more competitive with carbon monoxide at the heme iron.

Stagnant hypoxia is the inadequate delivery of oxygen to the tissues because of poor cardiac output, resulting from poor cardiac function, as in cardiogenic shock secondary to myocardial infarction, or hypovolemia from loss of intravascular volume.

Barcroft's fourth type of hypoxia is *histotoxic hypoxia* in which cellular poisoning impairs the ability to utilize oxygen. The most common example of this type of hypoxia in the ICU is cyanide poisoning from the excessive use of intravenous nitroprusside. Nitroprusside is broken down to release cyanide in the blood, which blocks the intracellular electron transport system resulting in the inability to use oxygen and thus metabolic acidosis.

OXYGEN MONITORING

Since oxygen is an essential part of the minute-to-minute survival of the cell, monitoring of oxygen becomes an important task in the ICU. Historically, clinicians have monitored oxygen partial pressure in the blood when attempting to assess cardiopulmonary function and oxygen delivery. Oxygen saturation was most often calculated, occasionally measured.

Leland Clark, a biochemist and physiologist, in 1954 developed the oxygen electrode so that oxygen partial pressure could be measured in

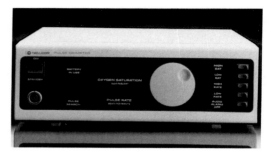

Figure 24.3. Pulse oximeter that uses both finger and nose probes with light-emitting diodes to continuously measure arterial oxygen saturation of hemoglobin.

a solution such as blood (32). The incorporation of the Clark electrode into a blood-gas machine capable of measuring blood P_{O_2}, P_{CO_2}, and pH revolutionized the simultaneously evolving concept of respiratory care, and now critical care.

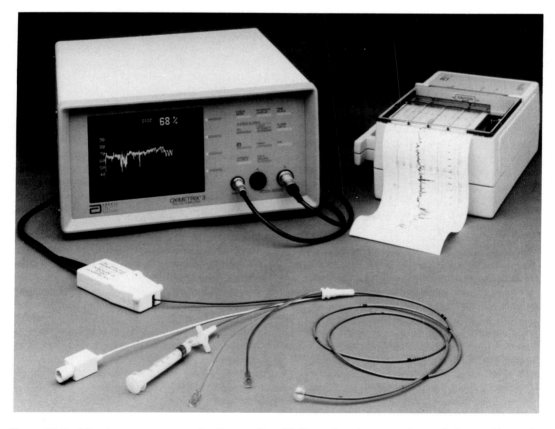

Figure 24.4. Mixed venous oxygen saturation monitor with fiberoptic pulmonary artery catheter used to continuously measure the oxygen saturation of blood in the pulmonary artery.

For over 25 years intensive care physicians have relied on intermittent measurements of partial pressure for adjusting oxygen therapy and respiratory care. Recently, the introduction of pulse oximeters has made oxygen therapy monitoring a process of recording continuous, real-time values rather than intermittent measurements. Oximeters read oxygen saturation or percentage of oxyhemoglobin in blood based on the Lambert-Beer law: the transmission of light is a logarithmic function of the density or concentration of the absorbent, since each absorbing molecule absorbs an equal fraction of a particular wavelength of the incident light (33).

The development of oximeters began in the 1930s, but not until the last 5 years, when new photodiodes and light-emitting diodes permitted miniaturization of ear and finger probes and instruments, did pulse oximetry find its place in the ICU (Fig. 24.3). Clinicians are now shifting their thinking from oxygen partial pressure to oxygen saturation as a monitor of the safety of oxygen delivery.

Spectrophotometry and oximetry via fiberoptic pulmonary artery catheters is now permitting the continuous evaluation of mixed venous blood oxygen saturation (Fig. 24.4). This technology uses reflectance spectrophotometry rather than the transmission spectrophotometry employed in the pulse oximeter.

As noted earlier, Svo_2 is an indicator of the adequacy of oxygen delivery to the tissues. If Hb concentration or cardiac output is low or $\dot{V}o_2$ is very high, blood returns to the right side of the heart after excessive oxygen extraction with a low Svo_2 (17). The etiology of the decreased Svo_2 is not immediately apparent, but an evaluation of arterial oxygenation, hemoglobin, and thermodilution cardiac output can quickly sort out the source of the increased oxygen extraction from the mixed venous blood.

The combined monitoring of arterial and mixed venous oximetry in the critically ill patient with questionable oxygen transport is a newly evolving standard of care in the ICU. Dual oximetry will certainly improve patient safety and make therapeutic decisions more accurate and expedient (31).

OXYGEN THERAPY

Oxygen has been used as a therapeutic agent in the practice of medicine since the late 1700s (23). It was originally discovered by Priestly.

Lavoisier explored its application to respiratory physiology and proved that it was absorbed by the lungs. Beddoes was responsible for the early work on the therapeutic applications of oxygen in the late 1700s and early 1800s. Not until Haldane's pioneering work using oxygen to treat patients with chlorine inhalation injuries during World War I was oxygen therapy accepted clinically (24). Later, both Meakins (26) and Barach (2) wrote about the use of oxygen in the treatment of lobar pneumonia, thereby establishing the foundation for respiratory therapy. Despite this 180-year history, oxygen is rarely recognized as a drug with specific therapeutic indications, an expected dose-response curve, and predictable complications when used in excessive dosage.

An odorless, tasteless, and colorless gas, oxygen has an atomic weight of 16, a molecular weight of 32, and a boiling point of $-183°C$, and is commercially prepared by the distillation of liquid air using the difference in boiling point between the oxygen and nitrogen components. The electron structure of oxygen gives the molecule a magnetic susceptibility, which is known as a paramagnetic property and is used in clinical oxygen analyzers. Oxygen also has a polarographic property that causes it to migrate to a cathode, resulting in a flow of electrons. This property is used in the oxygen electrode in blood-gas analyzers. Oxygen does not ignite or explode, but rather, supports combustion. An elevated oxygen concentration leads to more rapid oxidation of organic materials, making destruction by fire a greater risk.

Oxygen is clinically available in two forms: compressed gas in cylinders and liquid oxygen from a central hospital pipeline system. Cylinders are used less often, but are of historical interest because at one time they were the primary source of oxygen. Today, in modern hospitals, cylinders are used primarily during patient transport and as backup to a hospital pipeline system.

There are nine different sizes of oxygen cylinders. Design, construction, testing, marking, handling, filling, and transportation of compressed gases in cylinders are regulated by the Motor Carrier Safety Division of the Department of Transportation. Both the National Fire Protection Association (NFPA) and the Compressed Gas Association (CGA) publish standards on safe practices for compressed gas (14). In the United States, oxygen is stored in green cylinders as a compressed gas at a pressure of 1800–2400 pounds per square inch

(PSIG). These cylinders must be appropriately labeled and sealed with valves that are specific for oxygen. For the small oxygen cylinders (size E or less), a Pin-Index Safety System is used on the cylinder valve to assure that only an oxygen cylinder can be connected to oxygen yokes. For cylinders larger than size E, there is a similar safety protection based on a valve-threaded system. The various oxygen cylinders contain different amounts of compressed gas. A working knowledge of the volume of gas in each cylinder is helpful for planning transport of a patient (Table 24.3).

Most hospitals are now using central piping systems for delivery of oxygen to patient care areas because they are cost-effective and convenient. Safe practice guidelines for central pipeline systems are also available from the CGA and NFPA. One cubic foot of liquid oxygen delivers 860 cubic feet of gas. This fact alone markedly decreased the storage and delivery problems associated with cylinder gas.

Central pipeline systems deliver oxygen to the bedside at 50–55 PSIG. Again, as in the case of cylinders, there are noninterchangeable connectors at the patient bedside to assure the safe delivery of gas. The most common of these is the Diameter Index Safety System (DISS), which assures that only an oxygen flowmeter or oxygen high-pressure hose can be connected to an oxygen wall outlet from a hospital pipeline system.

Oxygen clearly is a therapeutic agent used in the management of critically ill patients. Yet, unlike the drugs that are commonly thought of as therapeutic agents, oxygen is also a normal part of daily physiologic functions. Oxygen should be classified with therapeutic agents such as electrolytes and blood products.

Oxygen administration in critically ill patients is divided into two very separate techniques, invasive and noninvasive. Noninvasive oxygen therapy includes the use of nasal prongs, face tents, and face masks with reservoir bags. This form of oxygen administration is intended for the patient with a small to moderate amount of $\dot{V}_A/\dot{Q}$ disturbance, as might be associated with pneumonia. The oxygen does not cure the pneumonia, but protects the patient from hypoxic complications associated with the pneumonia. This form of oxygen therapy has been recommended for pneumonia since the 1920s. Invasive oxygen therapy refers to either translaryngeal (oral or nasal) or tracheostomy tube administration of enriched oxygen mixtures. This oxygen therapy is given with humidity, PEEP, intermittent positive pressure breathing, or expiratory retard. This form of therapy has only a 25 to 30-year history, and specific indications are controversial. Invasive oxygen therapy also has a higher nosocomial infection rate than does any form of noninvasive oxygen therapy in critically ill patients.

Noninvasive oxygen therapy is divided into low-flow and high-flow systems (34). Low-flow systems deliver inadequate volumes of fresh gas to meet the inspiratory needs of the patient, and as a result, the patient's inspired gas includes variable quantities of room air. Probably the best example of this low-flow system is the nasal prong or nasal cannula system that delivers up to 6 liters/min of 100% oxygen. Flow rates greater than 6 liters/min are not recommended, because of patient discomfort and drying of the nasal mucosa. The nasal cannula oxygen delivery system fills the 50-ml anatomic reservoir in the adult patient's pharynx, while the patient pauses between breaths. When inspiration begins, the first 50 ml of an expected 400 to 500-ml tidal volume is 100% oxygen. The remaining 350–450 ml of the tidal volume is 100% oxygen diluted by room air. As a result, tracheal Fio_2 is dependent on tidal volume, respiratory rate, and inspiratory flow rate. One can roughly predict that 1 liter/min of nasal prong oxygen results in a tracheal Fio_2 of 0.24. Each additional liter per minute of 100% oxygen will increase this Fio_2 by about 0.04. Oxygen in higher flows can be delivered through a face mask with or without a reservoir bag to further increase Fio_2. Clinicians should carefully consider the value of trying to deliver more than 60% oxygen noninvasively to the trachea. The degree of respiratory failure requiring such levels almost always indicates a significant shunt that will not respond to oxygen therapy alone. PEEP

Table 24.3
Volumes of Various Gas Cylinders

Size of Cylinder	Liters of Gas	Duration of Use	
		At 5 liters/min	At 10 liters/min
A	76	15/min	8 min
B	196	39 min	20 min
D	396	1.3 hr	40 min
E	659	2.1 hr	1.1 hr
F	2062	6.8 hr	3.4 hr
M	3000	10.0 hr	5.0 hr
G	5331	17.7 hr	8.8 hr
H	5570	18.5 hr	9.2 hr
K	7500	25.0 hr	12.5 hr

must be employed, usually through an endotracheal tube. There is some interest among clinicians in delivering face mask PEEP, but the long-term place of this technique in the respiratory therapy armamentarium is unclear.

Other forms of low-flow oxygen delivery systems can be combined with humidity delivery. The usual nasal prong oxygen system goes through a bubble humidifier, which picks up very small amounts of water. On the other hand, a warm or room temperature nebulizer can deliver impressive volumes of particulate water and oxygen to either a face tent or face mask. These systems also require the adult patient to entrain room air at peak inspiratory flow rates, and as a result, are classified as "low-flow" systems, though the total flow is higher than with nasal prongs.

The best example of a clinically useful "high-flow" oxygen delivery system is a Venturi device. This system employs the Bernoulli principle to entrain air when gas flowing through an orifice creates a negative lateral wall pressure. For example, a 4 liters/min flow of 100% oxygen through a device calibrated to deliver an Fio_2 of 0.28 entrains 40 liters/min. This system delivers an accurate Fio_2 and the very high flow prevents the patient from diluting this accurate oxygen mixture by pulling in an indeterminate volume of air. A variety of accurate Fio_2 mixtures are available with the Venturi system.

Types of invasive oxygen delivery include ambient pressure spontaneous breathing, spontaneous PEEP, continuous positive airway pressure (CPAP), and mechanical ventilation in a variety of forms. All of these oxygen delivery systems should use a heated humidified gas source that delivers adequate particulate or molecular water to keep secretions thin and prevent occlusion of the endotracheal tube. Invasive oxygen therapy has a higher nosocomial infection rate than any form of noninvasive oxygen therapy (15).

OTHER THERAPIES

Improvement of oxygen delivery to the mitochondria of the cells must take many forms in the ICU besides the use of invasive and noninvasive oxygen administration. Attention must be directed not only to the partial pressure of oxygen in blood and the oxygen saturation of Hb, but to Hb concentration, cardiac output, $\dot{V}o_2$, matching of ventilation and perfusion, and atmospheric pressure.

As discussed earlier, 10 g has in the past been arbitrarily set as a minimally acceptable Hb in the critically ill patient. Because of critical illness–induced bone marrow suppression and frequent sampling of blood for analysis, many critically ill patients have to undergo transfusion on a regular basis. The recent introduction of recombinant human erythropoietin may eventually find a role in some ICU patients to maintain adequate Hb concentrations with less frequent transfusion therapy (16).

Some blood substitutes have been used with limited success in an attempt to find alternatives to Hb for oxygen delivery. One of these is a fluorocarbon emulsion that has been tested in this country, but not approved for routine use (35). Another substitute for blood transfusion would be the use of stroma-free hemoglobin or the use of synthetic erythrocytes to increase Do_2 (13).

One of the most effective techniques for optimizing oxygen delivery to the cells is by manipulating cardiac output, since each liter of cardiac output with 10 g of Hb will deliver 134 ml of oxygen per minute. Three techniques are used for optimizing cardiac output in the ICU. First, preload manipulation increases left ventricular end-diastolic volume and, as a result, increases cardiac output. Second, inotropic agents such as dobutamine and amrinone improve cardiac contractility. Third, afterload reduction is performed pharmacologically with agents such as nitroprusside, or mechanically with an intraaortic counterpulsation balloon.

If attempts to match Do_2 with $\dot{V}o_2$ have failed, as frequently occurs in malignant hyperthermia, hypothermia should be considered. Lowering body temperature reduces the need for oxygen delivery. This therapy is clearly helpful in malignant hyperthermia, and has also been used in other critical illnesses such as severe adult respiratory distress syndrome (ARDS) and head trauma, but has not achieved common acceptance (18).

Two old therapies, hyperbaric oxygen and extracorporeal membrane oxygenation (ECMO), are enjoying somewhat of a rebirth in certain specific areas. New single-patient hyperbaric chambers are now available at much lower cost than the original chambers. This therapy is indicated in anaerobic gas-producing infection and in carbon monoxide poisoning. ECMO is being used primarily in the management of respiratory failure in newborns.

Finally, there have been many attempts to improve matching of ventilation and perfusion in the lung in critically ill patients. Some drugs such as nitroprusside and nitroglycerine have been clearly shown to worsen matching of ventilation and perfusion, particularly in the face of pulmonary hypertension (6). A new drug, almitrine bismesylate, has been shown to improve $\dot{V}_A/\dot{Q}$ matching in chronic obstructive lung disease and, as a result, to improve oxygenation (5). This agent or other similar agents may find a role in the ICU to improve the uptake and distribution of oxygen from the lungs with lower and less toxic concentrations of oxygen.

OXYGEN TOXICITY

Oxygen, like all drugs used in large doses for prolonged periods of time, causes toxicity. The important aspects of excessive dosage are the absolute P_{IO_2} and the duration of dose. Inhalation of 100% oxygen at sea level (Pb = 760 mm Hg) for more than 12 hours results in chest pain, a sense of bronchial irritation, cough, dyspnea, painful deep breathing, and a fall in vital capacity (7).

The source of oxygen toxicity is reactive oxygen intermediates such as superoxide (O_2^-), H_2O_2, OH^-, and singlet oxygen. These products destroy cell membranes and are particularly active against lung cells such as macrophages and type I and type II alveolar cells (12). Reactive oxygen intermediates are normal body products that are used to kill phagocytosed bacteria. Only when abnormal concentrations or release of these intermediates occur does tissue damage result. The body strives to protect itself from such damage by natural body enzymes such as superoxide dismutase, which scavenges and detoxifies free radicals. Considerable research interest now centers on agents to protect against damage from oxygen intermediates, e.g., catalase, mannitol, vitamin E, and superoxide dismutase.

The best clinical recommendation is that critically ill patients can tolerate up to 24 hours of 100% oxygen. Injured lungs, such as occur in ARDS, seem more sensitive to oxygen toxicity, leading to active lung fibrosis (19). The present clinical recommendation is to use the lowest F_{IO_2} possible by maximizing PEEP.

RESPIRATORY STIMULANTS

Failure of central receptors to respond to carbon dioxide and/or hydrogen ion is a major cause of respiratory failure. This failure is seen in patients with metabolic alkalosis, chronic obstructive pulmonary disease (COPD), and the obesity hypoventilation syndrome. A variety of therapeutic agents are used to augment respiratory drive, most commonly, medroxyprogesterone acetate and doxapram. Both function by central stimulation.

Doxapram must be given by continuous intravenous infusion and can be effective in patients with COPD. Moser and associates (27) administered doxapram as a continuous intravenous infusion at a dose of approximately 3 mg/min to a group of patients with COPD who were known carbon dioxide retainers with a Pa_{CO_2} in excess of 50 torr. This therapy was done simultaneously with oxygen administration to see whether doxapram could blunt the occurrence of respiratory acidosis, which can occur in patients with COPD who are given oxygen. When compared with a control group, the patients on doxapram infusion clearly did not demonstrate the same increase in Pa_{CO_2}. Using this and other suggestive information, some clinicians attempt to use doxapram to aid in weaning patients with COPD from mechanical ventilation (21, 27).

Because doxapram is a general CNS stimulant, it has many side effects including hypertension, tachycardia, and arrhythmias. These side effects are particularly bothersome in patients with coronary artery disease and preclude the frequent use of this agent.

Progesterone has been tested in the obesity hypoventilation syndrome and COPD and found to be of some limited value. It must be given as an intramuscular injection or by mouth. Sutton and associates (38) examined the effect of medroxyprogesterone acetate, 20 mg sublingually every 8 hours, in a population of patients with obesity hypoventilation syndrome. They noted a fall in Pa_{CO_2} of 13 torr and an increase in Pa_{O_2} of 12.6 torr after progesterone was started in 10 patients. Other investigators have noted that 50 mg of progesterone intramuscularly caused an increase in breathing that peaked at 12 hours after the dose. The side effects of this drug are certainly less than for doxapram, and as a result, it possibly has greater clinical usefulness as a respiratory stimulant (38, 39).

References

1. Babior RM, Stossel TP: *Hematology: A Pathophysiological Approach.* New York, Churchill Livingstone, 1984, pp 21–36.
2. Barach AL: Recent advances in inhalation therapy in the treatment of cardiac and respiratory disease. *NY State J Med* 35:1095–1110, 1937.

3. Barcroft J: Physiological effects of insufficient oxygen supply. *Nature* 1920, pp 106–125.
4. Bartlett RH, Dechert RE, Mault JR, et al: Measurement of metabolism in multiple organ failure. *Surgery* 92:771–779, 1982.
5. Bell RC, et al: The effect of almitrine bismesylate on hypoxemia in chronic obstructive pulmonary disease. *Ann Intern Med* 105:342–346, 1986.
6. Bishop MJ, Cheney FW: Vasodilators worsen gas exchange in dog oleic-acid lung injury. *Anesthiology* 64:435–439, 1986.
7. Brodsky JB: Clinical aspects of oxygen. *Int Anesthiol Clin* 19:169–199, 1981.
8. Comroe JH Jr, Botelho S: The unreliability of cyanosis in the recognition of arterial anoxemia. *Am J Med Sci* 214:1–6, 1947.
9. Crystal RG: Idiopathic pulmonary fibrosis: clinical, histologic, radiographic, physiologic, scintigraphic, cytologic, and biochemical aspects. *Ann Intern Med* 85:769–788, 1976.
10. Curry S: Methemoglobinemia. *Ann Emerg Med* 11:214–221, 1982.
11. De V. Weir JB: New methods for calculating metabolic rate with special reference to protein metabolism. *J Physiol* 109:1–9, 1949.
12. Deneke SM, Fanburg BL: Normobaric oxygen toxicity of the lung. *N Engl J Med* 303:76–86, 1980.
13. Djordjevich L, Mayoral J, Miller IF, et al: Cardiorespiratory effects of exchange transfusions with synthetic erythrocytes in rats. *Crit Care Med* 15:318–323, 1987.
14. Dorsch JA, Dorsch SE: *Understanding Anesthesia Equipment: Construction, Care and Complications.* Baltimore, Williams & Wilkins, 1976, pp 1–25.
15. El-Naggar M, Sadagopan S, Levine H, et al: Factors influencing choice between tracheostomy and prolonged translaryngeal intubation in acute respiratory failure: a prospective study. *Anesth Analg* 55:195–201, 1976.
16. Eschbach JW, Egrie JC, Downing MR, et al: Correction of the anemia of end-stage renal disease with recombinant human erythropoietin. *N Engl J Med* 316(2):73–78, 1987.
17. Fahey PJ, Harris K, Vanderwarf C: Clinical experience with continuous monitoring of mixed venous oxygen saturation in respiratory failure. *Chest* 86:748–752, 1984.
18. Gronert GA, et al: Human malignant hyperthermia: awake episodes and correction by dantrolene. *Anesth Analg* 59:377–378, 1980.
19. Haschek WM, Reiser KM, Klein-Szanto AJ, et al: Potentiation of butylated hydroxytoluene–induced acute lung damage by oxygen. *Am Rev Respir Dis* 127:28–34, 1983.
20. Hegesh E, Hegesh J, Kaftory A: Congenital methemoglobinemia with a deficiency of cytochrome b_5. *N Engl J Med* 314:757–761, 1986.
21. Houser WC, Schleuter DP: Prolonged doxapram infusion in obesity-hypoventilation syndrome. *JAMA* 239:340–341, 1978.
22. Kellet PB, Copeland CS: Methemoglobinemia associated with benzocaine-containing lubricant. *Anesthesiology* 59:463–464, 1983.
23. Leigh JM: Early treatment with oxygen. *Anaesthesia* 29:194–208, 1974.
24. Leigh JM: The evolution of oxygen therapy apparatus. *Anaesthesia* 29:462–485, 1974.
25. Mansouri A: Review: methemoglobinemia. *Am J Med Sci* 289:220–209, 1985.
26. Meakins J: Observations on the gases in human arterial blood in certain pathological pulmonary conditions and their treatment with oxygen. *J Pathol Bacteriol* 24:70–90, 1921.
27. Moser KM, Luchsinger PC, Adamson JS, et al: Respiratory stimulation with intravenous doxapram in respiratory failure: a double-blind co-operative study. *N Engl J Med* 288:427–431, 1973.
28. Norfleet EA, Watson CB: Continuous mixed venous oxygen saturation measurement: a significant advance in hemodynamic monitoring? *J Clin Monit* 1:245–258, 1985.
29. Nunn JF: *Applied Respiratory Physiology.* London, Butterworths, 1977, pp 375–444.
30. Park CM, Nagel RL: Sulfhemoglobinemia: clinical and molecular aspects. *N Engl J Med* 310:1579–1584, 1984.
31. Rasanen J, Downs JB: Titration of continuous positive airway pressure by real-time dual oximetry. *Crit Care Med* 15:395, 1987.
32. Severinghaus JW, Astrup PB: History of blood gas analysis. IV. Leland Clark's oxygen electrode. *J Clin Monit* 2:125–139, 1986.
33. Severinghaus JW, Astrup PB: History of blood gas analysis. VI. *J Clin Monit* 2:270–288, 1986.
34. Shapiro BA, Harrison RA, Trout CA: *Clinical Application of Respiratory Care.* Chicago, Year Book, 1979, pp 133–152.
35. Shoemaker WC, Thompson WL, Holbrook PR: *Textbook of Critical Care.* Philadelphia, WB Saunders, 1984, pp 210–218.
36. Snyder JV, Pinsky MR: *Oxygen Transport in the Critically Ill.* Chicago, Year Book, 1987, pp 3–15.
37. Snyder JV, Pinsky MR: *Oxygen Transport in the Critically Ill.* Chicago, Year Book, 1987, pp 16–21.
38. Sutton FD Jr, Zwillich CW, Creagh CE, et al: Progesterone for outpatient treatment of Pickwickian syndrome. *Ann Intern Med* 83:476–479, 1975.
39. Tyler JM: The effect of progesterone on the respiration of patients with emphysema and hypercapnia. *J Clin Invest* 39:34–41, 1960.
40. Weissman C, Kemper M, Askanazi J, et al: Resting metabolic rate of the critically ill patient: measured versus predicted. *Anesthesiology* 64:673–679, 1986.
41. West JB: *Pulmonary Pathophysiology—The Essentials.* Baltimore, Williams & Wilkins, 1977, pp 169–183.
42. Zurick AM, Wagner RH, Starr NJ, et al: Intravenous nitrolglycerine, methemoglobinemia, and respiratory distress in a postoperative cardiac surgical patient. *Anesthesiology* 61:464–466, 1984.

25

Pharmacological Approach to Acute Seizures

Joseph A. Miller, M.D.
John M. Hallenbeck, M.D.

Seizures have been recognized as a major medical problem since the dawn of history, whereas effective therapy has been available only for the last several decades. It is the purpose of this chapter to review current thought regarding diagnostic and therapeutic modalities available for treatment of seizures, particularly in the setting of the intensive care unit (ICU), where extremely complex problems may occur because of coexisting medical and surgical illnesses.

The general area of seizure management in the uncomplicated patient has been exhaustively reviewed in several recent monographs and will be only briefly discussed here; emphasis will be placed on the management of acute seizures, especially status epilepticus, an aspect of seizure control undergoing rapid changes in diagnosis and therapy.

CLASSIFICATION OF SEIZURES

Any discussion of seizures must begin with at least a brief review of the major classification scheme now employed, the International Classification of the Seizures. This classification, which has been in use for nearly 20 years and has been accepted by most authorities in the Western world, has brought a significant degree of order to discussions of seizure disorders, permitting more effective communication about seizures. This has in turn facilitated a more rational approach to recommendations for diagnosis, therapy, and the determination of prognosis. Somewhat revised in 1980, the currently used version is given as Table 25.1.

In addition, a classification of the epilepsies has appeared, aimed at organizing the various recognizable syndromes producing seizures alone or in combination with other neurological and systemic manifestations. It should be recognized that this is only a preliminary clas-

Table 25.1
International Classification of the Seizures[a]

PARTIAL SEIZURES
Simple partial seizures (consciousness preserved)
  Motor
  Somatosensory
  Autonomic
  Psychic
Complex partial seizures (consciousness impaired)
  Beginning as simple partial seizures and
    progressing to impairment of consciousness
    With no other features
    Starting as elementary seizures as in the four types
     of simple partial seizures
    With automatisms
  With impairment of consciousness at onset
Partial seizures evolving to secondarily generalized
  seizures.

GENERALIZED SEIZURES
Absence seizures
  Absence seizures
  Atypical absence seizures
Myoclonic seizures
Clonic seizures
Tonic seizures
Tonic-clonic seizures
Atonic seizures

UNCLASSIFIED SEIZURES
Seizures that cannot be classified because of
  incomplete data.

[a] Abstracted from Commission on Classification and Terminology of the International League Against Epilepsy 1981.

sification and will undoubtedly undergo significant evolution as time progresses. Sufficient time has not passed to allow us to determine whether this is a useful classification.

DIAGNOSIS OF SEIZURE

When approaching any patient with seizures, the clinician must first address this

Table 25.2
Medical Illnesses Resembling Seizures[a]

Processes resembling generalized tonic-clonic seizures
   Syncope or syncope with myoclonic movements, "convulsive syncope"
   Hyperventilation with carpopedal spasm
   Narcolepsy with cataplexy
   Nonepileptic myoclonus
   Psychiatric processes

Processes resembling elementary partial seizures
   Paroxysmal choreoathetosis
   Complicated migraine
   Paroxysmal attacks in multiple sclerosis
   Nonepileptic segmental myoclonus
   Tourette syndrome
   Psychiatric processes

Processes resembling complex partial seizures
   Toxic metabolic encephalopathies
   Transient ischemic attacks
   Transient global amnesia
   Psychiatric processes

[a] This list is not meant to be all inclusive but rather to serve as an example of the various entities that can mimic seizures.

Table 25.3
Drugs Reported To Induce Seizures[a]

Aqueous iodinated contrast agents
Anticholinesterases
Antihistamines
Antidepressants
Antipsychotics
Baclofen
β-blockers
Bronchodilators[b]
Camphor
Cefazolin
Chlorambucil
Cocaine
Cycloserine
Cyclosporin A
Ergonovine
Folic acid
General anesthetics (including ketamine, halothane, enflurane, propanidid)
Hyperbaric oxygen
Hypoglycemic agents
Hyperosmolar parenteral solutions
Insulin[b]
Isoniazid[b]
Local anesthetics (lidocaine, procaine)[b]
Mefenamic acid
Methylxanthines
Metronidazole
Narcotic analgesics
Penicillins
Phencyclidine
Psychotropic agents[b]
Sympathomimetics

[a] Modified from Messing RO, Closson RG, Simon RP: Drug-induced seizures: a 10-year experience. *Neurology* 34: 1582–1586, 1984.
[b] Drugs associated with bouts of status.

question: Has the patient actually had a seizure? This is a frequently overlooked issue, and one that obviously plays a great role in the outcome of any therapeutic intervention. It is also a problem that is more vexing than is apparent at first glance; for example, in one study of a large number of patients with a single seizure 30% were ultimately found to have a cause completely unrelated to seizure disorder as it is currently understood. Thus, it is of paramount importance to consider the various processes that can mimic seizures. It is only too easy in the stressed circumstances of the emergency room (ER) or the ICU to overlook this issue, but perhaps in those areas it is of greatest importance because of the urgency of the decisions that must be made and the gravity of their consequences.

There is no simple algorithm for determining whether a patient has had a seizure, and indeed the question may be difficult to conclusively resolve even under the ideal circumstance of observation. However, several suggestions can be made. First and foremost a clear history is necessary. Length of history does not necessarily equate with quality, however, detail is of great importance. Several important areas to cover include questions regarding sensations preceding the suspected seizure, the patient's level of consciousness immediately prior to the event, and what the

patient was doing at the time of the seizure. Questions should also be directed at what time of day the seizure occurred, how quickly the seizure developed, what the individual did

Table 25.4
Anticonvulsant Drug Interactions[a]

Anticonvulsant	New Anticonvulsant	Effect on Serum Concentration of Original Anticonvulsant
Valproate	Phenobarbital	Decrease
	Phenytoin	Decrease
Carbamazepine	Phenobarbital	Decrease
	Phenytoin	Decrease
Phenytoin	Phenobarbital	Variable
	Valproate	Decrease
Phenobarbital	Phenytoin	Variable
	Valproate	Increase

[a] Adapted from Penry JK: *Diagnosis and Management of Epilepsy: Monotherapy of Primary Generalized Seizures.* New York, Biomedical Information Corporation, 1986.

during the seizure, and the patient's state after the event. Questions regarding variations in symptoms from spell to spell are useful, particularly when the event in question is a possible recurrent seizure. One must certainly be aware of various medical states that can mimic seizures, for example syncope. A partial list of other diseases that can be associated with seizure-like states is given as Table 25.2 Although it is beyond the scope of this discussion to deal with this subject in greater detail, it must be emphasized that failure to recognize the importance of this aspect of seizure care will doom subsequent efforts in a large number of cases. Finally, seizures triggered by medications represent another frequently neglected diagnostic consideration (3, 4). A partial list of drugs reported capable of at least aiding the induction of seizures is given as Table 25.3. Although about 2% of all seizures appear to be drug induced, it is difficult to determine how much drug induction of seizures contributes to the occurrence of seizures with other causes although the size of the list and the common nature of many of the agents listed suggests that contribution is a large one. It is also perhaps revealing to note that in those cases with strictly drug-induced seizures, about 50% have multiple fits.

DIFFERENTIATING BETWEEN PRIMARY GENERALIZED AND PARTIAL SEIZURES

Once a diagnosis of seizure has been made, several decisions must be reached. Principal among these is to identify what type of seizure has occurred. The major point of differentiation is between primary generalized and partial seizures, as the pharmacologic approach to each is different. It is at this point that understanding of the current classification of the seizures is useful.

Primary generalized seizures always begin without an aura and usually start in childhood and adolescence. For example, quite often confused with complex partial seizures, the absence attack can be clearly differentiated by recognizing its abrupt onset and the prompt return of consciousness at the end of an attack, whereas the complex partial seizure is almost always followed by a period of postictal diminution of awareness. More particularly, the electroencephalogram (EEG) is specifically abnormal in over 95% of patients with absence, demonstrating the classical three-per-second

spike and wave. Although complex partial seizures are fairly easily differentiated from absence they are often quite difficult to diagnose in and of themselves as their symptomatology is quite often complex and can be bizarre (7). Unfortunately, these seizures are also the most common type that occur in adults, and the EEG is a less useful diagnostic procedure than in absence attacks.

A similar difficulty arises in distinguishing *primary generalized tonic clonic seizures* from those arriving from spread of an epileptic focus. This fact is particularly true in cases in which there is no preceding aura or it is too brief to be recognized or remembered. In general, those generalized tonic-clonic seizures that have their onset in adulthood are more likely to be secondarily generalized, whereas a juvenile onset points to a primary generalized disorder. There are, however, no clear distinguishing features that allow precise differentiation, and often the true situation becomes clear only after treatment either blocks the tonic clonic seizures and partial seizures become evident or treatment for secondarily generalized seizures fails. Another feature that may help differentiation is the presence of an initial clonic phase to the seizure, which is a feature seen in primary generalized seizures.

Agents particularly suitable for treatment of partial seizures, including partial seizures that secondarily generalize, are carbamazepine and, currently as a secondary agent, Dilantin. Within the last several years carbamazepine has become recognized as the agent of first choice for treatment of partial seizures, eclipsing Dilantin and phenobarbital and its congeners in this regard. Presently there is controversy regarding the role of carbamazepine in treatment of primary generalized seizures. Several studies have indicated its efficacy in this regard is no different than that of Dilantin; however, another school of thought recommends valproate for this seizure type. A resolution of this debate awaits further experience. Carbamazepine has a half-life of 6–12 hours and must be administered in divided dosages daily. Adverse effects include drowsiness, vertigo, and nausea. Much has been made in the past of the hematologic toxicity of this agent, which apparently was initially overestimated and is now felt to be rare. Nevertheless, serious bone marrow depression can occur and surveillance for this problem is warranted, especially when the drug is first begun. Drug interactions of this and other agents are given in Table 25.4. Carbamazepine (and other anticonvulsants) may accelerate the metabolism of a number of other drugs, for example oral contraceptives; however, a detailed analysis of these effects is beyond the scope of this discussion. Carbamazepine is available only as an oral agent.

Dilantin, previously a drug of choice for partial seizures, has been relegated to a secondary role as it is associated with an excessive number of side effects and may be associated with a depression of cognitive function with long-term use. It nevertheless retains usefulness, especially in cases in which carbamazepine cannot be employed, and, as discussed below, it is an initial drug of choice for treatment of status. It should be noted that different preparations of phenytoin have varying bioavailability, resulting in different absorption times and thus apparently different half-lives. Thus, caution should be exercised when using generic sources. Also, phenytoin is available in both oral and parenteral forms; the latter may be used only intravenously, as intramuscular administration produces precipitation in the muscle with consequent grossly reduced bioavailability and a sterile muscle abscess. Dilantin, as mentioned, has several side effects ranging from gum hypertrophy to production of a pseudolymphoma. The drug interactions of this agent are also especially complex and often difficult to predict. There are several congeners of phenytoin, for example mephenytoin, which have a very limited usefulness because of increased toxicity and no advantages over phenytoin.

Phenobarbital was the first modern anticonvulsant to be introduced and has enjoyed a long history of use. Today it is beginning to lose favor as a primary anticonvulsant for any kind of seizure, primarily because of the severe, undiminishing sedation associated with this agent. However, as it is the only anticonvulsant, besides phenytoin, available in parenteral form in the United States, it continues to play a central role in the treatment of status epilepticus, for which it is quite effective. Phenobarbital has a very long half-life (up to 96 hours), which may be still further prolonged by agents such as valproate, further exacerbating its sedating effects. As it is the archetypical hepatic enzyme inducer, it is associated with a number of drug interactions (Table 25.4). A closely related agent, primidone, was popular for many years as an agent for partial seizures, although it too has decreased in use, as much of the anticonvulsant activity of this drug can be attributed to its metabolism to phenobarbital. Thus, its properties are essentially those

of phenobarbital, save that there is a more prolonged time to onset of action because of the metabolic processing required.

Agents for primary generalized seizures include valproate and ethosuximide. The former is the most recent anticonvulsant to have been introduced into the United States and is experiencing a gradual increase in use as the spectrum of seizure types for which it has been found effective expands. Presently it is the agent of choice for mixed primary generalized absence and tonic clonic seizures and for tonic clonic seizures. As mentioned above, it is recommended by many as the agent of choice for all tonic clonic seizures as it controls many such disorders where the traditional agents fail. There are several studies that show it to be at least as effective as ethosuximide in the treatment of absence seizures. Unfortunately, valproate is available only in oral form. The half-life of this agent is from 6 to 15 hours; the longer values are associated with the enteric-coated form, which delays absorption somewhat. The most common adverse effect of this agent is gastric irritation and the most serious is idiosyncratic hepatotoxicity, which is seen particularly in children under 12 years of age who are also receiving other anticonvulsants and which is felt to be the consequence of the hepatic production of metabolites of valproate toxic to the liver. The effect on valproate of adding other anticonvulsants is given in Table 25.4. The other drug currently employed for primary generalized seizures is ethosuximide, an agent effective only for absence. If other seizure types are present this agent should not be used and valproate should be employed, as any of the other anticonvulsants available will aggravate absence. Ethosuximide is also available only in oral form and in adults has a half-life of up to 50–60 hours. The most common side effects of this drug are nausea, vomiting, and, in higher dosages, headaches. The most serious side effect is an increased risk of a psychotic reaction, which is more common than generally realized. A listing of the pharmacokinetic properties of the various anticonvulsants is found in Table 25.5.

Although the distinction between seizure types may be difficult, the patient appearing in the emergency room must be treated and several strategies may be of assistance. If the suspected seizure is the first one, two considerations are paramount. The first is that of diagnosis of seizure disorder—not a minor consideration as the societal consequences are often very profound for the patient and the

Table 25.5
Pharmacokinetic Data on Antiepileptic Drugs

Drug	Half-life (hr)	Time to Reach Steady State (days)	Therapeutic Range (μg/ml)	Protein Binding (%)
Phenytoin	10–34	7–28	10–20	69–96
Carbamazepine	14–27	3–4	4–12	66–89
Phenobarbital	46–136	14–21	15–40	40–60
Valproate	6–15	1–2	50–125	80–95
Ethosuximide	20–60	7–10	40–100	0

Adapted from Penry JK: *Diagnosis and Management of Epilepsy: Monotherapy of Primary Generalized Seizures.* New York, Biomedical Information Corporation, 1986.

family. The second is that if a seizure has taken place in an adult, even though no focality can be found, it strongly suggests a focal origin and therefore raises the question of an underlying disease process; for example a structural lesion, a cerebral ischemic process, or a metabolic abnormality. Attention must be directed as much to that issue as to the seizure itself, and an immediate diagnostic evaluation is indicated. There is justification then to consider withholding anticonvulsants until that evaluation is completed.

The patient most commonly presenting to the ER will be one who has an established seizure disorder and who has had either a single recurrent seizure or a flurry of these. It is critical to distinguish the circumstances of the individual situation. Clearly, the patient who has an established seizure disorder and has well-documented infrequent isolated seizures requires only a careful examination to assure that no injury has resulted from the seizure and to eliminate the unlikely possibility that an intercurrent process triggered the seizure. The most common cause of such recurrent seizures is medication noncompliance, and the most common mistake to make under such circumstances is to change the patient's medication even though it may actually be the correct medication and in the correct dosage. Thus, it is most important to diligently question a patient about possible omission of doses, recalling that the patient may be reluctant at first to admit that noncompliance has occurred. Once these considerations have been made and it has been established that no significant underlying problem is present, it is usually best to simply maintain the patient on the present regimen of anticonvulsants, obtain a blood level of the anticonvulsant(s) being given (even if those levels are not immediately available), and arrange for follow-up on a routine basis. If there is indication for a change of anticonvulsants, this task can then be done in an orderly fashion.

On the other hand, the patient who has had a sudden flurry of seizures and then is brought to the ER represents a more significant problem and requires intervention as there is a risk that further seizures, and possibly even status epilepticus, may supervene. Of course, once again the common problems of medication noncompliance and underlying illness must be considered, as must the less common potential for drug interaction, in which concurrently administered medications (even anticonvulsants) can alter each other's metabolism and cause lowered serum levels of each other. This is especially a problem as these interactions occur on a somewhat unpredictable basis. Also, there is the possibility that the patient's seizure type has been incorrectly diagnosed and an ineffective anticonvulsant prescribed; this is a possibility more likely in the patient whose seizures are of recent onset or who has had a recent change in drug regimen. Thus, it is important to clearly review the basis for the patient's diagnosis. When that is accomplished, a decision can be made regarding anticonvulsant therapy. In the majority of cases requiring adjustment, it will be made in dosage rather than in the kind of anticonvulsant. If no explanation is found for the recurrences, the anticonvulsant appears appropriate for the seizures involved and there is no evidence, historical or otherwise of anticonvulsant toxicity, an increase of anticonvulsant (or, if the patient is on multiple anticonvulsants, the most appropriate one for the seizures involved) is indicated. This is simply a linear increase for almost all the agents currently used, with the sole exception of Dilantin. This agent exhibits nonlinear kinetics, such that in the therapeutic range small increases in dosage can produce dramatically large increases in blood levels. The situation is particularly confused in cases involving multiple anticonvulsants, and here it can be quite difficult to predict blood levels for a particular increase of medication. (This last factor is one of several that can be given in favor of monotherapy for epilepsy, i.e., the use of a single agent to control seizures.) A variety of schemes have been given for the rapid increase of anticonvulsant levels. Simply adding twice the difference between the old and new dosage to the old dosage of the anticonvulsant for one time and then continuing with the new dosage schedule is the method most often recommended to achieve that rapid increase. It should be recalled however that many of the currently employed anticonvulsants (particularly carbamazepine and valproate) when given in suddenly increased dosages produce transient symptoms of toxicity, particularly nausea and vomiting; as these medications must be given orally, those side effects will hardly promote compliance. In addition, following dosage changes, oral absorption of several of the anticonvulsants (e.g., carbamazepine) can be quite uncertain, which adds still further unpredictability. These potential pitfalls must be kept in mind when increasing anticonvulsants, especially in the outpatient setting. A compromise approach can be tried; when circumstances seem less urgent, one might simply increase the anticonvulsant employed to its new dosage level, with perhaps fewer toxic side effects. The relatively short half-lives of most of the agents currently used will result in increased blood levels in a short time. If this is too long a period, it may be advisable to consider that the patient is in status in a broad sense and begin parenteral agents. If the anticonvulsant in question is Dilantin, its relatively long half-life mandates that a parenteral approach be employed in any case, and the same applies to the other parenterally available agent, phenobarbital. Regardless, especially if outpatient treatment is elected, the patient must be carefully instructed about the possible complications mentioned above and the need to seek immediate follow-up should they occur.

STATUS EPILEPTICUS

Status epilepticus has been recognized for at least the last century and constitutes one of the true medical emergencies. There is a significant element of misunderstanding that surrounds the concept of status, and this problem is not helped by the existence of various defi-

nitions for the problem (2). For example, the World Health Organization (WHO) defines status epilepticus as any epileptic condition persisting long enough to constitute a permanent condition. Others have defined it as any seizure lasting longer than 30 minutes continually, or recurrent seizures without an intervening period of consciousness between events. It should be noted that none of these specify the kind of seizure involved, and indeed as several authors have pointed out, status epilepticus is a state not an illness in and of itself. Thus, any type of seizure can become continuous (elementary, complex partial, and generalized including tonic clonic, myoclonic, and absence). Perhaps as Leppik (10) has suggested, the most useful definition is to simply consider the appearance of three seizures in 24 hours as evidence of status, for the consequences of recurrent seizures are greater than the risks of treatment. This fact is specifically true of the most dangerous of the various forms of status, generalized tonic clonic. Other seizures that at least infrequently become continuous in adults include complex partial, elementary partial (Koshevnikov syndrome), and absence (see later sections in this chapter). Although generalized tonic clonic (GTC) status is easily recognized in the majority of cases, at times the seizures can become somewhat disorganized clinically, and thus may be difficult to diagnose if the seizures have been taking place for an extended period.

As in the case of isolated seizures, at times a variety of seizure-like entities can be mistaken for status. These may include a number of movement disorders, such as choreoathetosis and some forms of segmental myoclonus. Also, decorticate and decerebrate posturing, and a variety of rigors can be seen in obtunded patients, in whom the greatest difficulty arises in reaching the correct diagnosis. The key point regarding these seizure-like disorders is that none of these respond to anticonvulsants, which may lead ultimately to the use of greater and greater amounts of anticonvulsants to suppress them, resulting in patient toxicity. The key to recognizing seizure-like entities is often an awareness of the possibility of the diagnosis and the realization that the patient is not responding to treatment with anticonvulsant drugs. Still less frequently, the patient can present with psychogenic seizures, i.e., seizures without an organic basis. The EEG can also be of use in confirming that an epileptic condition does or does not exist; however, it is critical to realize that the usefulness of this diagnostic test depends on reliable interpretation of the data.

Precipitating Factors

Although it is surprising to many, the incidence of status is probably greater today than before the widespread use of anticonvulsants, probably because the inappropriate use of such drugs has been a major factor in precipitating status. The causes of status must be considered from a dual perspective: There must be both an underlying neurophysiologic cause for the seizure disorder and a precipitating factor that engendered the status. Several studies have considered this point; the most common causes have included underlying structural lesions such as metastatic and primary tumors. The latter most often involve low-grade gliomas such as astrocytomas, and these are more often found in the frontal area (9). Other processes predisposing to status include anoxic encephalopathy; Wernike's encephalopathy; drug abuse, including alcoholism; and various metabolic disorders influencing water and electrolytes, including calcium and magnesium. Vasculitis and other cerebrovascular disorders and particularly head injury are also numbered among the common underlying causes of status, as are meningeal and parenchymal infections of bacterial, fungal, and viral origin. In addition to these underlying etiologies, precipitating factors are usually present as well; for example, withdrawal from alcohol, withdrawal of anticonvulsants in a patient with a brain tumor and seizures, and so forth. These immediate causes vary from community to community, but a prevalent pattern of triggering factors can be characteristic of a given community, and thus, as Leppic has recommended, it is wise for the physician to be familiar with the mechanisms particularly common in the locality.

Failure to consider the aforementioned etiologic problems can severely impair the effectiveness of the therapeutic effort. For example, many metabolically induced seizures are quite resistant to anticonvulsants, and failure to correct that discrepancy can greatly prolong an episode of status. The consequences of status are evident both in the central nervous system and systemically. Despite full support for the metabolic stresses induced by status, including correction of hypoxia, etc., after a period of about 60 minutes, irreversible neuronal damage progressively appears, indicating that prolonged epileptic activity is capable of inducing damage to the brain directly and must be controlled (1). Clinical examples include the prolonged memory deficits seen in cases of complex partial status and permanent paralysis of the involved area following elementary partial status. Leppik (10) has also reviewed the systemic consequences of generalized tonic-clonic seizures, and they are detailed below. If these problems are sought and recognized, and current methods of treatment applied, survival of the patient will depend on the nature of the underlying pathology rather than the severity of the seizures themselves. This point even extends to patients with primary generalized seizures in status who may be expected to do well with prompt treatment.

Therapeutic Intervention for Control of Status

Although most authors agree that status epilepticus, particularly of the generalized tonic-clonic variety, requires prompt intervention, there is some considerable variation in the particulars of achieving that end. Porter has pointed out that status may be considered to exist in a bipolar form, consisting on the one hand of repetitive seizures continuing as the ER physician watches, and the more common history of a flurry of seizures in which the most recent seizure occurred shortly before the patient presented at the ER. Both require immediate intervention. In the case of repetitive seizures, there is often little or no time for casual contemplation of a plan, and a well-thought-out course of action must be developed ahead of time. This approach may even be extended to the point of having a specific team designated for response to a patient in status. Rothner and Morris (6) have described the following series of steps, which should be carried out in the sequence described next, but as close to simultaneously as possible.

It is essential that the airway be assured, and this goal takes absolute precedence. Early intubation should be considered to avoid aspiration and assure an adequate airway throughout the resuscitation. This point is important not only because of the usual concerns regarding mechanical obstruction but also because of the respiratory supressant effect of many anticonvulsants employed. Vital signs must be quickly monitored, and the patient protected from inadvertent injury, particularly head injuries. A brief history and physical examination should be obtained; this examination should emphasize a search for occurrence of prior seizures, a history of head injury, current major medical problems, alcoholism and drug abuse, and most especially the patient's anticonvulsant history if available. As well, the examination should be highly focused to include a determination of the vital signs and to seek evidence of head injury. Because of the side effects of status described below, continued observation of vital signs must be maintained, just as with a cardiac arrest. While the above is being done, blood studies are drawn, to include anticonvulsant levels even if there is no history of use of such agents, for the obvious reason that the history may simply not be available. Even if rapid anticonvulsant level determinations are not available, baseline studies for later comparison are of value. Also, blood for glucose, electrolytes (to include calcium), hepatic and renal functions should be monitored. Occasionally overlooked, a toxicological screen is important especially in cases where drug abuse is strongly suspected, not only because of concern regarding etiology for the status but also for possible interactions with the medications used to treat the status. An arterial blood gas should be drawn as well. Urinary catheterization should be performed for urinalysis and to monitor urinary output as significant fluid loads may accompany treatment. A secure intravenous access should be established; obviously, a large-bore catheter is appropriate. Fluid therapy should begin with a bolus of 50 ml of 50% glucose. As a history of alcohol abuse and therefore Wernike's encephalopathy is frequently found in patients in status, and as glucose infusion places such individuals at great risk of a worsening of their encephalopathy, infusion of 50 mg of thiamine is also indicated. At this point anticonvulsant therapy is begun.

ANTICONVULSIVE THERAPY

Benzodiazepines

Porter (5) has given useful guidance regarding the most effective approach to anticonvulsant administration at this stage. For those with continuous generalized tonic-clonic seizures, there is general agreement that immediate infusion of a benzodiazepine is appropriate. On the other hand, in the case of patients with repetitive seizures manifesting in-between periods of stupor, one has the option of avoiding the use of benzodiazepines and pro-

ceeding directly to administration of diphenlhydantoin (Dilantin). There are advantages to this course of action. Benzodiazepines are effective depressants of respiration and blood pressure and synergize with at least phenobarbital to worsen those effects, further complicating patient care in the likely event that barbiturates are subsequently administered. Moreover, in the case of drug-induced status, further supression of vital functions may occur with addition of benzodiazepines. Finally, the anticonvulsant effect of benzodiazepines is long outlived by the sedating effect, which can impede recovery of alertness after termination of the status. Indeed, if the seizures are sufficiently separated in time, administration of benzodiazepines may actually interfere with the primary therapeutic goal, long-term control of seizures with long-acting anticonvulsants. Thus use of benzodiazepines can be supported in the instance of a patient with seizures requiring immediate, urgent control but should not be used simply as an automatic reaction to every situation in which seizure control is sought.

Should it be necessary to resort to benzodiazepines, there are currently two choices available: diazepam and lorazepam. Traditionally, diazepam (Valium) has been used for this purpose, but in the last few years, a new agent, lorazepam, has come into vogue. Valium found favor initially because it distributes rapidly and quickly achieves therapeutic levels in the brain. That rapid distribution, along with other factors, unfortunately limits the usefulness of diazepam as its period of anticonvulsant action is only 30 minutes. This fact means that breakthrough seizures are likely, and thus, this medication must be followed up with a long-acting agent even if seizures stop with diazepam. A constant infusion with diazepam is no longer considered effective. The alternate agent, lorazepam, has a longer duration of central nervous system (CNS) action, and in a large study, it was found that 4 mg of lorazepam was as effective as 10 mg of diazepam. Lorazepam is available in parenteral form and is administered intravenously as a 4 to 8 mg bolus. However, as with diazepam, the anticonvulsant effect of lorazepam manifests tachyphylaxis; that is, repeated doses become progressively less effective in supressing seizures. Also, because of ethical considerations, it has not been possible to determine the duration of action of this agent, although early reports suggested a considerably longer effective period than diazepam. Regardless of that, however, as with diazepam, administration of a long-acting anticonvulsant on the heels of the benzodiazepine is mandatory for long-term seizure control.

Phenytoin

The anticonvulsant most often employed initially is phenytoin (10). The choice is based on its efficacy in controlling seizures, a nearly 50-year experience with the drug, ready penetration of the nervous system on parenteral administration, and a relative lack of CNS suppression, which allows quick recovery of consciousness in patients in whom it stops seizures. In animal preparations, significant anticonvulsant levels are achieved in the brain in a matter of minutes, and it is primarily for this reason that many authorities recommend that this agent be employed as the first-line anticonvulsant in the treatment of status. This fact is especially true in those cases in which seizures are interspersed by periods of quiescence or in circumstances that do not otherwise demand immediate intervention with benzodiazepines.

Phenytoin has the disadvantage of producing unwanted cardiovascular effects, such as hypotension and arrhythmias, especially with rapid administration. The rate of administration must be carefully regulated, and this problem limits the usefulness of this agent in circumstances requiring very rapid achievement of seizure control. (Of course, this agent must be given intravenously as it is quite alkaline and precipitates in muscle if given by that route.) Porter (5) also gives useful recommendations regarding administration of phenytoin:

1. An infusion rate of 50 mg/minute avoids the risks of cardiac arrhythmia and hypotension mentioned above, although young individuals otherwise in good health may be able to accept 100 mg/minute dosage without difficulty.
2. A cardiac monitor is useful, especially when more rapid infusion rates are used.
3. Frequent blood pressure determinations are indicated as a monitor for hypotension. If hypotension occurs, it is an obvious indication to decrease the rate of phenytoin administration.
4. Parenteral phenytoin, because of the necessity to bring it into solution with a highly alkaline vehicle, precipitates in neutral and acidic solutions, for example 5% dextrose. Prompt precipitation occurs under these

circumstances and may occur even in saline preparations, particularly after 30 minutes. (Precipitation in the bloodstream presumably does not occur because of the avid adsorption of phenytoin by albumin.) Added advantages of direct administration are that it overcomes the uncertainty of administration of medication by non-physician personnel and obtains prompt achievement of therapeutic blood levels; also, significant fluid loading is avoided at a time when cerebral and pulmonary edema are real concerns.
5. Achievement of adequate blood levels is critical to the efficacy of phenytoin. The blood level sought by most authorities is $25\mu g/ml$, and in most cases this is achieved by administering 18 mg/kg. Toxicity from overdosage is less of a concern than cardiotoxicity from too rapid administration, as the former is primarily ataxia and unlikely to represent a problem in a patient who is most likely to be bedridden.

If seizure control is obtained, it is important to recall that blood levels of medication will be maintained for about 12–24 hours, and daily maintenance will have to begin about 12–18 hours after the initial administration of phenytoin. This therapy should be monitored with blood level determinations, and further parenteral dosages are not infrequently required, particularly in those patients with underlying pathology producing depression of consciousness.

Phenobarbital

About 40–50% of patients with convulsive status will not respond to intravenous phenytoin, and one must resort to phenobarbital, the other effective anticonvulsant available for parenteral use. As with phenytoin, phenobarbital quickly (in minutes) achieves peak brain levels. This medication inevitably produces sedation and possibly respiratory depression in the dosages required for supression of seizures, and the rate of administration does not significantly alter this. Thus most authorities recommend that a large loading dose (6–8 mg/kg) be administered, or if divided dosages are employed, that 10–20 mg/kg be given over 60–90 minutes. This dose should be administered even if it is more than the amount necessary to interrupt the status. Daily maintenance will need to begin about 12–24 hours later, and serum drug levels should be measured to assure therapeutic levels are achieved. This fact is especially true if drug-drug interactions or altered elimination of this medication is possible, e.g., in liver or renal disease. It is also important to realize that phenobarbital is a sedating drug and inevitably results in depression of a patient's level of consciousness in the dosages given above, and can significantly depress respiration and blood pressure, especially when a benzodiazepine has been used. Should seizures persist after the recommended dosages of phenobarbital have been administered, larger amounts can be used sufficient to achieve barbiturate coma with a burst-suppression pattern. This therapy should be performed under EEG control. Obviously under these circumstances, careful control of the airway must be emphasized again, as well as careful monitoring of blood pressure. An objection can be raised that phenobarbital, as it is a potent depressant, could worsen an already dangerous situation; however, if DPH fails, there are really few effective, efficient alternatives available beyond phenobarbital.

Paraldehyde, Lidocaine, and Valproate

Other medications have been used occasionally for control of seizures, including paraldehyde, lidocaine, and valproate. Paraldehyde is an agent with a long tradition of use in status epilepticus and about which little is actually known with confidence. It is a potentially quite toxic substance that when aged or exposed to light and heat is converted to acetic acid, an obviously dangerous property for any parenteral form. Intravenous administration is accompanied by serious risk of hypotension and pulmonary edema; for this reason it is given rectally at times. The latter route has variable rates of absorption and is therefore unreliable especially in cases of severe status. If the intravenous route is chosen, a solution of 4% paraldehyde in saline is used with dosages of 0.1–0.3 mg/kg given over about 30 minutes, with follow-up slow infusion of similar concentrations of the medication to control further seizures. Although it is possible to maintain a patient on paraldehyde for several days, long-acting anticonvulsants must be used eventually, and there is an urgency to this move, as dependence on this agent may appear. Paraldehyde is also incompatible with many of the plastics used in intravenous tubing, etc. and this problem also places obvious restrictions on its use. The drawbacks resulting from the above problems have led to its recent

withdrawal from general availability, still further diminishing its applicability for treatment of status. There is evidence to suggest that in the case of seizures due entirely to alcohol withdrawal, paraldehyde may be a drug of choice since it appears to suppress the appearance of delirium tremens beside being an effective anticonvulsant. Dilantin has been shown to be ineffective for such seizures. Paraldehyde may also be useful in cases in which the patient is allergic to more traditional agents.

Lidocaine is an agent that also has not been thoroughly studied in status, and the drug is somewhat paradoxical for use in this problem as it is known to be a convulsant agent in large doses. There is, nonetheless, evidence that it is effective for both generalized status and elementary partial status although it has variable brain distribution. Dosages of this agent are not well defined, however, the largest study recommends a single dose of 2–3 mg/kg, with an infusion of 3–10 mg/kg/hour if seizures persist. It should not be injected at rates greater than 25–50 mg/minute. It is considered nonsedating.

Valproate in general has been considered an adjunctive medication for status. It is as yet not available as a parenteral drug. Enemas of valproate were used originally to overcome this problem, although this practice has been subsequently replaced by the employment of suppositories, containing crushed 200-mg tablets. Rectal absorption is rapid and complete; following doses of 400 mg of valproate peak values are reached in 3–4 hours. On a 6 hourly dosage schedule, therapeutic plasma levels are reached in 24–48 hours and are well maintained. In most studies, valproate has not been used alone, and withdrawal of the other anticonvulsant, usually phenytoin, has precipitated a worsening or recurrence of seizures. There is also reason to believe that simultaneous administration of benzodiazepines with valproate may, through determined mechanisms, worsen seizures. Thus, the current role of valproate appears to be as an adjunct to phenytoin, to potentiate its effect and to "cover" a patient until therapeutic phenytoin levels are reached; it is possible that valproate may directly potentiate the effect of phenytoin.

EEG MONITORING

Although the termination of status may often appear clinically easy to recognize, this finding may be deceiving and at times EEG seizures may persist, presumably with the progressing neuronal damage that can follow prolonged seizures. For this reason EEG monitoring is always indicated when available. This test may be begun at any time during the course of treatment and should not take precedence over other life-saving interventions. A detailed discussion of the changes seen on the EEG is beyond the scope of this discussion; nevertheless it is worth recognizing that there is increasing awareness that somewhat specific EEG changes take place during most episodes of generalized tonic-clonic status and that these, when recognized, can give useful information about the progress toward control. There is increasing agreement that control of an episode of status cannot be considered achieved until EEG evidence of seizure activity is stopped as well. More prolonged monitoring, when available, is useful after the bout of status is over to further assure that there is no recurrence of the problem, a particularly significant point in obtunded patients in whom unrecognized recurrent seizures are a potential problem.

Medical Complications

Although the primary interest to this point has been pharmacologic treatment of status, it is important to realize that there are a number of medical complications of generalized tonic-clonic status that must be recognized. Simon has enumerated a number of these (11). Hyperthermia occurs frequently in status and is felt to be the result primarily of increased motor activity. Temperatures of 107°F have been reported, and this finding tends to parallel the duration and severity of the status. These temperature elevations may occur independent of infection, although infection must be ruled out. Thus, heat stress must be considered a risk of status. Hypothermia has also been reported in status, and in the majority it has been the result of drug effects and metabolic derangements such as hypoglycemia and hypothyroidism.

Another frequently encountered problem is leukocytosis, which can range above 25,000 cells/mm^3 in the absence of any sign of infection. Up to 50% of patients demonstrate this effect, and it may manifest with either a polymorphonuclear or lymphocytic predominance. As Simon points out, there is rarely a shift toward immature forms, and that is a potential means of differentiating this phenomenon from a true infection. There may also

be a mild cerebrospinal fluid pleocytosis; this finding has been reported in 2–6% of patients and consists of cell counts not exceeding 80 cells/mm^3 with an initial polymorphonuclear predominance, although in days this count may tend to lymphocytosis. There may also be a slight elevation of CSF protein. Obviously, the critical point here is to rule out infection before the decision is made that the above mechanisms are in operation.

A significant acidosis as a result of lactate production also occurs, and up to one-half of patients have pH values less than 7.0 during status. The acidosis probably results from the vigorous muscle activity occasioned by the seizures, as it can be suppressed by motor paralysis. Although this acidosis would appear to increase the risk of development of a hyperkalemia and resultant cardiac arrhythmia, fortunately that does not seem to occur. There is also little evidence that the degree of acidosis correlates with the neurological outcome, and it rapidly resolves with cessation of seizures, and thus does not represent one of the potentially more serious effects of status.

Pulmonary edema can also occur with generalized tonic-clonic status: in one series over one-third of patients with status had this problem. It probably results at least in part from elevated pulmonary pressures that have been recorded in status. There, however, remains considerable uncertainty about the precise mechanism of this pulmonary edema. Pneumonia is also an unfortunately common accompaniment of status and can result from aspiration. The pulmonary vascular changes that accompany status may also contribute to this problem. Cardiac arrhythmias are common during status, and again extreme care must be used when administering anticonvulsants such as Dilantin.

The anoxia that can accompany status may also exacerbate underlying neurological dysfunction, and the medial temporal lobe and cerebellum are particularly susceptible. Recent work suggests that this problem may not be evident for as long as 24 hours or more following status, and reinforces the need for vigorous efforts to prevent anoxia during status.

Renal failure can also occur with resultant oliguria and uremia and may be associated with renal tubular necrosis and lower nephron nephrosis. The resultant hyperkalemia and azotemia obviously have the potential for increasing the likelihood of further seizures. Rhabdomyolysis is probably a significant factor in this issue, both from the vigorous muscle effort, and from pressure on dependent muscles after prolonged recumbency as in coma. The hyperpyrexia mentioned above may also contribute, with release of large amounts of myoglobin and resultant lower nephron nephrosis possibly leading to acute renal failure. The above factors associated with the profound sweating seen in status can lead to dehydration and marked electrolyte and osmolarity problems. This problem can be further worsened by alterations in blood glucose levels. Initially hyperglycemia may occur during an episode of status probably as the result of the profound sympathetic discharge that accompanies the event. The subsequent hypoglycemia that may follow is probably related to consumption of glucose by muscle and brain and by increased plasma insulin levels. Such a hypoglycemia might be harmful if sufficiently prolonged and could actually be a factor contributing to the precipitation of further seizures. As such it should be guarded against. Yet, hyperglycemia can also be harmful to the cerebrum under certain circumstances, for example during the course of a stroke; thus, the best advice that can be given is to maintain the blood glucose levels as close to the normal range as possible.

It is perhaps needless to say that primary causes of the deviations listed above must also be ruled out. It is also obvious that there are significant complexities in the treatment of tonic clonic status, and in general these require admission to an intensive care facility, at least until the status is controlled. There are certain exceptions to this rule, particularly patients who are otherwise known to be well but who are in status secondary to drug overdosage or other limited process; however, these are in the minority and the safest course is to admit the patient to an intensive care setting.

Postintervention Treatment

Also, the period following control of the status is critical. There is a natural tendency to consider the problem resolved when seizures have been controlled. This is a major error, and indeed, can be considered a fundamental point in the care of a patient with status. Aside from treatment of any underlying illnesses involved in the status, the major goal at this point is to establish a regimen that will both maintain control of the patient's seizure disorder and not result in toxicity. This approach will frequently require adjustments not only in dosage, but also in the kind of anticonvulsant administered. The major principles regarding anticonvulsant choice are the desirability of monotherapy and the recognition that nonsedating anticonvulsants are preferable. Both of the major anticonvulsants recommended in preceding sections (Dilantin and particularly phenobarbital) are sedating, and as a result it will almost certainly be preferrable to convert the patient to an oral monotherapy with the currently preferred agent for generalized tonic-clonic status, carbamazepine. This change must be done in a fashion that will not leave the patient uncovered by anticonvulsant therapy. Thus, one should begin with a carbamazepine dosage of about 200 mg four times a day, with the expectation that stable blood levels will be reached in 3–4 days. After that has been accomplished, an effort should be made to withdraw the most sedating agent, usually phenobarbital. This change can be done abruptly, as long as therapeutic levels of carbamazepine are maintained, for the long half-life of phenobarbital results in a gradual reduction of its blood level. Following this, withdrawal of Dilantin can be attempted as well.

An alternative anticonvulsant that can be employed for those patients with generalized tonic-clonic seizures is valproate, which is considered by some as a primary therapeutic agent for generalized seizures. Use of this agent in patients who are receiving phenobarbital must be approached with caution as valproate can significantly prolong the half-life of barbiturates, causing deep sedation and, potentially, coma. Also, many if not most tonic-clonic seizures in adulthood are secondarily generalized and valproate may not be effective in suppressing the underlying focal seizures. Thus, the circumstances surrounding the individual case require a tailored approach, and for that reason more specific recommendations cannot be made regarding long-term therapy. Since the treatment of seizure disorder is a long-term problem in which a strong patient-physician relationship must be developed, the involvement of the patient's primary-care giver should be sought if at all possible to allow coordinated long-term planning. Certainly the patient will require, even in the best of circumstances, observation in the hospital to recover from the effects of the status (which may produce significant depression for several days independent of medication effects and the underlying disease); during this time the careful monitoring of anticonvulsant levels should be undertaken and oral administration of anticonvulsants should be begun as soon as possible to achieve the basic goal of a course of therapy, the establishment of a therapeutically effective steady state of anticonvulsant medication. Oral loading dosages can be employed for this purpose, and, except for Dilantin, an initial dosage of twice the maintenance dosage can be tried, with the expectation that a therapeutic blood level will be established in 24 hours. This approach is more complicated than might be appreciated at first glance because of drug-drug interactions, making this an effort that must be guided by careful monitoring of blood levels. Also, it is frequently the case that initiation of large dosages can produce unwanted side effects, including gastrointestinal discomfort, particularly in the case of carbamazepine. Particular caution is warranted in the case of Dilantin, because the zero-order kinetics of this agent with drug levels in the therapeutic range make it particularly easy to overshoot into the toxic range. When circumstances permit, and this is a matter of judgement, consideration can be given to starting therapy at the maintenance dosage level, which may avoid many of the problems just stated.

NONCONVULSIVE STATUS AND ELEMENTARY PARTIAL STATUS

In addition to the most common form of status, generalized tonic-clonic status, several other forms of status are encountered, including nonconvulsive status and elementary partial status. Although these forms are not immediately life-threatening as is generalized tonic-clonic status, they are nevertheless associated with sufficiently significant complications that they also warrant immediate intervention. The first category is nonconvulsive status, and as the name implies, consists of seizures without a tonic-clonic component. The name was often taken to be synonymous with complex partial seizures, however, presently is considered to consist of two seizure types, complex partial seizures and adult onset absence status, sometimes called "petit mal". The latter is poorly named as the relation to the classic absence of childhood is problematical at best. The second category is elementary partial status.

Complex partial status is an entity that until recently was considered rare because few cases

had been reported (7, 12). Yet, at least one to two cases yearly can be expected in large referral centers, and recognition is important. Recognition of the various types of complex status that may occur usually requires specialized closed-circuit monitoring techniques. It is sufficient to say that complex partial status may be suspected when a patient manifests repeated episodes, usually with distinctive onset, of alterations of consciousness possibly associated with automatisms followed by a gradual progression toward recovery of full consciousness, if another episode does not intervene. There are clear-cut episodes, distinguishing this from the other likely diagnosis, adult onset absence status. In the case of the latter, there will more likely be a continued fluctuation of consciousness, with intervals of apparent relatively normal responsiveness grading into marked confusion, rather than a few distinct bouts of loss of consciousness.

The EEG can be of real value in differentiating complex partial status from absence status. It is again beyond the scope of this discussion to detail these, and the interested reader is referred to any of the several monographs listed among the references, that describe these in detail. The pertinence in differentiating these is based on the differences in anticonvulsants appropriate for each, and the recognition that improperly treated complex partial status have as a dire consequence the risk of prolonged memory deficit particularly. For this form of nonconvulsive status, initial treatment with lorazapam and then phenytoin as in generalized tonic-clonic status is appropriate; phenobarbital can be added if necessary, as in generalized status. This approach is appropriate as these seizures may easily secondarily generalize if not controlled. Determining that the seizures have stopped may be difficult, and, if available, the EEG may be of assistance. Adult onset absence status also responds to benzodiazepines, especially diazepam. That agent is used in dosages similar to the treatment of generalized tonic-clonic status, although the efficacy of lorazepam has not been established for this purpose. Following that, a maintenance anticonvulsant appropriate for absence seizures should be begun, for example, valproate. If that cannot be tolerated, and if the patient does not have generalized tonic-clonic seizures, ethosuximide can be used in the dosages given previously. If both of these are unsatisfactory, the third choice of anticonvulsant is Tegretol. For patients in whom a benzodiazepine fails to control the seizures, rectal valproate can be considered although the efficacy of this therapy has not been established. Dosages are as described previously for that agent.

The final entity to be considered is elementary partial status, sometimes called "epilepsia partialis continua." This condition usually consists of progressively spreading seizures that focally involve the motor cortex on one side, very often recruiting body parts in the order represented by the motor cortical homunculus (Jacksonian march), and that recur repeatedly. These seizures are often intermixed with myoclonias that may involve other parts of the body. The EEG often shows diffuse slowing and epileptiform rhythms may appear from a variety of foci, at times distant from the rolandic area, which is consistent with the observation that these focal seizures are associated with multifocal brain pathology. Treatment is aimed at preventing further spread of these seizures and discovering the underlying cause. Anticonvulsant therapy is similar to that for generalized tonic-clonic seizures, save that the urgency of administration is not so great, and if therapeutic levels of phenytoin do not control the seizures, most authorities agree that administration of phenobarbital should not produce blood levels exceeding the upper limits of the therapeutic range. Control of these seizures is often quite difficult and the toxicity of the agents used may exceed the risks from the focal seizures themselves.

References

1. Celesia G: Prognosis in convulsive status epilepticus. In Delgado-Escueta AV et al (eds): *Advances in Neurology Vol 34: Status Epilepticus*. New York, Raven Press, 1983, chap 5, pp 55–59.
2. Gastaut H. Classification of status epilepticus. In Delgado-Escueta AV et al (eds): *Advances in Neurology Vol 34: Status Epilepticus*. New York, Raven Press, 1983, chap 2, pp 15–35.
3. Klawans HL, Carvey PM, Tanner CM, Goetz, CG: Drug-induced myoclonus. In Fahn S et al (eds): *Myoclonus*. New York, Raven Press, 1986, pp 251–264.
4. Messing RO, Closson RG, Simon RP: Drug-induced seizures: a 10 year experience. *Neurology* 34:1582–1586, 1984.
5. Porter RJ: *Epilepsy: 100 Elementary Principles*. Philadelphia, WB Saunders, 1984.
6. Rothner AD, Morris HH: Generalized status epilepticus. In Luders H et al (eds): *Epilepsy: Electroclinical Syndromes*. New York, Springer Verlag, 1987, chap 10, pp 207–222.
7. Sharbrough FW: Complex partial seizures. In Luders H et al (eds): *Epilepsy: Electroclinical Syndromes*. New York, Springer Verlag, 1987, chap 12, pp 279–302.
8. Simon RP, Aminoff MJ: Electroencephalographic status epilepticus in fatal anoxic coma. *Ann Neurol* 20:351–355, 1986.
9. Hauser WA: Status epilepticus: frequency, etiology, and neurologic sequelae. In Delgaso-Esqueta AV (eds): *Advances in Neurology. Vol 34: Status Epilepticus*. New York, Raven Press, 1984, chap 1, 1984, pp 3–14.
10. Leppik IE, Patrick BK, Cranford RE: Treatment of acute seizures and status epilepticus with intravenous phenytoin. In Delgado-Esqueta AV et al (eds): *Advances in Neurology. Vol 34: Status Epilepticus*. New York, Raven Press, 1984, chap 45, pp 447–451.
11. Simon RP: Physiologic consequences of status epilepticus. *Epilepsia* 26 (Suppl 1):S58–S66, 1985.
12. Treiman DM, Delgado-Esqueta AV: Complex partial status epilepticus. In *Advances in Neurology. Vol 34: Status Epilepticus*. New York, Raven Press, 1984, chap 7, pp 69–81.

26

Analgesics

Frank Balestrieri, D.D.S., M.D.

PAIN SENSATION

Pain is defined as "an unpleasant sensory and emotional experience associated with actual or potential tissue damage, or described in terms of such damage" (64). Pain is a personal and subjective experience that each individual learns through life, as actual or potential tissue-damaging experiences are encountered. Pain is also an unpleasant experience with an associated emotional response. The emotional or psychologic state of the patient may result in pain in the absence of tissue damage or other pathology. The emotional or psychologic state of the patient may modify the character of the pain.

The nociceptor activity initiated by a noxious stimulus is not pain. Rather, pain is the conscious psychologic state, usually resulting from a noxious stimulus but not requiring one. It consists of sensory, emotional, and cognitive elements arising from very complex and, as yet, incompletely understood activities within the central nervous system.

Although pain is subjective and difficult to define, it is clear that critically ill patients experience pain. The critically ill not only are often subjected to major physical injury, but also suffer sleeplessness, noise, trauma, frequent handling, and fear. Our knowledge of patients' experiences during a critical illness is mostly anecdotal. Ian Donald, a gynecologist-obstetrician, described his own intensive care unit (ICU) experience following three heart operations (30, 31). He points out that the patient's state of mind is paramount and of more importance than the most powerful analgesics. Other factors that modify the experience of pain are past experience, knowledge of the postoperative routine, and fear. Donald stresses the importance of the preoperative anesthetist's visit, the need for sympathy from attendants,, and the importance of preventing pain or treating it early. Fortunately, he points out, the memory of pain fades mercifully and quickly. Similar anecdotal reports are those of Henschel (53) who describes his ICU experience with Guillain Barre syndrome, and Shovelton (110) who had a thymectomy for myasthenia gravis.

Larger and more controlled studies of patients' perception of pain (55, 69, 96, 104) indicate that pain is an important concern of those patients that remember their ICU time, but many remember only a part or none of their stay. Since there is no method of predicting which patients will remember the pain associated with an ICU experience, it is necessary for the staff involved in the patient's care to be alert to the signs and symptoms of pain and to render appropriate relief. The problem of what constitutes appropriate pain relief and how best to administer it has not been well studied or defined.

The treatment of postoperative surgical pain has received much attention, and present-day pain regimens have been widely criticized (41, 138). A number of studies document that the medical profession's attitude toward pain is, or may be perceived as, cruel and callous (21, 35–38, 129, 134). Effective pain management in the critical care setting requires effective use of narcotic analgesia (2, 59), better use established techniques of regional anesthesia, and further study and use of new techniques such as continuous narcotic infusions (14, 16, 74, 120) and epidural and intrathecal narcotic administration (10, 135, 136, 143).

PAIN MECHANISMS

Peripheral Receptors

Prior to the 19th century, Aristotle's view of pain as an emotion opposite to pleasure was widely accepted. With the work of Bell (8) and Magendie in the early 1800s, pain became recognized as a sensation. Cutaneous receptors

475

were described by von Frey (42), who proposed a specific receptive and transmission system for various cutaneous sensory modalities including pain. The opposite view, of functional nonspecificity of nerve endings, was proposed by Lele and Weddell (80). We now know that three categories of cutaneous receptors are present: mechanoreceptors, thermoreceptors, and nociceptors (62). These peripheral receptors have been classified on the basis of their morphology (63) and the correlation of structure with function (e.g., Pacinian corpuscles, Golgi-Mazzoni receptors, hair follicle receptors, Meissner corpuscles, Merkel "touch spots," and Ruffini endings). Nevertheless, there are no anatomic structures defined for most sensory cutaneous functions. One can classify nerve fibers and human peripheral receptors (25, 101, 105, 125) (Table 26.1). The cutaneous mechanoreceptors are supplied by large myelinated fibers, whereas the cutaneous nociceptors are supplied by fine myelinated (A δ) and unmyelinated (C) fibers. Animal studies indicate that the cutaneous nociceptors have two characteristic features: a progressive augmenting response to repeated or increasing noxious stimuli (sensitization) and a high threshold to all natural stimuli relative to other receptors in the same tissue (100). Sensitization is produced by a number of chemicals (56, 90) (bradykinin, histamine, serotonin, and a prostaglandin), and can be reduced by anti-inflammatory drugs such as indomethacin and aspirin (70, 75). Another study by Jansco et al. (67) suggests the possibility of a single

cutaneous receptor that responds to capsaicin, a chemical toxin, when applied to the skin. Treatment with capsaicin depletes the cutaneous nerve endings of substance P, an 11-amino-acid peptide. It is speculated that substance P may mediate noxious thermal and chemical stimuli, possibly at the first afferent synapse (57).

There are many peripheral receptors capable of transmitting noxious mechanical, thermal, and chemical stimuli. Peripheral receptors also demonstrate some specificity, but most are polymodal, that is, responding to more than one form of noxious event. It is clear that the exact mechanisms of peripheral cutaneous nociception are poorly understood and that more information is needed before interruption of nociceptive information at the periphery is possible. The function and relationship of muscle, joint, and visceral nociception is also quite unclear.

Peripheral receptors occur in association with nerve fiber innervation by the sympathetic nervous system. Increased sympathetic nervous system activity may increase the sensitivity of the various peripheral pain receptors. Indeed, increased sympathetic activity following surgery or trauma is thought to be the cause for the pain of reflex sympathetic dystrophy (causalgia). The pain of reflex sympathetic dystrophy is characterized by hyperalgesia over the affected limb, by dry skin, and by decreased activity of the limb due to severe pain. The pain and functional disability associated with this syndrome may be relieved by sequential

Table 26.1
Classification of Nerve Fibers and Peripheral Receptors with Conduction Velocities

Class	Function	Diameter (μm)	Conduction Velocity (m/sec)
A$_\alpha$	Motor	12–20	70–120
A$_\beta$	Pressure/touch	5–12	30–70
A$_\delta$	Proprioception	5–12	30–70
A$_\delta$	Pain/temperature (mechanical, heat and cold sensation)	1–4	12–30
B	Preganglionic autonomic (sympathetic)	1–3	14
C			
Cutaneous nociceptors	Pain/temperature (polymodal, mechanical, and cold sensation)	0.5–1	1.2
Cutaneous mechanoreceptors Type I Type II	Sense skin indentation		55
Meissner corpuscle	Sense skin indentation		55
Pacinian corpuscle	Sense pressure changes		50
Warm	Sense increased temperature		0.5

sympathetic blocks, by the application of lo-cally acting or centrally acting drugs that block the effect of norepinephrine at the sympathetic nerve ending, or by surgical sympathectomy.

CENTRAL MECHANISMS

The cell bodies of primary afferent fibers are located in the dorsal root ganglia and tri-geminal sensory ganglia. Normally, activity be-gins in the periphery, and the action potential travels past the dorsal root ganglia cells, which may depolarize, before entering the dorsal horn layers (81).

The dorsal roots provide the pathway by which axons from the peripheral somatic nerves enter the spinal cord. A dermatomal distribu-tion of the dorsal roots exists (26), and over-lapping of primary afferent fibers occurs within the dorsal horn (4). Axons in any given dorsal root may extend over five or more spinal cord segments. This fact implies that any point on the body is supplied by two adjoining dorsal roots. As the large and small fibers enter the dorsal horn, the large fibers separate and enter the dorsal columns, with collaterals entering the dorsal horn. The small fine fibers enter separately, forming a longitudinal tract bearing Lissauer's name (82). The dorsolateral fascic-ulus (Lissauer's tract) contains mainly fine pri-mary afferent fibers (15, 72) and fibers from the substantia gelatinosa (89).

The ventral roots also contain myelinated and unmyelinated sensory fibers (18, 19, 29). These fibers arise from the dorsal root ganglion cells and represent from 15% to 30% of axons in the ventral roots (87). The presence of these sensory fibers in the ventral roots may provide a portion of the explanation for the failure of dorsal rhizotomy to result in complete relief of pain.

The spinal cord comprises a central gray zone and an outer white zone. The central gray matter can be divided into 10 groups based on cell morphology (Fig. 26.1) (108). The cell groups I and VI are involved in sensory trans-mission and make up the dorsal horn.

The marginal zone of Waldeyer, lamina I, receives excitatory input from primary affer-ents, and receives inhibitory input from the substantia gelatinosa (94). The marginal zone cells respond to noxious mechanical, thermal and polymodal stimulation, as well as innoc-uous thermal change (76).

The cells of the substantia gelatinosa may be classified according to their projections: (a)

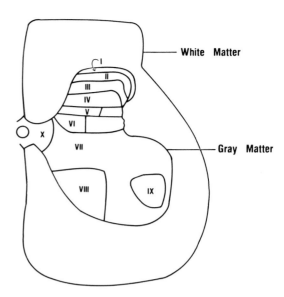

Figure 26.1. Spinal cord laminae. I, marginal zone; II and III, substantia gelatinosa; IV, V and VI, nucleus proprius; VII, VIII, IX and X, motor areas (Adapted from Rexed B: Cytoarchitectonic organization of the spinal cord in the cat. *Comp Neurol* 96:415–495, 1952.)

short axon cells that remain within the dorsal horn, (b) cells with axons that enter the tract of Lissauer or propriospinal pathways, (c) cells with two axons, (d) spinothalamic tract neu-rons (44, 48, 71, 141). Afferent input into the substantia gelatinosa is by way of collaterals of large primary afferents and fine primary afferents and their collaterals (15, 72, 77). Nu-merous complex synaptic connections occur in the region of the substantia gelatinosa, which functions as an integrator of sensory input (126).

The nucleus proprius (laminae IV, V and VI) responds to cutaneous stimulation from me-chanoreceptors and tactile receptors (narrow dynamic range), and pressure and pinching (wide dynamic range). Lamina VI cells re-spond to joint movement (132), and somatic and visceral input is received by other neurons in the nucleus proprius (52).

ASCENDING PATHWAYS OF THE SPINAL CORD

The spinothalamic and spinoreticular tracts are the most significant ascending pathways for the transmission of nociceptive input in humans. Axons from second-order neurons in laminae I, IV, V, and VI cross the midline to ascend as the lateral and ventral spinothalamic tracts (73). The spinothalamic tracts travel to the posterior thalamic nuclei and the ventroposterolateral nuclei of the thalamus and then to the cerebral cortex. They relay tactile information as well as nociception.

It is clear that mechanisms of pain transmission involve extremely complex connections in diverse areas of the central nervous system, many of which have yet to be defined.

NARCOTIC ANALGESICS

Analgesic medications are classified as strong or mild and subdivided into narcotic or nonnarcotic categories. Narcotics are either naturally occurring, semisynthetic, or synthetic (Table 26.2). Morphine, codeine, and papaverine (the only naturally occurring clinically significant narcotics) are obtained from the poppy plant, *Papaver somniferum*. Opium is the dried powdered mixture of alkaloids obtained from the unripe seed capsules of the poppy plant, which contains more than 20 pharmacologically active natural alkaloids. These alkaloids are of two chemical classes,

the phenanthrenes (morphine and codeine) and the benzylisoquinolines (papaverine).

The semisynthetic narcotics are derivatives of morphine. Codeine results from the etherification of one hydroxyl group, heroin from the esterification of both hydroxyl groups, and hydromorphone (Dilaudid) from oxidation of the alcoholic hydroxyl group to a ketone group, or saturation of a double bond on the benzene ring (50).

The synthetic narcotics resemble morphine but are usually entirely synthesized. They include the morphinians (levorphanol), the propionanilides (methadone, d-propoxyphene), the benzomorphans (pentazocine, phenazocine, cyclazocine), and the phenylpiperidines (meperidine, fentanyl, sufentanil, alfentanil).

MECHANISMS OF ANALGESIA

Morphine and other narcotic analgesics produce their major effects on the central nervous system and the gastrointestinal tract. The major effects of opiates include analgesia, mood changes (euphoria or dysphoria), drowsiness, respiratory depression, cough suppression, de-

Table 26.2
Classification and Dosage of Some Narcotic Agonists and Antagonists

Drug (Trade Name)	Dose (in 70-kg adult)		Dose Interval (hr)	Comparative Narcotic Potency
	i.v. (mg)	i.m./s.c. (mg)		
NATURAL ALKALOIDS OF OPIUM				
Morphine	2–10 (titrate)	5–10	2–4	1
Codeine	30–60	60–120	2–4	0.1
SEMISYNTHETIC DERIVATIVES				
Hydromorphone (Dilaudid)	0.5–1 (titrate)	2	3–4	5
Oxymorphone (Numorphan)	0.5 (titrate)	1	3–4	10
SYNTHETIC DERIVATIVES				
Meperidine (Demerol, etc.)	25–100 (titrate)	50–100	2–4	0.1
Methadone (Dolophine, etc.)	2–5 (titrate)	2–10	2–4	1.2
Pentazocine (Talwin)	10–30 (titrate)	30	3–4	0.25
Fentanyl (Sublimaze)	0.05–0.1 (titrate)	0.1	½–2	150
NARCOTIC ANTAGONISTS				
Naloxone (Narcan)	0.2–0.4	0.4	½–¾	
Nalorphine (Nalline)	5–10		p.r.n.	
Levallorphan (Lorfan)	1		p.r.n.	

creased gastrointestinal motility, nausea, vomiting, and alterations of endocrine and autonomic nervous system function. It is now clear that opiates act as agonists, interacting with saturable, stereospecific binding sites or receptors in the central nervous system and other sites (102, 112, 123, 151). These binding sites are unevenly distributed throughout the central nervous system. They are present in highest concentration in the limbic system (frontal and temporal cortex, amygdala, and hippocampus), thalamus, corpus striatum, hypothalamus, midbrain and spinal cord (111).

Narcotic analgesic compounds demonstrate stereospecific receptor binding and reversal of effects by narcotic antagonists. Structurally, narcotics are complex, three-dimensional compounds that usually exist as optical isomers (115). Usually only the levorotatory isomer is capable of producing analgesia, and a close relationship exists between the stereochemical structure of a narcotic and its activity (6). Significant variation in pharmacologic activity may result from conformational changes in the molecule produced by a changing pH (5). Most narcotics have a relatively rigid T-shaped conformation, an electron-rich hydroxyl or ketone group, a positively charged basic nitrogen, a quaternary carbon that is separated from the basic nitrogen by an ethane chain, and a flat benzene or 2-thienyl ring, which is 4.58 angstroms from the nitrogen (115).

It is now known that there is more than one type of opiate receptor, and that different receptors may be involved in different functions (45, 83, 86). Opiate receptors may differ in both their affinity for various opiates and opiate antagonists and thereby in their physiologic significance. Various classifications have been proposed to distinguish between receptor types. One classification separates receptors into high- and low-affinity groups. The high-affinity receptors mediate analgesia, whereas the low-affinity receptors are associated with respiratory depression (97, 98). Wood classifies opiate receptors into four groups: (a) the μ-receptor (morphine receptor), (b) the K-receptor (cyclazocine receptor), (c) the σ-receptor, and (d) the δ-receptor. The μ-receptor mediates supraspinal analgesia, respiratory depression, feelings of well-being, euphoria, and a morphine-type physical dependence. The σ receptor mediates feelings of dysphoria, hallucinations, mydriasis, hypotension, and respiratory stimulation. Finally, the δ-receptor mediates some of the in vitro pharmacological effects of the enkephalins and endorphins. There is also a claim for a possible fifth narcotic receptor, the E-receptor. The current classification of opioid-type drugs into agonists, antagonists, and agonists-antagonists type opioids has been based on this receptor concept.

TOLERANCE AND DEPENDENCE

Tolerance to some of the effects of narcotic analgesics may develop rapidly. It develops most quickly to the depressant actions (respiratory depression, sedation, analgesia), and more slowly to the excitatory effects. Tolerance is evident 4 hours after commencement of a morphine infusion in the experimental animal (20) and is likely after 6–8 consecutive administrations in humans. The mechanisms of tolerance are unclear (93). Cross tolerance occurs within members of the narcotic analgesics but does not extend to other central acting medications. Tolerance may be considerable; a narcotic addict may tolerate up to 500 times the clinical dose of morphine.

Physical dependence on opiates is of minor importance in patients receiving morphine for postoperative pain, or in those receiving opiates for relief of terminal cancer pain. Many physicians are unnecessarily reluctant to utilize therapeutically effective doses of opiates in acute pain, for fear of inducing severe physical dependence. Tolerance may be an early sign of physical dependence, but is usually associated with dependence. After a 1- to 2-week course of clinical doses of opiates, mild withdrawal symptoms may be detected, but in most patients the symptoms pass unnoticed. Should a narcotic antagonist or agonist-antagonist be administered, more severe withdrawal may be precipitated. The symptoms of withdrawal are generally opposite to the effects of the narcotic analgesics (e.g., diarrhea, hyperventilation, mydriasis) except for nausea and vomiting, which may be both an effect of opiates and a withdrawal symptom. Deaths have occurred during narcotic withdrawal but probably are not due to the withdrawal symptoms per se (46).

NARCOTIC AGONISTS

Morphine

Morphine (Fig. 26.2) is the prototype narcotic analgesic and the most widely used. It is

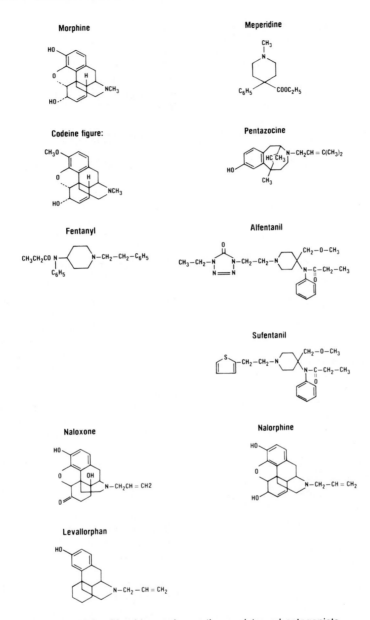

Figure 26.2. Morphine and narcotic agonists and antagonists.

examined here in detail and serves as a basis for understanding the pharmacology of other narcotic analgesics.

ABSORPTION

Morphine may be administered via the oral, subcutaneous, intramuscular, or intravenous routes. When given orally, as in Brompton's solution, a 10-mg dose in the average adult patient results in a plasma concentration of about 10 ng/ml within 15 minutes (11) (Fig. 26.3). Plasma concentration is maintained between 8 and 10 ng/ml for 45–60 minutes and then gradually decreases to about 1 ng/ml at 8 hours. Morphine is readily absorbed from the gut, but plasma levels are considerably lower after oral administration than after parenteral administration. This finding is secondary to uptake and metabolism of the morphine by the

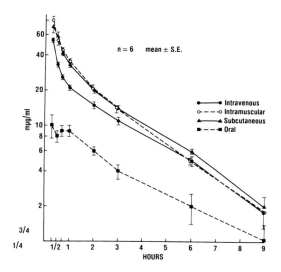

Figure 26.3. Plasma concentrations of unchanged morphine in volunteers after a dose of approximately 10 mg (5.75 mg/m²). (Adapted from Brunk SF, Delle M: Morphine metabolism in man. *Clin Pharmacol Ther* 16:51–57, 1974.)

liver and intestinal mucosa prior to reaching the central circulation (first-pass effect). There also exists an enterohepatic circulation for morphine that accounts for the observed second peak in plasma concentration in humans and animals that occurs about 30–40 minutes after oral ingestion (11, 65).

Subcutaneously administered morphine results in rapid absorption with plasma levels of unchanged morphine of about 70 ng/ml 15 minutes after injection of 10 mg in a 70-kg subject (11). The plasma levels decline progressively from the peak (Fig. 26.3).

Intramuscular injection also results in rapid absorption, with plasma concentrations of 80 ng/ml 15 minutes after administration. As with subcutaneous injection, plasma concentration decreases rapidly. Since muscle blood flow varies greatly in humans at rest (39), and even more so with activity, the rate of absorption varies. This fact explains the wide variations observed in time-to-peak plasma levels following intramuscular injection and the reports of poor pain control after intramuscular narcotic injections (3).

Intravenous injection of morphine bypasses the absorption process. Peak plasma levels are higher than by any of the other routes (11). Metabolism and distribution are more rapid since first-order kinetics operate. Plasma levels decrease rapidly, since there is no sustained

absorption phase. Plasma levels after 10 mg of intravenously administered morphine in 70-kg subjects are about 50 ng/ml 15 minutes after injection, which is lower than after intramuscular or subcutaneous administration (11). They subsequently remain lower for 3–4 hours (Fig. 26.3).

Morphine has been injected into the epidural and spinal subarachnoid spaces (136, 139). On the whole, the plasma levels of morphine are proportional to the dose, but there is wide variation (139). These routes of administration may provide a useful method of pain relief, especially in the ICU, where continuous epidural and subarachnoid catheters can be readily employed.

DISTRIBUTION

In addition to the central nervous system, morphine is readily taken up and concentrated by the parenchymal tissues of the lungs, kidney, liver, spleen, and muscle. The amount of morphine found in the brain is much smaller than that found in the parenchymal tissues. Morphine has a low oil/water partition coefficient and therefore penetrates cellular barriers more slowly and accumulates to a lesser degree in the lipid compartment. Morphine therefore tends to distribute more to tissues in which it is ionized, bound, or actively transported.

EXCRETION

Hepatic metabolism is by far the most important route for the elimination of morphine in humans and animals (92). Minor routes for excretion include the urine, bile, and saliva. Biotransformation of morphine occurs mainly by glucuronic acid conjugation. Morphine-3-glucuronide, the principle metabolite, is essentially not active due to its polarity and is readily excreted by both glomerular filtration and active tubular transport (11, 60).

RESPIRATORY SYSTEM

Morphine exerts a direct depressant effect on the medullary respiratory centers and affects the pontine centers involved in respiratory rhythmicity. Initially respiratory rate is affected more than tidal volume, but as the dose of morphine is increased, tidal volume and minute ventilation decrease and periodic breathing and apnea occur (47, 140). A 10-mg dose of morphine (0.15 mg/kg) decreases tidal

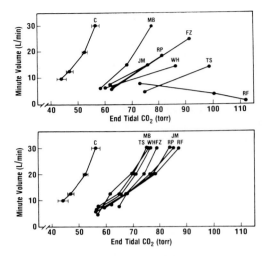

Figure 26.4. Naloxone reversal of morphine: $PaCO_2$/ventilation response curves after morphine 2 mg/kg. Curve C is the averaged control. *Top,* Before naloxone. *Bottom,* after antagonism by naloxone. (Adapted from Johnstone RE et al: Reversal of morphine anesthesia with naloxone. *Anesthesiology* 41:361–367, 1974.)

volume and respiratory rate while increasing resting $PaCO_2$ by about 3 torr in normal subjects (34). Respiratory depression is even more marked when evaluated in terms of the expected ventilatory response to hypercarbia (34, 114). At higher doses of morphine (e.g., 2 mg/kg) not only is the $PaCO_2$ ventilation response curve displaced to the right, but the slope is reduced (Fig. 26.4) and can be partially reversed by naloxone (68). The administration of large doses of morphine for cardiac surgical operations may prolong the postoperative length of assisted ventilation. This effect is particularly important for patients undergoing valve replacement and is not observed in patients having myocardial revascularization procedures (7). These observed differences are likely due to different rates of excretion of morphine, secondary to the overall lower cardiac indices and therefore lower hepatic and renal blood flows in patients that have valve surgery (118).

Although patients demonstrate respiratory depression after morphine administration, they usually increase their tidal volume and respiratory rate on command if they are still conscious, demonstrating that voluntary respiratory control remains intact. Morphine may be dangerous in those critically ill patients with respiratory compromise (e.g., asthma, COPD, severe pneumonia,, restrictive lung disease) and should be used cautiously. Morphine also has central antitussive properties and may in-

terfere with pulmonary toilet in the critically ill patient.

CARDIOVASCULAR SYSTEM

The effect of morphine on the circulation depends upon several factors, including the patient's illness, dose, route of administration, position, activity of the patient, and the presence of other cardiovascular active medications. Clinical doses of morphine (0.1–0.2 mg/kg) in normal supine patients has little effect, but postural hypotension may occur due to peripheral vasodilation and venous pooling. With larger doses used in cardiovascular anesthesia (1–2 mg/kg) the cardiovascular system is stable so long as ventilation, oxygenation and blood volume are maintained. Lowenstein et al. (84) administered 1 mg/kg of morphine to eight healthy normal patients and to seven patients with aortic valve disease. Minimal cardiovascular effects were observed in the normal patients, and the patients with valve disease showed increases in cardiac index, stroke index, and pulmonary artery and central venous pressures and a decrease in systemic vascular resistance. Morphine may improve myocardial dynamics in patients with elevated left ventricular end diastolic pressures by dilating venous capacitance vessels. Intravenous injections of morphine (0.5–1 mg/kg) during cardiopulmonary bypass decreases peripheral vascular resistance within 2 minutes by about 50% (58) (Fig. 26.5). This is followed by a

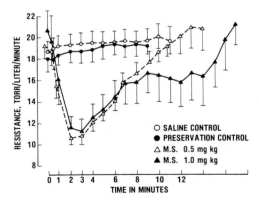

Figure 26.5. Peripheral vasculature resistance and morphine. Morphine, 0.5 mg/kg and 1 mg/kg, decreased peripheral vascular resistance in humans, whereas the injection of saline solution or the preservatives in morphine solution did not ($P < 0.01$). Data points are means ± SE. (Adapted from Hsu HO et al: Morphine decreases peripheral vascular resistance and increases capacitance in man. *Anesthesiology* 50:98–102, 1979.)

return to control levels after about 10 minutes. Hypotension following morphine administration can be treated by rapid infusion of fluids to increase the intravascular volume.

The vasodilation observed with morphine is attributed to (a) histamine release, (b) direct vasodilation, and (c) neural mediation. Histamine is reported to play a major role in morphine-induced vasodilation, and a dose-dependent increase in plasma histamine levels is associated with a decrease in mean arterial pressure (124). Meperidine and codeine also increase plasma histamine levels, whereas methadone and probably fentanyl do not (124). Morphine also has direct vasodilator properties (85) and may decrease central α-adrenergic activity.

The peripheral vascular and analgesic effects of morphine are beneficial in pulmonary edema, congestive heart failure, and myocardial infarction. Morphine causes a rapid decrease in pulmonary artery flow and pressure and left ventricular end diastolic pressure, and results in increased myocardial contractility (Fig. 26.6) (130). Vismara et al. (131) have given intravenous injections of morphine (0.1 mg/kg) to patients with congestive heart failure and pulmonary edema. They attribute the beneficial effects of morphine to splanchnic pooling, decreased preload and afterload, and decreased work of breathing. Morphine attenuates the sympathetic efferent discharge associated with pulmonary edema and the pain of myocardial ischemia (145, 146). Morphine (4–8 mg every 5–15 minutes until pain relief or respiratory depression occurs) remains the drug of choice for the treatment of pain associated with myocardial infarction or ischemia.

Morphine and other narcotics have a negative chronotropic effect and act by central effects and by a direct effect on the sinoatrial node (121, 127). Morphine in analgesic doses

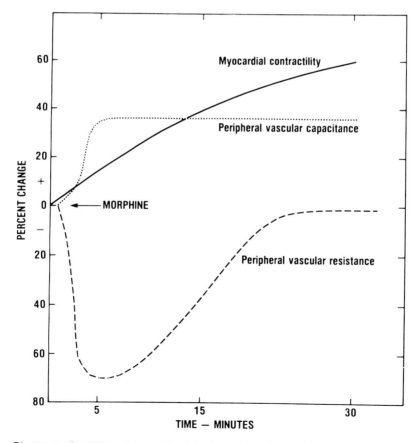

Figure 26.6. Diagrammatic representation of the interdependent effects of morphine upon the contractile state of the heart and upon the peripheral vascular bed. (Adapted from Vasko JS et al: Mechanisms of action of morphine in the treatment of experimental pulmonary edema. *Am J Cardiol* 18:876–883, 1966.)

(0.1–0.2 mg/kg, intravenously administered) has little effect on the sinus node (128) and may protect against ventricular fibrillation (27). In higher doses such as those used for anesthesia, morphine, and other narcotics may decrease heart rate. Fentanyl (5–10 μg/kg, intravenously administered) decreases heart rate by 60–70% of control (107).

Morphine should be used with caution in patients with a history of blood loss or other illness associated with a reduced intravascular volume, due to the likelihood of hypotension. Sudden postural changes should be avoided and adequate intravenous access should be present so that fluids can be administered rapidly should hypotension occur. Because of an increased risk of hypotension, morphine should be used with caution in patients with cor pulmonale and when phenothiazines are also in use.

GASTROINTESTINAL TRACT

Narcotic substances were used for the relief of dysentery and diarrhea long before their use as analgesics. Morphine delays gastric emptying time mainly by its action on the stomach and duodenum (13). Morphine and meperidine in equianalgesic doses have the same qualitative effects on the GI tract: that is, diminished propulsive activity and an increase in resting tone and incidence of spasm (13). Meperidine effects peak at 1–1½ hours, while morphine effects are prominent at 4 hours. Morphine also decreases intestinal motility in the terminal ileum (23), and diminishes activity in the colon. These effects account for the constipating effects of morphine and other narcotics. These effects are of little concern in healthy subjects, but in patients with ulcerative colitis and possibly other diseases of the GI tract, narcotics may have serious deleterious effects. Garrett et al. (43) studied patients with ulcerative colitis and found marked hypermotility and increased tone. In their retrospective analysis of 18 patients with ulcerative colitis who developed toxic megacolon, they found that 17 of the 18 had symptoms associated with recent narcotic administration. Morphine also decreases secretions of the salivary glands, stomach, pancreas, and biliary tract. When given alone, morphine (0.2 mg/kg to 15 mg) causes a 20% increase in splanchnic blood flow and 13% decrease in splanchnic vascular resistance (78). This effect is mainly due to arteriolar dilatation, which may be of advantage in patients with compromised intestinal blood flow.

Morphine has been linked to biliary spasm and symptoms of biliary colic (12). Equianalgesic doses of morphine (0.125 mg/kg), meperidine (1.0 mg/kg), fentanyl (1.25 μg), and pentazocine (0.15 mg/kg) given intraoperatively increase common bile duct pressures by 52.7%, 61.3%, 99.5% and 15% after injection, respectively. Whether or not all narcotics uniformly increase biliary pressure is not clear, but any abnormal cholangiogram or other study of the biliary tree obtained in association with narcotic administration should be suspect.

RENAL CONSIDERATIONS

In unstressed surgical patients, morphine (0.11 mg/kg) is associated with a decrease in glomerular filtration rate, but no alteration in urine volume or composition (28). The addition of anesthesia with nitrous oxide further decreases glomerular filtration rate and urine output. Although ADH may be a factor, the major effect appears to be a renal hemodynamic one, via decreased cardiac output, sympathetic stimulation, and vasoconstriction. The addition of surgical stress to nitrous oxide-narcotic anesthesia may result in very high plasma ADH levels (103). Patients with renal failure may accumulate morphine and demonstrate an enhanced narcotic effect.

OTHER CONSIDERATIONS

It is frequently stated that elderly patients are more sensitive to the CNS effects of narcotic analgesics. Berkowitz et al. (9) noted that serum levels of morphine are about 1.5 times higher in patients over 50 years of age than in younger patients at 2 minutes after an intravenous injection of 10 mg/70 kg. The differences in plasma morphine concentrations were less at 5 minutes and absent at 10 minutes. Factors causing the higher serum morphine levels have not been identified, but a slower titration of narcotic analgesics to obtain the desired effect is advised in those over 50 years of age.

Only free morphine is capable of penetrating biologic membranes and reaching its site of action. Approximately one-third of unchanged morphine is bound to albumin in normal humans, with a much lower amount bound to globulin (95). Protein-bound morphine is pharmacologically inactive, but the complex can readily dissociate. Alkalosis increases the percentage of morphine bound to plasma proteins. For each increase in pH of 0.2 unit, the percentage of protein-bound morphine increases by 3% (95), and likewise a decrease in pH releases more free active morphine. The percentage of morphine bound to protein is also directly related to protein concentration and to other drugs which compete for albumin binding. Therefore, in the critically ill patient on numerous medications and with a low albumin, normal doses of morphine may have a much greater effect. Morphine has also recently been reported as a cause of immune thrombocytopenia (17).

DOSAGE AND ADMINISTRATION

Morphine is available as the salts, morphine sulfate and morphine hydrochloride. The optimal dose is stated as up to 10 mg/70 kg of body weight via subcutaneous or intravenous routes. The dose should be modified according to the disease and age of the patient. Subsequent doses should be titrated depending on the analgesic effect and side effects observed. Intravenous is the preferred route of administration in the ICU. Administration by continuous intravenous infusion (51) can sustain effective blood levels and pain relief, and avoid periods of depressed level of consciousness associated with peak blood levels after intramuscular or subcutaneous injections. Table 26.2 lists dosage and duration of action of narcotic agonists and antagonists used parenterally.

CODEINE

Codeine is an alkaloid of opium and considered a mild analgesic. Codeine is two-thirds as effective orally as parenterally, both as a respiratory depressant and analgesic. Codeine is metabolized in the liver and about 10% is demethylated to form morphine, which may be responsible for codeine's major analgesic effect, since codeine itself has an exceptionally low affinity for the opioid receptor (66). Codeine sulfate is usually given by mouth in a dose of 15–60 mg, and may be given by intramuscular injection.

HYDROMORPHONE (SEMISYNTHETIC)

Hydromorphone (Dilaudid) is a semisynthetic modification of morphine. It is five times

as potent as morphine and can be given orally or parenterally. It has no advantages over morphine in the intensive care setting.

MEPERIDINE (SYNTHETIC)

Meperidine, a synthetic analgesic, is a piperidine derivative whose major actions are similar to morphine. Meperidine is lipophilic and exhibits a close correlation between its plasma levels and the intensity of its analgesic and ventilatory depressant actions (2, 120).

Meperidine demonstrates a dose-dependent cardiac depressant action especially at doses above 5 mg/kg (117). Meperidine is metabolized in the liver to normeperidine, a potent CNS stimulant, and convulsions in humans have been attributed to the N-demethylated metabolites after large doses (122). This factor may be significant if meperidine is taken orally (first-pass effect) or administered in the presence of renal failure, or if meperidine and chlorpromazine are given together (116). Besides the toxic interaction of meperidine with chlorpromazine, it also should not be given with monoamine oxidase (MAO) inhibitors (33).

FENTANYL

Fentanyl is a synthetic opioid related to the phenylpiperidines. Fentanyl is approximately 7000 times more lipophilic than morphine (54). Fentanyl penetrates biologic membranes quite rapidly and has a rapid onset of action. There exists an extremely close relationship between brain and plasma concentrations and between plasma fentanyl levels and its intensity of effect (88). Fentanyl is considered 75–200 times more potent than morphine. This fact is due in part to its ready access to the brain, and may also be due to a greater activity at opioid receptors (54). Fentanyl is highly protein bound in both the plasma (67%) and in the brain (90%) and has a high affinity for fat such that prolonged exposure may result in its accumulation in fat and a prolonged recovery. Fentanyl demonstrates a proportional, dose-related increase in its duration of action, and this factor explains why initial doses are of short duration of action, whereas repeated doses increase the concentration and duration of action (61). In equianalgesic doses fentanyl and morphine produce approximately the same degree of respiratory depression. Due to its minimal effect on the cardiovascular system (119), short duration of action and rapid effect, fentanyl is a very useful analgesic for use during potentially painful procedures (e.g., placement of vascular catheters, balloon pumps, and endotracheal tubes). Addition of diazepam or other sedative to fentanyl may result in decreased cardiac output, blood pressure, and peripheral vascular resistance (119). Fentanyl is usually administered intravenously, with 1-3–μg/kg being the usual dose for analgesia. Up to 10 μg/kg may be given in the absence of other sedative, analgesic medications if ventilation is controlled. Fentanyl is supplied for injection as 50 μg/ml and is also available in a fixed combination with droperidol (fentanyl 50 μg with droperidol 2.5 mg in 1 ml).

ALFENTANIL AND SUFENTANIL

Sufentanil was synthesized in 1974 as a result of manipulation of fentanyl structure. Sufentanil has recently been released for clinical use and is 5–10 times more potent than fentanyl. In the tail withdrawal reflex in rats, sufentanil is 4521 times as potent as morphine, and there is minimal effect on the cardiovascular system (32). Sufentanil is highly protein bound (92.5%), predominantly to the α-$_1$-acidic glycoprotein. It is highly lipophilic and has a faster onset of action than that of fentanyl. Sufentanil has a shorter elimination half-life (148 minutes), and this combined with its somewhat lesser volume of distribution may explain the reported shorter duration of respiratory depression with sufentanil than with fentanyl. The clearance and hepatic extraction ratio of sufentanil are similar to those of fentanyl, and, as with fentanyl, the effect of small doses is likely to be terminated by redistribution to the peripheral compartment. With larger doses, as with fentanyl, the plasma concentrations of sufentanil may not be rendered subtherapeutic by redistribution. When this redistribution occurs, hepatic biotransformation is the limiting factor for termination of the clinical effect.

Alfentanil is another new fentanyl derivative, which has only recently been released for clinical use. Alfentanil is approximately one-fourth as potent as fentanyl, but has a faster onset and shorter duration of action than fentanyl. Alfentanil is significantly less lipophilic than fentanyl and has a significantly smaller volume of distribution at steady state. Alfentanil is highly bound to plasma proteins (92%),

and is approximately 10% ionized at a pH of 7.4. Alfentanil is rapidly metabolized by the liver, but the clearance of alfentanil is less than that of fentanyl; however, the small volume of distribution of alfentanil at steady state results in an elimination half-life considerably less than that of fentanyl (1.5 vs. 3.5 hrs). In the intensive care unit, alfentanil may be a highly useful medication for performing short procedures in either spontaneously breathing patients or in intubated patients. For short procedures, a bolus of 8–20 μg/kg may provide analgesic protection against hemodynamic responses to the stress associated with performing needed procedures. Should the procedure last longer than 20–30 minutes, incremental doses of 3–5 μg/kg given as a bolus or 0.5–1 μg/kg/minute by continuous infusion, titrated to patient response, may be useful in continued alleviation of the stress associated with surgical or other procedures.

NARCOTIC AGONIST-ANTAGONISTS

Pentazocine is a benzomorphan derivative with both agonist and weak opioid antagonist activity. In equianalgesic doses pentazocine produces a similar degree of respiratory depression as morphine (e.g., 30 mg of pentazocine and 10 mg of morphine). Increasing the dose beyond 30 mg does not result in a proportionate increase in respiratory depression (113), and respiratory depression is maximal at 60 mg of pentazocine. Pentazocine may cause an elevation of mean arterial pressure, left ventricular end-diastolic pressure and mean pulmonary artery pressure, resulting in an increase in myocardial work load (70). Pentazocine has weak opioid antagonist properties. It will not reverse the respiratory depression of other "pure" agonists, but may precipitate opioid withdrawal in patients receiving narcotics on a regular basis. For the above reasons pentazocine has little use in the critical care setting.

Butorphanol and nalbuphine are two other mixed agonist-antagonist medications with strong analgesic properties. Their use in the intensive care setting is presently under investigation.

ANTAGONISTS

The narcotic antagonists comprise nalorphine, levallorphan, and naloxone. Nalorphine and levallorphan have both antagonist and agonist actions, whereas naloxone is a pure antagonist.

In the absence of opioid drugs naloxone produces almost no clinical effect. Naloxone antagonizes the effects of both the narcotic agonists and agonist-antagonists. Narcotic reversal with naloxone has been associated with ventricular tachycardia and fibrillation in patients following cardiac surgery (91), and cause premature ventricular contractions, increased heart rate, increased cardiac output, and increased mean blood pressure and decreased stroke volume in animals anesthetized with morphine (99). It is clear that the acute withdrawal of narcotic anesthesia in the wide variety of postoperative patients presenting to intensive care units (e.g., cardiac surgical patients, neurosurgical patients, general surgical patients) could result in disastrous hemodynamic effects. Furthermore naloxone may have specific agonist effects of its own (24, 40), and until further data are available careful titration of naloxone in small increments for the purpose of known narcotic reversal is advised.

Naloxone may be used very effectively to reverse the respiratory effects of narcotics, however, the duration of action of a single bolus of intravenously administered naloxone is short; its half-life is about 20 minutes (1). Prolonged reversal of narcotic anesthesia has been reported with intramuscular injection of naloxone; however, due to the unreliable uptake of intramuscular medications, this route is not advised. Repeated boluses or a continuous closely monitored infusion will more reliably prevent renarcotization of postoperative patients while avoiding abrupt narcotic reversal.

References

1. Anderson R, Dobloug I, Refstad S: Postanesthetic use of naloxone hydrochloride after moderate doses of fentanyl. *Acta Anaesth Scand* 20:255–258, 1976.
2. Austin KL, Stapleton JV, Mather LE: Relationship between blood meperidine concentrations and analgesic response: a preliminary report. *Anesthesiology* 53:460–466, 1980.
3. Austin KL, Stapleton JV, Mather LE: Multiple intramuscular injections: a major source of variability in analgesic response to meperidine. *Pain* 8:47–62, 1980.
4. Basbaum AI, Clanton CH, Fields HL: Three bulbospinal pathways from the rostral medulla of the cat: an autoradiographic study of pain modulating systems. *J Comp Neurol* 178:209–224, 1978.
5. Beckett AH: Analgesics and their antagonists: some steric and chemical considerations. Part I. The dissociation constants of some tertiary amines and synthetic analgesics, the conformations of methadone-type compounds. *J Pharm Pharmacol* 8:848–853, 1956.
6. Beckett AH, Casey AF: Synthetic analgesics, stereochemical considerations. *J Pharm Pharmacol* 6:986–989, 1954.
7. Bedford R, Woolman H: Postoperative respiratory effects of morphine and halothane anesthesia: a study of patients undergoing cardiac surgery. *Anesthesiology* 43:1–9, 1975.
8. Bell C: Idea of a New Anatomy of the Brain Submitted for the Observation of His Friends. London, 1811.
9. Berkowitz BA, Cerreta K, Spector S: Influence of physiologic and pharmacological factors on the disposition of morphine as determined by radioimmunoassay. *J Pharmacol Exp Ther* 191:527–534, 1974.
10. Bromage PR, Camporessi E, Chestnut D: Epidural narcotics for postoperative analgesia. *Anesth Analg* 59:473–480, 1980.
11. Brunk SF, Delle M: Morphine metabolism in man. *Clin Pharmacol Ther* 16:51–57, 1974.
12. Butsch WL, McGowan JW: Clinical studies on the influence of certain drugs in relation to biliary pain and to the variations in intrabiliary pressure. *Surg Gynecol Obstet* 63:451–456, 1936.
13. Chapman WP, Rowlands EN, Jones CM: Multiple-balloon kymographic recording of the comparative action of demerol, morphine and placebos in the motility of the upper small intestine in man. *N Engl J Med* 243:171–177, 1950.
14. Charkravarty K, Tucker W, Rosen M, et al: Comparison of buprenorphine and pethidine given intravenously on demand to relieve post-operative pain. *Br Med J* 2:895–897, 1979.
15. Chung K, Langford LA, Applebaum AE, et al: Primary afferent fibers in the tract of Lissauer in the rat. *J Comp Neurol* 184:587–598, 1979.
16. Church JJ: Continuous narcotic infusions for relief of postoperative pain. *Br Med J* 1:977–979, 1979.
17. Cimo PL, Hammond JJ, Moake JL: Morphine-induced immune thrombocytopenia. *Arch Intern Med* 142:832–834, 1982.
18. Coggeshall RE, Coulter JD, Willis WD: Unmyelinated fibers in the ventral root. *Brain Res* 57:229–233, 1973.
19. Coggeshall RE, Coulter JD, Willis WD: Unmyelinated axons in the ventral roots of the cat lumbosacral enlargement. *J Comp Neurol* 153:39–58, 1974.
20. Cox BM, Ginsburg M, Osman OH: Acute tolerance to narcotic analgesic drugs in rats. *Br J Pharmacol* 33:245–256, 1968.
21. Cronin M, Redfern PA, Utting JE: Psychometry and postoperative complaints in surgical patients. *Br J Anaesth* 45:879–886, 1973.
22. Cuello AC, Delfiacco MD, Paxinos G: The central and peripheral ends of the substance-P-containing sensory neurones in the rat trigeminal system. *Brain Res* 152:499–500, 1978.
23. Daniel EE, Sutherland WH, Bogoch A: Effects of morphine and other drugs on motility of the terminal ileum. *Gastroenterology* 36:510–523, 1959.
24. Dashwood M, Feldbert W: A pressor response to naloxone. Evidence for release of endogenous opioid peptides. *J Physiol* 281;30P–31P, 1978.
25. de Jong RH, Nace RA: Nerve impulse conduction and cutaneous receptor responses during general anesthesia. *Anesthesiology* 28:851–855, 1967.
26. Denny-Brown D, Kirk EJ, Yangagisawa N: The tract of Lissauer in relation to sensory transmission in the dorsal horn or the spinal cord in the macaque monkey. *J Comp Neurol* 151:175–200, 1973.
27. DeSilva RA, Verrier RL, Lown B: Protective effect of the vagotonic action of morphine sulfate on ventricular vulnerability. *Cardiovasc Res* 12:167–172, 1978.
28. Deutsch S, Bastron RD, Pierce EC, et al: The effects of anesthesia with thiopentone, nitrous oxide, narcotics and neuromuscular blocking drugs on renal function in normal man. *Br J Anaesth* 41:807–815, 1969.

29. Dimsdale JA, Kemp JM: Afferent fibers in ventral roots in the rat. *J Physiol (Lond)* 187:25P–32P, 1966.
30. Donald I: At the receiving end, a doctor's personal recollections of valve replacement. *Scott Med J* 2:1129–1131, 1969.
31. Donald I: At the receiving end, a doctor's personal recollection of second time valve replacement. *Scott Med J* 21:49–57, 1976.
32. Dubois-Primo J, Dewatchter B, Massaut J: Analgesic anesthesia with fentanyl and sufentanil in coronary surgery. *Acta Anaesthesiol Belg* 2:113–126, 1979.
33. Eade NR, Renton KW: Effect of monoamine oxidase inhibitors on the N-demethylation and hydrolysis of meperdine. *Biochem Pharmacol* 19:2243–2250, 1970.
34. Eckenhoff J, Helrich M: The effects of narcotics, thiopentone and nitrous oxide upon respiration and the respiratory response to hypercapnia. *Anesthesiology* 19:240–253, 1958.
35. Editorial: Attitude to pain. *Br Med J* 3:261, 1975.
36. Editorial: Pain relief after thoracotomy. *Lancet* 1:576, 1976.
37. Editorial: Postoperative pain. *Anesth Intensive Care* 4:95, 1976.
38. Editorial: Postoperative pain. *Br Med J* 2:664, 1976.
39. Evans FF, Proctor JD, Fratkin MJ: Blood flow in muscle groups and drug absorption. *Clin Pharmacol Ther* 17:44–47, 1975.
40. Faden AI, Holaday JW: Opiate antagonists: a role in the treatment of hypovolemic shock. *Science* 205:317–318, 1979.
41. Freed DLJ: Inadequate analgesia at night. *Lancet* 1:519–520, 1975.
42. Frey M von: Untersuchungen uber die Sinnesfunctionen der Menschlichen Haut. Erste Abhandlung: Druckempfindung und Schmerz. *Berl scahs Gess Wiss math phys KL* 23:175–183, 1896.
43. Garrett JM, Sauer WG, Moertel CG: Colonic motility in ulcerating colitis after opiate administration. *Gastroenterology* 53:93–100, 1967.
44. Giesler GJ, Canon JT, Urca G, et al: Long ascending projections from substantia gelatinosa rolandi and the subjacent dorsal horn in the rat. *Science* 202:984–986, 1978.
45. Gilbert PE, Martin WR: The effects of morphine- and nalarphine-like drugs in the non-dependent, morphine-dependent and cyclazocin-dependent chronic spinal dog. *J Pharmacol Exp Ther* 198:66–82, 1976.
46. Glaser FB, Ball JC: Death due to withdrawal from narcotics. In Ball JC, Chambers CD: *The Epidemiology of Opiate Addiction in the United States.* Springfield, IL, Charles C Thomas, 1970, pp 263–287.
47. Glynn CJ, Mather LE, Cousins MJ, et al: Spinal narcotics and respiratory depression. *Lancet* 2:356–357, 1979.
48. Gobel S: Neurons with two axons in the substantia gelatinosa layer of the spinal trigeminal nucleus of the adult cat. *Brain Res* 88:333–338, 1975.
49. Goldstein AL: Opiate peptides (endorphins) in pituitary and brain. *Science* 193:1081–1086, 1976.
50. Goodman LS, Gilman A (eds): *The Pharmacological Basis of Therapeutics,* ed. 6. New York, Macmillan, 1980, p. 496.
51. Greenblatt DJ: Predicting steady state concentrations of drugs. *Annu Rev Pharmacol Toxicol* 19:347–356, 1979.
52. Hancock MB, Foreman RD, Willis WD: Convergence of visceral and cutaneous input into spinothalamic tract cells in the thoracic spinal cord of the cat. *Exp Neurol* 47:240–248, 1975.
53. Henschel EO: The Guillain-Barre syndrome, a personal experience. *Anesthesiology* 47:228–231, 1977.
54. Herz A, Teschenmacher HJ: Activities and sites of antinociceptive action of morphine-like analgesics and kinetics of distribution following intravenous, intra-

cerebral and intraventricular application. *Adv Drug Res* 6:79–119, 1971.
55. Hewitt PB: Subjective follow-up of patients from a surgical intensive therapy ward. *Br Med J* 4:669–673, 1970.
56. Hodge CJ, Woods CI, Delatizky J: Noradrenalin, serotonin, and the dorsal horn. *J Neurosurg* 52:674–685, 1980.
57. Hokfelt T, Ljungdahl A, terenius L, et al: Immunohistochemical analysis of peptide pathways possibly related to pain and analgesia: enkephalin and substance P. *Proc Natl Acad Sci* 74:3081–3085, 1977.
58. Hsu HO, Hickey RF, Forbes AR: Morphine decreases peripheral vascular resistance and increases capacitance in man. *Anesthesiology* 50:98–102, 1979.
59. Hug CC: Improving analgesic therapy. *Anesthesiology* 53:441–443, 1980.
60. Huc CC, Mellett, Carfruny EJ: Stop-flow analysis of the renal excretion of tritium-labeled dihydromorphine. *J Pharmacol Exp Ther* 150:259–269, 1965.
61. Hug CC, Murphy MR: Fentanyl disposition in cerebrospinal fluid and plasma and its relationship to ventilatory depression in the dog. *Anesthesiology* 50:342–349, 1979.
62. Iggo A: Peripheral and spinal "pain" mechanisms and their modulation. In Bonica JJ, Albe-Fessard: *Advances in Pain Research and Therapy.* New York, Raven Press, 1976, pp 381–394.
63. Iggo A: Is the physiology of cutaneous receptors determined by morphology? *Prog Bain Res* 43:15–31, 1976.
64. International Association for the Study of Pain Subcommittee on Taxonomy: Pain terms: a list with definitions and notes on usage. *Pain* 6:249–252, 1979.
65. Iwamoto K, Klaassen CD: First-pass effect of morphine in rats. *J Pharmacol Exp Ther* 200:236–244, 1977.
66. Jaffe JH, Martin WR: Opioid analgesics and antagonists. In Goodman LS, Gilman A: *The Pharmacological Basis of Therapeutics,* ed 6. New York, Macmillan, 1980, p 506.
67. Jansco N, Jansco-Gabor A, Szolcsanyi J: The role of sensory nerve endings in neurogenic inflammation induced in human skin and in the eye and paw of the rat. *Br J Pharmacol* 33:32–39, 1974.
68. Johnstone RE, Jobes DR, Kennell EM: Reversal of morphine anesthesia with naloxone. *Anesthesiology* 41:361–367, 1974.
69. Jones J, Hoggart B, Withey J, et al: What the patients say: a study of reactions to an intensive care unit. *Intensive Care Med* 5:89–92, 1979.
70. Juan H: Prostaglandins as modulators of pain. *Gen Pharmacol* 9:403–409, 1978.
71. Kerr FWL: Pain: a central inhibitory balance theory. *Mayo Clin Proc* 50:685–690, 1975.
72. Kerr FWL: Neuroanatomical substrates of nociception in the spinal cord. *Pain* 1:325–356, 1975.
73. Kerr FWL: The ventral spinothalamic tract and other ascending systems of the ventral funiculus of the spinal cord. *J Comp Neurol* 159:335–356, 1975.
74. Keeri-Szanton M, Heaman S: Postoperative demand analgesia. *Surg Gynecol Obstet* 134:647–651, 1972.
75. King JS, Gallant P, Myerson V, et al: The effects of antiinflammatory agents on the responses and the sensitization of unmyelinated (c) fiber polymodal nicoceptors. In Zotterman Y: *Sensory Functions of the Skin in Primates with Special Reference to Man.* Oxford, UK, Pergamon Press, 1976, pp 441–461.
76. Kumazawa T, Perl ER: Excitation of marginal and substantia gelatinosa neurons in the primate spinal cord: indications of their place in dorsal horn functional organization. *J Comp Neurol* 177:417–434, 1978.
77. La Motte C: Distribution of the tract of Lissauer and the dorsal root fibers in the primate spinal cord. *J Comp Neurol* 177:529–561, 1978.

78. Leaman DM, Levenson L, Zelis R, et al: Effect of morphine on splanchnic blood flow. *Br Heart J* 40:569–571, 1978.

79. Lee G, De Maria A, Amsterdam EA, et al: Comparative effects of morphine, meperidine and pentazocine on cardiocirculatory dynamics in patients with acute myocardial infarction. *Am J Med* 60:949–955, 1976.

80. Lele PP, Weddell G: Sensory nerves of the cornea and cutaneous sensibility. *Exp Neurol* 1:334–359, 1959.

81. Light AR, Perl ER: Central termination of identified cutaneous sensibility. *Exp Neurol* 1:334–359, 1959.

82. Lissauer H: Bietrag zum faserverlauf in hinterhorn des menschlichen ruckenmarkes und verhalten desselben bei tabes dorsalis. *Arch Psychiat Nervenkrankh* 17:377–382, 1886.

83. Lord JAH, Waterfield AA, Hughes J, et al: Endogenous spinal peptides: Multiple agonists and receptors. *Nature* 267:495–500, 1977.

84. Lowenstein E, Hallowell P, Levine FH, et al: Cardiovascular response to large doses of intravenous morphine in man. *N Engl J Med* 281:1389–1393, 1969.

85. Lowenstein E, Whiting RB, Bittar DA, et al: Local and neurally mediated effect of morphine on skeletal muscle vascular resistance. *J Pharmacol Exp Ther* 180:359–367, 1972.

86. Martin WR, Eades CG, Thompson JA, et al: The effects of morphine and nalorphine like drugs in the non-dependent and morphine-dependent chronic spinal dog. *J Pharmacol Exp Ther* 197:517–532, 1976.

87. Maynard CW, Leonadr RB, Coulter JD, et al: Central connections of ventral root afferents as demonstrated by the HRP method. *J Comp Neurol* 17:601–608, 1977.

88. McClain DA, Hug CC: Intravenous fentanyl kinetics. *Clin Pharmacol Ther* 17:21–30, 1975.

89. Merrill EG, Wall PD, Yaksh TL: Properties of the two unmyelinated fibre tracts of the central nervous system: laterla Lissauer tract and parallel fibres of the cerebellum. *J Physiol (Lond)* 284:127–145, 1978.

90. Messing RB, Lytle LD: Serotonin-containing neurons: their possible role in pain and analgesia. *Pain* 4:1–21, 1977.

91. Michaelis LL, Hickey PR, Clark TA: Bentricular irritability associated with the use of naloxone hydrochloride. *Ann Thor Surg* 18:608–614, 1974.

92. Misra AL: Metabolism of opiates. In Adler MW, Manara, L, Samanin R: *Factors Affecting the Action of Narcotics.* New York, Raven Press, 1978, pp 297–343.

93. Mule SJ: Physiologic disposition of narcotic agonists and antagonists. In Clonet DH et al: *Narcotic Drugs: Biochemical Pharmacology.* New York, Plenum Press, 1971, pp 99–121.

94. Narotzky RA, Kerr FWL: Marginal neurons of the spinal cord: types, afferent synaptology and functional considerations. *Brain Res* 139:1–20, 1978.

95. Olsen GD: Morphine binding to human plasma proteins. *Clin Pharmacol Ther* 17:31–35, 1975.

96. Paiement B, Boulanger M, Jones CW, et al: Intubation and other experiences in cardiac surgery: the consumer's views. *Can Anaesth Soc J* 26:173–180, 1979.

97. Pasternak GW, Childers SR, Snyder SH: Opiate analgesia: evidence for mediation by a subpopulation of opiate receptors. *Science* 208:514–516, 1980.

98. Pasternak GW, Zhang A, Tecott L: Developmental differences between high and low affinity opiate binding sites: their relationship to analgesia and respiratory depression. *Life Sci* 27:1185–1190, 1980.

99. Patschke D, Eberlein HJ, Hess W, et al: Antagonism of morphine with naloxone in dogs: Cardiovascular effects with special reference to the coronary circulation. *Br J Anaesth* 49:525–533, 1977.

100. Perl ER: Sensitization of nociceptors and its relation to sensitization. In: Bonica JJ, Albe-Fessard DG: *Advances in Pain Research and Therapy.* New York, Raven Press, 1976, pp 17–28.

101. Perl ER, Kumazawa T, Lynn B, et al: Sensitization of high threshold receptors with unmyelinated (c) afferent fibers. *Prog Brain Res* 43:263–277, 1976.

102. Peter CB, Snyder SH: Opiate receptor: its demonstration in nervous tissue. *Science* 179:1011–1014, 1973.

103. Philbin DM, Coggins CH: Plasma antidiuretic hormone levels in cardiac surgical patients during morphine and halothane anesthesia. *Anesthesiology* 49:95–98, 1978.

104. Phillips GD, Austin KL, Runciman WB, et al: Deaths in intensive care: analysis and prediction. *Med J Aust* 1:424–426, 1980.

105. Price DD, Dubner R: Neurons that observe the sensory discriminative aspects of pain. *Pain* 3:307–338, 1977.

106. Radnay PA, Brodman E, Mankikar D, et al: The effect of equianalgesic doses of fentanyl, morphine, meperidine and pentazocine on common bile duct pressure. *Anaesthesist* 29:26–29, 1980.

107. Reitan JA, Stengert KB, Wymore ML, et al: Central vagal control of fentanyl-induced bradycardia during halothane anesthesia. *Anesth Analg* 57:31–36, 1978.

108. Rexed B: Cytoarchitectonic organization of the spinal cord in the cat. *J Comp Neurol* 96:415–495, 1952.

109. Sar M, Stumpf WC, Miller RJ, et al: Immunohistochemical localization of enkephalin in rat brain and spinal cord. *J Comp Neurol* 182:17–27, 1978.

110. Shovelton DS: Reflections on an intensive therapy unit. *Br Med J* 1:737–738, 1979.

111. Simon EJ, Hiller JM: The opiate receptors. *Annu Rev Pharmacol Toxicol* 18:371–384, 1978.

112. Simon EJ, Hiller JM, Edelman J: Stereospecific binding of the potent narcotic analgesic ^{3}H-etorphine to rat brain homogenate. *Proc Natl Acad Sci* 70:1947–1949, 1973.

113. Sinclair DC: Cutaneous sensation and the doctrine of specific energy. *Brain* 78:584–614, 1955.

114. Smith T, Stephen G, Zeigler L: Effects of premedicant drugs on respiration and gas exchange in man. *Anesthesiology* 28:883–890, 1967.

115. Snyder SH: Opiate receptors and internal opiates. *Sci Am* 236:44–56, 1977.

116. Stambaugh JE, Wainer IW: Drug interaction: meperidine and chlorpromazine, a toxic combination. *J Clin Pharmacol* 21:140–146, 1981.

117. Stambaugh JE, Wainer IW, Stanstead JK, et al: The clinical pharmacology of meperidine; comparison of routes of administration. *J Clin Pharmacol* 16:245–256, 1976.

118. Stanley T, Lathrop G: Urinary excretion of morphine during and after valvular and coronary artery surgery. *Anesthesiology* 46:166–169, 1977.

119. Stanley TH, Webster LR: Anesthetic requirements and cardiovascular effects of fentanyl-oxygen and fentanyl-diazepam-oxygen anesthesia in man. *Anesth Analg* 57:411–416, 1978.

120. Stapelton JV, Austin KL, Mather LE: A pharmacokinetic approach to postoperative pain: continuous infusion of pethidine. *Anaesth Intensive Care* 7:25–32, 1979.

121. Stein EA: Morphine effects on the cardiovascular system of awake freely behaving rats. *Arch Int Pharmacodyn* 223:54–63, 1976.

122. Szeto HH, Inturrisi CE, Houde R, Saals, et al: Accumulation of normeperidine, an active metabolite of meperidine, in patients with renal failure or cancer. *Ann Intern Med* 86:738–741, 1977.

123. Terenius L: Stereospecific interaction between narcotic analgesics and a synaptic plasma membrane fraction of rat cerebral cortex. *Acta Pharmacol Toxicol* 32:317–320, 1973.

124. Thompson WL, Walton RP: Elevation of plasma histamine levels in the dog following administration of

muscle relaxants, opiates, and macromolecular polymers. *J Pharmacol Exp Ther* 143:131–136, 1966.

125. Torebjork HE: Afferent C units responding to mechanical thermal and chemical stimuli in human nonglabrous skin. *Acta Physiol Scand* 92:374–390, 1974.

126. Trevino DL: Integration of sensory input in laminae I, II, and III of the cat's spinal cord. *Fed Proc* 37:2234–2236, 1978.

127. Urthaler F, Isobe JH, Gilmour KE, et al: Morphine and autonomic control of the sinus node. *Chest* 64:203–212, 1973.

128. Urthaler F, Isobe JH, James TN: Direct and vagally mediated chronotropic effects of morphine studied by selective perfusion of the sinus node of awake dogs. *Chest* 68:222–228, 1975.

129. Utting JE, Smith JM: Postoperative analgesia. *Anaesthesia* 34:320–332, 1979.

130. Vasko J, Henney R, Oldham HN: Mechanisms of action of morphine in the treatment of experimental pulmonary edema. *Am J Cardiol* 18:876–883, 1966.

131. Vismara LA, Leaman DM, Zelis R: The effects of morphine on venous tone in patients with acute pulmonary edema. *Circulation* 54:335–337, 1976.

132. Wall PD: The laminar organization of the dorsal horn and effects of descending impulses. *J Physiol (Lond)* 188:403–423, 1967.

133. Wall PD: The gate control theory of pain mechanisms. A re-examination and restatement. *Brain* 101:1–18, 1978.

134. Wallace PGM, Norris W: The management of postoperative pain. *Br J Anaesth* 47:113–120, 1975.

135. Wang JK: Analgesic effect of intrathecally administered morphine. *Reg Anesth* 2:8, 1977.

136. Wang JK, Nauss LA, Thomas JE: Pain relief by intrathe-cally applied morphine in man. *Anesthesiology* 50:149–151, 1979.

137. Watson SJ, Barchas JP: Anatomy of the endogenous opoid peptides and related substances: the enkephalins, β-endorphin, β-lipotropin and ACTH. In Beers RF, Bassett EG: *Mechanisms of Pain and Analgesic Compounds*. New York, Raven Press, 1979, pp 227–237.

138. Watts GT: Inadequate analgesia. *Lancet* 1:678, 1975.

139. Weddell SJ, Ritter RR: Epidural morphine: serum levels and pain relief. *Anesthesiology* 53:S419, 1980.

140. Weil J, McCullough R, Kline J, et al: Diminished ventilatory response to hypoxia and hypercapnia after morphine in normal man. *N Engl J Med* 292:1103–1106, 1975.

141. Willis WD, Leonard RB, Kenshalo DR: Spinothalamic tract neurons in the substantia gelatinosa. *Science* 202:986–988, 1978.

142. Wood M: Narcotic analgesics and antagonists. In Wood M, Wood A: *Drugs and Anesthesia*. Baltimore, Williams & Wilkins, 1982, pp 163–197.

143. Yaksh TL, Rudy TA: Analgesia mediated by a direct spinal action of narcotics. *Science* 192:1357–1358, 1976.

144. Yaksh TL, Rudy TA: Narcotic analgesics: CNS sites and mechanisms of action as revealed by intracerebral injection techniques. *Pain* 4:299–359, 1978.

145. Zelis R, Flaim JH: Effects of morphine on reflex arteriolar constriction induced in man by hypercapnia. *Clin Pharmacol Ther* 22:172–178, 1977.

146. Zelis R, Mansour EJ, Capone RJ, et al: The cardiovascular effects of morphine: the peripheral capacitance and resistance vessels in human subjects. *J Clin Invest* 54:1247–1258, 1974.

27

Psychopharmacology in the ICU

Edwin H. Cassem, M.D.
C. Raymond Lake, M.D., Ph.D.
William F. Boyer, M.D.

This chapter concerns the diagnosis and pharmacologic treatment of emotional disorders in the intensive care unit (ICU). Emphasis is on commonly used drugs, although some newer, alternative forms of therapy are mentioned. Problems are divided into delirium/psychosis, anxiety, and depression. In some patients two or all three of these may coexist. As in every other medical specialty, the treatment depends on the diagnosis.

APPROACH TO THE PATIENT

When confronted by a patient with disturbed thought, feeling, and/or behavior, the physician should decide whether the illness or its treatment has produced these symptoms or whether the patient has, in addition to a medical illness, developed a psychiatric disorder. Psychiatric symptoms frequently accompany physical illness and often resolve when the physical condition is effectively treated and is getting better. Table 27.1 lists illnesses that are associated with psychiatric symptoms.

Of all organic causes of altered mental status in intensive care settings, drugs are probably the most common contributor. Table 27.2 lists the drugs associated with psychiatric symptomatology. Some, like lidocaine, are predictable in their ability to cause an encephalopathic state, and the relationship is clearly dose related. Others, like the antibiotics, are

Table 27.1
Physical Illnesses Associated with Psychiatric Symptoms[a]

Illness	Anxiety	Despondency	Delirium or Psychosis
Circulatory			
Cerebral insufficiency or anoxia	+	+	+
Paroxysmal atrial tachycardia	+		
Coronary insufficiency	+		
Hypertensive encephalopathy		+	+
Electrolyte Disturbance			
Hypernatremia	+ (hyperactivity, irritability)		
Hyponatremia		+	+
Hyperkalemia			
Hypokalemia	+	+	+
Hypercalcemia		+	+
Hypocalcemia	+		+
Hypomagnesemia	+	+	+
Hypophosphatemia	+		
Endocrine			
Hyperfunction or hypofunction of thyroid, parathyroid or pituitary	+	+	+
Pancreas:			
Pancreatitis		+	+
Carcinoma	+	+	
Hyperinsulinism (any cause)	+	+	+
Diabetes mellitus	+	+	+

Table 27.1

Illness	Anxiety	Despondency	Delirium or Psychosis
Adrenals:			
Addison's or Cushing's disease	+	+	+
Pheochromocytoma	+		+
Hyperaldosteronism		+	
Gastrointestinal			
Ulcerative colitis		+	
Regional enteritis		+	
Whipple's disease		+	
Postgastrectomy		+ (fatigue, weakness)	
Hematologic			
Anemia	+	+	
Polycythemia vera	+	+	+
Thrombocytopenia (TTP)			+
Hepatic			
Cirrhosis		+	
Failure			+
Infections (other)			
Malaria	+	+	+
Pneumonia	+	+ (especially viral)	+ (especially bacterial)
Infectious mononucleosis	+	+	+
Brucellosis	+	+	
Tuberculosis	+	+	+
Viral hepatitis	+	+ (especially in convalescence)	
Subacute bacterial endocarditis			+
Septicemia			+
Malignancies (other)			
Disseminated carcinomatosis		+	
Lymphomas		+	+
Carcinoid	+	+	+
Other (especially oat cell)		+	+
Neurological			
Parkinson's disease		+ (may be early dementia)	
Stroke, space-occupying lesion, encephalitis, neurosyphilis, multiple sclerosis, Wilson's disease, Huntington's chorea	+	+	+
Partial complex seizures (temporal lobe epilepsy, right hemisphere focus)		(especially nondominant hemisphere focus)	(especially dominant hemisphere focus)
Post concussive syndrome	+	+	+
Polyneuritis	+		
Combined systems disease	+		
Posterolateral sclerosis	+		
Meningitis			+
Normal pressure hydrocephalus			+
Nutritional (deficiency)			
B$_6$, B$_{12}$, folic acid, niacin, thiamine, ascorbic acid		+	+
Renal			
Nephritis	+		
Uremia			+
Rheumatic or Collagen Vascular			
Systemic lupus	+	+	+
Rheumatoid arthritis, polyarteritis nodosa, temporal arteritis	+		
Other			
Acute intermittent porphyria		+ (between attacks)	+
Sarcoidosis		+	
Amyloidosis		+	

[a] Data from references 26, 47, 50, 51, 86, 89, 90, 105, 106, 107, 108.

Table 27.2
Medications with Psychiatric Side Effects

Drug	Anxiety	Despondency	Delirium or Psychosis
Analgesics + Antiinflammatories (nonsteroidal)			
Morphine + congeners		+	+
Meperidine, especially normeperidine		+	+
Pentazocine		+	+
Salicylates (severe abuse)			+
Acetaminophen			+
Fenoprofen	+	+	+
Indomethacin		+	+
Naproxen		+	
Phenylbutazone		+	
Propoxyphene		+	
Tolmetin sodium			+
Zomepirac sodium		+	+
Ibuprofen		+	+
Sulindac		+	+
Anticonvulsants			
Barbiturates	+	+	+
Hydantoins		+	+
Primidone		+	+
Sodium valproate		+	+
Succinimides (ethosuximide, phensuximide, methsuximide)	+	+	+
Antibiotics, Antifungals, Anthelminths			
Ampicillin		+	
Sulfonamides		+	
Clotrimazole		+	+
Cycloserine		+	+
Dapsone		+	+
Ethionamide		+	+
Griseofulvin		+	
Isoniazid			+
Metronidazole		+	
Nitrofurantoin		+	
Nalidixic acid		+	
Para-aminosalicylic acid			+
Quinacrine			+
Streptomycin		+	
Ketaconazole	+		
Aminoglycosides		+	+
Amodiaquine		+	+
Amphotericin-B		+	+
Cephalosporins		+	+
Chloramphenicol		+	+
Chloroquine		+	+
Colistin sulfate		+	+
Ethambutol HCl		+	+
Rifampin		+	+
Tetracycline		+	+
Ticarcillin		+	+
Flucytosine		+	+
Thiabendazole			+
Anticholinergics (numerous drugs)	+	+	+
Antihistamines			
Cimetidine	+	+	+
Promethazine		+	+
Ranitidine	+	+	+
Antineoplastics			
Fluorouracil		+	+
Aminoglutethimide		+	+
Vinblastine		+	

Table 27.2

Drug	Anxiety	Despondency	Delirium or Psychosis
Vincristine		+	+
Azathioprine		+	
Asparaginase		+	
Bleomycin		+	
Mithramycin		+	
Trimethoprim		+	
Azacytadine		+	+
Cytabarine (high dose)		+	+
Dacarbazine		+	+
Methenamine		+	+
Methotrexate (high dose)		+	+
Procarbazine		+	+
Tamoxifen		+	+
Interferon		+	+
Interleukin 2	+	+	+
Etopside		+	
Cyclosporine		+	+
Antivirals			
Acyclovir	+	+	+
Azidothymidine (AZT)	+	+	+
Suramin		+	
Endocrine			
Adrenocorticosteroids (including ACTH)	+	+	+
Estrogens	+	+	+
Oral hypoglycemics			+
Thyroid	+	+	+
Sympatholytics (e.g., methysergide)	+	+	
Sympathomimetics (including theophylline preparations)			
Vitamins			
A	+		+
B complex	+	+	
D		+	
Folic acid			+
Other			
Baclofen	+		
Diphenoxylate	+		
Disulfiram		+	+
Metrizamide	+		+
Orphenadrine		+	
Halothane	+		
Coumarin			+
Antiparkinsonians			
Anticholinergic (e.g., procyclidine)	+	+	+
Amantadine		+	+
Bromocriptine		+	+
Carbidopa	+	+	+
Levodopa	+	+	+
Cardiovascular			
Antiarrhythmics			
Lidocaine	+	+	+
Procainamide		+	+
Disopyramide	+	+	+
Mexiletine	+	+	+
Quinidine			+
Digitalis			+
Antihypertensives			
Carbonic anhydrase inhibitors			+
Ethacrynic acid			+
Furosemide		+	+
Hydrochlorothiazide		+	+

Table 27.2

Drug	Anxiety	Despondency	Delirium or Psychosis
Spironolactone			+
β-Blockers		+	+
Ganglionic blockers (mecamylamine, pentolinium, trimethaphan)			+
Rauwolfia alkaloids	+	+	+
Guanethidine		+	+
Methyldopa		+	+
Hydralazine	+	+	+
Clonidine	+	+	+
Prazosin		+	+
Calcium blockers		+	+
Narcotic Antagonists		+	+

very rare causes of delirium and usually occur only in someone whose brain is already vulnerable, as in a patient with a low seizure threshold. The number of drugs that can be involved either in direct toxic reactions or in toxic effects because of drug interactions are numerous, potentially bewildering, and constantly changing. Certain sources provide regular reviews of published summaries and updates (80).

DELIRIUM AND PSYCHOSIS

The term "ICU psychosis" is a popular diagnosis often applied to patients exhibiting abnormal behavior in an ICU. In fact, the occurrence of acute functional psychosis in an ICU is rare. The term implies that the environmental features of critical care settings are themselves capable of inducing psychosis. The rationale given for this entity is usually either sensory deprivation or sensory monotony. In point of fact, use of this diagnosis usually indicates that the etiology of a delirium is simply unknown. Hence, making the diagnosis of a functional psychosis has more risks than benefits because it tends to discourage a thorough differential diagnosis.

Diagnosis

Making a psychiatric diagnosis must begin by excluding organic factors that could cause symptoms in the realm of thought, emotion, and/or behavior. Throughout such an evaluation, it is helpful to have in mind a systematic schema for exclusion of organic causes of these psychiatric abnormalities. Figure 27.1 presents a decision tree or quasi-algorithm, according to which the diagnosis and treatment of specific abnormalities in the ICU can proceed. Usually the diagnostic and therapeutic considerations contained in the summary algorithm have already been considered by the ICU physicians and failure to reach any specific answer may be the reason that a psychiatric diagnosis has been entertained. Even at the point when that question is raised, however, it is the obligation of the physician to reconsider all organic possibilities that may have caused the psychiatric symptoms of the patient. Sometimes the psychiatric symptomatology is so bizarre or so offensive, as when a belligerent, delirious patient strikes a nurse, that the prior diagnostic efforts are disrupted and left incomplete.

The most common organic syndrome is delirium. Patients are typically older and have no previous psychiatric history. Delirium is usually preceded by a "lucid interval" of 1–3 days in which no abnormality is noted in the patient, and thereafter the abrupt onset of agitation signals that delirium is present. Delirium may include disordered or incoherent speech, sensory misperceptions (hallucinations, illusions, or misidentifications), psychomotor retardation or agitation, alterations in the sleep-wake cycle, irritability, fluctuations in arousal and somnolence, with variable disturbance in orientation, concentration, and memory. Therefore, the physician who suspects delirium should test the full range of the patient's cognitive functions (orientation, short-term memory, calculations, naming, repetition, praxis, and ability to think abstractly). Delirium usually worsens when external stimuli are reduced, characteristically at night. Prior dementia and any other CNS disturbance in-

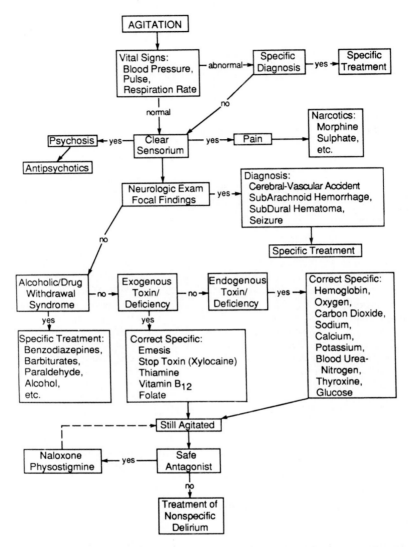

Figure 27.1. Decision tree for diagnosis and treatment of abnormalities in ICU setting. (From Cassem NH: The setting of intensive care. In Hackett TP, Cassem NH (eds): *MGH Handbook of General Hospital Psychiatry,* ed 2. Littleton MA, PSG Publishing Co., 1987, pp 362.)

creases the likelihood of delirium in the ICU setting. As Tables 27.1 and 27.2 indicate, specific diseases and drugs may be the culprit or make a contribution to the disturbances in the patient's mental state. Anticholinergic agents can be devastating, and some elderly patients who receive eye drops may absorb more because of corneal abrasions or simply absorb the drops through the tear ducts. Adrenocortical steroids, in doses of 40 mg/day or more of prednisone or its equivalent, will produce abnormalities in 5% of patients and when it reaches 80 mg/day in nearly 20% of patients. Analgesics may be culprits; none more than

meperidine, whose first metabolic product, normeperidine, causes tremors, myoclonus, delirium and ultimately seizures (59). Not only are medications potentially toxic in themselves, but withdrawal states must always be considered. Patients may be heavy drinkers who have ceased to drink on their admission to hospital, or in other instances simply stopped agents to which they were habituated, such as barbiturates, meprobamate, and alprazolam (9, 10, 15). A critical review of the literature on postcardiotomy delirium concluded that cardiac status, the severity of physical illness, the complexity of the surgical procedure, and preoperative organic brain disease are the determining factors in the prediction of this disturbance (28). It is not possible to discuss each one of the headings in the two tables. Often several factors coincide to cause some sort of decompensation in the patient and a final encephalopathic state.

Patients with chronic functional psychoses such as schizophrenia or manic-depressive disorder may also be patients in an ICU. Schizophrenic patients are known to do well clinically under such settings. Patients with stable manic-depressive psychosis maintained on lithium may be less stable, and a psychiatric consultation should be sought if abnormalities arise while the patient is in the ICU.

Nonpharmacological Intervention

Drugs are not the only way to reduce the risk of physical harm to the patient or others. Most ICU nurses are extremely proficient in their efforts to make the ICU a nonthreatening place to the patient, orienting them to time and place, and trying to manipulate the lighting so as to help reinstate normal biologic rhythms. Physical restraints are usually necessary in agitated patients to protect vital indwelling arterial or venous catheters, Foley catheters, intraaortic balloon pumps, pacing wires, chest tubes, nasogastric and feeding tubes, and other devices that assist the patient. A night light, clock, window, radio, and artifacts from home are helpful, but when agitation begins, it is usually the sign that these items have failed. Family presence at the bedside can be very reassuring to the patient and in some cases a family member's presence at night may be sufficient to keep the patient out of difficulty. It is always helpful for the physician to assess the patient's medication and care schedules to see that the longest possible period of uninterrupted sleep at night can be obtained (69).

When the patient has delusions, it is seldom helpful to manage it on intellectual grounds. If patients have delusional explanations for how they got to the ICU, it does not help to agree with them. If they believe that there is a plot to kill them, they must be reassured that this is not the case, but argument of the facts or attempted proofs are not helpful. A calm, reassuring stance wherein the physician listens to patient but repeatedly reassures them that they are in the ICU and that everything is being done to help them is probably best. Talking should not delay treatment.

Drug Treatment

Good fortune sometimes rewards a careful diagnostic search with a specific etiology. If this is the case, and one of the conditions in Figure 27.1 is realized, specific treatment can proceed. Occasionally, a history of heavy alcohol use emerges and treatment of alcohol withdrawal can proceed. In such circumstances, management with benzodiazepines is preferred.

Sometimes it is clear that a drug is causing the confusional state but stopping or reducing it is not possible. For example, in a patient with life-threatening ventricular irritability for whom a high rate of lidocaine infusion seems essential, there may be no way that one can immediately reduce the dosage even though the etiologic connection with agitation is clear. In such a case, treatment of nonspecific delirium, specifically with intravenous haloperidol, can proceed while lidocaine is being given. However, the CNS derangement will not cease until the drug is reduced to a nontoxic level or stopped.

Occasionally, one may want to establish the diagnosis of an anticholinergic psychosis by intravenously administering physostigmine in a dose of 0.5–2 mg parenterally. Caution is essential for patients in critical care settings; however, because the cholinergic reaction to intravenously administered physostigmine can cause profound bradycardia and hypotension, thereby multiplying the complications instead of reducing them. It should be noted, on the other hand, that a continuous intravenous infusion of physostigmine has been successfully used to manage a case of anticholinergic poisoning (113). If one were to use an intravenous injection of 1 mg of physostigmine, protection against excessive cholinergic reaction can be provided by preceding this injection with an intravenous injection of 0.2 mg of glycopyrrolate. This anticholinergic agent does not cross the blood-brain barrier and should protect the patient from the peripheral cholinergic actions of physostigmine.

Antipsychotic Pharmacokinetics

An intramuscular dose of an antipsychotic is about 1.5 times as potent as the equivalent oral dose. These drugs are quickly and reliably absorbed after intramuscular administration, reaching peak blood levels in as little as 10–20 minutes (22, 81). Maximum blood levels are obtained more rapidly after deltoid than after gluteal injection (77). There is considerable interindividual variation in antipsychotic blood levels following an equal oral dose. Antipsychotics are absorbed primarily in the jejunum (71) and peak blood levels are attained in roughly 2–6 hours (52). Cholestyramine, gel acids, and anticholinergic agents may inhibit absorption (9). Hence, an oral antipsychotic should precede these agents whenever possible. Liquid concentrates are the best absorbed of oral forms, but also can form an insoluble precipitate with milk, fruit juice, coffee or tea, with which they are frequently mixed. Chlorpromazine (CPZ) undergoes extensive metabolism by enzymes in the gut wall.

Antipsychotics are metabolized by the liver and excreted in both the urine and bile (8). There is significant enterohepatic circulation (81). CPZ is predicted to have over 100 metabolites, many of which are active (77). Estimates of the half-life of CPZ in the body range from 2 to 60 days, although the longer estimate is probably more accurate (23). Haloperidol, by contrast, has no active metabolites and its half-life is between 12 and 36 hours (34). For comparison, mean half-lives of the oral preparation and the intramuscular and intravenous routes are 24, 21, and 14 hours, respectively. The long half-lives of antipsychotic drugs mean that once-a-day dosing is rational for chronic maintenance use. Acute treatment of delirium requires more frequent dosing.

Choice of Drug

There are some helpful guidelines in choosing an antipsychotic. These include side effect profile (other than sedation), available dosage forms, and history of response in the patient or family member (3). Side effect information is summarized in Table 27.3.

There is no convincing evidence that one antipsychotic is more effective than another for particular psychotic symptoms (77), nor is there substantial data that a drug with more sedative side effects is better for agitated patients than a more "activating" drug that is assumed to be useful in treating someone who is withdrawn, although these unproven hypotheses are often adhered to in clinical practice (3, 25, 78).

Potency refers to the amount of drug needed to achieve a certain level of antipsychotic effect. The higher the potency, the less that is

needed for the same clinical effect. In general, the lower a drug's potency, the more likely it is to produce sedative, anticholinergic, and hypotensive effects; whereas the higher potency drugs are more likely to produce neurologic (extrapyramidal) side effects. In most medically ill patients, undue sedation, hypotension, and anticholinergic effects are more troublesome than an extrapyramidal reaction. Such a reaction, although distressing, is rarely life threatening. These include those rare situations that involve the respiratory muscles (5, 49, 57, 85).

Low-potency drugs are usually more anticholinergic and therefore more likely to exacerbate delirium. The effect of CPZ on blocking total peripheral resistance can be devastating and severe hypotension can result. CPZ is more painful than, for example, haloperidol, when injected intramuscularly. Among the low-potency antipsychotic drugs, thioridazine and mezoridazine both have quinidine-like side effects with significant potential for causing serious ventricular arrhythmias (64, 104).

Table 27.3 contains dosage recommendations for treatment of delirium with various antipsychotic drugs. The best guide to the dose and drug required for schizophrenia or manic-depressive disorder is the patient's treatment history. In this situation a psychiatric consultation is indicated. In general, whereas a schizophrenic may require 10–30 mg of haloperidol or its equivalent daily, a delirious patient may be calmed down by as little as 0.5 mg of haloperidol, especially if the patient is elderly.

Haloperidol is the recommended agent, mostly because of the extensive experience with this agent over other high-potency neuroleptic drugs. Its effect on blood pressure, pulmonary artery pressure, heart rate, and respiration are milder than those of the benzodiazepines, making it an excellent agent for severely ill patients with impaired cardiorespiratory status (6, 111). Although haloperidol can be administered orally or parenterally, acute delirium with extreme agitation requires parenteral medication. Intravenous administration is preferable to intramuscular administration for the following reasons:

1. Drug absorption may be poor in distal muscles if a patient's delirium is associated with circulatory compromise or borderline shock.
2. The agitated patient is commonly paranoid

Table 27.3
Psychoactive Drugs[a]

Drugs	Dosage Forms Available[b]	Usual Dose Range for Agitation	Comments
ANTIPSYCHOTICS			
Low potency			
		(up to QID)	
Chlorpromazine	t, c, i, s	25–100	See text
Thioridazine	t, c	25–100	Similar to chlorpromazine; drug most frequently associated with ECG changes
Mid-potency			
Perphenazine	t, c, i	4–12	Moderately sedating
High potency			
Trifluoperazine	t, c, i	1–5	
Haloperidol	t, c, i	1–10	Often recommended for medically ill patients
Molindone	t, c	2–10	Virtually no hypotensive effects
Loxapine	t, c	2–10	Metabolized to amoxapine, an antidepressant
SEDATIVE/HYPNOTICS			
Benzodiazepines (BDZs)			
Long-acting			
		(up to QID)	
Diazepam	t, i	2–10	Only BDZ with proven muscle relaxant, anticonvulsant and analgesic properties
Chlordiazepoxide	t, i	5–25	This drug and diazepam have rarely been associated with increased hostility and rage
Clorazepate	t	3.25–15	Like diazepam and chlordiazepam, useful for alcohol withdrawal
Flurazepam	t	15–30	Used only for sleep; cumulative effects sometimes responsible for undue sedation or disorientation
Short-acting			
Oxazepam	t	10–30	Especially well tolerated by patients with liver disease and the elderly
Lorazepam	t, i	2–24	Strong amnesic effect; used to sedate ventilator patients, same as above
Temazepam	t	30	Marketed as a hypnotic; molecularly similar to oxazepam
Alprazolam	t	0.5–2	May have significant antidepressant effects
Non-benzodiazepines			
Propranolol	t, i	30–120	Affects autonomic symptoms of anxiety; little if any effect on psychic symptoms
Phenobarbital	t	15–30	Barbiturates are noted for inducing respiratory failure
Secobarbital	t	30–50	
Chloral hydrate	t, c	250	
Hydroxyzine	t, c	100	Ineffective unless given in large doses

[a] Data from references 3, 8, 9, 10, 12, 52, 62, 63, 67, 68, 76, 88, 97, 124.
[b] Dosage forms: t = tablets, c = oral concentrate, i = injectable, s = suppositories.

and repeated, painful intramuscular injections may increase the patient's sense of being attacked by enemy forces.

3. Intramuscular injections can complicate interpretations of muscle enzyme studies if such studies are important clinically and if enzyme fractionation cannot solve the source of elevation.

4. Finally, and most important, intravenously administered haloperidol is less likely to produce extrapyramidal side effects.

In contrast to the immediate observable sedation produced by intravenous diazepam, intravenous haloperidol has a mean distribution time of 11 minutes in normal volunteers; this may be even longer in critically ill patients. Because of this unusually long distribution time there is no reason for giving an intravenous bolus of haloperidol slowly. A rapid push of the dose is safe.

The initial bolus dose of haloperidol varies from 0.5 to 20 mg: 0.5–2 mg for mild agitation, 2–5 mg for moderate agitation, and 10 or more mg for severe agitation. The only time a consultant would use a higher initial dose is when the patient has already been treated with reasonable doses of haloperidol unsuccessfully. To allow for haloperidol's delayed onset, doses are usually staggered by at least a 30-minute interval. If a 5-mg dose does not calm an agitated patient after 30 mintues, 10 mg should be administered. Partial control of agitation usually is not adequate and only prolongs the delirium. Therefore, it is recommended that haloperidol be given every 30 minutes until the patient is calm. Agitation will respond first, followed closely by hallucinations and extreme anxiety. Delusions, if present, usually take the longest to disappear.

After calm is achieved, agitation should be the sign for a repeat dose. Ideally, the total dose of haloperidol on the second day should be a fraction of that on day 1. After complete lucidity has been achieved, the patient needs to be protected from delirium only at night, by small doses of haloperidol (0.5–3 mg), which can be given orally. This therapy is seldom necessary for more than 2 or 3 nights. As in the treatment of delirium tremens, the consultant is advised to stop the agitation completely at the outset rather than barely keeping up with it over several days. The maximum total intravenous dose of haloperidol to be used as an upper limit has not been established, although single-bolus intravenous doses of 150 mg have been administered, inasmuch as 945 mg total dose has been used in a 24-hour period (114).

Hypotensive episodes following the administration of intravenous haloperidol are rare and almost invariably caused by hypovolemia. Ordinarily this problem is easily checked in ICU patients who have indwelling pulmonary artery catheters, but since agitation is likely to return, volume replacement is necessary before administering further doses. There are no local caustic effects on veins. Intravenous haloperidol is generally safe for epileptics and patients with head trauma. Although intravenous haloperidol may be used without mishap in patients receiving epinephrine drips, after very large doses of haloperidol a pressor other than epinephrine, such as norepinephrine, should be used to avoid unopposed β-adrenergic activity.

Intravenous haloperidol does not block the dopamine-mediated increase in renal blood flow. It also appears to be the safest agent for patients with chronic obstructive pulmonary disease.

Combining haloperidol with a benzodiazepine in the treatment of a nonspecific delirium may at times be quite helpful. When, for example, repeated doses of haloperidol fail to give a therapeutic response, another agent, preferably lorazepam or midazolam, can be tried. Adams has recommended a regular treatment regimen with alternating doses of haloperidol (10 mg) and lorazepam (1 mg) for the treatment of nonspecific delirium (1).

Although there is now extensive experience with intravenous administration of haloperidol (14, 29, 83, 114), the Food and Drug Administration (FDA) has not given approval for the administration of the drug by the intravenous route. Protecting the patients from extrapyramidal side effects makes this route extremely attractive. The less frequent appearance of these extrapyramidal effects after intravenous administration in medically ill patients may be due to the fact that many of the medically ill patients are receiving other medications that are protective, especially the benzodiazepines and β-blockers; or that patients with psychiatric disorder, especially schizophrenia, are more susceptible to extrapyramidal side effects of the drugs; or that the patients are elderly and therefore at a very low risk for acute dystonia and akathisia. The lack of these effects in medical patients continues to be documented clinically (82).

Alternative agents to haloperidol have been sought. Droperidol, an agent already approved for intravenous administration by the FDA, is a far more potent α-adrenergic antagonist than haloperidol, and it is far more likely to lead to difficulties with hypotension, particularly when it is combined with other agents. One such reaction has been noted in several instances when droperidol was used as an intravenous antiemetic for cancer patients simultaneously receiving oral tetrahydrocannabinol. Intravenous diazepam is used routinely to treat agitated states, particularly delirium tremens, as are intravenous chlordiazepoxide and lorazepam. Any one of these intravenous benzodiazepines may be a useful adjunct in the treatment of acute nonspecific delirium. Intravenous alcohol is also extremely effective in the treatment of alcohol withdrawal states. Its disadvantage is that it is toxic in itself to both liver and brain, although its use can be safe if these organs do not already show extensive damage (and sometimes safe even when they do). A 5% solution of alcohol mixed with 5% dextrose and water, run at 1 ml/minute, brings a calming effect amazingly quickly. Other parenteral neuroleptic drugs for treatment of agitation are thiothixene, trifluoperazine hydrochloride, and fluphenazine.

Midazolam maleate is available in the United States for intravenous sedation. It acts even faster than diazepam and is 3–4 times as potent. Its rapid onset, short elimination half-life (from 1–4 hours), and amnestic potency make it an ideal short-term sedative and anesthetic agent. Clinical experience with this agent is still not sufficient to evaluate its usefulness for the treatment of acute delirium. Respiratory depression and hypotension have both been reported with midazolam; the latter was particularly severe when the drug was combined with large doses of fentanyl citrate.

FEAR AND ANXIETY

Diagnosis

Admission to an intensive care setting is invariably associated with a life-threatening disease. Even after the fear of death has ceased to haunt their consciousness, patients may fear that they will be maimed by the illness or by its treatments. This fear may assume many guises; verbosity, outbursts of anger, paranoia, and silent withdrawal are all behaviors typically produced by fear.

If the patient has a past history of a specific anxiety disorder, such as panic disorder, agoraphobia, a specific phobia such as claustrophobia, or obsessive-compulsive disorder, a psychiatric consultation is indicated. All of these specific disorders can in their own way interfere with the patient's treatment and recovery.

Nonpharmacologic Intervention

Anxiety is treated both by medication and by quiet reassurance. Much more is often gained by listening to the patient rather than by specific questioning, especially to open-ended questions about fears. Clarification, explanation, and reassurance are highly effective when fear stems from threatening or erroneous misconceptions about disease or the ICU itself. After false ideas have been corrected, it is important to mention positive aspects of the treatment plan. For example, the cardiac patient might be assured that myocardial healing is complete in 5–6 weeks, and that normal activities will be resumed along with an exercise program. Even when the prognosis is grave, the calm statement of the treatments planned to counteract and contain the patient's suffering is of value to the anxious patient. The more ominous the prognosis, the more important it is to encourage the patient to specify the fear, so that specific and valid reassurances (e.g., that medication can control pain) can be given. False reassurance is not recommended because it robs the physician of credibility and therefore the ability to reassure the patient later in the illness.

When an anxiety persists despite explanations, further questions such as, "Have you ever known anyone with these symptoms (or this disease)?" or, "What is your idea of a heart attack (pulmonary embolus, recovery)?" can be used to uncover misconceptions. When a family member has died of the same condition, his or her age at death may figure heavily in the patient's fear; often patients expect that fate will take them at the same age.

Equanimity has perhaps the most soothing effect on the patient. Anxious patients have a way of making people who take care of them anxious, and a vicious circle may develop. A calm person can break that deleterious interaction.

Drug Treatment

Unless panic has begun to encroach on rationality, the drugs of choice are the benzodiazepines (Table 27.4). If the patient's condition is one in which autonomic lability may be a hazard (e.g., myocardial infarction), routine prescription of one of these agents is recommended whether or not the patient looks anxious. Even when autonomic lability is not a hazard, the anxiety that accompanies severe acute medical illness is the most common in-

Table 27.4
Side Effects of Psychotropic Drugs, Presentation and Management

Organ System	AP	TCA	BDZ	Presentation	Management
Central Nervous System					
Dystonias	Common	Rare		Sudden, dramatic muscle contractions, especially upper trunk, head and neck; young males most susceptible; occurs early in treatment; may be precipitated by emotional stress	Benadryl 50, benztropine 2–10 mg, p.o., i.m. or i.v., for prophylaxis same dose b.i.d.-q.i.d.
Pseudo-parkinsonism	Common	Very rare		Indistinguishable from Parkinson's disease; occurs especially in elderly; mostly with high potency APs	Benadryl 50 mg or benztropine 1–2 mg p.o. q.d.-q.i.d.
Akathisia	Common	Rare		Mostly with high potency APs; vague sense of need to move; can be confused with psychotic agitation	Reduce dose, change or stop AP; can give propranolol 10 mg b.i.d. or t.i.d.
Seizures	Rare	Rare		Possibly more common with low potency APs, especially in high doses, and patients with known seizure disorder	Reduce dose, stop AP, or raise dose of anticonvulsant
Tremor		Rare		More common with stimulating TCAs, e.g., imipramine, desipramine	Usually requires no treatment
Hematologic					
Leukopenia/ agranulocytosis	Rare	Rare	Very rare	Rapid onset of sore throat and fever; periodic WBC counts of little value	Stop drug, routine management
Gastrointestinal					
Jaundice	Rare	Very rare	Very rare	Most often with low potency APs in first month of treatment	Stop drug, management routine

Data from references 15, 27, 33, 43, 55, 58, 72, 75, 77, 112.
AP, antipsychotic; TCA, tricyclic antidepressant; BDZ, benzodiazepine.

dication for the prescription of benzodiazepines. The benzodiazepines have a wide therapeutic margin, about 10 times that of the barbiturates (21); little tendency to induce hepatic enzymes; few interactions with other drugs; little effect on respiratory cardiovascular status in well patients; and relatively low potential for dependency or addiction, with the exception of alprazolam (35).

Of the benzodiazepines available, diazepam probably produces the high blood level most rapidly and is of particular value for the patient who needs to feel tranquilization quickly. If the tranquilizers are given routinely to all patients, about 8% of them will complain of feeling sedated (18). Some of these patients may be reacting to a drug's rapid absorption and would better tolerate the slow, steady accumulation of one of the less lipid-soluble benzodiazepines, such as oxazepam or prazepam.

Clorazepate and prazepam are two long-acting benzodiazepines that are not active in their original form. They both have the same active metabolite, n-desmethyldiazepam, which is the only metabolite that produces psychotropic effects. However, clorazepate produces high blood levels within the first hour, whereas prazepam enters the system slowly. These differences are due to the lipophilic nature of the two drugs. By 4 hours, the concentration of desmethyldiazepam is essentially the same for both of these agents (48). According to this rationale, a clinician would choose diazepam, clorazepate, lorazepam, or alprazolam if the patient wanted to experience tranquilization quickly. Oxazepam, prazepam, and temazepam are better for the patient who prefers to get the benefits slowly and imperceptibly. When using longer-acting agents such as diazepam, whose half-life varies between 20 and 60 hours, the physician can assume that saturation has been attained after 2 or 3 days and administered only at bedtime or twice-daily dose thereafter. However, if the patient's anxiety responds best to the impacts of repeated dosing, three or four divided doses a day may remain clinically preferable. In fact, the latter is the most common way of prescribing the agent for both inpatients and outpatients. Parenteral forms of chlordiazepoxide, diazepam, and midazolam are available, but intramuscular absorption of the first two agents is erratic and less complete than absorption of oral doses. For this reason, oral or cautious intravenous administration is recommended. Chlordiazepoxide, diazepam, and alprazolam can, on rare occasions, produce paradoxical hostility or rage (10, 102). Hence, oxazepam, lorazepam, or temazepam may be more appropriate if the patient already seems hostile.

Among the short-acting benzodiazepines—oxazepam, lorazepam, temazepam, alprazolam, triazolam, and midazolam—only lorazepam and midazolam are currently available for parenteral use and, for this reason, have special value in critical care units. Otherwise, the major advantage of the first three (oxazepam, lorazepam, temazepam) is that they have no active metabolites and therefore do not accumulate in the blood. These shorter-acting agents are metabolized by glucuronidation, a metabolic process well preserved not only in the elderly but in patients with impaired hepatic function. Since both advanced age and impaired liver function are associated with increased benzodiazepine half-lives (65, 99) these agents are very useful for these types of patients.

A general rule is to prescribe the simplest and shortest-acting effective drug, for example, 15 mg of oxazepam 3 or 4 times a day. With the physician's permission, the nurse can hold this drug if it seems excessive or report it if the patient seems undermedicated. One of the most sensitive measures of the dose's adequacy is the perception of the ICU nurse. The nurse, who attends the patient for an entire 8-hour shift, is generally able to see whether the patient appears to be growing more anxious or has begun to sleep all the time and is becoming harder to arouse and engage.

Slow accumulation of benzodiazepine metabolites is a problem worth worrying about. It is especially likely with flurazepam, diazepam, and all agents in which desmethyldiazepam is a metabolite. In addition, since the metabolism of these agents requires oxidative processes, patients with hepatic impairment are even more likely to accumulate excessive doses. There are those who maintain that flurazepam, despite its long half-life, is the most effective sleeping medication available to them. This claim appears to be correct in some cases, but one must still be vigilant for effects of accumulation.

Drug Interactions

Benzodiazepines interact rarely with few compounds. All sedatives/hypnotics have added effects with CNS depressants. Disulfiram decreases the clearance of chlordiazepoxide, although these two drugs are unlikely to be administered concurrently in an ICU (36). Cimetidine may increase the clearance of benzodiazepines (53), but can also potentiate the sedative effects and double the plasma levels of diazepam (98). The dose of benzodiazepines, except for the three short-acting agents metabolized by glucuronidation, should be less in patients receiving cimetidine.

Other Agents

If the patient's fear is sufficiently intense to impair reason, or if the patient appears to be in a state of panic or transient psychosis, an antipsychotic drug is the agent of choice. Panicked individuals are barely in control; the benzodiazepines can sometimes further compromise an already diminished ability to cope. The preferred neuroleptic is again haloperidol, which can be administered in oral or parenteral form.

Special Situations

In some patients anxiety may inhibit weaning from the mechanical ventilator. Multimodal treatment of this anxiety often begins with a benzodiazepine such as lorazepam, administered prior to weaning periods or a neuroleptic such as haloperidol if the patient appears to be in a near panic state. Persons who suffer acute and chronic respiratory failure and therefore require prolonged mechanical ventilation may become so anxious when the weaning process begins that psychiatric assistance is requested. Even though the patient is physically ready for weaning, anxiety can transiently increase metabolic demands and cardiac work until further weaning becomes impossible.

Most behavioral exercises for relaxation encourage the subject to take slow, deep, easy breaths. This is one of the quickest and surest ways of inducing relaxation for most people, but it is precisely what patients with respiratory problems cannot do and precisely what makes them so anxious. The multimodal treatment of their anxiety usually begins with a drug, as mentioned above. Patient themselves can indicate whether the drug has been effective or which drug is more helpful. In some cases it may be possible to use a mixture of nitrous oxide if the respiratory specialist or anesthesiologist is present to administer it. Hypnosis or relaxation techniques are often helpful in distracting the patient from the weaning process. When these are used, the instruction to breathe easily is best omitted from the hypnotic suggestion; the patient should be encouraged to concentrate either on a tranquil scene such as a beach or a single concept (mantra) (10). Since despondency and major depression, as well as anxiety, can impede weaning, the treatments for depression may apply here as well.

DEPRESSIVE DISORDERS

Diagnosis

In any serious illness the mind sustains an injury of its own, as though the illness (for example, myocardial infarction) produced an ego infarction.

Despondency

This psychic damage, called "despondency", is distinct from depression, which is a major affective disorder. Even when recovery of the diseased organ is complete, recovery of self-esteem appears to take somewhat longer,

and despondency tends to become a serious problem in ICU patients the longer they stay in a unit (18). In uncomplicated myocardial infarction patients, the myocardial scar is fully formed in 5–6 weeks, but recovery of psychological well-being often requires 2–3 months.

Despondency is a mixture of dread, sadness, bitterness, and despair, which causes patients to see themselves as broken, scarred, or even ruined. Working relationships seem jeopardized. Disappointment with what has and has not been accomplished haunts the individual, who now may feel old and a failure. The disease may not have killed the patient, but the patient may feel it has crippled his or her career and personal aspirations.

Concerns of this kind become apparent rather early in acute illness and may prompt concern even by the second or third day of hospitalization.

Feeling better is the best antidote for illness-induced acute despondency. In the interim, the patient should be encouraged, but never forced, to express any concerns about the damage done by the illness. Some patients are upset merely to find such depressive concerns in their consciousness and even worry that this signals a "nervous breakdown." It is essential to let them know that such concerns are normal emotional counterparts to physical illness, that fluctuate in their intensity and usually disappear gradually as health returns. It is also reassuring for patients to hear about any rehabilitation plans while they are still in the recovery phase.

When progress is slow and intangible, minor interventions can sometimes be helpful. For example, getting a patient with severe congestive heart failure out of bed and into a reclining chair not only relieves cardiovascular strain but also provides reassurance and boosts confidence.

Major Depression

There are various types of depression, but pharmacologic help is required only in those mood states that meet specific diagnostic criteria, i.e., major depression, depression with mania or manic symptoms, and depression with psychotic symptoms. The diagnostic criteria for a depressive episode are as follows:

1. Depressed mood most of the day, nearly every day;
2. Markedly diminished interest or pleasure in all, or almost all, activities;

3. Significant weight loss or weight gain when not dieting, or decrease or increase in appetite;
4. Insomnia or hypersomnia;
5. Psychomotor agitation or retardation;
6. Fatigue or loss of energy;
7. Feelings of worthlessness or excessive or inappropriate guilt;
8. A diminished ability to think or concentrate or indecisiveness;
9. Recurrent thoughts of death (not just fear of dying), recurrent suicidal ideation without a specific plan, or a suicide attempt or a specific plan for committing suicide.

Ordinarily, the patient must possess at least five of these nine symptoms for a duration of 2 weeks to qualify for the diagnosis of major depression. Even if a patient has not been in the ICU this long, he or she may have been depressed prior to admission.

The presence of a distinguishable loss or life event is not necessary for a diagnosis of major depression. The patient may actually deny being depressed, ascribing symptoms of fatigue, anorexia, and sleep disturbance to the medical condition. When it is not clear whether an individual symptom like anorexia or fatigue is due to the primary medical illness or to a superimposed depression, the recommendation is to take an inclusive approach and count every symptom that actually is present, regardless of etiology. The true concern with every ICU patient is that, even though the treatment of the primary medical illness has been maximized, something is retarding the process of the patient towards recovery. Unless there is confidence that the patient does not meet criteria for depression, a drug trial is warranted.

Drug Treatment

A wide variety of agents is available to treat major depression. There is no reason why all of these drugs might not, at some time or other, help a depressed patient in an ICU. The drugs include polycyclic antidepressants, monoamineoxidase inhibitors (MAOI), lithium, carbamazepine, and psychostimulants. The following approach is recommended in the ICU setting.

Psychostimulants

If the patient is lethargic, hard to mobilize, listless, and seems to show no investment in a caretaking regimen, an excellent safe choice for treatment would be to start with a psychostimulant: either 5 mg of dextroamphetamine sulfate once a day or 5 mg of methylphenidate. These drugs can be extremely helpful in mobilizing a person who appears to be physiologically recovering from a long illness but lacks motivation. They are helpful both therapeutically and diagnostically. If, for example, one is not sure whether an element of major depression exists, one excellent way to probe for this is with a test dose of a psychostimulant (41).

For example, a patient could be given 5 mg of dexedrine once in the morning. If the patient shows considerable brightening, one can assume there is a significant component of major depression and treatment should continue. There is no need to switch to a tricyclic or conventional antidepressant immediately. Some patients improve with psychostimulant therapy alone, become mobilized, and achieve recovery. Other patients require the addition of a traditional antidepressant. Dexedrine is administered once a day, usually first thing in the morning, in order to prevent the side effect of insomnia. The dose is increased daily until a beneficial effect is seen or an unwanted side effect (such as feeling tense) appears. The half-life of dexedrine varies from 7 to 30 hours, and some patients may need it twice, e.g. 8 AM and noon. Methylphenidate, whose half-life varies from 2 to 4 hours, needs to be given at least twice and sometimes three times daily. Patients tolerate these drugs well. In medically ill patients, the incidence of tachycardia, elevated blood pressure, or increased agitation even in demented patients has been mild (121). Nearly 90% of the patients who responded to stimulants reached their maximum response by the second day. The advantage, of course, is that one does not have to wait 2–3 weeks for treatment response to occur.

Pharmacokinetics of Polycyclic Antidepressants

The polycyclic antidepressants (PCAs) are molecularly similar to the phenothiazines. The PCAs are well absorbed early, generally reaching peak concentration in 2–6 hours. Anticholinergics and antacids may impede absorption. They are highly lipophilic and are rapidly taken up by the brain and peripheral tissues. PCAs are metabolized in the liver through oxidation and glucuronidation. They are excreted primarily in the urine, but there is significant enterohepatic circulation (93). Estimates to their half-lives generally range from 12–24 hours and the commonest method of dosing is once a day at bedtime.

Choice of Drug

The few clear reasons for selecting one PCA over another involve side effects more than specific depressive symptoms. A more sedating agent, e.g., doxepin, is often recommended for patients with severe insomnia, whereas a less sedating agent such as desipramine is used more commonly with a withdrawn, psychomotor retarded patient. It is important to remember that none of these agents appears to be superior to any other in the overall treatment of depression, but the side effect profile of each drug provides a reasonable rationale for its selection. This side effect profile (Table 27.5) and a history of previous response by the patient or family member can provide a relative indication for a particular drug.

The PCAs have three major side effects, which if understood, provide the ICU physician with an excellent knowledge of what to expect from each drug.

ORTHOSTATIC HYPOTENSION

The potency for the various PCAs is listed in Table 27.5. In general, the tertiary amines (the top four PCAs) are more likely to cause an orthostatic fall in blood pressure than are secondary amines (the next three drugs). For reasons not clearly understood, imipramine is the tricyclic most commonly associated with orthostatic mishaps, such as falling and sustaining a fracture or head injury. Ordinarily in the ICU the patients are bedridden and orthostatic effects are not as worrisome. The orthostatic effect appears earlier than the therapeutic effect and will be objectively verifiable at roughly half the therapeutic plasma level for imipramine. The clinical consensus is that nortriptyline is the PCA least likely to cause orthostatic hypotension clinically.

ANTICHOLINERGIC EFFECTS

Urinary retention, constipation, dry mouth, confusional states, and tachycardia are the commonest unwanted side effects of the PCAs. The increase in heart rate is a sinus tachycardia resulting from the ability of these drugs to oppose vagal tone in the heart. Amitriptyline is the most anticholinergic of the PCAs, with protriptyline a rather close second. These two agents will regularly cause tachycardia in

Table 27.5
Antidepressant Drugs

	Relative Potencies for Producing Certain Clinical Effects			Cardiac Conduction/ Arrhythmia	Target Dose (mg/day)	Dosage Range (mg/day)	Therapeutic Plasma Level (ng/ml)
	Sedative	Orthostatic	Anticholinergic				
Tricyclic Agents							
Doxepin	High	Moderate	Moderate	Yes	200	25–400	
Amitriptyline	High	Moderate	Highest	Yes	150	25–300	
Imipramine	Moderate	High	Moderate	Yes	200	50–400	≥200
Trimipramine	High	? Moderate	Moderate	Yes	150	50–300	
Protriptyline	Lowest	Low	High	Yes	30	5–60	
Nortriptyline	Moderate	Lowest	Moderate	Yes	100	25–150	50–150
Desipramine	Lowest	Low	Moderate	Yes	150	75–300	≥125
Other Cyclic Agents							
Amoxapine	Moderate	Low	Moderate	Lower	200	50–300	
Maprotiline	Moderate	Low	Moderate	Lower	150	50–200	
Trazodone	Moderate	Moderate	Very Low	Lower	200	50–600	
Benzodiazepine							
Alprazolam	High	None	None	None	3	0.5–10	
MAOI							
Phenelzine	Low	High	None	Very rare	60	30–90	
Tranylcypromine	Low	High	None	Very rare	30	10–60	
Isocarboxazid	Low	Moderate	None	Very rare	30	10–60	
Psychostimulants							
Dextroamphetamine	None	None	None	Rare	10	2.5–30	
Methylphenidate	None	None	None	Rare	20	5–60	

medically ill patients, and one should check the heart rate as the dose is increased. If significant tachycardia results, another agent may have to be used. Many hospitalized patients, particularly those with ischemic heart disease, are already being treated with β-adrenergic blockers, such as propranolol, which will usually protect the patient from developing a significant tachycardia from the antidepressant.

Among all the PCAs, trazodone is unique in its relative freedom of anticholinergic potency. While switching from imipramine to desipramine to avoid urinary retention is seldom successful, trazodone may be used with no further retentive problems.

CARDIAC CONDUCTION EFFECTS

All PCAs appear capable of producing cardiac arrhythmias. The mechanism for most of them is related to their ability to prolong ventricular depolarization. This action tends to produce on the electrocardiogram (ECG) a lengthening of the PR and QRS intervals, as well as the QT interval, corrected for heart rate (QTc). This effect makes the PCAs resemble the class IA antiarrhythmic drugs such as quinidine and procainamide hydrochloride (39). In practical terms, the depressed patient with ventricular premature contractions, when started on an antidepressant such as imipramine, is likely to experience a therapeutic reduction in ventricular irritability.

Ordinarily this property does not pose a problem for medically ill patients who do not already have disease in the conduction system. Conditions that are most worrisome, therefore, are patients with impaired conduction in the His Purkinje system such as bifascicular block, bundle branch block with prolonged PR, alternating bundle branch block, second- or third-degree atrioventricular block. First-degree heart block and right bundle branch block ordinarily present little problem with PCAs, especially if the patient is stable. The patient with unstable atrial fibrillation is always a concern. Cardiology consultation will almost always be present for these patients. Electrolyte abnormalities, particularly hypokalemia or hypomagnesemia, increase the danger of arrhythmia and require careful monitoring. There is some evidence that the hydroxymetabolites of the traditional tricyclics are more specifically related to the production of slowing in HV conduction (122). Amoxapine has been singled out because patients who overdosed on that agent, despite having suffered seizures, coma, and acute renal failure, manifested no cardiac toxicity. But atrial flutter/fibrillation has been reported in patients taking amoxapine. Trazodone has also been defended in a thorough review by Ayd as having fewer cardiotoxic effects. Even though trazodone is said not to prolong conduction in the His Purkinje system, aggravation of preexisting ventricular irritability has been reported with its use. Clinical caution must therefore be maintained.

If a patient were to have a serious conduction disease, either a psychostimulant or alprazolam might be helpful for depression and will be less likely to produce cardiac conduction disturbances.

The Question of Myocardial Depression

Persons have been concerned about the ability of PCAs to depress left ventricular function. Left ventricular ejection fractions were measured before and during imipramine, doxepin, and nortriptyline treatment of cardiac patients with major depression. These tricyclics showed no adverse effects on ventricular function even in patients who demonstrated impaired ventricular function before treatment (38, 95). In fact, the use of PCAs has also been found to be safe in patients with congestive heart failure (39, 100).

Clinical Use

A reasonable plan for an ICU patient is to start at 10–25 mg/day of a PCA and increase toward the recommended therapeutic dose. All or most of the dose can be given at bedtime, even if the drug is not especially sedating, e.g., desipramine. Insomnia responds first to the medication, often on the very first night. If no improvement is noted in 7–10 days on the therapeutic dose, further increases are in order. Imipramine, desipramine, and nortriptyline have reliable plasma levels that can be reassuring, especially if one wants to keep the patient in therapeutic range for a 3- to 4-week period of time. These values (Table 27.5) are, respectively, equal to or greater than 200 ng/ml, equal to or greater than 125 ng/ml, and 50–150 ng/ml.

SUMMARY

Psychiatric problems are a frequent occurrence in an ICU, and most often they probably come and go without anyone having taken

Table 27.6
Psychotropic Drugs

Chemical	Trade
Antipsychotics	
Chlorpromazine	Thorazine, Promapar, Chlor-PZ
Thioridazine	Mellaril
Perphenazine	Trilafon
Trifluoperazine	Stelazine
Haloperidol	Haldol
Molindone	Moban, Lidone
Loxapine	Loxitane, Daxolin
Benzodiazepine Sedative/Hypnotics	
Diazepam	Valium
Chlordiazepoxide	Librium
Clorazepate	Tranxene, Azene
Prazepam	Centrax
Flurazepam	Dalmane
Oxazepam	Serax
Lorazepam	Ativan
Alprazolam	Xanax
Temazepam	Restoril
Triazolam	Halcion
Midazolam	Versed
Antidepressants	
Imipramine	Tofranil, Antipress, Imavate, Jamimine, Presamine, Ropramine, SK-Pramine
Desipramine	Norpramin, Pertofrane
Amitriptyline	Elavil, Endep, Amitril, Rolavil
Nortriptyline	Pamelor, Aventyl
Doxepin	Sinequan, Adapin
Trimipramine	Surmontil
Amoxapine	Asendin
Maprotiline	Ludiomil
Trazodone	Desyrel
Phenelzine	Nardil
Tranylcypromine	Parnate
Isocarboxazid	Marplan
Dextroamphetamine	Dexedrine
Methylphenidate	Ritalin

notice of their presence. At other times, however, appearance of a psychiatric disorder may prolong and complicate the patient's ICU stay or even threaten the patient's very existence. When abnormalities of thought, feeling, and behavior arise, it is important to diagnose the cause of these problems and prescribe the proper treatment. Drug interactions and knowledge of pharmacokinetics and reasonable dosage schedules allow for effective use of psychotropic drugs in the critically ill patient. Trade names of drugs mentioned in this chapter are given in Table 27.6.

References

1. Adams F, Fernandez F, Andersson BS: Emergency pharmacotherapy of delirium in the critically ill cancer patient. *Psychosomatics* 27:33–37, 1986.
2. Anderson WH: Differential diagnosis of acute psy-chosis. In Manschreck TC: *Psychiatric Medicine.* New York, Elsevier/North Holland, 1979.
3. Atkinson K, Biggs J, Darveniza P, et al: Cyclosporine-associated central-nervous-system toxicity after allo-geneic bone-marrow transplantation. *N Engl J Med* 310:527, 1984.
4. Aubree JC, Lader MH: High and very high dosage antipsychotics. *J Clin Psychiatry* 41:341–350, 1980.
5. Ayd FJ: Guidelines for using intramuscular haloperi-dol for rapid neuroleptization. In Ayd FJ: *Haloperidol Update: 1959–1980.* Baltimore, Avd Medical Communications, 1980.
6. Ayd FJ, Intravenous haloperidol therapy. *Int Drug Ther Newslett* 13:20–23, 1978.
7. Ayd FJ, Jr. Trazodone cardiac effects. *Int Drug Ther Newslett* 20:29–32, 1985.
8. Baldessarini RJ: Drugs effective in the treatment of psychiatric disorders. In Gilman AG, Goodman LS, Gilman A: *Goodman and Gilman's The Pharmacological Basis of Therapeutics,* ed 6. New York, Macmillan, 1980.
9. Ban T: *Psychopharmacology for the Aged.* New York, Karger, 1980.
10. Benson HA, *The Relaxation Response.* New York, William Morrow & Co, 1975.
11. Borison RL, Amantadine-induced psychosis in a geriatric patient with renal disease. *Am J Psychiatry* 136:111–112, 1979.
12. Brophy JJ: Psychiatric disorders. In Krupp MA, Chatton MJ: *Current Medical Diagnosis and Therapy.* Los Altos, CA, Lange, 1980.
13. Byrd GJ: Acute organic brain syndrome associated with gentamycin therapy. *JAMA* 238:53–54, 1977.
14. Cassem EH, Hackett TP: Psychiatric medicine in intensive care settings. In Manschreck TC: *Psychiatric Medicine.* New York, Elsevier/North Holland, 1979.
15. Cassem N: Cardiovascular effects of antidepressants. *J Clin Psychiatry* 43:22–28, 1982.
16. Cassem NH, Depression. In: TP Hackett and NH Cassem (eds.), *MGH Handbook of General Hospital Psychiatry,* ed 2. Littleton, MA, PSG Publishing Co, 1987, pp 227–260.
17. Cassem NH, Hackett TP: Psychiatric consultation in a coronary care unit. *Ann Intern Med* 75:9–14, 1971.
18. Cassem NH, Psychiatric problems. In Parrillo JE (ed): *Current Therapy in Critical Care Medicine.* Philadelphia, Decker, Inc, 1987, pp 331–340.
19. Cassem NH, The setting of intensive care. In Hackett TP, Cassem NH (eds): *MGH Handbook of General Hospital Psychiatry,* ed 2. Littleton, MA, PSG Publishing Co, 1987, pp 353–379.
20. Cohen S: *The Drug Abuse Problem.* New York, Harvorth Press, 1981.
21. Cole JO: Drug treatment of anxiety. In Cole JD: *Psychopharmacology Update.* Lexington, MA, Collamore Press, 1980.
22. Cressman WA, Blanchine JR, Slotnick VB, et al: Plasma level profile of haloperidol in man following intramuscular administration. *Eur J Clin Pharmacol* 7:99–103, 1974.
23. Davidson J, Turnbull CD: The effects of isocarboxazid on blood pressure and pulse. *J Clin Psychopharmacol* 6:139–143, 1986.
24. Davis JM: Antipsychotic drugs. In Kaplan HI, Freedman AM, Sadock BJ: *Comprehensive Textbook of Psychiatry,* ed 3. Baltimore, Williams & Wilkins, 1980.
25. Devaul RA, Hall RCW: Hallucinations. In Hall RCW: *Psychiatric Presentations of Medical Illness.* New York, Spectrum Publications, 1980.
26. Director KL, Muniz CE: Diazepam in the treatment of extrapyramidal symptoms: a case report, *J Clin Psychiatry* 43:160–161, 1982.
27. Dubin WR, Field HL, Gastfriend DR: Postcardiotomy delirium: a critical review. *J Thor Cardiovasc Surg* 77:586–594, 1979.

28. Dudley DL, Rowlett DB, Loebel PJ: Emergency use of intravenous haloperidol. *Gen Hosp Psychiatry* 1:240–246, 1979.

29. Dysken MW, Merry W, Davis JM: Anticholinergic psychosis. *Psychiatr Ann* 8:30–40, 1978.

30. Eisendrath SJ, Sweeney MA: Toxic neuropsychiatric effects of digoxin at therapeutic serum concentrations. *Am J Psychiatry* 144:506–507, 1987.

31. Ekholm S, Fischer H: Neurotoxicity of metrizamide. *Arch Neurol* 42:24–25, 1985.

32. Eikayam U, Frishman W: Cardiovascular effects of phenothiazines. *Am Heart J* 100:397–401, 1980.

33. Forsman A, Ohman R: Pharmacokinetic studies on haloperidol in man. *Curr Ther Res* 20:319–336, 1976.

34. Fyer HA, Liebowitz MR, Gorman JM, et al: Discontinuation of alprazolam treatment in panic patients. *Am J Psychiatry* 144:303–308, 1987.

35. Gaultieri CT, Powell SF: Psychoactive drug interactions. *J Clin Psychiatry* 39:720–729, 1978.

36. Georgotas A, McCue RE, Friedman E, et al: Electrocardiographic effects of nortriptyline, phenelzine, and placebo under optimal treatment conditions. *Am J Psychiatry* 144:798–801, 1987.

37. Giardina E,-GV, Bigger JT, Jr. Johnson LL: The effect of imipramine and nortriptyline on ventricular premature depolarization and left ventricular function (abstract). *Circulation* 64(Suppl)4:316, 1981.

38. Glassman AH: Cardiovascular effects of tricyclic antidepressants. *Ann Rev Med* 35:503–511, 1984.

39. Glassman AH, Johnson LL, Giardina E,-GV, et al: The use of imipramine in depressed patients with congestive heart failure. *JAMA* 250:1997–2001, 1983.

40. Goff DC: The stimulant challenge test in depression. *J Clin Psychiatry* 47:538–543, 1986.

41. Goff DC, Garber HJ, Jenike MA: Partial resolution of ranitidine-associated delirium with physostigmine: case report. *J Clin Psychiatry* 46:400–401, 1985.

42. Goldman LS, Hudson JI, Weddington WW: Lupus-like illness associated with chlorpromazine. *Ann J Psychiatry* 137:1613–1614, 1980.

43. Good MI, Shader RI: Behavioral toxicity and equivocal suicide associated with chloroquine and its derivatives. *Am J Psychiatry* 134:798–801, 1977.

44. Good MI, Shader RI: Lethality and behavioral side effects of chloroquine. *J Clin Psychopharmacol* 2:40–47, 1982.

45. Goodwin JS, Regan M: Cognitive dysfunction associated with naproxen and ibuprofen in the elderly. *Arthritis Rheum* 25:1013–1015, 1982.

46. Granacher RP: Agitation in the elderly. *Postgrad Med* 72:83–96, 1982.

47. Greenblatt DJ: Pharmacokinetic comparisons. *Psychosomatics.* 21(Suppl):9–14, 1980.

48. Greenberg D, Murray GB: Hyperventilation as a variant of tardive dyskinesia. *J Clin Psychiatry* 42:401–403, 1981.

49. Hall RCW: Anxiety. In Hall RCW: *Psychiatric Presentations of Medical Illness.* New York, Spectrum Publications, 1980.

50. Hall RCW: Depression. In Hall RCW: *Psychiatric Presentations of Medical Illness.* New York, Spectrum Publications, 1980.

51. Harvey SC: Hypnotics and sedatives. In Gilman AG, Goodman LS, Gilman A: *Goodman and Gilman's The Pharmacological Basis of Therapeutics,* ed 6, New York, Macmillan, 1980.

52. Holllister LE: Polypharmacy: which drug combinations make sense? *Hosp Community Psychiatry* 33:433–435, 1982.

53. Hotson JR, Langston JW: Disulfiram-induced encephalopathy. *Arch Neurol* 33:141–142, 1976.

54. Intil TM, Soldatos C: Epileptogenic side effects of psychotropic drugs: practical recommendations. *JAMA* 244:1460–1463, 1980.

55. Jacobsen FM, Sack DA, James SP: Delirium induced by verapamil. *Am J Psychiatry* 144:248, 1987.

56. Jan MW, Bitar AH: Respiratory dyskinesia. *Psychosomatics* 23:764–765, 1982.

57. Johnson AL, Hollister LE, Berger PA: The anticholinergic syndrome: diagnosis and treatment. *J Clin Psychiatry* 42:313–317, 1981.

58. Kaiko RF, Foley KM, Grabinski PY, et al: Central nervous system excitatory effects of meperidine in cancer patients. *Ann Neurol* 13:180–185, 1983.

59. Kane JM, Smith JM: Tardive dyskinesia: prevalence and risk factors, 1959–1979. *Arch Gen Psychiatry* 39:473–481, 1982.

60. Katon W, Raskind M: Treatment of depression in the medically ill elderly with methylphenidate. *Am J Psychiatry* 137:963–965, 1980.

61. Katz IR, Greenberg WH, Barr GA, et al: Screening for cognitive toxicity of anticholinergic drugs. *J Clin Psychiatry* 46:323–326, 1985.

62. Kaufman MW, Murray GB, Cassem NH: Use of psychostimulants in medically ill depressed patients. *Psychosomatics* 23:817–819, 1982.

63. Kaufman MW, Murray GS: The use of d-amphetamine in medically ill depressed patients. *J Clin Psychiatry* 43:463–464, 1982.

64. Kiriike N, Maeda Y, Nishiwaki S, et al: Iatrogenic torsade de pointes induced by thioridazine. *Biol Psychiatry* 22:99–103, 1987.

65. Klotz U, Avant GR, Hoyumpa A, et al: The effects of age and liver disease on the disposition and elimination of diazepam in adult men. *J Clin Invest* 55:347–359, 1975.

66. Knox SJ: Severe psychiatric disorders in postoperative period: five-year survey of Belfast Hospitals. *J Ment Sci* 107:1078, 1961.

67. Koepke HH, Lion JR, Gold RL, et al: Multicenter controlled study of oxazepam in anxious elderly outpatients. *Psychosomatics* 23:641–645, 1982.

68. Kolin IS, Linet OI: Double-blind comparison of alprazolam and diazepam for subchronic withdrawal from alcohol. *J Clin Psychiatry* 42:169–173, 1981.

69. Kornfeld DS: Psychiatric problems of an intensive care unit. *Med Clin North Am* 55:1353–1363, 1971.

70. Kulig K, Rumeck BH, Sullivan JB, Jr. et al: Amoxapine overdose: Coma and seizures without cardiotoxic effects. *JAMA* 248:1092–1094, 1982.

71. Lader M: *Introduction to Psychopharmacology.* Kalamazoo, Mich., Upjohn Co., 1980.

72. Lader MH, Petursson H: Benzodiazepine derivatives—side effects and dangers. *Biol Psychiatry* 16:1195–1201, 1978.

73. Linn L, Kahn RL, Coles R: Patterns of behavior disturbances following cataract extraction. *Am J Psychiatry* 110:281–289, 1953.

74. Lipowski ZJ: Delirium updated. *Comp Psychiatry* 21:190–197, 1980.

75. Resource Exchange, 1982. Lowry MR, Dunner FJ: Seizures during tricyclic therapy *Am J Psychiatry* 137:1461–1462, 1980.

76. Lydiard RB: Temazepam [Restoril]—a new short acting benzodiazepine hypnotic. *Biol Ther Psychiatry* 4:37–38, 1981.

77. Mason A, Granacher RP: *Clinical Handbook of Antipsychotic Drug Therapy.* New York, Brunner/Mazel, 1980.

78. May PRA, Goldberg SC: Prediction of schizophrenic patients' response to pharmacotherapy. In Lipton MA, DiMascio AD, Killam KF: *Psychopharmacology: A Generation of Progress.* New York, Raven Press, 1978.

79. McGrath PJ, Blood DK, Stewart JW, et al: A comparative study of the electrocardiographic effects of phenelzine, tricyclic antidepressants, mianserin, and placebo. *J Clin Psychopharmacol* 7:335–339, 1987.

80. Medical Letter. Drugs that cause psychiatric symptoms. *Med Letter* 28:81–86, 1986.

81. Menuck M, Voineskos G: Rapid parenteral treatment of acute psychosis. *Comp Psychiatry* 22:351–361, 1981.
82. Menza MA, Murray GB, Holmes VF, Rafels WA: Decreased extrapyramidal symptoms with intravenous haloperidol. *J Clin Psychiatry* 48:278–280, 1987.
83. Moeller H, Kissling W, Lang C, et al: Efficacy and side effects of haloperidol in psychotic patients: oral versus intravenous administration. *Am J Psychiatry* 139:1571–1575, 1982.
84. Moore DP: Rapid treatment of delirium in critically ill patients. *Am J Psychiatry* 134:1431–1432, 1977.
85. Murray GB: Atrial fibrillation/flutter associated with amoxapine: Two case reports. *J Clin Psychopharm* 5:124–125, 1985.
86. Nadelson T: The psychiatrist in the surgical intensive care unit: postoperative delirium. In Guggenheim FG, Nadelson C: *Major Psychiatric Disorders*. New York, Elsevier Biomedical, 1982.
87. Newman G: Intermittent recurring psychoses. In Hall RCW: *Psychiatric Presentations of Medical Illness*. New York, Spectrum Publications, 1980.
88. Noyes R: Beta-blocking drugs and anxiety. *Psychosomatics* 23:155–169, 1981.
89. Paykel ES, Fleminger R, Watson JP: Psychiatric side effects of anti-hypertensive drugs other than reserpine. *J Clin Psychopharmacol* 2:14–39, 1982.
90. Peterson LG, Perk M: Psychiatric presentations of cancer. *Psychosomatics* 23:601–604, 1982.
91. Pluss JL, DiBella NJ: Reversible central nervous system dysfunction due to tamoxifen in a patient with breast cancer. *Ann Intern Med* 101:652, 1984.
92. Pratt TH: Rifampin-induced organic brain syndrome. *JAMA* 241:2421–2422, 1979.
93. Preskorn SH, Irwin HA: Toxicity of tricyclic antidepressants—kinetics, mechanism, intervention: a review. *J Clin Psychiatry* 43:151–156, 1982.
94. Pumariega AJ, Muller B, Rivers-Bulkeley N: Acute renal failure secondary to amoxapine overdose. *JAMA* 248:331–341, 1982.
95. Raskind M, Veith RC, Barnes R, et al: Cardiovascular and antidepressant effects of imipramine in the treatment of secondary depression in patients with ischemic heart disease. *Am J Psychiatry* 139:1114–1117, 1982.
96. Richelson E: The pharmacology of antidepressants. *J Psychopathol* 1987.
97. Rickels K: Discussion. *Psychosomatics* 21:26–32, 1980.
98. Risch SC, Green GP, Janowsky DS: Interfaces of psychopharmacology and cardiology—part two. *J Clin Psychiatry* 42:47–59, 1981.
99. Roberts RK, Wilkinson GR, Branch RA, et al: Effect of age and parenchymal liver disease on the disposition and elimination of chlordiazepoxide. *Gastroenterology* 75:419–485, 1978.
100. Roose SP, Glassman AH, Giardina E,-GV, et al: Nortriptyline in depressed patients with left ventricular impairment. *JAMA* 256:3253–3257, 1986.
101. Roose SP, Glassman AH, Giardina EGV, et al: Tricyclic antidepressants in depressed patients with cardiac conduction disease. *Arch Gen Psychiatry* 44:273–275, 1987.
102. Rosenbaum JF, Woods SW, Gross JE, et al: Emergence of hostility during alprazolam treatment. *Am J Psychiatry* 141:792–793, 1984.
103. Sadeh M, Brahman J: Effects of anticholinergic drugs on memory in Parkinson's disease. *Arch Neurol* 39:666–667, 1982.
104. Salama AA: Complete heart block associated with mesoridazine in lithium combination. *J Clin Psychiatry* 48:123, 1987.
105. Scully JH: *Psychiatric Problems in Surgery*. Nutley, N.J., Roche Products, 1982.
106. Seymour-Shove R: Labile hypertension presenting as effective disorder. *Br J Clin Pract* 35:124–127, 1981.
107. Shader RI, Greenblatt DJ: Management of anxiety in the elderly: the balance between therapeutic and adverse effects. *J Clin Psychiatry* 43:8–15, 1982.
108. Sherwin I, Peron-Magnan P, Bancard J, et al: Prevalence of psychosis in epilepsy as a function of the laterality of the epileptogenic lesion. *Arch Neurol* 39:621–623, 1982.
109. Silberman EK, Reus VI, Jimerson DC, et al: Heterogeneity of amphetamine response in depressed patients. *Am J Psychiatry* 138:1302–1307, 1981.
110. Snavely SR, Hodges GR: The neurotoxicity of antibacterial agents. *Ann Intern Med* 101:92–104, 1984.
111. Sos J, Cassem NH: Managing postoperative agitation. *Drug Therapy* 10:103–106, 1980.
112. Sovner R, McGorril S: Stress as a precipitant of neuroleptic-induced dystonia. *Psychosomatics* 23:707–709, 1982.
113. Stern TA, Continuous infusion of physostigmine in anticholinergic delirium: Case Report. *J Clin Psychiatry* 44:462–464, 1983.
114. Tesar GE, Murray GB, Cassem NH: Use of high-dose intravenous haloperidol in the treatment of agitated cardiac patients. *J Clin Psychopharmacol* 5:344–347, 1985.
115. Tesar GE, Rosenbaum JF, Biederman J, et al: Orthostatic hypotension and antidepressant pharmacotherapy. *Psychopharmacol Bull* 23:182–186, 1987.
116. Thornton TL: Delirium associated with sulindac. *JAMA* 243:1630–1631, 1980.
117. Wade JC, Meyers JD: Neurologic symptoms associated with parenteral acyclovir treatment after marrow transplantation. *Ann Intern Med* 98:921–925, 1983.
118. Walker WR: Phenothiazine therapy and latent organic brain syndrome. *Psychiatr Ann* 8:452–456, 1978.
119. Weddington WW, Jr: Delirium and depression associated with amphotericin B. *Psychosomatics* 23:1076–1078, 1982.
120. Weisman AD, Hackett TP: Psychosis after eye surgery. Establishment of a specific doctor-patient relationship and treatment of "black-patch" delirium. *N Engl J Med* 258:1284–1289, 1958.
121. Woods S, Tesar G, Murray GB, et al: Psychostimulant treatment of depressive disorders secondary to medical illness. *J Clin Psychiatry* 47:12–15, 1986.
122. Young RC, Alexopoulos GS, Shamoian CA, et al: Plasma 10-hydroxy-nortriptyline and ECG changes in elderly depressed patients. *Am J Psychiatry* 142:866–868, 1985.
123. Zaret BS, Cohen RA: Reversible valproic acid-induced dementia: a case report. *Epilepsia* 27:234–240, 1986.
124. Zavodnick S: Atrial flutter with amoxapine: A case report. *Am J Psychiatry* 138:1503–1505, 1981.

28

Anticoagulants in Critical Care Medicine

John J. Nanfro, M.D.

Maintaining normal hemostatic integrity is a central issue in the management of the critically ill. Optimal hemostasis requires a complex interaction of the vascular endothelium, platelets, and coagulation factors. This well-balanced system may be perturbed by an underlying systemic disorder or a therapeutic intervention. It is essential that the clinician involved in the care of critically ill patients understand the normal physiology of hemostasis. This information enables one to manage a hemorrhagic or thrombotic disorder. This chapter reviews the aspects of normal hemostatic events, pathologic states, and finally the pharmacology of anticoagulants and related substances.

NORMAL HEMOSTASIS

Vascular injury may occur in a direct or an indirect manner. Initially when the vascular endothelium is damaged, vasoconstriction occurs promptly. The exposed collagen fibrils in the subendothelial region attract circulating platelets (Fig. 28.1). The platelets adhere to the collagen fibrils closing the endothelial defect and undergo significant metabolic changes that promote continued hemostasis (87, 97, 102). Upon exposure to the collagen, the platelet begins a release reaction from the dense core granules generating serotonin and adenosine diphosphate (ADP). The release of these substances promotes aggregation by attracting further circulating platelets to the damaged endothelial collagen-platelet complex. Plasma coagulation factors in close association with the platelet membrane, as well as factors in other platelet organelles (alpha granules) are also activated (85). The contact factors (XII, XI) are activated by collagen and ADP and subsequently lead to the formation of activated factor X (X_a) in the common pathway of the coagulation schema. X_a in the presence of ac-

tivated factor V (V_a) and calcium convert prothrombin (II) to thrombin (IIa). The generated thrombin converts fibrinogen to fibrin monomer and fibrin monomers subsequently bind to each other. Thrombin also activates many other factors, including factor XIII (fibrin stabilizing factor), V, VIII, and protein C. The soluble fibrin monomer is stabilized to an insoluble polymer by the action of factor XIII_a.

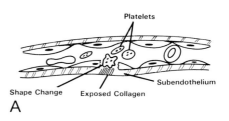

A

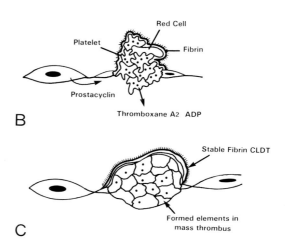

B

C

Figure 28.1. *A,* Blood vessel is injured, collagen exposed, and platelets undergo prompt shape change. *B,* Platelet plug forms, and coagulation schema results in fibrin formation in association with platelet plug. *C,* Hemostatic plug becomes organized.

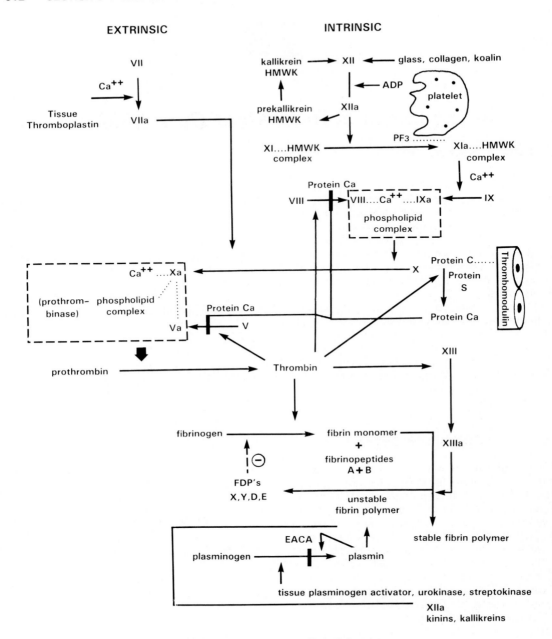

Figure 28.2. The coagulation-fibrinolytic schema.

Thrombin also promotes contraction of the platelet mass by its action on platelet acto-myosin. This action further controls the hemostatic defect. If fibrin polymerization were inadequate, the initial platelet plug would disaggregate.

The coagulation schema is outlined in Figure 28.2. The initiating vascular injury may be traumatic, vasculitic, or related to endotoxin.

The intrinsic pathway requires the presence of adequate concentrations of coagulation factors, calcium, and phospholipid. High-molecular-weight kininogen (HMWK) and prekallikrein (PK), released during vascular injury, augment the initial contact activation and formation of XII$_a$. Platelets and endothelium act as a matrix upon which the coagulation complex forms. Each coagulation factor is activated by an enzymatic reaction, which results in a functional factor in close apposition to cofactors. The extrinsic pathway predominately involves factor VII. This factor is activated by tissue thromboplastin as well as XIIa. Kinins are generated during inflammatory states and by the activation of factor XII. These substances promote tissue contraction, hypotension, and vascular permeability.

The fibrin clot must be controlled by the fibrinolytic system (10, 66) or diffuse thrombosis develops. This system is activated by factor XIIa, the kallikreins and tissue plasminogen activator. The resulting reaction converts plasminogen to plasmin. Plasmin may also be formed by exogenous compounds such as streptokinase. Plasmin converts fibrin to fibrin degradation products (FDPs) and dissolves clot. The FDPs inhibit further conversion of fibrinogen to fibrin by thrombin (Fig. 28.2). The procoagulant system (intrinsic and extrinsic) must be complemented by the fibrinolytic system to maintain normal hemostasis. Altera-

tions in either limb may result in hemorrhage or thrombosis. Plasmin and factor XIIa generate the formation of complement. Complement components promote chemotaxis and the release of leukotrienes contained within leukocytes. During the inflammatory response associated with sepsis, many of these factors circulate and promote localized fibrin deposition in the form of disseminated intravascular coagulation (DIC). Circulating antiplasmins can inactivate the fibrinolytic system. An absence of the antiplasmins may result in hemorrhage. There are also circulating inhibitors of the procoagulants. The predominant inhibitor is antithrombin III. This serine protease is referred to as "heparin cofactor." Antithrombin III naturally inhibits thrombin activity and to a lesser degree, factors XIIA and XA. However, in the presence of heparin, this activity is markedly increased and coagulation is prevented (Fig. 28.3).

Platelets are critical for adequate coagulation (Fig. 28.4). Platelet-released—ADP activates

PLATELET PHYSIOLOGY

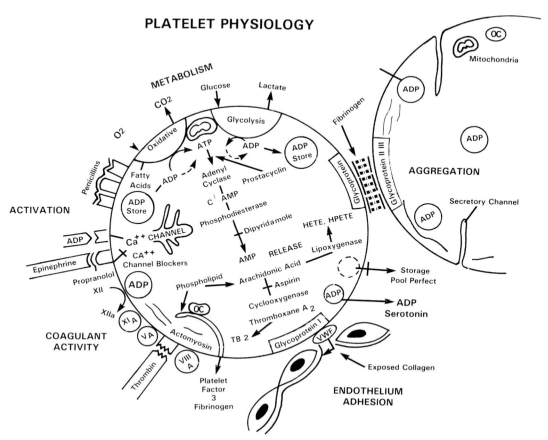

Figure 28.3. Platelet physiology and function.

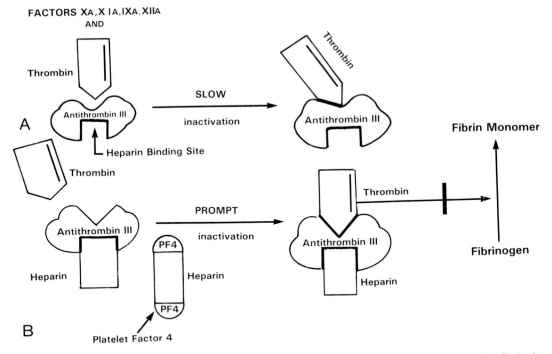

FACTORS X_A, X I_A, IX_A, XII_A

Figure 28.4. *A,* Thrombin interacts with antithrombin III and slow inactivation of thrombin occurs. *B,* In the presence of heparin, antithrombin undergoes a molecular alteration and promptly inactivates thrombin.

factors XII and XI in the presence of collagen. Platelets release phospholipid and platelet factor 4 (PF4), which alters heparin function. Platelets also liberate fibrinogen, factors V and VIII. Platelets store the phospholipid platelet factor 3 (PF3), which is necessary for modulation of the intrinsic pathway. The platelets act as a substrate for complex coagulation reactions.

Platelet metabolism is also critical to adequate hemostasis and platelet function. Platelets passively absorb glucose and produce lactic acid, with the energy thus formed stored as adenosine triphosphate (ATP). Lipid degradation provides energy as well. Glucose and lipids may be stored in granules in the platelet cytosol. When the release reaction and aggregation occurs, the platelet metabolic rate markedly escalates. ATP is converted to ADP and cyclic AMP. ADP is a critical component of the platelet release reaction. Stored ADP is localized in the dense core granules of the platelets. The platelet metabolic machinery attempts to maintain stores of the adenosine phosphates for catabolism and the release reaction.

Prostaglandins play a critical role in platelet function (64, 74). The exposure to collagen

and subsequent release of thrombin initiates metabolism of arachidonic acid. Arachidonic acid is converted enzymatically into the eicosatrienoic acids (HPETE and HETE). These components are involved in prostaglandin feedback mechanisms and the inflammatory response. The enzyme cyclooxygenase, promotes the production of the prostaglandins PGI$_2$ (prostacyclin) and thromboxane A$_2$ (TXA$_2$). TXA$_2$ is a potent platelet-aggregating agent and promotes further release of ADP. TXA$_2$ causes profound vasoconstriction and may play a role in coronary vasospasm and other vasosopastic events. PGI$_2$ is produced by the endothelium in contact with the platelet and is a vasodilating substance that counteracts TXA$_2$ activity. The relative quantities of TXA$_2$ and PGI$_2$ are currently believed to play a role in thrombotic thrombocytopenic purpura (TTP), DIC, and some antiplatelet drug activity. The byproducts of arachidonic acid metabolism are actively being studied for potential use in treating thrombotic events.

Coagulation factors may critically affect platelet function. Thrombin acts on platelets by promoting aggregation, release, and clot retraction. The von Willebrand's-factor VIII complex associates with the vessel wall and platelet. These complex associations point out the necessity of intact components of hemostasis: vessels, platelets, coagulation factors, and the fibrinolytic system. In the critical care setting, each of these elements may be perturbed. Vessels may be disrupted by trauma, surgery, toxic damage to the endothelium, or a vasculitic process. Platelets may be diminished in number by decreased production or increased destruction. This thrombocytopenia may be due to sepsis, surgery, endotoxins, or autoimmune phenomenon. Coagulation factors may be dysfunctional or inadequately produced as in hepatic disease. Rarely, patients in the intensive care unit may present with a previously undiagnosed congenital coagulopathy. Finally, thrombotic events may occur secondary to systemic disease or on the basis of alterations in the fibrinolytic system.

TESTS OF HEMOSTASIS

Tests of hemostasis are performed by drawing venous blood into commercially available test tubes containing either an anticoagulant [(EDTA, citrate, oxalate) which binds calcium and prevents clot formation] or heparin [which promptly binds to antithrombin 3 (AT^{III}) preventing coagulation via thrombin modification]. The tubes may also be siliconized to prevent activation of contact factors. Platelet function tests are performed on fresh platelet-rich plasma.

Microscopic review of the peripheral blood smear from a patient in the intensive care unit with a coagulopathy is imperative. Information obtained may be useful in clinical management and helpful in determining etiology. For example, one may note a diminished platelet count from the hematology lab. A review of the peripheral smear will rule out artifactual platelet "satelliting" and clumping. The presence of schistocytes supports microangiopathy in patients with burns, severe organ trauma, TTP, or DIC. Microangiopathy implies fibrin deposition and may support early use of heparin as well as fresh-frozen plasma.

A normal platelet count is between 150,000 and 400,000 thrombocytes per cubic milliliter. An increase or decrease in the count may result in hemorrhage or thrombosis depending on platelet function. A bleeding time (Simplate II) by the technique of Ivy-Mielke is the most widely used means of assessing platelet function (79, 54). The bleeding time progressively prolongs as the platelet count falls below

$100,000/ml^3$. Performing a bleeding time on patients with platelets less than $50,000/mm^3$ is rarely of benefit unless one is using the bleeding time to assess a therapeutic manipulation to improve platelet function. The most important clinical utility of the bleeding time is in patients with normal platelet counts. Bleeding times greater than 9 minutes imply a qualitative defect, either congenital or acquired. Bleeding times are often used to evaluate platelet function following cardiopulmonary bypass, or in bleeding patients with liver or renal dysfunction (3). Platelet aggregometry is reserved for the outpatient setting and is not of great utility in the ICU (16).

The more common tests in critical care are the coagulation tests. These include the prothrombin time (PT), activated partial thromboplastin time ($_aPTT$), thrombin time (TT), whole-blood clotting time (WBT), and a measure of fibrin degradation products (FDP). The prothrombin time is performed by adding a source of tissue thromboplastin to plasma and observing the time required for a clot to form. The test screens the integrity of the extrinsic limb of coagulation (II, V, VII, X, fibrinogen) and is reported as a time compared with control values. A prolonged PT suggests a deficiency of these factors, the presence of heparin, FDPs, or low or dysfunctional fibrinogen. To perform the $_aPTT$ one adds a contact agent (kaolin, ellagic acid) to plasma and observes the time necessary for clot to form. This screens the intrinsic schema (II, V, VIII, IX, X, XI, XII, fibrinogen). A prolonged $_aPTT$ suggests the same defects as the PT (except factor VII). In addition, $_aPTT$ detects a deficiency of VIII, IX, XI, XII, prekallikrein, and HMWK. The PT and $_aPTT$ do not detect deficiency of factor XIII, low level FDPs, or fibrinolytic defects. A routine admission PT or PTT may be unnecessary if an adequate history and physical examination rule out a hemorrhage or thrombotic process. The critical care setting differs however, in that these tests are generally monitored serially. The severity of the systemic illness and drugs used in the ICU may affect the PT and $_aPTT$ and result in altered hemostasis. The thrombin time is performed by adding measured amounts of thrombin to plasma and measuring time to clot formation. The test therefore does not rely on the presence of endogenous thrombin. Thrombin acts on fibrinogen to cleave fibrinopeptides A and B and promotes fibrin monomer polymerization. Abnormal fibrinogens (produced in liver disease), fibrin split products or a low fibrinogen may prolong the thrombin time. Renal disease, autoimmune disorders, and hepatic dysfunction may also result in a prolonged thrombin time. Heparin is a significant cause of a prolonged thrombin time. This abnormality may be present secondary to indwelling arterial catheters, right atrial catheters, or hemodialysis. It may be difficult to distinguish systemic DIC from a heparin effect. Reptilase time (RT) (venom of Bothrops Atrox) cleaves fibrinopeptide A from fibrinogen and is unaffected by the presence of heparin (22). Thus, a prolonged TT with a normal RT suggests heparin. Whereas, a prolonged RT suggests FDPs, dysfibrinogenemia, or low fibrinogen.

Other tests that may be used in an attempt to distinguish DIC from primary fibrinolysis and include the euglobulin clot lysis and the protamine paracoagulation tests. These tests must be interpreted in light of the peripheral blood smear and clinical setting. This point is important since ε-aminocaproic acid (EACA) is used in the treatment of primary fibrinolysis, while it is contraindicated in DIC. FDPs are measured by a semiquantitative test of latex agglutination.

BLEEDING

The manifestation of inadequate hemostasis, regardless of the cause, is bleeding. In the critical care setting, the control of bleeding is imperative. Many of these patients are monitored with right atrial and pulmonary artery flotation catheters and arterial "lines". Loss of blood exacerbates volume control and promotes hypotension. Hypotension leads to end organ dysfunction. The management of these patients must be aggressive, not only in regard to cardiopulmonary, central nervous system (CNS), hepatic, and renal support, but also in maintaining hemostasis. Disorders of hemostasis are common and may go undetected unless bleeding is apparent. Bleeding may be grossly evident from the gastrointestinal tract or a surgical wound. The possibility of occult blood loss must be considered in patients with hypotension or a decreasing hematocrit. Patients should have hemostasis parameters studied if invasive procedures (such as lumbar puncture, thoracentesis, pericardiocentesis, bronchoscopy with biopsy, and Swan-Ganz catheterization) are to be performed. Baseline studies should include PT, $_a$PTT, platelet count, hemoglobin, and hematocrit. Tamponade of the bleeding site may control acute bleeding.

However, the evacuation of blood in the setting of a coagulopathy or platelet disorder may result in continued bleeding unless the abnormalities are corrected. A knowledge of the interaction of medications with the hemostatic system is critical.

QUANTITATIVE AND QUALITATIVE PLATELET DISORDERS

Platelet abnormalities occur in many intensive care patients. Surgical units tend to see thrombocytopenia due to the dilutional effects of red cell transfusion, or decreased production due to sepsis and drugs. Qualitative disorders may also be seen, either as acquired or previously undetected congenital disorders (28, 75). Medical intensive care units tend to see a much broader range of platelet abnormalities both quantitative and qualitative.

Quantitative abnormalities must first be confirmed by a review of the peripheral smear. Relying on an automated counter valve may result in premature calls to the blood bank for platelet support. In the bleeding patient, an incorrect assumption of thrombocytopenia as the cause for hemorrhage may be made. Platelet transfusions will not correct a significant coagulopathy or a wound requiring surgical intervention. Having confirmed thrombocytopenia on the examination of the blood smear, one must determine etiology (Table 28.1). The presence of petechiae suggests thrombocytopenia.

Patients may have decreased platelet production caused by exposure to a toxin such as

Table 28.1
Causes of Thrombocytopenia

Viral Infections
    CMV, HTLV III, rubella, adenovirus, mumps
Vaccines
    Rubella, rubeola
Nonimmune Platelet Destruction
    Infection, shock, surgery, DIC, malignancy,
        obstetrical complications, cardiac prostheses,
        burns, vasculitis, TTP, HUS
Immune Thrombocytopenia
    Idiopathic, alloantibodies, collagen vascular
        disorders, viral infections, malignancy, drug
        mediated (Quinidine)
Radiation
Aplastic Anemia
Preleukemia, Leukemia, Neoplastic Involvement of
    Marrow
Drug-induced Myelosuppression (Benzene,
    mycotoxin)

benzene (24). In these patients one should avoid platelet transfusion to prevent allosensitization. If the aplastic patient is not bleeding, platelets are not indicated on a prophylactic basis. Patients with irreversible decreased platelet production should not be transfused platelets unless actively bleeding. If patients have decreased production because they have received cytotoxic agents, or drugs such as cimetidine or heparin, platelets can be given for bleeding or counts less than 20,000. In general, it is the precipitous reduction of the platelet count as seen in cytotoxic therapy that is associated with severe life-threatening bleeding. Patients who have received intensive chemotherapy for acute leukemia may occasionally be transferred to the ICU for fluid management, or for treatment of respiratory failure, hyperuricemia or septic shock. Sepsis may induce transient bone marrow failure and decreased production of all bone marrow—generated cellular elements. Platelet replacement therapy for circulating platelet counts less than 20,000/ml^3 may benefit these patients. Performing a bleeding time in thrombocytopenic patients is of minimal clinical benefit. Corticosteroids are generally not used to treat chemotherapy-induced thrombocytopenia as they may exacerbate gastrointestinal bleeding, and promote vascular fragility without increasing the platelet count. For these patients, strict bed rest, avoidance of drugs that alter platelet function or reduce the platelet count are indicated. Invasive procedures are avoided unless clinically indicated and supported by platelet transfusion and adequate surgical technique. Intramuscular injection and vigorous dental care are also contraindicated. Thrombocytopenia due to decreased production from leukemia and induction chemotherapy is common. Platelets are given prophylactically to these patients for counts less than 20,000/ml^3. If this is difficult to attain then at least for counts less than 10,000/ml^3. Intubation or mechanical ventilation of such patients is exceedingly difficult and excessive bleeding may occur into the respiratory tract regardless of intervention. The use of ϵ-aminocaproic acid (EACA) to decrease bleeding in this setting is not without risk.

Increased destruction of platelets may also be noted in sepsis (70). Platelet transfusions are withheld unless the platelet count gets low or bleeding occurs. Autoimmune disorders may cause thrombocytopenia by different mechanisms (8, 60, 62). An examination of the bone marrow is usually required. Increased platelet destruction on an immune basis is treated with corticosteroids (e.g., prednisone 100 mg daily or an intravenous equivalent). Corticosteroids may also be used for drug-induced thrombocytopenias. If the platelet count has not corrected within 2 weeks other measures are indicated. Patients may be treated with intravenous immunoglobulin 0.4 g/kg/day for 5 days and subsequently splenectomy, or splenectomy alone (41, 95). The mechanism of action of intravenous immunoglobulin on immune thrombocytopenia is unclear but presumptively involves macrophage inhibition. The clinical situation dictates which of these approaches is appropriate. Platelet transfusions are contraindicated for the treatment of immune thrombocytopenia except for acute uncontrolled bleeding or the need for surgical intervention. Platelet sequestration may occur in hypersplenism due to chronic lymphocytic leukemia. Splenectomy may be indicated if tests with ^{51}chromium red blood cell labeling documents sequestration and the clinical condition merits such an approach. Giant hemangioma may be another site of platelet sequestration.

During cardiopulmonary bypass, platelets are altered to a degree that depends on the type of oxygenator used (2). Platelets may be sequestered by the pump or may be reduced by heparin therapy and/or by dilutional effects. Platelet dysfunction may also develop because of platelet degranulation. A review of the peripheral blood smear and bleeding time may help to determine the etiology. Bleeding postpump usually occurs from the sternotomy drain. The cardiothoracic surgeon and hematologist monitor these parameters, as well as the rate of bleeding. Rapid bleeding suggests the need for prompt surgical reexploration. A slow stable bleed allows time for evaluation of other causes. If the PT, $_a$PTT, TT, platelets, and bleeding time are normal, then surgical reexploration is indicated for hemodynamic instability.

Thrombocytopenia is frequently caused by drugs (Table 28.2). Quinine derivatives, such as quinidine, are a common cause of drug-related thrombocytopenia. The treatment is prompt discontinuation of the offending agent. The abnormality usually corrects within a few days. The use of a short course of prednisone at 100 mg daily may be of benefit, as this disorder is often immunologically mediated. Patients with the acquired immune deficiency syndrome have a high rate of marrow dysfunction with thrombocytopenia (91, 100). Trimethoprim sulfamethoxazole often worsens this

Table 28.2
Some Drugs That Cause Thrombocytopenia[a]

ANTIMICROBIALS
  Chloramphenicol
  Sulphonamides
  Amphotericin
  Quinacrine
  Pyrimethamine
  Streptomycin
  Tetracycline
  Penicillins
  Cephalosporins
  INH
ANTICONVULSANTS
  Diphenylhydantoin (Dilantin)
  Primidone (Mysoline)
  Trimethadione (Tridione)
  Ethosuximide (Zavontin)
  Mephenytoin (Mesantoin)
  Carbamazepine (Tegretol)
  Paramethadime
DIURETICS
  Thiazides
  Furosemide
  Acetazolamide
  Ethacrynic Acid
ORAL HYPOGLYCEMICS
  Tolbutamide (Orinase)
  Chlorpropamide (Diabinase)
CHEMICALS
  Arsenicals
  Benzene
RHEUMATOLOGIC MEDICATIONS
  Aspirin
  Phenylbutazone
  Indomethacin
  Gold salts
  Colchicine
  Phenacetin
TRANQUILIZERS
  Meprobamate
  Chlorpromazine
  Chlordiazepoxide
  Chloral hydrate
  Alcohol
OTHERS
  Allopurinol
  Cimetidine
  Estrogens
  Lipid infusions
  Cytotoxic agents
  Corticosteroids
  Heparin
  Inferferon
  Quinidine

[a] May be due to an immune mechanism or decreased production.

Table 28.3
Drugs That Cause a Qualitative Platelet Defect

Alteration of Prostaglandin Metabolism (A)
  Aspirin
  NSAID (Indomethacin, Ibuprofen)
  Corticosteroids
  Sulfinpyrazone
  Furosemide
  Vitamin E
Alteration of Surface Receptors (C)
  Penicillins (Carbenicillin, Ticarcillin)
  Cephalosporins
  β-Lactams (Moxalactam)
  Nitrofurantoin
  Ristocetin
Alteration of Epinephrine Receptors (E)
  α-Blockers (Phentolamine)
  β-Blockers (Propranolol)
  Ca^{++} Channel Blocker (Verapamil)
Phosphodiesterase Inhibitors (B)
  Dipyridamole?
  Xanthines (Theophylline, Caffeine)
  Papaverine
Membrane Stabilizers (D)
  Anesthetics (Xylocaine)
  Tricyclics
  Antihistamines (Diphenhydramine)
Other
  Dextran
  Heparin
  Ethanol
  Glyburide
  Clofibrate
  Reserpine
  Methylsergide
  Glyceryl Guaiacolate
  Phenothiazines
  Fish oils
  Amiodarone

phenomenon. The treatment of these patients is similar to patients with idiopathic thrombocytopenic purpura.

Qualitative platelet defects may be caused by numerous drugs or systemic disorders (Tables 28.3 and 28.4). Collagen vascular disorders, such as systemic lupus erythematosis, may cause a prolonged bleeding time. Uremia may induce a qualitative defect. This thrombopathy may be corrected by the use of cryoprecipitate, desmopressin (dDAVP), or conjugated estrogens (42, 55, 58). Aspirin acetylates serine residues on platelet cyclooxygenase preventing the formation of TXA_2. This action of aspirin results in a prolongation of the bleeding time. The alternate products, HETE and HPETE, are produced. Aspirin blocks cyclooxygenase for the life of the platelet or approximately 7–10 days. With no further aspirin therapy there is a gradual improvement in the bleeding time that coincides with the generation of new platelets. At higher doses, aspirin inhibits endothelial prostacyclin synthetase and prevents generation of PGI_2. At lower doses (less than 300 mg) aspirin pre-

Table 28.4
Acquired Qualitative Platelet Defects

Drugs[a]
Aged Platelets
Antiplatelet Antibodies
Cardiopulmonary Bypass
Myelodysplastic Syndromes
Acute Leukemia
Myeloproliferative Syndromes
Acquired Storage Pool Defect
Acquired von Willebrand's Disease
Hepatic Dysfunction
Uremia
Paraproteinemias
Disseminated Intravascular Coagulation

[a]See Table 28.5.

vents TXA_2 generation, which results in decreased aggregation, release, and vasoconstriction (71). This observation explains the theoretic utility of aspirin in vasospastic disorders or fixed atheromatous lesions. However, with the inhibition of PGI_2 at higher doses, this effect may be negated. Nonsteroidal antiinflammatory drugs such as indomethacin and ibuprofen inhibit cyclooxygenase, but not irreversibly. The inhibition of platelet aggregation depends on the half-life of the nonsteroidal drugs. Choline magnesium trisalicylate maintains the antiarthritic effect of aspirin and in some studies did not alter platelet aggregation. This compound may be useful in arthritics predisposed to a bleeding diathesis.

Some antibiotics may alter platelet function, predominating by altering response to aggregating agents. Classically, this platelet dysfunction occurs with carbenicillin and, to a lesser degree, with ticarcillin and other penicillins (66). Should the patient be predisposed to bleeding for other reasons these agents are best avoided. Many drugs may affect platelet function alone or in conjunction with other drugs. A bleeding time and platelet aggregometry are useful measures of this effect.

Congenital qualitative disorders are occasionally seen in the ICU in patients without a past history of bleeding (75). Von Willebrand's disease is a complex disorder involving a protein complex (VWF-VIII). Many variants exist and it is critical that the specific subtype of von Willebrand's disease be defined. The use of agents such as arginine vasopressin (dDAVP) may precipitate fatal thrombotic events if used in certain von Willebrand variants. In general, it is appropriate to use cryoprecipitate in suspected von Willebrand's disease unless the dDAVP-responsive subtype has been previously diagnosed. Aspirin-like thrombopathy or poorly defined qualitative platelet disorders may occasionally respond to low-dose prednisone (63). The severe qualitative disorders, such as Glanzmann's or Bernard-Soulier, are best treated with platelet transfusion for bleeding events. If surgical intervention is planned in these patients, platelets should be administered prophylactically. ε-Aminocaproic acid can be used to diminish postoperative bleeding.

When a patient presents with either a quantitative or qualitative platelet disorder, procoagulant activity should be studied as well. Disorders such as DIC, liver disease, and renal disease may affect both hemostatic parameters. For adequate hemostasis, it is necessary to correct platelet abnormalities as well as coagulation defects.

COAGULATION DISORDERS

In the critical care unit, bleeding due to a coagulopathy is a common event. Coagulopathy is most often due to an acquired rather than congenital defect. Patients with gastrointestinal bleeding may be heavily transfused, resulting in dilutional effects on platelets and coagulation factors. It is important to address platelet and coagulation factor replacement routinely in the massively transfused patient. One should prophylactically replace with FFP after 4–6 U of red cells have been administered and monitor the platelet count, PT, and $_a$PTT.

The clinician should first assess the site of bleeding. Purpura, ecchymoses, and hemarthroses suggest coagulation defects. The laboratory tests obtained should include a hematocrit, PT, $_a$PTT, platelet count, and review of the peripheral blood smear. If these tests are all normal and the bleeding is accounted for by a surgical wound, packed red cell transfusion therapy as needed is initiated. However, if the bleeding is unusual (i.e., protracted bleeding from mucous membranes, intravenous sites, urinary tract, joints, skin), a more thorough investigation is indicated. Blood oozing from multiple sites is very suggestive of DIC or primary fibrinolysis. The clinician should obtain hepatic and renal function test parameters, which may suggest an etiology of the coagulopathy (90).

If the PT and $_a$PTT are prolonged, a thrombin time and a 1:1 dilution of the PT and PTT (with a mix of the patient's and normal plasma) are recommended. A 1:1 mixture with normal plasma corrects the PT and $_a$PTT if there is an absence of a coagulation factor. If these tests do not correct, an inhibitor is implied (e.g., FDPs, heparin, lupus anticoagulant VIII or IX inhibitors). First, one must rule out inadvertent administration of heparin. The RT should be normal in the setting of heparin effect. A normal thrombin time and a normal 1:1 mix of the PT, $_a$PTT implies a defect above the level of thrombin either in the common, intrinsic, or extrinsic pathway. In DIC, the platelet count would be low unless there is a chronic compensated consumptive coagulopathy secondary to liver disease, primary fibrinolysis, or underlying neoplasia.

Disseminated intravascular coagulation is a common event in the critically ill patient and often a therapeutic dilemma. It represents an uncontrolled stimulation of the coagulation schema by various causes (Table 28.5) (21). The coagulation cascade proceeds unabated, consuming factors and platelets in the process. Often, the bone marrow of the ICU patient is suppressed and does not adequately respond to bleeding and thrombocytopenia with increased megakaryopoiesis. Liver disease may compound this process, resulting in the inability to produce coagulation factors. The fibrinolytic system is activated by the kallikreins and other inflammatory byproducts. Generated plasmin degrades the fibrinogen and fibrin to the degradation products (FDPs). The FDPs subsequently inhibit coagulation at multiple points of the cascade. If fibrin deposition

Table 28.5
Precipitating Events for Disseminated Intravascular Coagulation

Pancreatitis
Prostatic Surgery
Cardiopulmonary Bypass
Extensive Surgery
Trauma
Burns
Obstetrical Complications (Eclampsia, Placenta Previa)
Cavernous Hemangioma
Heat Stroke
Peritoneovenous Shunts
Aneurysmal Rupture
Snake Venoms
Activated Concentrates of K-Dependent Factors
Acute Leukemia (Promyelocytic)
Mitomycin
Neoplasia
Liver Disease
Viral Infections
Systemic Vasculitis
Rhabdomyolysis

in the vasculature is diffuse, red cell fragmentation or microangiopathic changes may be seen in the peripheral smear. Fibrinogen levels decrease markedly. The acute inflammatory state may have induced high fibrinogen levels; hence, the relative value must be taken into account. Thrombotic events may occur because of the stimulus to coagulation. The titer of the FDP by latex agglutination may correlate with the severity of DIC. Chronic DIC as seen in liver disease and neoplasia may have low levels of FDPs without frank bleeding. However, these patients are at risk of conversion to high-grade DIC with the proper stimulus (surgery, shock, sepsis, and chemotherapy). Because of diffuse fibrin deposition, organ dysfunction may progress to hepatic, renal and CNS dysfunction. This fibrin deposition may further release products of inflammation, compounding the fibrinolytic and procoagulant dysfunction. Tests of DIC have been described and are useful in monitoring a response to therapy.

The treatment of DIC is aimed primarily at the elimination of the precipitating cause. Rhabdomyolysis and associated shock are best treated with intense fluid and electrolyte management. Hemodialysis may be required if acute renal failure occurs. Should bleeding occur, the use of fresh-frozen plasma (FFP) and platelet transfusions are indicated. These components are given to control bleeding; one should attempt to maintain platelet counts greater than $20,000/mm^3$ and normalize the PT and $_a$PTT if possible. Gestational causes of DIC are best treated by removing the thromboplastic products, fetal or placental. If bleeding persists, FFP and platelets with heparin coverage may be used. However, in a patient suffering from irreversible liver disease or a terminal neoplastic disorder, the overvigorous use of these products is expensive and may limit their use in other critically ill patients. The ICU team must assess the utility of such component therapy on an individual basis. Patients requiring surgical intervention in the setting of DIC should be supported with FFP and platelets. Sepsis is a common cause of DIC in the critically ill patient. Treatment involves aggressive cardiopulmonary support, antimicrobials and monitoring of hemostasis. If bleeding is occurring from intravenous sites, an initial trial of FFP and platelets are indicated; however, should DIC persist, some hematologists would recommend a trial of heparin.

Heparin use remains a controversial therapy in the management of DIC (29). The use of heparin is established for specific entities, contraindicated in some patients, and often a final intervention to reverse DIC in others. A sound indication for the use of heparin includes acute promyelocytic leukemia. There are some hematologists who have successfully induced acute promyelocytic leukemia patients into complete remission without the use of heparin. They achieved this goal by closely monitoring clinical hemostasis, fibrinogen levels, platelets, PT, and PTT. However, since most patients with promyelocytic leukemia, and occasionally monocytic leukemia, have large amounts of thromboplastic material released into the circulation during induction, heparin is recommended. In acute leukemia, the dose of heparin generally recommended is lower than the dose used for pulmonary embolus and other cases of DIC (14, 15). In general, patients are given 100–200 U/kg/day by continuous infusion: a bolus is not given. Heparin may be used in cases of gestational DIC in which the excessive bleeding persists after removal of the thromboplastic material. One parameter used to determine benefit from heparin is review of the peripheral blood smear. The presence of microangiopathy and thrombocytopenia supports intravascular fibrin deposition. The use of heparin may prevent further fibrin deposition, decrease the microangiopathy, and increase the platelet count. Heparin is often augmented with the use of FFP and platelets. In a burn patient with DIC, heparin may be of benefit. Heparin is generally contraindicated in cases of surgical bleeding with DIC. These cases must be treated by surgical intervention, if feasible. Brisk bleeding from a peptic ulcer in an ICU patient with DIC is not benefited by heparin use. Finally, patients with intractable DIC, in which the underlying cause is adequately treated, can be given a trial of heparin. Occasionally, the hemostatic parameters may correct. In these situations, heparin is given as a 5000- to 10,000-U bolus followed by 1000–1200 U/hour; however, lower doses, as for promyelocytic leukemia, have also been used. The heparin dose is adjusted based upon the fibrinogen concentration, FDP level and platelet count, as well as the peripheral blood smear. As the fibrinogen level and platelets increase and FDPs decrease, the dose of heparin may be decreased, and the need for component replacement diminishes. The use of Amicar (ϵ-aminocaproic acid) in DIC is generally contraindicated, as there is a risk of EACA-induced diffuse thrombosis.

Primary fibrinolysis is a rare entity (48). A secondary fibrinolytic state may be seen in the continuum of DIC. The common causes of primary fibrinolysis are prostatic surgery, malignancy, and, rarely, sepsis. The ability to distinguish primary fibrinolysis from DIC with the secondary state may be difficult. In the proper clinical setting of primary fibrinolysis, one sees bleeding, a relatively normal platelet count, elevated FDPs, fibrin monomer, minimal microangiopathy, low fibrinogen, and a positive euglobulin clot lysis. The treatment of primary fibrinolysis is with Amicar (EACA), with close hemostatic monitoring.

Coagulopathy may be due to an individual factor or to a combination of factor defects. The vitamin K-dependent factors (II, VII, IX, X,) are markedly affected by alterations in vitamin K metabolism (72). If there is a deficiency of vitamin K or an interfering substance (warfarin), these factors are not produced and a coagulopathy results. These factors are synthesized in the liver, and liver disease represents a common cause of coagulopathy (49). Vitamin K must be provided to ICU patients as part of their nutritional support. In normal individuals, the gastrointestinal tract bacterial flora provide adequate amounts of vitamin K. If an antimicrobial is used, the gut may be sterilized, inadequate vitamin K production occurs, and vitamin K replacement therapy becomes necessary. If acute bleeding has developed, patients should be given oral or intravenous vitamin K replacement, as well as FFP to replace vitamin K–dependent factors while hepatic synthesis resumes.

Calcium replacement must also be addressed in ICU patients. As the exogenous source of calcium diminishes and bone reabsorption occurs, patients may develop diminished ionized calcium stores. Calcium is critical to the function of the coagulation cascade. Lipid must also be provided for adequate platelet production of the necessary phospholipids. Although hypocalcemia and decreased phospholipid production play an insignificant clinical role in coagulopathy, they may certainly compound decreased hepatic synthesis of coagulation factors. Patients with severe liver disease may not adequately respond to vitamin K replacement and may respond only to FFP. Patients with severe viral hepatitis progressing to atrophy are monitored for the production of vitamin K–dependent factors by determination of the PT and $_a$PTT. These tests as well as factor assays are sensitive measures of hepatic synthetic abilities.

Acquired anticoagulants may be seen in collagen vascular disease, viral illness, chronic factor replacement and idiopathic causes (13, 33). Factor VIII inhibitors usually occur in the setting of hemophilia A with prolonged factor replacement (104). However, occasionally during pregnancy, childhood or in the elderly, inhibitors to factor VIII develop spontaneously. The anticoagulant may result in a severe bleeding event requiring intervention. The administration of greater than 75 U/kg/12 hours of factor VIII with corticosteroids (prednisone 60–100 mg), plasmapheresis, or the use of activated procoagulant (IXa) may be necessary. Lupus anticoagulant represents an inhibitor to the phospholipid and is manifested by a prolonged $_a$PTT (5, 65). It occurs in children, the elderly and in collagen vascular disease. It is associated with thrombotic events in the hospitalized patient and spontaneous abortion. Lupus anticoagulant production may decrease following the administration of corticosteroids (I recommend 30 mg prednisone daily). In healthy outpatients, lupus anticoagulant represents a laboratory phenomenon, and its clinical importance is still being defined. Endogenous inhibitors to factor IX may develop and are treated in a way similar to factor VIII inhibitor. In liver disease with decreased production of vitamin K–dependent factors, procoagulants induced by vitamin K absence (PIVKA) may form. PIVKA represent the K-dependent precursors that lack a second carboxyl moiety introduced on a glutamine residue. Hence, each vitamin K–dependent factor has its own PIVKA antecedent. Some of the PIVKAs inhibit the coagulation schema. Hypotension with a dysfunctional liver may result in PIVKA formation and precipitate a coagulopathy. Coumadin may also allow for the expression of PIVKA. As previously mentioned, fibrin degradation products also act as inhibitors to coagulation. Plasmin converts fibrinogen to fibrinopeptide fragments X, Y, D, and E. Fragments X and Y are extremely efficient inhibitors of fibrin polymerization. These fragments result in the prolongation of the PT, $_a$PTT, TT, and RT. The FDPs may also adversely effect platelet function.

The maintenance of hemostasis in the critically ill patient involves an extremely complex interaction between cellular components, proteins, and exogenous factors. Most cases of platelet disorders and coagulopathies in the ICU are multifactorial. They require an understanding of the physiological aspects of hemostasis and appropriate intervention.

THROMBOSIS

In general, the endothelium is thromboresistant and normally nonreactive to platelets, coagulation factors, or the fibrinolytic system (99). However, in the ICU patient the endothelium may be damaged, resulting in decreased thromboresistance. The result may be a thrombotic event such as a superficial phlebitis or a massive pulmonary embolus. Patients in the ICU for a systemic disease may be predisposed to recurrent thrombotic events. These patients may be best managed by prophylactic measures to reduce the risk of thrombosis. Major thrombotic events are life threatening and result in ICU admission. Arterial thrombosis can be induced by mechanical, toxic, or immune-mediated events. Small vessel thrombosis may be a platelet and endothelium-mediated event. Disorders such as TTP, hemolytic uremic syndrome, malignant hypertension, and eclampsia are examples. Antiplatelet drugs such as aspirin, dipyridamole, or heparin have been used with some success in small vessel disease. Endotoxic shock can induce endothelial injury and subsequent microangiopathy in experimental models. Venous thrombosis was originally defined by Virchow. The etiology has not been altered since that time. Trauma and stasis remain the predominant cause of venous thrombotic events.

HYPERCOAGULABILITY

Hypercoagulability is an ill-defined state that lags behind bleeding disorders in clinical comprehension. This clinical state represents the predisposition of patients to thromboembolic phenomenon (46, 83). There are idiopathic as well as defined hypercoagulable disorders (Table 28.6). The best example of hypercoagulability is Antithrombin^{III} (AT^{III}) deficiency (98). This may be congenital or acquired. AT^{III} is the predominant circulating anticoagulant, inhibiting thrombin and controlling exuberant hemostasis. Patients with AT^{III} deficiency experience recurrent deep venous thrombosis and pulmonary emboli. It is inherited as an autosomal dominant disorder (86). The incidence in the general population may be as high as one in 2000. Thromboembolic events in AT^{III} deficiency are treated initially with heparin, followed by long-term oral anticoagulation. As expected, heparin resistance is seen in this deficiency state. To document AT^{III} deficiency, one must measure AT^{III} levels. Patients with

Table 28.6
Hypercoagulable States

Congenital	Acquired
Antithrombin III deficiency	Malignancy
Protein C deficiency	Estrogens
Protein S deficiency	Activated procoagulant
Dysfibrinogenemia	complex
Factor XII deficiency?	Pregnancy
Dysplasminogenemia	Lupus anticoagulant
Low plasminogen	Nephrotic syndrome
Homocystinuria	Hepatic dysfibrinogenemia
Sickle cell disease	Vasculitis
	Diabetes mellitus
	Paroxysmal nocturnal
	hemoglobinuria
	Thrombotic
	thrombocytopenic
	purpura
	Venous stasis
	Myeloproliferative
	syndromes

systemic diseases may acquire AT^{III} deficiency. Severe liver disease prevents the synthesis of AT^{III} and compounds dysfunction of platelets and deficiency of coagulation factors with low-grade DIC. Patients with the nephrotic syndrome may excrete large amounts of AT^{III} in the urine and are predisposed to renal vein occlusion and other thrombotic events (43).

Protein C deficiency is another cause of thromboembolism and dermal necrosis associated with coumadin use (12, 26). Protein C is a vitamin K–dependent factor converted to protein Ca (activated protein C) by the action of thrombin. Protein S, a protein Ca cofactor, may also predispose to venous thrombosis when deficient. Protein Ca is an anticoagulant that inactivates factors V_a and VIII_a. Inactivation may not occur initially with warfarin sodium therapy. Protein C–deficient patients are treated with chronic warfarin sodium therapy. However, when initiating the warfarin sodium serious skin necrosis involving the breast and the extremities may occur. Coumadin acutely lowers protein C levels commensurate with factor VII, prior to factors X, IX, II. In suspected or documented cases of protein C deficiency it is recommended that lower starting doses of warfarin sodium (2.5–5 mg/day) be initiated.

Other causes of hypercoagulability include disorders in the fibrinolytic system. Dysfibrinogenemia in liver disease and the lupus anticoagulant may cause thromboses. Acquired hypercoagulable states are seen in malignancy (Trousseau's syndrome), pregnancy, estrogen usage, paroxysmal nocturnal hemoglobinuria, myeloproliferative syndromes, and diabetes

mellitus (37). Many ICU patients may in fact have acquired hypercoagulability compounded by venous stasis and endothelial trauma. The key to proper management is to maintain vascular integrity. Other patients develop thromboembolic events without known hypercoagulability. These events include deep venous thrombosis, pulmonary emboli, and cerebrovascular and cardiovascular thromboembolic events.

PULMONARY EMBOLISM AND DEEP VENOUS THROMBOSIS

Pulmonary embolus is a serious life-threatening event in most patients (80); however, if diagnosed promptly and treated effectively, the outcome is favorable. It remains, a leading undiagnosed acute illness. It is estimated that it is the third most common cause of death in the United States (greater than 600,000 cases/ year) and the incidence is increasing. The increased incidence relates to the increasing age of the population, increase in oral estrogen use, more extensive surgery, increase in malignancy, and increased awareness of the disorder. The difficulty in diagnosis correlates with the lack of pathognomonic physical findings, lab data, and noninvasive diagnostic parameters. More than 90% of pulmonary emboli arise from DVT in the pelvis and thighs. Air, tumor, amniotic fluid and fat emboli are much less common.

Deep venous thrombosis (DVT) occurs in patients at prolonged bed rest. Patients with stasis due to congestive heart failure, recent myocardial infarction, immobilization, hypotension, and malignancy are at significant risk. Most patients with DVT are older than age 60. DVT in younger patients should lead one to consider AT^{III} deficiency. The incidence of DVT as detected by ^{125}I-fibrinogen scanning is 30% in myocardial infarction and as high as 50% in hip surgery. Surgery to the abdomen and thorax predisposes the patient to a high risk of DVT due to endothelial damage, stasis, and immobilization. Venous stasis is central to the development of DVT. If an inflammatory process ensues, the thrombosis may be clinically detected; however, in approximately 50% of cases DVT may be silent. The factors predisposing to embolization are unclear. The tests used to diagnose DVT are institution dependent and include Doppler, plethysmography, ^{125}I-fibrinogen scanning, and venography (38, 39). Venography remains the definitive test.

The clinical utility of the venogram decreases with previous episodes of DVT, and one must occasionally rely on clinical impression.

Pulmonary embolus is a serious complication of DVT. Most pulmonary emboli are multiple (85%). The embolus itself contains those materials previously discussed under "Hypercoagulability", such as platelets, fibrin, and thromboxane. Arterial blood gases are useful but not diagnostic. Patients who have pulmonary embolism may have a $PaO_2 > 90$ mmHg and patients with a $PaO_2 < 80$ mmHg may not have had an embolus. The alveolar-arterial O_2 gradient is a much more useful parameter. Ventilation-perfusion ($\dot{V}/\dot{Q}$) scans require strict interpretation to determine probability of an embolus. Pulmonary angiography remains the standard diagnostic test for pulmonary embolus (40). The patients undergoing a $\dot{V}/\dot{Q}$ scan are assigned a probability. This probability, as well as the clinical condition, dictate the need for angiography. With a normal $\dot{V}/\dot{Q}$ scan, the frequency of pulmonary embolus is extremely low. With multiple subsegmental defects and mismatch on $\dot{V}/\dot{Q}$, the odds of a pulmonary embolus are approximately 90%. The intermediate or indeterminate results require pulmonary angiograms. Angiography should be performed within 24–48 hours of a suspected embolus; otherwise, the activated fibrinolytic system may alter clot consistency and appearance. The angiogram should reveal luminal filling abnormalities or vessel cutoff. False-negative results are extremely rare at most centers.

The therapy of DVT or pulmonary embolus is well established (27, 30, 31, 78). Prophylactic heparin may be given to high risk patients. The prophylactic heparin dose is 5000 units every 8–12 hours. Therapeutic heparin is usually given as a 5000- to 10,000-U intravenous bolus followed by the continuous infusion of 1000–1200 U/hour. DVT or pulmonary embolus should be initially treated with heparin or a heparin derivative. The dose of heparin should be adjusted to maintain the $_aPTT$ or the Lee-White clotting time at 1½–2½ times normal or 2 or 3 times normal, respectively. Bleeding occurs in 3–8% of patients receiving heparin depending on the presence of other underlying disorders such as liver disease and malignancy. Elderly females are statistically at an increased risk for bleeding (25). Aspirin and other antiplatelet drugs are contraindicated. Platelet counts should be monitored at least every 2–3 days while the patient is on

heparin in order to detect heparin-associated thrombocytopenia. If the pulmonary embolus is acute and life threatening, patients should also be given oxygen and dopamine for circulatory support, if necessary. If these measures are unsuccessful and a massive pulmonary embolus is suspected, fibrinolytic therapy or embolectomy are indicated. The pulmonary embolus should be confirmed by angiography prior to the use of streptokinase or urokinase therapy. Recent surgery, peptic ulcer, cerebrovascular accident, or history of hemorrhagic event are relative contraindictions to fibrinolytic therapy. Active bleeding is an absolute contraindication to this therapy. Arterial blood gas monitoring and other invasive techniques should be kept to a minimum. Tamponade must be maintained at all intravenous-access sites. Streptokinase is given as 250,000 IU over 30 minutes, followed by 100,000 IU/hour. This is continued for 24–72 hours. Most centers employ streptokinase for 24–48 hours, then initiate heparin. The agents are not administered simultaneously. Patients are usually discontinued from streptokinase for 3–4 hours prior to heparin initiation. The thrombin time (TT) and occasionally the FDP level are used to monitor streptokinase activity.

Thrombin time is maintained at two to three times normal, and heparin should not be instituted until the TT is less than two times normal. The use of streptokinase or urokinase requires clinical experience in thrombotic disorders. The clinical utility of streptokinase continues to increase. Coumarin derivatives are used after heparin therapy to prevent recurrent thromboembolic disease. Patients may be started on warfarin, once stable on heparin therapy. The coumarin derivatives require 2–7 days to adequately anticoagulate. The prothrombin time is maintained at 1½–2½ times normal (35). Warfarin is continued from 6 weeks to 6 months depending on the severity of the thromboembolic process and underlying disease process. Patients with congenital or acquired hypercoagulable states may require life-long warfarin therapy and require counseling on drug interactions. Low-dose heparin is not effective in preventing recurrent DVT.

If properly treated, DVT and pulmonary embolus have a favorable outcome (36). Patients with prior thromboembolic disease are predisposed to recurrence and should be counseled regarding prophylactic measures. These patients should avoid immobilization, avoid crossing the legs, and employ elastic compression stockings. The same measures may be carried out in patients with prolonged ICU stays, adding passive leg exercise.

RENAL VEIN THROMBOSIS

Renal vein thrombosis may be unilateral or bilateral. It may be associated with nephrotic syndrome, paroxysmal nocturnal hemoglobinuria, malignancy, or congestive heart failure. Oliguria and renal failure may result from bilateral thromboses, necessitating dialysis. The treatment may require thombectomy, if no improvement with conventional anticoagulants are seen. Heparin resistance may be present because of low AT^{III} levels. Higher doses of heparin may be required to reach the therapeutic range of the $_a$PTT.

MYOCARDIAL INFARCTION

Recent studies in the field of myocardial infarction have led to the conclusion that coronary artery thrombosis is critical to the development of ischemic events. The known risk factors to coronary artery disease (e.g., smoking, hyperlipidemia, obesity, and diabetes mellitus) may alter platelet function and the fibrinolytic system (18, 23). The major physiologic activator of fibrinolysis is tissue plasminogen activator (tpa). Recent data suggest that reduced levels of tpa may be due to a circulating inhibitor. Pharmacologic manipulation of tpa may alter the outcome of myocardial infarction patients. Coronary angioscopy has documented that unstable angina may be related to thrombi in association with atheromatous plaques refractory to medical management (89). This pathophysiologic information has led to the use of anticoagulants, antiplatelet agents, and fibrinolytic therapy in patients with myocardial disease. However, studies have been slow to document significant survival advantage of such therapeutic intervention.

The use of anticoagulants to alter the course of myocardial ischemia is not recommended. An exception is crescendo angina. In this disorder, therapeutic heparin may be beneficial (92). For large infarctions the risk of pericardial bleeding with tamponade has been a concern, although this risk is not as common as might be expected. The presence of a pericardial rub is considered to be a contraindiction to the use of heparin. Heparin has been rec-

ommended on a prophylactic basis at low dose (5000 U every 8–12 hours) for patients felt to be at risk for DVT or pulmonary embolus. Patients with congestive heart failure, marked peripheral edema, and those confined to bed are at particular risk. Patients with chronic atrial fibrillation, ventricular aneurysms, and massive cardiomegaly may present on coumadin because of a history of recurrent thromboembolic disease. The drug is usually maintained during the early infarction period, avoiding the higher therapeutic range. It is critical to keep in mind the cardiac medications that alter coumadin action or binding. The role of coumadin and heparin in reducing infarct size or affecting overall survival remains unanswered despite a number of trials.

There is widespread use of aspirin, dipyridamole, sulfinpyrazone, and other antiplatelet drugs in clinical practice despite conflicting evidence showing benefit. Studies have revealed a trend towards benefit in reducing the incidence of reinfarction with these agents. However, the use of these antiplatelet drugs is generally not recommended in this setting. Doses of aspirin used in some trials have been those that would reduce both platelet TXA$_2$ and endothelial prostacyclin levels. Proper dosage and scheduling of aspirin remain to be established. Experimental data in animal models would suggest that coronary artery thrombosis and atherogenesis may be altered by the use of antiplatelet drugs or fish oils. Recent data suggest that platelet inhibition of prostaglandin synthesis may require continued blood levels of aspirin and that a slow-release formulation may be more appropriate. The patients found most likely to benefit from low-dose (300 mg) aspirin are those with recurrent bouts of unstable angina. Postmortem studies of these patients have shown fresh thrombi in association with atheromata.

Thrombolytic therapy in myocardial infarction has become routine in critical care patients. Coronary angiography during early infarction or unstable angina reveals thrombi in the coronary arteries. In laboratory animals, fibrinolytic therapy has resulted in reperfusion and reduction in infarct size. In human trials, intracoronary perfusion with streptokinase has resulted in increased patency of obstructed coronary arteries (67). However, improvement in survival and left ventricular function as a result of thrombolytic therapy have not been demonstrated. Because of the difficulty of intracoronary streptokinase, the intravenous route has been advocated (84). Some early trials have not shown benefit from thrombolytic therapy, perhaps because of the delays in the initiation of streptokinase. If streptokinase is administered early in myocardial infarction (within hours) progressive ischemic damage may be avoided. However, bleeding of a severe nature may occur. Routine use of streptokinase in myocardial infarction awaits confirmation by larger definitive trials. Compared with intravenous streptokinase, newer formulations such as acylated streptokinase, plasminogen activator, or tissue plasminogen activator may prove to be of benefit with a lower incidence of complications.

CEREBROVASCULAR THROMBOEMBOLIC DISEASE

The mechanisms described for coronary vasospasm, ischemia, and thrombosis are similar in the cerebral circulation (69). Cerebrovascular accidents may be thrombotic or hemorrhagic. In the event of a cerebrovascular accident, an emergent computer tomography scan with contrast is generally performed. If this scan is indicative of thrombosis, lumbar puncture does not reveal frank blood or xanthochromia, the patient does not have marked meningeal findings, and neurologic examination is progressive, a trial of heparin is usually indicated. Heparin is used intravenously at conventional therapeutic doses. Subsequent cerebral angiography may detect a surgically amenable lesion. The role of the fibrinolytic system in cerebral vessels is less well defined than in coronary vessles and the role of thrombolytic therapy is not defined. The use of antiplatelet drugs has not been of therapeutic benefit in the management of thrombotic stroke.

Transient ischemic attacks (TIA) result from atheromatous material or small emboli dislodging from major vessels in the neck and lodging in the brain. Antiplatelet drugs are used in the management of TIAs. Their use relates to the shift in the thromboxane A2/prostacylin balance in favor of dimished thrombosis and atherogenesis. In a large trial of aspirin and sulfinpyrazone (200 mg four times a day), it was concluded that aspirin (325 mg four times a day) significantly reduced the incidence of stroke in men with a history of cerebral or retinal ischemic attacks. The same study revealed a decreased incidence of coronary death. Other trials have shown benefit to both sexes and no added benefit from

dipyridamole (100–200 mg four times a day). Some investigators feel that women may benefit as well as men from the use of aspirin. Trials on low-dose versus high-dose aspirin are pending. There is currently a trend to use low-dose aspirin, because conceptually bleeding and gastric irritation may be less. Low-dose aspirin may not impair prostacyclin production.

Hemorrhagic stroke implies different pathologic events than thrombotic processes. In this setting, a cerebral bleed has recurred and will progress unless adequate hemostasis occurs. The diagnosis may be confirmed by an early CT scan of the head and lumbar puncture. Altered hemostatic integrity may be detected by studying the platelet count, PT, and $_a$PTT. A drug history should be obtained to rule out drugs that may compromise hemostasis. Drugs that promote bleeding are absolutely contraindicated in the treatment of hemorrhagic stroke. Rebleeding is a frequent complication of hemorrhagic stroke and theoretically may be prevented with antifibrinolytic therapy. The antifibrinolytic agent available for stabilizing cerebral clot is ϵ-aminocaproic acid (EACA). This drug can reduce the incidence of rebleeding and may improve overall survival in hemorrhagic stroke. However, the routine use of EACA in stroke remains controversial. Other trials have concluded that antifibrinolytic therapy does not alter the outcome of subarachnoid hemorrhage. One of the problems in proving efficacy of antifibrinolytic therapy is the inability to monitor EACA therapy. One proposed method is cerebrospinal fluid FDP levels, but this method may be tedious (82). When used, a loading dose of 5 g of EACA is given and followed by a continuous intravenous infusion at 2 g/hour. Complications include thrombosis and cerebral rebleeding.

PHARMACOLOGY OF DRUGS EFFECTING HEMOSTASIS AND THROMBOSIS

Anticoagulants have been in clinical use for over 40 years in the management of thromboses. Numerous trials have documented their efficacy. More recent studies have attempted to reduce complications and maintain therapeutic effect. The utility of anticoagulants is established for the treatment of systemic thromboembolic disease, prosthetic cardiac valves, mitral valve disease, and atrial fibrillation (51). There are other areas in which the

Table 28.7
Dosage and Route of Administration of Anticoagulants, Antiplatelet Drugs, and Related Compound

Drug	Route	Loading Dose	Maintenance Dose	Test Monitored
Heparin	i.v.	5–10,000 USP U i.v.	1000–1200 USP U/hr by continuous infusion	$_A$PTT
	s.c.		5000 USP U every 8–12 hours	$_A$PTT
Protamine	i.v.	1 mg/100 U of heparin[a]		
Streptokinase	i.v.	250,000 U over 30 min	100,000 U/hr for 24–48 hours[b]	TT, FDP, $_A$PTT
Urokinase	i.v.	4400 U/kg	4400 U/kg/hr	TT, FDP, $_A$PTT
ε-aminocapriotic acid (Amicar)	i.v.	4–5 g	1 g/hr i.v.	Clinical response
	p.o.	5 g	1 g/hr	
Warfarin	p.o.	5–10 mg/day	2–5 mg/day	PT
Aspirin	p.o.		150–1300 mg/day	
Dipyridamole	p.o.		200–400 mg/day	

[a] Calculated based on $t_{1/2}$ and dose of heparin given.
[b] Follow by therapeutic heparin when streptokinase or urokinase has been discontinued 3 hr.

benefit needs to be documented. Although doses are not totally agreed upon, a table of accepted doses is included (Table 28.7).

HEPARIN AND HEPARIN-LIKE SUBSTANCES

Heparin prolongs clotting in vivo or in vitro. Knowledge of the action of heparin remains incomplete because of its heterogeneous nature (20). Heparin is a naturally occurring mucoitin polysulfuric acid consisting of equal amounts of hexuronic acid and acetylated glycosamine with sulfuric acid ester groups. The heterogeneous molecule has a significant electronegative charge. Naturally occurring heparin is stored within mast cells. The exact role of endogenous heparin is unclear, but it is thought to affect platelet function and coagulation factors. Isoelectric focusing of heparin has detected 21 components. These components differ in their affinity for AT^{III} and PF 4. The anticoagulant effect of heparin results from the cumulative effect of these components. Recently, attempts have been made to separate these components, resulting in a more specific mode of action with decreased complications. Further description of these derivatives follows.

The commercial source of heparin is the lungs or intestinal mucosa of domestic animals. The heparins obtained in this fashion have different potency and must be standardized. The biologic effect is analyzed by comparing the activity of the preparation with a USP reference standard. The standard heparin is used to prevent clotting of citrated sheep plasma to which calcium has been added. The USP guidelines state that sodium heparin must contain no less than 120 USP units/mg but allows the manufacturer a 10% margin of error. The heparin available in the United States is labeled with activity in units and weight of heparin. In clinical use, 1 unit of heparin activity is equivalent to 0.01 mg of sodium heparin. The USP-standard heparin sodium injection may contain an antimicrobial agent and materials to prevent absorption. The most common preparation is 10,000 U (100 mg) in 10 ml water; more concentrated solutions are available.

Heparin is an ineffective anticoagulant via the oral or rectal route; it must be given parenterally. Intramuscular injections are painful and should be avoided. Heparin is usually given intravenously or subcutaneously. Depot injections have been given, but absorption is erratic and clinically unreliable. Following intravenous administration, 20–25% of the dose is recovered active in the urine. Radiolabeled heparin has revealed uptake of heparin within mast cells and subsequent storage. The heparin may bind to plasma proteins or may be degraded in the liver.

Heparin inhibits blood coagulation by a number of mechanisms (7). The predominant effect at therapeutic levels is to act in conjunction with AT^{III} as an inhibitor of activated coagulation factors. AT^{III} inhibits factors XII_a, XI_a, IX_a, X_a and II_a at a serine residue. AT^{III} in combination with the serine residue irreversibly undergoes esterfication at an arginyl site. The binding site on AT^{III} for heparin is in a lysine residue. Heparin promotes a conformational change allowing for enhanced binding to activated factors, in particular XII_a, X_a, and thrombin. Factors XI_a and IX_a are relatively insensitive to the heparin-AT^{III} complex. A second cofactor, heparin cofactor II may also act like an antithrombin (93). Heparinoids may act via heparin cofactor II. Heparin also inhibits the activation of prothrombin by X_a. Heparin affects platelet aggregation in a nonspecific manner and heparin-induced bleeding may be on the basis of altered platelet function (57). Low-molecular-weight heparin (enoxaparin) has a high affinity for AT^{III} compared with high-molecular-weight fractions (34).

Low-molecular-weight heparins are as effective as unfractionated standard heparin in preventing deep venous thrombosis in animal models. In one trial, patients were given 30 mg enoxaparin subcutaneously twice a day compared with placebo. This therapy was effective in preventing DVT in patients undergoing elective hip surgery and resulted in few complications. Enoxaparin may have less antiplatelet effect and hence less bleeding complications.

Heparin can be used in either a prophylactic regimen or the therapy of DVT or pulmonary embolus (32). Low-dose subcutaneous heparin is usually given in a dose of 5000 U 2 hours preoperatively, then 5000 U every 8–12 hours postoperatively for the period of decreased ambulation. This method is extremely effective in preventing calf and proximal vein thromboses; hence, pulmonary emboli are decreased in incidence. Prophylactic low-dose heparin is the treatment of choice in most high-risk surgical and medical patients. This group of patients includes those with prolonged bed rest, congestive heart failure, and general surgery patients. In extremely high-risk patients, such as those undergoing hip surgery and amputations, a higher dose may be required. Recently, low-molecular-weight heparin was shown in a randomized trial to prevent DVT in hip surgery and to be more effective than placebo (with fewer complications)(94). The risk of bleeding with low-molecular-weight heparin is considered low. Prophylactic low-dose heparin in conjunction with dihydroergotamine (Embolex) was found to be effective as well, but a consensus has not been reached regarding its use (0.5 mg dihydroergotamine/5000 U heparin intravenous 2 hours preoperatively, then every 12 hours for 5 days).

The presence of platelet dysfunction, primary coagulopathy, or a neurosurgical procedure are contraindications to low-dose heparin. Most patients on low-dose heparin are not monitored with laboratory tests. However, in patients undergoing elective hip surgery, if the $_a$PTT is maintained between 31.5 and 36 seconds with heparin therapy for 8 days postoperatively, the incidence of DVT, and bleeding are statistically reduced. The final recommendations regarding high-risk patients await larger trials.

For patients with DVT or pulmonary embolus, treatment with heparin is routine. Untreated pulmonary embolus has a mortality rate approaching 25%. Thromboembolism is treated with a constant infusion of intravenous heparin. Patients are given an intravenous bolus of heparin 5000–10,000 USP units followed by a continuous infusion of 1000–1200 U/hour (20,000 U of heparin in 500 ml of $\frac{2}{3}$ dextrose, $\frac{1}{3}$ saline at 30 ml/hour). The dose is adjusted in an attempt to reach an endpoint of $1\frac{1}{2}$–$2\frac{1}{2}$ times the $_a$PTT control. Heparin is usually administered for 7–10 days. Oral anticoagulants are begun on day 4 or 5 from the start of heparin. The therapy of heparin and warfarin should overlap by 4–5 days. This dual therapy potentially counteracts the thrombotic potential of inducing protein C deficiency.

The complications of heparin therapy are often overstated and perhaps have led to decreased usage. Heparin-induced bleeding usually occurs at large heparin doses and may be life threatening. The risk of heparin-induced hemorrhage is from 1% to 33%. Prophylactic low-dose heparin has a very low rate of bleeding complications in most patients. Heparin-induced bleeding can be reversed with protamine sulfate. Protamines are low-molecular-weight proteins containing large amounts of arginine. These compounds are strongly basic and are derived from fish. Protamine functions as an anticoagulant but is not as potent as heparin. Five milliliter vials of protamine contain 50 mg per vial of the basic protein. Protamine sulfate is given intravenously and forms a stable salt with heparin, which inactivates the conformational change of AT^{III}. This effect occurs within 5 minutes of administration. Patients may develop a hypersensitivity reaction; the role of fish allergy has not been defined. The appropriate dose of protamine depends on the heparin dose administered. To reverse recent heparin administration, an intravenous dose of 1 mg of protamine for every 100 USP U of heparin, is given slowly over 10 minutes to prevent hypotension. Heparin has a plasma half-life of 60 minutes and 50 mg (maximum dose, may be repeated based on normalization of the $_a$PTT) of protamine reverses 15,000 U of heparin.

If 30 minutes have elapsed since administration of heparin, 25 mg of protamine may be given; if 60 minutes have elapsed then 12.5 mg of protamine sulfate is given. One attempts to err on a lower dose of protamine to avoid overdosing and exacerbating bleeding. The dose of protamine may need to be repeated as heparin may dissociate from the salt complex. The $_a$PTT may be monitored to determine decreasing heparin effect. Another complication of heparin therapy is thrombocytopenia (45, 88). This adverse reaction is an idiosyncratic reaction and the frequency of this drug-induced problem is less than 6%. The likelihood of heparin-induced thrombocytopenia is independent of the route of administration; however, the source of heparin does affect the frequency of this problem. Thrombocytopenia is seen more frequently with bovine lung than porcine intestinal mucosa heparin (1). Thrombocytopenia generally occurs 6–12 days after initiation of heparin therapy, but may occur throughout the course of therapy. Platelet-associated immunoglobulin has been implicated as the cause of heparin-related thrombocytopenia; however, the immunoglobulin is not a universal finding (57). Heparin-associated thrombocytopenia is thought to be immune mediated. Occasionally patients may also develop thrombotic complications (11). Patients with heparin-induced thrombocytopenia should avoid a similar heparin source if retreatment is required (44). Patients are begun on oral anticoagulants and heparin is stopped as soon as possible. Platelet counts are carefully monitored during this period.

Heparin is rarely associated with an anaphylactic reaction (53). Patients with a history of hypersensitivity should be given a test dose. Patients with hypersensitivity or heparin-induced thrombocytopenia may be considered for low-molecular-weight heparin. Theoretically, the antigenic stimulus is not a component of this formulation. Osteoporosis is a rare complication of heparin therapy. This complication occurs in women who are treated with 20,000 U/day for more than 6 months. Heparin also has an antichylomicronemic action, the significance of which is unknown. This action is being studied with regard to the development of atherosclerotic lesions.

Heparin has been a critical therapeutic tool for many years and will remain so. Continued research into its mode of action, clinical utility, components, and complications are imperative.

ORAL ANTICOAGULANTS

The first oral anticoagulants were synthesized approximately 40 years ago. The first compound was bishydroxycoumarin. Other derivatives have since been synthesized, including sodium warfarin (Coumadin). These compounds are similar in structure to vitamin K. Sodium warfarin is the only product currently used because of its reliable pharmacokinetics. The half-life of warfarin is about 35 hours. The metabolism and excretion rates vary among individuals. Many systemic disorders and drugs alter the absorption, metabolism, excretion and plasma binding of warfarin (Table 28.8). Approximately 99% of warfarin is bound to plasma albumin. Only the free warfarin is biologically active. Hence, drugs that alter warfarin binding affect free warfarin and its biologic action.

These vitamin K antagonists inhibit the effect of vitamin K on posttranslational liver synthesis of factors II, VII, IX, and X; protein C; and protein S. This inhibition results in the formation of inactive compounds referred to

Table 28.8
Drugs or Disease States That Affect Warfarin Action

POTENTIATION
Drugs
  Androgens, chloral hydrate, chloramphenicol, clofibrate, glucagon, indomethacin, neomycin, acetaminophen, allopurinol, diazoxide, disulfiram, ethacrynic acid, heparin, 6-mercaptopurine, α-methyldopa, MAO inhibitors, nalidixic acid, sulfinpyrazone, thyroid drugs, tolbutamide, sulfa drugs, phenylbutazone, phenytoin, quinidine, salicylates, thyroxine, alcohol, anesthetics, metronidazole, cimetidine.

Disease States
  Collagen vascular disorders, congestive heart failure, hepatitis, hyperthyroidism, vitamin K deficient diet, malignancy, malabsorption, narcotic abuse.

INHIBITION
Drugs
  Barbiturates, glutethimide, griseofulvin, haloperidol, corticosteroids, estrogens, meprobamate, colchicine, rifampin, tetracyclines, carbamazepine, alcohol, cholestyramine.

Disease States
  Hereditary resistance to coumadin, hypothyroidism.

previously as PIVKA. Vitamin K promotes carboxylation of factors II, VII, IX, and X; protein C; and protein S to the active procoagulant or anticoagulant. The activated factors have reactive sites for calcium and phospholipid. The vitamin K antagonists inhibit the cyclic conversion of vitamin K and its 2, 3 epoxide. This action results in increased amounts of the vitamin K epoxide compared with vitamin K. The nonepoxide is necessary for activation of vitamin K–dependent factors.

Protein C is converted to its active form by the action of thrombin. Protein C binds to thrombomodulin on the endothelium, markedly increasing its conversion by thrombin to active protein C_a. Protein C_a inhibits factors V_a and VIII_a. The thrombin bound to thrombomodulin is rendered ineffective in further activating factors V and VIII. This functions as an important anticoagulant system. This system is affected by the action of warfarin. Hence, thrombotic potential exists if the anticoagulant protein C is not synthesized. The anticoagulant effect of warfarin is first seen at 24 hours by suppression of factor VII. However, it is not until 96 hours when factors II, IX, and X are inhibited, that maximal effect is seen. Protein C activity is also reduced concomitantly with factor VII. This fact has clinical importance in patients with underlying protein C deficiency (105). After warfarin has been initiated the prothrombin time begins to prolong at 24 hours because of loss of factor VII activity. Because of the risks of rapidly reducing protein C, smaller starting doses are recommended. Warfarin is begun with a 4–5 day overlap with heparin therapy for deep venous thrombosis or pulmonary embolus. This overlap prevents the thrombogenic risk of reducing protein C_a acutely.

Vitamin K antagonists are monitored with the prothrombin time (19). In general, the doses of vitamin K antagonists are adjusted to maintain the PT at 1½–2½ times control. However, the effect of these agents on the PT is still being studied. The source of tissue thromboplastin may alter the relationship of PT to control values. The controls used to adjust the warfarin sodium dose may differ depending on the source of tissue thromboplastin. One must inquire as to the methods for standardizing the control values.

The use of oral anticoagulants in unstable angina has not been established in well-designed studies. In patients with cerebrovascular disease there is evidence that suggests that oral anticoagulants may be of benefit in progressive thrombotic stroke. In patients with cardiac disease (congestive heart failure, cardiomyopathy) anticoagulant therapy can prevent reembolization to the cerebral circulation. Patients with mitral valve disease with resultant or chronic atrial fibrillation clearly benefit from long-term anticoagulation. Patients with prosthetic valves in the mitral position are at high risk of embolization; aspirin alone in these patients is not of benefit. Combining warfarin with antiplatelet drugs in these patients decreases embolization compared with warfarin alone; however, in combining warfarin and aspirin, bleeding episodes are increased. Clearly, a safer prophylactic measure is necessary. One should avoid the combination of warfarin sodium and aspirin since the plasma kinetics of warfarin sodium are altered by aspirin.

Persantine does not have a similar effect. Hence, patients who experience embolization while on Coumadin may benefit from the addition of dipyridamole.

The complications of oral anticoagulant therapy, particularly bleeding, can be life threatening. Clinicians must be aware of the numerous drug interactions. The bleeding complications relate to the dosage of the oral anticoagulants, the underlying systemic disease, particularly hepatic dysfunction, and other factors such as trauma, surgery, and drugs. Minor bleeding occurs in 18% of patients in large anticoagulation clinics; major bleeding occurs in less than 5% of patients. Minor bleeding is predominately from mucous membranes and includes epistaxis and gingival bleeding. When evaluating patients with bleeding as a result of receiving sodium warfarin, one promptly orders a PT, $_a$PTT, and platelet count. If PT is in the therapeutic range, another cause of bleeding should be sought. Bleeding due to coumadin is managed with vitamin K as well as the administration of FFP. Occasionally one encounters patients who have inadvertently or purposefully ingested Coumadin. Coumadin and PIVKA levels may be used for documentation of occult usage; the activity of factors II, VII, IX, and X may also be measured.

In Coumadin overdose, if the PT and $_a$PTT are markedly prolonged and bleeding is uncontrolled, prompt administration of FFP is indicated. Vitamin K can be given intravenously slowly at a dose of 10–25 mg (rate no faster than 1 mg/minute). The response of the PT is used to determine the frequency of subsequent doses of vitamin K. The preferred route of administration of vitamin K is subcutaneous or intramuscular; however, with a markedly prolonged PT this route of administration may be contraindicated. Intravenously administered vitamin K has resulted in anaphylaxis and anaphylaxis precautions (epinephrine, antihistamines, steroids at the bedside) are necessary even with slow administration. The PT is affected within 1–2 hours of vitamin K administration.

If the PT is only marginally outside the therapeutic range (two to three times) and no bleeding is present, Coumadin is discontinued and the patient observed. If the PT is further prolonged, 2.5–5 mg of vitamin K may be given. If the bleeding occurs in the setting of acute DVT and further use of Coumadin is contraindicated, subcutaneous heparin for the duration of therapy (3–6 months) is indicated.

Numerous drugs alter the pharmacokinetics of warfarin (Table 28.8). These drug alterations result in varying levels of vitamin K–dependent factors. The production of these vitamin K–dependent factors directly relates to the plasma level of free warfarin. The plasma level of warfarin may be dependent on the rate of biotransformation or the binding of warfarin to plasma proteins. The liver microsomal enzyme system inactivates the coumarin derivative. A drug that increases activity of this system biodegrades warfarin at an increased rate. This biodegradation necessitates increasing the warfarin dose in order to maintain the anticoagulant effect. If this class of drug is stopped suddenly, warfarin levels markedly increase and hemorrhagic complications may ensue. Drugs that induce activation of the liver microsomal enzyme system include phenobarbital, chloral hydrate, haloperidol, and griseofulvin. These drugs decrease the plasma warfarin level. Some drugs may inhibit the microsomal enzyme system and increase warfarin levels. Warfarin promptly binds to plasma proteins upon administration. Salicylates, diphenylhydantoin and phenylbutazone displace warfarin from plasma proteins and increase free warfarin levels. Certain antibiotics such as chloramphenicol and neomycin interfere with the synthesis of vitamin K by inhibiting bacterial intestinal flora and may potentiate the warfarin effect. Warfarin responsiveness is increased with anabolic steroids and thyroxine.

Certain disease states may also alter warfarin action. Thyrotoxicosis enhances the mode of action of warfarin, predisposing to bleeding. Congestive heart failure prolongs the warfarin half-life. Neoplastic diseases may be associated with decreased production of vitamin K–dependent factors. Acute viral hepatitis is associated with a hypoprothrombinemic state, if hepatic dysfunction is significant. Warfarin compounds the reduced levels of factors II, VII, IX, and X in these patients. Patients on vitamin K–deficient diets may be more susceptible to a warfarin effect.

An important clinical entity seen with Coumadin therapy is dermal necrosis (59, 61). Coumadin causes other dermatological reactions as well. Bleeding into the skin with ecchymoses and purpura are commonly seen. Urticaria, macules, and papules are seen in patients allergic to Coumadin. Dermal skin necrosis is a very rare, severe complication of warfarin therapy that occurs about 1 week after therapy has begun. Dermal necrosis begins as macules and papules and progresses to hemorrhagic bulli, and finally skin sloughing occurs. The lesions are seen in areas of adipose tissue, (e.g., breasts, buttocks and thighs). The histopathology reveals dermal vein fibrin deposition. Some of the cases have been associated with protein C deficiency. Treatment consists of warfarin withdrawal, prompt heparin therapy, and local skin care. The syndrome of Coumadin dermal necrosis has proved to be fatal in some patients.

ANTIPLATELET DRUGS

The action of platelets and endothelium in maintaining hemostasis has been described (68, 101, 102). Salicylates were first used therapeutically in 1763. Aspirin-induced prolongation of bleeding was first noted in 1954. This observation has been subsequently confirmed, and the use of aspirin to alter hemostasis has become commonplace. The predominant effect of aspirin is the acetylation of cyclooxygenase and subsequent inhibition of TXA_2 synthesis. Nonsteroidal antiinflammatory drugs act by a similar mechanism. Eicosatrienoic acid has recently been introduced to alter platelet function and reduce atherogenesis. Eicosatrienoic acid causes platelets to produce thromboxane A_2, an ineffective aggregating compound, and endothelium to produce prostaglandin I_3, a potent antiaggregating agent. Dipyridamole is a coronary vasodilator that is found to alter platelet function; the mode of action is still unclear. Dipyridamole inhibits adhesion of platelets to the subendothelium. The mechanism has been attributed to increased platelet cyclic AMP. Aspirin synergistically acts with dipyridamole to prevent platelet aggregation. Xanthines, such as theophylline, inhibit platelet phosphodiesterase and increase platelet cyclic AMP.

Antibiotics such as penicillin, carbenicillin, and ticarcillin inhibit platelet responsiveness by coating platelets and blocking binding sites on which aggregating substances act. These drugs also interfere with the release reaction. This phenomenon may have clinical importance in the critically ill patient with uncontrolled bleeding. Propranolol and other β-blockers inhibit second-wave aggregation by ADP and epinephrine. Propranolol also effects platelet clot retraction. Clofibrate, used in the treatment of hyperlipidemia, can inhibit aggregation to epinephrine and ADP. Other drugs known to inhibit platelet function include corticosteroids, furosemide, cyproheptadine, hydroxychloroquine, and heparin.

THROMBOLYTIC THERAPY

Streptokinase and urokinase activate the fibrinolytic system by complexing with plasminogen and forming plasmin (17, 81). Streptokinase is the most widely employed plasminogen activator, probably because of cost. Urokinase is isolated from human urine, is costly, and has a shorter half-life.

The action of streptokinase varies in individual patients. However, its utility in patients with pulmonary embolus, DVT, and early myocardial infarction is unquestioned. Patients treated for DVT with streptokinase have rapid clot resolution and increased reversal of altered hemodynamics in response to pulmonary embolus when compared with heparin. Thrombolytic therapy can also clear microthrombi from the pulmonary circulation. Thrombolytic therapy may, in the case of DVT, preserve venous valvular function. The National Institutes of Health have strongly endorsed the use of streptokinase for treatment of thromboembolic disease. Streptokinase has been advocated for *early* treatment of pulmonary emboli as well as proximal deep vein thrombosis. The diagnosis of thromboembolic disease should be confirmed by venogram or pulmonary angiogram. For thrombolytic therapy to be considered, the duration of thromboembolic disease should be less than 1 week, since clot organization has begun by this time. The action of streptokinase on organized clot is limited.

Contraindications to streptokinase use include active bleeding, a cerebrovascular accident, or surgery less than 2 months prior to therapy. Other traumatic events such as organ biopsy, pregnancy, and pericardiocentesis are relative contraindicactions. Invasive techniques should be avoided while the patient is receiving streptokinase. For each patient considered for streptokinase, a risk-versus-benefit algorithm should be established.

Streptokinase is prepared from group C streptococci; hence, allergic reactions may occur due to development of neutralizing antibodies. The molecular weight of streptokinase is 47,000 and the half-life is approximately 10–12 minutes. Streptokinase is prepared in sodium chloride or dextrose and should be stored at 2–4°C if not used immediately.

Patients are given 250,000 U of intravenous streptokinase over 30 minutes, then begun on 100,000 U/hour continuous infusion for 24–72 hours. If patients have had a recent streptococcal infection, higher doses may be needed to overcome blocking antibodies. However, more than 90% of patients respond to the loading dose. Should inadequate response to streptokinase be noted, urokinase may be used. Urokinase 4400 U/kg is given intravenously over 10 minutes followed by 4400 U/kg/hour for 24 hours. Laboratory monitoring is used to ensure that systemic fibrinolysis is occurring. If the systemic clots are less than 7 days old, prompt lysis should be seen and improvement detected by impedance plethysmography, Doppler, or pulmonary hemodynamics. It is important to document lysis because if patients are refractory to fibrinolytic therapy, reembolization may occur. Monitoring the thrombin time, euglobulin clot lysis, fibrinogen, and FDPs have all been employed. Prolongation of the PT and $_a$PTT also reflect the presence of plasmin-generated FPDs. If no evidence of fibrinolysis is detected, streptokinase should be discontinued and heparin begun promptly. Heparin is not begun simultaneously with thrombolytic therapy because of the increased risk of bleeding. When the TT is less than two times normal, heparin is begun at conventional continuous infusion doses (1,000–1,200 U/hour). Treatment with heparin is continued for 7–10 days and overlapped for 4–5 days with warfarin.

While the patient is receiving streptokinase, it is best to avoid antiplatelet drugs, invasive techniques, intramuscular injections, or physical handling. Bleeding is the major complication of thrombolytic therapy. In one series, only 4% of patients required transfusion and there were no fatalities from bleeding. In order to prevent bleeding complications, one gives attention to meticulously avoiding trauma. Minor bleeding can be managed with an ϵ-aminocaproic acid soaked pledget and compression. If major bleeding does occur, thrombolytic therapy should be stopped. Because of the short half-lives of thrombolytics, this approach is usually successful. If transfusion is needed, packed RBCs with use of cryoprecipitate or FFP may be in order. In episodes of severe bleeding, an oral dose of ϵ-aminocaproic acid has been given in 5-g courses every 4–6 hours, or 1–2 g/hr by continuous infusion after a loading dose of 5 g.

Febrile reactions occur in 20% of patients receiving streptokinase; skin allergic reactions are reported in 5% of patients. Febrile reactions are managed with acetaminophen. Allergic phenomenon can be treated with corticosteroids and antihistamines. Repeat therapy with thrombolytic therapy is usually avoided for 6 months.

Streptokinase has been administered intravenously to patients with early myocardial infarction (within 3 hours). Patients were given 750,000 U of streptokinase over 30 minutes, followed by heparin infusion and oral nitrates. Long-term anticoagulation was maintained with oral anticoagulants. Given in this manner, severe bleeding occurred in only 2 of 53 patients. Reduction in the infarct size and subsequent myocardial preservation were documented. Further randomized trials are indicated to determine effects on long-term survival.

PHARMACOLOGICAL AGENTS EMPLOYED TO ENHANCE HEMOSTASIS

Antifibrinolytic therapy is currently available in the form of ϵ-aminocaproic acid (56), which is used clinically to counteract excessive fibrinolysis. ϵ-Aminocaproic acid (EACA) is a synthetic monoaminocarboxylic acid with properties similar to lysine, is readily absorbed from the gastrointestinal tract, and is water soluble. EACA promptly distributes to the intravascular and extravascular spaces. Peak circulating EACA levels are seen within 2 hours of oral administration and excretion is mainly via the kidneys. Greater than 50% is cleared in 24 hours, and 1 g of EACA inhibits the activation of plasminogen to plasmin. EACA competively inhibits plasminogen conversion by its effect on the arginine-lysine moiety.

EACA at high dose also exerts an antiplasmin effect. EACA can be employed in cases of primary fibrinolysis, altered hemostasis following cardiac surgery, amegakaryocytic thrombocytopenia and after prostatic surgery. EACA has also been used to decrease factor requirements in hemophiliacs undergoing surgical or dental procedures. EACA should not be administered in the presence of active disseminated intravascular coagulation. Adverse reactions to EACA include myopathy (rarely rhabdomyolysis) and thrombosis, particularly in the setting of consumptive coagulopathy.

Thrombin is available only for topical use. It is used when a surgical wound continues to ooze and ligation or pressure is unsuccessful. Allergic reactions to thrombin have been reported. Thrombin may be used in conjunction with a gelatin sponge. Sclerosing agents such as sodium tetradecyl sulfate have been employed for bleeding esophageal varices. Upon injection, this compound acts by irritating the endothelium and causing prompt thrombus formation. The risk of extensive thrombosis exists and requires use by experienced gastroenterologists.

In summary, hemorrhage and thrombosis are frequent complications in the ICU setting. These events require knowledge of the pathophysiology in order to elect proper therapeutic management. The hematologist may be of assistance to the critical care team in this regard.

References

1. Bell WR, Royall RM: Heparin-associated thrombocytopenia: a comparison of three heparin preparations. N Engl J Med 303:902–907, 1980.
2. Bick RL: Hemostasis defects associated with cardiac surgery, prosthetic devices, and other extracorporeal circuits. Sem Thromb Hem 11:249–279, 1985.
3. Bick RL: Alterations of hemostasis associated with cardiopulmonary bypass: pathophysiology, prevention, diagnosis, and management. Sem Thromb Hemostasis 3:59–82, 1979.
4. Bick RL: Clinical relevance of antithrombin III. Sem Thromb Hem 8:276–284, 1982.
5. Branch DW, Scott JR, Kochenour N, et al: Obstetric complications associated with the lupus anticoagulant. N Engl J Med 313:1322–1326, 1985.
6. Brown C, Natelson E, Bradshaw M, et al: The hemostatic defect produced by carbenicillin. N Engl J Med 291:265–270, 1976.
7. Buchanan MR, Boneu B, Ofosu F, et al: The relative importance of thrombin inhibition and factor X_A inhibition to the antithrombotic effects of heparin. Blood 65:198–201, 1985.
8. Burns T, Saleem A: Idiopathic thrombocytopenic purpura. Am J Med 75:1001–1007, 1983.
9. Cains J, Gent M, Singer J, et al: Aspirin, sulfinpyrazone or both, unstable angina. N Engl J Med 313:1369–1375, 1985.

10. Castellino FJ: Biochemistry of human plasminogen. *Sem Thromb Hem* 10:18–23, 1984.

11. Cimo PL, Moake J, Weinger R: Heparin-induced thrombocytopenia. *Amer J Heme* 6:1298–1304, 1979.

12. Clouse LH, Comp PC: The regulation of hemostasis. The Protein C System. 314:1298–1304, 1986.

13. Cohen A, Philips T, Kessler C: Circulating coagulation inhibitors in the acquired immunodeficiency syndrome. *Ann Int Med* 104:175–180, 1986.

14. Cordonnier C, Vernant JP, Brun B, et al: Acute promyelocytic leukemia in 57 previously untreated patients. *Cancer* 55:18–25, 1985.

15. Daly P, Schriffer C, Wiernik P: Acute promyelocytic leukemia—clinical management of 15 patients. *Am J Heme* 347–359, 1980.

16. Day HJ, Rao A: Evaluation of platelet function. *Sem Hem* 23:89–101, 1986.

17. Duckert F: Thrombolytic therapy. *Sem Thromb Hem* 10:87–102, 1984.

18. Eichner E: Platelets, carotids and coronaries. *Am J Med* 77:513–523, 1984.

19. Errichetti A, Holden A, Ansell J: Management of oral anticoagulant therapy. *Arch Int Med* 144:1966–1968, 1984.

20. Fareed J: Heparin, its fractions, fragments and derivatives. *Sem Thromb Hem* 11:1–8, 1985.

21. Feinstein D: Diagnosis and management of disseminated intravascular coagulation: the role of heparin therapy. *Blood* 60:284–287, 1982.

22. Fekete L, Bick R: Laboratory modalities for assessing hemostasis during cardiopulmonary bypass. *Sem Thromb Hem* 3:83–89, 1976.

23. Fuster V, Chesebro J: Antithrombotic therapy: role of platelet-inhibitor drugs. *Mayo Clin Proc* 56:102–112, 1981.

24. Gardner F, Bessman J: Thrombocytopenia due to defective platelet production. *Cli Hem* 12:23–38, 1983.

25. Gore J, Appelbaum J, Greene H, et al: Occult cancer in patients with acute pulmonary embolism. *Ann Int Med* 96:556–560, 1982.

26. Griffin JH: Clinical studies of protein C. *Sem Thromb Hem* 10:162–167, 1984.

27. Halkin H, Goldberg J, Modan M, et al: Reduction of mortality in general medical in-patients by low dose heparin. *Ann Int Med* 96:561–565, 1982.

28. Hardisty R: Hereditary disorders of platelet function. 12:153–173, 1983.

29. Harlan J: Thrombocytopenia due to non-immune platelet destruction. 12:39–68, 1983.

30. Hattersby P, Mitsuoka C, King J: Sources of error in heparin therapy of thromboembolic disease. *Arch Int Med* 140:1173–1175, 1980.

31. Hattersby P, Mitsuoka C, King J: Heparin therapy for thromboembolic disorders. 11:1413–1416, 1983.

32. Hayes A, Baker WH: heparin prophylaxis trials of venous thrombosis. A critical review. *Sem Thromb Hem* 11:222–226, 1985.

33. Herbst K, Rapaport S, Kenoyer D, et al: Syndrome of an acquired inhibitor of factor VIII responsive to cyclophosphamide and prednisone. 95:575–578, 1981.

34. Hirsch J, Ofosu F, Buchanan M: Rationale behind the development of low molecular weight heparin derivatives. *Sem Thromb Hem* 11:13–16, 1985.

35. Hirsch J: Mechanism of action and monitoring of anticoagulants. *Sem Thromb Hem* 12:1–11, 1986.

36. Hirsch J: Effectiveness of anticoagulants. *Sem Thromb Hem* 12:21–37, 1986.

37. Hirsch J: Hypercoagulability. *Sem Thromb Hem* 14:409–422, 1977.

38. Huisman M, Buller M, Ten Cate J: Serial impedance plethysmography for suspected deep venous thrombosis in outpatients. *N Engl J Med* 314:823–828, 1986.

39. Hull R, Hirsch J, Sackett D, et al: Replacement of venography in suspected venous thrombosis by impedance plethysmography and ^{125}I fibrinogen leg scanning. *Ann Int Med* 94:12–15, 1981.

40. Hull R, Hirsch J, Carter C, et al: Pulmonary angiography, ventilation lung scanning, and venography for clinically suspected pulmonary embolism with abnormal perfusion lung scan. *Ann Int Med* 98:891–899, 1983.

41. Imbach P: A multicenter european trial of intravenous immune globulin in immune thrombocytopenic purpura in childhood. *Vox Sang.* 49(Suppl):25–31, 1985.

42. Janson P, Jubelner S, Weinstein M, et al: Treatment of the bleeding tendency in uremia with cryoprecipitate. *N Engl J Med* 303:1318–1322, 1980.

43. Kaufmann R, Veltkamp J, Van Tilburg N, et al: Acquired AT III deficiency and thrombosis in the nephrotic syndrome. *Am J Med* 65:607–613, 1978.

44. Kalton J, Levine M: Heparine-induced thrombocytopenia. *Am J Med* 12:59–61, 1986.

45. King D, Kelton J: Heparin-associated thrombocytopenia. *Ann Int Med* 100:535–540, 1984.

46. Kitchens C: Concept of hypercoagulability: a review of its development, clinical application and recent progress. *Sem Thromb Hem* 11:293–312, 1985.

47. Knapp H, Reilly I, Alessandrini P, et al: In vivo indexes of platelet and vascular function during fish-oil administration in patients with atherosclerosis. *N Engl J Med* 314:937–942, 1986.

48. Kwaan H: The role of fibrinolysis in disease processes. *Sem Thromb Hem* 10:71–79, 1984.

49. Lechner K, Niessener H, Thaler E: Coagulation abnormalities in liver disease. *Sem Thomb Hem* 4:40–52, 1977.

50. Lerner W, Caruso R, Faig D, et al: Drug-dependent and non drug-dependent antiplatelet antibody in drug-induced immunologic thrombocytopenic purpura. *Blood* 66:306–311, 1985.

51. Levine M: Risks and benefits of anticoagulant therapy. *Sem Thomb Hem* 12:67–71, 1986.

52. Levine M, Hirsch J: Hemorrhagic complications of anticoagulant therapy. *Sem Thromb Hem* 12:39–57, 1986.

53. Levine M: Nonhemorrhagic complications of anticoagulant therapy. *Sem Thromb Hem* 12:63–66, 1986.

54. Lind S: Prolonged bleeding time. *Am J Med* 77:305–312, 1984.

55. Livio M, Manmucci P, Vigano C, et al: Conjugated estrogens for the management of bleeding associated with renal failure. *N Engl J Med* 315:731–735, 1986.

56. Lucas O, Albert T: Episilon aminocaproic acid in hemophiliacs undergoing dental extractions. a concise review. *Oral Surg* 51:115–120, 1981.

57. Lynch D, Howe S: Heparin-associated thrombocytopenia antibody binding specificity to platelet antigens. *Blood* 66:1176–1181, 1985.

58. Mannucci P, Remuzzi G, Pusineri F, et al: DDAVP shortens the bleeding time in uremia. *N Engl J Med* 308:8–12, 1983.

59. Marcinak E, Wilson H, Marlar R: Neonate purpura fulminans: a genetic disorder related to the absence of protein C in blood. *Blood* 65:15–20, 1985.

60. Martin J, Morrison J, Files J: Autoimmune thrombocytopenic purpura: current concepts and recommended practices. *Am J Obstet Gynecol* 150:86–97, 1984.

61. McGehee W, Klotz T, Epstein D, et al: Coumarin necrosis associated with hereditary protein C deficiency. *Ann Int Med* 101:59–60, 1984.

62. McMillan R: Immune thrombocytopenia. *Clin Hem* 12:69–88, 1983.

63. Mielke C, Levine P, Zucker S: Preoperative prednisone therapy in platelet function disorders. *Thrombosis Res* 21:655–662, 1981.

64. Moncada S, Vane T: Arachidonic acid metabolites and

interactions between platelets and blood vessel walls. *N Engl J Med* 300:1142–1148, 1979.

65. Mueh T, Herbst K, Rapaport S: Thrombosis in patients with the lupus anticoagulant. *Ann Int Med* 156–159, 1980.
66. Mulberty S: Fibrinolysis: an overview. *Sem Thromb Hem* 10:1–5, 1984.
67. O'Neill W, Timmis G, Bourdillon P: A prospective randomized clinical trial of intracoronary streptokinase versus coronary angioplasty for acute myocardial infarction. *N Engl J Med* 314:812–818, 1986.
68. Packham M, Mustard J: The role of platelets in the development and complications of atherosclerosis. *Sem Hem* 23:8–26, 1986.
69. Pizzo S, Petruska D, Doman K, et al: Releasable vascular plasminogen activator and thrombotic strokes. *Am J Med* 79:407–411, 1985.
70. Poskitt T, Poskitt P: Thrombocytopenia of sepsis. *Arch Int Med* 145:891–894, 1985.
71. Preston F, Whipps S, Jackson C, et al: Inhibition of prostacyclin and thromboxane A_2 after low-dose aspirin. *N Engl J Med* 304:76–79, 1981.
72. Prydz H: Vitamin K-dependent clotting factors. *Sem Thromb Hem* 4:1–10, 1977.
73. Ramirez-Lassepas M: Antifibrinolytic therapy in subarachnoid hemorrhage caused by ruptured intracranial aneurysm. *Neurology* 31:316–322, 1981.
74. Ramwell P: Biologic importance of arachadonic acid. *Arch Int Med* 141:275–278, 1981.
75. Rao A, Holmsen H: Congenital disorders of platelet function. *Sem Hem* 23:102–118, 1986.
76. Rao A, Walsh P: Acquired qualitative platelet disorders. *Clin Hem* 12:201–238, 1983.
77. Robertson RM, Robertson D, Roberts J, et al: Thromboxane A_2 in vasotonic angina pectoris. *N Engl J Med* 304:998–1003, 1981.
78. Rooke T: Heparin and the in-hospital management of deep venous thrombosis: cost considerations. *Mayo Clinic Proc* 61:198–204, 1986.
79. Roper-Drewinko P, Drewinko B, Corrigan G: Standardization of platelet function tests. *Am J Hem* 11:183–203, 1981.
80. Rosenow E, Osmandsan P, Brown M: Pulmonary embolism. *Mayo Clinic Proc* 56:161–178, 1981.
81. Sasahara A, Sharma V, Trow D: Clinical use of thrombolytic agents in venous thromboembolism. *Arch Int Med* 142:684–688, 1982.
82. Sawaya R, Sonnino V, McLaurin R, et al: Monitoring of antifibrinolytic therapy following subarachnoid hemorrhage. *J Neurosurg* 58:699–707, 1983.
83. Schafer A: The hypercoagulable states. *Ann Int Med* 102:814–828, 1985.
84. Schroder R, Neuhaus K, Leizorovicz A, et al: A prospective trial of intravenous streptokinase in acute myocardial infarction. *N Engl J Med* 314:1465–1471, 1986.
85. Seegers WH: Basic principles of blood coagulation. *Sem Thromb Hem* 7:180–198, 1981.
86. Shapiro ME, Rodvien R, Bauer K, et al: Acute aortic

thrombosis in antithrombin III deficiency. *JAMA* 245:1759–1761, 1981.
87. Shattil S, Bennett J: Platelets and their membranes in hemostasis: physiology and pathophysiology. *Ann Int Med* 94:108–118, 1980.
88. Sheridan D, Carter C, Kelton J: A diagnostic test for heparin induced thrombocytopenia. *Blood* 67:27–30, 1986.
89. Sherman C, Litrack F, Grundfest W, et al: Coronary angioscopy in patients with unstable angina Pectoris. *N Engl J Med* 315:913–919, 1986.
90. Straub PW: Diffuse intravascular coagulation in liver disease? *Sem Thromb Hem* 4:29–39, 1977.
91. Stricker R, Abrams D, Corash L, et al: Target platelet antigen in homosexual men with immune thrombocytopenia. *N Engl J Med* 313:1375–1380, 1985.
92. Telford A, Wilson C: Trial of heparin versus atenolol in prevention of myocardial infarction in intermediate coronary syndrome. *Lancet* 1225–1226, 1981.
93. Tollefson D, Peska C: Heparin cofactor II activity in patients with disseminated intravascular coagulation and hepatic failure. *Blood* 66:769–774, 1985.
94. Turpir A, Levine M, Hirsch J: A randomized trial of a low molecular weight heparin (enoxaprin) to prevent deep vein thrombosis in patients undergoing elective hip surgery. *N Engl J Med* 315:925–929, 1986.
95. Uchino H, Yasunaga K, Akatsuka: A cooperative clinical trial of high dose immunoglobulin therapy in 177 cases of idiopathic thrombocytopenic purpura. *Thromb Haemostas* 51:182–185, 1984.
96. VonDem Borne AK, Pegels J, VanDer Stadt R: Thrombocytopenia associated with bold therapy: a drug-induced autoimmune disease? *Br J Hem* 63:509–516, 1986.
97. Vermylin J, Badenhorst P, Deckmyn H, et al: Normal mechanisms of platelet functions. *Clin Hem* 12:107–151, 1983.
98. Vikydal R, Korringer C, Kyrle PA, Et al: The prevalence of hereditary antithrombin III deficiency in patients with a history of venous thromboembolism. *Thromb Haemostas* 1985.
99. Wall R, Harker L: The endothelium and thrombosis. *Ann Rev Med* 31:361–371, 1980.
100. Walsh C, Krigel R, Lennette E, et al: Thrombocytopenia in homosexual patients. *Ann Int Med* 103:542–545, 1985.
101. Wautier J, Caen JP: Pharmacology of platelet suppressive agents. *Sem Thromb Hem* 5:293–315, 1979.
102. Weiss HJ: Platelet physiology and abnormalities of platelet function. *N Engl J Med* 293:531–588, 1975.
103. Weiss HJ: Antiplatelet therapy. *N Engl J Med* 298:1344–1407, 1978.
104. White III G, McMillan C, Blatt P, et al: Factor VIII inhibitors: a clinical overview. *Am J Hem* 13:335–342, 1982.
105. Zauber N, Stark MW: Successful warfarin anti-coagulation despite protein C deficiency and a history of warfarin necrosis. *Ann Int Med* 104:659–660, 1986.

29

Antineoplastics

Antonella Surbone, M.D.
Charles Myers, M.D.

Cancer is the second leading cause of death in the United States, and 1 of 4 Americans will be diagnosed as having cancer. Even though a trend toward a slight decrease in incidence and in mortality has been recently reported by the National Cancer Institute in November 1986, it still remains one of the most common problems that health workers have to face in their daily practice.

As our understanding and our therapeutic efforts and results improve, a larger group of patients can be treated on an outpatient basis. However, during the course of their disease and therapy and in the terminal phase, cancer patients often require "critical care".

As the present book is dedicated to the clinical pharmacology in the critically ill patient, we will only briefly describe the generalities about antineoplastic agents. Our effort will be to describe (a) how cancer chemotherapy can lead to critical and/or emergency situations and how to deal with them, and, (b) how the critical care patient has to be managed, when a specific antitumor therapy (in this case chemotherapy) is required.

Cancer patients, no matter how critical and often hopeless their situation is, do not differ from other medical or surgical patients. Once a decision has been made with the patient concerning how far to go with the therapies, there is no room for any fear or hesitation and all the general principles stated elsewhere in this text have to be applied. It is, however, true that the care of a cancer patient is particularly delicate and demands special attention and effort. In fact, we are dealing with a very debilitating spectrum of diseases (impaired nutrition and immunity), often silently involving vital organs and affecting a large number of persons in advanced age who already have preexisting medical problems. Moreover, because cancer can sometimes be cured by aggressive therapy, cancer treatment modalities are often pushed to severe, even life-threatening levels.

CHEMICAL PROPERTIES

We will only briefly describe the properties of cancer drugs and will focus on their side effects, while we refer the readers to the classical textbooks for more extensive information. Antineoplastic drugs can be classified as:

Alkylating agents;
Antimetabolites;
Antitumor antibiotics;
Plant alkaloids;
Miscellaneous agents.

In addition hormones, antiretrovirus agents, and biological response modifiers can be considered part of the antitumor agents, but these are not covered here.

Alkylating Agents

Alkylation is a reaction involving the substitution of an alkyl group for an H atom on biologically important macromolecules. All useful drugs in this category are bifunctional and thus cross link DNA. These lesions are also responsible for their most worrisome toxicity, carcinogenicity. They are erratically absorbed by the gastrointestinal tract and cyclophosphamide requires hepatic activation.

NITROGEN MUSTARD
(MECHLORETHAMINE)

Nitrogen mustard (HN_2) was the first nonhormonal drug to show significant antitumor activity in humans. Its main use is as a component of the MOPP combination for Hodgkin's disease (which gives a >90% response rate in the early stages). The clinical pharmacology of nitrogen mustard is unclear due to its rapid hydrolysis in plasma. It is usually given intravenously, although it has been administered by the intracavitary and topical routes (e.g., treatment of mycosis fungoides).

Toxicity includes nausea and vomiting, myelosuppression, and tissue irritation. The nadir of myelosuppression occurs at 7–14 days with recovery by 28 days. The drug may produce phlebitis, venous thrombosis, and tissue necrosis if extravasation occurs during an intravenous injection and it is extremely irritating for the skin.

MELPHALAN

Melphalan is generally used in ovarian cancer and multiple myeloma, in which case it is given orally, even though it has a variable bioavailability. The predominant toxicities consist of nausea, vomiting, and myelosuppression. Leukopenia and thrombocytopenia occur 14–21 days after intermittent doses although the myelosuppression can be delayed and cumulative, extending its nadir periods to 4–6 weeks. There are ongoing trials that are using this drug intravenously and at high dose, as an induction treatment for bone marrow transplantation in solid tumors. This regimen needs careful hydration and antiemetic therapy.

CHLORAMBUCIL

Chlorambucil is another mechlorethamine derivative structurally similar to melphalan. This drug has a relatively limited spectrum of clinical use (e.g., chronic lymphocytic leukemia, myeloma, macroglobulinemia, and carcinoma of the ovary). As with some of the other alkylating agents, drug-induced interstitial pneumonitis may rarely occur with long-term use (19).

BUSULFAN

Busulfan is an alkylating agent, unrelated to the mechlorethamine derivatives, that is used primarily for the treatment of chronic granulocytic leukemia. It is administered orally and is extensively metabolized to inactive compounds prior to renal excretion. Due to the lack of a sensitive assay, the pharmacokinetics of this drug are still poorly understood.

The most important busulfan-induced toxicities consist of myelosuppression and lung damage (interstitial pneumonitis). Myelo-suppression is usually predictable but may be long-lasting and even permanent after very high doses or long-term therapy (65). Granulocyte nadir occurs at 11–30 days with recovery occurring over 24–54 days. Busulfan-induced pneumonitis is relatively uncommon (4–12%) but more frequent in patients who are receiving cumulative doses of greater than 500 mg (see "Management of Side Effects) (16). Busulfan can also induce diffuse hyperpigmentation.

CYCLOPHOSPHAMIDE

Cyclophosphamide (CTX) is a cyclic phosphamide ester of mechlorethamine that is metabolized by the liver to active alkylating compounds. It is the most commonly used alkylating agent and has a wide spectrum of activity (e.g., acute leukemia, lymphoma, myeloma, breast, lung and ovarian cancer, sarcomas). Oral and intravenous routes are both commonly used. High-dose intravenous therapy is used in the most common preparation regimens for bone marrow transplant. Although the metabolism of CTX has been well studied, its pharmacokinetics are not entirely clear (6, 21, 33). CTX undergoes a series of complex metabolic transformations that yield products, such as phosphoramide mustard, that are cytotoxic, and acrolein, which is irritating to the bladder and may be responsible for the cystitis. These metabolites, normally excreted by the kidneys, accumulate in renal insufficiency and are thought to be responsible for an increased incidence in systemic toxicity.

CTX commonly causes nausea, vomiting, and alopecia. Myelosuppression, consisting primarily of leukopenia and occasionally thrombocytopenia, represents the dose-limiting toxicity. The nadir occurs at 7–14 days with recovery usually by 21 days. Sterile hemorrhagic cystitis, while infrequent, may also become a dose-limiting factor.

The onset of symptoms and signs of hemorrhagic cystitis usually occurs in close proximity to drug administration but may occasionally become apparent several months after CTX has been discontinued. Bleeding may persist for months but is rarely life threatening. Obviously, infectious cystitis has to be excluded. Adequate hydration (2000–3000 ml/day) before and during therapy is mandatory and represents the best prophylaxis. Patients receiving very high doses (e.g., 50 mg/kg) may require bladder irrigation during and following the period of drug administration.

Acute CTX-related cystitis is an indication to stop the drug until the cystitis had cleared. It can then generally be restarted at 50% of the original dose and then increased to 75%, if no cystitis recurs. However, occasionally it may be necessary to switch to another alkylating agent. Once hemorrhagic cystitis is detected, continuous irrigation of the bladder to prevent intravesicular clot formation and blood transfusions to replace blood loss are often necessary. More severe cases do not respond to these conservative measures and require critical care, with possible bladder fulguration (61), intravesical formalin instillation (73), intravenous vasopressin (60), or even urinary diversion (36), and rarely cystectomy. Investigational approaches include the use of such agents as N-acetylcysteine (51), 2-mercaptoethane sulfonate (15), and possibly disulfiram (38) to prevent the development of cystitis and thus increase the therapeutic index of cyclophosphamide and isophosphamide. There is one report of busulfan-induced hemorrhagic cystitis (49) and another of Adriamycin enhancing previous cyclophosphamide-induced bladder injury (30).

Both cyclophosphamide and isophosphamide can produce a syndrome of inappropriate antidiuretic hormone secretion (SIADH). The site of action of high-dose cyclophosphamide is thought to be renal (37). The diagnosis of SIADH is made when other causes of dilutional hyponatremia are excluded and when use of diuretic therapy is not implicated. The combination of hyponatremia and low plasma osmolality with urinary osmolality higher than plasma and continuous excretion of sodium should alert the clinician to the possibility of this diagnosis. Clinically, patients with dilutional hyponatremia may be asymptomatic or else manifest typical symptoms of water intoxication ranging from lethargy and stupor to functional psychosis and coma. When unrecognized and untreated, SIADH may result in death (39). In the case of symptomatic cases of SIADH due to drug treatment, it is probably wise to suspend chemotherapy until simple fluid restriction (500 ml/24 hours) results in resolution of the symptoms and normalization of plasma electrolytes. Severely affected patients may require more aggressive intervention with the administration of hypertonic saline and diuretics intravenously. Careful monitoring of plasma and urine osmolalities and of body weight is necessary to avert further iatrogenic complications. Vincristine, through an unclear mechanism of action, can also give rise to an SIADH syndrome. Mild dilutional hyponatremic patients who are asymptomatic should be carefully monitored for signs of deterioration, but a case can be made for continuation of chemotherapy even if vincristine or cyclophosphamide are components of the regimen (50). The most important point in the management of such cancer patients is to consider the possibility that these drugs may be cause of reversible CNS disturbances and not assume a priori that all neurological symptoms are always due to the primary disease process.

At high doses, CTX can also cause cardiac toxicity and rare instances of interstitial pneumonia have also been reported, following long-term, low-dose CTX therapy. The cardiac toxicity can present as a hemorrhagic myocarditis, pericarditis and/or congestive heart failure.

NITROSOUREAS

The commonly used nitrosoureas consist of carmustine (BCNU), lomustine (CCNU), semustine (methyl-CCNU), and streptozotocin. They are fairly lipid soluble, chemically reactive compounds that show activity against the lymphomas, gliomas, melanoma, and gastrointestinal cancers. BCNU at high doses is now used in some of the induction regimens for bone marrow transplant. They have variable degrees of alkylating and carbamylating activity. Streptozotocin differs from other nitrosoureas in that it has a sugar moiety, which is probably responsible for an enhanced uptake by the β cells of the pancreas. In addition to its direct cytotoxic effect, streptozotocin decreases the concentration of nicotinamide adenine dinucleotide (NAD) in the islet cells of the pancreas. The clinical pharmacology of these agents is not well understood, but each is characterized by a rapid disappearance from plasma that probably reflects their extreme chemical reactivity. Despite the fact that a number of longer-lived metabolites are formed, even less is known about these compounds.

BCNU, CCNU, and methyl-CCNU share similar toxicities: They can all produce nausea and vomiting and delayed bone marrow suppression. The leukocyte and platelet count nadirs occur at about 3–5 weeks and usually recover in 6–8 weeks. This myelosuppression may be cumulative after repeated treatment courses. Interstitial pneumonitis and pulmonary fibrosis can occasionally occur after BCNU and rarely after CCNU, methyl-CCNU, and streptozotocin treatments (6, 34). Pulmonary toxicity usually occurs after repeated courses of therapy and is particularly frequent in BCNU-treated patients when cumulative doses of greater than 100–1400 mg/m² are reached. Renal toxicity is also cumulative, occurring after larger doses of methyl-CCNU and less frequently after CCNU or BCNU treatments (59, 71). A cumulative dose of more than 1500 mg/m² should be avoided and therapy should be discontinued when these complications arise.

Streptozotocin has a somewhat different pattern of toxicity than the other nitrosoureas in that it can produce severe dose-limiting nausea and vomiting but is much less myelosuppressive. Renal toxicity of streptozotocin is the most frequent dose-limiting toxicity and may lead to azotemia, Fanconi's syndrome and permanent tubular damage and fibrosis. Patients treated with streptozotocin are to be monitored for proteinuria or a decline in creatinine clearance, and drug treatment must be temporarily discontinued should these features occur. Liver dysfunction can occur but is usually mild and reversible. Although streptozotocin is effective against islet cell carcinomas of the pancreas and produces diabetes in animals, it is not diabetogenic in humans, and only reversible abnormalities of the glucose tolerance have been noted in some patients.

CIS-PLATINUM

Cis (II)-platinum diaminedichloride (cis-DDP) is the first inorganic compound to show important antineoplastic activity. The cytotoxicity of cis-DDP may be related to the formation of interstrand and intrastrand DNA crosslinks and DNA protein complexes.

It is effective in the treatment of testicular tumors, ovarian cancer, squamous cell carcinoma of the head and neck, osteogenic sarcoma, and bladder cancer and has recently shown activity against lymphomas as well.

Plasma disappearance of platinum species after an intravenous bolus is biphasic, with an initial half-life of 25–79 minutes and a terminal half-life of 58–73 hours (26). This long terminal half-life is probably the result of metal binding to plasma proteins (protein binding 90%), since the terminal half-life of free (unbound or filterable) platinum is fairly short (half-life of 23–54 minutes) (57). The kidney is responsible for most of the excretion of cis-DDP and its chemical products. However, most of the active drug is not cleared by the kidney, but rather, by binding to plasma proteins and tissue constituents. Cis-DDP can also be administered intraperitoneally, and concentra-tions 20 to 30-fold higher than the plasma concentration can be achieved by this route (17, 42).

Similar toxicities have been observed for the intravenous and the intraperitoneal route. Nausea and vomiting are extremely intense and prolonged. Aggressive antiemetic therapy must be started before the first dose and continued on a regular basis, until therapy is completed. Myelotoxicity peaks at the third week, but generally does not represent a limiting factor, except for heavily pretreated patients. Cis-DDP can produce rare anaphylactic reactions and liver enzyme elevations. However, there are three main toxic effects that can be severe and require careful management and knowledge:

1. *Ototoxicity.* Even if eighth nerve damage is not acute and therefore does not lead to dose reduction, the common occurrence of this side effect (clinically manifested by a symmetrical, bilateral, high frequency hearing loss, sometimes accompanied by tinnitus) must be remembered and patients need frequent audiology follow-up. The need for hearing aids is common after prolonged high-dose therapy, in patients older than 45 and whenever there is a preexisting hearing problem.

2. *Peripheral neuropathy.* With high-dose cis-DDP, it is not rare to see patients who acutely develop a peripheral neuropathy and have to stop therapy because of it (45). Neuropathy usually presents with distal sensory loss; with paresthesias of the hands and feet; and with severe diminution of vibration, position, pin-prick, and light touch sensation (corresponding to abnormal nerve conduction and segmental demyelinization).

3. *Nephrotoxicity.* Renal toxicity is multifactorial in origin and has both a tubular and vascular component (48, 76). Toxicity can be averted by maintaining a high urine output, through sustained hydration and induced diuresis. Moreover, renal toxicity appears to be greatly reduced if the cis-DDP itself is administered in hypertonic saline (55). We have used hydration, starting 12 hours before the administration of cis-DDP, consisting of 250 ml/hour of NS with 20 mEq of K^+ per liter, and ending 24 hours after the last dose of drug. The cis-DDP is mixed in 250 ml of 3% saline and infused over 30 minutes. Furosemide (Lasix), 20 mg intravenously is administered to all patients prior to administering Cis-DDP, and then as needed. Because of the severe hypomagnesemia, related to tubular damage, that many patients experience (with consequent

neurological abnormalities and frequently accompanied by Ca^{++} disturbances, including tetany), in some centers Mg^{++} (7 mEq/liter) is added prophylactically. In any case, Mg^{++} must always be monitored and oral or intravenous replacement promptly given.

Attention should be paid to the selection of other drugs which may also be nephrotoxic, since patients receiving drug combinations may be at greater risk for developing acute renal failure (35). As most of the active drug is cleared via binding rather than renal clearance, plasma pharmacokinetics is minimally altered by renal failure and modification of drug dosage is thus not required to avoid systemic toxicity. However, modification of drug dosage might be indicated in the face of renal failure to prevent additional kidney damage or impaired recovery.

Last, cis-DDP is unstable and solutions must be fresh. It also reacts with aluminum and therefore steel needles need to be used.

PLATINUM ANALOGUES

As cis-DDP is the most active single agent in the treatment of ovarian cancer and has shown remarkable activity in other solid tumors, many efforts have been made in order to develop less toxic agents. Cyclobutane dicarboxylate platinum (CBDCA) (25, 63) is a new cisplatin analog that appears to have activity similar to cis-DDP but does not require hydration, since it is not nephrotoxic. CBDCA also does not have neurotoxic or emetic effects. However, it is dose-limited by myelotoxicity, which manifests as profound and prolonged thrombocytopenia, often requiring transfusion therapy.

Antimetabolites

ANTIFOLATES

Tetrahydrofolates, reduced forms of folic acid, are required for the synthesis of purines and pyrimidines and hence are useful targets for antimetabolite drugs. Antifolates inhibit the formation of tetrahydrofolate from dihydrofolates and thus interfere with DNA synthesis. Although several antifolates have been studied, methotrexate (MTX), which inhibits dihydrofolate reductase (DHFR), is by far the most commonly used drug in this class. MTX is used in the treatment of acute leukemia, lymphoma, breast cancer, lung cancer, sarcoma, choriocarcinoma, and squamous cell carcinoma of the head and neck. The drug penetrates the cell membrane via a carrier-mediated, energy-dependent transport system and then binds stoichiometrically to its target enzyme, DHFR. An excess concentration of free drug is required for its activity. MTX blocks thymidylate synthesis at a concentration of $1 \times 10^{-8}M$ and inhibits the synthesis of purines at free drug concentrations higher than $1 \times 10^{-7}M$ (4).

Inside the cell, MTX is conjugated with glutamic acid. The polyglutamates formed represent the retained form of MTX, probably responsible for both delayed effects and toxicity. Several mechanisms of resistance account for the lack of activity of MTX in drug resistant cells: altered transport, altered target protein (DHFR), gene amplification, altered polyglutamation, salvage pathways. Of these, the altered transport across the membrane and increased DHFR can be overcome by increasing the MTX concentration. Leucovorin, 5-formyl-tetrahydrofolic acid, is a reduced folate that is able to reverse the cytotoxicity of MTX. Several mechanisms appear to be involved in this rescue. Leucovorin supplies reduced folate, the production of which is blocked by MTX. Membrane transport of MTX and folates is by a bidirectional process carrier that exhibits counter transport. Thus, as leucovorin enters the cell treated with MTX, MTX must be countertransported out of the cell. In addition, leucovorin and its metabolites have complex effects on cellular biochemistry, so as to lessen the need for reduced folates. The net effect is that leucovorin rescues both bone marrow and gastrointestinal mucosa from MTX toxicity. Leucovorin appears to be less effective in rescuing certain tumors. Since leucovorin and MTX share a common transport system across the cell membrane, to prevent toxicity the dose of leucovorin must be increased as the MTX concentration increases. Leucovorin rescue is difficult above a MTX concentration of $1 \times 10^{-5}M$.

The product of drug concentration and duration of exposure $(C \times T)$ are critical determinants of the cytotoxicity produced by MTX. Since MTX is a cell cycle–specific drug, prolongation of exposure at a given drug concentration increases the likelihood of cell kill since more cells will enter the critical "S" phase with time (58).

Methotrexate has a distribution volume that equals the total body water (TBW) and is found in all body fluids, including the CSF (explaining the attempts for intravenous use in meningeal carcinomatosis) and third-space fluid accumulations. MTX is loosely bound to proteins (albumin) and is excreted by the kidneys. MTX clearance equals the creatinine clearance. The initial phase of drug disappearance from plasma has a half-life of 2–3 hours, whereas the terminal phase plasma half-life is 8–10 hours (72, 81).

During the first 12 hours, 40–100% of administered MTX is excreted and the initial half-life is dependent on renal function. High urinary concentrations of MTX during the first 12 hours following administration can lead to precipitation of MTX in the form of 7-OH-MTX and consequent renal damage.

The second phase of MTX elimination starts at a MTX plasma concentration which is above the threshold for bone marrow and gastrointestinal toxicity. Elimination can be affected by acute renal damage during the initial phase or by the presence of third-space fluid accumulations. Thus, MTX administration, especially at high dose, must be closely monitored in every patient, even in the absence of preexisting renal function abnormalities.

Patients with normal renal function should be adequately hydrated to ensure prompt renal elimination. Patients receiving moderate and high dose MTX infusions (> 500–1000 mg/m^2) should receive at least 3000 ml of fluid per day and have their urine alkalinized (urine pH$>$7) with oral or intravenous sodium bicarbonate (e.g., 50–100 mEq sodium bicarbonate per liter of intravenous fluid). This approach will lessen the incidence of renal toxicity by preventing the precipitation of MTX and 7-OH-MTX in the renal tubules, and thus averts delayed drug elimination (43).

Patients receiving high doses of MTX, as well as those with abnormal renal function or third-space fluid accumulation, should have their plasma MTX levels monitored 48 hours after the dose is given and should receive intravenous leucovorin.

If plasma MTX levels are greater than 5×10^{-7}M at 48 hours after administration, drug elimination is likely to be slower than usual and the risk of drug toxicity increases. In this situation, the administration of folinic acid (leucovorin) to circumvent the MTX-induced metabolic block is needed until nontoxic MTX levels are attained ($<5 \times 10^{-8}$M). For plasma MTX levels at 48 hours of between 5×10^{-7} and 1×10^{-6}M, leucovorin 15 mg/m^2 every 6 hours for 8 doses should be given. If MTX levels are higher than 2×10^{-6}M, leucovorin 200 mg/m^2 every 6 hours for eight doses

should be given. Determination of plasma MTX levels should then be repeated every 24 hours and the folinic acid (leucovorin) rescue continued at the appropriate dose until the MTX level is below 5×10^{-8}M. If these approaches are not done, marked toxicity and sometimes death will result.

The major toxic effects of MTX are myelosuppression, mucositis, and renal dysfunction. Mucositis usually appears within 3–7 days and myelosuppression within 7–10 days of drug administration. These toxicities usually reverse after 14–21 days unless drug elimination is impaired. Although careful attention to hydration and alkalinization of urine during high dose MTX infusions usually prevents renal toxicity, it may still occur in patients with slow drug elimination (detected by plasma MTX monitoring). Renal toxicity is manifested by an abrupt rise in serum creatinine and BUN and a fall in urine output. Neither peritoneal dialysis nor hemodialysis are very useful in increasing MTX clearance (1, 41).

Other less common toxicities include hepatic dysfunction (usually subclinical), hepatic fibrosis and cirrhosis (usually after long-term oral therapy), interstitial pneumonitis (usually self-limited), and acute hypersensitivity. MTX-induced pneumonitis needs to be differentiated from neoplasm, infection, radiation pneumonitis or other nononcologic conditions.

Methotrexate may also produce neurologic damage, when given intrathecally for meningeal carcinomatosis, which can be acute (arachnoiditis), subacute (paraplegia), or chronic (delayed necrotized leukoencephalopathy).

In conclusion, when administering MTX consider the following:
1. Variations in renal function. MTX may cause renal damage which is manifested by a rise in BUN and a decrease in urine output. In practice, the urinary output should always be maintained$>$100 ml/hr and the urinary pH$>$7.0. Patients should be monitored for fluid overload.
2. Leucovorin must be given when the plasma MTX level is above 5×10^{-8}M.
3. Presence of third-space fluid collections that can cause prolonged elevations of plasma drug levels. This is a frequent cause of delayed toxicity and requires special monitoring of the MTX plasma level even after low-dose MTX. Evacuation of an effusion before and after therapy may be of value (vide infra).

4. Substances that compete with MTX for tubular secretion. Weak acids can decrease the tubular secretion of MTX; therefore, probenecid, penicillin and other antibiotics must be used carefully. Also salicylates and nonsteroidal antiinflammatory agents are associated with prolonged and enhanced MTX levels in the plasma (77).

Trimetrexate is a MTX analog that differs from the parent compound in that it is more lipophylic and crosses the cell membrane by passive diffusion, not requiring carrier-mediated transport. This drug is less nephrotoxic than MTX, and its administration does not require hydration. Trimetrexate is also a promising new antiparasitic agent, active against Pneumocystis carinii pneumonia and toxoplasmosis in immunocompromised patients allergic to sulfonamides (5, 27). It also requires leucovorin rescues so as to avoid severe bone marrow toxicity.

Fluoropyrimidines

The commonly used fluoropyrimidines include 5-fluorouracil (5-FU) and 5-fluorodeoxyuridine (FUdR). These drugs act primarily by inhibiting thymidylate synthase and by incorporation into RNA. They share similar qualitative toxicities and are used in the treatment of gastrointestinal and breast cancer, adenocarcinoma of the lung, and ovarian cancer. 5-FU if discussed as it is the most frequently used drug in this class.

5-Fluorouracil is extensively incorporated into the RNA and its metabolite, fluorodeoxyuridine monophosphate (FdUMP) inhibits thymidylate synthase, leading to a block in pyrimidine synthesis (4). Both actions are possible because the small size of the fluorine atom allows 5-FU to substitute for the natural uracil-metabolite.

5-Fluorouracil is administered by a variety of routes and schedules (i.e., oral, intravenous, intraarterial, intraperitoneal) (20, 52). Standard doses are 300–400 mg/m^2 administered intravenously every day for 5 days, repeated every 3–4 weeks, or 10–12 mg/kg intravenously administered weekly. The bioavailability of 5-FU after oral administration is erratic and hence it is generally given either as an intravenous bolus or infusion. When used in conventional doses, the plasma half-life is 10–20 minutes although when used at very high doses its elimination becomes nonlinear (K_m ~ 15μM) (20). Approximately 90% of a conventional dose of 5-FU is eliminated by metabolism (occuring primarily in the liver) with less than 5% of the unchanged parent compound appearing in urine. 5-FU doses should probably be adjusted in patients with hepatic dysfunction even if the bulk of 5-FU metabolism probably occurs via extrahepatic pathways. At present, there is still no clear understanding of the relationship between the clinical pharmacokinetics of 5-FU, the antitumor efficacy, and the toxicity. 5-FU concentrations may persist in malignant effusions but the influence of this accumulation on antitumor efficacy and toxicity is not clearly understood.

The major toxicities of 5-FU are gastrointestinal and hematologic. After a continuous intravenous infusion, mucositis and diarrhea may become dose limiting. Following an intravenous bolus, myelosuppression is dose limiting. The leukocyte and platelet nadirs usually occur within 7–14 days of administration and recover within 3 weeks. Other less common toxicities include acute neurologic damage (somnolence, ataxia) and a syndrome of chest pain, cardiac enzyme elevations in plasma and ECG changes consistent with myocardial ischemia.

5-Fluorouracil has now been tried in combination with high-dose intravenous leucovorin both in breast cancer and colon cancer. The rationale for this combination is that there is in vitro evidence that an excess folate concentration increases the tightness of the binding of the active metabolite of 5-FU to its target enzyme, thymidylate synthase. With this combination, a higher incidence of severe leukopenia and mucositis has been seen.

CYTOSINE ARABINOSIDE

Cytosine arabinoside (Ara-C) is an analogue of the nucleoside deoxycytidine and acts through inhibition of DNA polymerase (by its Ara-CTP metabolite) and incorporation into DNA, which is cell cycle dependent. It is phosphorylated by a kinase and deaminated by both human cytidine and deoxycytidine deaminase. An increase in the deaminases and a decrease in the kinase are major determinants of resistance to Ara-C.

While it has a limited spectrum of antitumor activity, Ara-C is a very useful antineoplastic drug with demonstrated efficacy in the treatment of acute nonlymphocytic leukemia and of refractory lymphomas (70, 71).

Ara-C is not effective when given orally because it is rapidly inactivated by deamination in gut and liver. When given intravenously, Ara-C is rapidly eliminated from plasma with an initial half-life of 7–20 minutes and a terminal disappearance phase of 0.5–2.6 hours (40); however, considerable interindividual variability has been reported. Since systemic clearance of Ara-C is rapid and its mode of action is phase specific, it is often given as a continuous intravenous infusion over 5–7 days to maintain a cytotoxic blood concentration for sufficient time to allow a reasonable proportion of the tumor population to enter the sensitive phase of the cell cycle. Within the usual dose range of 50–200 mg/m^2, its elimination is linear although with very high doses the elimination kinetics may become zero-order, resulting in delayed drug clearance (58). Higher doses have also been used. The toxicity of Ara-C in normal tissues is related to $(C \times T)$ product. For example, a bolus dose of Ara-C of 4.2 g/m^2 is well tolerated, whereas a dose of 1 g/m^2 given as a 48-hour infusion produces severe myelosuppression (32). Myelosuppression and gastrointestinal epithelial injury are the major toxic side effects produced by Ara-C. With the use of the conventional 5–7 day infusions for acute leukemia, myelosuppression begins during the first week of treatment and may last for 7–14 days. Gastrointestinal toxicity includes mucositis (particularly after prolonged infusion), nausea, vomiting, diarrhea, and reversible hepatic dysfunction. Transfusion-related hepatitis should be differentiated from the hepatitis produced by Ara-C. Hepatitis requires cessation of therapy in <20% of patients. Because of its good penetration through the blood-brain barrier (47), Ara-C is used to treat meningeal involvement. When used intravenously in high dose, it can cause severe CNS toxicity, mainly in the form of cerebellar damage. Therapy in this case should be stopped and supportive treatment promptly started. Ara-C is given intrathecally, at a standard dose of 70 mg (for an adult) q 4 days in buffered solution. Intrathecal Ara-C can occasionally produce headaches, meningismus, vomiting, parathesias, paraplegia, fever, and, rarely, generalized seizures (29, 66).

Ara-C can also cause skin toxicity (rash and folliculitis) and conjunctivitis. Both respond to topical steroids. Because of its use in refractory lymphomas and in acute leukemias and because of its use at high dose, Ara-C is frequently administered in an ICU and for this reason the critical care staff should be familiar with the drug.

PURINE ANALOGUES: 6-MERCAPTOPURINE AND 6-THIOGUANINE

The two most commonly used purine analogs are 6-mercaptopurine (6-MP) and 6-thioguanine (6-TG). Despite extensive clinical experience in the use of these drugs, there is still some controversy regarding the exact mechanism of their antineoplastic action. While both agents interfere with purine biosynthesis, only 6-TG is incorporated into DNA (46). Both drugs are most commonly used in the treatment of acute leukemia; phase II trials of 6-MP in refractory lymphomas are ongoing.

These drugs are usually given orally, although they can be given intravenously. Both show variable and incomplete absorption after oral administration. Standard doses are 100 mg of 6-MP, administered orally for 5 consecutive days every 3–4 weeks, and 100 mg of 6-TG, administered intravenously for 5 days every 3–4 weeks. It is recommended that an oral dose of 6-MP be reduced to 25% of the standard dose when given concurrently with allopurinol. This adjustment is not required after intravenous administration of 6-MP, since the major effect of allopurinol is to modulate the first-pass extraction of oral 6-MP trough the liver and the gastrointestinal mucosa (85). 6-TG can be used without dose modification in the presence of allopurinol. The plasma half-lives are short after intravenous administration for both drugs (20–60 minutes for 6-MP and 25–240 minutes for 6-TG). Each of these agents undergoes metabolic clearance via different metabolic pathways.

The toxicities of the two drugs are similar. Each agent can produce nausea, vomiting, and myelosuppression. The nadir for myelosuppression usually occurs after 7–14 days and recovery ensues within 21 days. Stomatitis and diarrhea can occur after high doses. Jaundice and hepatitis may occasionally be dose limiting, although these problems usually occur after chronic drug therapy or with continuous infusion. Other hepatotoxic drugs should be avoided while these purine analogs are being used. A very high incidence of hepatotoxicity has been reported with the use of a combination of doxorubicin (Adriamycin) and 6-MP, while the same dose of 6-MP administered alone is generally without such side effects. Dose reduction is necessary in cases of severe hepatotoxicity.

Antitumor Antibiotics

BLEOMYCIN

Bleomycin, a mixture of fungal peptides from *Streptomyces verticillus*, has demonstrated activity against testicular carcinoma, squamous cell carcinoma and in various lymphomas. Of particular interest is the lack of bone marrow toxicity with this agent, which enables it to be incorporated into multidrug regimens without exacerbating myelosuppression.

The cytotoxicity is thought to be related to bleomycin's ability to cause chain scission and fragmentation of DNA strands. This occurs via generation of highly reactive oxygen-free radicals from a Fe(II)-bleomycin complex (75). While cytotoxicity has been demonstrated throughout the cell cycle (78), there is some suggestion of enhanced cell kill during both G_1 and M phases (79).

Following intravenous bolus administration, the elimination of bleomycin from plasma shows a biphasic decline, with an initial half-life of 24 minutes and a terminal half-life of 2–4 hours (3, 24). The drug is widely distributed in tissues and particularly high concentrations are found in skin, kidney, and bladder. Clearance of the drug is principally via the kidneys and correlates with creatinine clearance. The terminal half-life of bleomycin is prolonged in renal failure (24). Bleomycin has also been administered by prolonged intravenous infusion because clinical experience has shown that this approach minimizes toxicity.

Regional injection of bleomycin into pleural and peritoneal spaces have achieved high drug concentrations locally along with a 10-fold lower plasma drug concentration (2). Similarly, urinary bladder instillation with bleomycin is effective local therapy for transitional cell carcinoma in patients with limited disease (12). The major adverse effects from bleomycin use are pulmonary and skin toxicities. Pulmonary toxicity can take a subacute or chronic course and appears to be dose related; it involves 3–5% of patients receiving total doses less than 450 mg of bleomycin, whereas 10% of patients receiving a higher dose develop pulmonary fibrosis.

Skin toxicity due to bleomycin may manifest as pruritus, erythema, hyperkeratosis, vesiculation, and frank ulceration. The hands are most frequently involved, but skin over other joints, pressure areas, and areas of previous irradiation are also commonly affected. Alopecia, nail changes, and pigmentation are minor changes that are commonly seen, but do not normally warrant cessation of bleomycin therapy. Other toxic manifestations include nausea, vomiting, hyperpyrexia, headache, and Raynaud's phenomenon.

ANTHRACYCLINES

Anthracyclines, a subgroup of the rhodomycin antibiotics produced by various streptomyces species, are characterized structurally by a tetracycline ring linked to a sugar moiety. This group of agents include some of the most active antitumor agents used in clinical oncology. Doxorubicin (Adriamycin) and daunorubicin have demonstrated activity against leukemias and a wide variety of solid tumors. DNA intercalation has been postulated as a possible mechanism of action, but it seems clear now that the major determinant of activity, toxicity, and resistance is the formation of free radicals.

Doxorubicin is converted to a semiquinone free radical in a reaction mediated by microsomal cytochrome P-450 reductase (67). In the presence of oxygen, the semiquinone radical reverts back to the parent compound and generates superoxide. In turn, superoxide may lead to the formation of hydrogen peroxide and hydroxyl radicals, all of which are capable of inflicting damage on cells. (Damage to cell membrane and/or to DNA could result in cell death.) This process can lead to lipid peroxidation, which has been correlated with dose-limiting cardiotoxicity in clinical studies. The demonstration that anthracycline-iron chelates are associated with increased oxygen radical-mediated membrane damage and with cell lysis in both in vitro (53) and in vivo (44) studies lends support to the importance of membrane binding of this group of compounds for their tumoricidal effects.

Following intravenous bolus administration, the plasma doxorubicin concentration declines in a triexponential fashion, with half-lives ranging from 8–24 minutes, 1.5–10 hours, to 24–48 hours (10, 18). The drug is metabolized by aldo-keto reductase to doxorubicinol and by cytochrome P-450 reductase to the aglycone.

Cardiomyopathy, which is related to the total cumulative dose, is the dose-limiting toxicity for Adriamycin (see "Management of Side Effects"): a dose of 550 mg/m^2 should not be exceeded, and, even below that dose, every patient should be carefully monitored for cardiac toxicity.

Nausea and vomiting are prominent. The drug is a vesicant and must be given by the intravenous route. Myelosuppression and hepatic toxicity often occur and can be dose limiting. Adriamycin has a radiation recall effect, consisting of skin toxicity that occurs when the drug is administered after radiation therapy. Enhancement of the local skin toxicity during radiation therapy also occurs and Adryamicin should therefore be avoided when radiation is being given.

ADRIAMYCIN ANALOGUES

Because of the high antitumor activity of Adriamycin, its analogues are being evaluated for similar antitumor efficacy. Studies are ongoing to assess the efficacy and toxicity of aclacinomycin A, 4′ epiadriamycin, and several others compounds. It seems that 4-deoxy-adriamycin lacks emesis and alopecia, but the most promising analog appears to be 4-epirub-icine, because of lesser cardiotoxicity.

MITOMYCIN C

Mitomycin C is a product of *Streptomyces caespitosus*. It has a broad spectrum of antitumor activity. It alkylates and cross-links DNA and induces microsomal lipid peroxidation. Mitomycin C can be used as a single agent at a dose of 10–20 mg/m^2 for 6–8 weeks, in solid tumors refractory to other therapies (breast cancer and sarcomas) and is part of combination chemotherapy regimens for gastrointestinal malignancies and lung cancer. Following intravenous bolus, mitomycin C is rapidly distributed and has an initial plasma half-life of 30–45 minutes (65).

It causes severe myelotoxicity with delayed pancytopenia and can lead to irreversible marrow aplasia. It also has lung and kidney toxicity and can increase Adriamycin cardiotoxicity. It induces severe nausea, vomiting and stomatitis and is a vesicant.

ACTINOMYCIN D

Actinomycin D is an antibiotic synthesized by streptomyces species that has demonstrated antitumor activity in Wilms' tumor, Ewing's sarcoma, choriocarcinoma, neuroblastoma, rhabdomyosarcoma, and in both Hodgkin's and non-Hodgkin's lymphomas.

While the antitumor mode of action is not clearly understood, it is thought to be related to the ability of actinomycin D to intercalate into DNA. At low doses, actinomycin D inhibits DNA-directed RNA synthesis, whereas at higher drug concentrations it inhibits both DNA and protein synthesis (64).

Following an intravenous bolus administration, actinomycin D is rapidly distributed and has an initial half-life of approximately 5 minutes; however, the terminal plasma half-life in humans is 36 hours.

Actinomycin D (50 µg/kg) is generally administered in an intermittent schedule every 3 weeks (9). The dose-limiting toxicity of actinomycin D is myelosuppression, with granulocyte and platelet nadirs occurring 10 days after treatment. Early gastrointestinal toxicity is manifested within hours of treatment by nausea, vomiting, and diarrhea and usually subsides after 24 hours. Late toxicity involves mucous membrane damage throughout the gastrointestinal tract and includes oral mucositis. Some patients develop acneiform skin lesions.

Radiation recall, a phenomenon in which skin previously exposed to irradiation demonstrates ultrasensitivity when actinomycin D is administered, is a problem with this drug and increased skin sensitivity to actinomycin D has been demonstrated even when radiation exposure preceded drug exposure by 2 years. The severity of the recall reaction ranges from mild erythema to frank desquamation. Indeed, therapeutic advantage has been taken of this radiosensitizing effect of actinomycin D in the treatment of Wilms' tumor and Ewing's sarcoma.

MITHRAMYCIN

Mithramycin, a fermentation product of *Streptomyces plicatus*, has proven antitumor activity against testicular carcinoma as well as a calcium lowering activity in both normocalcemic and hypercalcemic patients. Because of the severe side effects (diffuse intravascular coagulation, thrombocytopenia, renal failure, nausea and vomiting, skin toxicity), the drug is now obsolete as a cancer drug and is only used as a last resort in hypercalcemic patients.

Plant Alkaloids

VINCRISTINE, VINBLASTINE, AND VINDESINE

Vincristine, vinblastine, and vindesine are alkaloids derived from the periwinkle plant, *Vinca rosea*. These compounds share a common structure that comprises a linkage of two complex rings, and individual compounds are distinguishable by small side chain substitutions which result in considerable differences in the pharmacokinetic behavior of each drug. These compounds have a common mode of antitumor action because of their ability to bind to tubulin. Among its many known functions, tubulin plays an integral part in spindle formation, which enables chromosomal integration during cell division. The inhibition of spindle formation leads to metaphase arrest of cells undergoing mitosis (14).

Following intravenous bolus administration, elimination of vincristine from plasma is initially very rapid; it has a distribution half-life of less than 1 minute and subsequent clearance with half-lives of approximately 8 minutes and $2\frac{1}{2}$ hours (8). Vinblastine and vindesine also have triphasic plasma elimination profiles with half-lives of 3–4 minutes, 60–100 minutes, and 20 hours, and hence their effects are considerably prolonged compared to vincristine (54). Both vincristine and vinblastine have very large volumes of distribution, which indicates extensive tissue binding, but cerebrospinal fluid penetration is minimal. Vincristine depends on hepatic metabolism and hepatobiliary secretion for its elimination. While it is thought that the majority of a dose of vinblastine is metabolized prior to elimination from the body, the organ primarily responsible for its metabolism has not been conclusively established. Caution is advised in the use of either drug in the presence of obstructive jaundice and hepatic failure since the hepatic route of elimination of metabolites appears to be quantitatively most important.

Vincristine is administered as an intravenous bolus in weekly doses of 1–1.4 mg/m². Vinblastine is similarly administered in doses ranging from 0.1 to 0.3 mg/m².

The dose-limiting toxicity for vincristine is peripheral neuropathy, manifesting as symmetric loss of deep tendon reflexes. Development of paraesthesias affecting wrist and ankle joints has also been described. Diplopia, facial nerve palsy, and hoarseness are the result of drug-induced cranial nerve lesions. The auto-nomic nervous system may also be affected, and this involvement manifests as sphincter dysfunction, abdominal cramps, paralytic ileus, and, rarely, as postural hypotension.

Vincristine is a very potent antitumoral agent and it seems that its activity plays an important role in several combination chemotherapy regimes. Based on its efficacy and on the importance of dose-intensity in achieving responses, it is our opinion that the cutoff of 2 mg recommended by many oncologic centers should be reconsidered.

In our experience, doses of 1.4 mg/m² have been given without any major toxicity. We think that careful observation of the patient and the appropriate drug reduction based on the toxicity, if any, is of more value than establishing an arbitrary limit and, in fact, this has been the standard practice in the Hodgkin's disease protocols of the National Cancer Institute.

Less common side effects of vincristine include dysphagia, Raynaud's phenomenon, and, rarely, a syndrome of inappropriate antidiuretic hormone secretion (SIADH). Vincristine overdose causes severe myelosuppression and SIADH. SIADH is one of the major causes of death in cases of vincristine overdose.

Vinblastine toxicity differs from that of vincristine, in that the most important dose-limiting toxicity for vinblastine is myelosuppression. The nadir is reached 7–10 days following drug administration. Vinblastine can cause a life-threatening paralytic ileus when given in excess dose. Mucositis is another troublesome and dose-limiting side effect of vinblastine.

Both vincristine and vinblastine are associated with alopecia and both cause an acute local reaction after extravasation.

EPIPODOPHYLLOTOXINS

VM-26 and VP-16 are glycosidic derivatives of podophyllotoxin, a plant extract of the May Apple. These agents have antitumor effects against small cell carcinoma of lung testicular tumors, and various lymphomas. They share a complex multitier structure and they both act by causing metaphase arrest of dividing cells (e.g., they prevent cells from entering mitosis). In addition, they trigger topoisomerase II–dependent cleavage of DNA.

Following an intravenous bolus injection of VP-16, plasma elimination of the drug is triphasic with half-lives of 0.5, 3.8, and 26.7 hours (22). Although details of the metabolic fate of VP-16 are still uncertain, approximately

45% of a dose may be recovered in urine (60–70% as unchanged drug) and 15% in feces. Plasma elimination of VM-26 has a terminal half-life of 11–38.5 hours (23). Neither drug penetrates the cerebrospinal fluid very well. An oral preparation of VP-16 has been investigated in patients with small cell lung cancer; its oral bioavailability is 80% of an intravenously administered equidose. VP-16 has antitumor activity in refractory lymphomas and has recently been used in combination with CDDP. VP-16 is also used as a single agent in treating Kaposi's sarcoma.

The dose-limiting toxicity of each agent is leukopenia, with a lesser effect on platelet count. Nausea and vomiting are usually severe. VP-16 infusion can cause bradycardia and/or hypotension, which can generally be controlled by stopping the infusion and restarting it at a slower rate. However, in rare instances, this may become an emergency problem and require ICU admission.

Miscellaneous Agents

HEXAMETHYLMELAMINE

Hexamethylmelamine (HMM) and pentamethylmelamine (PMM) are structural analogues of the alkylating agent triethylenemelamine and have demonstrated antitumor activity against cancers of lung, breast, and ovary and lymphomas. The exact mechanism of antitumor action of the methylmelamine remains to be defined, but is probably alkylation.

HMM is largely insoluble in water and hence administration is limited to the oral route. HMM is rapidly and extensively metabolized, since over 90% of the dose is excreted in urine as various demethylated metabolites (84).

Given the completeness of gastrointestinal absorption and the rapidity of its metabolism, the large variability in plasma HMM concentrations (>100-fold) may be due to interindividual differences in the rate of gastrointestinal absorption and in activity of the microsomal P-450 enzyme system. The plasma half-life varies from 4.7 to 10.2 hours. Nausea and emesis are common side effects of HMM administration and become dose-limiting with total doses of 200 mg/kg regardless of the period of administration. Myelosuppression is seen in nearly 50% of patients in most trials, with the nadir in cell counts occurring 6 weeks after initiation of therapy. Neurotoxicity is a major complication and occurs in 25% of pa-

tients following prolonged HMM therapy; both the central and peripheral nervous systems are affected. Ataxia, gait, and proprioceptive disturbances are among the more frequent manifestations. Psychiatric manifestations such as depression and hallucinations may also occur.

HYDROXYUREA

Hydroxyurea is a structural analogue of urea, and antitumor activity has been noted in several mammalian tumor systems. Used primarily in chronic myeloid leukemia (CML), hydroxyurea has an advantage over busulphan in that its leukopenic effects are rapid in onset and rapidly reversed upon cessation of therapy. The mechanism of antitumor action is due to is potent inhibitory effect on ribonucleotide reductase, an enzyme that plays a key role in DNA synthesis. Hydroxyurea exerts its maximal antitumor effect in the S- phase of the cell cycle. The drug is synergistic with radiation therapy. Fragmentation and translocation of metaphase chromosomes and breaks in DNA have been documented in cell culture systems (80), and this could represent an alternate mechanism of action.

Kinetic analysis following intravenous bolus administration demonstrates a plasma elimination half-life of approximately 4 hours (7). Following oral administration, peak concentrations are achieved in 1.5–2 hours, and the plasma elimination half-life is about 3 hours. The major elimination route is thought to be renal, so dose reduction is advised in patients with reduced renal function.

Mild nausea and emesis commonly accompany hydroxyurea therapy, while mucositis and gastrointestinal ulceration are less common. Dermatologic reaction are common with long-term therapy; they manifest as increased pigmentation, skin scaling, nail changes, and partial alopecia.

PROCARBAZINE

Procarbazine is a substituted hydrazine compound with proven antitumor activity in lymphoma. Its mechanism of action is not understood, but abundant evidence exists that procarbazine is a prodrug and requires metabolic activation for its antitumor activity.

Biologic effects ranging from DNA alkylation to inhibition of key enzymes in carbohydrate metabolism are reported for this drug, but the importance of each of these effects to the drug's antitumor action is not clear. Microsomal metabolism however, is thought to be very important. Because of a lack of a specific and sensitive assay for procarbazine, knowledge of its pharmacokinetic behavior is limited.

Procarbazine is given orally (100 mg/m²/day) for 10–14 days. Moderate degrees of anorexia and nausea along with mild to moderate leukopenia and thrombocytopenia occur with this regimen. Neurotoxicity is a less frequent complication of oral treatment; however, intravenous administration of procarbazine is complicated by peripheral paresthesia and drowsiness. Depression following procarbazine treatment may be related to its ability to inhibit monoamine oxidase activity. Avoidance of tyramine in the diet is mandatory so as to avert a hypertensive crisis. Similarly, avoidance of alcohol during procarbazine therapy is advised, since disulfiram-like reactions involving headache, facial flushing, profuse sweating, and nausea have been reported. Hypersensitivity reactions involving skin rash and occasionally lung infiltrates are also seen, although coadministration of steroids may control these side effects. Azospermia frequently occurs. Procarbazine is a carcinogen and can contribute to the induction of secondary malignancies.

DACARBAZINE

Dacarbazine (DTIC) is a synthetic antitumor agent. Activity has been documented in malignant Hodgkin's disease, melanoma, and certain sarcomas. It owes its antitumor activity to its alkylating properties. Indirect evidence of the importance of N-demethylation on the plasma half-life of DTIC suggests that hepatic metabolism plays a key role in the elimination of the parent compound (69). The importance of the kidneys in the elimination of the parent compound is uncertain, but considerable amounts of various metabolites are found in the urine following treatment with DTIC.

Severe nausea and emesis are frequently dose limiting and dose reduction is associated with amelioration of these symptoms. Tolerance to these toxic symptoms develops with multiple dosing and allows for some escalation in dose. With a daily dosage regimen of 250 mg/m² for 5 days, modest leukopenia and thrombocytopenia develop with a nadir at 15–20 days. Higher doses are associated with protracted nausea and emesis. There is one report of increased cardiac toxicity in children with malignant melanoma when treated with a chemotherapeutic regimen which includes DTIC

and Adriamycin. In animals, DTIC is carcinogenic and teratogenic.

L-ASPARAGINASE

The antitumor effect of L-asparaginase (discovered in the serum of guinea pig) is due to inhibition of protein synthesis as a result of depletion of L-asparagine. Dose-response curves for L-asparaginase have been reported for childhood lymphoblastic leukemia (31). Resistance to L-asparaginase may arise by either derepression of the enzyme, L-asparagine synthetase, or else by simple selection of a cell line that naturally expresses this enzyme.

Normal plasma concentrations of asparagine (110^{-5}M) are in excess of that required to maintain the viability of cells, so that large doses of L-asparaginase need to be administered to inhibit cell growth. The antitumor effect of L-asparaginase depends upon the specific affinity for L-asparagine and upon the plasma clearance of the enzyme. Both affinity for substrate and plasma half-life of L-asparaginase vary depending upon its source. Patients who have an immune reaction to the enzyme also show a reduction in its plasma half-life.

L-asparaginase is thought to be distributed mainly in the intravascular space, but penetration of the blood-brain barrier occurs with a concomitant antileukemic effect. Toxicity of L-asparaginase is the result of either the immune response to injection of foreign protein or to the inhibition of protein synthesis in normal tissue. Hypersensitivity reactions range from mild urticaria to life-threatening anaphylaxis and vary in their time course from immediate to delayed responses. For this reason, L-asparaginase must always be administered in a controlled setting, with the availability at the bedside of epinephrine and hydrocortisone. When given in a polychemotherapeutic regimen containing immune-suppressing agents, such as 6MP, the severity of the allergic reaction seems to be decreased. Other toxic effects are liver damage, with hypoalbuminemia and decreases in clotting factors (sometimes followed by a hemorrhagic diathesis); acute pancreatitis, and temporary clouding of cerebral functions.

MITOTANE

Mitotane is an isomer of dichlorobis(p-chlorophenyl)ethane (DDD) and appears to exert a direct toxic effect on the metabolism and survival of adrenal cortical cells, affecting their mitochondria. It also decreases steroid secretion, probably interfering with the anabolic pathways of steroid synthesis, and causes an alteration of peripheral metabolism of cortisol and androgens. It has a very long half-life and plasma levels can be detectable after 10 weeks, while metabolites persist in the urine even after 18 months.

Mitotane is used, with minor success, in advanced adrenal carcinoma. Its toxicity is mainly related to the gastrointestinal tract (diarrhea), but about 40% of patients also experience neurotoxicity (vertigo and drowsiness). The possibility of acute hypoadrenalism is, of course, present.

M-AMSA

Amsacrine is a synthetic acridine, that intercalates into DNA. It has some antitumor activity against refractory lymphomas. Its toxicities are mainly myelosuppression and cardiotoxicity, with the possibility of ventricular fibrillation.

MITOXANTRONE

Mitoxantrone belongs to the family of aminoanthraquinones and probably acts similarly to anthracyclines. It has antitumor activity in breast cancer, where it can be used (up to a total dose of 100 mg/m²) in patients pretreated with Adriamycin (59).

DEOXYCOFORMYCIN

Deoxycoformycin (DCF) is an irreversible inhibitor of adenosine deaminase, an enzyme essential for purine nucleoside metabolism, which is found both in normal and malignant B and T cells. T cells have higher adenosine deaminase activity and DCF appears to be more specific towards T-cell malignancies. It has antitumor activity against lymphomas, hairy cell leukemia, and T and B cell and adult T cell leukemia/lymphoma. During phase I trials, severe neurotoxicity (including coma) were observed. At lower doses, however, no CNS side effects have been observed. It causes conjuctivitis (often indistinguishable from a herpetic infection) and transient liver toxicity.

BIOLOGICAL RESPONSE MODIFIERS AND HORMONES

Hormones and biological response modifiers (e.g., antibodies, IL$_2$-LAK) are now under investigation as antitumor therapies, but we will not discuss them here as it would be beyond the scope of this chapter. However, it seems worth mentioning two situations that may result in ICU admission:

1. Hypocortisolism may develop from inappropriate aminoglutethamide therapy. Aminoglutethimide is used to treat breast cancer and produces a chemical castration. It is given together with steroid replacement, but sometimes patients fail to take the steroids properly.
2. Hyperpyrexia may develop from interferon therapy. Interferon is now used for treatment of hairy cell leukemias and for Kaposi's sarcoma. It produces myelosuppression and can cause violent fever, generally responsive to antipyretics.

MANAGEMENT OF SIDE EFFECTS

The amount of drug received (dose intensity) by the patient is a major determinant of the antitumor response and every attempt should

Table 29.1
Antineoplastic Drugs and Renal Dysfunction

Drug	Renal Toxicity	% Dose for GFR of	
		>50 ml/min	<50 ml/min
Methotrexate	yes, high dose	50–100	50–75
cis-Platinum	yes	50–100[a]	0–50[a]
Cyclophosphamide	yes (bladder)	100	50–75
Bleomycin	no	75–100	50–75
Streptozotocin	yes	75–100	50–75
Mithramycin	yes	75–100	50–75
Mitomycin C	yes	50–100[a]	0–50[a]
Lomustine	yes	no[b]	no[b]
Semustine	yes	no[b]	no[b]

[a] Modify dose to avoid further kidney damage, not to lessen systemic toxicity.
[b] Renal toxicity is a late complication and not predictable.

Table 29.2
Renal Dysfunction in Patients with Cancer

Tumor Involvement of the Urinary Tract
    Kidney parenchyma invaded (leukemia, lymphoma)
    Ureteral obstruction
Tumor Products Toxic to the Kidney
    Paraprotein
    Uric acid
    Calcium
Drug Toxicity
    Methotrexate
    Cis-platinum
    Streptozotocin
    Mitomycin C
    Nitrosoureas
Radiation Therapy
    Acute and chronic radiation nephritis
Other Drugs Given to Cancer Patients
    Aminoglycosides
    Amphotericin B

be made to administer full doses whenever it is possible. However, some patients require special evaluation and occasionally an initial dose reduction. This is true for very old persons, who have a poor performance status and with preexisting organ damage. In addition, cells that divide more rapidly are the ones more affected by chemotherapy and therefore gastrointestinal symptoms, myelosuppression, and alopecia are the most universal adverse effects.

Dose reductions may be required in the presence of liver and kidney function abnormalities and we suggest some empirical guidelines. Since routine therapeutic monitoring of antineoplastic drugs, other than methotrexate, is not generally available, the proposed guidelines are empirical, although based on the known clinical pharmacology of the individual antineoplastic drugs (Tables 29.1 and 29.2).

Renal Dysfunction

Drugs that are eliminated by renal pathways have their doses reduced in patients with renal dysfunction to prevent drug accumulation and hence toxicity. As most anticancer drugs are given intermittently, long-term accumulation is usually not a problem. However, small changes in drug clearance associated with a single intravenous injection may lead to toxicity, since most antineoplastic drugs have a low toxic therapeutic index. Therefore, the usual concept of not changing the loading dose does not apply to this group of drugs. No specific dosage nomograms exist, although rough guidelines, usually based on creatinine clearance, have been published (Table 29.1). In addition, several anticancer drugs can themselves be nephrotoxic (Table 29.2) and produce increased systemic toxicity as a result of reduced drug clearance (e.g., methotrexate). Finally, the patients with cancer may have renal dysfunction as a result of their underlying disease (Table 29.2)

Hepatic Dysfunction

Prediction of the degree of altered drug pharmacokinetics is often difficult in the individual with underlying liver disease or hepatic metastases, and routine liver function tests are often not very helpful nor specific. One of the drugs that is usually reduced based an liver

Table 29.3
Cancer Drugs and Hepatic Dysfunction

Drug	Liver Toxicity	% Dose if bilirubin is:		
		1.5	3–5	>5
Doxorubicin[a]	no			
Daunomycin[a]	no			
Vincristine	no	50	25	omit
Vinblastine	no	50	25	omit
VP-16, VM-26	no	50	25	omit
Nitrosoureas[b]	yes			
Ara-C	yes			
6-Mercaptopurine	yes	50	25	omit
Methotrexate	yes	50	25	omit
Mithramycin	yes			
L-Asparaginase	yes			

[a]Older literature and some protocols have specified dose modification for bilirubin. There is no clear correlation between bilirubin and drug clearance nor between bilirubin and toxicity.
[b]In animal models, coadministration of nitrosoureas and doxorubicin can result in acute liver necrosis.

function tests is Adriamycin, even though it is unclear how its pharmacokinetics are actually affected by alterations in hepatic metabolism. Moreover, despite the fact that dose adjustments are routinely made on the basis of serum bilirubin values (Table 29.3), this liver function test is not an accurate indication of the liver's ability to clear the drugs. In addition, although hepatic cirrhosis will modify the pharmacokinetics of a number of drugs, this may not be the case for Adriamycin. Because of the problems in attempting to quantitate hepatic drug clearance, some empirical guidelines are suggested for the patient with hepatic dysfunction (Table 29.3). Finally some antineoplastic drugs are hepatotoxic themselves although in most cases the degree of liver function abnormalities are mild and reversible. The use of high-dose therapies increases the frequency and the severity of hepatotoxicity (e.g., methotrexate or cyclophosphamide).

Pulmonary Toxicity

Bleomycin, busulfan, cyclophosphamide, methotrexate, nitrosoureas, and mitomycin C can induce lung lesions. An early recognition of the process can lead to the suspension of the drug and can be life saving.

With busulfan, patients usually present with cough, dyspnea, fever, diffuse pulmonary infiltrates, and hypoxemia. These symptoms are usually progressive, with death occurring in several months. It is unclear whether high-dose steroids are of benefit. It is important to consider causes of respiratory distress other than that due to neoplastic lung involvement (or its therapy) in these patients, as some may be reversible with appropriate treatment. Toxicity results in a chronic interstitial pneumonitis and generally follows long-term therapy, appearing 4–10 years after the beginning of the treatment.

Chronic pneumonitis is a rare event with cyclophosphamide and consists of an intraalveolar fibrosis.

Methotrexate has been reported to cause an acute interstitial pneumonitis, characterized by fever and eosinophilia. Patients present with acute symptoms, which need prompt differentiation from Pneumocystis carinii and viral pneumonia. High-dose steroids seem to be effective, but no standard therapy has been established. The process is generally reversible. It appears to be a hypersensitivity reaction, but some patients have received additional meth-

otrexate without further pneumonitis episodes.

Nitrosoureas give rise to an interstitial pneumonia that is followed by fibrosis, is lethal in 60–80% of cases, and is dose-related, appearing after a cumulative dose of >1400 mg/m². It is probably due to direct epithelial damage.

Mitomycin C causes an interstitial pneumonitis/alveolitis in 3–5% of patients. It is often reversible by stopping the drug and instituting steroid therapy.

The drug that most commonly causes lung damage is bleomycin. Early clinical symptoms are nonspecific (e.g., nonproductive cough), and disabling dyspnea may develop rapidly without any prior symptoms. Auscultation of the chest may demonstrate fine basilar rales and chest radiography may show diffuse basilar infiltrates in the absence of clinical symptoms. Pulmonary function tests may be of some value in predicting those at risk for developing toxicity. Differentiation between bleomycin-induced lung injury and pulmonary infection (especially Pneumocystis carinii) can often only be resolved by open lung biopsy. Respiratory failure is more common in the early postoperative period in patients who have had bleomycin treatment previously. While severe pulmonary fibrosis is associated with hypoxemia, oxygen therapy must be undertaken with some caution in view of the oxygen–free radical mechanism of toxicity postulated for bleomycin. The role of corticosteroids in amelioration of the bleomycin-induced pulmonary damage remains unproven; however, isolated reports of clinical improvement suggest that a trial of corticosteroid therapy may be of benefit. Predisposing factors for toxicity include age, chronic pulmonary diseases such as emphysema and pneumoconiosis, previous radiation therapy to the chest, and excessive dosage of BLM (>200–250 mg/m²) and of nitrosoureas.

In summary, there are two types of lung toxicity: an acute form (e.g., methotrexate pneumonitis) and a chronic form, presenting initially as an interstitial process and ending in irreversible fibrosis. All efforts must be made to detect them early in order to stop the drug that is responsible.

Cardiac Toxicity

The drug most often responsible for cardiac toxicity is Adriamycin. Toxicity can be acute or chronic. Acutely, approximately 50% of all patients treated with Adriamycin demonstrate

ECG changes. These ECG changes include sinus tachycardia, premature atrial or ventricular contractions, and variable ST-T wave changes, which usually revert back to baseline within days or weeks of drug administration. However, serious arrhythmias such as complete heart block and ventricular tachycardia may develop with this drug and may explain isolated reports of sudden death. Another serious side effect of doxorubicin therapy, which manifests within days of initiation of treatment, is the "pericarditis-myocarditis" syndrome (12). This syndrome manifests as low output cardiac failure with pericarditis. Acute cardiotoxicity can be also observed with 5-fluorouracil infusion (ischemia), M-amsacrine infusion (ventricular fibrillation), and with high-dose cyclophosphamide (hemorrhagic mycarditis-pericarditis).

Chronically, Adriamycin causes a cardiomyopathy. Symptoms and signs are clinically indistinguishable from other causes of heart failure and respond poorly to digitalis. Most patients can be successfully managed by rest, afterload reduction and careful attention to fluid and electrolyte problems. Cardiotoxicity is dose dependent and the incidence of symptomatic cardiac failure is 1.5–2.2% below 550 mg/m^2, but increases to 36% for patients who have received more than 550 mg/m^2.

Pathologic cardiac damage is diagnostic (11). Lipid peroxidation via oxygen free radicals appears to be the mechanism responsible for the cardiomyopathic damage. Free radical scavengers such a tocopherol (vitamin E) lessen both the extent of lipid peroxidation and the incidence of cardiomyopathy in animals. Adriamycin-induced free radical injury is dependent upon iron; recently, coadministration of the metal chelator ICRF 187 with Adriamycin has shown some efficacy in preventing the chronic cardiomyopathy in humans. Furthermore, relative to other tissues, cardiac muscle has a very low catalase concentration and hence is unable to detoxify hydrogen peroxide. Doxorubicin, which reduces the activity of glutathione peroxidase in cardiac tissue, renders the heart defenseless against lipid peroxidation by reactive oxygen species. In addition, doxorubicin can bind to cardiolipin, a phospholipid found in the cell membrane and in mitochondria. Since mitochondria are the major source of ATP in the heart, these observations may be cogent to the cardiomyopathic effects of doxorubicin. Predisposing factors for cardiotoxicity include age, dose schedule (cardiotoxicity is less when Adriamycin is administered in low weekly doses), previous mediastinal radiation, and previous heart disease.

It is important to remember that potassium abnormalities can also contribute to the acute cardiac toxicity and that this electrolyte needs careful monitoring in all cancer patients on chemotherapy.

Myelosuppression

Cytotoxicity from antineoplastic agents is unfortunately not restricted to tumor cells but also affects normal tissue, particularly those with high cell turnover rates such as gastrointestinal mucosa and bone marrow. Bone marrow toxicity is predictable in that granulocytes (half-life approximately 6 hours) are most markedly suppressed, with platelets ($t_{1/2} = 7–10$ days) and erythrocytes ($t_{1/2} = 120$ days) being less affected. Drugs that exert their cytotoxicity by arresting cell cycling at a particular phase (DNA synthesis or S phase, mitosis or M phases, or resting phases G_0 and G_1) are known as phase specific, cycle-active agents that have characteristic myelosuppressive patterns (Table 29.4). Drugs in the more heterogeneous group, which can be classed as cycle active but phase nonspecific, are less predictable in their myelosuppressive effects (Table 29.5).

Nitrosoureas represent an unusual group of agents whose cytotoxic action does not depend for their cytotoxic effect upon cells being in cycle and the characteristic myelosuppressive patterns are prolonged, with white cell nadirs occurring at 3–6 weeks and recovery occurring at 7–12 weeks following administration. The severity of myelosuppression is a function of the dose and schedule and, for methotrexate, of the use of leucovorin rescue. Patient factors such as age, disease infiltration of bone marrow, previous chemotherapy or radiotherapy,

Table 29.4
Myelosuppression by Cancer Drugs: Phase-Specific

Drug	Myelosuppression (days)	
	Nadir	Recovery
Methotrexate	7–14	14–21
6-Mercaptopurine	7–14	14–21
5-Fluorouracil	7–14	20–24
Cyclophosphamide	7–14	14–21
Vinblastine	4–9	7–21
Ara-C	7	14
Hydroxyurea	7	14

Table 29.5
Myelosuppression by Cancer Drugs:
Phase Nonspecific

Drug	Myelosuppression (days)	
	Nadir	Recovery
Busulphan	11–30	24–54
Chlorambucil	8–15	24–28
Adriamycin	7–14	21–24
Mithramycin	5–10	10–18
Mitomycin	28–42	42–56
Procarbazine	25–36	35–50
Cis-platinum	14	21

and nutritional status may also influence severity and rate of recovery from myelosuppression.

Myelosuppression can also present as anemia and thrombocytopenia. Severe anemia is unusual with most treatment regimens, so that other common causes such as hemolysis or nutritional factors should be considered. Thrombocytopenia, while often seen in patients treated with anticancer drugs, does not usually cause severe hemorrhages. However, platelet transfusion can be effective in such cases. Different opinions exists regarding the management of thrombocytopenia, as transfusion therapy can lead to the development of antibodies. However, given the high fatality rate of hemorrhage in patients with less than 20,000/mm³ platelets, we recommend transfusing the patients when their platelets fall below 20,000/mm³. To reduce the risk of antibody formation, blood products should preferably be irradiated.

Patients whose cytopenia is due to bone marrow involvement need full-dose chemotherapy, since the chances for recovery increase proportional to the adequacy of therapy. Age, per se, is not a limiting factor and dose reduction should be evaluated based on the degree, if any, of functional impairment of vital organs (liver, kidney, and heart), and not based on age alone. Previous chemotherapy can have drastic effects on the marrow function. However, in cases of relapse or progression of the disease, the probability of bone marrow involvement by tumor is high. Cytopathological evaluation of the marrow should be undertaken by deciding on dose modification. Previous radiotherapy to the mediastinum usually indicates dose reduction. Dosage can then be escalated if no major toxicity is observed. Radiotherapy to the pelvis has similar implications, whereas small-field radiotherapy to other areas does not necessarily

imply any need for dose reduction. Careful individual evaluation is deserved by the patient who has undergone total body irradiation for bone marrow transplant.

The nutritional status of the patient can be reconstituted through hyperalimentation and does not represent a contradiction to full-dose therapy.

When a combination chemotherapy regimen is formulated and drugs are given on different days of a cycle, a certain degree of myelosuppression from the previously given drugs is expected. Therefore, dose modification generally applies only to day 1. However, there are exceptions, and guidelines are always given for any chemotherapy regimen. One drug that almost invariably creates major dilemmas is methotrexate. In fact, it is very often given in the last part of the cycle, when the patient is already leukopenic, and is often administered at high dosage. However, because of the availability of folinic acid, which reverses the myelosuppression due to methotrexate, there is no need for any dose reduction. Methotrexate can be safely administered to every patient, no matter how high the dose and how low the white blood cell and platelet count, provided that appropriate leucovorin rescue is given (e.g., until the plasma MTX level is $<10^{-8}$ M). If the patient has an active infection and is receiving antibiotics, at the time the MTX is due, then no chemotherapy should be given until the acute infection resolves. Moreover, special consideration should be paid to the type of antibiotic, knowing that most of them are weak acids and can therefore interfere with MTX clearance.

Fever

How should we respond to fever in a patient on chemotherapy? We will not go into the details of proper antimicrobial therapy, which can be found in other sections of this book, but we will discuss some practical guidelines.

Fever can be of different origins (e.g., tumor, drug related, infection) but one must search for an infectious cause. This means that every patient should have appropriate cultures (e.g., blood, urine, throat, stool, and vaginal), in addition to a complete physical examination. Some oncologists recommend avoiding routine internal rectal exams because of the risk of contamination in the neutropenic patient, but this remains a controversial point. It is also important to obtain a complete blood count and chest x-ray. Arterial blood gases are needed when pneumonitis is suspected as a source of the fever. Intravenous lines or catheters should be changed and cultured. Third-space fluid collections should be tapped and cultured. This approach is mandatory if the patient is neutropenic (<1000 cells).

If the absolute neutrophil count is >1000 and the temperature is <38.5°C and there is no evidence of a source of infection, the patient must be carefully followed, but no antibiotic therapy should be started. The temperature must be taken every 4 hours. Patients should avoid antipyretics. Patients on steroid therapy should be kept under strict observation and the antipyretic effect of steroids should be considered. Women must be told to avoid using tampons, and all patients must be told to avoid using suppositories.

If the absolute neutrophil count is <1000 in the febrile patient, the patient needs to be hospitalized and intravenous broad spectrum antibiotics should be started. The optimal regimen and duration of therapy has not been standardized. Outside research settings, a three-drug regimen (a cephalosporin, an aminoglycoside, and ticarcillin) should be immediately instituted and continued until neutrophils are >1000 and fever has subsided. Vancomycin should be added if central line–related sepsis is suspected. Clindamycin should be added in cases of severe mucositis. The use of granulocyte transfusions, initially thought to be of therapeutic value in the neutropenic patient deteriorating after 2–3 days, has now been abandoned in almost every oncologic center. Fungal infections are a common cause of morbidity and mortality in the neutropenic patient, and they should be suspected and appropriately treated in case of persistent fever.

The management of septic shock in the cancer patient does not differ from that in any other patients. Oxygen therapy, however, should be minimized in patients receiving bleomycin.

Third-Space Fluid Accumulation

Many cancer patients develop pleural effusions, pericardial effusions, and ascites during the course of their disease. Malignant effusions present two management problems. The first is the prevention of recurrent fluid accumulation once drainage has been accomplished (e.g., thoracentesis, paracentesis). The second is the problem associated with systemic drug therapy in the face of a potential drug reservoir.

This occurs particularly in patients receiving methotrexate who develop significant toxicity (even after moderate doses), as a result of the slow continued egress of the drug from the third-space fluid collections.

Malignant effusions tend to reaccumulate, often at a very fast rate. Generally, the first step would be an attempt to control the underlying disease with systemic therapy. If this fails, the next step is intracavitary treatment. This is accomplished following drainage and when adhesion between the two serosal surfaces is obtained. After prolonged drainage (24–48 hours) of the pleural effusion and x-ray evidence of reexpansion of the lung, different substances can be instilled into the pleural space in 100 ml of normal saline: the most commonly used agent is bleomycin (60–90 mg/m^2 once a week until regression), which gives a 40–60% response and produces toxicity (fever and local pain) in about 10% of cases. Thiotepa, mechlorethamine, 5-FU, Adriamycin, and cis-platinum may also be used. Tetracyclines can be used, 500 mg in 50 ml NS, often in combination with bleomycin.

For peritoneal and pericardial effusions, the use of intracavitary therapy has not given the same results as for pleural effusions, but all agents previously mentioned can be tried. For ascites, they are diluted in 500 ml normal saline and instilled through a temporary catheter or a permanent Tenkhoff. For pericardial and peritoneal effusions, radioactive isotopes (^{158}Au and ^{32}P) can be used instead of cytotoxic agents.

If drug therapy fails, the next step is external radiation therapy (3000–5000 rad in 3 weeks for pleural effusions, 3000 rad in about 4 weeks to the porta hepatis for peritoneal effusions and 2500–3500 rad in 3–4 weeks for pericardial effusions). Surgery is the last step.

A completely different but not less challenging problem is the pharmacological approach to a patient with a malignant effusion, who is to receive treatment with systemic chemotherapy. The most common situation is the need to administer methotrexate to patients with third-space fluid collections. MTX penetrates third-space fluids and tends to have a slower clearance, as compared with the plasma clearance. This leads to a "sustained release" into the bloodstream, with consequent prolonged high plasma levels and the almost invariable occurrence of unexpected toxicity. To avoid severe MTX toxicity, the effusion should be drained before MTX is administered and again if it has reaccumulated by 24 hours. In the presence of an effusion that can not be drained, MTX plasma levels should be monitored for prolonged periods of time and leucovorin rescue should be administered, guided by the MTX plasma level (until it is $<10^{-8}$M).

We believe that if the previous guidelines can be strictly followed, there is no need for dose modification. A difference of opinion exists among oncologic centers regarding this problem, but in our experience no major complications have occurred and full-dose therapy is generally of benefit to patients at that stage of disease. It is conceivable that a similar situation occurs for other drugs too.

Tumor Lysis Syndrome and Metabolic Complications

Tumor lysis syndrome represents the acute occurence of hyperuricemia, hyperkalemia, hyperphosphatemia, and hypocalcemia as a consequence of the rapid destruction of a tumor mass. It happens with a certain frequency in leukemias and aggressive lymphomas (mainly Burkitt's), but can also be seen in solid tumors (e.g., embryonal rhabdomyosarcoma, embryonal cancer of the testis, and choriocarcinoma in women). Prophylaxis with adequate hydration, urine alkalinization, and use of allopurinol is generally efficacious, together with careful monitoring of electrolytes. When established, tumor lysis syndrome can lead to renal failure and lactic acidosis. There can also be hyperphosphatemia with secondary hypocalcemia (and tetany) and hyperkalemia.

Another metabolic complication frequently observed is hypercalcemia, which is often unresponsive to standard management and requires the use of hydrocortisone, calcitonin, and mithramycin. Hypocalcemia and hypomagnesemia can also present acutely and generally respond to replacement therapy (see Chapter 32).

Drug Extravasation

The intravenous administration of several antineoplastic drugs may produce phlebitis or severe local tissue necrosis if they are extravasated. The treatment of local phlebitis is conservative and includes the use of heat, analgesics, and avoidance of the involved vein for a long enough time to allow resolution of the inflammation and preserve vein patency. The management of drug extravasation is less clear as there are only a few controlled clinical

trials. Extravasation probably occurs during 1–2% of chemotherapy infusions. This may produce a local chemical cellulitis as well as extensive tissue necrosis and fibrosis. This potentially serious complication can be prevented if the drug is infused in a vein with a free-flowing intravenous administration. If possible, areas such as the hand, wrist, or antecubical fossa, which have little subcutaneous tissue (for highly vesicant or reactive drugs), should be avoided.

Several classes of drugs can produce local tissue injury. Vesicant properties are reported for Actinomycin D, Adriamycin (doxorubicin), daunorubicin, mitomycin C, nitrogen mustard (mechlorethamine), mithramycin, streptozotocin, vinblastine, and vincristine. In addition, phlebitis is reported as a result of VM-26, dacarbazine, BCNU, and m-AMSA administration although they may not have severe vesicant properties. The anthracycline drugs Adriamycin and daunorubicin produce the most severe local tissue damage, as they may cause ulcers that are slow to heal (this problem is associated with persistence of the drug in the ulcer crater for months after extravasation).

If drug extravasation occurs during the administration of a vesicant drug, several guidelines have been proposed although none have been universally accepted. Treatment should begin immediately after extravasation occurs. The injection should be stopped by the needle left in place. An attempt should be made to withdraw several milliliters of blood to decrease the local drug concentration. In addition, a small-gauge needle can be used in an attempt to aspirate any subcutaneous fluid blebs that may contain drug. The intravenous needle should then be removed and various antidotes injected locally. After extravasation of Actinomycin D, Mitomycin C, and nitrogen mustard, 4 ml of 10% sodium thiosulfate has been used successfully. After extravasation of Adriamycin, daunorubicin, carmustine, vincristine, and vinblastine 4–5 ml of 8.4% sodium bicarbonate have been tried. For the management of anthracycline (Adriamycin or daunorubicin) extravasation there have been several experimental approaches reported. The local injection of dexamethasone 1 mg (1 ml of 4 mg/ml solution) may be useful in decreasing local inflammation. In addition, DMSO, isoproterenol, and propranolol used locally may decrease the severity of local damage although these approaches require further validation (25, 72). The local use of N-acetylcysteine may actually increase the severity of Adriamycin-induced ulcers (25). Finally, cold compresses applied locally may be a useful adjunct. In our institution, we have found the combined use of cold compresses and steroid injection to effectively eliminate problems following Adriamycin extravasation. Ulcers resulting from anthracycline extravasation should be seen by a plastic surgeon as early as possible, since they may require local tissue debridement and skin grafting.

Nausea and Vomiting

Different categories of antiemetics are available and a combination of various drugs (e.g., phenothiazines or high-dose metoclopramide with steroids and benzodiazepines) may be more effective than a single agent. The use of lorazepam (Ativan), which has the property of inducing a certain degree of amnesia, should be considered. When the antineoplastic drug administered is strongly emetic (CDDP, HN_2, Adriamycin, DTIC, Actinomycin D, Streptozotocin, VP_{16}), antiemetic therapy should not be given on an as-needed basis but rather on an around-the-clock basis. In outpatients, the use of long-acting preparations of oral antiemetics, starting the day before the chemotherapy is begun, can also be of value.

References

1. Ahmad S, Shen F, Bleyer WA: Methotrexate-induced renal failure and ineffectiveness of peritoneal dialysis. *Arch Intern Med* 138:1146, 1978.
2. Alberts DS, Chen MSG, Lui R, et al: Bleomycin pharmacokinetics in man. I. Intravenous administration. *Cancer Chemother Pharmacol* 1:177, 1978.
3. Alberts DS, Chen MSG, Mayersohn M, et al: Bleomycin pharmacokinetics in man. II. Intracavitary administration. *Cancer Chemother Pharmacol* 2:127, 1979.
4. Allegra CJ, Curt GA, Baram J et al: Antimetabolites. In Pinedo, Chabner: *Cancer Chemotherapy*. Amsterdam, Elsevier, 1986.
5. Allegra CJ, Drake JC, Swan J et al: Preliminary results of a phase I-II trial for the treatment of *Pneumocystis carinii* pneumonia using a potent lipid-soluble dihydrofolate reductase inhibitor, trimetrexate. *Proceedings and Abtracts of the 26th Interscience Conference on Antimicrobial and Antibiotic Chemotherapy*. Washington, DC: American Society for Microbiology, 1986, p 224.
6. Bagley CM, Bosllick FW, DeVita VT: Clinical pharmacology of cyclophosphamide. *Cancer Res* 33:226, 1973.
7. Belt RJ, Haas CD, Kennedy J, et al: Studies of hydroxyurea administered by continuous infusion. *Cancer* 46:455, 1980.
8. Bender RA, Castle MC, Margelith DA, et al: The pharmacokinetics of ^3H vincristine in man. *Clin Pharmacol Ther* 22:430, 1977.
9. Benjamin RS, Hall SW, Burgess MA: A pharmacokinetically based phase I-II study of single dose actinomycin-D (NSC 3053). *Cancer Treat Rep* 60:209, 1976.
10. Benjamin RS, Riggs NR, Bachur NR: Plasma pharmacokinetics of Adriamycin and its metabolites in humans with normal hepatic and renal function. *Cancer Res* 37:19, 1974.
11. Billingham ME, Mason JW, Bristow MA, et al: Anthracycline cardiomyopathy monitored by morphological changes. *Cancer Treat Rep* 62:865, 1978.
12. Bracken RB, Johnson DE, Rodriquez L, et al: Treatment of multiple superficial tumors of bladder with intravesical bleomycin. *Urology* 9:161, 1977.
13. Bristow MR, Thompson PD, Martin RP: Early anthracycline cardiotoxicity. *Am J Med* 65:823, 1978.
14. Bruchovsky N, Owen AA, Becker AJ, et al: Effects of vinblastine on the proliferative capacity of L cells and their progress through division cycle. *Cancer Res* 25:1232, 1965.
15. Bryant BM, Jarman M, Ford HT, et al: Prevention of isophosphamide-induced urothelial toxicity with 2-mercaptoethanesulfonate sodium (mesnum) in patients with advanced carcinoma. *Lancet* 2:657, 1980.
16. Burns WA, McFarland W, Mathews MJ: Busulfan-induced pulmonary disease: report of a case and review of the literature. *Am Rev Respir Dis* 101:408, 1970.
17. Casper ES, Kelsen DP, Alcock NW et al: Ip cisplatin in patients with malignant ascites: pharmacokinetic evaluation and comparison with the iv route. *Cancer Treat Rep* 67; 235–238, 1983.
18. Chan KK, Cohen JL, Gross JF, et al: Prediction of Adriamycin disposition in cancer patients using a physiologic pharmacokinetic model. *Cancer Treat Rep* 62:1161, 1978.
19. Cole SR, Myers JJ, Klatsky AU: Pulmonary disease with chlorambucil therapy. *Cancer* 41:455, 1978.
20. Collins JM, Dedrick RL, King FG, et al: Non-linear pharmacokinetic models for 5-fluorouracil in man: intravenous and intraperitoneal routes. *Clin Pharmacol Ther* 28(2):235, 1980.
21. Colvin M, Padgett CA, Fenselau C: A biologically active metabolite of cyclophosphamide. *Cancer Res* 33:915, 1973.
22. Creaven PJ, Allen LM: EPEG, a new antineoplastic epipodophyllotoxin. *Clin Pharmacol Ther* 18:221, 1975.
23. Creaven PJ, Allen LM: PTG, a new antineoplastic epipodophyllotoxin. *Clin. Pharmacol Ther* 18:227, 1975.
24. Crooke ST, Luft F, Broughton A, et al: Bleomycin serum pharmacokinetics as determined by radioimmunoassay and a microbiological assay in a patient with compromised renal function. *Cancer* 39:1430, 1977.
25. Curt GA, Grygrel JJ, Corde BJ et al: A phase I and pharmacokinetic study of diamminecyclobutane-dicarboxylate platinum (NSC 241240) *Cancer Res* 43:4470–4473, 1984.
26. DeConti RC, Toftness BR, Lange RC, et al: Clinical and pharmacological studies with cisdiamminedichloroplatinum (II). *Cancer Res* 33:310, 1973.
27. DeVita VT, Broder S, Fauci AS et al: Developmental therapeutics and the acquired immunodeficiency syndrome: NIH Conference. *Ann Intern Med* 106:568–581, 1987.
28. Dorr RT, Albert DS: Pharmacological antidotes to experimental doxorubicin skin toxicity: a suggested role for beta-adrenergic compounds. *Cancer Treat Rep* 65:1001, 1981.
29. Eden OB, Goldie W, Wood T, et al: Seizures following intrathecal cytosine-arabinoside in young children with acute lymphoblastic leukemia. *Cancer* 42:53, 1978.
30. Ershler WB, Gilchrist KW, Citrin DL: Adriamycin enhancement of cyclophosphamide-induced bladder injury. *J Urol* 121:123, 1980.
31. Ertel IJ, Nesbitt ME, Hammond D, et al: Effective dose of L-asparaginase for induction of remission in previ-

ously treated children with acute lymphocytic leukemia: a report from Children's Cancer Study Group. *Cancer Res* 39:3895, 1979.

32. Frei E III, Bickers JN, Hewlett JS, et al: Dose, schedule and antitumor studies of arabinosyl-cytosine (NSC-63878). *Cancer Res* 29:1325, 1969.
33. Friedman OM, Myles A, Colvin M: Cyclophosphamide and related phosphoramide mustards: current status and future prospects. In Rosowsky A: *Advances in Cancer Chemotherapy*. New York, Marcel Dekker, 1979.
34. Ginsberg SJ, Comis RL: The pulmonary toxicity of antineoplastic drugs. *Semin Oncol* 9:34, 1982.
35. Gonzales-Vitale JC, Hayes DM, Cvitkovic E, et al: Acute renal failure after cis-dichlorodiammineplatinum (II) and gentamicin cephalotin therapies. *Cancer Treat Rep* 62:693, 1978.
36. Golin AL, Benson RC: Cyclophosphamide hemorrhagic cystitis requiring urinary diversion. *J Urol* 118:110, 1977.
37. Green TP, Mirkin BL: Prevention of cyclophosphamide-induced antidiuresis by furosemide infusion. *Clin Pharmacol Ther* 29:634, 1981.
38. Hacker MP, Newman RA, Ershler WB: The prevention of cyclophosphamide-induced cystitis in mice by disulfiram. *Res Commun Chem Pathol Pharmacol* 35:145, 1982.
39. Harlow PJ, DeClerk YA, Shore NA, et al: A fatal case of inappropriate ADH secretion induced by cyclophosphamide therapy. *Cancer* 44:896, 1979.
40. Ho DHW, Frei E III: Clinical pharmacology of 1-b-D-arabinofuranosyl cytosine. *Clin Pharmacol Ther* 12:944, 1971.
41. Howell SB, Che BBF, Wung WE, et al: Long duration intracavitary infusion of methotrexate with systemic leucovorin protection in patients with malignant effusions. *J Clin Invest* 67:1161, 1978.
42. Howell SB, Pfeifle CE, Wung WE et al: Intraperitoneal cisplatin with systemic thiosulfate protection. *Ann Intern Med* 97:1085–1092, 1982.
43. Jacobs SA, Stoller RG, Chabner BA, et al: 7-hydroxymethotrexate as a urinary metabolite in human subjects and rhesus monkeys receiving high dose methotrexate, *J Clin Invest* 57:534, 1976.
44. Kappus M, Muliawan H, Scheulen ME: In vivo studies of adriamycin-induced lipid peroxidation and effects on ferrous ions. In Homstedt B et al: *Mechanism of Toxicity and Hazard Evaluation*. New York, Elsier/North Holland, 1980, p 635.
45. Legha SS, Dimery IW: High-dose cisplatinum administration without hypertonic saline: observation of disabling neurotoxicity. *J Clin Oncol* 3: 1873–1876, 1985.
46. LePage GA, Whitecar GP: The pharmacology of 6-thioguanine in man. *Cancer Res* 31:1627, 1971.
47. Lopez JA, Nassif E, Vannicola P, et al: Central nervous system pharmacokinetics of high-dose cytosine-arabinoside. *J Neuro-Oncol* 3:119–122, 1985.
48. Madias NE, Harrington JT: Platinum nephrotoxicity. *Am J Med* 65:307–314, 1978.
49. Millard RJ: Busulfan-induced hemorrhagic cystitis. *Urology* 18:143, 1981.
50. Minna JD, Bunn PA: Endocrinologic manifestations of malignancy. In DeVita VT et al: *Cancer: Principles and Practice of Oncolgy*. Philadelphia, JB Lippincott, 1982, p 1478.
51. Morgan RL, Donley PJ, Harrison EF, et al: Protective effect of N-acetylcysteine on the urotoxicity produced by oxazaphosphorine without interference with anticancer activity. *Eur J Cancer Clin Oncol* 18:113, 1982.
52. Myers CE: The pharmacology of the fluoropyrimidines. *Pharmacol Rev* 33:1, 1981.
53. Myers CE, Gianni L, Simone CB, et al: Oxidative destruction of erythrocytes ghost membranes catalyzed by doxorubicin-iron complex. *Biochemistry* 21:1708, 1982.
54. Owellen RJ, Hartke CA, Haines FO: Pharmacokinetics

and metabolism of vinblastine in humans. *Cancer Res* 37:2597, 1977.
55. Ozols RF, Corden BF, Jacob J, et al: High-dose cisplatin in hypertonic saline. *Ann Intern Med* 100:19, 1984.
56. Ozols RF, Ostchega Y, Myers CE et al: High dose cisplatin in hypertonic saline in refractory ovarian cancer. *J Clin Oncol* 3:1246–1250, 1985.
57. Patton TF, Himmelstein KJ, Belt R, et al: Plasma levels and urinary excretion of filterable platinum species following bolus injection and IV infusion of cis-dichlorodiammineplatinum (II) in man. *Cancer Treat Rep* 63:1359, 1979.
58. Pinedo HM, Zarharko DS, Bull JM, et al: The relative contribution of drug concentration and duration of exposure to mouse bone marrow toxicity during continuous methotrexate infusion. *Cancer Res* 37:445, 1977.
59. Posner LE, Dukart G, Goldberg J et al: Mitoxantrone; an overview of safety and toxicity. *Invest New Drugs* 3:123–126, 1985.
60. Powis G, Ames MM, Kovach JS: Dose-dependent pharmacokinetics and cancer chemotherapy. *Cancer Chemother Pharmacol* 6:1, 1981.
61. Pyeritz RE, Droller MJ, Bender WL, et al: An approach to the control of massive hemorrhage in cyclophosphamide-induced cystitis by intravenous vasopressin: a case report. *J Urol* 120:253, 1978.
62. Rabinovitch HH: Simple innocuous treatment of massive cyclophosphamide hemorrhagic cystitis. *Urology* 13:610, 1979.
63. Reed E, Yuspa SH, Zwelling LA, et al: Quantitation of cis-dismminedichloroplatinum(II) (cisplatin)-DNA-intrastrand adducts in testicular and ovarian cancer patients receiving cisplatin chemotherapy. *J Clin Invest* 77:545–550, 1986.
64. Reich E, Franklin RM, Shatkin AJ, et al: Action of actinomycin D on animal cells and tissues. *Proc Natl Acad Sci* 48:1230, 1962.
65. Reich SD: Clinical pharmacology of mitomycin C. In Carter SK, Crooke ST: *Current Status and New Developments*. New York, Academic Press, 1979, p 243.
66. Saiki JH, Thompson S, Smith F, et al: Paraplegia following intrathecal chemotherapy. *Cancer* 29:370, 1972.
67. Sato S, Iwaizumi M, Handa K, et al: Electron spin resonance study on the mode of generation of free radicals of daunomycin, adriamycin, and carboquine in NADPH microsomal system. *Gann* 68:603, 1977.
68. Schilsky RL: Renal and metabolic toxicities of cancer chemotherapy. *Semin Oncol* 9:75, 1982.
69. Skibba JL, Beal DD, Ramirez G, et al: N-demethylation of the antineoplastic agent 4(5) (3,3-dimethyl-1-triazene)-imidazole-5-carboxamide by rats and man. *Cancer Res* 30:147, 1970.
70. Spriggs DR, Griffin J, Wisch J, et al: Clinical pharmacology of low-dose cytosine arabinoside. *Blood* 65:1087, 1985.
71. Spriggs DR, Robbins G, Takvorian T, et al: Continuous infusion of high dose 1-b-D-arabinofuranosylcytosine: a phase I and pharmacological study. *Cancer Res* 45:3932, 1985.
72 Stoller RG, Jacob SA, Drake JC, et al: Pharmacokinetics of high dose methotrexate (NSC-740). *Cancer Chemother Rep* 6:19, 1975.
73. Stein M, Leiter E: Uncontrollable hemorrhage secondary to bladder carcinoma and cyclophosphamide cystitis. *NY State J Med* 10:56, 1978.
74. Stuart JJ, Crocker DL, Roberts HR: Treatment of busulfan-induced pancytopenia. *Arch Intern Med* 136:1181, 1976.
75. Sugiura Y, Kikuchi TK: Formation of superoxide and hydroxy radicals by bleomycin and iron (II), *J Antibiot (Tokyo)* 31:1310, 1978.
76. Swainson CP, Colls BM, Fitzharris BM et al: Cis-platinum and distal renal tubule toxicity. *N Z Med J* 98:375–379, 1895.

77. Thyss A, Milano G, Kubar J et al: Clinical and pharmacokinetic evidence of a life-threatening interaction between methotrexate and ketoprofen. *Lancet* I:256–258, 1986.

78. Tobey RA: Arrest of Chinese hamster cells in G2 following treatment with the antitumor drug bleomycin. *J Cell Physiol* 79:259, 1972.

79. Twentyman PR, Bleehen NM: The sensitivity of bleomycin in spleen colony formating units in the mouse. *Br. J. Cancer* 28:66, 1973.

80. Walker IG, Yatscoff RW, Sridhar R: Hydroxyurea: induction of breaks in template strands of replicating DNA. *Biochem Biophys Res Commun* 77:403, 1977.

81. Wang Y, Suton WW, Romsdahl MM, et al: Age-related pharmacokinetics of high-dose methotrexate in patients with osteosarcoma. *Cancer Treat Rep* 63:405, 1979.

82. Weiss RB, Poster DS: The renal toxicity of cancer chemotherapeutic agents. *Cancer Treat Rev* 9:37, 1982.

83. Wolgemuth RL, Myers CA, Luce JK, et al: Doxorubicin extravasation ulceration: animal model development and testing for potential antidotes. *Proc Am Assoc Cancer Res* 23:171, 1982.

84. Worzalla JF, Kaiman BD, Johnson BM, et al: Metabolism of hexamethylmelamine-ring ^{14}C in rats and man. *Cancer Res* 34:2669, 1974.

85. Zimm S, Narang PK, Riccardi R, et al: The effect of allopurinol on the pharmacokinetics of oral and parenteral 6-mercaptopurine. *Proc Am Assoc Cancer Res* 23:210, 1982.

30

Corticosteroids

Robert Chin, Jr., M.D.

The corticosteroids are a group of compounds that are essential for normal homeostasis and the endocrine response to stress. They are classified by their major physiological action into the glucocorticoids, the mineralocorticoids, and the sex hormones. In caring for the critically ill patient the first two have the most importance; therefore, this chapter concentrates on the pharmacology and clinical uses of the glucocorticoids and mineralocorticoids.

THE HYPOTHALAMUS-PITUITARY-ADRENAL AXIS

The glucocorticoid system involves a governing body (hypothalamus and pituitary), secretory cells (adrenal gland), and target tissues. Corticotropin releasing hormone (CRH) is secreted into a portal system of blood vessels by the hypothalamus and transported to the anterior pituitary gland. CRH stimulates pituitary corticotrophs to secrete adrenocorticotrophic hormone (ACTH). ACTH, in turn, stimulates the adrenal gland to release glucocorticoids. This "regulatory" system is subject to stimulatory and inhibitory input ("positive" and "negative" feedback) (Fig. 30.1).

The free cortisol concentration modulates ACTH release. Decreased plasma cortisol levels lead to an increase in ACTH secretion and a subsequent rise in the cortisol level. Elevated cortisol levels feedback "negatively" on the HPA axis and decreases ACTH release. This servomechanism maintains the plasma cortisol concentration within a normal range (Fig. 30.1).

Exogenous glucocorticoid therapy, however, suppresses the normal function of the HPA axis. In order for the axis to recover, a plasma cortisol nocturnal nadir must occur, which in turn causes ACTH release and adrenal stimulation. Therefore, when a patient has received glucocorticoids for more than 2 weeks, a ta-

pering regimen is required to allow the HPA axis to recover its normal function. The tapering time is usually proportional to the length of time on systemic steroid therapy. Sudden withdrawal may precipitate adrenal crisis or an exacerbation of the underlying disease. The glucocorticoid dosage is progressively lowered and changed from divided daily doses to a single AM dose in order to simulate the normal cortisol circadian rhythm. For example, if a patient is receiving dexamethasone (a long-acting glucocorticoid preparation), 2 mg every 6 hours, the dose may be reduced to 1 mg every 6 hours, and then to a single daily dose. Using an equivalency chart (Table 30.1) one can then change the steroid to an equally po-

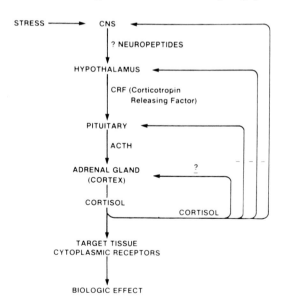

Figure 30.1. The glucocorticoid system. The various levels of influence on corticosteroid production are depicted. Cortisol provides negative feedback at multiple levels to maintain homeostasis. This system operates to produce the optimum level of cortisol required by the organism.

559

Table 30.1
Properties of Commonly Prescribed Corticosteroids[a]

Agent	Dose (mg)	Mineralocorticoid Potency[b]	Glucocorticoid Potency[a]	Duration of Action (hr)
Dexamethasone	0.75	0	25	72
Methylprednisolone	4.0	0.5	5	36
Prednisolone	5.0	0.8	4	24
Prednisone	5.0	0.8	4	24
Cortisol	20.0	1.0	1	8
Hydrocortisone	25.0	1.0	0.8	8
Cortisone	25.0	1.0	0.8	8

[a] From Chernow B: Hormonal and metabolic considerations in critical care medicine. In *Critical Care: State of the Art.* Fullerton, CA, Society of Critical Care Medicine, 1982, vol 3, pp J1.
[b] The higher the number in this column, the more likely it is that the use of the agent will cause metabolic alkalosis.
[c] The higher the number in this column, the more likely the agent will cause suppression of hypothalamic corticotropin-releasing factor (CRF) and pituitary ACTH.

tent amount of a short-acting steroid, e.g., hydrocortisone 75 mg each morning. This allows for a nocturnal cortisol nadir and an ACTH surge. The hydrocortisone dosage is then progressively lowered to 20–30 mg daily and can then be discontinued when the AM plasma cortisol concentration is >10 Ug/dL and/or the

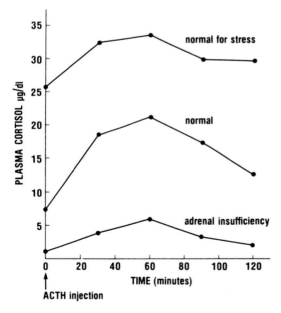

Figure 30.2. The ACTH stimulation test. If synthetic ACTH (250 μg of Cortrosyn) is given at time zero, normally a rise in plasma cortisol of at least 7 μg/dl should occur and the cortisol level should rise to ≥18 μg/dl by 60 minutes. In stress, the response is exaggerated. It is blunted in adrenal insufficiency. (From Chernow B.: Hormonal and metabolic considerations in critical care medicine. In *Critical Care: State of the Art.* Fullerton, CA., Society of Critical Care Medicine, 1982)

ACTH stimulation test is normal (Fig. 30.2). Alternate day therapy with a relatively short-acting glucocorticoid further allows the HPA axis to recover, but does not accelerate the recovery phase after suppression (1, 32). The rapidity of the tapering schedule depends on the continuing control of the underlying disease, the duration and the dose of glucocorticoid therapy, and a previous history of any prior glucocorticoid therapy.

There exists a diurnal rhythm to ACTH and cortisol secretion that is linked to an individual's sleep-wake habits. ACTH and cortisol secretion rise sharply during the 3rd–5th hour of sleep, reach a maximum just after awakening, and then fall through the day to a nadir around the hour of sleep. This rhythm is seen in normal subjects (Fig. 30.3), but may be lost in the critically ill (88) and in those with Cushing's disease (hypercortisolism). The significance of the loss of diurnal cortisol secretion in the critically ill remains unclear.

The hypothalamus-pituitary-adrenal (HPA) axis responds to stresses such as surgery, trauma, hypoglycemia, and sepsis. These stresses override normal regulatory influences and lead to sustained increases in ACTH secretion and plasma cortisol concentrations. The maximum stress-induced output of cortisol is thought to be 200–300 mg/day, with corresponding circulating plasma levels of greater than 60 ug/dl (1650 nmol/liter) (114). The normal daily production of cortisol is estimated to be 13–20 mg (10). The stress response of the HPA axis is likely to be mediated through the CNS. Plasma cortisol levels in critically ill patients are usually elevated above 20 ug/dl (552 nmol/liter), but exhibit a wide baseline range as well as the response to ACTH (31a).

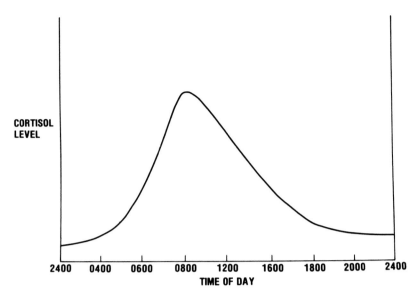

Figure 30.3. The diurnal rhythm of cortisol secretion. Cortisol levels peak in the early morning just after awakening, then fall to a minimum in the evening hours. Therefore, "normal" cortisol levels depend on the time of day samples are drawn and the state of "stress" the patient is in.

However, McKee and Finlay found 18 of 57 severely stressed patients to have cortisol levels less than 13 ug/dl (293 nmol/liter) within 24 hours of death (70a). In a later correspondence, they suggested that those patients with levels less than 13 ug/dl (350 nmol/liter) drawn at 8 AM may benefit from "replacement" doses of hydrocortisone, 100 mg twice daily, if a subsequent synthetic ACTH stimulation test did not elicit a positive response (70a). Low premorbid cortisol levels may be the consequence of overwhelming stress and subsequent adrenal failure (10). The reported incidence of adrenal insufficiency in the critically ill patient, though, appears quite variable, ranging from 0 to 28% (60a). Baseline levels as well as stimulatory testing should be done if adrenal insufficiency is suspected.

PHARMACOLOGY OF ACTH

ACTH is synthesized as a prohormone (pro-ACTH) in the anterior pituitary gland and then is enzymatically cleaved intracellularly to the final product, ACTH. Pro-ACTH is a component of β-lipotropin which also contains the amino acid sequences of β-MSH; α, β, and γ endorphins; and the enkephalins (51) (Fig. 30.4). β-Lipotropin is affected by the same feedback loops as ACTH (51). ACTH is a 39 amino acid polypeptide whose α-component (amino acids 1–24) is responsible for its biological activity, whereas its β-subunit (amino acids 25–39) is considered the antigenic determinant (47). A shortened peptide (α-1–24-corticotropin) consisting of the biologically active α component is clinically available and can be used in place of ACTH, lessening the potential antigenic complications (55). Because of this property, α-1–24-corticotropin has supplanted biological ACTH as the diagnostic agent of choice. Naturally occurring ACTH, derived from mammal pituitaries, is still available in a lyophilized powder as well as in a repository form; 0.25 mg of corticotropin is equivalent to 25 USP units of animal derived ACTH.

The secretion of cortisol, the major endogenous glucocorticoid, by the adrenal cortex is promoted by ACTH via a cAMP mechanism and the activation of phospholipase A. These second messenger systems cause the release of free cholesterol in the adrenal gland and stimulate uptake of cholesterol from plasma lipoproteins. Cholesterol, in the mitochondria, is converted to pregnenolone, the first intermediate in adrenal corticosteroid synthesis (55). ACTH stimulates both steroid synthesis as well as release of preformed steroids (55, 103). The promotion of cortisol production by ACTH is also accompanied by increased synthesis of

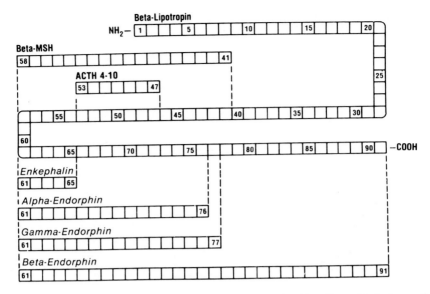

Figure 30.4. The relation between ACTH and β-lipotropin, the endorphins, the enkephalins, and β-MSH are depicted. (From Guillemin R: β-lipotropin and endorphins: implications of current knowledge. In Krieger DT, Hughes, JC (eds): *Neuroendocrinology*. Sunderland, MA, Sinauer Associates, Inc., 1980, p 69.)

other adrenocorticosteroids including corticosterone, aldosterone, and several weak androgens. In addition, ACTH causes an increase in adrenal blood flow (103), adrenal hypertrophy, and the depletion of adrenal ascorbic acid—the clinical importance of this fact is unknown (55).

ACTH increase lipolysis, causes insulin resistance, and increases skin pigmentation (55). These effects usually occur with large supraphysiologic doses. ACTH is rapidly metabolized by intravascular degradation (48), with a plasma half-life of roughly 15 minutes (55).

ACTH is rarely used therapeutically due to the widespread availability of the its end products, the corticosteroids. Requirements for parenteral injection, an inconsistent cortisol response to ACTH, the absence of benefit in HPA axis recovery after ACTH therapy, and the lack of distinct advantages over the corticosteroid preparations have led to its limited use. However, the use of ACTH versus a glucocorticoid agent should not be considered as equivalent since ACTH also stimulates the adrenal secretion of mineralocorticoids and androgens as well as glucocorticoids, and the combination of effects may be different from use of glucocorticoids alone (55). The major use of ACTH or corticotropin today is in the diagnosis of adrenal insufficiency.

CHARACTERIZATION OF THE CORTICOSTEROIDS

The adrenal cortex is histologically divided into three zones: the outer (zona glomerulosa), the middle (zona fasciculata), and the inner (zona reticularis). The zona glomerulosa excretes aldosterone, the major adrenal mineralocorticoid; whereas the zona fasciculata and zona reticularis synthesize the glucocorticoids and the sex hormones (androgens, progestins, and estrogens). The layers are characterized by the presence or absence of certain key enzyme systems in the biosynthetic pathway of the adrenocortical steroids (Fig. 30.5) that lead to a relatively segregated production of the hormones. The initial substrate in corticosteroid synthesis is cholesterol. Most of the cholesterol is derived from circulating sources (60–70%) (e.g., low-density lipoproteins), although the adrenal cortex does have a limited ability to produce it form acetate (55). The major adrenal steroids include cortisol, corticosterone, 11-deoxycorticosterone, aldosterone, and the androgens. Corticosteroids are not stored in the adrenal gland, and secretion rates are directly related to the rate of synthesis (55).

Corticosteroids act by binding to cytoplasmic receptors (55). The hormone-receptor complex then migrates into the nucleus and

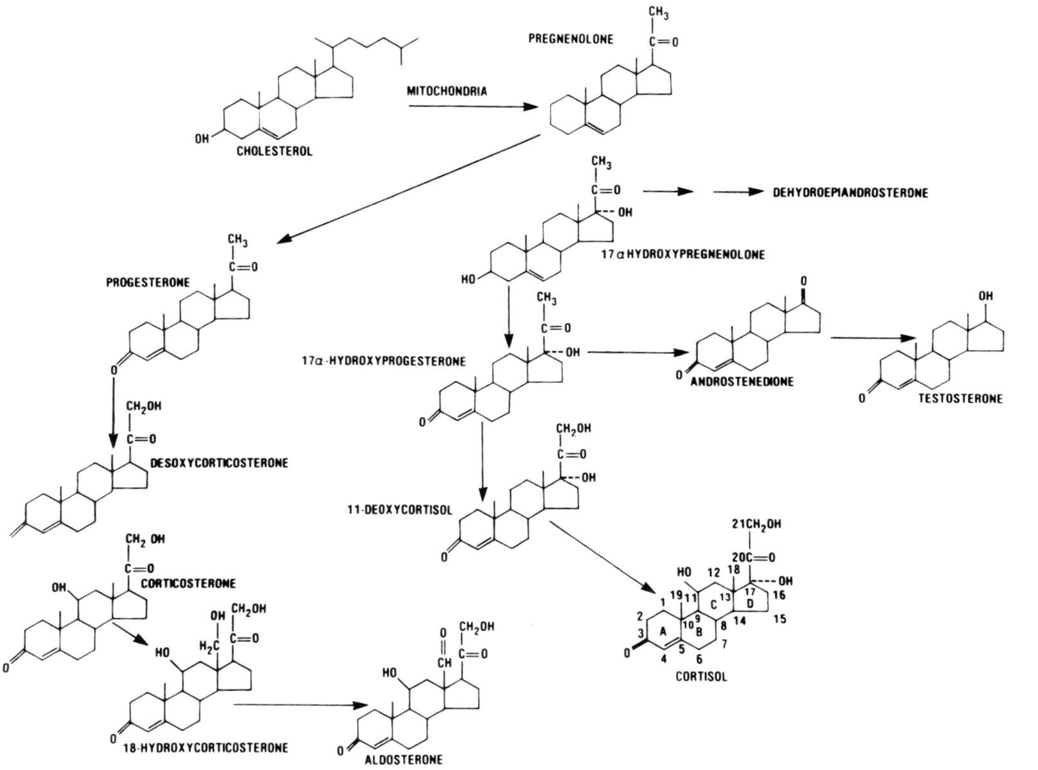

Figure 30.5. The biosynthetic pathway of the corticosteroids. Cholesterol is the precursor of the various endogenous corticosteroids. Pregnenolone is the first intermediate. The pathway pregnenolone then enters to form cortisol, aldosterone, or testosterone is determined by the presence or absence of certain key enzymes in each of the different zones of the adrenal. Cortisol is the major endogenous glucocorticoid. Modification in its structure as shown alters its properties quantitatively in terms of potency and half-life, or qualitatively (e.g., mineralocorticoid vs. glucocorticoid, vs. androgen activity).

associates with the nuclear chromatin leading to specific transcription of DNA and production of new messenger RNA (55). This process directs the synthesis of specific proteins. Because new protein synthesis is involved, a lag time exists between drug administration and the phenotypic expression. This fact is clinically demonstrated in obstructive airway disease, where beneficial steroid effects are delayed approximately 4 hours after initiation of therapy (26). Certain effects, however, have a faster response (e.g., ACTH suppression) and may be mediated by other mechanisms [e.g., changes in membrane-based Ca^{++} transport (78), activation of preformed proteins (78), and increased cellular cAMP (28)].

The corticosteroids are characterized by three 6-carbon rings and one 5-carbon ring with a side chain for a total of 18–21 carbon atoms (Fig. 30.5). The C4-5 double bond and C3 ke-

tone group are required for adrenocorticoid activity. Modifications at the other carbon groups alter anti-inflammatory and carbohydrate (CHO) regulating properties, sodium retention properties, change bioavailability, metabolism, membrane penetration, and affinity for the cell receptors.

A corticosteroid is classified as a glucocorticoid or mineralocorticoid based on its predominant effects on either glucose metabolism (the former) or sodium retention (the latter) (Table 30.1). Glucocorticoid activity promotes hepatic gluconeogenesis and glycogen deposition. Further, amino acids released by the induction of peripheral protein catabolism are converted by the liver into glucose molecules, which causes a negative nitrogen balance (55). Peripheral utilization of glucose is blocked, except in the liver, heart, brain, and red blood cells (55, 103). Consequently, blood glucose levels and urinary nitrogen excretion increase. The antiinflammatory action of the corticosteroids are invariably tied to their relative effects on glucose metabolism. Both require an oxygen group at C-11 in ring C (Fig. 30.5). Modifications of the sterol nucleus, which increase antiinflammatory properties, also cause a concomitant increase in carbohydrate and protein metabolism (31, 55).

Glucocorticoids also affect lipid metabolism by suppressing lipolysis and lipogenesis (103). Truncal obesity, "moon facies", and "buffalo humps" occur in Cushing's syndrome (hypercortisolism). The mechanism behind these changes are unknown, but it is speculated that lipogenesis from secondary increases in circulating insulin levels in response to the steroid-induced hyperglycemia and a general increase in appetite lead to the overall obesity seen (104). A differential response of adipose tissue to the effects of insulin and the glucocorticoids leads to the central obesity (55). The lipolytic effects of epinephrine, norepinephrine, and other adipokinetic agents in fat tissue may be facilitated by glucocorticoid potentiation of the tissue's response to cAMP (55).

The major action of the mineralocorticoids is to enhance ion transport in secretory cells. The principal target of the mineralocorticoids is the renal tubular cell. Sodium reabsorption is facilitated while potassium and hydrogen ion excretion are increased. Addison's disease, or primary adrenocortical failure, is a corticosteroid deficient state characterized by hyponatremia because of renal sodium loss and decreased free water excretion (a cortisol action), hyperkalemia, and extracellular volume contraction. Although glucocorticoid activity is also missing, the disturbances in fluid and electrolyte balance pose the most immediate life-threatening problems and the predominant presenting picture. Other secretory cells (e.g., salivary glands, sweat glands, and exocrine, pancreatic, and gastrointestinal cells) are also affected by mineralocorticoid activity and can contribute to fluid and electrolyte changes.

The secretion of the principal mineralocorticoid, aldosterone, is primarily regulated by potassium balance and the renin-angiotensin axis with only limited influence from ACTH. Therefore, in secondary adrenocorticoid insufficiency (where only ACTH input is lost) major problems with fluid and electrolyte balance are generally not encountered and it is unusual to require extra mineralocorticoid replacement.

The corticosteroids, although defined by their effects on glucose metabolism or the maintenance of fluid and electrolyte balance, also have other effects. They have effects on the cardiovascular system, the central nervous system, skeletal muscle, lymphoid tissue, blood cells, the supportive tissue cells, and the immune system. These effects are expanded on in later sections dealing with either the salutary or detrimental effects of glucocorticoids. The sex hormones are not discussed other than to mention that progesterone can increase minute ventilation and has been used in alveolar hypoventilation syndromes.

GLUCOCORTICOID PHARMACOLOGY

There are several synthetic glucocorticoid compounds available. The relative advantages of each depend on the desired clinical effect, the glucocorticoid/mineralocorticoid potency, the duration of action, and the mode of administration.

Oral glucocorticoid preparations are well absorbed in patients with intact gastrointestinal function. Intravenous administration assures systemic delivery and results in rapid increases in concentrations of the steroid in body fluid. Intramuscular or subcutaneous injections are used primarily as depot forms and result in prolonged absorption and longer duration of activity. The advantage of inhalational, topical, rectal, or intraarticular preparations is their ability to deliver high levels of antiinflammatory drug to local areas, minimizing deleterious systemic effects. However, with the use of plastic occlusive dressings over topically applied glucocorticoid products (with larger doses, or prolonged usage) clinically significant absorption can occur. HPA axis suppression has been reported with increased dosing of inhalational beclamethasone (108).

Circulating corticosteroids are carried reversibly and competitively bound to plasma proteins and in a free metabolically active state (8%) (10). Eighty percent of endogenous cortisol is bound to corticosteroid binding globulin [CBG, or transcortin] and 10% to other plasma proteins including albumin (8). CBG, which is produced by the liver, has a high affinity for cortisol but a low capacitance and is saturated at a plasma cortisol level concentration of 40 μg/dl (8). Above this level, an increased fraction is bound to albumin (low affinity, large capacitance) and more circulates in the free state. Because the free fraction is responsible for the biological activity of cortisol, hypoproteinemia can lead to a higher incidence of "cushingoid" side effects when these patients are placed on glucocorticoid therapy (8, 67). In addition, since the clearance of corticosteroids is primarily hepatic, liver dysfunction with decreased enzyme activity and protein synthesis (e.g., cirrhotics) can also contribute to the increased frequency of side effects (8). The bound cortisol acts as a reservoir for the free hormone since equilibrium between the two states is quickly reached (10). The normal HPA axis is remarkably sensitive to changes in the free cortisol level and can maintain normal homeostasis provided there is no iatrogenic interference.

Based on studies of the metabolism of cortisol, the corticosteroids are converted intrahepatically and extrahepatically into biological inactive metabolites through reduction of the C4-5 double bound or hydroxylation of the C3 ketone group (Fig 30.5) (55). Conjugation of these products with either a sulfate or glucuronic acid then occurs and these water-soluble metabolites are subsequently excreted via the kidneys (55) along with small amounts of unchanged cortisol (103). Structural changes in the hormone can result in slower metabolism and extend the drug's half-life and potency. Cortisone and prednisone require a reduction of the C-11 ketone group for biological activity. Other influences such as concomitant drug therapy can affect clearance, and rapid intravenous bolus administration can lead to early saturation of CBG with an increased fraction of unbound hormone available for activity and clearance (58). Thus, the volume of distribution, the kinetics of the enzyme clearance systems and the functional state of the tissues responsible for metabolism all contribute to the overall clearance rate. However, the half-life of the corticosteroid present in the plasma or tissues does not correlate with the biological or physiological half-life. This fact is because the biological activity of corticosteroids follows second messenger activation and new protein synthesis. This system is associated with delayed onset and prolonged activity that does not directly correlate with plasma levels of the corticosteroids. The durations of physiologic action of the major commercial preparations are listed in Table 30.1.

Different glucocorticoids have different avidity for the cytoplasmic steroid receptors and this fact, in part, contributes to their relative strengths. Dexamethasone and prednisolone have eight times and two times, respectively, the affinity of cortisol for these receptors (7).

On a cellular level, there is also heterogeneity of receptor numbers and responsiveness in different cell populations (55). Other factors such as route and rapidity of administration, time after administration, clearance, and the bioassays used to evaluate activity also influence the overall quantification of relative strengths of specific glucocorticoids (74, 104). Mineralocorticoid activity is measured by its ability to sustain life in adrenalectomized animals and its effects on sodium retention; whereas glucocorticoid activity is judged by the amount of liver glycogen deposited, which parallels its lymphoid tissue involution and antiinflammatory actions (55). Thus, the relative potencies of the various corticosteroid compounds may be only rough guides to their biological activities.

Consideration of the aforementioned kinetics and the relative glucocorticoid to mineralocorticoid activity is important in the choice of a steroid. An agent with increasing mineralocorticoid activity increases the risk of steroid-mediated metabolic alkalosis and sodium and fluid retention. The former can be significant in the treatment of patients with chronic obstructive lung disease. Many of these patients develop a metabolic alkalosis while on glucocorticoid therapy and compensate to maintain a normal pH with alveolar hypoventilation, which leads to hypercapnia and a respiratory acidosis (20–22). These effects may impair weaning from the ventilator. A preparation, such as methylprednisolone, with less mineralocorticoid activity may be preferable to cortisol in many of these instances. Fluid and sodium retention is a major concern in states already characterized by fluid overload such as congestive heart failure, the nephrotic syndrome and cirrhosis, and where any further sodium and fluid retention might aggravate the condition being treated, such as increased intracranial pressure secondary to cerebral edema; again prednisolone or dexamethasone is preferred in these situations. Conversely, hydrocortisone is preferable to methylprednisolone in acute adrenal crisis, since the former provides needed mineralocorticoid activity. In active liver disease, prednisolone is preferred over prednisone, because of the latter's requirement for hepatic hydroxylation to gain agonist activity (6). In addition, abnormal liver function may require lower doses of a glucocorticoid for the desired effect because of decreases in hepatic clearance and protein binding secondary to hypoproteinemia (6, 65).

Drug interactions between steroids and other

medications are important. Estrogens can increase CBG levels and total plasma cortisol (55). Troleandomycin, a macrolide antibiotic, reportedly extends the beneficial action of methylprednisolone, which allows lower doses to be used in asthma (98). Drugs such as phenytoin, barbiturates, and rifampin increase the clearance of synthetic corticosteroids by induction of hepatic microsomal enzymes (20, 35, 103). Corticosteroid therapy lessens the anticoagulation produced by ethylbiscoumacetate (18) and can augment renal clearance of salicylates (63). In addition, hydrocortisone prolongs the half-life of nortriptyline (106).

STEROID PREPARATIONS

There are many commercially available steroid preparations for topical, aerosol, intravenous, intramuscular, subcutaneous, rectal, and oral administration. Because of their wide range of clinical applicability, both proven and empirical, they are invariably encountered by most physicians. A short summary of the most commonly used products in the critical care setting follows.

Hydrocortisone

Hydrocortisone is the synthetic equivalent to cortisol, the principal endogenous glucocorticoid. Because of this fact, it is assigned the relative glucocorticoid activity of 1.0 and is the standard with which other glucocorticoids are compared. The quality that separates it from the other major glucocorticoid agents is its mineralocorticoid activity (approximately 1% that of aldosterone) (8). It is therefore the glucocorticoid of choice in the physiologic replacement of corticosteroids (20 mg in the AM and 10 mg in the PM) in primary adrenocortical failure. This same property hinders its use as an antiinflammatory agent because of the fluid and electrolyte disorders it can engender. It is available in intravenous and oral forms with different ester conjugates [sodium succinate, sodium phosphate, and cypionate; the latter is poorly soluble and used only orally (114)]. It also can be used in topical (skin and ophthalmological), rectal, depot, and intravaginal forms. Its plasma half-life is 80–115 minutes (6) and it has a relatively short duration of action of 8 hours.

Cortisone

Cortisone is the 11-keto form of cortisol. It is essentially equivalent to hydrocortisone but requires hepatic hydroxylation at C-11 to form cortisol, its active metabolite, and as a result is 25% less potent (114). It is unsuitable for local use because it is inactive in its native state.

Prednisolone

A double bond in position C1-C2 increases the glucocorticoid activity of prednisolone relative to its mineralocorticoid activity. This quality allows lower doses to be given compared with cortisol, for the same antiinflammatory response, with less sodium retention. The unsaturated bond in C1-C2 also slows the metabolism of the drug (55). Its plasma half-life is 115–252 minutes (6) and the duration of action is 24 hours. The half-life may be significantly prolonged in renal failure (61). It has four times the glucocorticoid potency of cortisol but only 0.8 times the mineralocorticoid action. It is available in oral, topical, and parental forms (conjugated with either acetate, sodium phosphate, or tebutate esters) (55).

Methylprednisolone

This congener of prednisolone has a methyl group added to C-6 that further increases its antiinflammatory activity. The plasma half-life is between 78 and 188 minutes (6) and its duration of action is 24–36 hours. Methylprednisolone has five times the glucocorticoid activity of cortisol and 0.5 times the mineralocorticoid potency. It is the most common intravenous steroid used in this country today. It is available in intravenous (acetate or sodium succinate esters), oral, and depot forms.

Prednisone

Hepatic hydroxylation of the C-11 keto group is necessary to convert prednisone from a weak steroid antagonist to a potent agonist. It has a relative activity similar to that of prednisolone. The plasma half-life is 160 minutes and the duration of action is 24 hours. It is well absorbed from the gastrointestinal tract (114).

Dexamethasone

Dexamethasone is a flourinated hydrocarbon with a flourine atom at C-9, a double bond between C-1 and C-2, and a methyl group at C-16 distinguishing it from cortisol. Each of these modifications serves to increase the antiinflammatory action and decrease the mineralocorticoid activity. Available in the parenteral (acetate or sodiumphosphate ester), oral, and topical form, it has 25 times the glucocorticoid strength of cortisol and negligible mineralocorticoid activity. The plasma half-life is 110–120 minutes and duration of action is 72 hours (6). However, in renal failure the clearance may be increased, whereas in hepatic dysfunction it is prolonged (61). It is best utilized in situations where a strong antiinflammatory agent is required, but fluid or sodium retention is undesirable (e.g., cerebral edema secondary to tumor). A disadvantage is its long duration of action, which extends HPA axis suppression and makes it a poor choice when recovery of the HPA axis is wanted.

Deflazacort

Deflazacort is a new product and is not currently available on the U.S. market. It reportedly has less hyperglycemic and osteoporotic effects than equivalent antiinflammatory doses of prednisone (1.2mg = 1mg). Further studies on this drug should be forthcoming (14).

Triamcinolone, Betamethasone, Flunisolide, and Beclomethasone

These are halogenated glucocorticoids with increased antiinflammatory activity as compared with cortisol. Triamcinolone, Betamethasone, and flunisolide are flourinated, whereas beclomethasone is chlorinated. They are long-acting agents. Triamcinolone can be used in an oral, parenteral, topical, or inhalational form. Beclomethasone dipropionate's major use is as an inhaled drug to control asthma, which enables the reduction of systemic doses. The usual daily dose is 400 μg/day (2–4 puffs four times a day, each puff equals approximately 40 μg). In terms of HPA axis suppression, 500–600 μg/day of inhaled beclomethasone is equivalent to 20 mg of oral prednisone administered on alternate days (100).

BENEFICIAL EFFECTS OF GLUCOCORTICOID THERAPY

Glucocorticoids have therapeutic benefits in a wide array of clinical disorders (Table 30.2). Other than adrenal replacement therapy, the antiinflammatory and/or immunosuppressive actions are their principal desired qualities. Although the proposed mechanism for this action has been rather well defined, the clinical relevancy of these mechanisms is not known with certainty.

The key to glucocorticoid antiinflammatory activity is an alteration of the immune response to activating stimuli. Changes in the migratory patterns and compartmentalization of the immune cells may be partly responsible for this effect. Glucocorticoids accelerate the release of granulocytes from marrow stores, but reduce their departure from the intravascular space to sites of inflammation and extend their half-lives (80). Granulocytic adherence to endothelial cells as well as granulocytic production of plasminogen activator are lessened (55). Plasminogen activator, through the formation of plasmin, may allow easier migration of neutrophils into areas of inflammation by hydrolysis of fibrin laid down by the inflammatory response (55). Binding of complement and IgE and IgG antibodies to inflammatory cell receptors sites is also diminished (78). The end result is a neutrophilic granulocytosis but reduced migration and accumulation at inflammatory sites. However, chemotaxis and phagocytosis of the polymorphonuclear cells (PMNS) does not seem to be affected (89). Steroid-induced granulocytosis may be differentiated from the leukocytosis associated with infections by review of the peripheral blood smear. Shoenfield and associates showed that an increase in premature white cell forms (bands) of >6% and the appearance of toxic granulations favored the diagnosis of infection (90). Clinically, fever is also suppressed by glucocorticoid therapy, the result of reduced leukocyte pyrogen production [demonstrated in vitro (40)] and/or the inhibition of interleukin-1 release, an endogenous pyrogen, from monocytes (10). The contribution of steroid-induced granulocytic lysosomal stabilization to their antiinflammatory effects is unclear. Most authors believe that steroid influence on the migratory patterns of inflammatory cells and the release of their mediators (such as prostaglandins and their derivatives) are the more significant effects.

Table 30.2
Clinical Applications of Glucocorticoid Therapy in Critical Care

Cardiovascular	*Hematological*
Shock States	Hemolytic anemias
Anaphylactic	Idiopathic thrombocytopenic purpura
Septic[a]	*Infections*
Hypovolemic[a]	Septic shock[a]
Mixed[a]	*Malignancy*
Altered Immune States	Multiple myeloma
Collagen-vascular diseases	Lymphomas
Systemic lupus erythematosus	Acute lymphocytic leukemias
Polymyositis/dematomyositis	Breast Cancer
Rheumatoid arthritis	*Neonatalogy*
Mixed connective tissue disease	Neonatal respiratory distress syndrome (antenatal)
Disorders characterized by a predominant	*Neurological*
vasculitis	Multiple sclerosis[a]
Sarcoidosis	Cord compression
Hypersensitivity reactions	Cerebral edema (vasogenic edema)
Drug and contrast dye reactions	Myasthenia gravis
Serum sickness	Guillain-Barre[a]
Urticaria	*Ophthalmological*
Allergic rhinnitis	Acute uveitis
Bee stings	Choroiditis
Anaphylaxis	Optic neuritis
Dermatological	*Pulmonary*
Pemphigus	Asthma/reversible obstructive disease
Pemphigoid	Adult respiratory distress syndrome[a]
Erythema multiforme	Interstitial pneumonitis
Toxic epidermolysis necrosis	Vasculitic disorders of the respiratory tract, e.g.
Contact dermatitis	Wegener's granulomatosis, Churg-Strauss,
Endocrine	Goodpasture's syndrome, etc.
Adrenal insufficiency: primary and secondary	Bronchiolitis obliterans
Hypercalcemia	Nitrous dioxide gas exposure
Gastrointestinal	*Renal*
Inflammatory bowel disease	Cetain glomerulonephritis syndromes
Crohn's disease	*Transplant*
Ulcerative colitis	Transplant rejection

[a] Areas of controversy in the clinical efficacy of glucocorticoid therapy

In contrast, steroids cause the circulating mononuclear, eosinophilic, and basophilic populations to fall, with a maximum lymphocytopenia occurring 4–6 hours after administration and recovery occurring by 24 hours (41). Pharmacological doses of glucocorticoids result in a striking reduction in thymic weight and spleen and peripheral lymph node size in corticosteroid-sensitive species (e.g., mouse, rat, and rabbit) (23). Cell cultures of chromium-tagged mouse thymus cells admixed with cortisol succinate undergo cell lysis; however, human (corticosteroid resistant species) thymus cells do not (23). Although a certain minority of human lymphocytes have been shown to be sensitive to destruction in the presence of steroids, it is doubtful that cytolysis significantly contributes to the lymphocytopenia seen in humans (28). Cellular redistribution of recirculating intravascular lymphocytes into the extravascular space

(probably bone marrow) is primarily responsible for the observed lymphocytopenia (28). Both B- and T-cell lymphocytes are affected; but the T-cells more so perhaps because the subcellular rate of metabolism of cortisol is greater in the B cell than the T cell (28). The changes in the migratory patterns may be mediated through steroid-induced changes on the lymphocyte surface (28, 41).

Lymphocytic function is affected by glucocorticoid therapy. Clinically, delayed hypersensitivity is impaired with the subsequent development of anergy. Various theories have been proposed to explain this phenomena. The most recent data suggest that interference with soluble mediators (e.g., lymphokines, macrophage inhibition factor) released from activated lymphocytes alters the recruitment of other lymphocytes and cells (e.g., macrophages) (41). T-cell processing of antigen is normal after steroid administration, but lymphocyte migration and attraction to an inflammatory site is not (116). Proliferation of lymphocytes after a stimulus is also reduced both in vitro and in vivo, as is interleukin-1 stimulation of interleukin-2 production (28). Interleukin 1 is a macrophage-derived mediator that contributes to the activation of T cells upon antigen presentation; interleukin 2 is a T-cell growth factor and required for cytotoxic T-cell development (117). Corticosteroid effects on the humoral system and B-cell function are less clear. Studies have shown that serum IgG levels, but not IgE (15, 41) and complement (4, 41) levels are diminished after steroid administration. Fauci and Cupps suggest that the glucocorticoid effects on monocytes, T lymphocytes, and on B-cells all can influence the B-lymphocyte response (28). Inhibition of immune complex movement across basement membranes in rabbits by steroids has also been reported (41). The reticuloendothelial system is impaired with less than optimum removal of opsinized and nonopsinized substances (4, 5). Circulating monocytes and tissue macrophages are reduced in number (89). Although phagocytosis is intact, the intracellular killing of microorganisms is abnormal.

Eosinopenia also occurs and is likely to be secondary to redistribution of these cells as opposed to destruction, and follows the same time course as for lymphocytopenia (89). The mechanisms of steroid influence and its importance on eosinophilic migration, and basophilic and mast cell function (particularly histamine release) in type I immediate allergic reactions (anaphylaxis) are not fully understood. The clinical efficacy of steroids in allergic responses may be based more on its effects on the late phases of the allergic response rather than their effects on the immediate phase (89).

Local factors induced by glucocorticoid treatment may also modify the inflammatory response. Stabilization of the microcirculation via decreased endothelial adherence of PMNs (89) and vasoconstriction through augmentation of adrenergic activity (40) interferes with the increased capillary permeability brought on by acute inflammation, reducing plasma and protein exudation (50). Furthermore the release of vasoactive kinins is blocked by steroids and this action may lessen the local immune response to a stimulus (25). This combined with the action on the effector cells (PMNs, lymphocytes, eosinophils, basophils, and monocytes/macrophages), as described

above, limits the normal inflammatory response.

The vast array of effects leading to the antiinflammatory capability of the glucocorticoids may be all tied to a group of cellular proteins called "lipocortins" (lipomodulin, macrocortin) that are regulated by the presence of steroid activity (46). The lipocortins block phospholipase A, an enzyme responsible for the liberation of arachidonic acid from membrane phospholipids. Through both the cyclooxygenase and lipoxygenase pathways, arachidonic acid is the common precursor of the prostaglandins, leukotrienes, and platelet activating factor, which are proposed mediators of inflammation. Phospholipase A also plays a role in the signal translation by the PMNs that enables them to respond to a stimulus (46). Changes induced by steroids in membrane-bound Ca^{++} may also affect mediator release (78). The relative contributions of these effects to the overall immunosuppresive effects of steroids is speculative, but they provide a cellular and subcellular theoretical model for this action. By interfering with the normal immune response to an antigen/stimulus and the resultant cell mediator release, glucocorticoids may interrupt the cascade that promulgates the inflammatory response.

The glucocorticoids can be tumorcidal in certain tumor cell lines (lymphoproliferative malignancies), but the mechanism is unknown. Steroid efficacy in the treatment of other tumors (breast carcinoma, juvenile hemangiomas) is also puzzling, but perhaps related to steroid-induced inhibition of cellular growth and in breast cancer through adrenocorticoid suppression of androgen production (12, 55, 104).

The cardiovascular system in Addison's disease is characterized by a hypodynamic state. Corticosteroid replacement returns the cardiac function to normal, but it is not clear whether this action is due to glucocorticoid activity or mineralocorticoid activity with reestablishment of a normal volume status. The independent actions of glucocorticoids on cardiac inotropy and/or chronotropy, and smooth muscle vascular tone are not fully elucidated. They could play a "helper" role in the interactions of other vasoactive hormones (e.g., catecholamines) with their target organs. Hypertension is commonly seen in hypercortisol states and is not necessarily related to mineralocorticoid effects. The mechanism of action of glucocorticoids when used in suprapharmacologic doses in shock states is equally unclear. Fauci postulates that selective vasoconstriction of certain capillary beds through a direct action or potentiation of α-adrenergic drugs stabilizes the cardiovascular system and possibly increases cardiac inotropy and cardiac output, which preserves capillary wall integrity and arrests tissue destruction (40). An alternate theory is that ACTH and β-lipotropin, the parent compound of the endorphins and enkephalins (Fig. 30.4), are secreted simultaneously by the pituitary gland in response to sepsis, hemorrhage, or other stresses. Their secretion may be inhibited by elevated levels of glucocorticoid activity (51). This fact is important because endogenous opioid peptides such as endorphins are released during a shock state and may contribute to hypotension (110). Blockage of prostaglandin synthesis [e.g., prostacyclin (PGI_2), a vasodilator] may also preserve vascular tone (10).

A delayed bronchodilatory effect is seen in severe asthmatics after glucocorticoid therapy (89). Mechanisms that may be responsible for these effects include an increased sensitivity to β-adrenergic agents by up-regulation of β-receptors with an increase in their numbers and sensitivity; an antiinflammatory effect that reduces cellular infiltrates and exudates, especially in the late phase of asthma; a reduction in target tissue responsiveness to inflammatory mediators (e.g., histamine, platelet-activating factor, leukotrienes, and cyclooxygenase prostaglandin derivatives) (78); an inhibition of mucous production (69); a decrease in epithelial cell permeability (89); a decrease in IgE receptor binding (114); and altered Ca^{++} transmembrane movement, decreasing smooth muscle reactivity (78). However, glucocorticoids should not be used alone in obstructive pulmonary disease but as an adjunct to xanthine and β-adrenergic bronchodilators (81, 100).

Glucocorticoids may reduce circulating calcium levels in hypercalcemic patients. Reduced calcium absorption from the intestines, inhibition of 1,25 dihydroxycholecalciferol (vitamin D) production, increased renal excretion of calcium, and redistribution of calcium from the extracellular into intracellular space contribute to the lowering of the serum calcium (6, 55). These effects are best observed in the hypercalcemia associated with sarcoidosis and are less effective in hypercalcemia secondary to increased parathormone levels. The use of glucocorticoids with calcitonin lengthens the calcium-lowering effects of the latter (9).

The most apparent and least controversial indication for corticosteroid use is in adrenocorticoid hormone replacement therapy. The corticosteroids have a variety of complex interactions with many of the other endogenous hormones and other organ systems that maintain homeostasis and a normal response to stress. The musculoskeletal system appears to be dependent on the physiological presence of steroid activity for normal function (55). Glucocorticoids have a "permissive" function in the sympathetic nervous system and cross the blood-brain barrier to interact with the central nervous system (103). Maintenance of the plasma glucose for nutritional needs of the CNS and erythrocytes and fluid and electrolyte balance depends on corticosteroid influences.

CLINICAL COMPLICATIONS OF GLUCOCORTICOID THERAPY

The side effects of therapy (Table 30.3) can be divided into those expected to occur with physiologic doses, those with pharmacologic doses, and those that are unexpected. They can be further subdivided into those seen with acute therapy and those with more chronic therapy. Proper steroid choice, dosage, dosing interval, and length of therapy along with an intelligent choice of endpoints of therapy can minimize the complications. Some toxicities are so entangled with the disease process being treated, that it is difficult to ascertain an independent effect from the glucocorticoids. Although the intensivist is more concerned with the side effects of acute glucocorticoid therapy, the metabolic changes induced by chronic therapy must be anticipated and recognized.

There is little danger in a short course of high-dose steroid therapy, even in the critically ill patient, but since not all the facts are known regarding corticosteroid actions, there may be unknown deleterious effects. Massive rapid bolus doses of 1 g or greater have been associated with sudden death and cardiovascular collapse when given concurrently with furosemide (70, 97). Although it is not known what the exact reason for this problem is (e.g., rapid electrolyte shifts), it is prudent to give large doses slowly. Glucose intolerance with glycosuria, metabolic alkalosis, sodium and fluid retention, the risk of peptic ulceration, psychosis and an impairment of host immune defenses are troublesome, but are more related to long courses of therapy rather than one- or two-dose therapy.

Table 30.3
Deleterious Effects of Glucocorticoid Therapy[a]

Cardiovascular
  Cardiovascular collapse and sudden death
    associated with rapid intravenous administration
  Hypertension
  Fluid and sodium retention with edema
  Hypokalemic metabolic alkalosis
  Accelerated atherosclerosis leading to coronary
    vascular disease
Musculoskeletal
  Proximal myopathy
  Osteoporosis of trabecular bones
  Aseptic necrosis of bones
Gastrointestinal
  Peptic ulceration, hemorrhage, and perforation
  Pancreatitis
  Intestinal perforation
Central Nervous System
  Psychiatric disturbances
    Mild euphoria
    Psychosis
    Dementia
  Pseudotumor cerebri
Ophthalmological
  Ocular hypertension
  Subcapsular cataracts
  Infectious keratitis
  Delayed healing of the cornea
Dermatological
  Hirsutism
  Atrophy of the skin and subcutaneous tissue
  Acne
  Striae
  Telangiectasias
Hematological and Immunological
  Neutrophilic granulocytosis
  Monocytopenia
  Eosinopenia
  Erythrocytosis and thrombocytosis
  Suppression of immune and inflammatory
    response (immunosurveillance)
    Effects on circulating inflammatory cells
    Effects on the local mediators including
      prostaglandins
    Effects on the reticuloendothelial system
Hypersensitivity Reactions
  ACTH
  Glucocorticoid preparations
Metabolic and Endocrinological
  Glucose intolerance (hepatic gluconeogenesis,
    glycogen deposition, and inhibition of peripheral
    glucose utilization)
  Increased appetite and weight gain
  Altered lipid metabolism and deposition
  Peripheral protein catabolism
  Impaired skeletal growth in children
  Poor wound healing
  Secondary amenorrhea
  HPA suppression leading to secondary adrenal
    insufficiency

[a] Adapted from Melby JC: Systemic corticosteroid
therapy: pharmacology and endocrinologic considerations. *Ann Intern Med* 81:505, 1974.

Many of the complications seen with glucocorticoid therapy are magnified with higher doses and longer duration of therapy. Steroid myopathy involving the proximal musculature, commonly develops after prolonged therapy (weeks to months), and for the most part is reversible with the cessation of therapy. Muscle enzymes (CPK, aldolase) (32, 55) are not elevated and can be used to distinguish it from a primary myositis (e.g., polymyositis). In those requiring chronic therapy, one report suggests that isokinetic exercise may be able to partially reverse the muscle wasting and atrophy (57). Although an increased incidence of osteoporosis has not been consistently found in all patients receiving chronic glucocorticoid treatment, those receiving pharmacological doses for long periods of time and those with predisposing disorders (e.g., rheumatoid arthritis, low calcium intake, immobilization, and the perimenopausal female) are most likely to develop this problem. A study of asthmatics, over the age of 40, on daily or alternate-day glucocorticoid therapy for at least 1 year compared with an age-matched group of asthmatics who did not require long-term steroid therapy found that while 11% of the steroid group had multiple fractures (usually vertebral compression or rib fractures associated with tussive episodes), no fractures where seen in the nonsteroid group (2). The mean daily steroid dose in the fracture group was 30 mg of prednisone. A prospective study done by the same group on 30 patients (age 20–70) showed that 42% receiving long-term steroids had similar fractures, but no fractures were seen in those that did not require such therapy (2). Although bone density studies done on the radius by photon absorptiometry revealed that trabecular, but not cortical, bone mass was reduced in the chronic steroid group, no significant correlation could be found between bone density and dose or duration of steroid therapy (2). Therefore, despite earlier studies suggesting less of an association (86), it is reasonable to encourage regular exercise and to add supplemental oral calcium (1.5–2 g/day) and estrogen therapy (in females, conjugated estrogens 0.625 mg/day), unless otherwise contraindicated, to those in the high-risk categories. Preventive measures in males (who appear at less risk than females), including vitamin D supplementation, calcitonin therapy, and the use of fluoride, require further clarification before recommendations can be made. Aseptic necrosis of the bone is also linked to chronic steroid therapy, occurring in approximately 1% of a steroid-dependent population (32, 85), with a higher incidence (14–50%) occurring in selected populations such as patients with systemic lupus erythematosis (SLE) (115). Sites at risk for aspetic necrosis include the femoral heads, knees, and shoulders. Higher daily steroid doses, Cushingoid changes, and Raynaud's phenomena are associated with an increased incidence of ischemic necrosis in patients with SLE (115).

The frequency of steroid-induced peptic ulceration of the gastrointestinal tract remains contraversial, but 40 mg of prednisone for greater than 2 weeks probably predisposes to ulcer formation. Conn and Blitzer in 1976 (27) reviewed a number of studies but did not find a significant increase in the incidence of peptic ulceration, hemorrhage, and/or perforation in a steroid-treated group compared with controls. A divergence between the groups did appear when the total dose of steroids was considered (with greater than 1 g of prednisone, the ulcer rate was 5.3% in contrast to 2.5% in the placebo group). Although Conn did not find a proclivity toward peptic ulceration in his retrospective study, he emphasized that ". . . one must not conclude that steroids are in no way associated with the development of peptic ulcer . . ." (27); individual cohorts treated with steroids such as those with cirrhotic or nephrotic disease and those receiving large total doses of steroids may indeed have an increased tendency toward ulceration (27). Messer and associates in 1983 reexamined the literature and found an increased incidence of peptic ulceration and gastrointestinal hemorrhage in patients receiving corticosteroid treatment (76). Proposed avenues for the pathogenesis of steroid-related ulcers include increased acid production (as documented in dogs) (42), decreased mucus production by the gastric lining cells (42, 75) and a defective capacity of the mucosal cells to repair and regenerate themselves (42). Recently, certain classes of prostaglandins (PGE_2) have been noted to exhibit a "cytoprotective" effect on gastric cells. Since glucocorticoids appear capable of blocking prostaglandin formation through inhibitory action on Phospholipase A, this action may cause the gastric cells to lose their prostaglandin cytoprotection. This behavior is particularly important in critically ill patients who are already at risk for stress ulceration. The addition of antacids (54), sucralfate, or perhaps enteral feedings (84) may protect the gastric cell lining.

Pancreatitis occurs with an increased frequency in those on steroid therapy, but is not a common clinical problem. A direct relationship between corticosteroids and intestinal perforation remains unproven since reported cases have occurred in patients with inflammatory bowel disease (32).

Psychiatric disturbances seen with glucocorticoid therapy range from mild euphoria to frank psychosis and dementia (107). These reactions are reversible with discontinuation of the steroid and are not necessarily related to the pretreatment psyche (32). Larger doses (≥ 40 mg of prednisone/day) are associated with a higher frequency of psychiatric problems. Onset of the mental disturbances usually occurs within 10 days of starting therapy (118). Lithium prophylaxis may help prevent the development of steroid-induced psychosis if continued therapy is required (49). Dexamethasone may cause less problems in this regard than either cortisol or prednisone (44). Uncommon cases of pseudotumor cerebri have been reported in children and adults on glucocorticoid therapy (31, 59, 109). Ocular hypertension and posterior subcapsular cataracts are ophthalmological manifestations of chronic therapy; the former is reversible with the cessation of therapy, but the latter is not. Additionally, topical ophthalmological preparations can lead to fungal keratitis, worsening of herpes keratitis, and delayed healing of the cornea. Hirsutism, thinning of the skin with atrophy, poor wound repair, acne, striae, and telangiectasias are common skin complications of steroid administration.

The effects of glucocorticoids on the hematologic and immune systems have already been discussed. Neutrophilic granulocytosis, monocytopenia, and eosinopenia are common laboratory findings. An elevation in the circulating erythrocyte and platelet levels may also be seen (103). Due to the reduction in immune surveillance, especially in the cell-mediated response, infections with bacteria, viruses, fungi, and parasites (especially Pneumocystis carnii) complicate long-term therapy. Fauci and associates (41) reported that the incidence and frequency of infections rose with higher doses of steroids in patients with SLE. Potential problems from steroid therapy also result from the masking of the usual signs of inflammation (rubor, calor, dolor, and tumor) and delaying early recognition of a clinically significant infection. The frequency of reactivation tuberculosis with steroid therapy remains unclear. However, in at least asthmatics on chronic steroid therapy, there appears to be no increase in reactivation tuberculosis (34). Additionally, only one of 25 patients with chronic active hepatitis treated with steroids in Hong Kong (where tuberculosis is likely to be more endemic than in the United States) developed tuberculosis (66). Still, it is suggested that isoniazid (INH) 300 mg/day for 1 year, be given prophylactically to chronic steroid patients who have a known positive PPD skin test and have not been previously treated (38, 39). Cutaneous anergy is common while on daily doses of prednisone, developing within a few days of therapy and resolving after 10–14 days of steroid cessation (40).

Hypersensitivity to commercial glucocorticoid products is known (47, 105) but can vary with different products (e.g., hydrocortisone vs. prednisone vs. dexamethasone) (73). Some patients may require desensitization (24).

Normal metabolism is markedly altered by steroid therapy. Skeletal growth is impaired in children on chronic therapy. Switching to alternate-day administration allows some improvement. Because of the effect of the steroid on glucose metabolism and stimulation of glucagon secretion (68), hyperglycemia is commonly encountered, but the development of ketosis or acidosis associated with absolute insulin deficiency is rare. Treatment strategies consist of dietary manipulation and insulin therapy and do not differ from those of non-steroid-induced diabetes mellitus. Control of the hyperglycemia is especially imperative in the critically ill patient so as to avoid glucosuria (with a wasting of calories) and an osmotic diuresis, which interferes with the accurate assessment of the hourly urine output. Exogenous glucocorticoid therapy may also contribute to the abnormal glucose production and utilization seen in burn patients (113). The Cushingoid appearance (moon facies, buffalo hump, and centripetal obesity) is a result of altered lipid metabolism. Abnormal fat accumulation can also be seen in the mediastinum (thoracic lipomatosis; easily distinguished by computer tomography scan (64) from other malignant causes) or can imitate a pericardial effusion (79). Weight gain and an increased appetite are typically seen with chronic therapy. In addition, it has been speculated that accelerated atherosclerosis may be a complication of long-term steroid administration leading to an increased mortality from cardiovascular disease (80).

Fluid and salt retention occurs because of excessive mineralocorticoid activity. This effect is greater with the preparations that have a high mineralocorticoid-glucocorticoid ratio. Sodium retention at the expense of hydrogen ion excretion can lead to a metabolic alkalosis and consequently hypercapnia due to respiratory compensation (20–22). This effect can cause difficulty in weaning patients from the ventilator. Edema and hypertension because of augmented fluid and sodium retention can also be seen. Substitution of an agent with less mineralocorticoid activity such as prednisone or dexamethasone may ameliorate the problem (22).

Glucocorticoid use in human pregnancy is relatively safe. Although animal data have suggested an increased prevalence of fetal wastage and cleft palates in corticosteroid-treated rats (30, 101), a recent report found no fetal malformations, neonatal deaths, or maternal death in 56 women with severe asthma requiring systemic glucocorticoids and/or inhaled steroids (45). Neonatal adrenal insufficiency is also a rarity despite maternal use of pharmacological doses of steroids (30). Poor penetration of prednisone and/or prednisolone through the placenta may account for this observation (101). Despite this fact, careful monitoring of the newborn for signs of adrenal insufficiency is indicated because of its potential devastating effects but ease of treatment. Glucocorticoids are excreted in breast milk and nursing infants should be observed for hypercortisol effects (40).

An important consequence of exogenous glucocorticoid therapy is adrenal insufficiency caused by HPA axis suppression. Although numerous studies have been performed regarding this aspect, the data are difficult to interpret because of the heterogeneity of the patient populations, the steroid dose, the frequency of administration, the length of therapy, and the means used to assess adrenal insufficiency (6). It is clear, however, that prolonged therapy with glucocorticoids will cause suppression of the HPA axis for several months to a year after withdrawal of therapy (50) and is often asymptomatic. The hypothalamic-pituitary axis recovers first with the return of a normal diurnal secretion of ACTH. This ACTH secretion is followed by recovery of the adrenal gland (50, 104). The exogenous administration of ACTH does not hasten the recovery (55, 40). Streck and Lockwood (96) reported a reduced response to synthetic ACTH for up to 5 days after stopping a brief 5-day course of prednisone, 25 mg orally twice a day. A course of prednisone (30 mg/day) given for more than 1 week will suppress the HPA axis for a period of time. Larger doses over longer periods of time may suppress the normal axis for up to a year (40). Certainly those currently on glucocorticoids should also be considered to have HPA suppression.

Symptoms of secondary adrenal insufficiency due to HPA axis suppression may be more subtle (e.g., malaise, lethargy, fatigue, hypoglycemia, and hypothermia) than those of classic Addison's disease (primary adrenal failure). There is an absence of both major fluid and electrolyte disturbances (e.g, hypotension, hyperkalemia, and dehydration) and increased skin pigmentation. Adequate physiologic replacement with an agent containing both glucocorticoid and mineralocorticoid activity (hydrocortisone 30–40 mg/day in two divided doses) corrects both states although mineralocorticoid activity may not be absent in secondary adrenal insufficiency due to the preservation of aldosterone secretion.

Even with normal HPA axis function, occasional patients may experience steroid-withdrawal symptoms consisting of anorexia, malaise, nausea with emesis, headache, lethargy, orthostatic hypotension, myalgias, and weight loss (6, 30). Laboratory testing in these patients shows "normal" plasma cortisol levels and normal responses to stimulatory testing (6, 30). The reason for these symptoms is unknown, but it is important not to confuse them with documented adrenal insufficiency with low basal and stimulated cortisol levels, because simple education and counseling may be all that is required to deal with the problem. A physical dependence on higher levels of glucocorticoids may exist, requiring reinstitution of physiologic dosages and a slower and longer tapering schedule (40). Not only is HPA axis suppression a problem after stopping corticosteroid administration, but reactivation of the primary disease process for which therapy was initiated further complicates the process. Both respond to restarting the medication at physiological doses or at the last dose that controlled the disease manifestations and a more protracted tapering schedule.

Secondary adrenal insufficiency is often asymptomatic and not manifested clinically until a stress situation (e.g., surgery, general anesthesia, trauma, or critical illness) disastrously intervenes; therefore, provocative testing may be necessary to detect patients with suspected impairments in the HPA axis. The insulin tolerance test is a standard method for testing the HPA axis, but is hazardous in critically ill patients. A safe and practical test, though less sensitive, is the Cosyntropin (ACTH) stimulation test (11). A baseline cortisol level is drawn, then 250 μg of Cosyntropin (1–24 corticotropin) is injected intravenously. A rise in the plasma cortisol level of at least 7 μg/dl and an absolute level above 18 μg/dl at 60 minutes occurs with an intact axis. In adrenal insufficiency, the response curve is blunted, while it is exaggerated in stress situations (Fig. 30.2). Although the cosyntropin test should discriminate normal from abnormal adrenocorticol function in terms of glucocorticoid activity, it does not necessarily pinpoint the locus of pathology (20). This simplified test may also miss patients with inadequate ACTH-cortisol response to physiological stress. Thus, a subnormal test is more informative than a normal one (11, 82, 29). An insulin tolerance test producing hypoglycemic stress, a metyrapone test (enzymatic blocker of the biosynthetic cascade for cortisol synthesis), a 3-day cosyntropin test, or ACTH and aldosterone levels may be required to localize (primary vs. secondary) the site of adrenal insufficiency. Because obtaining the results of these tests is time consuming in the critically ill patient, prednisolone or dexamethasone and other supportive measures (fluid and electrolyte replacement) should be administered coincident with testing. Plasma cortisol levels measured by the radioimmunoassay have little cross reactivity with other synthetic steroids (103). If mineralocorticoid activity is also felt to be absent, hydrocortisone and/or 9-α-fludrocortisol (0.05–0.1 mg/day orally) should be administered after drawing blood for hormonal levels.

Surgery and general anesthesia normally increase glucocorticoid secretion. Thus, preoperative patients who are suspected of adrenal insufficiency (previous or current steroid therapy) should undergo provocative testing. If time does not permit diagnostic procedures, then patients presently on steroids or who have been on glucocorticoids within the preceding 6 months to 1 year for at least 1 week, and those with known adrenal insufficiency (primary or secondary) should be provided with stress coverage [Table 30.4 (111)]. In acute stress situations, the total steroid dose should be equivalent to 200–300 mg of hydrocortisone per day. Recent evidence supports the concept that the amount of glucocorticoid "stress coverage" should be titrated to the degree of stress (20a). If mineralocorticoid activity is required,

Table 30.4
Recommended Steroid Coverage for Preoperative Patients with First- or Second-Degree Adrenocortical Insufficiency[a]

Day	Hydrocortisone Sodium Succinate or Equivalent
Preoperative day 1	25 mg at 1800 and 2400, i.v. or i.m.
Day of operation	100 mg i.v. during surgery
Postoperative	100 mg i.v. q8hr times 24 hr
	50 mg i.v. q8hr times 24 hr ⎫ may be switched to p.o. if the patient is able
	25 mg i.v. q8hr times 24 hr ⎭ to tolerate oral medications.

[a] Modified from White VA, Kumagai LF: Preoperative endocrine and metabolic considerations. Symposium on medical evaluation by the preoperative patient. *Med Clin North Am* 63:1321, 1979.

it is important to choose an agent that has both glucocorticoid and mineralocorticoid activities, such as hydrocortisone.

Since the unwanted effects are inexorably tied to the welcomed effects, a healthy respect for the balance between the two is paramount. These drugs can both be lifesaving and life-threatening in the critically ill patient.

MINERALOCORTICOIDS

Mineralocorticoids are defined by their action on ion transport (8). Aldosterone and deoxycorticosterone (DOC) are the major endogenous mineralocorticoids. About 55% of aldosterone is carried bound to protein, chiefly albumin, but the free form is the active form (103). DOC is over 95% bound to plasma proteins and therefore under normal physiological conditions, contributes little to the overall mineralocorticoid activity despite its potency in the free state (103). Cortisol has approximately 1% of the affinity of aldosterone for the mineralocorticoid receptor but circulates freely in the blood stream at concentrations 15–750 times higher than aldosterone (8). Thus, cortisol may participate in normal fluid and electrolyte balance. Aldosterone is cleared hepatically and has a circulating half-life of 15 minutes (103).

The kidney is the major target organ for the mineralocorticoids, and excess or depleted states are reflected by abnormal renal fluid and electrolyte homeostasis. However, the gastrointestinal tract, salivary glands and sweat glands are also affected. Like glucocorticoids, the mineralocorticoids bind to a cytosol receptor, inducing DNA transcription and the production of specific proteins. After a delay of up to 2 hours (8), reabsorption of sodium ions in exchange for potassium and hydrogen ions occurs in the distal renal tubules. In the ab-

sence of mineralocorticoid activity (e.g., primary adrenal insufficiency), hyperkalemia, hyponatremia, extracellular dehydration, and metabolic acidosis ensues (8). Conversely, in an excess state (Conn's syndrome or primary hyperaldosteronism), hypokalemia, fluid retention with hypertension, and metabolic alkalosis are seen.

Control of aldosterone secretion is regulated by the renin-angiotensin system, β-adrenergic stimulation, blood pressure, and the extracellular potassium level. Salt depletion and/or hypotension stimulate renin release by the kidney's juxtaglomerular cells. Through a series of enzymatic cleavages, angiotensin II is produced. This product increases aldosterone biosynthesis after binding to receptors in the zona glomerulosa and altering intracellular Ca^{++} transport and phospholipid metabolism. Angiotensin II also exerts a trophic effect on the zona glomerulosa. The role of ACTH in aldosterone secretion is not well understood. Administered ACTH results in a nonsustained rise in aldosterone (102), but ACTH suppression by dexamethasone does not impair basal aldosterone levels or its response to sodium depletion (8). Hypophysectomized animals can survive without salt therapy, and the zona glomerulosa is the zone least affected by the withdrawal of ACTH (55). Potassium balance affects aldosterone secretion both through the renin-angiotensin pathway and independently. Hyperkalemia amplifies production of aldosterone, whereas hypokalemia diminishes production. Dopamine is said to inhibit aldosterone secretion, especially in sodium-depleted individuals, whereas dopamine antagonists (e.g., metaclopramide) have the opposite effect (10, 103). The overall secretion rate of aldosterone is a combination of the various influences that affect its secretion.

Aldosterone causes an alteration in sodium permeability, increases the energy stores (ATP) for the Na^+/K^+ pump, effects the Na^+/K^+ pump itself so as to augment sodium reabsorption, and establishes an electrical gradient promoting potassium and hydrogen ion excretion (8, 103). In this regard, kaliuresis is tied to sodium delivery to the distal tubule (8). Clinically, the use of the urine Na^+/K^+ ratio can reflect the level of aldosterone activity. A low ratio indicates a high aldosterone state, and a high ratio indicates the reverse.

Therapeutic uses of exogenous mineralocorticoids are limited to primary adrenal insufficiency, hyporenin-hypoaldosteronism, and primary orthostatic hypotension. The primary commercial mineralocorticoid (excluding hydrocortisone) is 9-α-fludrocortisone (fludrocortisone acetate). It is usually administered in doses of 0.05–0.1 mg a day orally (up to 0.4 mg/day in hyporenin-hypoaldosteronism). It has 125 times the mineralocorticoid activity of cortisol (86). Deoxycorticosterone and aldosterone, because of rapid hepatic clearance, are not suitable for oral use; however, deoxycorticosterone is available in the parenteral form as an acetate or pivalate ester. In primary adrenal dysfunction, hydrocortisone sometimes can provide a sufficient amount of mineralocorticoid activity; however, additional fludrocortisone is often needed.

Antagonists of aldosterone such as spironolactone have wider clinical application. By competitive inhibition (competitive binding to the aldosterone cystol receptors without agonist activity), spironolactone promotes a diuresis, sodium loss, and potassium retention. It is used in the management of hypertension, edematous states (especially those associated with excessive aldosterone activity, e.g., cirrhosis, nephrosis, and congestive heart failure), and in certain hypokalemic states. Since 10% of the filtered sodium load reaches the distal tubule where aldosterone has its action, spironolactone is not a potent diuretic and its effects are dependent on the filtered sodium load and state of aldosterone activity. It is available only in the oral form and the average daily dose is 100–200 mg/day in divided doses. Edematous states usually require the higher doses. Side effects include hyperkalemia, gynecomastia, and androgen-like effects (55).

Newer agents such as captopril and enalapril are angiotensin-converting enzyme inhibitors that work by preventing the conversion of angiotensin I into angiotensin II, a powerful vasoconstrictor and a stimulator of aldosterone. They are of use in the management of hypertension and cardiac failure; the latter is a cause of secondary hyperaldosteronism.

CLINICAL USES OF CORTICOSTEROIDS

The spectrum of clinical indications for steroid therapy is immense (Table 30.2). The basis for the use of glucocorticoids in many of these conditions resides in its abilities to alter the immune response and inflammation; hence a decrease in tissue and cellular destruction and dysfunction. Other aspects of corticosteroid activity are capitalized on in special circumstances; physiological replacement in adrenocorticol insufficiency, decreased calcium absorption and increased renal excretion in hypercalcemia, and tumor control in certain malignant cell lines. Steroid use is also at times empirical, based on anecdotal evidence and theoretical grounds without substantial scientific evidence.

Doses to achieve clinical remission in a disease process vary from replacement doses of 30 mg of hydrocortisone per day for adrenocortical failure to suprapharmacological doses of 1–2 g of intravenous prednisolone for transplant rejection (Table 30.5). If steroids are to be used, a sufficient amount should be given to induce a clinical remission based on predetermined clinical signs and symptoms. The difficulty is in determining the minimum adequate dose to obtain the anticipated end result. The usual doses employed to control hypersensitivity or autoimmune disorders (connective tissue diseases, vasculitidies, etc.) are in the range of 40–100 mg or 1 mg/kg of pred-

Table 30.5
Usual Dosages of Glucocorticoids

Treatment	Dose Equivalent
Physiologic glucocorticoid replacement	Hydrocortisone 20 mg in the AM; 10 mg in the PM p.o.
Mineralocorticoid replacement	Fludrocortisone acetate 0.1 mg p.o. every 24–48 hr
Anti-inflammatory	Prednisone 40–100 mg p.o. every day *or* Prednisolone 40–100 mg i.v. every day
Suprapharmacologic	Prednisolone ≥ 1 g i.v. bolus or in divided doses every day

nisone equivalent per day. Higher doses, pulse doses and more frequent administration (divided daily doses) may be required initially to control an acute inflammatory process before being able to taper back to a single daily dose. Even some rather chronic disorders (SLE or temporal arteritis) may require twice (or more) daily doses to achieve and maintain remission. Once control has been obtained, dropping to the lowest single daily dose or alternate-day therapy if possible will provide maximum benefit with the lowest risk of side effects (especially of HPA axis suppression). It is important before embarking on steroid treatment to maximize adjunctive therapy and establish specific endpoints.

Acute attacks of asthma are characterized by bronchial smooth muscle contraction (bronchoconstriction), airway inflammation, and mucous plugging. Through reduction in inflammatory mediator release, mucous secretion (78), migration of inflammatory cells, potentiation of response to β-adrenergics (78), alteration in ventilation/perfusion mismatches (78), and direct effects on smooth muscle reactivity by way of membrane bound Ca^{++} (78), glucocorticoids are considered by many a mainstay in the treatment of status asthmaticus along with other nonsteroidal bronchodilators. The dose and frequency of administration, though, is more of a debatable subject. Fanta et al. (36) suggest a 2-mg/kg bolus of hydrocortisone followed by a 0.5-mg/kg/hr continuous infusion for 24 hours as the initial regimen in acute asthma. However, no correlation between plasma cortisol levels and spirometric lung function was found (36). Haskell et al. demonstrated that 40 and 120 mg of methylprednisolone intravenously every 6 hours were effective in relieving status asthmaticus, whereas 15 mg was not (53). They favored the use of the higher dose because of a more rapid response within the first 3 days (53). Others note no differences between low versus high doses (15 mg vs. 125 mg of methylprednisolone) after 7 days of treatment (99). At least 1 mg/kg of methylprednisolone every 6 hours appears to be the most agreed upon initial regimen (114) although larger doses may be required if there is no subsequent improvement. The time course of response to steroids is usually on the order of 4–6 hours (78); therefore, the decision to employ steroids should be made as early as possible. After control is established, converting to a single daily dose, usually in the AM and gradual

tapering is indicated. Long-term systemic glucocorticoid therapy, though, may be required in some patients (33). Inhaled, topically administered steroid preparations are available for use in those with stable disease but who require steroids to minimize symptoms and exacerbations. Inhaled steroids allow freedom from systemic therapy, with its attendant complications and reduction in systemic doses. Devices, such as spacers for metered-dose inhalers (MDI), improve topical lung deposition by reducing droplet size and velocity. They are especially helpful in those who have difficulty in coordinating the use of the MDI with their breathing pattern. These devices may also limit complications such as oral thrush.

The use of steroids in chronic obstructive pulmonary disease (COPD) is less clear than in the asthmatic. However, since most have some "reversible" obstructive component during an exacerbation, a trial of glucocorticoids is indicated if there is not an adequate response to conventional bronchodilators (β-adrenergics and theophylline). Albert has shown a beneficial effect with methylprednisolone, 0.5 mg/kg every 6 hours intravenously, in the first 72 hours in patients with chronic bronchitis and acute respiratory insufficiency (3). Longer-term glucocorticoids may also be of benefit in the stable COPD patient (72). However, in both asthma and chronic obstructive pulmonary diseases, objective improvement (e.g., spirometric values) is important because not all show a significant response (e.g., primary emphysematous patients with little or no bronchitic component) and some chronic asthmatics are resistant to steroid therapy (17). Therefore, these individuals should not be subjected to the risks of corticosteroid therapy.

Probably the most desired and controversial benefit of suprapharmacological doses of glucocorticoids in the critically ill patient is in the treatment of septic shock and the adult respiratory distress syndrome (ARDS). Glucocorticoids have been reported to have the ability to disaggregate clumps of granulocytes (52, 93); stabilize lysosomal enzymes and capillary membranes, which minimizes capillary permeability (13); improve oxygenation by altering ventilation/perfusion mismatches (78); increase cardiac contractility (56); antagonize complement (56), and reduce complement mediated granulocytic aggregation (93); diminish coagulopathy (56); antagonize endotoxin effects (56); decrease the local inflammatory response and release of mediators including the prostaglandin derivatives (77, 46); alter the migratory patterns of inflammatory cells; reduce toxic oxygen radical release (52); and vasoconstrict the capillary bed either directly or indirectly through the potentiation of the adrenergic system (40). In 1976, a prospective study by Schumer (119) indicated that methylprednisolone (30 mg/kg) or dexamethasone (3 mg/kg) given once or twice in 24 hours reduced mortality from 38.4% to 10.5% in sepsis. In 1984, Sprung et al. (95) conducted a prospective, controlled study of sepsis. They found that methylprednisolone (30 mg/kg) and dexamethasone (6 mg/kg) given as a 10–15 minute infusion (either once or twice, 4 hours later), were more likely to reverse shock, but the overall survival rate was similar in both groups (steroid treated, 23%; and control, 31%). These survival rates were much lower than Schumer (119) reported, but more in line with other studies and clinical practice (95). Other clinical and animal studies have been less conclusive (83). Despite the initial enthusiasm in the 1970s, the mortality from septic shock and ARDS remains high and favor has shifted away from steroid use. Animal studies (though not always applicable to human trials) suggest that earlier administration of glucocorticoids (e.g., at the time of challenge with endotoxin or *Escherichia coli*) does improve survival. In Sprung's study an average of 17.5 ± 5.4 hours passed between the onset of shock and the first dose of glucocorticoid therapy. Perhaps the cascade of events that may have been responsive to steroid therapy had already been initiated. Although it was noted in Sprung's study that those who had received steroids within 4 hours of shock had a higher reversal of shock, the overall mortality was not changed (95). Two more recent well-designed cooperative clinical trials with a combined total of 605 patients concluded that high-dose corticosteroids (methylprednisolone sodium succinate 30 mg/kg in four doses every 6 hours or 30 mg/kg as the initial dose followed by 5 mg/kg/hour for 9 hours given within 2 hours of the studies' definition of sepsis) had no benefit in the treatment of sepsis (10, 60a). Mortality secondary to infectious complications was noted to be even higher in the steroid cohort than the control group in one of the trials (60a). Additionally, though large doses of glucocorticoids given in a short course have been generally free of major complications, there have been reports of cardiac arrhythmias with sudden death after rapid bolus intravenous administration (70, 97) and aggravation of acute

lung damage with prednisolone given during the early phase of repair (62).

The data suggesting efficacy of glucocorticoids in ARDS mirror those of septic shock. Most of the studies dealing with the use of steroids in ARDS are combined with their use in septic shock. In Sprung's study there appeared to be no significant reduction in the cases of ARDS in either of the steroid-treated groups compared with the control group (27% vs. 15%, respectively) (95). Glucocorticoids also have not been efficacious in the treatment of acid aspiration or fresh-water drowning, both of which can lead to ARDS (83). However, Cheyney et al. (19) reported that methylprednisolone increased the resolution of oleic acid embolism–induced pulmonary injury in dogs. Sibbald et al. (92) reported reduced accumulation of radiolabeled serum albumin into pulmonary edema fluid in patients with septic ARDS given methylprednisolone. Schonfeld et al. published a study showing that prophylactic methylprednisolone (7.5 mg/kg every 6 hours times 12 for a total dose of 90 mg/kg) prevented the fat emboli syndrome (a predisposing cause of ARDS) in patients with long bone fractures (91). Glucocorticoids have also been shown to increase surfactant synthesis (87). These studies suggest a salutary effect of glucocorticoids in ARDS. Recently, the Severe Sepsis Study Group, in a follow-up to their negative evaluation of the value of methylprednisolone in sepsis, concluded that methylprednisolone sodium succinate given early in the course of sepsis not only did not halt the development of ARDS but increased the mortality rate of the syndrome (52% in those treated with methylprednisolone compared with 22% in the controlled group) (108a). Early enthusiasm for corticosteroids has now given way to other agents such a prostaglandin agonists and antagonists, antioxidants, heavy metal chelators, oxygen radical scavengers, niacin, and surfactant replacement (60) in the treatment of acute lung injury. To date the overall data do not support a beneficial role for glucocorticoids in either septic shock or ARDS.

In the treatment of cerebral edema (vasogenic edema) secondary to tumor, an initial dose of dexamethasone (10 mg) followed by 4 mg every 6 hours is generally recommended (44). Dexamethasone is particularly well suited in this case because of its minimal fluid-retaining properties, although this has not been proven clinically. The extension of the use of dexamethasone to other forms of cerebral edema such as that seen after intracerebral hemorrhage (mixed vasogenic and cytotoxic edema) is not warranted and may be harmful (120). Hypercalcemia secondary to lymphoma, myeloma, and metastatic solid tumors usually responds to initial doses of 50–100 mg of prednisolone given intravenously every 8 hours (112). Hypercalcemia due to sarsoidosis is very sensitive to glucocorticoids and can be treated with lower oral doses.

In adrenal crisis, prompt therapy is lifesaving. Corticosteroid replacement is essential; dexamethasone (10 mg), methylprednisolone (50 mg) or hydrocortisone (200–300 mg) are given intravenously over 10–20 minutes (20). Fluid replacement with isotonic saline should be instituted simultaneously. Hypertonic saline should be avoided since this fluid worsens intracellular dehydration and may precipitate coma (20). Since hypoglycemia occurs, administration of 5% dextrose in normal saline is preferred (20). Sodium bicarbonate is rarely needed to correct the metabolic acidosis, and the hyperkalemia usually resolves with mineralocorticoid and fluid replacement. For maintenance therapy, hydrocortisone may be given in 100-mg dosages every 6–8 hours or as a continuous drip of 200 mg over 16 hours. At this dose further mineralocorticoid activity is generally not needed; however, with smaller hydrocortisone doses or with other glucocorticoids, fludrocortisone (0.1–0.2 mg/day orally) may be required (94). If hypothyroidism coexists with hypoadrenalism (e.g., Schmidt's syndrome), corticosteroid replacement should occur first, so as to avoid aggravation of the adrenal insufficiency by thyroid hormone replacement.

After control of the disease process is accomplished, the lowest possible dose to maintain a remission should be used and adjunctive

Table 30.6
Schedule for Glucocorticoid Withdrawal[a]

Step	Interval	Observation	Result	Glucocorticoid Dose
I.	Variable	Underlying disease	Clinical improvement	Variable
II.	Variable	Underlying disease	Stable	Switch from divided doses to single daily doses. Gradual decrements to the equivalent of 20 mg/day of hydrocortisone
			Decline in status or signs and symptoms of steroid withdrawal	Raise dosage for flare ups of disease; supplement for stress; recontinue tapering when disease is quiescent
III.	4 wk	8 AM plasma cortisol	Plasma cortisol: <10 μg/dl	When tapered to the equivalent of 20 mg of hydrocortisone per day, start hydrocortisone at 20 mg/day and then taper by 2.5 mg/day once/week to 10 mg each morning and continue this dosage; supplement for stress
			Plasma cortisol: >10 μg/dl	Stop maintenance hydrocortisone Supplement for stress
IV.	4 wk to indefinite	8 AM Cortrosyn 250 μg test[b]	When plasma cortisol increment is <6 μg/dl or maximum <18 μg/dl at 60 min (or both)	Supplement for stress
V.	4 wk to indefinite	8 AM Cortrosyn 250 μg test[b]	When plasma cortisol increment is >6 μg/dl and maximum >18 μg/dl at 60 min	Stop supplementation for stress
VI.	Indefinite	Routine		As indicated

[a] Adapted from Byyny RL: Withdrawal from glucocorticoid therapy. *N Engl J Med* 295:30, 1976.
[b] See Fig. 30.3 for explanation of the ACTH (Cortrosyn: synthetic ACTH) stimulation test.

therapy maximized. If the requirement for steroid therapy is short lived, a rapidly tapering schedule can be instituted (Table 30.6). If chronic therapy is required and the disease is amenable to alternate day therapy, it should be considered. It is initiated by doubling the daily maintenance dose and giving it as a single dose in the morning every other day. The dose is reduced in daily decrements of 5–10 mg over a gradual period until a 20-mg-every-other-day dose is reached. The dose is then reduced by 2.5 mg every other day until the requirement for therapy has resolved or the disease flares (40). Once the process has flared, doubling the last dose given usually suppresses the disease activity although full doses are occasionally again required. After reinduction of remission, weaning back to alternate-day therapy can be attempted and a slower tapering schedule begun. This type of regimen allows recovery of the HPA axis and reduction in some of the undesirable effects (1, 32).

SUMMARY

Corticosteroid activity is required for the normal homeostasis of day to day living. Stress situations increase the demand for this activity and the HPA axis responds accordingly. Corticosteroid therapy in patients with a normal HPA axis provides therapeutic benefit in many circumstances but oftentimes does not cure the disease but ameliorates the pathophysiology until more definitive therapy can take place or the inciting insult is removed. It has revolutionized the care of patients in many instances but has not fulfilled all the early promises.

In the critical care patient, one encounters advantages and disadvantages in both acute and chronic steroid therapy. The intensivist needs to be aware of the benefits, the shortcomings, and controversies in steroid therapy. They have wide application but should not be given without an appreciation of their adverse effects. Refinement in our knowledge of the pharmacology and physiology of steroids may introduce broader application with more specific effects and finer definition of their benefits and toxicities.

References

1. Ackerman GL, Nolan CM: Adrenocortical responsiveness after alternate-day corticosteroid therapy. N Engl J Med 278:405, 1968.
2. Adinoff AD, Hollister JR: Steroid-induced fractures and bone loss in patients with asthma. N Engl J Med 309:265, 1983.
3. Albert RK, Martin TR, Lewis SW: Controlled clinical trial of methylprednisolone in patients with chronic bronchitis and acute respiratory insufficiency. Ann Intern Med 92:753, 1980.
4. Atkinson JP, Frank MM: Effect of cortisone therapy on serum complement components. J Immunol 111:1061, 1973.
5. Atkinson, JP, Schreiber AD, Frank MM: Effects of corticosteroids and splenectomy on immune clearance and destruction of erythrocytes. J Clin Invest 52:1509, 1973.
6. Axelrod L: Glucocorticoid therapy. Medicine 55:39, 1976.
7. Ballard PL, Carter JP, Graham BS, et al: A radioreceptor assay for the evaluation of the plasma glucocorticoid activity of natural and synthetic steroids in man. J Clin Endocrinol Metab 41:290, 1975.
8. Baxter JD, Tyrell JB: The adrenal cortex. In Felig P et al: Endocrinology and Metabolism, New York, McGraw-Hill, 1981, pp 385–510.
9. Binstock ML, Mundy GR: Effect of calcitonin and glucocorticoids in combination on the hypercalcemia of malignancy. Ann Intern Med 93:269, 1980.
10. Bondy PK: Disorder of the adrenal cortex. In Wilson JD, Foser DW (eds): Williams Textbook of Endocrinology, 7th ed. Philadelphia, WB Saunders, 1985, p 816–880.
10a. Bone RC, Fisher CJ, Clemmer TP et al: A controlled clinical trial of high-dose methylprednisolone in the treatment of severe sepsis and septic shock. N Engl J Med 317:653, 1987.
10b. Bone RC, Fisher CJ, Clemmer TP et al: Early methylprednisolone treatment for septic syndrome and the adult respiratory distress disease syndrome. Chest. 92:1032, 1987.
11. Borst G, Michenfleder JHJ, O'Brian JT: Discordant cortisol response to exogenous ACTH and insulin-induced hypoglycemia in patients with pituitary disease. N Engl J Med 306:1462, 1982.
12. Brennan MJ; Corticosteroids in the treatment of solid tumors: symposium on steroid therapy. Med Clin North Am 57:1225, 1973.
13. Brigham KL, Bowers RE, Mckeen CR: Methylprednisolone prevention of increased lung vascular permeability following endotoxemia in sheep. J Clin Invest 67:1103, 1981.
14. Bruno A, Cavallo-Perin P, Cassader M, Pagnano G: Deflazacort vs. prednisone. Effect on blood glucose control in insulin-treated diabetics. Arch Int Med 147:679, 1987.
15. Butler WT, Rossen RD: Effect of corticosteroids on immunity in man. I. Decreased serum IgG concentration caused by 3 or 5 days of high dose methylprednisolone. J Clin Invest 52:2629, 1973.
16. Byyny RL: Withdrawal from glucocorticoid therapy. N Engl J Med 295:30, 1976.
17. Carmichael J, Paterson IC, Diaz P, Crompton GK, Kay AB, Grant IWB: Corticosteroid resistance in chronic asthma. Br Med J 282:1419, 1981.
18. Chatterjea JB, Salmon L: Antagonistic effect of ACTH and cortisone on the anticoagulant activity of ethyl biscoumacetate. Br Med J. 2:790, 1954.
19. Cheyney FW, Huang TH, Gronka, R: Effects of methylprednisolone on experimental pulmonary injury. Ann Surg 190: 236, 1979.
20. Chernow B: Hormonal and metabolic considerations in critical care medicine. In Critical Care: State of the Art. Fullerton, CA, Society of Critical Care Medicine, 1982, vol 3, p J1.
20a. Chernow B, Alexander HR, Smallridge RC, et al: Hormonal responses to graded surgical stress. Arch Intern Med 147: 1273–1278, 1987.

21. Chernow B, Zwillich CW: Is hypercapnia complicating metabolic alkalosis, a rare clinical entity? *Chest* 70:421, 1976.

22. Chernow B, Vernoski BK, Saloga GP, et al: Dexamethasone causes less steroid-induce alkalemia than methylprednisolone or hydrocortisone. *Critical Care Med* 12:384, 1984.

23. Claman HN: Corticosteroids and lymphoid cells. *N Engl J Med* 287:388, 1972.

24. Clee MD, Ferguson J, Browning MCK, Jung RT, Clark RA: Glucocorticoid hypersensitivity in an asthmatic patient: Presentation and treatment. *Thorax* 40:477, 1985.

25. Cline MJ, Melmon KL: Plasma kinins and cortisol; A possible explanation of the anti-inflammatory action of cortisol. *Science* 153:1135, 1966.

26. Collins JV, Clark TJH, Brown D, et al: The use of corticosteroids in the treatment of acute asthma. *Q J Med* 44:259, 1975.

27. Conn HO, Biltzer BL: Nonassociation of adrenalcorticosteroid therapy and peptic ulcer. *N Engl J Med* 294:473, 1976.

28. Cupps TR, Fauci AS: Corticosteroid-mediated immunoregulation in man. *Immunol Rev* 65:133, 1982.

29. Cunningham SK, Moore A, McKenna J: Normal cortisol response to corticotropin in patients with secondary adrenal failure. *Arch Intern Med* 143:2276, 1983.

30. David DS, Grieco MH, Cushman P: Adrenal glucocorticoids after twenty years, a review of their clinically relevant consequences. *J Chronic Dis* 22:637, 1970.

31. Dhuly RG, Lauler DP, Thorn GW: Pharmacology and chemistry of adrenal glucocorticoids: Symposium of steroid therapy. *Med Clin North Am* 57:1155, 1973.

31a. Drucker D, Shandling M: Variable adrenocortical function in acute medical illness. *Crit Care Med* 13:477, 1985.

32. Dujovne CA, Azarnoff DL: Clinical complication of corticosteroid therapy: symposium on steroid therapy. *Med Clin North Am* 57:1331, 1973.

33. Dykewicz M, Greenberger PA, Patterson R, Halwig M: Natural history of asthma in patients requiring long-term systemic corticosteroids. *Arch Intern Med* 146:2369, 1986.

34. Editorial: Tuberculosis in corticosteroid treated asthmatics. *Br Med J* 2:266, 1976.

35. Elias AN, Gwinup G: Effects of some clinically encountered drugs on steroid synthesis and degradation. *Metabolism* 29:583, 1980.

36. Fanta CH, Rossing TH, McFadden ER: Glucocorticoids in acute asthma. A critical controlled trial. *Am J Med* 74:845, 1983.

38. Farer LS: Chemoprophylaxis: Kock centennial supplement. *Am Rev Resp Dis* 125:102, 1982.

39. Farer LS: Chemoprophylaxis against tuberculosis. *Clin Chest Med* 1:203, 1980.

40. Fauci AS: Glucocorticoid therapy: In Wyngaarden JB and Smith LH (eds): *Cecil Textbook of Medicine*, 17th ed. Philadelphia, WB Saunders, 1985, p 111–116.

41. Fauci AS, Dale DC, Lalow JE: Glucocorticoid therapy: Mechanisms of action and clinical considerations. *Ann Intern Med* 84:304, 1976.

42. Fenster KF: The ulcerogenic potential of glucocorticoids and possible prophylatic measures: Symposium on steroid therapy. *Med Clin North Am* 57:1289, 1972.

43. Finlay WE, Mckee J: Serum cortisol levels in severely stressed patients. *Lancet* 1:414, 1982.

44. Fishman RA: Brain edema. *N Engl J Med* 293:706, 1975.

45. Fitzsimons R, Greenberger PA, Patterson R: Outcome of pregnancy in women requiring corticosteroids for severe asthma. *J Allergy Clin Immunol* 78:349, 1986.

46. Flower RJ: The mediators of steroid action. *Nature* 320:20, 1986.

47. Foresman O, Mulder J: Hypersensitivity to different ACTH peptides. *Acta Med Scand* 193:557, 1973.

48. Frohman LA: Diseases of the anterior pituitary. In Felip P et al: *Endocrinology and Metabolism*. New York, McGraw-Hill, 1981, p 151.

49. Goggans FC, Weisberg LJ, Koran LM: Lithium prophylaxis of prednisone psychosis: a case report. *J Clin Psychiatry* 44:3, 1983.

50. Graber AL, Ney RL, Nicholson WE et al: Natural history of pituitary-adrenal recovery following long-term suppression with corticosteroids. *J Clin Endocrinol Metab* 25:11, 1965.

51. Guillemin R, Bargo T, Rossier J, et al: Beta-endorphin and adrenocorticotropin are secreted concomitantly by the pituitary gland. *Science* 197:1367, 1977.

52. Hammerschmidt DE, White JG, Craddok, PR et al: Corticosteroids inhibit complement-induced granulocyte aggregation: four possible mechanisms for their efficacy in shock states. *J Clin Invest* 63:798, 1979.

53. Haskell RJ, Wong BM, Hansen JE: A double-blind, randomized clinical trial of methylprednisolone in status asthmaticus. *Arch Intern Med* 143:1324, 1983.

54. Hastings Pr, Skillman JJ, Bushnell LS et al: Antacid titration in the prevention of acute gastrointestinal bleeding. A controlled, randomized trial in 100 critically ill patients. *N Engl J Med* 298:1041, 1978.

55. Haynes RC, Murad F: Adrenocorticotropic hormone; adrenocortical steroids and their synthetic analogs; inhibitors of adrenocortical steroid biosynthesis. In Gilman AG, Goodman LS, Rall TW, Murad F (eds): *The Pharmacological Basis of Therapeutics*, 7th ed. New York, Macmillan, 1985, pp 1459–1489.

56. Hess ML, Hastillo A, Greenfield LJ: Spectrum of cardiovascular function during gram-negative sepsis. *Prog Cardiovasc Dis* 23:279, 1981.

57. Horber FF, Scheidegger JR, Grunig BE, Frey J FJ: Evidence that prednisone-induced myopathy is reversed by physical training. *J Clin Endocrinol Metab* 61:83, 1985.

58. Hsueh WA, Pas-Guevara A, Bledsoe T: Studies comparing the metabolic clearance rate of 11 beta, 17, 21-trihydroxypregn-1,4-diene-3,20-dione (prednisolone) after oral 17,21-dihydrooxypregn-1,4-diene-3,11,20-trione and intravenous prednisolone. *J Clin Endocrinol Metab* 48:748, 1979.

59. Ivey KJ, Dennssesten L: Pseudotumor cerebri associated with corticosteroid therapy in an adult. *JAMA* 208:1698, 1969.

60. Jacobs ER, Bone RC: Therapeutic implications of acute lung injury. *Crit Care Clin* 2:615, 1986.

60a. Jurney TH, Cockrell JL, Lindberg JS, Lamiell JM, Wade CE: Spectrum of serum cortisol response to ACTH in ICU Patients. *Chest* 92:292, 1987.

61. Kawai S, Ichikawa Y, Homma M: Differences of metabolic properties among cortisol, prednisolone, and dexamethasone in liver and renal diseases: Accelerated metabolism of dexamethasone in renal failure. *J Clin Endocrinol Metab* 60:848, 1985.

62. Kehrer JP, Klein-Szanto AJP, Sorensen EMB, Pearlman R, Rosner MH: Enhance acute lung damage following corticosteroid treatment. *Am Rev Respir Dis* 130:256, 1984.

63. Klinenberg JR, Miller R: Effect of corticosteroids on blood salicylate concentrations. *JAMA* 194:601, 1965.

64. Koener JH and Sun DC: Mediastinal lipomatosis secondary to steroid therapy. *AJR* 98:461, 1966.

65. Kozower N, Veatch L, Kaplan MM: Decrease clearance of prednisolone, a factor in the development of corticosteroid side effects. *J Clin Endocrinol Metab* 38:407, 1974.

66. Lam KC, Lai CL, Trepo C, et al: Deleterious effect of prednisolone in HBsAg-positive chronic active hepatitis. *N Engl J Med* 304:380, 1981.

67. Lewis GP, Jusko, Burke CW, et al: Prednisone side effects and serum protein levels. *Lancet* 2:778, 1971.

68. Marco J, Colle C, Roman D, et al: Hyperglucagonism induced by glucocorticoid treatment in man. *N Engl J Med* 288:128, 1973.

69. Marom Z, Shelhamer, Alling D, Lainer M: The effects of corticosteroids on mucous glycoprotein secretion from human airways in vitro. *Am Rev Respir Dis* 129:62, 1984.

70. McDougal BA, Whittier FC, Cross DE: Sudden death after bolus steroid therapy for acute rejection. *Transpl Proc* 8:493, 1976.

70a. McKee JI, Finlay WE: Cortisol replacement in severely stressed patients (letter). *Lancet* 1:484, 1986.

71. Melby JC: Systemic corticosteroid therapy: pharmacology and endocrinologic considerations. *Ann Intern Med* 81:505, 1974.

72. Mendella LA, Manfreda J, Warren CP, Anthonisen NR: Steroid response in stable chronic pulmonary disease. *Ann Intern Med* 96:17, 1982.

73. Mendelson LM, Meltxer EO, Hamburger RN: Anaphylaxis-like reactions to corticosteroid therapy. *J Allergy Clin Immun* 54:125, 1974.

74. Meikle AW, Tyler F: Potency and duration of action of glucocorticoids: effects of hydrocortisone, prednisone, and dexamethasone on human pituitary-adrenal function. *Am J Med* 63:200, 1977.

75. Menguy R, Masters YF: Effect of cortisone on mucoprotein secretion by gastric antrum of dogs: pathogenesis for steroid ulcer. *Surgery* 54:19, 1963.

76. Messer J, Reitman D, Sacks HS, Smith H, Chalmers TC: Association of adrenocorticosteroid therapy and peptic ulcer disease. *N Engl J Med* 309:21, 1983.

77. Moore PK, Hoult JRS: Anti-inflammatory steroids reduce tissue prostaglandin synthetase activity and enhance prostaglandin breakdown. *Nature* 288:269, 1980.

78. Morris HG: Mechanisms of glucocortiocoid action in pulmonary disease. *Chest* 88(Suppl):133S, 1985.

79. Mulrow CD, Corey GR: Pericardial pseudoeffusion due to steroid-induced lipomatosis. *North Carolina Med J* 46:179, 1985.

80. Nashel DJ: Is atherosclerosis a complication of long-term corticosteroid treatment? *Am J Med* 80:925, 1986.

81. Nassif EG, Weinberger M, Thompson R, et al: The value of maintenance theophylline in steroid dependent asthma. *N Engl J Med* 304:71, 1981.

82. Newmark SR: Can the pituitary release adrenocorticotrophic hormone during stress. *Arch Int Med* 143:2248, 1983.

83. Nicholson DP: Glucocorticoids in the treatment of shock and the adult respiratory distress syndrome. *Clin Chest Med* 3:121, 1982.

84. Pingleton SK: Gastrointestinal hemorrhage. In Bone RC (ed): Park Ridge, American College of Chest Physicians, 1984; 82–97.

85. Richards JM, Santiago SM, Klausutermyer WB: Aseptic necrosis of the femoral head in corticosteroid-treated pulmonary disease. *Arch Intern Med* 140:1473, 1980.

86. Robbins JJ, Santle PD: Corticoids in osteoporosis. *Ann Intern Med* 74:1013, 1971.

87. Rooney SA: The surfactant system and lung phospholipid biochemistry. *Am Rev Respir Dis* 131:439, 1985.

88. Sainsberg JRC, Stoddard JC, Watson MJ: Plasma cortisol levels: a comparison between sick patients and volunteers given intravenous cortisol. *Anaesthesia* 36:16, 1981.

89. Schleimer RP: The mechanisms of antiinflammatory steroid action in allergic diseases. *Ann Rev Pharmacol Toxicol* 25:381, 1985.

90. Schoenfeld Y, Gurewich Y, Gallant LA, et al: Prednisone-induced leukocytosis: influence of dosage, method and duration of administration on the degree of leukocytosis. *Am J Med* 71:773, 1981.

91. Schonfeld SA, Polysongsang Y, DiLisio R, et al: Fat embolism prophylaxis with corticosteroids. A prospective study in high-risk patients. *Ann Intern Med* 99:438, 1983.

92. Sibbald WJ, Anderson RR, Reid B, et al: Alveoli-capillary permeability in human septic ARDS: Effect of high-dose corticosteroid therapy. *Chest* 79:133, 1981.

93. Skubitz KM, Craddock PR, Hammershmidt DE, et al: Corticosteroid block binding of chemotactic peptide to its receptor in granulocytes and cause disaggregation of granulocyte aggregates in vitro. *J Clin Invest* 67:1103, 1981.

94. Smith SJH, MacGregor GA, Markandu ND, et al: Evidence that patients with Addison's disease are undertreated with fludrocortisone. *Lancet* 1:11, 1984.

95. Sprung CL, Caralis PV, Marcial EH, et al: The effects of high-dose corticosteroids in patients with septic shock. A prospective, controlled study. *N Engl J Med* 311:1137, 1984.

96. Streck WK, Lockwood DH; Pituitary adrenal recovery following short-term suppression with corticosteroids. *Am J Med* 66:910, 1979.

97. Stubs SS, et al: Intravenous methylprednisolone sodium succinate: adverse reactions reported in association with immunosuppressive therapy. *Transpl Proc* 5:1145, 1976.

98. Szefler SJ, Rose JQ, Ellis EF, et al: The effect of troleandomycin on methylprednisolone elimination. *J Allergy Clin* 66:447, 1980.

99. Tanaka RM, Santiago SM, Kuhn GJ, et al: Intravenous methylprednisolone and adults in status asthmaticus: comparison of two dosages. *Chest* 82:438, 1982.

100. Toogood JH: Steroid and cromolyn for treatment of chronic asthma. *Chest* 82S:42S, 1982.

101. Turner ES, Greenberger PA, Patterson RP: Management of the pregnant asthmatic patient. *Ann Intern Med* 6:905, 1980.

102. Tucci Jr, Espiner EA, Jagger PL, et al: ACTH stimulation of aldosterone secretion in normal subjects and in patients with chronic adrenocortical insufficiency. *J Clin Endocrinol Metab* 27:568, 1967.

103. Tyrrell JB, Baxter JD: Disorders of the adrenal cortex. In Wyngaarden JB, Smith LH (eds): *Cecil Textbook of Medicine*, 17th ed. Philadelphia, WB Saunders, 1985, pp 1300–1320.

104. Tyrell JB, Baxter JD: Glucocorticoid therapy. In Felig P et al: *Endocrinology and Metabolism*. New York, McGraw-Hill, 1981, pp 559.

105. VanArsdel PP: Drug allergy, an update. symposium on clinical allergy. *Med Clin North Am* 65:1089, 1981.

106. VanBahr C, Sjoquist F, Orrenius S: The inhibitory effect of hydrocortisone and testosterone in plasma disappearance of nortriptyline in the dog and perfused rat liver. *Eur J Pharmacol* 9:106, 1970.

107. Varney NR, Alexander B, MacIndoe JH: Reversible steroid dementia in patients without steroid psychosis. *Am J Psychiatry* 143:3, 1984.

108. Vaz R, Sencor B, Morris M, et al: Adrenal effects on beclomethasone inhalation therapy in asthmatic children. *J Pediatr* 100:660, 1982.

108a. The Veterans Administration Systemic Sepsis Cooperative Study Group: Effect of high-dose glucocorticoid therapy on mortality in patients with clinical signs of systemic sepsis. *N Engl J Med* 317:659, 1987.

109. Walker AE, Adamkiewicz JJ: Pseudotumor cerebri associated with plonged corticosteroid therapy: report of four cases. *JAMA* 188:779, 1964.

110. Weissglas IS: The role of endogenous opiates in shock: Experimental anc clinical studies in vitro and in vivo. *Adv Shock Res* 10:87, 1983.

111. White VA, Kumagai LF: Preoperative endocrine and metabolic considerations. Symposium on medical evaluation of the preoperative patient. *Med Clin North Am* 63:132, 1979.

112. Whyte MP: Mineral, parathyroid and metabolic bone diseases. In Orland MJ, Saltman RJ (eds): *Manual of*

Medical Therapeutics, 25th ed. Boston, Little, Brown Co., 1986, pp 360–363.

113. Wolfe R: Carbohydrate metabolism in the critically ill patient. Implications for nutritional support. *Crit Care Clin* 3:11, 1987.

114. Ziment I: Steroids. *Clin Chest Med* 7:341, 1986.

115. Zizic TM, Maroux C, Hungerford DS, Dansereau J-V, Stefens MB: Corticosteroid therapy associated with ischemic necrosis of bone in systemic lupus erythematosus. *Am J Med* 79:596, 1985.

116. Weston WI, Mandel MJ, Yeckley Ja, et al: Mechanism of cortisol inhibition of adoptive transfer of tuberculin sensitivity. *J Lab Clin Med* 82:366, 1973.

117. Paul WE: Introduction: The immune system. In Wyngaarden JB, Smith LH (eds): *Cecil Textbook of Medicine*, 17th ed. Philadelphia, WB Saunders, 1984, pp 1846–1852.

118. Perry PJ, Tsuang MT, Hwang MH: Predniosolone psychosis: clinical observations. *Drug Intell Clin Pharm* 18:603, 1984.

119. Schumer W: Steroids in the treatment of clinical septic shock. *Ann Surg* 184:333, 1976.

120. Poungvarin N, Bhoopat W, Viriyavejakul A, et al: Effects of dexamethasone in primary supratentorial intracerebral hemorrhage. *N Engl J Med* 316:1229, 1987.

31

Catecholamines and Other Inotropes

Arno L. Zaritsky, M.D.
Bart Chernow, M.D., F.A.C.P., F.C.C.P.

Management of the critically ill patient often necessitates the use of one or more inotropic agents to maintain adequate tissue perfusion. Catecholamines and other sympathomimetics are the most important group of inotropic agents currently available; however, a number of new, noncatecholamine agents are being used in critically ill patients. This chapter reviews the pharmacology of both catecholamines and the new inotropes, arminone and milrinone. Adrenergic receptor physiology and endogenous catecholamine responses in the critically ill patient are highlighted, and the cardiovascular actions and clinical indications for these agents are reviewed.

Clinical use of inotropes requires an understanding of several important pharmacologic principles. These have been discussed in detail in chapters 1 and 2 but are reviewed briefly here. Whenever a drug is administered to a patient, its clinical actions are due to a complex interaction between the concentration of drug in the plasma, elimination from the body, diffusion to its site of action, and the response of the target tissue to the drug. Plasma drug concentration is modified by changes in the drug dose and pharmacokinetics, whereas the tissue response is influenced by changes in receptor and tissue responsiveness.

Pharmacokinetics is the mathematical expression of the time course of all processes leading to drug distribution and elimination. This time course is typically determined by quantifying drug concentration in the plasma compartment, although this approach may not be ideal since inotropic drug action occurs in the tissue. In the critical care setting, most inotropic agents are administered by continuous intravenous infusion, making the kinetics relatively simple. Pharmacodynamics is the relationship between drug concentration (again, usually measured in plasma samples) and drug

effect. In the case of inotropic agents, measurable drug-induced physiologic action may be a change in cardiac output, blood pressure, and heart rate. When used clinically, the pharmacodynamic effects of inotropes are not related to the drug plasma concentration in a simple manner, since the patient's illness may influence the net hemodynamic effect observed.

In patients with circulatory shock, for example, drug within the plasma compartment may not be distributed to the active site because of poor perfusion. As the patient's clinical condition changes, the pharmacokinetics and pharmacodynamics of administered inotropes may also change, necessitating frequent reassessment of the patient and adjustment of the infusion rate. In the discussion of individual inotropes that follows, statements regarding hemodynamic effects observed with specific infusion doses should be recognized as being relative and that individual adjustment is needed for each patient.

ADRENERGIC RECEPTORS

The actions of catecholamines are determined by their binding at three major classes of receptors: α-adrenergic, β-adrenergic, and dopaminergic (DA) receptors. There are two subtypes of each of these receptors, termed α_1 and α_2, β_1 and β_2, and DA_1 and DA_2 (103, 138). Three of the four types of α- and β-adrenergic receptors mediate their cellular effects through stimulation (β-receptors) or inhibition (α_2-receptors) of adenylate cyclase activity. The α_1-receptor transduces the signal from receptor-agonist binding by increasing transcellular calcium flux through a recently described mechanism that results from phosphoinositol turnover at the cell membrane (117, 118).

Adrenergic receptor density on the cell surface is dynamic; the density of receptors can

Table 31.1
Disease and Conditions Altering Receptor Density on Effector Cells[a]

Disease or Condition	Receptor Altered	Change
Congestive heart failure	β (heart)	Increased[b]
Sepsis	α (liver, vasculature)	Decreased
Myocardial ischemia	β (heart)	Decreased
Myocardial ischemia	α (heart)	Increased
Asthma[c]	β (lung, leukocytes)	Decreased
Cystic fibrosis	β (leukocytes)	Decreased
Fetal and neonatal life	α, β (heart, platelets, leukocytes)	Decreased
Agonist administration	α, β (heart, platelets, leukocytes)	Decreased
Antagonist administration	α, β (heart, platelets, leukocytes)	Increased
Hyperthyroidism	β (heart)	Increased
Hypothyroidism	β (heart)	Decreased
Glucocorticoids	β (heart, leukocytes)	Increased

[a] From Zaritsky A, Eisenberg, MG: Ontogenetic considerations in the pharmaco-therapy of shock. In Chernow B, Shoemaker WC (eds): *Critical Care: State of the Art,* vol 7. Society of Critical Care Medicine, Fullerton, CA, 1986, pp 485–534.
[b] β-Adrenergic receptors are decreased in severe heart failure.
[c] If on β-agonist therapy for asthma.

be modulated by a number of disease states or conditions (Table 31.1). Changes in receptor density can have important implications in the pharmacotherapy of the patient with circulatory shock. Down-regulation (a decrease in the number of receptors on the cell surface) of β-adrenergic receptors in the myocardium of patients with chronic congestive heart failure results in decreased catecholamine sensitivity (21). In endotoxic shock, β-adrenergic receptors are down regulated in the liver, which may partially mediate the glucose dyshomeostasis seen in sepsis (149), and α_1-adrenergic receptor density and responsiveness is diminished in the peripheral vasculature (98), accounting for a portion of sepsis-mediated adrenergic vascular unresponsiveness (28). Similarly, adrenergic receptor density may be altered by ontogenetic influences (158). Infants have diminished catecholamine responsiveness; a portion of this phenomenon is probably due to diminished numbers and/or responsiveness of adrenergic receptors. (158).

Even when adrenergic receptor density is normal or increased, altered catecholamine-induced inotropic, chronotropic, or peripheral vascular effects may be noted because of postreceptor influences. This circumstance is observed, for example, in neonatal and young dogs (123), and following either chronic exposure to catecholamines or chronic blockade of α- or β-adrenergic receptors (115). β-Adrenergic receptors have two agonist-affinity states; changes being regulated by guanine nucleotides (115), and those affinity changes being modulated by small changes in plasma cate-

cholamine concentration (49). Differences in receptor affinity produce variations in adrenergic responsiveness, although our understanding of the β-adrenergic receptor coupling mechanism is currently limited. It is likely that changes in receptor affinity have important implications in the actions of exogenous or endogenous catecholamines. For example, repeated or prolonged exposure of the β-adrenergic receptor to an agonist results in an attenuated response that is partly mediated by altering the coupling state of the receptor (140).

ENDOGENOUS CATECHOLAMINE RESPONSE

The neurohumoral response to critical illness has important effects on the pharmacodynamics of inotropes. Besides altering adrenergic receptor affinity state and cell density as outlined above, endogenous catecholamines exert vasoactive effects: stimulating heart rate and cardiac contractility, modulating peripheral vascular tone, and partly mediating the metabolic changes characteristic of critical illness (27). When an inotrope is administered to a critically ill patient, the net hemodynamic effect reflects the pharmacodynamic action of the drug and the modifying influence of the patient's endogenous catecholamine response.

The majority of plasma norepinephrine is derived from synaptic nerve clefts. Norepinephrine is the neurotransmitter of the sympathetic nervous system; it is released from sympathetic nerves and acts locally. The concentration of norepinephrine in the plasma is used as a marker of sympathetic nerve activity (59), although it is influenced by the rate of norepinephrine release, the rate of norepinephrine reuptake by the sympathetic nerve, the rate of metabolic degradation at the effector site, and the rate of metabolic clearance from the plasma. Esler (48) has shown that a normal plasma norepinephrine concentration may be associated with an increased rate of norepinephrine release balanced by an increased rate of metabolic clearance. Plasma norepinephrine (and epinephrine) concentrations are also influenced by the site of sampling; epinephrine is increased and norepinephrine decreased in forearm arterial versus venous blood. (14). Therefore, caution should be used in the interpretation of plasma norepinephrine concentrations as a reflection of sympathetic nervous system activity. Finally, elevations in plasma norepinephrine concentration reflect neuronal activity and are *not* equivalent to norepinephrine infusions since circulating norepinephrine concentrations must exceed 1800 pg/ml to produce a clinically measurable hemodynamic effect (130), and these endogenous plasma concentrations are unusual in most stress states.

The release of norepinephrine from sympathetic nerves is controlled by a complex interplay between presynaptic receptors (for catecholamines, acetylcholine, angiotensin and other mediators) (129) and modulation by such other factors as pH, adenosine concentration, and prostaglandin E_2 (PGE_2) that can either increase or decrease norepinephrine release (129, 137). Many of these hormonal or metabolic systems are abnormal in critical illness and may modulate the local release and action of catecholamines.

Circulating epinephrine is largely derived from the adrenal gland and a small contribution is derived from other chromaffin tissue. Unlike norepinephrine, epinephrine functions as a circulating hormone; small changes in concentration can produce significant alterations in hemodynamic effects (31). Normal plasma epinephrine concentrations are in the range of 24–74 pg/ml; concentrations of 75–125 pg/ml produce increases in heart rate and systolic blood pressure (31).

Despite the limitations in the interpretation of plasma catecholamine concentrations noted above, it is apparent that the sympathetic nervous system functions as an important homeostatic mechanism to maintain blood pressure and cardiac output in response to shock and other stresses, and that this response can be approximately quantitated by measurement of plasma catecholamine concentrations.

Myocardial infarction (12) hemorrhagic hypotension (26), trauma (35, 70), and cardiopulmonary arrest (155), to name a few, are all associated with substantial increases in circulating norepinephrine and/or epinephrine concentrations. The extent of plasma catecholamine elevation has been correlated with the severity of congestive heart failure (32) and with the severity of injury early after trauma (35). This type of assessment may prove to be a useful means of assessing the severity of illness in critically ill patients. The increase in plasma catecholamines in critical illness may function in concert with other counter-regulatory hormones to mediate some of the hemodynamic and metabolic alterations characteristic of stress (53), although the degree of correlation between plasma catecholamine concentrations and cardiac effects is unclear (156). Thus, endogenous catecholamine responses to critical illness influence the net hemodynamic response (pharmacodynamics) of exogenously administered catecholamines.

SPECIFIC INOTROPIC AGENTS

Epinephrine

PHARMACOLOGY

As noted previously, epinephrine is an important endogenous hormone (Fig. 31.1) that is largely produced and released from the adrenal gland in response to stress. The direct cardiac effects of epinephrine are mediated through β_1-adrenergic receptors. Epinephrine shortens systole more than diastole, in part by increasing conduction through the atrioventricular (AV) node and Purkinje system. It accelerates transmission through the SA node directly, and accelerates ectopic foci. Although epinephrine therapy may increase coronary blood flow, particularly in patients with coronary artery disease, epinephrine often increases myocardial oxygen demand more than oxygen delivery so that a mismatch occurs (127). In addition, it decreases the refractory period of ventricular muscle, predisposing the myocardium to arrhythmias.

When epinephrine is infused, its hemodynamic actions are determined by the infusion rate: at low rates (0.005–0.02 μg/kg/minute in adults) epinephrine principally stimulates β-

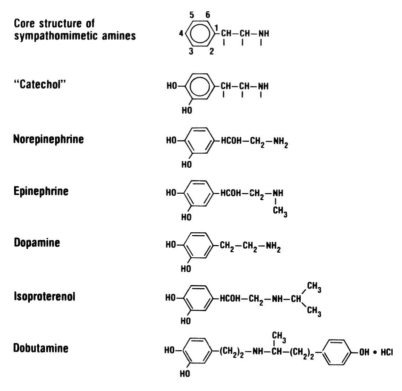

Figure 31.1. Chemical structure of the catecholamines. (From Chernow B, Rainey TG, Lake CR: Endogenous and exogenous catecholamines in critical care medicine. *Crit Care Med* 10:409–416, 1982.)

adrenergic receptors, resulting in peripheral vasodilation and increased heart rate and contractility. The net hemodynamic effects are to widen the pulse pressure, decrease systemic and pulmonary vascular resistance, and increase stroke volume, left ventricular stroke work, and cardiac output, provided that the patient's circulating blood volume is adequate. As the infusion rate is increased, more α-adrenergic mediated effects are seen, resulting in increased systemic vascular resistance, elevation of blood pressure, and variable effects on cardiac output (the latter action is dependent on the myocardium's ability to maintain stroke volume as afterload is increased).

Similar epinephrine-induced actions are seen in pediatric patients, although the dosage ranges are substantially different (based on infusion rate/weight). Thus, infusions up to 0.3 μg/kg/ minute in infants and children often produce a predominant β-adrenergic effect with little evidence of increased systemic vascular resistance.

Epinephrine has important effects on the respiratory system. Activation of β_2-adrenergic

receptors in bronchial smooth muscle results in bronchodilation, which combined with an inhibition of mast cell degranulation (mediated through β_2-adrenergic stimulation) has beneficial effects in asthma (7). Epinephrine is particularly important in the asthmatic patient since sympathetic nervous innervation of bronchial smooth muscle is scant (83), and, therefore, β-adrenergic mediated bronchodilation is largely determined by the amount of circulating epinephrine (148).

Epinephrine is a potent renal artery vasoconstrictor that limits its usefulness in patients with shock. Infusions as low as 0.035 μg/kg/ minute induce a 10% fall in renal plasma flow in humans (60). A portion of epinephrine's vasoconstrictive effect is also probably mediated by increased renin activity following direct stimulation of β-adrenergic receptors of the juxtaglomerular apparatus (69). The net effect is to reduce renal blood flow and urine output. Despite these limitations, in patients with low cardiac output, epinephrine may increase urine output by increasing cardiac output and therefore renal blood flow (33).

Infusion of epinephrine to achieve plasma concentrations seen with exercise or stress causes plasma glucose, lactate, β-hydroxybutyrate, and free fatty acid concentrations to rise (31, 131), and serum potassium (22, 141) and phosphorus (18) concentrations to fall. The former are mediated by increased gluconeogenesis from the liver (131), skeletal muscle insulin resistance (13), and inhibition of insulin release (31). Epinephrine concentrations up to 1000 pg/ml do not alter plasma alanine, glucagon, growth hormone, or cortisol levels (31). Epinephrine-induced hypokalemia occurs through a β_2-adrenergic mechanism; mean plasma potassium falls 0.8 mEq/liter in response to epinephrine concentrations achieved during myocardial infarction (22, 141). Coincident with the decline in potassium, T-wave flattening and QT_c prolongation were observed (141). These electrophysiologic effects in combination with epinephrine-induced hypokalemia may predispose the critically ill patient to serious dysrhythmias. Similar decreases in plasma potassium are seen with the use of other β_2-agonists, such as agents used in asthma or to inhibit labor (80).

INDICATIONS AND DOSE

Epinephrine infusions are most frequently used in pediatric patients; in adults, their potential toxicity in patients with coronary artery disease limits their utility. The recommended infusion rate in adults to produce principally a β-adrenergic effect is 0.005–0.02 μg/kg/minute (27). In pediatric patients, infusion rates of 0.05–0.3 μg/kg/minute are recommended in the treatment of cardiogenic or septic shock (160). Epinephrine may be particularly useful when combined with afterload reduction in cardiogenic shock, (10) and is preferable to dopamine in pediatric patients in whom catecholamine stores may be depleted (see "Dopamine", Table 31.2).

In the treatment of acute asthma, epinephrine may be administered subcutaneously in a dose of 0.01 mg/kg, up to 0.3 mg every 15–20 minutes. It is also administered subcutaneously in the treatment of acute allergic, local reactions (e.g., to bee stings), and may be administered intravenously (5–10 ml of the 1:10,000 solution) in the treatment of anaphylaxis. In cardiac arrest, epinephrine is the most effective pharmacologic agent (see Chapter 10) and may be administered intravenously (0.01 mg/kg) or endotracheally.

ADMINISTRATION AND TOXICITY

Epinephrine (adrenaline) is available in several forms: prediluted in syringes (1:10,000 concentration; 0.1 mg/ml) for use in cardiac arrest and anaphylaxis and in vials for subcutaneous administration (1-ml vials) and the preparation of intravenous infusions (30-ml vials) Tables 31.3 and 31.4).

The pharmacokinetics of epinephrine have been examined in a number of studies but always in normal adult volunteers (14, 31). Epinephrine is rapidly cleared from the plasma at mean rates of 35–89 ml/kg/minute, depending on the site of sampling and the rate of epinephrine infusion (14, 31). Clearance is largely by the liver and kidney, which contain

Table 31.2
Suggested Uses of Catecholamines by Age[a]

Condition	Infant	Child	Adult
Cardiogenic shock	EPI or Dobut DA[a]	Dobut DA or EPI	Dobut or DA EPI NE
Septic shock	EPI or Dobut DA	Dobut EPI or DA	Dobut or DA NE or EPI
Hypovolemic shock	Not Indicated	Not Indicated	Not Indicated
Shock from bradycardia	EPI or ISO	EPI or ISO	ISO or EPI
Anaphylactic shock	EPI	EPI	EPI
Decreased renal blood flow or urine output	DA	DA	DA

DA, dopamine; EPI, epinephrine; Dobut, dobutamine; NE, norepinephrine; ISO, isoproterenol.
[a] Listed in order of preference.
[b] DA at low infusion rates (1 to 2 μg/kg/minutes) may be used in combination with other catecholamines in shock to help maintain renal blood flow. DA is relatively contraindicated in patients with pulmonary artery hypertension. From Zaritsky A, Eisenberg MG: Ontogenetic considerations in the pharmacotherapy of shock. In Chernow B, Shoemaker WC (eds): *Critical Care: State of the Art,* vol. 7. Fullerton, CA, Society of Critical Care Medicine, 1986, pp 485–534.

Table 31.3
Prescribing Infusions of Synthetic Catecholamines: Deriving Concentrations

Catecholamine	How Supplied	Diluent	Concentration
Epinephrine (Adrenalin chloride)	1 mg (1 ml) dosette ampules of 1:1000 epi; also in 30-ml vial of 1 mg/ml[a]	250 ml of either D_5W or 0.9% NaCl	4 μg/ml
Norepinephrine (Noradrenaline)	4-mg ampule of NE bitartrate; each ampule has 4 ml of fluid with 1 mg NE/ml[a]	250 ml of either D_5W, 0.9% NaCl or 0.45% NaCl	16 μg/ml
Dopamine	200-mg ampules (5 ml) of dopamine HCl (40 mg/ml); also available in 400-mg (10 ml) prefilled syringe.[a,b]	250 ml of D_5W or 0.9% NaCl	800 μg/ml
Dobutamine	250-mg lyophilized vials of dobutamine HCl which also contain 250 mg of mannitol; reconstitute with 10–20 ml of sterile water or D_5W; also in premixed solution– 400 mg/5 ml.[a,b]	250 ml of either D_5W or 0.9% NaCl	1000 μg/ml
Isoproterenol	1-mg ampule of 1:5000 isoproterenol HCL; each ampule has 1 mg/5 ml of fluid[a]	250 ml of either D_5W or 0.9% NaCl	4 μg/ml

[a] Protect ampules from light.
[b] Avoid use with alkaline solutions.

substantial concentrations of the enzymes catechol-O-methyl transferase and monoamine oxidase (78). This clearance results in a short half-life (about 2 minutes), which requires a continuous infusion to maintain hemodynamic effects. Perhaps more important is the degree of interindividual variation in epinephrine clearance reported in normal adults. In critical illness, greater variation in clearance would be expected, emphasizing the importance of individual titration of the infusion rate.

Epinephrine is also well absorbed from the tracheobronchial tree, although the plasma concentration and hemodynamic effects are about 1/10 those seen with a similar dose given intravenously (25). Endotracheal administration is reserved for patients in cardiac arrest or severe anaphylaxis in whom vascular access is not readily available. To improve absorption by this route, it is important to deliver the drug deeply into the airway, which may be accomplished by administration through a small feeding tube or other suitable catheter followed by flushing with air and manual hyperventilation (62, 116).

Epinephrine should preferably be administered through a central venous line, or at least a secure peripheral catheter, since infiltration from peripheral venous administration can result in local ulceration. If infiltration occurs and is recognized early, local injection of the site with 5–10 ml of phentolamine in 10–15 ml of saline may be effective. The epinephrine infusion rate should be controlled by a constant infusion pump to avoid inadvertent boluses. Epinephrine is compatible with a number of intravenous solutions (Table 31.3);

Table 31.4
Preparation of Catecholamine Infusions in Children

Catecholamine	Preparation	Dose
Isoproterenol Epinephrine Norepinephrine	0.6 mg × body weight (kg), added to diluent to make 100 ml	Then 1 ml/hr delivers 0.1 μg/kg/min
Dopamine Dobutamine	6 mg × body weight (kg), added to diluent to make 100 ml	Then 1 ml/hr delivers 1 μg/kg/minute

From Zaritsky A, Chernow B: Use of catecholamines in pediatrics. *J Pediatr* 105:341–350, 1984.

alkaline solutions should be avoided as diluents for epinephrine and other catecholamines that are inactivated at the higher pH.

Epinephrine-induced toxicities include restlessness, fear, throbbing headache, tachycardia, tachydysrhythmias (PVCs, ventricular tachycardia, and ventricular fibrillation), severe hypertension with secondary cerebral hemorrhage, and anginal pain resulting from an increase in myocardial oxygen demand relative to myocardial oxygen delivery.

Norepinephrine

PHARMACOLOGY

Norepinephrine is the neurotransmitter of the sympathetic nervous system and is the biosynthetic precursor of epinephrine, differing only by a methyl group on its amino terminus (Fig. 31.1). It possess both α- and β-adrenergic receptor activity; low-infusion doses produce mainly β-adrenergic effects: cardiac contractility, conduction velocity, and chronotropy increase with little change in peripheral vascular resistance. More commonly, in the doses used during hypotensive shock, mixed α- and β-adrenergic effects occur. Peripheral vascular resistance is increased by α_1-adrenergic mediated vasoconstriction. Cardiac contractility, cardiac work and stroke volume all increase if the augmentation in afterload is tolerated by the ventricle. Chronotropy is generally blunted by baroreceptor-mediated vagal effects to slow the heart rate in response to norepinephrine-induced increase in blood pressure.

As with epinephrine, norepinephrine is a potent renal and splanchnic vasoconstrictor, which limits its clinical usefulness (63). It vasoconstricts the pulmonary as well as the systemic vascular bed and should be used with caution in patients with pulmonary artery hypertension. Norepinephrine infusion at 5.0 μg/minute in normal adults elevates blood glucose, glycerol, β-hydroxybutyrate, and acetoacetate (130); the metabolic effects of infusions in critical illness have not been reported.

INDICATIONS AND DOSE

Norepinephrine has limited usefulness in critically ill patients; its major indication is to elevate blood pressure in hypotensive patients who have failed to respond to adequate volume resuscitation and other, less potent, inotropes. The most frequent clinical condition

generating this state is septic shock, and norepinephrine can help maintain perfusion pressure in this setting (29).

Norepinephrine may also be useful in myocardial infarction shock, since the major determinant of myocardial oxygen delivery is the diastolic blood pressure–left ventricular end diastolic pressure gradient (105). The goal should be to increase mean arterial pressure to 70–80 torr, at which time coronary blood flow improves (105). Use of a potent vasoconstrictor must be balanced against the increase in ventricular afterload, which heightens myocardial oxygen demand; therefore, norepinephrine should only be considered a temporizing measure. Intraaortic balloon counterpulsation is one of therapeutic approaches that is supplanting norepinephrine in hypotensive, cardiogenic shock patients since it has the advantage of both increasing diastolic coronary perfusion and decreasing ventricular afterload.

An additional concern with norepinephrine is renal vasoconstriction compromising renal function. Low-dose dopamine ameliorates the vasoconstrictive action of norepinephrine in dogs. (126). The clinical combination of dopamine and norepinephrine may therefore provide both the desired increase in coronary perfusion pressure and the maintenance of adequate renal function.

Initial norepinephrine infusion rate of 2 μg/minute is typical and is subsequently increased until the desired change in blood pressure is achieved. In pediatric patients, norepinephrine infusions may be prepared as seen in Table 31.4; initial infusion rates are 0.05–0.1 μg/kg/minute and are subsequently titrated up to 1.0 μg/kg/minute.

ADMINISTRATION AND TOXICITY

Norepinephrine bitartrate (Levophed bitartrate) is available in 4-ml ampules of 1 mg/ml (Table 31.3). Intravenous infusions are constituted by adding 4 mg of norepinephrine to 250 or 500 ml of 5% dextrose in water or normal saline, which produces final concentrations of 16 or 8 μg/ml, respectfully. Norepinephrine is rapidly cleared from the plasma following intravenous administration; its average half-life is 2–2.5 minutes, although substantial interindividual variation has been noted (50). Norepinephrine is cleared by enzymatic degradation in the liver and kidney and by uptake and degradation in neuronal and nonneuronal effecter organ sites.

Norepinephrine infusions should preferably be given through a central vein. Careful monitoring of arterial pressure, perfusion, and renal function is necessary during norepinephrine infusions to prevent organ ischemia and excessive increases in ventricular afterload. Inadvertent boluses may precipitate profound hypertension, which may result in myocardial infarction or cerebral hemorrhage (150). Infiltrated infusions may produce local skin necrosis and ulceration, and if recognized early should be treated with phentolamine injunction (see "toxicity" under "Epinephrine"). Anxiety, respiratory difficulty, palpitations, angina, and transient headaches also occur.

Norepinephrine may also be added to gastric lavage solutions used in the treatment of acute gastrointestinal bleeding, with 16 mg of norepinephrine added to 200 ml of iced saline (40).

Isoproterenol

PHARMACOLOGY

Isoproterenol is a synthetic, N-alkylated catecholamine similar in structure to epinephrine (Fig. 31.1). It is a potent β-adrenergic agonist and therefore has potent effects on the heart; it stimulates an increase in cardiac contractility, heart rate, and conduction velocity. It also shortens arteriovenous nodal conduction and may incite either ventricular or atrial dysrhythmias. Stimulation of peripheral β_2-adrenergic receptors results in vascular smooth muscle relaxation, while systemic vascular resistance and diastolic blood pressure fall. Since β_2-adrenergic vascular receptors are most prevalent in the skeletal muscle vascular bed, cardiac output may be redirected from the splanchnic bed to the skeletal muscle bed producing a "splanchnic steal" (65).

The net hemodynamic effect produced by isoproterenol infusion is an increase in cardiac output, provided circulating blood volume is adequate. When circulating blood volume is low, vasodilation may impair venous return and cardiac output may fall. Pulse pressure increases because of a rise in systolic pressure generated by enhanced cardiac contractility and the fall in diastolic blood pressure mediated by peripheral vasodilation. Much of the increase in cardiac output is often related to the change in heart rate, rather than an increase in stroke volume, particularly in pediatric patients (43, 65).

Isoproterenol also relaxes pulmonary vascular and bronchial airway smooth muscle; pulmonary vascular resistance falls and bronchospasm may be reversed. By overcoming hypoxic pulmonary vasoconstriction, isoproterenol can increase intrapulmonary shunt and may result in a fall in arterial oxygen tension when used in patients with parenchymal lung disease.

Since heart rate and contractility are increased, myocardial oxygen demand is enhanced. At the same time, isoproterenol-induced decreases in diastolic filling time and diastolic coronary perfusion pressure may impair myocardial oxygen supply, which results in myocardial ischemia (104).

Isoproterenol does not produce the same degree of hyperglycemia as epinephrine, probably because β-adrenergic stimulation enhances insulin release, whereas α_2-adrenergic stimulation seen with epinephrine inhibits insulin release (114).

INDICATIONS AND DOSE

Once a popular inotrope, isoproterenol has fallen out of favor because of its propensity to produce myocardial ischemia and excessive tachycardia and because more selective inotropes are available. Isoproterenol may be used to treat hemodynamically significant bradycardia, particularly in the setting of heart block but should only be considered a temporizing measure until more definitive therapy, such as cardiac pacing, is obtained (135). In bradycardic pediatric patients, low-dose epinephrine infusion may be useful and has the advantage of maintaining diastolic coronary perfusion pressure better than isoproterenol.

Isoproterenol has been effective in pediatric patients with status asthmaticus (41) and those with pulmonary artery hypertension (100). Indeed, isoproterenol has been used to help assess the reversibility of pulmonary hypertension in pediatric patients prior to surgery in certain forms of congenital heart disease, as well as to reduce pulmonary artery pressure in the postoperative period (92, 100). Finally, isoproterenol may be used as an inotrope, although other agents that have fewer side effects are available. In adults with coronary artery disease, isoproterenol should be avoided since myocardial ischemia is likely (104).

Infusions are usually begun at 0.01 μg/kg/minute and are adjusted to produce the desired hemodynamic effect. In pediatric patients, infusions may be conveniently prepared as seen in Table 31.4. Initial infusion rates are 0.05–0.1 μg/kg/minute. As with other catecholamines, infusions should be administered through a secure intravenous line using a calibrated infusion pump, and the patient's heart rate and blood pressure should be carefully monitored.

ADMINISTRATION AND TOXICITY

The parenteral form of isoproterenol (Isuprel HCl) is available in 5-ml vials containing 1 mg (1:5,000 solution; Table 31.3). For adults, one vial (1 mg) is added to 250 ml of saline or D_5W giving a concentration of 4μgml.

After intravenous administration, isoproterenol is rapidly cleared from the plasma; it has a half-life of about 2 minutes (57). It is largely cleared in the liver and to a lesser extent it is taken up by effecter organs throughout the body. It is also well absorbed from the tracheobronchial tree and is thus available in an aerosol form for treatment of asthma, although more selective β-$_2$-adrenergic agonists, such as metaproterenol and albuterol, have largely replaced aerosolized isoproterenol.

The major side effects of isoproterenol are tachycardia and tachydysrhythmias, particularly ventricular tachycardia. As noted previously, angina and myocardial infarction may result from the unfavorable action of isoproterenol on myocardial oxygen demand relative to oxygen delivery (104, 105), and has been reported in pediatric patients treated for status asthmaticus (81). Palpitation, headache, and flushing of the skin are common; whereas nausea, tremor, dizziness, and weakness are less common side effects.

Dopamine

PHARMACOLOGY

Dopamine is the immediate precursor of norepinephrine in the endogenous catecholamine biosynthetic pathway and differs from norepinephrine by the absence of a β-hydroxyl group (Fig. 31.1). Dopamine also serves as a neurotransmitter in both the central and peripheral nervous systems (82). In the latter, it appears to modulate autonomic activity at sympathetic ganglia, alter gastrointestinal activity, decrease aldosterone synthesis, and release (134) and increase renal blood flow (38, 82). When infused in pharmacologic concentrations, dopamine has complex actions because of its mixed direct and indirect sympathomimetic actions.

Unlike the other catecholamines, dopamine's hemodynamic effects are attributed to dopamine-stimulated release of norepinephrine from sympathetic nerves, as well as direct stimulation of α-, β- and DA receptors (42, 55). Pretreatment of dogs with reserpine to deplete endogenous norepinephrine stores suggests that as much as 50% of dopamine's hemodynamic action may be produced by norepinephrine release (42). In clinical studies, dopamine infusions increase plasma norepinephrine in a dose-dependent manner (77), and dopamine's hemodynamic effect is less pronounced than that observed with a direct-acting catecholamine, such as dobutamine, in clinical conditions characterized by myocardial norepinephrine depletion (30, 90).

When infused at 2–5 μg/kg/minute in normal subjects, dopamine increases cardiac contractility and cardiac output with little change in heart rate, blood pressure, or systemic vascular resistance (54, 55). Doses up to 10 μg/kg/minute in normal subjects further increase cardiac output, with small increases in heart rate and blood pressure (54). Renal blood flow and urine output increase at doses of 0.5–2.0 μg/kg/minute secondary to selective action at dopaminergic receptors (85); sodium excretion is enhanced by the increase in renal flow and dopamine-mediated inhibition of proximal tubular sodium reabsorption (112). Further improvement in renal function may occur at higher infusions rate related to improved global cardiac output. At infusion rates in excess of 10 μg/kg/minute an increasing α-adrenergic effect may be seen with increases in systemic vascular resistance and subsequently mean arterial pressure (122). The salutary effect of dopamine on renal blood flow may be lost at higher doses due to predominant α-adrenergic effects. (55).

In patients with pulmonary hypertension, dopamine infusions may lead to further increases in mean pulmonary artery pressure (67, 136), and dopamine enhances hypoxic pulmonary vasoconstriction (100). In the absence of pulmonary hypertension, dopamine increases pulmonary blood flow with little change in mean pulmonary artery pressure or pulmonary capillary wedge pressure (55). Dopamine constricts capacitance veins that may raise pulmonary capillary wedge pressure (84, 96); serious consequences may then result by increasing myocardial wall tension, and therefore myocardial oxygen demand, and by worsening hydrostatic pulmonary edema. (90).

Dopamine has several metabolic effects that may be important in the critically ill patient. Dopamine receptors located in the zona glomerulosa of the adrenal cortex decrease aldosterone secretion (151). Conversely, dopamine receptor blockade (for example, following the administration of metoclopramide) increases plasma aldosterone concentration (24). Dopamine inhibits thyroid-stimulating hormone (TSH) and prolactin release (157); the former blunts the response to thyroxine-releasing hormone (TRH), making discrimination between the patient with hypothyrodism and the one with the euthyroid-sick syndrome more difficult. Insulin secretion is also inhibited by a direct action of dopamine on pancreatic islet cells (161), although the clinical importance of this effect during dopamine infusion is unclear.

INDICATIONS AND DOSE

In cardiogenic shock due to myocardial infarction, a mean dopamine infusion rate of 17.2 μg/kg/minute was required to raise mean arterial pressure to 65–70 torr (106). In this study, dopamine infusion also increased heart rate, mean arterial pressure and cardiac index, and decreased pulmonary capillary wedge pressure (PCWP), central venous pressure (CVP), and systemic vascular resistance (SVR). Myocardial oxygen extraction significantly increased along with lactate production, indicating that the improvement in cardiac performance was at the expense of an increase in myocardial oxygen demand. Holzer et al. (68) also studied dopamine administration in cardiogenic shock. Survivors had improved cardiac output, urinary flow, PCWP, and heart rate at mean infusions of 9.1 μg/kg/minute, whereas nonsurvivors failed to show beneficial effects at mean infusion rates of 17.1 μg/kg/minute. Nonresponse to dopamine may have been because these patients were more acidotic.

Combined administration of dopamine and dobutamine may have advantages over the administration of either agent alone in cardiogenic shock (121). Dopamine alone (15 μg/kg/minute) consistently increased mean arterial pressure but also increased PCWP, had variable effects on stroke index, and reduced PaO₂. Dobutamine alone (15 μg/kg/minute) failed to increase mean arterial pressure, but

more consistently improved stroke volume. The combination of dopamine and dobutamine (7.5 μg/kg/minute each) had the most beneficial effects: mean arterial pressure, cardiac index, and stroke volume index all increased with no change in PCWP, mean pulmonary artery pressure, or PaO_2 (121). All three infusion combinations increased intrapulmonary shunt. This effect is common to inotropes that increase cardiac output, and is due to improved perfusion of poorly ventilated lung segments (72). Dopamine, however, caused hypoxemia, probably due to an increase in PCWP (90).

As in cardiogenic shock, dobutamine is superior to dopamine in chronic heart failure (90). Based on animal studies, dopamine's inotropic response is attenuated because myocardial norepinephrine stores are depleted in chronic cardiac failure (30). In addition, dopamine loses its inotropic effect after 24 hours of infusion in experimental myocardial infarction, presumably because of depletion of myocardial norepinephrine stores, and dopamine accentuates myocardial norepinephrine release, which may more rapidly deplete stores (93). Dopamine does not influence infarct size (6, 93), whereas dobutamine decreases the area of ischemic infarction (93).

After coronary artery bypass grafting, dopamine has frequently been used to support the circulation. Dopamine had increasing inotropic action during a 24-hour observation period after bypass graft (143), unlike the response seen in experimental myocardial infarction (93). Despite this beneficial effect, when compared with dobutamine, dopamine produces a relatively smaller enhancement of left ventricular contractility and it increases myocardial oxygen demand (142). Differences in the hemodynamic response to dopamine and dobutamine in the postoperative period may be related to the state of the ventricle (39). In normal ventricles, dobutamine had a greater chronotropic response; in volume-loaded ventricles, both drugs had similar effects on heart rate and cardiac output, but dobutamine caused a greater reduction in systemic vascular resistance and pulmonary vascular resistance (39). Neither agent (at 5 μg/kg/minutes) produces a hemodynamic effect in the pressure-loaded ventricle. Dobutamine appears to be superior to dopamine in the postoperative period.

In septic shock, dopamine is effective in improving cardiac output, although intrapulmonary shunting may increase as well (119). The latter can be prevented by the application of positive end-expiratory pressure (PEEP) (119). Since many septic patients are hypotensive, dopamine has the advantage of increasing systemic vascular resistance, and therefore blood pressure, and may be preferable over dobutamine in this clinical setting (153). An additional advantage of dopamine is its beneficial effect on urine output (37). Despite these advantages, dopamine has the disadvantage of increasing PCWP and pulmonary artery pressure in septic patients (37, 119).

Dopamine's major clinical benefit is that it causes a selective increase in renal and splanchnic blood flow. A low-dose infusion (1–4 μg/kg/minute) augments urine output following cardiopulmonary bypass (36), and in patients with oliguria and critical illness (111). Dopamine may also antagonize the vasoconstrictive action of norepinephrine and other adrenergic vasoconstrictors (126). In experimental studies, it improves blood flow and protein synthesis in the postischemic liver (66).

In pediatric patients, the pharmacodynamic effects of dopamine are further complicated by ontogenetic changes in response (158). In experimental animal studies, the more immature the animal, the smaller the relative hemodynamic response compared with adults (23, 42). Clinical studies reveal more consistent salutary effects of dopamine in premature neonates: infusions of 0.5–2 μg/kg/minute improve urine output, sodium excretion, and creatinine clearance (144), and dose-dependent improvement in blood pressure and cardiac output is seen at infusion rates between 2–8 μg/kg/minute (110). Recommendations for the use of dopamine and other catecholamines in pediatric patients are seen in Table 31.2.

Infusion rates of 0.5–2 μg/kg/minute result in selective dopaminergic actions on the renal and splanchnic vasculature. With infusion rates between 5–10 μg/kg/minute β-adrenergic effects usually dominate: infusions between 10–20 μg/kg/minute have mixed α- and β-adrenergic effects, whereas infusions in excess of 20 μg/kg/minute have predominant α-adrenergic effects.

ADMINISTRATION AND TOXICITY

Dopamine is available in a number of commercial formulations (Table 31.3). In adults, 200 mg may be diluted in 250 ml of diluent (e.g., D_5W), producing a final dopamine concentration of 800 μg/ml. In pediatric patients, infusions are prepared as seen in Table 31.4.

As with other catecholamines, dopamine should not be mixed in an alkaline solution.

After intravenous administration, dopamine is rapidly cleared from the plasma by a biphasic process and has a terminal elimination half-life of 9 minutes. Steady state plasma clearance of dopamine (50–70 ml/kg/minute) is similar in both adults and infants (73, 110).

Nausea, emesis, and tachyarrhythmias are the most frequent side effects (64). Anginal pain, myocardial ischemia (93), serious hypertension, and profound vasoconstriction may occur (56, 93). In patients dependent on hypoxic ventilatory drive, dopamine may depress ventilation and worsen hypoxemia (108).

Dobutamine

PHARMACOLOGY

Dobutamine was developed after the catecholamine molecule was systematically modified in the search for an agent that would have selective inotropic activity with little peripheral vascular effect (145). Dobutamine has a large substitution on the amino terminus of the catecholamine molecule (Fig. 31.1), and it is the only catecholamine administered as a racemic mixture of the (+)- and (−)- isomers. This racemic mixture provides dobutamine with its characteristic β_1-adrenergic selectivity: the (−)-isomer is an α-adrenergic agonist and the (+)-isomer acts as a competitive α-adrenergic receptor antagonist (125). The (+)-isomer is also the more potent form at the β-adrenergic receptor, although both isomers produce inotropic and chronotropic actions (125).

Dobutamine's hemodynamic effect is dependent on drug dose. At the usual infusion rates (5–15 μg/kg/minute) dobutamine's predominant effect is on the heart with an increase in contractility and a relatively smaller increase in heart rate. Dobutamine's comparatively selective inotropic action is probably multifactorial and attributed partly to the presence of both β_1- and β_2-adrenergic receptors in the sinoatrial node, which produce chronotropic effects, and dobutamine's higher affinity for the β_1-adrenergic receptor (152). Attenuated α-adrenergic effects in the peripheral vasculature are further balanced by a modest β_2-adrenergic effect so that peripheral vascular resistance is little changed (88). Dobutamine generally lowers central venous and pulmonary wedge pressure and has little effect on pulmonary vascular resistance. Like other inotropes, dobutamine can increase intrapulmonary shunt by augmenting cardiac output and thus perfusion of poorly ventilated lung regions (71).

Dobutamine does not have a selective vascular action, and significant metabolic side effects have not been reported. Although it lacks a selective renal vascular effect, dobutamine often enhances urine output by improving cardiac output and thus renal perfusion (87).

Unlike dopamine, dobutamine's pharmacologic action does not depend upon releasable stores of norepinephrine (125). Dobutamine loses its hemodynamic effect during prolonged infusion (146), presumably because of down-regulation of receptors, but dobutamine maintains its hemodynamic effect much better than dopamine during continuous infusion since the latter depletes myocardial norepinephrine stores (97).

INDICATIONS AND DOSE

Dobutamine is indicated in clinical conditions where increased contractility with little effect on peripheral vascular resistance is desired. This setting most often occurs in normotensive patients with congestive heart failure (88). In patients with congestive heart failure, dobutamine increases stroke volume and cardiac output, while reducing the elevated filling pressure accompanying this clinical state (5, 87). When used in lower dosages (2–10 μg/kg/minute), little change in heart rate is seen (88). In patients with very poor myocardial function and higher baseline plasma norepinephrine concentrations, however, dobutamine's effect on cardiac index is attenuated (34).

In patients with myocardial failure and non-obstructed coronary arteries, dobutamine improves coronary blood flow and myocardial oxygen supply equal to, or in excess of, the increase in myocardial oxygen demand elicited by its positive inotropic action (94). Supplementation of myocardial perfusion may partly explain dobutamine's ability to produce sustained improvement of cardiac function in patients with congestive heart failure following short-term infusions (89). In one study, a 72-hour dobutamine infusion improved endomyocardial ATP/creatinine ratio and the ultrastructural appearance of mitochondria (147).

Dobutamine generally improves the balance between myocardial oxygen supply and demand in patients with myocardial failure resulting from coronary artery disease (88). Patients with myocardial infarction also benefit from dobutamine infusion, even those having hypotension prior to therapy (76, 120). Patients with hypotensive cardiogenic shock, however, may not be improved by dobutamine since it has relatively less peripheral vascular action, and dopamine may be superior in this setting (52, 88).

In postoperative cardiovascular surgical patients, dobutamine improves stroke volume and decreases ventricular filling pressures with less positive chronotropy than observed with dopamine (61). In addition, dobutamine has a more beneficial effect on myocardial blood flow than dopamine (51). In patients following a heart transplant, myocardial sympathetic innervation is destroyed. Since dobutamine's inotropic action does not depend on myocardial stores of norepinephrine, it should be a better inotrope than dopamine, and indeed this finding has been observed (46).

Because dobutamine lacks clinically important vasoconstrictive effects, it may be disadvantageous in the patient with septic shock and hypotension. Dobutamine should ideally be reserved for septic patients with combined ventricular dysfunction and elevated filling pressures (71, 88).

Dobutamine is also a useful inotropic agent in pediatric patients with a variety of clinical conditions: cardiovascular failure (128), postoperative cardiovascular surgery (11), and septic shock (113). Clinical studies suggest that dobutamine is most useful in children >12 months of age since the cardiac index in younger patients failed to increase and PCWP rose in response to 10 μg/kg/minute of dobutamine (113). Depending on the clinical state, dobutamine-induced increases in cardiac index may be entirely due to increases in heart rate with little change in stroke volume (11, 19).

Initial infusion rates of dobutamine are the same in adult and pediatric patients: 2–5 μg/kg/minute. Maximal beneficial effects are generally observed with 10–15 μg/kg/minute; higher infusion rates increase the risk of drug-induced toxicity (88).

ADMINISTRATION AND TOXICITY

Dobutamine (Dobutrex) is supplied in 250-mg vials (Table 31.3). One vial is usually diluted into 250 ml of an appropriate diluent, achieving a final drug concentration of 1000 μg/ml. A good correlation exists between dobutamine dose, plasma concentration, and hemodynamic effects (88). Dobutamine is rapidly cleared and has a plasma half-life of 2.37 ± 0.7 minutes in patients with congestive heart failure (75). The drug is cleared by cathechol-O-methyl transferase and rapid redistribution from the plasma compartment.

With drug infusion, steady state plasma concentration is achieved in about five half-lives, thus like the other catecholamines, maximal effect is seen approximately 10 minutes after starting or changing the infusion rate. As with the other catecholamines, dobutamine should preferably be administered into a central venous site using a continuous infusion pump.

Dysrhythmias are the most frequent toxic side effect, although they are less frequent than with dopamine or isoproterenol (132). Other side effects include excessive tachycardia, headaches, anxiety, tremors, and excessive increases or decreases in blood pressure (88).

Amrinone and Milrinone

PHARMACOLOGY

The bipyridine, amrinone, was discovered in the search for positive inotropic drugs with a better therapeutic/toxic ratio than digoxin. Amrinone possesses positive inotropic and, to a lesser extent, chronotropic actions on the heart and has potent vasodilator properties (3, 47). Amrinone has recently been approved by the Food and Drug Administration (FDA) for intravenous administration but is not useful orally. Milrinone is a methyl carbonitrile derivative of amrinone that is orally effective and produces few side effects. The addition of a methyl group to the carbon-3 atom (Fig. 31.2) greatly increases the efficacy of the compound. Based on studies in isolated animal hearts, milrinone is 10–30 times more potent than amrinone (4).

Pharmacologically, these compounds differ from the catecholamines and the cardiac glycosides. They possess a unique structure, unlike any of the other inotropic agents (Fig. 31.2). Although their mechanism of action is still not completely understood, they do not stimulate either α- or β-adrenergic receptors nor provoke the release of either histamine or prostaglandins (1, 2). Unlike cardiac glycosides, the bipyridines do not inhibit cell membrane sodium-potassium ATPase (1, 2) but do share a similar pharmacologic action with methylxanthines (3); both inhibit phosphodiesterase resulting in an increase in intracellu-

AMRINONE

5-Amino [3,4'-Bipyridine]
-6(1H)-one

MILRINONE

1,6-Dihydro-2-methyl-6-oxo-
[3,4'-bipyridine]-5-carbonitrile

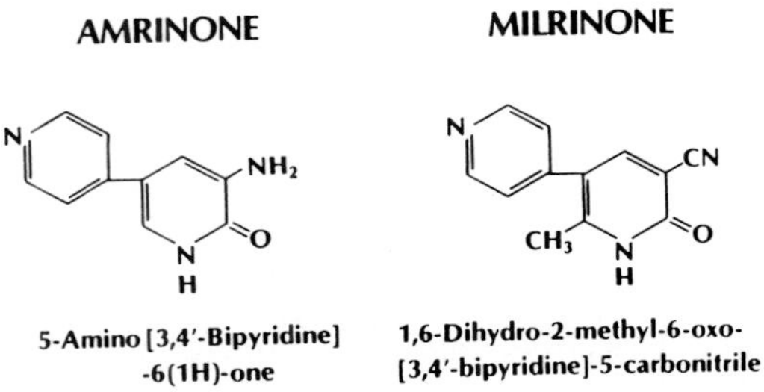

Figure 31.2. Chemical structure of amrinone and milrinone.

lar cyclic AMP (cAMP), although it is unlikely that the inotropic action of the bipyridines is simply due to phosphodiesterase inhibition (3). Finally, like most other inotropic agents, the bipyridine's inotropic action is characterized by an increase in intracellular calcium concentration (102), which can be attenuated by pretreatment with calcium channel blockers (3). Unlike catecholamines and other drugs whose inotropic effect is mediated only by increasing cAMP concentration, amrinone also appears to prolong the release and/or delay the reuptake of calcium by the sarcoplasmic reticulum (102).

Amrinone increases cAMP concentrations in vascular smooth muscle, relaxing tone (99) and thus decreasing peripheral and pulmonary vascular resistance, and dilating coronary vessels (157). Based on studies in isolated tissue, the potency of these drugs in vascular tissue is 10–100 times greater than their inotropic action (102).

In intact animals and humans, the bipyridines increase cardiac contractility, stroke volume, heart rate, and cardiac output. Although the bipyridines decrease systemic vascular resistance, systemic blood pressure is unchanged with low doses because the drug-induced increase in stroke volume compensates for the fall in resistance (3, 9). In the pulmonary vascular bed, pulmonary systolic and diastolic blood pressures usually decline (3, 9). The bipyridines are particularly beneficial in cardiac failure since they reduce afterload by peripheral vasodilation and increase cardiac contractility, often without an increase in myocardial oxygen consumption (8). The net hemodynamic effect is dose related: increasing doses produce greater afterload reduction and increased contractility, although with little further increase in cardiac output in intact dogs (3).

Complicating the pharmacology of amrinone

and milrinone is the observation of species-dependent and age-dependent differences in their inotropic effects (17). In newborn puppies, amrinone administration induces a significant *decrease* in both peak myocardial tension developed and the rate of myocardial tension development, which changed to a positive inotropic effect by 3 days of age and increased in magnitude thereafter (16). These effects are not a result of developmental changes in the effects of amrinone on phosphodiesterase (17). It is speculated that the observed ontogenetic differences are related to inadequate development of the T-tubule-sarcoplasmic reticulum system in the newborn (3, 86). Supporting this theory is the observation that amrinone has negative inotropic effects in adult Purkinje fibers, another tissue that lacks a T-tubular system (124).

Both amrinone and milrinone are largely eliminated by renal excretion (79); milrinone's half-life in normal volunteers is approximately 50 minutes (139) compared with 2 hours in patients with congestive heart failure (45). Even with drug-induced improvement in cardiac function, however, milrinone kinetics remain constant for up to 30 days with oral administration (45). Studies with amrinone reveal a mean half-life of 3.6 hours, with somewhat slower elimination seen in patients with congestive heart failure (5–8 hours) (44, 45). The relatively slow elimination observed in sicker patients has potential therapeutic implications since a continuous infusion (as currently recommended) of amrinone or milrinone may result in progressive increase in drug plasma concentrations over several hours.

INDICATIONS AND DOSE

Most of the clinical data on these drugs are derived from studies in either normal populations or patients with chronic congestive heart failure, and little data are available in patients with acute, critical illness.

When compared with dobutamine, milrinone has similar beneficial effects on stroke volume and cardiac output in normal subjects; a greater portion of the improved stroke volume observed with milrinone results from afterload reduction (20). In addition, milrinone decreases myocardial oxygen demand while enhancing cardiac output. Monrad and co-workers (101) compared milrinone to dobutamine and nitroprusside in patients with advanced congestive heart failure. All three drugs consistently improved cardiac output, but do-

butamine increased myocardial oxygen consumption and heart rate, whereas nitroprusside produced a much greater fall in blood pressure. Milrinone had little effect on heart rate or blood pressure; myocardial oxygen consumption was unchanged and pulmonary capillary wedge pressure was lowered (101). Sonnenblick et al. (133) demonstrated in patients with severe heart failure (left ventricular ejection fraction of 9–37%) that milrinone exhibited a moderate positive inotropic and potent vasodilating action; mean cardiac index increased from 1.75 to 2.36 liter/minute/m². Similar findings have been described with amrinone (8).

In patients with heart failure, amrinone augments dP/dt without significant changes in heart rate or blood pressure (58). Both amrinone and milrinone reduce left ventricular filling pressure, mean pulmonary artery pressure, right atrial pressure, and pulmonary and systemic vascular resistances (58, 74). The magnitude of these changes is variable depending on the underlying clinical state of the patient and the dosage regimen employed. Thus, milrinone and amrinone appear to have ideal hemodynamic properties in patients with severe heart failure: cardiac index is enhanced and filling pressure is reduced with minimal effect on myocardial oxygen demand.

Individual variation in the peripheral vascular and myocardial response makes it difficult to select the correct dose of either drug in critically ill patients. Since the half-life of amrinone and milrinone is substantially longer than that with either catecholamines or intravenous vasodilators used in cardiogenic shock, it is probably preferable to individually titrate an inotrope and vasodilator rather than use an agent, such as milrinone, that possesses both activities. By virtue of their vasodilator action, both amrinone and milrinone may also result in clinically important hypotension (74), which could compromise diastolic coronary filling in the patient with cardiogenic shock.

With the above considerations in mind, the recommended dosage for amrinone is an initial intravenous loading dose of 0.75 mg/kg over 3–5 minutes, followed by a second equal bolus 30 minutes later if required. The bolus should be followed by a continuous intravenous infusion of 5–10 μg/kg/minute with the total daily dose not exceeding 10 mg/kg (58). After an intravenous bolus, peak effects are seen in several minutes; with an intravenous infusion alone, peak effects occur at about 7 hours (58). Milrinone is not currently approved for intravenous infusion, and dosage recommendations are therefore not available.

ADMINISTRATION AND TOXICITY

Amrinone lactate (Inocor) is available as a solution of 100 mg in 20-ml vials. The drug is generally diluted in normal or half-normal saline to a concentration of 1–3 mg/ml. Glucose-containing solutions should not be used since a slow chemical interaction occurs when amrinone is mixed in dextrose. This interaction does not preclude the coinfusion of amrinone with dextrose-containing solutions using a Y-connector.

Neither drug is approved for use in infants or children, and caution against the use of amrinone in newborns is raised because of observed negative inotropic effects in neonatal puppies (15), although positive inotropic effects have been reported in lambs (95).

The relatively long half-life, and thus slow attainment of a new steady state with changes in continuous infusion rate of amrinone, make it less attractive in the critical care setting. There is no information about drug excretion in patients with renal failure, and amrinone should be used cautiously, if at all, in this population.

Several studies in adults with chronic congestive heart failure report small, statistically insignificant, increases in ventricular ectopy during long-term therapy with either amrinone or milrinone (91, 107). Thus, these agents may be safer than currently used inotropes that have much greater arrhythmogenic potential.

Intravenous amrinone produces reversible thrombocytopenia in approximately 4% of patients (79); the frequency increases with total daily doses in excess of 24 mg/kg. Elevation of liver enzymes has been reported with long-term but not short-term use (79). In addition, oral long-term therapy has produced numerous side effects, especially gastrointestinal disturbances and thrombocytopenia, which preclude its clinical use (109).

SUMMARY

The pharmacology of catecholamines and bipyridines have been reviewed in this chapter. These compounds possess potent myocardial and peripheral vascular actions that may be used in critically ill patients to maintain cardiac function and manipulate peripheral and pulmonary vascular tone. Optimal use of these potent and useful drugs requires an understanding of their pharmacology, and the influence of critical illness on the hemodynamic actions resulting from their administration. In pediatric applications, age-related changes in drug kinetics or dynamics may occur, further complicating their administration to infants and children and emphasizing the need to individually titrate the infusion rate to observed hemodynamic changes.

References

1. Alousi AA, Canter JM, Montenaro MJ, et al: Cardiotonic activity of milrinone, a new and potent cardiac bipyridine, on the normal and failing heart of experimental animals. *J Cardiovasc Pharmacol* 5:792, 1983.
2. Alousi AA, Farah AE, Lesher GY, et al: Cardiotonic activity of amrinone-Win 4080 [5-amino- 3.4'-bipyridin-6(1H)-one]. *Circ Res* 45:666, 1979.
3. Alousi AA, Johnson DC: Pharmacology of the bipyridines: amrinone and milrinone. *Circulation* 73(Suppl 3):3–10, 1986.
4. Alousi AA, Stankus GP, Stuart JC, et al: Characterization of the cardiotonic effects of milrinone, a new and potent cardiac bipyridine on isolated tissue from several animal species. *J Cardiovasc Pharmacol* 5:804, 1983.
5. Andy JJ, Curry CL, Ali N, et al: Cardiovascular effects of dobutamine in severe congestive heart failure. *Am Heart J* 94:175, 1977.
6. Arnold JMO, Braunwald E, Sandor T, et al: Inotropic stimulation of reperfused myocardium with dopamine: Effects on infarct size and myocardial function. *J Am Coll Cardiol* 6:1026, 1985.
7. Assem ESK, Schild HO: Inhibition by sympathomimetic amines of histamine release induced by antigen in passively sensitized human lung. *Nature* 224:1028, 1969.
8. Benotti JR, Grossman W, Braunwald E, et al: Effects of amrinone on myocardial energy metabolism and hemodynamics in patients with severe congestive heart failure due to coronary disease. *Circulation* 62:23, 1980.
9. Benotti JR, Grossman W, Braunwald E, et al: Hemodynamic assessment of amrinone. A new inotropic agent. *N Engl J Med* 299:1373, 1978.
10. Benzing G III, Helmsworth JA, Schreiber JT, et al: Nitroprusside and epinephrine for treatment of low output in children after open-heart surgery. *Ann Thorac Surg* 27:523, 1979.
11. Berner M, Rouge JC, Friedli B: The hemodynamic effect of phentolamine and dobutamine after open-heart operations in children: influence of the underlying heart defect. *Ann Thorac Surg* 35:644, 1983.
12. Bertel O, Buhler FR, Baitsch G, et al: Plasma adrenaline and noradrenaline in patients with acute myocardial infarction. *Chest* 82:64, 1982.
13. Bessey PQ, Brooks DC, Black PR, et al: Epinephrine acutely mediates skeletal muscle insulin resistance. *Surgery* 94:172, 1983.
14. Best JD, Halter JB: Release and clearance rates of epinephrine in man: Importance of arterial measurements. *J Clin Endocrinol Metab* 55:263, 1982.
15. Binah O, Banilo P, Rosen MR: Development changes in the effects of amrinone on cardiac contraction. *Am J Cardiol* 49:993, 1982.
16. Binah O, Legato MJ, Danilo P Jr, et al: Developmental changes in the cardiac effects of amrinone in the dog. *Circ Res* 52:747, 1983.

17. Binah O, Sodowick B, Vulliemoz Y: The inotropic effects of amrinone and milrinone on neonatal and young canine cardiac muscle. *Circulation* 73(Suppl 3):3–46, 1986.

18. Body J-J, Cryer PE, Offord KP, et al: Epinephrine is a hypophosphatemic hormone in man. *J Clin Invest* 71:572, 1983.

19. Bohn DJ, Poirier CS, Edmonds JF, et al: Hemodynamic effects of dobutamine after cardiopulmonary bypass in children. *Crit Care Med* 8:367, 1980.

20. Borow KM, Neumann A, Lang RM: Milrinone versus dobutamine: contribution of altered myocardial mechanics and augmented inotropic state to improved left ventricular performance. *Circulation* 73(Suppl 3):3–153, 1986.

21. Bristow MR, Ginsburg R, Minobe W, et al: Decreased catecholamine sensitivity and β-adrenergic receptor density in failing human hearts. *N Engl J Med* 307:205, 1982.

22. Brown MJ, Brown DC, Murphy MB: Hypokalemia from beta₂-receptor stimulation by circulating epinephrine. *N Engl J Med* 309:1414, 1983.

23. Buckley NM, Brazeau P, Frasier ID: Cardiovascular effects of dopamine in developing swine. *Biol Neonate* 43:50, 1983.

24. Carey RM, Thorner MO, Ortt EM: Dopaminergic inhibition of metoclopramide-induced aldosterone secretion in man. *J Clin Invest* 66:10, 1980.

25. Chernow B, Holbrook P, D'Angona DS Jr, et al: Epinephrine absorption after intratracheal administration. *Anesth Analg* 63:829, 1984.

26. Chernow B, Lake CR, Barton M, et al: Sympathetic nervous system sensitivity to hemorrhagic hypotension in the subhuman primate. *J Trauma* 24:229, 1984.

27. Chernow B, Rainey TG, Lake CR: Endogenous and exogenous catecholamines in critical care medicine. *Crit Care Med* 10:409, 1982.

28. Chernow B, Roth BL: Pharmacologic manipulation of the peripheral vasculature in shock: Clinical and experimental approaches. *Circ Shock* 18:141, 1986.

29. Chernow B, Roth BL: Pharmacologic support of the cardiovasculature in septic shock. In Sibbald WJ, Sprung CL (eds): *Perspectives on Sepsis and Septic Shock.* Fullerton, CA, Society of Critical Care Medicine, 1986, pp 173.

30. Chidsey CA, Braunwald E, Morrow AG, et al: Myocardial norepinephrine concentration in man: effects of reserpine and of congestive heart failure. *N Engl J Med* 269:653, 1963.

31. Clutter WE, Bier DM, Shah SD, et al: Epinephrine plasma metabolic clearance rates and physiologic thresholds for metabolic and hemodynamic actions in man. *J Clin Invest* 66:94, 1980.

32. Cohn JN, Levine TB, Olivari MT, et al: Plasma norepinephrine as a guide to prognosis in patients with chronic congestive heart failure. *N Engl J Med* 311:819, 1984.

33. Coffin LH Jr, Ankeney JL, Beheler EM: Experimental study and clinical use of epinephrine for treatment of low cardiac output syndrome. *Circulation* 33(Suppl 1):78, 1965.

34. Colucci WS, Wright RF, Jaski BE, et al: Milrinone and dobutamine in severe heart failure: differing hemodynamic effects and individual patient responsiveness. *Circulation* 73(Suppl 3):175, 1986.

35. Davies CL, Newman RJ, Molyneux SG, et al: The relationship between plasma catecholamines and severity of injury in man. *J Trauma* 24:99, 1984.

36. Davis RF, Lappas DG, Kirklin JK, et al: Acute oliguria after cardiopulmonary bypass: renal functional improvement with low-dose dopamine infusion. *Crit Care Med* 10:852, 1982.

37. DeLaCal MA, Miravalles E, Pascual T, et al: Dose-related hemodynamic and renal effects of dopamine in septic shock. *Crit Care Med* 12:22, 1984.

38. Dinerstein RJ, Jones RT, Goldberg LI: Evidence for dopamine-containing renal nerves. *Federation Proc* 42:3005, 1983.

39. DiSesa VJ, Brown E, Mudge GH Jr, et al: Hemodynamic comparison of dopamine and dobutamine in the postoperative volume-loaded, pressure-loaded, and normal ventricle. *J Thorac Cardiovasc Surg* 83:256, 1982.

40. Douglas HD Jr: Levarterenol irrigation: control of massive gastrointestinal bleeding in poor risk patients. *JAMA* 230:1653, 1974.

41. Downes JJ, Wood DW, Harwood I, et al: Intravenous isoproterenol infusion in children with severe hypercapnia due to status asthmaticus. *Crit Care Med* 1:63, 1973.

42. Driscoll DJ, Gillette PC, Ezrailson EG, et al: Inotropic responses of the neonatal canine myocardium to dopamine. *Pediatr Res* 12:42, 1978.

43. Driscoll DJ, Gillette PC, Fukushige J, et al: Comparison of the cardiovascular action of isoproterenol, dopamine and dobutamine in the neonatal and mature dog. *Pediatr Cardiol* 1:307, 1980.

44. Edelson J, LeJemtel TH, Alousi AA, et al: Relationship between amrinone plasma concentration and cardiac index. *Clin Pharmacol Ther* 29:723, 1981.

45. Edelson J, Stroshane R, Benziger DP, et al: Pharmacokinetics of the bipyridines amrinone and milrinone. *Circulation* 73(Suppl 3):145, 1986.

46. Edwards H, Olafsson O, Hyman AI, et al: Dobutamine in the rejecting transplanted heart. *Crit Care Med* 9:498, 1981.

47. Einzig S, Rao GH, Pierpont ME, et al: Acute effects of amrinone on regional myocardial and systemic blood flow distributions in the dog. *Can J Physiol Pharmacol* 60:811, 1982.

48. Esler M, Leonard P, O'Dea K, et al: Biochemical quantification of sympathetic nervous activity in humans using radiotracer methodology: fallibility of plasma noradrenaline measurements. *J Cardiovasc Pharmacol* 4:S152, 1982.

49. Feldman RD, Limbird LE, Nadeau J, et al: Dynamic regulation of leukocyte β-adrenergic receptor-agonist interactions by physiological changes in circulating catecholamines. *J Clin Invest* 72:164, 1983.

50. FitzGerald GA, Hossman V, Hamilton CA, et al: Interindividual variation in kinetics of infused norepinephrine. *Clin Pharmacol Ther* 26:669, 1979.

51. Fowler MB, Alderman EL, Oesterle SN, et al: Dobutamine and dopamine after cardiac surgery: greater augmentation of myocardial blood flow with dobutamine. *Circulation* 70(Suppl 1):103, 1984.

52. Francis GS, Sharma B, Hodges M: Comparative hemodynamic effects of dopamine and dobutamine in patients with acute cardiogenic circulatory collapse. *Am Heart J* 103:995, 1982.

53. Gelfand RA, Matthews DE, Bier DM, et al: Role of counterregulatory hormones in the catabolic response to stress. *J Clin Invest* 74:2238, 1984.

54. Goldberg LI: Dopamine-clinical uses of an endogenous catecholamine. *N Engl J Med* 291:707, 1974.

55. Goldberg LI, Hsuh Y, Resnekov L: Newer catecholamines for treatment of heart failure and shock: an update on dopamine and a first look at dobutamine. *Prog Cardiovasc Dis* 19:327, 1977.

56. Goldbrauson F, Lurie L, Vance RM, et al: Multiple extremity amputations in hypotensive patients with dopamine. *JAMA* 243:1145, 1980.

57. Goldstein DS, Zimlichman R, Stull R, et al: Plasma catecholamine and hemodynamic response during isoproterenol infusions in humans. *Clin Pharmacol Ther* 40:233, 1986.

58. Goldstein RA: Clinical effects of intravenous amrinone in patients with congestive heart failure. *Circulation* 73(Suppl 3):191, 1986.

59. Goldstein DS: Plasma norepinephrine as an indicator

of sympathetic neural activity in clinical cardiology. *Am J Cardiol* 48:1147, 1981.

60. Gombos EA, Hulet WH, Bopp P, et al: Reactivity of renal and systemic circulations to vasoconstrictor agents in normotensive and hypertensive subjects. *J Clin Invest* 41:203, 1962.

61. Gray R, Shah PK, Singh B, et al: Low cardiac output states after open heart surgery: comparative hemodynamic effects of dobutamine, dopamine and norepinephrine plus phentolamine. *Chest* 80:16, 1981.

62. Greenberg MI, Spivey WH: Comparison of deep and shallow endotracheal administration of dionosil in dogs and effect of manual hyperventilation. *Ann Emerg Med* 14:209, 1985.

63. Greenway CV, Stark RD: Hepatic vascular bed. *Physiol Rev* 51:23, 1971.

64. Guller B, Fields AI, Coleman MG, et al: Changes in cardiac rhythm in children treated with dopamine. *Crit Care Med* 6:151, 1978.

65. Halloway EL, Stinson EB, Derby GC, et al: Action of drugs in patients early after cardiac surgery. I. Comparison of isoproterenol and dopamine. *Am J Cardiol* 35:656, 1975.

66. Hasselgren P-O, Biber B, Fornander J: Improved blood flow and protein synthesis in the postischemic liver following infusion of dopamine. *J Surg Res* 34:44, 1983.

67. Holloway El, Palumbo RA, Harrison DC: Acute circulatory effects of dopamine in patients with pulmonary hypertension. *Br Heart J* 37:482, 1975.

68. Holzer J, Karliner JS, O'Rourke RA, et al: Effectiveness of dopamine in patients with cardiogenic shock. *Am J Cardiol* 32:79, 1973.

69. Insel PA, Snavely MD: Catecholamines and the kidney: Receptors and renal function. *Ann Rev Physiol* 43:625, 1981.

70. Jaattela A, Alho A, Avikainen V, et al: Plasma catecholamines in severely injured patients: a prospective study on 45 patients with multiple injuries. *Br J Surg* 62:177, 1975.

71. Jardin F, Sportiche M, Bazil M, et al: Dobutamine: a hemodynamic evaluation in septic shock. *Crit Care Med* 9:329, 1981.

72. Jardin F, Eveleigh MC, Gurdjian F, Margairaz A: Venous admixture in human septic shock. *Circulation* 60:155, 1978.

73. Jarnberg P-O, Bengtsson L, Ekstrand J, et al: Dopamine infusion in man. Plasma catecholamine levels and pharmacokinetics. *Acta Anaesth Scand* 25:328, 1981.

74. Jaski BE, Fifer MA, Wright RF, et al: Positive inotropic and vasodilator actions of milrinone in patients with severe congestive heart failure: dose-response relationship and comparison to nitroprusside. *J Clin Invest* 75:643, 1985.

75. Kates RF, Leier CV: Dobutamine pharmacokinetics in severe heart failure. *Clin Pharmacol Ther* 24:537, 1978.

76. Keung ECH, Siskind SJ, Sonnenblick EH, et al: Dobutamine therapy in acute myocardial infarction. *JAMA* 245:144, 1981.

77. Kho TL, Henquet JW, Punt R, et al: Influence of dobutamine and dopamine on hemodynamics and plasma concentrations of noradrenaline and renin in patients with low cardiac output following acute myocardial infarction. *Eur J Clin Pharmacol* 18:213, 1980.

78. Kopin IJ: Catecholamine metabolism (and the biochemical assessment of sympathetic activity). *Clin Endocrinol Metab* 3:525, 1977.

79. Kullberg MP, Freeman GB, Biddlecome C, et al: Amrinone metabolism. *Clin Pharmacol Ther* 29:394, 1981.

80. Kung M, White JR, Burki NK: The effect of subcutaneously administered terbutaline on serum potassium in asymptomatic adult asthmatics. *Am Rev Respir Dis* 129:329, 1984.

81. Kurland G, Williams J, Lewiston NJ: Fatal myocardial toxicity during continuous intravenous isoproterenol

therapy of asthma. *J Allergy Clin Immunol* 63:407, 1979.

82. Lackovic Z, Relja M: Evidence for a widely distributed peripheral dopaminergic system. *Federation Proc* 42:3000, 1983.

83. Laitinen A, Partanen M, Hervonen N, et al: Electron microscopic study on the innervation of the human lower respiratory tract: evidence of adrenergic nerves. *Eur J Respir Dis* 67:209, 1985.

84. Lang P, Williams RG, Norwood WI, et al: The hemodynamic effects of dopamine in infants after corrective cardiac surgery. *J Pediatr* 96:630, 1980.

85. Lee MR: Dopamine and the kidney. *Clin Sci* 62:539, 1982.

86. Legato MJ: Cellular mechanisms of normal growth in the mammalian heart. II. A quantitative and qualitative comparison between the right and left ventricular myocytes in the dog from birth to five months of life. *Circ Res* 44:263, 1979.

87. Leier CV, Hebran PT, Huss P, et al: Comparative systemic and regional hemodynamic effects of dopamine and dobutamine in patients with cardiomyopathic heart failure. *Circulation* 58:466, 1978.

88. Leier CV, Unverferth DV: Dobutamine. *Ann Intern Med* 99:490, 1983.

89. Liang C-S, Sherman LG, Doherty JU, et al: Sustained improvement in patients with congestive heart failure after short-term infusion of dobutamine. *Circulation* 69:113, 1984.

90. Loeb HS, Bredakis J, Gunnar RM: Superiority of dobutamine over dopamine for augmentation of cardiac output in patients with chronic low output cardiac failure. *Circulation* 55:375, 1977.

91. Ludmer PL, Baim DS, Gauthier DF, et al: Effect of milrinone on complex ventricular arrhythmias in congestive heart failure. *Circulation* 72(Suppl 3):405, 1985.

92. Lupi-Herrera E, Sandoval J, Seonane M, et al: The role of isoproterenol in the preoperative evaluation of high blood pressure high resistance ventricular septal defect. *Chest* 81:42, 1982.

93. Maekawa K, Liang C-S, Hood WB Jr: Comparison of dobutamine and dopamine in acute myocardial infarction. *Circulation* 67:750, 1983.

94. Magorien RD, Unverferth DV, Brown GP, et al: Dobutamine and hydralazine: comparative influences on positive inotropy and vasodilation on coronary blood flow and myocardial energetics in nonischemic congestive heart failure. *J Am Coll Cardiol* 1:499, 1983.

95. Mammel MC, Einzig S, Kulik TJ, et al: Pulmonary vascular effects of amrinone in conscious lambs. *Pediatr Res* 17:720, 1983.

96. Marino RJ, Romagnoli A, Keats AS: Selective venoconstriction by dopamine in comparison with isoproterenol and phenylephrine. *Anesthesiology* 43:570, 1975.

97. MacCannel KL, Giraud GD, Hamilton PL, et al: Haemodynamic response to dopamine and dobutamine infusions as a function of duration of infusion. *Pharmacology* 26:29, 1983.

98. McMillan M, Chernow B, Roth BL: Hepatic alpha$_1$-adrenergic receptor alteration in a rat model of chronic sepsis. *Circ Shock* 19:185, 1986.

99. Meisheri KD, Plamer RF, van Breemen C: The effects of amrinone on contractility, Ca^{2+} uptake and cAMP in smooth muscle. *Eur J Pharmacol* 61:159, 1980.

100. Mentzer RM Jr, Alegre CA, Nolan SP: The effects of dopamine and isoproterenol on the pulmonary circulation. *J Thorac Cardiovasc Surg* 71:807, 1976.

101. Monrad ES, Baim DS, Smith HS, et al: Milrinone, dobutamine and nitroprusside: comparative effects on hemodynamics and myocardial energetics in patients with severe congestive heart failure. *Circulation* 73(Suppl 3):3–168, 1986.

102. Morgan JP, Gwathmey JK, DeFeo TT, et al: The effects of amrinone and related drugs on intracellular calcium

in isolated mammalian cardiac and vascular smooth muscle. *Circulation* 73(Suppl 3):65, 1986.

103. Motulsky HJ, Insel PA: Adrenergic receptors in man. *N Engl J Med* 307:18, 1982.

104. Mueller HS, Ayres SM, Gregorry JJ, et al: Hemodynamics, coronary blood flow and myocardial metabolism in coronary shock: response to L-norepinephrine and isoproterenol. *J Clin Invest* 49:1885, 1970.

105. Mueller HS: Treatment of acute MI. In Shoemaker WC, Thompson WL (eds): *Critical Care Medicine: State of the Art,* vol. 3. Fullerton, CA, Society of Critical Care Medicine, 1982, pp G1.

106. Mueller HS, Evans D, Ayres SM: Effect of dopamine on hemodynamics and myocardial metabolism in shock following acute myocardial infarction in man. *Circulation* 57:361, 1978.

107. Naccarelli GV, Gray EL, Dougherty AH, et al: Amrinone: electrophysiologic and hemodynamic effects in patients with congestive heart failure. *Am J Cardiol* 54:600, 1984.

108. Olson LG, Hensley MJ, Saunders NA: Ventilatory responsiveness to hypercapnic hypoxia during dopamine infusion in humans. *Am Rev Respir Dis* 126:783, 1982.

109. Packer M, Medina N, Yushak M: Hemodynamic and clinical limitations of long-term inotropic therapy with amrinone in patients with severe chronic heart failure. *Circulation* 70:1038, 1984.

110. Padbury JF, Agata Y, Baylen BG, et al: Dopamine pharmacokinetics in critically ill newborn infants. *J Pediatr* 110:293, 1987.

111. Parker S, Carlon GC, Isaacs M, et al: Dopamine administration in oliguria and oliguric renal failure. *Crit Care Med* 9:630, 1981.

112. Pelayo JC, Fildes RD, Eisner GM, et al: Effects of dopamine blockade on renal sodium excretion. *Am J Physiol* 245:F247, 1983.

113. Perkin RM, Levin DL, Webb R, et al: Dobutamine: a hemodynamic evaluation in children with shock. *J Pediatr* 100:977, 1982.

114. Porte D Jr: Sympathetic regulation of insulin secretion. *Arch Intern Med* 123:252, 1969.

115. Post G: New insights into receptor regulation. *J Appl Physiol* 57:1297, 1984.

116. Ralston SH, Voorhees WD, Babbs CF: Intrapulmonary epinephrine during prolonged cardiopulmonary resuscitation: Improved regional blood flow and resuscitation in dogs. *Ann Emerg Med* 13:79, 1984.

117. Rasmussen H: The calcium messenger system (Part I). *N Engl J Med* 314:1094, 1986.

118. Rasmussen H: The calcium messenger system (Part II). *N Engl J Med* 314:;1164, 1986.

119. Regnier B, Kapin M, Gory G, et al: Hemodynamic effects of dopamine in septic shock. *Intensive Care Med* 3:47, 1977.

120. Renard M, Bernard R: Clinical and hemodynamic effects of dobutamine in acute myocardial infarction with left heart failure. *J Cardiovasc Pharmacol* 2:543, 1980.

121. Richard C, Ricome JL, Rimailho A, et al: Combined hemodynamic effects of dopamine and dobutamine in cardiogenic shock. *Circulation* 67:620, 1983.

122. Robie NW, Goldgerg LI: Comparative systemic and regional hemodynamic effects of dopamine and dobutamine. *Am Heart J* 90:340, 1975.

123. Rockson SG, Homcy CJ, Quinn P: Cellular mechanisms of impaired adrenergic responsiveness in neonatal dogs. *J Clin Invest* 67:319, 1981.

124. Rosenthal J, Ferrier G: Inotropic and electrophysiologic effects of amrinone on untreated and digitalized ventricular tissues. *J Pharmacol Exp Ther* 221:188, 1982.

125. Ruffolo RR Jr, Spradlin TA, Pollock GD, et al: Alpha- and beta-adrenergic effects of the stereoisomers of dobutamine. *J Pharmacol Exp Ther* 219:447, 1981.

126. Schaer GL, Fink MP, Parrillo JE: Norepinephrine alone vs. norepinephrine plus low-dose dopamine: enhanced renal blood flow with combination pressor therapy. *Crit Care Med* 13:492, 1985.

127. Schechter E, Wilson MF, Kong Y-S: Physiologic responses to epinephrine infusion: The basis for a new stress test for coronary artery disease. *Am Heart J* 105:554, 1983.

128. Schranz D, Stopfkuchen H, Jungst B-K, et al: Hemodynamic effects of dobutamine in children with cardiovascular failure. *Eur J Pediatr* 139:4–7, 1982.

129. Shepherd JT, Vanhoutte PM: Local modulation of adrenergic neurotransmission. *Circulation* 64:655, 1981.

130. Silverberg AB, Shag SD, Haymond MW, et al: Norepinephrine: hormone and neurotransmitter in man. *Am J Physiol* 234:E252, 1978.

131. Soman VR, Shamoon H, Sherwin RS: Effects of physiologic infusion of epinephrine in normal humans: relationship between the metabolic response and β-adrenergic binding. *J Clin Endocrinol Metab* 50:294, 1980.

132. Sonnenblick EH, Frishman WH, LeJental TH: Dobutamine. A new synthetic cardioactive sympathetic amine. *N Engl J Med* 300:17, 1979.

133. Sonnenblick EH, Grose R, Strain J, et al: Effects of milrinone on left ventricular performance and myocardial contractility in patients with severe heart failure. *Circulation* 73(Suppl 3):162, 1986.

134. Sowers JR, Brickman AS, Sowers DK, et al: Dopaminergic modulation of aldosterone secretion in man is unaffected by glucocorticoids and angiotensin blockage. *J Clin Endocrinol Metab* 52:1078, 1981.

135. Standards and Guidelines for Cardiopulmonary Resuscitation and Emergency Cardiac Care. *JAMA* 255:2841, 1986.

136. Stephenson LW, Edmunds LH, Raphaely R, et al: Effects of nitroprusside and dopamine on pulmonary arterial vasculature in children after cardiac surgery. *Circulation* 60(Suppl 1):106, 1979.

137. Stjarne L, Brundin J: Frequency dependence of ^{3}H-noradrenaline secretion from human vasoconstrictor nerves: modification by factors intering with alpha- or beta-adrenoceptor or prostaglandin E_2 mediated control. *Acta Physiol Scand* 101:199, 1977.

138. Stoof JC, Kebabian JW: Two dopamine receptors: biochemistry, physiology, and pharmacology. *Life Sci* 35:2281, 1984.

139. Stroshane RM, Koss RF, Biddlecome CE, et al: Oral and intravenous pharmacokinetics of milrinone in human volunteers. *J Pharm Sci* 73:1438, 1984.

140. Strulovici B, Cerione RA, Kilpatrick BF, et al: Direct demonstration of impaired functionality of a purified desensitized β-adrenergic receptor in a reconstituted system. *Science* 225:837, 1984.

141. Struthers AD, Whitesmith R, Reid JL: Metabolic and haemodynamic effects of increased circulating adrenaline in man. *Br Heart J* 50:277, 1983.

142. Trigt PV, Spray TL, Pasque MK, et al: The comparative effects of dopamine and dobutamine on ventricular mechanics after coronary artery bypass grafting: a pressure dimension analysis. *Circulation* 70(Suppl I):I–112, 1984.

143. Trigt PV, Spray TL, Pasque MK, et al: The influence of time on the response to dopamine after coronary artery bypass grafting: assessment of left ventricular performance and contractility using pressure/dimension analyses. *Ann Thorac Surg* 35:3, 1983.

144. Tulassay T, Seri I, Machay T, et al: Effects of dopamine on renal functions in premature neonates with respiratory distress syndrome. *Int J Pediatr Nephrol* 4:19, 1983.

145. Tuttle RR, Mills J: Dobutamine. Development of a new catecholamine to selectively increase cardiac contractility. *Circ Res* 36:185, 1975.

146. Unverferth DV, Blanford M, Kates RE, et al: Tolerance

to dobutamine after a 72-hour continuous infusion. *Am J Med* 69:262, 1980.

147. Unverferth DV, Magorien RD, Altschuld R, et al: The hemodynamic and metabolic advantages gained by a three-day infusion of dobutamine in patients with congestive cardiomyopathy. *Am Heart J* 106:29, 1983.

148. Warren JB, Dalton N: A comparison of the bronchodilator and vasopressor effects of exercise levels of adrenaline in man. *Clin Sci* 64:475, 1983.

149. Watters JM, Wilmore DW: Metabolic responses to sepsis and septic shock. In Sibbald WJ, Sprung CL, (eds): *Perspectives on Sepsis and Septic Shock.* Fullerton, CA, Society of Critical Care Medicine, 1986, p 97.

150. Weiner N: Norepinephrine, epinephrine, and the sympathomimetic amines. In Gilman AG, Goodman LS, Rall TW, Murad F (eds): *The Pharmacologic Basis of Therapeutics.* New York, Macmillan, 1985, pp 145.

151. Whitfield L, Sowers JR, Tuck ML, et al: Dopaminergic control of plasma catecholamine and aldosterone response to acute stimuli in normal man. *J Clin Endocrinol Metab* 51:724, 1980.

152. Williams RS, Bishop T: Selectivity of dobutamine for adrenergic receptor subtypes. *J Clin Invest* 67:1703, 1981.

153. Wilson RF, Sibbald WJ, Jaanimagi JL: Hemodynamic effects of dopamine in critically ill septic patients. *J Surg Res* 20:163, 1976.

154. Wortsman J, Frank S, Cryer PE: Adrenomedullary response to maximal stress in humans. *Am J Med* 77:779, 1984.

155. Young MA, Hintze TH, Vatner SF: Correlation between cardiac performance and plasma catecholamine levels in conscious dogs. *Am J Physiol* 248:H82, 1985.

156. Zaloga GP, Smallridge RC: Thyroidal alterations in acute illness. *Semin Resp Med* 7:95, 1985.

157. Zannad F, Juillere Y, Royer RJ: The effects of amrinone on cardiac function, oxygen consumption and lactate production of an isolated, perfused working guinea pig heart. *Arch Int Pharmacodyn Ther* 263:264, 1984.

158. Zaritsky AL, Eisenberg MG: Ontogenetic considerations in the pharmacotherapy of shock. In Chernow B, Shoemaker WC (eds): *Critical Care: State of the Art,* vol 7. Fullerton, CA, Society of Critical Care Medicine, 1986, pp 485.

159. Zaritsky A, Chernow B: Use of catecholamines in pediatrics. *J Pediatr* 105:341, 1984.

160. Zern RT, Foster LB, Blalock JA, et al: Characteristics of the dopaminergic and noradrenergic systems of the pancreatic islets. *Diabetes* 28:185, 1979.

32

Divalent Ions: Calcium, Magnesium, and Phosphorus

Gary Paul Zaloga, M.D., F.A.C.P., F.A.C.N.
Bart Chernow, M.D., F.A.C.P.

Calcium (Ca^{2+}), magnesium (Mg^{2+}), and phosphorus (PO_4) are divalent ions that are essential for normal body function. Disorders involving these ions are common in critically ill patients due to their underlying illnesses and the effects of administered drugs. This chapter discusses the pharmacology, homeostasis, causes, clinical features, and treatment of disorders involving these ions. The emphasis is placed upon those disorders most commonly seen in the critical care setting.

CALCIUM

Ca^{2+} is important in humans for both structural and biochemical integrity. The normal adult body contains approximately 1000–1400 g of Ca^{2+} of which 99% is in the skeleton and 1% is in the soft tissues and extracellular spaces. Ca^{2+} is the most abundant electrolyte in the human body. Skeletal Ca^{2+} supports and protects body tissues and serves as a storehouse, providing Ca^{2+} for physiologic requirements when dietary Ca^{2+} is unavailable. Loss of skeletal Ca^{2+} with aging (e.g., osteoporosis) is responsible for loss of height and fractures.

Ca^{2+} movement into the cell and release from intracellular sites is vital for the coupling of receptor-stimulated cell surface events to cellular responses (i.e., stimulus-response coupling). Ca^{2+} is required for muscle contraction (e.g., excitation-contraction coupling), hormonal and neurotransmitter secretion (i.e., stimulus-secretion coupling), cell division, cell motility, axonal flow, enzyme activity, cell membrane structure, and blood coagulation. It also plays a vital role in the cardiac action potential and is essential for cardiac pacemaker automaticity.

Measurement of Blood Calcium

Ca^{2+} circulates in the blood in three forms: an ionized fraction (50%), a protein bound (mostly to albumin) fraction (40%), and a diffusible but nonionized fraction in chelates with other circulating ions (10%). It is the ionized fraction that is thought to be physiologically active and homeostatically regulated. A determination of the total serum calcium concentration is the measurement that is performed in most hospital laboratories. However, alterations in the amount of protein present, the percentage of Ca^{2+} bound to protein, and the amount of Ca^{2+} bound in chelates may affect the total Ca^{2+} value independent of the ionized Ca^{2+} concentration (94, 109, 132, 133, 135).

A variety of factors can alter the serum total and ionized Ca^{2+} levels (15, 133). Protein bound Ca^{2+} (primarily albumin) represents a large proportion (40%) of the total serum Ca^{2+} concentration. Thus, alterations in a patient's serum albumin concentration can change that person's total serum Ca^{2+} measurement. Critically ill patients with low serum albumin levels characteristically have a low total serum Ca^{2+} value, while serum ionized Ca^{2+} measurements may be normal (135). On the other hand, a normal total serum Ca^{2+} level in the face of hypoalbuminemia may indicate ionized hypercalcemia. Elevations in serum protein levels (e.g., from albumin infusions, venostasis as a consequence of prolonged tourniquet use during phlebotomy, and rarely, myeloma) may also raise the total serum Ca^{2+} value and mask hypocalcemia.

Blood pH alters Ca^{2+} binding to serum proteins: acute acidosis decreases protein binding (increases the serum ionized Ca^{2+} concentration) while alkalosis increases protein binding (decreases ionized Ca^{2+}). Measurement of the total serum Ca^{2+} concentration in critically ill patients with acid-base changes may therefore give deceiving results. For example, a patient being therapeutically hyperventilated (e.g., in an attempt to reduce cerebral blood flow following head injury) may develop ionized hypocalcemia, without abnormalities in the total serum Ca^{2+} concentration, due to an alkalosis-induced increase in Ca^{2+} binding to proteins. Patients given bicarbonate for control of metabolic acidosis can also develop acute ionized hypocalcemia. Shifts in ionized Ca^{2+} induced by changes in arterial pH are usually small; however, occasionally, they may be associated with clinically important hypocalcemia. Patients most susceptible to hypocalcemia are those with an underlying abnormality in parathyroid hormone (PTH) and vitamin D metabolism.

Free fatty acids (FFA) constitute a major metabolic fuel for the body and are carried in the circulation bound to the albumin molecule. We (143) and others (3) have found that FFAs increase Ca^{2+} binding to albumin. Serum FFA levels increase during critical illness due to illness-induced elevations in plasma concentrations of epinephrine, glucagon, growth hormone, and corticotropin, as well as decreases in serum insulin concentrations. Elevations in FFA levels, sufficient to alter calcium binding, may also occur after the administration of heparin sodium, intravenous lipids, epinephrine, norepinephrine, isoproterenol, or with alcohol ingestion. These pharmacologic agents are commonly used in critically ill patients. Normal individuals have serum FFA concentrations of approximately 250 μmol/liter. Values of FFAs increase to 400–600 μmol/liter after an overnight fast and may rise to 1000 μmol/liter after prolonged fasting (72 hours). Severely stressed patients (e.g., those with acute pancreatitis, diabetic ketoacidosis, sepsis, or acute myocardial infarction) may have serum levels of 3000 μmol/liter. Increases in serum FFA levels in acutely ill and stressed patients may alter the distribution of Ca^{2+} between bound and unbound states. Alterations in Ca^{2+} binding occur in patients with acute pancreatitis, after heparin administration and after intravenous lipid administration (132, 143). FFAs may act as modulators of free Ca^{2+} levels in various pathologic states.

The timing and technique of venipuncture are important in the interpretation of serum Ca^{2+} values. Postprandial increases in serum Ca^{2+} levels of 1–2 mg/dl may occur. Postprandial increases in serum Ca^{2+} are higher and more prolonged in hyperabsorptive states such as hyperparathyroidism, vitamin D excess, and hypothyroidism. To avoid these changes, one should measure serum Ca^{2+} in the fasting state.

Changes in the concentration of chelating ions (e.g., phosphate, bicarbonate, albumin, and citrate) may also lower the circulating ionized Ca^{2+} level. Citrate is used as a blood preservative and anticoagulant. Citrate-induced decreases in ionized Ca^{2+} are usually transient, and without hemodynamic effect in most blood transfusion situations. Howland et al. (61) studied 100 patients who received blood during a variety of surgical procedures. Mean ionized Ca^{2+} levels decreased from 4.06 to 3.22 mg/dl (1.01 to 0.80 mmol/liter) while patients were receiving an average of 18.6 ml of blood per minute. Twenty of the 100 (20%) patients who received blood at this rate had ionized Ca^{2+} levels that fell below 2.5 mg/dl (0.62 mmol/liter) and 10 of the 100 patients (10%) had levels below 2 mg/dl (0.50 mmol/liter). Only one patient (1%) developed hypocalcemia-induced cardiovascular problems (e.g. hypotension). Kahn et al. (68) studied 53 patients undergoing a variety of surgical procedures. Serum-ionized Ca^{2+} levels decreased from a mean of 4.14 to 3.04 mg/dl (1.03 to 0.76 mmol/liter) during transfusion of blood at an average rate of 0.5 ml/kg/minute. However, hemodynamic variables remained stable throughout the period of observation, and ionized Ca^{2+} values returned to normal after discontinuation of the transfusion.

Decreases in ionized Ca^{2+} values during blood transfusion correlate with elevations in circulating citrate levels and speed of transfusion. Denlinger et al. (39) administered citrated blood to anaesthetized patients at rates of 50, 100, and 150 ml/70 kg/minute and found decreases in serum-ionized Ca^{2+} levels of 14%, 31%, and 41%, respectively. After a 5-minute blood transfusion period, ionized Ca^{2+} values returned to normal within 15 minutes, and this normalization correlated with metabolism of the citrate.

The metabolism of citrate is affected by tissue perfusion, acid-base status, and the activity of the rate limiting enzyme, aconitase, which is present in muscle, kidney, and liver. When transfusion rate exceeds citrate metabolism, citrate levels rise and ionized Ca^{2+} levels fall. Citrate may also chelate Mg^{2+}, causing hypomagnesemia, which in turn may accentuate hypocalcemia. Thus, when citrate clearance is impaired (e.g., in hypothermia or with renal or hepatic disease) or blood transfusion is rapid, plasma citrate levels may rise and cause clinically important hypocalcemia and cardiovascular insufficiency. The effect of citrate and other chelators on Ca^{2+} is accentuated in patients with underlying defects of the parathyroid–vitamin D axis. Similar decreases in ionized Ca^{2+} levels may occur after volume resuscitation with albumin, after intravenous injection of radiocontrast media, and after the intravenous administration of phosphates (132).

Heparin is capable of chelating with Ca^{2+}; however, heparin dosages capable of causing Ca^{2+} chelation are not obtained in vivo. However, adding heparin to syringes used to collect blood samples for measurement of ionized Ca^{2+} can significantly lower the ionized Ca^{2+} concentration. Thus, samples used for measurement of plasma or blood Ca^{2+} should use the smallest amount of heparin that will adequately anticoagulate blood. The amount of heparin added should be standardized and each laboratory performing ionized Ca^{2+} measurements should use their own normal values.

The serum-ionized Ca^{2+} value may be altered during hemodialysis, depending on the calcium concentration of the dialysate (58, 90, 132). Patients with renal failure are vulnerable to the hypocalcemic effects of dialysis because they have an impaired ability to hydroxylate vitamin D within the kidney and mobilize calcium. Maynard et al. (90) showed that the drop in blood pressure induced by hemodialysis was reduced when a high Ca^{2+} dialysate was used. Henrich et al. (58) demonstrated that ionized Ca^{2+} values during dialysis were key factors affecting left ventricular contractility, an increase in ionized Ca^{2+} being associated with improved contractility. These studies indicate that the Ca^{2+} composition of the dialysate baths can affect hemodynamics during dialysis. In fact, we have seen hypotensive episodes when critically ill patients were dialyzed against low Ca^{2+} baths. Currently, we recommend use of a high Ca^{2+} bath (7.5 mg/dl) in critically ill patients, unless the patient is hypercalcemic.

Many attempts have been made to mathematically correct the total serum Ca^{2+} concentration for alterations in circulating albumin levels and pH. Despite these attempts, total serum Ca^{2+} and calculated ionized Ca^{2+} levels have been poor predictors of the physiologically active ionized Ca^{2+} fraction (78, 135).

We have found abnormally low total and calculated ionized Ca^{2+} values in 50–60% of critically ill patients (135). However, when ionized Ca^{2+} levels were directly measured, only about 10% of critically ill patients have hypocalcemia. Despite high sensitivity, total serum and calculated ionized Ca^{2+} values lack specificity in predicting ionized hypocalcemia. On the other hand, an elevated total serum Ca^{2+} level in a critically ill patient is usually indicative of ionized hypercalcemia, whereas a normal total serum Ca^{2+} measurement is strong evidence against ionized hypocalcemia (135). We have found that the amount of Ca^{2+} bound to albumin varies widely between patients (e.g., 40–60%) and that alterations in binding that result from blood pH and FFA changes are significantly different between normal and sick patients (implying differences in the physicochemical properties of their binding proteins) (135, 143). At present, we believe that the serum-ionized Ca^{2+} level remains the best measure of Ca^{2+} delivery in critically ill patients, and we recommend that all centers caring for critically ill patients measure ionized Ca^{2+} concentrations. When ionized Ca measurements are not available, an ultrafilterable Ca^{2+} level may be substituted (142). Ultrafilterable Ca^{2+} levels can be easily measured by passing a plasma or serum sample through a small filter, which prevents the passage of protein through it. The Ca^{2+} in the ultrafiltrate can be measured in the hospital laboratory.

Different laboratories have different ways of measuring serum-ionized Ca^{2+} levels. Many laboratories correct the serum pH to 7.4 to correct for losses in carbon dioxide that may have occurred between the time of blood drawing and Ca^{2+} measurement. Since many critically ill patients have alterations in serum pH, we do not correct the pH to 7.4. In addition, we have found that present methods for correcting the pH to 7.4 work poorly in critically ill patients. We are extremely careful to collect our blood samples anaerobically and measure the ionized Ca^{2+} level immediately after drawing.

Calcium Homeostasis

The daily recommended oral dietary intake of Ca^{2+} is 1000–1500 mg. Thirty to 35% of this intake is absorbed primarily in the small intestine by both active (vitamin D–dependent) and passive (concentration–dependent) absorption. Loss of Ca^{2+} via the gastrointes-

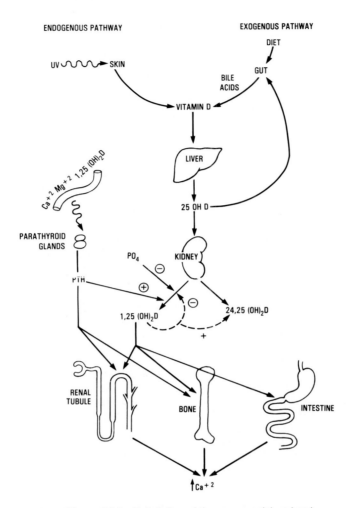

Figure 32.1 Regulation of the serum calcium level.

tinal tract (150–200 mg/day) and urine (150 mg/day) is balanced by gastrointestinal absorption.

The serum Ca^{2+} concentration is maintained within normal limits by the combined effects of PTH and vitamin D (Fig. 32.1). Dietary Ca^{2+} is usually not required, since these hormones can maintain a normal serum Ca^{2+} level via their skeletal effects. However, with chronic Ca^{2+} deficiency the skeletal Ca^{2+} mobilizing response to PTH or 1,25-dihydroxyvitamin D is diminished and predisposes the patient to hypocalcemia. This decrease in PTH and vitamin D responsiveness results from receptor desensitization due to high levels of the hormones and depletion of the mobilizable pool of Ca^{2+} in bone (85). A deficiency in either

hormone, however, may lead to hypocalcemia. Deficiency in PTH may result from parathyroid gland damage (as may occur after neck surgery) or from parathyroid gland suppression. The parathyroid glands may be suppressed by hypercalcemia, hypomagnesemia, hypermagnesemia, or 1,25-dihydroxyvitamin D. PTH increases bone resorption and renal tubular Ca^{2+} reabsorption, and promotes intestinal Ca^{2+} absorption by stimulating the renal conversion of 25-hydroxyvitamin D to 1,25-dihydroxyvitamin D (85). The action of PTH on bone osteoclasts may be mediated through an intermediary monocyte rather than by direct action (85).

Vitamin D can enter the body through the gastrointestinal tract (dietary vitamin D) or can be synthesized in the skin under the influence of ultraviolet light. Either source is sufficient to maintain normal vitamin D levels. However, when sunlight exposure is minimal and dietary intake is poor, vitamin D deficiency may develop. These circumstances are commonly found in elderly, debilitated, and chronically ill patients. Many of these patients are admitted to intensive care units and under the increased metabolic demands of severe illness may be unable to maintain normal serum Ca^{2+} levels. Vitamin D is a fat soluble vitamin, and its absorption is dependent on intact lipolytic activity, biliary secretion, and functional intestinal mucosa. Thus, diseases of the pancreas, liver, biliary system, or intestine may cause vitamin D malabsorption and deficiency (137).

Vitamin D is 25-hydroxylated in the liver and then 1-hydroxylated in the kidneys to 1,25-dihydroxyvitamin D, the active form of the vitamin. Vitamin D's renal hydroxylation is stimulated by both PTH and hypophosphatemia and is suppressed by hyperphosphatemia, acidosis, and 1,25-dihydroxyvitamin D (negative feedback). Synthesis of 25-hydroxyvitamin D within the liver is poorly regulated, and its measurement serves as a good indicator of dietary/skin vitamin D supply. Disease of the kidneys or liver can disrupt Ca^{2+} homeostasis by impairing vitamin D activation. Intestinal and renal tubular Ca^{2+} absorption and bone resorption is stimulated by 1,25-dihydroxyvitamin D. The osteoclast action of 1,25-dihydroxyvitamin D may result from the recruitment and differentiation of precursor cells (85) rather than by action on mature cells.

Thyroid hormone also has effects on the skeleton that affect Ca^{2+} homeostasis. Hyperthyroidism increases bone resorption and may cause hypercalcemia. Hypothyroidism causes a decrease in bone resorption and may cause hypocalcemia.

Hypocalcemia

CAUSES

Hypocalcemia develops when Ca^{2+} leaves the vascular space or is chelated faster than it can be replaced. A frequent underlying problem in critically ill patients who become hypocalcemic is their impaired ability to mobilize skeletal Ca^{2+} because of PTH or vitamin D deficiency. Table 1 lists various causes of hypocalcemia.

Table 32.1
Causes of Hypocalcemia

Hypoparathyroidism
  Primary
  Secondary
    After neck surgery
    Radioiodine
    Metastasis
    Hemochromatosis
  Neonatal
Hypomagnesemia or Hypermagnesemia
Hyperphosphatemia
  Iatrogenic
  Tumor lysis
  Rhabdomyolysis
Chelators
  Citrate (e.g., blood)
  Albumin
  Radiocontrast dye
Vitamin D deficiency
  Dietary
  Malabsorption
  Renal insufficiency
  Pseudohypoparathyroidism
Pancreatitis
Sepsis
Hungry bone syndrome
Fat embolism syndrome
Toxic shock syndrome
Burns
Hypothyroidism
Drugs
  Albumin
  Aminoglycosides
  Calcitonin
  Cis-platinum
  Citrate
  Diphosphonates
  EDTA
  Estrogens
  Ethylene glycol
  Gallium nitrate
  Heparin
  Loop diuretics
  Magnesium
  Mithramycin
  Phenobarbital
  Phenytoin
  Phosphates
  Protamine
  Radiocontrast dye
  Sodium fluoride
  Sodium sulfate
  WR-2721

Hypoparathyroidism

Primary (usually autoimmune) hypoparathyroidism is rarely seen, whereas secondary hypoparathyroidism after neck surgery is a common cause of hypocalcemia (98). Hypocalcemia is usually seen when surgery involves removal of a parathyroid adenoma, total or near-total thyroidectomy, or bilateral neck surgery for cancer. Hypocalcemia may occur immediately or 1–2 days after surgery and is transient (lasting less than 5 days) unless permanent parathyroid damage has occurred. Parathyroid insufficiency may result from gland suppression after removal of an adenoma, interference with parathyroid blood supply, or intraoperative release of calcitonin (11). Watson et al. (125) found a close correlation between decrements in serum Ca^{2+} and increases in calcitonin after thyroidectomy; however, no significant changes in PTH levels were observed, which suggests that calcitonin release accounted for the fall in serum Ca^{2+}. Serum Ca^{2+} returned to normal as calcitonin levels fell. With convalescence, there is resolution of edema or revascularization, which results in the reestablishment of parathyroid gland integrity.

Most patients who develop hypocalcemia after neck surgery remain asymptomatic; however, occasionally patients may develop paresthesias, laryngeal spasm, or tetany. We recommend that the serum-ionized Ca^{2+} level be monitored every 12 hours in patients after neck surgery—more frequently if hypocalcemic symptoms develop—until the serum-ionized Ca^{2+} level begins to rise (indicating recovery of the parathyroid glands). Symptomatic or severely hypocalcemic (ionized $Ca^{2+} < 3$ mg/dl) patients should receive supplemental Ca^{2+}. When Ca^{2+} is replaced in these patients, it is important that the Ca^{2+} level be maintained in the low normal ranges so as not to suppress the recovering parathyroid glands. Postoperative hypoparathyroidism may manifest itself late after neck surgery (months to years), and patients at risk should have their serum-ionized Ca^{2+} levels serially monitored. Other patients may have latent hypoparathyroidism after neck surgery, which manifests itself only with stress. Thus, critically ill patients with a previous history of neck surgery should have a serum Ca^{2+} determination performed.

Overt hypoparathyroidism rarely occurs after radioiodine treatment for thyroid disease (98); however, a significant number of these patients may have latent hypoparathyroidism, as measured by a diminished PTH response to ethylene diaminetetraacetic acid (EDTA)-induced hypocalcemia. The serum Ca^{2+} should be monitored in these patients during stress in order to avoid hypocalcemia. Infrequent causes of hypoparathyroidism are metastasis to the parathyroid glands and iron deposition due to hemochromatosis.

Two types of hypocalcemia have been described in newborn infants. The first occurs early after birth (1–3 days) and is called "early neonatal hypocalcemia". It is attributed to parathyroid immaturity and/or physiologic maternal hyperparathyroidism (causing neonatal parathyroid gland suppression) and usually resolves within the first week of life. Neonates have lower serum Ca^{2+} concentrations compared with older infants; the limits for pathologic hypocalcemia have been set at 8 mg/dl in full-term infants and 7 mg/dl in premature infants (98). Predisposing factors for neonatal hypocalcemia include prematurity, maternal diabetes mellitus, perinatal complications, and birth asphyxia. Late-onset neonatal hypocalcemia occurs 6–8 days after birth and is associated with hyperphosphatemia and hypomagnesemia. These infants frequently present with metabolic convulsions and the hypocalcemia likely results from high PO_4 intake (due to milk). High-serum PO_4 levels decrease the serum Ca^{2+} concentration by increasing Ca^{2+} deposition in bone. Hypomagnesemia results from decreased intestinal Mg^{2+} absorption. The hypomagnesemia augments the hypocalcemia via inhibition of PTH secretion and skeletal resistance. Other causes of hypoparathyroidism in infants include maternal hyperparathyroidism and excessive Ca^{2+} or vitamin D intake in the mother (both agents cross the placenta).

Postoperative hypocalcemia may also occur in patients after parathyroid or thyroid surgery, unrelated to hypoparathyroidism. After removal of the stimulus for elevated bone turnover (such as PTH or thyroid hormone) high rates of bone formation may develop and result in a lowering of the serum Ca^{2+} concentration ("recalcification hypocalcemia" or "tetany"). The incidence and severity of symptoms depends on the degree of postoperative bone involvement. These patients also frequently develop hypomagnesemia and hypophosphatemia.

Magnesium

Mg^{2+} abnormalities are common in critically ill patients and may cause hypocalcemia (7, 26, 30, 79, 110, 138, 142). The serum Mg^{2+} level influences both PTH secretion and action. Mild hypomagnesemia stimulates PTH secretion, whereas severe hypomagnesemia

$(Mg^{2+} < 1.0$ mg/dl) and hypermagnesemia inhibit PTH secretion. Hypomagnesemia also impairs PTH action at its receptor (i.e., skeletal resistance) and causes vitamin D resistance (11, 92, 93, 110). Since Mg^{2+} is an important cofactor for the activation of adenylate cyclase, it is possible that severe Mg^{2+} deficiency leads to an impairment of the adenylate cyclase receptor resulting in deranged PTH release and skeletal resistance. A variety of diseases and medications can cause hypomagnesemia and hypermagnesemia (see "Magnesium"). Hypomagnesemic hypocalcemia responds poorly to calcium therapy alone but does respond to Mg^{2+} repletion.

Phosphate

Hyperphosphatemia (see "Phosphorus") may cause hypocalcemia as a result of calcium precipitation, inhibition of bone resorption, and suppression of renal 1-hydroxylation of vitamin D (25, 29). The most common causes of this syndrome in the ICU include PO_4 administration (e.g. during the treatment of diabetic ketoacidosis),, tumor lysis syndromes following chemotherapy, renal failure, and rhabdomyolysis. Hypocalcemia during rhabdomyolysis is complex and appears to result from a combination of factors which include tissue Ca^{2+} deposition, hyperphosphatemia, impaired 1,25-dihydroxyvitamin D synthesis, and skeletal resistance to PTH (131). The serum PO_4 level should be measured in all hypocalcemic patients, since administration of Ca^{2+} to these patients may increase Ca precipitation and cause further harm. The hypocalcemia in hyperphosphatemic patients is treated by lowering the serum PO_4 level.

Chelators

Chelators are anions that are capable of forming complexes with Ca^{2+}. The most common chelators causing hypocalcemia in critically ill patients are citrated blood, albumin, and radiocontrast dyes.

Vitamin D Deficiency

Vitamin D deficiency is being increasingly recognized as an important cause of hypocalcemia in patients in the ICU. Approximately 20% of the hypocalcemic patients that we see in the ICU have a defect in the vitamin D axis. Many of these patients are chronically ill, malnourished, and have minimal sunlight expo-sure. They have low-serum 25-hydroxyvitamin D levels, suggestive of dietary vitamin D deficiency. Vitamin D deficiency may also occur in patients with a normal dietary intake as a result of gut malabsorption, defects in fat digestion, impaired biliary secretion or disrupted intestinal integrity (e.g. gastrectomy, gastrojejunostomy, celiac disease, Crohn's disease, intestinal bypass surgery, pancreatic insufficiency, hepatobiliary disease) (137). Excessive amounts of vitamin D bound to its transport protein may be lost in the urine of patients with the nephrotic syndrome.

Acquired defects in the hepatic 25-hydroxylase enzyme have not been shown to cause pathologic vitamin D deficiency (e.g., hypocalcemia). Although hypocalcemia is found in patients with advanced liver disease, the primary cause for low vitamin D levels appears to be malabsorption (failure of biliary secretion) rather than failure of hydroxylation.

Other patients have renal insufficiency with deficiency of the renal 1-hydroxylase system, which is responsible for the production of 1,25-dihydroxyvitamin D. These vitamin D–deficient patients frequently have normal serum Ca^{2+} levels as outpatients; however, they are unable to mobilize sufficient Ca^{2+} to maintain normal circulating levels during critical illness. Pseudohypoparathyroidism (11) is a rare disorder that results from resistance to PTH. Resultant suppression of the 1-hydroxylase system leads to deficiency of 1,25-dihydroxyvitamin D and hypocalcemia.

Pancreatitis

Hypocalcemia is commonly seen in patients with acute pancreatitis and is associated with a poor prognosis (64, 133). The exact etiology of the hypocalcemia in pancreatitis is uncertain. Saponification of Ca^{2+} is inadequate to explain the degree and length of hypocalcemia. PTH has been reported to be elevated (55), normal (53, 108), or decreased (33, 53). Bone and kidney can respond to exogenous PTH when it is given to patients with pancreatitis (108). Although this observation rules out complete end-organ resistance to PTH, it does not rule out partial PTH resistance. Analysis of the data on hypocalcemia in pancreatitis suggests that there are at least two groups of patients who develop hypocalcemia in this disorder. The majority have relative hypoparathyroidism (11) with normal or low PTH during hypocalcemia, whereas the remainder have appropriately increased levels of PTH. The group with elevated PTH levels may suffer from a defect in the vitamin D axis or from tissue resistance to PTH or vitamin D. In one study (55), serum 1,25-dihydroxyvitamin D levels were measured in six pancreatitis patients with hypocalcemia. In these patients serum vitamin D levels were low when the patients were admitted (during hypocalcemia) but increased in parallel with increases in PTH during recovery. Pancreatitis-associated hypomagnesemia and renal failure may also contribute to hypocalcemia.

Sepsis

The hypocalcemia occurring in patients with sepsis appears to have multiple causes (134). Some patients have dietary vitamin D deficiency, while others have acquired parathyroid gland insufficiency, renal 1-hydroxylase insufficiency, or peripheral resistance to 1,25-dihydroxyvitamin D (134). Renal 1-hydroxylase deficiency usually occurs when renal insufficiency accompanies sepsis.

Hungry Bone Syndromes

Hypocalcemia may occur after parathyroidectomy or thyroidectomy in patients with "overactive glands". These patients have accelerated bone resorption and formation. When the stimulus for resorption is removed at surgery, bone formation may exceed mineral supply and hypocalcemia results. The hypocalcemia is usually accompanied by hypophosphatemia and hypomagnesemia. Increased bone formation and hypocalcemia may also occur during osteoblastic metastasis from prostate, breast, and lung malignancies (11).

Fat Embolism Syndrome

Hypocalcemia is occasionally seen in trauma patients with fat embolism. The hypocalcemia probably results from a combination of Ca^{2+} chelation and increases in protein binding of Ca^{2+} induced by release of fatty acids. Transient episodes of ionized hypocalcemia associated with respiratory distress, in a patient after trauma, suggests the presence of this syndrome.

Miscellaneous

Hypocalcemia is associated with the toxic shock syndrome. Although circulating calcitonin levels are elevated in this syndrome, the exact pathogenesis of the hypocalcemia remains undefined (132). Ionized hypocalcemia occurs in patients with burns; however, the etiology remains to be defined. Hypothyroidism affects Ca^{2+} homeostasis by decreasing bone turnover and may also cause hypocalcemia. Hypothyroid patients usually have elevated levels of PTH and 1,25-dihydroxyvitamin D (133). A large number of drugs have been reported to cause hypocalcemia although clear documentation of ionized hypocalcemia is lacking with many. Listed in Table 32.1 are those drugs in which a clear association with hypocalcemia has been documented. Phosphates, citrate, magnesium, radiocontrast dye, albumin and heparin have already been discussed. Aminoglycosides, cis-platinum, and loop diuretics may cause hypocalcemia by producing hypomagnesemia. Cis-platinum also can inhibit bone resorption (24, 76, 77). EDTA and sodium sulfate (57) are potent Ca^{2+} chelators and have been used clinically to treat hypercalcemia. Mithramycin (117), calcitonin (116), estrogens, protamine (103), gallium nitrate (124), and diphosphonates (65, 66, 113) decrease bone resorption and are also used to treat hypercalcemia. WR-2721 is a radioprotective agent that inhibits PTH secretion (49, 50). Anticonvulsants such as phenytoin and phenobarbital have been associated with hypocalcemia and reduced bone mass. Although they increase the hepatic metabolism of vitamin D, this effect does not appear to be adequate to explain the hypocalcemia. These anticonvulsant drugs may also decrease intestinal Ca^{2+} absorption and reduce PTH-induced bone resorption (11). Ethylene glycol intoxication causes hypocalcemia, presumably by oxalate (a metabolic product of ethylene glycol metabolism) complexing with Ca^{2+} (120). Sodium fluoride forms an insoluble salt with Ca^{2+} (54) and may induce hypocalcemia when taken in large doses (as may be used in the treatment of osteoporosis).

CLINICAL MANIFESTATIONS

Hypocalcemia may present with a variety of clinical signs and symptoms (Table 32.2) that relate to increased neuronal irritability (133). Cardiovascular manifestations are the most commonly encountered features of hypocalcemia seen in critically ill patients. Patients may develop hypotension, cardiac insufficiency, bradycardia, arrhythmias (e.g. ventricular fibrillation), and failure to respond to drugs that act through calcium-related mechanisms

Table 32.2
Clinical Manifestations of Hypocalcemia

Cardiovascular
  Hypotension
  Cardiac insufficiency
  Bradycardia
  Arrhythmias
  Insensitivity to catecholamines and digitalis
ECG
      QT and ST interval prolongation
      T wave inversion
Respiratory
  Laryngeal spasm
  Apnea
  Bronchospasm
Neuromuscular
  Tetany
  Chvostek's and Trousseau's signs
  Muscle spasm
  Paresthesias
  Seizures
  Weakness
  Extrapyramidal manifestations
Psychiatric
  Anxiety
  Dementia
  Depression
  Irritability
  Psychosis
  Confusion
Miscellaneous
  Coarse, dry, scaly skin
  Brittle nails
  Thin brittle hair
  Cataracts

(e.g. digoxin, catecholamines, glucagon) (23, 28, 31, 34, 40, 48). Hypocalcemia should always be considered in patients with hypotension that responds poorly to fluids and/or to pressor agents. Restoration of a normal circulating Ca^{2+} level may restore vascular tone and improve cardiac contractility. Ca^{2+} may also be an effective inotropic agent in patients with advanced cardiac disease (18, 48) who have β-adrenergic receptor down-regulation as a result of chronic sympathetic stimulation. In some patients, digitalis may be ineffective, at normal levels, in controlling supraventricular arrhythmias (31) and catecholamines and glucagon (28) may be ineffective in raising blood pressure or heart rate due to hypocalcemia. Agents that decrease cellular Ca^{2+} availability (e.g. β-adrenergic blockers and slow calcium channel antagonists) may exacerbate hypocalcemia-induced cardiac insufficiency. Hypocalcemia may inconsistently cause Q-T and S-T interval prolongation; however, these ECG changes can not be relied upon to exclude a diagnosis of hypocalcemia.

Hypocalcemia may also present as laryngo-spasm or bronchospasm in critically ill patients. We have treated patients who were doing well and were extubated after surgery who required reintubation as a result of hypocalcemia-induced laryngospasm. The laryngospasm resolved with Ca^{2+} repletion.

Tetany and muscle spasms are the classical sign of hypocalcemia, but these signs may be absent in hypocalcemic ICU patients. Chvostek's and Trousseau's signs are nonspecific indicators of hypocalcemia. Chvostek's sign is present in 25% of normal adults while Trousseau's sign is present in 4% of the normal population (11). In addition, Trousseau's sign may be negative in 30% of subjects with hypocalcemia. Anticonvulsant drugs, sedation, and paralyzation may eliminate signs of neuronal irritability. The intubated, sedated or paralyzed patient may be unable to express symptoms such as anxiety and paresthesias. Psychiatric manifestations of hypocalcemia (Table 32.2) are nonspecific and are frequently seen in critically ill patients as a result of their illness.

We routinely monitor serum-ionized Ca^{2+} levels in all critically ill patients and treat all patients with hypocalcemic symptoms or severe hypocalcemia. Life-threatening arrhythmias develop when the ionized Ca^{2+} level approaches 2.0–2.5 mg/dl, and thus we recommend that all patients with an ionized Ca^{2+} concentration below 3.0 mg/dl should receive treatment (Zaloga GP, Flemming S; unpublished data).

TREATMENT

Patients with suspected hypocalcemia should have an ionized Ca^{2+} measured to confirm the diagnosis (Fig. 32.2). Once confirmed these patients should have a blood sample sent for measurement of serum magnesium and phosphorus levels. Blood samples should be saved for plasma PTH and vitamin D levels, should these tests later become necessary (Fig. 32.2).

Acute symptomatic hypocalcemia is a medical emergency that necessitates intravenous Ca^{2+} therapy (Table 32.3). Initial therapy in adults consists of the administration of a Ca^{2+} bolus (100–200 mg of elemental Ca^{2+} over 10 minutes) followed by a maintenance infusion of 1 to 2 mg/kg/hour of elemental Ca^{2+}. A 100–200 mg bolus of elemental Ca^{2+} will usually raise the serum total Ca^{2+} by 1 mg/dl, with levels returning to baseline by 30 minutes after injection. To maintain levels above baseline a continuous infusion or intermittent boluses of

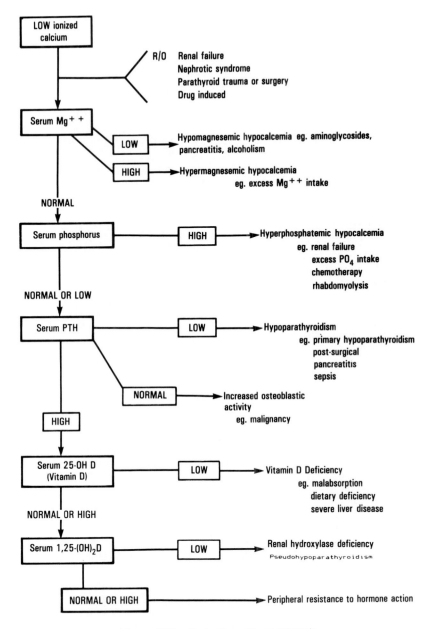

Figure 32.2 Evaluation of hypocalcemia.

Ca^{2+} are necessary. The serum Ca^{2+} usually normalizes in 6–12 hours with this regimen, and the maintenance rate may need to be decreased to 0.3–0.5 mg/kg/hour. Serum Mg^{2+} and PO_4 levels should be measured and restored to normal values. Administration of Ca^{2+} to hyperphosphatemic patients may cause Ca^{2+} precipitation. Hypomagnesemic and hypermagnesemic hypocalcemia responds poorly to Ca^{2+} therapy, but does respond to normalization of the serum Mg^{2+} level. Potassium deficiency protects the patient from hypocalcemic tetany and arrhythmias, and correction of the hypokalemia without correction of the hypocalcemia may provoke these disorders (54). Administration of drugs that may be aggravating hypocalcemia (e.g., furosemide) should be discontinued or another drug substituted if

Table 32.3
Calcium Preparations

	Size	Contents[a]
Parenteral		
Ca^{2+} Gluconate (10%)	10 ml	93 mg Ca^{2+} (4.6 mEq)
Ca^{2+} Gluceptate	5 ml	90 mg Ca^{2+} (4.5 mEq)
Ca^{2+} Chloride (10%)	10 ml	272 mg Ca^{2+} (13.6 mEq)
Oral		
Ca^{2+} Carbonate, e.g., Os-cal 500	tablets	500 mg Ca^{2+}
Ca^{2+} Gluconate	tablets	500 mg Ca^{2+}
Ca^{2+} Lactate	tablets	650 mg Ca^{2+}
Ca^{2+} Glubionate e.g., Neo-calglucon	syrup	115 mg Ca^{2+}/5 ml

[a] Elemental Ca^{2+}

possible. Intravenous Ca^{2+} preparations are irritating to veins and Ca^{2+} should be diluted in 50–100 ml of 5% dextrose in water. Ca^{2+} chloride should never be injected into tissues; however, Ca^{2+} gluceptate may be given intramuscularly when intravenous access is not possible (54). Ca^{2+} salts should not be administered with bicarbonate, since the two precipitate. Ca^{2+} must be administered cautiously to patients receiving digitalis, since hypercalcemia predisposes to digitalis toxicity. Adequacy of treatment can be monitored at the bedside by following Chvostek's and Trousseau's signs, the ECG, and hemodynamic parameters. Optimal therapy requires frequent monitoring of the serum Ca^{2+}, Mg^{2+}, PO_4, potassium, and creatinine levels. Once serum Ca^{2+} is stable in the low normal range the patient may be started on enteral Ca^{2+} (Table 32.3). Most patients require 2–4 g of calcium per day in divided doses. Ca^{2+} carbonate is converted in the stomach to a soluble calcium salt by hydrochloric acid. It is ineffective in patients with achlorhydria (11).

Table 32.4
Vitamin D Preparations

	Ergocalciferol (Vit D2)	Calcifediol (250HD)	Dihydrotachysterol (1-OHD)	Calcitriol (1,25(OH)2D)
Concentration in serum	10 ng/ml	30 ng/ml		0.03 ng/ml
Physiological dose (μg/day)	10	5	20	0.5
Pharmacological dose (μg/day)	1200	50	200–800	0.25–1
Onset of maximal effect (days)	30	15	15	3
Dosage forms	Tablets 625 μg 1250 μg Solution 8000 U/ml Oil for inject 500,000 U/ml	Capsules 20 μg 50 μg	Tablets 125 μg 200 μg 400 μg Solution 200 μg/ml	Capsules 0.25 μg 0.50 μg
Commercial products	Calciferol	Calderol	Hytakerol	Rocaltrol
Serum half-life (days)	30	15		0.2
Time for reversal of effect (days)	17–60	7–30	3–14	2–10
Advantages	Low cost, prolonged action, parent compound	Liver disease	Renal disease, hypoparathyroidism	Renal disease, liver disease, hypoparathyroidism, rapid onset, rapid offset
Disadvantages	Instability, long toxicity	Expense	Expense	Expense

When Ca^{2+} alone is insufficient in normalizing the serum Ca^{2+} concentration, vitamin D metabolites (Table 32.4) may be added (54). Vitamin D is rarely required during the period of critical illness while the patient is in the ICU. It is usually reserved for chronic treatment of hypocalcemia. The principal effect of vitamin D is to increase gut Ca^{2+} absorption, although it also has effects on bone resorption. The earliest calciferol metabolite that is deficient should be administered first. This approach allows the body to regulate activation of the vitamin and replenishes other vitamin D metabolites, which may have some, as yet unknown, physiologic function. When the 1-hydroxylase enzyme is deficient (as in renal failure) or when patients are resistant to ergocalciferol, they may respond to 1,25-dihydroxyvitamin D. This analogue is more potent than other vitamin D metabolites (Table 32.4), has a quicker onset of action, and a greater tendency to induce hypercalcemia and hypercalciuria, but a shorter duration of toxicity. Vitamin D requirements vary and must be adjusted based on disease activity, interacting drugs, and dietary Ca^{2+} intake. Hypercalciuria with its attendant problems (e.g., nephrocalcinosis and renal stones) may occur before eucalcemia is reached. In these situations, a thiazide diuretic can be helpful in reducing Ca^{2+} excretion. Serum Ca^{2+} and PO_4 levels and urinary Ca^{2+} excretion should be measured at regular intervals. The therapeutic goal is to restore the serum Ca^{2+} to near normal levels (which alleviate symptoms) and avoid complications (e.g., hypercalcemia and hypercalciuria).

Definitive treatment of hypocalcemia involves recognition and correction of the underlying disorder. Frequently, however, acute measures are required to stabilize the serum Ca^{2+} level in safe ranges before addressing the primary problem.

Hypercalcemia

CAUSES

Hypercalcemia occurs when Ca^{2+} enters the vascular space faster than it can be excreted or sequestered. The most common causes (Table 32.5) of hypercalcemia seen in the critical care setting are malignancy, hyperparathyroidism, immobilization, iatrogenic Ca^{2+} administration, hypercalcemia of renal failure, and posthypocalcemic hypercalcemia.

Table 32.5
Causes of Hypercalcemia

Malignancy
Hyperparathyroidism
Immobilization
Iatrogenic calcium administration
Renal causes
   Chronic renal failure
   Recovery from acute renal failure
   After renal transplantation
Posthypocalcemic hypercalcemia
Hypocalciuric hypercalcemia
   Familial
   Hypothyroidism
   Lithium
   Thiazides
   Adrenal insufficiency
   Bartter's syndrome
Granulomatous disease
   Sarcoidosis
   Histoplasmosis
   Coccidiomycosis
   Tuberculosis
Hyperthyroidism
Acquired immune deficiency syndrome (AIDS)
Phosphorus depletion syndrome
Multiple endocrine neoplasia syndromes
Pheochromocytoma
Acromegaly
Drug Induced
   Calcium
   Estrogens or progestins for malignancy
   Lithium
   Milk-alkali syndrome
   Theophylline
   Thiazides
   Vitamin D or A

Malignancy

Hypercalcemia occurs in approximately 10–20% of patients with malignancy because of direct tumor osteolysis of bone and from the secretion of humoral substances that stimulate bone resorption (11). Humoral bone resorbing substances include PTH-like substances (12, 20, 118), 1,25-dihydroxyvitamin D (17, 139), osteoclast activating factor (97), and prostaglandins (115). PTH-like substances cross react in the radioimmunoassay for PTH but are not identical to PTH. They are presently thought to be responsible for most instances of humoral hypercalcemia of malignancy and most likely represent a heterogenous group of molecules. These molecules stimulate bone resorption, and frequently are capable of stimulating the renal adenylate cyclase system and inhibiting phosphate resorption, similar to PTH. They have little activity on the renal 1-hydroxylase enzyme that is responsible for the renal synthesis of 1,25-dihydroxyvitamin D. Tumor synthesis of 1,25-dihydroxyvitamin D is a less common cause of hypercalcemia but has been described in patients with lymphoma (17) and Hodgkin's disease (139). Osteoclast activating factor, a lymphokine released by stimulated peripheral blood leukocytes, may be released into the circulation in neoplasia of lymphoid origin (e.g., multiple myeloma, lymphoma, and leukemia) and, like 1,25-dihydroxyvitamin D, is antagonized by glucocorticoids. Hypercalcemia due to prostaglandins are a rare cause of hypercalcemia, usually occur with solid tumors, and may respond to cyclooxygenase inhibitors. Tumor-related hypercalcemia occurs most commonly with breast, lung, kidney, prostate, and hematologic malignancies. Primary hyperparathyroidism also occurs with a higher frequency in hypercalcemic patients with malignancy (11).

Hyperparathyroidism

Primary hyperparathyroidism is found in the general population with a prevalence that ranges from 0.03% to 0.1% (52, 133). The most common causes of primary hyperparathyroidism are single adenomas (75–87%), hyperplasia of multiple glands (12–22%), and carcinoma of the parathyroid glands (3%). Hypercalcemia in hyperparathyroidism results from the combined effects of both increased PTH and 1,25-dihydroxyvitamin D on the bone, intestine, and kidneys. Many hyperparathyroid patients are asymptomatic and the hypercalcemia is noted only when a serum Ca^{2+} level is measured for other reasons. Most of these patients do not require emergency treatment for their hypercalcemia, but some type of treatment is frequently required to prevent accelerated bone loss. Surgery remains the only definitive treatment for patients with hyperparathyroidism, although some patients may have slight decreases in plasma Ca^{2+} and decreased bone turnover with estrogen or progestogen therapy (47, 60). Estrogens and progestins appear to work by antagonizing PTH action upon the skeleton. When one encounters a patient with hyperparathyroidism due to glandular hyperplasia, a search for other endocrine tumors should be sought as part of the multiple endocrine neoplasia syndromes (e.g. tumors of the pituitary, pancreas, adrenal, and thyroid).

Immobilization

Immobilization hypercalcemia occurs following immobilization in patients with rapid bone turnover. The patients most at risk are children, adolescents, postfracture patients, patients with Paget's disease of bone, and patients with underlying malignancy or hyperparathyroidism. Patients with renal failure are also at risk due to their inability to excrete an increased Ca^{2+} load. Most immoblized patients have increased urinary Ca^{2+} and PO_4 levels but only a few develop hypercalcemia (133). Serum PTH and 1,25-dihydroxyvitamin D levels are usually suppressed and hypercalcemia probably results from a relative increase in osteoclastic activity. Symptoms relate to the degree of hypercalciuria and hypercalcemia. The primary therapeutic modality in these patients is mobilization. Quiet standing for a few hours a day is superior to supine bed exercise. Serum Ca^{2+} levels may also be reduced by saline diuresis, calcitonin, oral phosphates, and diphosphonates. Dietary Ca^{2+} restriction has little effect since most circulating Ca^{2+} is derived from bone.

Renal-Related Causes

Hypercalcemia is occasionally seen in patients with uremia and may be iatrogenic, resulting from excess Ca^{2+} or vitamin D supplementation, from the use of high Ca^{2+} dialysate, or from immobilization. These patients are prone to hypercalcemia because they lack the ability to excrete Ca^{2+} through the kidneys and many have a defect in bone mineralization. Patients with secondary hyperparathyroidism may become hypercalcemic after the institution of dialysis. Dialysis may render the bone more responsive to PTH or may lead to hypercalcemia by lowering PO_4 levels. Other causes of hypercalcemia in these patients include the use of Ca^{2+}-containing cation exchange resins, PO_4 depletion with aluminum hydroxide compounds, or the use of thiazide diuretics. Hypercalcemia may also occur during the recovery phase of acute renal failure or following renal transplantation (11). The cause of hypercalcemia in these patients relates to the presence of secondary hyperparathyroidism, reduction in circulating PO_4 concentrations, tapering of steroids, and perhaps increased sensitivity of bone to PTH during resolution of uremia (11). Hyperplastic parathyroid glands usually involute within 6 months of renal transplantation. At times hyperplastic glands may persist and parathyroidectomy may be necessary to avoid renal graft dysfunction (11).

Posthypocalcemic Hypercalcemia

Transient hypercalcemia is not uncommonly seen in patients after a period of hypocalcemia (45). The hypercalcemia most likely results from increased PTH and 1,25-dihydroxyvitamin D levels that were stimulated by the hypocalcemia. Hypocalcemia resolves faster than the Ca^{2+} mobilizing hormones can readjust, resulting in a transient period of rebound hypercalcemia. A review of six cases of transient hypercalcemia of unknown etiology in our ICU revealed a period of hypocalcemia preceding the hypercalcemia in each case. The hypercalcemia resolved without treatment in all cases.

Hypocalciuric Hypercalcemia

Hypercalcemia may occur in patients associated with decreased urinary Ca^{2+} excretion. The hypercalcemia appears to result from the combination of altered parathyroid gland function and altered ion transport in the kidneys. Marx and associates (84) described the inherited syndrome of familial hypocalciuric hypercalcemia (FHH). This disease rarely causes symptoms and is usually discovered when a serum Ca^{2+} level is obtained for other reasons. Serum Ca^{2+}, PTH, 1,25-dihydroxyvitamin D, and urinary cyclic adenosine monophosphate levels (an index of PTH activity) overlap with normal and hyperparathyroid patients; however, urinary Ca^{2+} excretion is less than 150 mg/day and the Ca^{2+}/creatinine ratio is less than 0.01. These patients generally do well without treatment and do not develop bone disease. Hypocalciuric hypercalcemia may also occur in patients with hypothyroidism (140), with lithium therapy, after thiazide administration, with adrenal insufficiency, and with Bartter's syndrome.

Granulomatous Disease

Hypercalcemia (10–20%) and hypercalciuria (30–50%) are commonly seen in patients with sarcoidosis (11, 52). Most hypercalcemic sarcoid patients have an abnormal chest radiograph, abnormal pulmonary function tests, increased bone turnover, and increased gut absorption of Ca^{2+}. Parathyroid function is suppressed; however, these patients produce excess amounts of 1,25-dihydroxyvitamin D within their granuloma (9, 36, 89). Lymphocytes in granulomata associated with histo-plasmosis, coccidiomycosis, tuberculosis (1), silicone injections, and berylliosis are also capable of producing excessive amounts of active vitamin D metabolites and hypercalcemia. The hypercalcemia in these patients improves with glucocorticoids.

Miscellaneous

Thyroid hormone has direct effects on the skeleton, increasing bone turnover and Ca^{2+} release. Although severe hypercalcemia is rare in patients with hyperthyroidism, mild asymptomatic hypercalcemia is frequently encountered (11). PTH and 1,25-dihydroxyvitamin D levels are suppressed in these patients. Hypercalcemia in patients with hyperthyroidism may respond to calcitonin, glucocorticoids, propranolol, and lowering of thyroid hormone levels. Hypercalcemia associated with suppressed PTH and 1,25-dihydroxyvitamin D levels also may occur in patients with the acquired immune deficiency syndrome (AIDS) and probably results from increased bone turnover (136). Phosphorus depletion may occur in patients given phosphate-binding antacids. Stimulation of 1,25-dihydroxyvitamin D synthesis may lead to increased gut Ca^{2+} absorption and bone resorption and thereby cause hypercalcemia. Catecholamines may increase PTH secretion and stimulate bone turnover. In fact, hypercalcemia is occasionally seen in patients with pheochromocytoma (11). These patients may respond to therapy with β-adrenergic blockers. Growth hormone can enhance the formation of 1,25-dihydroxyvitamin D and hypercalcemia has been reported in patients with acromegaly (11). Patients with breast cancer may rarely develop progressive hypercalcemia after receiving treatment with estrogens or progestins, as a result of tumor necrosis with release of bone-resorbing substances. A variety of drugs may cause hypercalcemia (Table 32.5). Vitamin D or A administration increases bone turnover and causes hypercalcemia. Vitamin D also increases intestinal Ca^{2+} absorption. Hypervitaminosis D- or A-induced hypercalcemia responds to glucocorticoid administration. The milk-alkali syndrome (102, 120) consists of hypercalcemia, alkalosis, and renal impairment and is seen in patients who ingest excessive amounts of Ca^{2+} and alkali (e.g. Ca^{2+} carbonate or milk plus sodium bicarbonate for treatment of peptic ulcers). The alkali lowers the urine solubility for Ca^{2+}, decreases Ca^{2+} excretion, and may cause progressive hypercalcemia and renal insufficiency. Ca^{2+} depresses PTH secretion and increases renal bicarbonate reabsorption, further worsening alkalosis. Thiazides and lithium enhance renal Ca^{2+} resorption and decrease renal Ca^{2+} excretion (11). Lithium may also stimulate parathyroid gland activity. Theophylline causes an elevation of the serum Ca^{2+} level that is mediated through adrenergic mechanisms and is compatible with enhancement of PTH action (91). Serum Ca^{2+} levels fall after the administration of beta-adrenergic blockers.

CLINICAL MANIFESTATIONS

Hypercalcemia causes a variety of effects on multiple organ systems (Table 32.6). Ca^{2+} may form stones within the kidneys or disrupt tubular or glomerular function. Reduction in glomerular filtration results from volume depletion and a reduction in the ultrafiltration coefficient (11). Impairment of sodium reabsorption results from inhibition of sodium-potassium ATPase in the ascending limb of Henle and distal tubules. Ca^{2+} antagonism of antidiuretic hormone activity within the kidney can lead to a state of nephrogenic diabetes insipidus (impaired renal concentration), progressive dehydration, and further hypercalcemia. Neuromyopathic manifestations are common and may contribute to the failure to wean a hypercalcemic patient from the ventilator. Neuropsychiatric changes are frequent but are not specific for hypercalcemia.

The cardiovascular effects of hypercalcemia include hypertension and arrhythmias. These may respond to Ca^{2+} channel antagonists (141). Electrocardiographic changes are not reliable indicators of the degree of hypercalcemia and QT shortening is seen in only a minority of cases (43). Hypercalcemia increases cardiac sensitivity to digitalis and may lead to digitalis-related toxicity. Ca^{2+} administration in rats decreases cardiovascular responses to epinephrine (Zaloga GP, Willey SC, Malcolm D, Chernow B, Holaday J; unpublished data). Ca^{2+} may work in this situation by inhibiting adenyl cyclase activity. The clinical implications of this work await further studies in humans.

Anorexia is common in hypercalcemic patients. These patients are also prone to the development of pancreatitis and peptic ulcer disease. Skeletal disease may occur secondary to direct tumor invasion or secretion of bone-resorbing substances. Hypomagnesemia may result from Ca^{2+}-induced inhibition of Mg^{2+}

Table 32.6
Clinical Features of Hypercalcemia

Cardiovascular
  Hypertension
  Arrhythmias
  Digitalis sensitivity
  Catecholamine resistance
  QT shortening
Urinary system
  Nephrocalcinosis
  Nephrolithiasis
  Tubular dysfunction
    Renal tubular acidosis
    Impaired Na reabsorption
    Free water loss
  Glomerular disorders
  Interstitial nephritis
Gastrointestinal
  Peptic ulcers
  Pancreatitis
  Constipation
  Anorexia
  Nausea/vomiting
Neuromuscular
  Weakness, atrophy
  Hyporeflexia
Neuropsychiatric
  Depression
  Personality change
  Psychomotor retardation
  Memory impairment
  Psychosis
  Disorientation
  Obtundation
  Coma
  Seizures
  EEG abnormalities
Skeletal
  Osteopenia
  Osteitis fibrosa cystica
Miscellaneous
  Skin necrosis
  Corneal calcification
  Conjunctivitis
  Pruritis
  Decreased bronchial clearance of secretions
  Hypomagnesemia

reabsorption in the renal tubules (11). The threshold for the development of hypercalcemic symptoms varies; however, most asymptomatic patients have a total serum Ca^{2+} level below 12 mg/dl (with a normal albumin concentration). Factors such as the rapidity with which the serum Ca^{2+} rises, accompanying renal failure, electrolyte disturbances, cardiovascular status, and the general state of debilitation of the patient can alter the threshold for symptoms. The most common causes of death as a result of hypercalcemia relate to renal failure, arrhythmias, and central nervous system impairment.

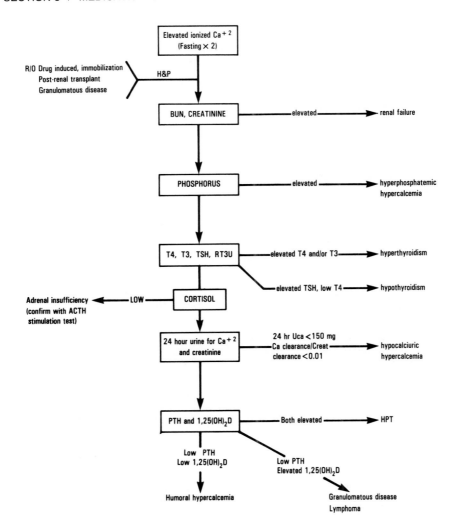

Figure 32.3 Evaluation of hypercalcemia.

EVALUATION

Hypercalcemia should be documented by measuring a fasting serum calcium level (Fig. 32.3) to exclude exogenous causes of hypercalcemia (e.g., orally or intravenously administered Ca^{2+}). Once established, a careful history, physical examination, and review of the patient's chart, including drugs, may uncover the cause of the hypercalcemia in most cases. Renal function and phosphate levels should be measured to rule out renal causes. Measurement of thyroid hormone and TSH concentrations can detect hypothyroidism or hyperthyroidism. A 24-hour urine collection for Ca^{2+} and creatinine determinations helps to separate hypocalciuric from hypercalciuric

syndromes. Frequently, one must differentiate between primary hyperparathyroidism and malignancy (Table 32.7). The best tests that distinguish between these two entities are PTH and 1,25-dihydroxyvitamin D measurements. PTH is elevated in primary hyperparathyroidism and normal or low in patients with hypercalcemia of malignancy. The 1-hydroxylase enzyme is stimulated by PTH and 1,25-dihydroxyvitamin D levels are usually high in patients with hyperparathyroidism. On the other hand, 1,25-dihydroxyvitamin D values are low in malignancy unless due to rare tumors that contain a 1-hydroxylase enzyme. PTH and factors released from certain tumors are both capable of raising nephrogenous cAMP levels (85). An elevated nephrogenous cAMP level

Table 32.7
Primary Hyperparathyroidism Versus Hypercalcemia of Malignancy

	Hyper-parathyroidism	Malignancy
Clinical course	Chronic	Acute
Serum Ca^{2+}	<12.5 mg/dl	>12.5 mg/dl
Serum Cl	>102 mEq/liter	<102 mEq/liter
Serum PO_4	Normal or low	Normal or high
Cl/PO_4	>33	<33
Acid-base	Hyperchloremic acidosis	Metabolic alkalosis
Renal calculi	Frequent	Rare
Osteitis fibrosa	Present	Absent
Urinary Ca^{2+}	High	Very high
PTH	Elevated	Low or normal
1,25(OH)2D	High	Low
TmP/GFR	Low	Variable
Nephrogenous cAMP	High	Variable

cannot distinguish between hypercalcemia due to hyperparathyroidism or malignancy; however, low levels can help to exclude hyperparathyroidism. A careful search for malignancy using chest roentgenograms, bone and liver scans, and computed tomography scanning may also help to establish a definitive diagnosis. If no malignancy can be found after a careful search and laboratory data are compatible with primary hyperparathyroidism, then neck exploration should be performed. In high-risk patients, selective venous catheterization with analysis of serum for PTH or nuclear medicine scanning may help to localize the site of overactive parathyroid tissue.

TREATMENT

Definitive treatment of hypercalcemia lies in the correction of the cause (e.g., surgery for hyperparathyroidism or chemotherapy, surgery or radiotherapy for malignancy); however, while evaluation is taking place it may be necessary to treat the patient to avoid complications and symptoms of hypercalcemia. Ca^{2+} enters and exits the circulation from the gastrointestinal, skeletal or renal routes. The goal of therapy is to minimize Ca^{2+} entry and maximize Ca^{2+} exit. General measures of treatment (Table 32.8) include hydration, correction of electrolyte abnormalities, removal of offending drugs, dietary Ca^{2+} restriction, and mobilization of the patient. Concomitant electrolyte disturbances (e.g. potassium, Mg^{2+}, PO_4) are common in patients with hypercalcemia. Aldinger and Samaan (5) found a 16.9% incidence of hypokalemia in patients with primary hyperparathyroidism and a 52.3% incidence in patients with hypercalcemia of malignancy. Serum potassium levels were lowest in patients with the highest serum Ca^{2+} concentrations. Hypokalemia or hypomagnesemia increase the arrhythmogenic potential of hypercalcemia. Diuresis may further lower the serum Mg^{2+} and potassium concentrations.

Renal Ca^{2+} excretion can be enhanced with the use of saline (inhibits proximal tubule reabsorption) and furosemide (inhibits distal Ca^{2+} reabsorption) (Table 32.8). Sodium competes with Ca^{2+} in the kidney and inhibits its reabsorption. In addition, expansion of intravascular volume dilutes the Ca^{2+} concentration in the blood and promotes renal flow. Furosemide and saline are adjusted to main-

Table 32.8
Treatments of Hypercalcemia: Alternatives

General Measures
  Hydration
  Remove offending drugs
  Dietary Ca^{2+} restriction
  Treat underlying disorder
  Mobilization
Increase Renal Ca^{2+} Excretion
  Saline: 2–3 liters over 3–6 hr, maintain urine output >200–300 ml/hr
  Furosemide: 10–40 mg i.v. every 2–4 hr
  Dialysis
Decrease Bone Resorption
  Calcitonin: 1–2 MRC U/kg i.v. or i.m. every 6 hours
  Mithramycin: 25 μg/kg i.v. over 4 hours every 2–7 days
  Glucocorticoids: Hydrocortisone 3 mg/kg/day in divided doses every 6 hours or prednisone 40–60 mg/day
  Indomethacin: 25 mg p.o. every 6 hours
  Etidronate disodium: 7.5 mg/kg/day i.v. in 250-ml saline over 2 hours for 1–4 days or 5–10 mg/kg/day p.o.
  Cis-platinum: 100 mg/m^2 over 24 hours
  Gallium nitrate: 200 mg/m^2/day by continuous infusion for 5–7 days
Ca^{2+} Chelators
  Phosphates
    p.o.: 500–1000 mg every 6 hours
    i.v.: 50 mM PO_4 over 8–12 hours
    Rectal: Phosphosoda 5 ml every 6 hours; Fleets enema 100 ml twice daily
  EDTA: 10–50 mg/kg over 4 hours
  Sodium citrate
  Sodium sulfate
Ca^{2+} Antagonists
  Verapamil 5–10 mg i.v.
  Nifedipine 10–20 mg sublingually
PTH Antagonists
  WR-2721 430–910 mg/m^2 over 20–60 minutes

tain a urine output of 200–300 ml/hour. Sodium, Mg^{2+}, PO_4, and potassium should be monitored and replaced as necessary. Central hemodynamic monitoring may be necessary in patients with heart or renal disease. Ca^{2+} may also be removed from the plasma with dialysis (22) in patients with oliguric renal disease. Hemodialysis can clear up to 682 mg of Ca^{2+} per hour as compared with 124 mg/hour for peritoneal dialysis and 82 mg/hour for forced diuresis (22).

Ca^{2+} may be lowered by agents which decrease bone resorption (Table 32.8). These agents work best in patients with hyperresorptive diseases such as hyperparathyroidism, Paget's disease, and malignancy. Calcitonin (116) inhibits osteoclastic bone resorption and can be given to patients with hyperphosphatemia and before hydration is complete. It is particularly useful in treating patients with congestive heart failure or renal failure in whom large quantities of saline or PO_4 cannot be used. A hypocalcemic effect (average decrease of 2–3 mg/dl) may be seen in 6–10 hours. Calcitonin has low toxicity but occasionally may cause nausea, vomiting, abdominal cramps, skin rash, flushing, and diarrhea. The major disadvantages of calcitonin are its unpredictability (25% do not respond) and drug resistance. Calcitonin resistance frequently develops in patients after 48–72 hours of use as a result of receptor down-regulation and uncoupling of adenyl cyclase (11); resistance may be delayed by the coadministration of glucocorticoids (20–40 mg prednisone every 6 hours) or oral phosphates. Discontinuation of the drug for 24–48 hours can also restore effect.

Osteoclastic bone resorption may be decreased by mithramycin (117) (Table 32.8). This drug is almost always effective but takes 12–24 hours to produce a hypocalcemic effect, and its maximal hypocalcemic effect occurs at 5–7 days. If a response is not seen within 24–48 hours the dose may be repeated until a response is seen. Hypocalcemia may be seen following its use and it has renal, hepatic, and hematologic toxicities (especially thrombocytopenia).

Cisplatinum is able to lower serum Ca^{2+} levels in cancer-associated hypercalcemia in animals (76) and humans (77). Lad et al. (77) treated 13 patients with severe cancer-induced hypercalcemia refractory to rehydration within a 24-hour infusion of cisplatinum (100 mg/m^2 of body surface area). Nine patients achieved normocalcemia. The maximal lowering oc-

curred 10 days after treatment and persisted for a mean duration of 38 days. Cisplatinum inhibits PTH and tumor extract-induced osteolysis in vitro in the mouse calvarium bone resorption assay (24), suggesting that it controls hypercalcemia by inhibiting bone resorption. Gallium nitrate (124) is an antitumor compound that decreases Ca^{2+} resorption from bone and causes hypocalcemia. Warrell et al. (124) treated 10 patients with cancer-related hypercalcemia with gallium nitrate (200 mg/m^2/day by continuous infusion for 5–7 days). Total serum Ca^{2+} concentrations decreased from 13.8 mg/dl to 8.0 mg/dl. Gallium nitrate produced few side effects although nephrotoxicity has been reported. Nausea and myelosuppression do not occur.

Glucocorticoids decrease osteoclastic bone resorption, inhibit osteoclast activating factor, block prostaglandin synthesis, and antagonize vitamin D action. They are the agents of choice in vitamin D excess states and in treating hypercalcemia due to granulomatous disease (e.g., sarcoidosis). Glucocorticoids are also effective in control of hypercalcemia in patients with multiple myeloma and lymphoid malignancies. They are ineffective in patients with hyperparathyroidism.

Indomethacin has been used to treat hypercalcemia in patients with some tumors that produce prostaglandins (e.g. hypernephroma and lung cancer). Propranolol has been used to treat hypercalcemia in patients with pheochromocytoma. Hypercalcemia in patients with hyperthyroidism responds to treatment of the thyroid disease. Diphosphonates decrease bone resorption by binding to hydroxyapatite and by inhibiting osteoclast function (65, 66, 113). Etidronate disodium (113), 7.5 mg/kg/day administered intravenously reduced Ca^{2+} to normal in 3 days in 19 of 26 patients with hypercalcemia of malignancy (mean decrease in Ca^{2+} of 2.2 mg/dl). It is the only diphosphonate approved for clinical use in the United States. We have also used this agent orally with some success. Side effects may occasionally occur and include nausea, vomiting, diarrhea, hyperphosphatemia, renal dysfunction, and defective bone mineralization. Oral and intravenous dichloromethylene diphosphonate is also effective in lowering serum Ca^{2+} levels in patients with malignancy and hyperparathyroidism (11, 65, 66). However, this drug is not approved for use in the United States. Large doses of protamine cause acute hypocalcemia in animals by blocking efflux of Ca^{2+} from bone (100). Further studies are needed to examine its potential clinical utility in control of hypercalcemia due to diseases associated with increased bone turnover.

Chelators (e.g., phosphates and EDTA) are indicated for the management of life-threatening hypercalcemic emergencies when an immediate lowering of the ionized Ca^{2+} level is required (Table 32.8). Phosphates (oral, rectal, or intravenous) are extremely effective agents for lowering circulating Ca^{2+}. They work by binding and precipitating Ca^{2+}, inhibiting bone resorption, and decreasing renal activation of vitamin D. Their major disadvantage is the potential for extraskeletal calcification in vital structures (e.g., heart, retina, and kidney). Orally and rectally administered phosphates are safer than intravenously administered phosphates but require several days for maximal effect. Intravenous phosphates work rapidly (maximal effect 6–24 hours) but should not be given in doses exceeding 50 mM over 6–8 hours. Serum Ca^{2+} may fall from 1 to 6 mg/dl depending upon the dose of PO_4 administered. Patients should be well hydrated and blood pressure and electrolytes should be monitored closely. Phosphates are contraindicated in the hyperphosphatemic hypercalcemic patient and should be withheld if the total serum $Ca^{2+} \times PO_4$ product exceeds 60–70. EDTA (ethylenediamine tetraacetic acid) forms complexes with Ca^{2+} as well as Mg^{2+} and is excreted in the urine. It is very effective in lowering circulating Ca^{2+} levels. Hydration is important so as to minimize renal toxicity. It is best given centrally and should be diluted in saline. A dose of EDTA of 50 mg/kg usually lowers the serum Ca^{2+} concentration by 2–3 mg/dl. Infusion of albumin, sodium citrate (19), or sodium sulfate (57) can also be used to acutely lower the ionized Ca^{2+} level. However, these agents have not been tested in clinical trials for the treatment of hypercalcemia and should not be used as primary therapy.

The chemoprotective and radioprotective agent, WR-2721, lowers serum Ca^{2+} when administered to patients with malignancy (49, 50). Reduction of PTH secretion plays a role in the hypocalcemic action of WR-2721, and this agent has been used to treat refractory hypercalcemia in a patient with parathyroid cancer (50). Further studies are needed before widespread use of this agent is recommended. Conjugated estrogens (1.25 mg daily) and norethindrone (5 mg daily) may lower serum Ca^{2+} and inhibit bone resorption by antagonizing PTH in patients with mild hyperparathyroidism (60, 83).

Ca^{2+} may have toxic life-threatening effects upon the cardiovascular system (e.g., arrhythmias, heart block, and cardiac arrest). These effects may be antagonized by calcium channel blockers such as verapamil (141) while awaiting definitive therapy.

Saline, furosemide, phosphates, EDTA, sodium citrate, sodium sulfate, and dialysis have a rapid hypocalcemic effect (within hours) and should be used for life-threatening hypercalcemic emergencies. WR-2721 and protamine are experimental agents that also work within hours of administration. Calcitonin and mithramycin work within 1–3 days of administration while glucocorticoids, prostaglandin inhibitors, gallium nitrate, diphosphonates, and cis-platinum take 4–7 days to elicit a hypocalcemic effect.

MAGNESIUM

Magnesium is the second most common intracellular cation, next to potassium. It is essential for the activity of many metabolic pathways and is vital to a number of enzyme systems. It is required for the activity of phosphatases, which are essential for splitting high-energy ATP bonds and providing energy for the sodium-potassium ATPase pump, proton pump, calcium ATPase pump, neurochemical transmission, muscle contraction, glucose-fat-protein metabolism, oxidative phosphorylation, and DNA synthesis (104). Mg^{2+} is also required for the activity of adenylate cyclase.

The total body content of Mg^{2+} in the average adult is 2000 mEq, about 50–60% of which is in the skeleton and 20% in muscle (104). Less than 1% of total body Mg^{2+} is found in the serum, and thus, serum levels may not accurately reflect intracellular stores (79). The total serum Mg^{2+} concentration ranges from 1.7 to 2.4 mg/dl (1.4–2.0 mEq/liter) in normal adults and is composed of three fractions: a protein-bound fraction (30%), a chelated fraction (15%), and an ionized fraction (55%). It is the ionized fraction that is physiologically active and homeostatically regulated. Although no reliable method is clinically available for the measurement of ionized Mg^{2+} concentrations, a simple filter method is available for measuring ultrafilterable (ionized plus chelated) levels (142). Ultrafilterable levels adjust the Mg^{2+} concentration for variations in serum protein levels.

The normal dietary intake of Mg^{2+} is approximately 25–30 mEq/day (0.3–0.4 mEq/kg/day), which is close to the amount required to maintain Mg^{2+} balance (16). Mg^{2+} is ubiquitous in foods, and dietary Mg^{2+} deficiency is rare unless food intake is severely limited. Mg^{2+} is absorbed in the small intestine and excreted in the urine and stool (104). Normally 30–40% of dietary Mg^{2+} is absorbed; however, this amount may increase during deficiency states. Gut Mg^{2+} absorption occurs by both a vitamin D dependent and independent mechanism. Mg^{2+} homeostasis is primarily regulated in the kidney by tubular reabsorption (35, 88, 104, 111, 123). The kidneys possess a remarkable ability to conserve Mg^{2+} and can decrease excreted Mg^{2+} to less than 1–2 mEq/day in deficiency states. Failure of the kidneys to conserve Mg^{2+} during hypomagnesemia suggests that the cause is renal Mg^{2+} wasting. Mg^{2+} reabsorption in the renal tubule is enhanced by PTH, vitamin D, extracellular fluid depletion, Mg^{2+} depletion, hypothyroidism, and hypocalcemia (104). Renal Mg^{2+} excretion is increased by extracellular fluid expansion, hypermagnesemia, hypercalcemia, loop and osmotic diuretics, PO_4 depletion, metabolic acidosis, and protein and alcohol intake (104). However, the majority of reabsorption is independent of hormonal influences. Urinary Mg^{2+} reabsorption is linked to reabsorption of Ca^{2+} and sodium and renal loss of either of these electrolytes causes Mg^{2+} loss. A tubular maximum (Tm) for Mg^{2+} reabsorption occurs at serum concentrations of 1.5–2.0 mg/dl. This Tm is close to the normal serum Mg^{2+} concentration and small changes in the serum level rapidly alter renal Mg^{2+} excretion. Thus, in Mg^{2+} overload, the kidneys can rapidly excrete excess Mg^{2+}. During correction of Mg^{2+} deficiency, despite cellular Mg^{2+} depletion, much of the administered Mg^{2+} is lost in the urine and repletion usually takes 5–7 days (e.g., to replete intracellular stores). With a normal functioning kidney, obligate loses of Mg^{2+} in stool, sweat, urine, and secretions amount to about 0.3 mEq/kg/day.

Although PTH and vitamin D can increase renal and gastrointestinal absorption of Mg^{2+}, this ion also has potent effects upon the parathyroid glands (7, 26, 30, 79, 110, 138). Hypermagnesemia and severe hypomagnesemia decrease PTH secretion, whereas mild hypomagnesemia stimulates secretion. Hypomag-

nesemia may also impair end-organ response to PTH (79, 110).

Hypomagnesemia

CAUSES

Hypomagnesemia usually occurs when Mg^{2+} losses exceed dietary intake and usually results from a defect in renal Mg^{2+} conservation or excessive stool losses (Table 32.9). Since there is an obligate daily Mg^{2+} loss, severe malnutrition or inadequate supplementation in parenteral nutrition or intravenously administered fluids may also cause hypomagnesemia. Hypomagnesemia may also develop when Mg^{2+} requirements are increased but intake remains constant (e.g., in pregnancy). Decreased gut absorption of Mg^{2+} and/or excessive stool losses may occur in a variety of diseases (e.g., inflammatory bowel disease, gastroenteritis, pancreatic insufficiency, fistulas, short bowel syndromes, ileal bypass, intestinal resection, and cholestatic liver disease). Hypomagnesemia results from a combination of reduced mucosal surface area, increased intestinal secretion, and formation of insoluble Mg^{2+} soaps in the stool due to complexing with unabsorbed fat. Secretions from the lower gastrointestinal tract are richer in Mg^{2+} (10–14 mEq/liter) than secretions from the upper tract (1–2 mEq/liter).

Acute hypomagnesemia can result from internal redistribution of Mg^{2+}. Mg^{2+} shifts into cells following the administration of glucose or amino acids (13, 16). This shift is more pronounced when intracellular Mg^{2+} depletion is coupled to an anabolic state, as may occur with refeeding after starvation or protein-calorie malnutrition, with administration of parenteral nutrition to depleted patients, and with insulin treatment of hyperglycemic disorders. Increased catecholamines from endogenous or exogenous sources, correction of acidosis, and hungry bone syndromes may also lower the serum Mg^{2+} levels by shifting Mg^{2+} into cells.

A large number of diseases may disrupt renal conservation of Mg^{2+} and result in hypomagnesemia. However, when advanced renal disease develops, hypermagnesemia usually occurs. Medications that alter renal Mg^{2+} conservation (Table 32.9) include the diuretics, aminoglycoside antibiotics, amphotericin B, cisplatinum, cardiac glycosides, calcium,

Table 32.9
Causes of Hypomagnesemia

Gastrointestinal Losses
  Reduced absorption
    Malabsorption
    Laxative abuse
    Fistulas
    Prolonged NG suction
  Reduced Intake
    Malnutrition
    Hyperalimentation
    Prolonged i.v. therapy
Drug-Induced Losses
  Diuretics
    Furosemide
    Thiazides
    Mannitol
    Glucose
    Urea
  Aminoglycosides
  Amphotericin B
  Cis-platinum
  Carbenicillin
  Thyroid hormone
  Digoxin
  Calcium
  Ethanol
  Insulin[a]
  Saline
  Citrate (blood)
  Catecholamines[a]
Renal Losses
  Renal disease
    Glomerulonephritis
    Tubular disorders
    Interstitial nephritis
    Diuretic phase of ATN
  Hypercalcemia
  Hyperaldosteronism
  Hyperthyroidism
  PO_4 deficiency
  Diabetic ketoacidosis
  SIADH
Miscellaneous Losses
  Lactation
  Pregnancy
  Severe sweating
  Hungry bone syndrome[a]
  Burns
  Sepsis
  Hypothermia
  Cardiopulmonary bypass
  Administration of glucose, amino acids, and insulin[a]
  Mg^{2+} free dialysis
  Refeeding after starvation[a]

[a]Redistribution of Mg^{2+}.

and saline (79). Aminoglycosides cause hypomagnesemia in 38% of patients receiving a standard intravenous course (138). Cardiac glycosides may cause hypomagnesemia by blocking the action of the sodium-potassium ATPase pump in the renal tubule. This effect is important in view of the fact that hypomagnesemia may also potentiate digitalis toxicity. Thyroid hormone excess causes loss of Mg^{2+} in the urine because of increases in glomerular filtration and may also shift Mg^{2+} intracellularly. Citrate (found in blood products) can lower the serum ionized Mg^{2+} concentration by chelation.

Hypomagnesemia is frequently encountered in patients admitted to the hospital for ethanol withdrawal. Although acute ethanol intake results in increased renal Mg^{2+} excretion, chronic ethanol exposure has no lasting effect. Hypomagnesemia in alcoholic patients results primarily from poor dietary intake, ketosis, emesis, diarrhea, and hyperaldosteronism. Many alcoholic patients have a normal serum Mg^{2+} level on admission, which decreases during hospitalization because of metabolic changes induced during hospitalization (e.g., insulin secretion induced by dextrose infusion and anabolism). These patients may benefit from careful monitoring of the serum Mg^{2+} concentration. Despite the occurrence of hypomagnesemia in many patients with delirium tremens, there are no convincing data to suggest a cause-and-effect relationship. Mg^{2+} supplementation has not been shown to prevent delirium tremens.

CLINICAL MANIFESTATIONS

Signs and symptoms of Mg^{2+} deficiency (Table 32.10), like hypocalcemia, relate to increased neuronal irritability and tetany. Symptoms are rare when the total serum Mg^{2+} concentration is above 1.5 mg/dl and most symptomatic patients have levels below 1.0 mg/dl. Most symptomatic patients with hypomagnesemia have concomitant hypocalcemia or hypokalemia, and it is unclear whether hypomagnesemia alone causes symptoms (70). Hypomagnesemic patients may complain of muscle spasms, paresthesias, and weakness. Correction of hypomagnesemia can improve respiratory muscle strength (94). Central nervous system effects range from coma, disorientation, apathy, and depression to irritability and seizures.

Cardiovascular consequences of Mg^{2+} depletion may include heart failure, coronary artery spasm, arrhythmias, and hypotension (13, 21, 63). Hypomagnesemia increases cardiac sensitivity to the effects of digitalis and pressor agents (16) and can lead to toxicity at

Table 32.10
Clinical Manifestations of Hypomagnesemia

Cardiovascular
 Heart failure
 Arrhythmias
 Coronary artery spasm
 Vasospasm
 Hypertension
 Digitalis sensitivity
 Decreased pressor response
 ECG: Prolonged PR and QT interval, ST
  depression, Tall peaked T-waves (early),
  Broadening and decreased amplitude of T
  waves (late), wide QRS (late)
Gastrointestinal
 Dysphagia
 Anorexia
 Nausea
 Abdominal cramps
Neuromuscular
 Tetany
 Muscle spasm, tremor
 Seizures
 Confusion, disorientation
 Obtundation, coma
 Ataxia, nystagmus
 Apathy
 Depression
 Paresthesias
 Irritability
 Weakness
 Psychosis
Miscellaneous
 Hypokalemia
 Hypocalcemia
 Hypophosphatemia

lower serum digitalis levels (10). This effect may result from the synergistic effects of magnesium and digitalis on the cardiac sodium-potassium pump. Mg^{2+} deficiency is thought to lead to increased vascular tone and reactivity by modulating uptake, content, and distribution of Ca^{2+} in the smooth muscle cell (13). Hypomagnesemia may contribute to vasospasm and hypertension. Standard antiarrhythmic therapy and defibrillation may be ineffective in controlling ventricular arrhythmias associated with Mg^{2+} deficiency (63).

Hypomagnesemia may cause hypokalemia and intracellular potassium depletion. Repletion of intracellular and extracellular potassium may be impaired unless concurrent Mg^{2+} deficits are simultaneously treated (13, 16, 127, 128). Hypomagnesemic hypokalemia results from impaired renal potassium conservation due to diminished activation of the sodium-potassium adenosine triphosphatase pump and altered cell membrane permeability to potassium (126, 138). Hypomagnesemia-induced hypocalcemia results from impaired PTH se-

cretion, end-organ resistance to PTH, and vitamin D resistance (7, 92, 93, 110). Impaired Mg^{2+} dependent adenyl cyclase generation of cyclic AMP may be responsible for some of these effects (13). These patients present with clinical features of hypocalcemia (Table 32.2). Hypocalcemia may be difficult to correct until Mg^{2+} is replaced.

EVALUATION

Hypomagnesemia is usually diagnosed when the serum Mg^{2+} level is below normal limits. However, since Mg^{2+} is 30% protein bound, low total serum levels may occur in patients with hypoalbuminemia despite the occurrence of normal ionized concentrations (142). There is an easy method for normalizing serum Mg^{2+} for alterations in serum protein values through the use of protein retaining filters (142). Mg^{2+} is primarily an intracellular ion, and circulating levels may not always reflect the status of the intracellular environment. However, most patients with chronic hypomagnesemia have Mg^{2+} depletion (16). At present, we remain dependent upon the serum level, until new methods become available for assessing intracellular Mg^{2+} activity.

Measurement of urine Mg^{2+} excretion (24-hour urine measurement) is helpful in separating renal from nonrenal causes of hypomagnesemia. Normal kidneys are capable of decreasing Mg^{2+} excretion to 1–2 mEq/day in deficiency states. High urinary Mg^{2+} excretion (>3 mEq/day) in the presence of a low-serum Mg^{2+} level suggests increased renal loss of Mg^{2+} as the mechanism for Mg^{2+} depletion. Low urinary Mg^{2+} excretion (<1–2 mEq/day) in the presence of hypomagnesemia suggests renal conservation of Mg^{2+} and a Mg^{2+} deficient state because of decreased intake, redistribution, or nonrenal losses. If Mg^{2+} depletion is suspected in patients with a normal serum Mg^{2+} concentration and low Mg^{2+} excretion (e.g., intact renal Mg^{2+} conservation), a Mg^{2+} load test can be helpful. After a baseline 24-hour urine collection, 30 mmol of Mg^{2+} sulfate is administered in 500 ml of 5% dextrose in water over 12 hours; urine is collected for 24 hours from the beginning of the infusion. Individuals with normal Mg^{2+} scores excrete more than 60–80% of the administered load within 24 hours, whereas Mg^{2+} deficient patients excrete less than 50% (13, 14, 16). Decreased fractional Mg^{2+} excretion occurs in Mg^{2+} deficiency as a result of enhanced reabsorption of Mg^{2+} in the renal tubules because of resetting of Mg^{2+} transport (104). This test should be used with caution in patients with renal insufficiency, disturbances in cardiac conduction, or advanced respiratory insufficiency. Careful review of the clinical situation and medications usually reveals the cause.

TREATMENT

Mg^{2+} deficiency is treated by the administration of Mg^{2+} supplements (Table 32.11). Mild deficiency may be treated with diet alone. Mg^{2+} requirements range from 0.3 to 0.4 mEq/kg/day orally or 12–30 mEq/day during parenteral nutrition. These requirements assume no unusual losses and must be augmented accordingly. For maintenance intravenous therapy or parenteral nutrition, we give the sulfate salt so as to provide needed sulfate ions as well (27). Overt or severe hypomagnesemia ($Mg^{2+} < 1$ mg/dl) should be treated with intravenous Mg^{2+} (35, 44, 56, 79, 111). We recommend giving an initial dose of 600 mg of elemental Mg^{2+} over 3 hours followed by a maintenance dose of 600–900 mg of elemental Mg^{2+} per 24 hours. In emergency situations the loading dose of Mg^{2+} should not exceed 15 mg/minute, and the patient should receive continuous ECG monitoring to avoid cardiac toxicity (see "Hypermagnesemia"). Replacement therapy should be carried out over 5–7 days to allow time for intracellular stores to be replenished. Mg^{2+} sulfate may be given intravenously, however, it is painful. During therapy, patients require monitoring of the serum Mg^{2+} level, neurologic status, respiratory status, renal function, ECG, and blood pressure. Patellar reflexes should be monitored at the bedside during Mg^{2+} repletion, and therapy stopped if the reflexes become suppressed. If the patient is hypocalcemic, we prefer to use the chloride salt, since the sulfate salt can chelate with Ca^{2+} and further lower its level. If the patient has renal insufficiency, replacement should be closely guided by the serum Mg^{2+} level so as to avoid toxicity. Hypocalcemia may occur during therapy if the patient develops hypermagnesemia.

Once the patient is stable, Mg^{2+} can be replaced by the oral route (Table 32.11). Mg^{2+} oxide is the preferred Mg^{2+} preparation. Mg^{2+}-containing antacids are poorly absorbed and should not be used to replace Mg^{2+} unless other preparations are not available.

Magnesium and the Heart

Intractable ventricular arrhythmias associated with hypomagnesemia may respond to Mg^{2+} therapy (16, 42, 63, 82). Mg^{2+} therapy has also been useful in suppressing ventricular tachycardia and fibrillation in patients with ischemic heart disease who have normal serum Mg^{2+} levels (2, 62). Abraham et al. (2) treated a group of patients with acute myocardial infarction with Mg^{2+} sulfate (2.4 g administered intravenously over 20 minutes daily for 3 days). Potentially lethal arrhythmias were reduced from 34.8% to 14.6%, when compared with placebo. We have used Mg^{2+} sulfate (1 g administered intravenously over 20 minutes every 6 hours) effectively in the ICU to treat refractory ventricular tachycardias and ventricular fibrillation. Mg^{2+} depletion interferes with the sodium-potassium ATPase and causes ionic imbalance and electrical instability. Mg^{2+} administration prolongs the effective refractory period, depresses conduction, increases the membrane potential (makes it more negative), and can control ventricular tachyarrhythmias. Thus, when ventricular fibrillation or malignant ventricular arrhythmias cannot be controlled with conventional antiarrhythmic drugs,

Table 32.11
Magnesium Supplements[a]

Parenteral	

Mg^{2+} Chloride
    1 g = 118 mg Mg^{2+} = 9 mEq
	Loading: 600 mg elemental Mg^{2+} in D5W over
	    3 hours
	Maintenance: 600–900 mg Mg^{2+} per day

Mg^{2+} Sulfate
    1 g = 98 mg Mg^{2+} = 8 mEq
	Same as for Mg^{2+} Chloride
	(intramuscularly: 200 mg every 4 hours for 24 hours
	    then 100 mg every 4 hours)

Enteral	
Mg^{2+} Oxide tablets tablet = 111 mg Mg^{2+} = 9 mEq	20–80 mEq/day in divided doses
Mg^{2+} Gluconate tablets 500 mg tablet = 32 mg Mg^{2+} = 2.4 mEq	20–80 mEq/day in divided doses

[a] 1 mEq = 0.5 mmol = 12.3 mg Mg^{2+}

we recommend infusing Mg^{2+}. Iseri et al. (62) give 16 mEq slowly over 1 minute followed by 80 mEq over the next 5 hours. Potassium chloride at 10 mEq/hour is also infused since there is evidence that Mg^{2+} and potassium depletion frequently occur together. It may be necessary to continue a maintenance infusion of Mg^{2+} to prevent recurrence of arrhythmias. We usually aim for a serum Mg^{2+} concentration of 3–4 mg/dl.

Intravenous administration of Mg^{2+} (50 mmol $MgCl_2$ in 1000 ml isotonic dextrose at 100 ml/hour for 6 hours followed by 22 ml/hour for 18 hours) has been reported to reduce both mortality and arrhythmias (106) when given to patients with acute myocardial infarction. Placebo (n = 74) and Mg^{2+} treated (n = 56) patients had similar admission serum Mg^{2+} levels. However, 4 weeks after myocardial infarction the patients given Mg^{2+} had a lower mortality (7% versus 19%). The proportion of patients requiring treatment for arrhythmias was also lower (21% versus 47%). In another study, Rasmussen et al. (105) found that patients with acute myocardial infarctions dropped their serum Mg^{2+} concentrations over the first 32 hours after infarction. The drop appeared to result from an extracellular to intracellular shift in Mg^{2+}. Kafka et al. (67) noted a 6% incidence of hypomagnesemia in patients with acute myocardial infarction, whereas Dyckner (41) reported a 46% incidence. Hypomagnesemia was associated with a higher frequency of major ventricular arrhythmias. Kafka et al. (67) also found a 17% incidence of hypokalemia in their patients with myocardial infarction. Ventricular arrhythmias occurred in all patients with both hypokalemia and hypomagnesemia.

Whang and colleagues (129) found a 19% incidence of hypomagnesemia and 9% incidence of hypokalemia in patients receiving digitalis. Hypomagnesemia and hypokalemia are important since both predispose to digitalis toxicity (13, 63, 114). Mg^{2+} deficiency may also enhance digoxin uptake by myocardial cells (51). Iseri et al. (63) reported the efficacy of intravenously administered Mg^{2+} in treating hypomagnesemic patients with toxic reactions to digitalis and recurrent ventricular tachycardia. Mg^{2+} responsive ventricular arrhythmias may also occur in normomagnesemic patients receiving digitalis (32, 62). A decrease in serum Mg^{2+} after cardiopulmonary bypass surgery has been reported (21). Suppression of cardiac arrhythmias after heart surgery may be assisted by Mg^{2+} therapy.

Magnesium and Bronchospasm

Relief of dyspnea and stridor after Mg^{2+} infusion has been observed on occasion. The Mg^{2+} ion has an inhibitory action on smooth muscle contraction, histamine release from mast cells, and on acetylcholine release from cholinergic nerve terminals (6, 101). Okayama et al. (101) studied the bronchodilating effect of Mg^{2+} sulfate infusion (0.5 mmol/minute for 20 minutes) in 10 patients with mild asthma. Serum Mg^{2+} concentration rose from 2.1 mg/dl (0.86 mmol/l) to 5.1 mg/dl (2.08 mmol/l) with this dose. Mg^{2+} infusion decreased respiratory resistance by 30%, improved forced vital capacity by 17%, and improved forced expiratory volume at 1 second by 18%. There were no adverse effects on blood pressure or heart rate. The magnitude of these effects were similar to those found with albuterol inhalation. These authors also administered Mg^{2+} to three patients with severe asthma who were treated with dexamethasone, aminophylline, and inhaled albuterol. They noted an improvement in wheezing, dyspnea, and sputum expectoration. More studies (prospective, blinded, and randomized) are needed before this therapy can be recommended, but Mg^{2+} infusion may provide yet another new drug for the treatment of reactive airway disease. Extreme caution must be used since hypermagnesemia can depress neuromuscular and cardiovascular function.

Hypermagnesemia

Spontaneous hypermagnesemia is rare in clinical practice and most cases result from iatrogenic causes (27, 30, 79, 96, 111). The most common etiology of hypermagnesemia is the administration of Mg^{2+} containing antacids, enemas, or parenteral nutrition to patients with renal insufficiency. Other causes of hypermagnesemia include hypothyroidism, Addison's disease, lithium intoxication, familial hypocalciuric hypercalcemia, and the administration of Mg^{2+} to patients with premature labor or preeclampsia/eclampsia. Hypermagnesemia may also occur in infants born to mothers who received Mg^{2+} for these problems.

Hypermagnesemia diminishes neuromuscular transmission and can depress skeletal muscle function and cause neuromuscular blockade (Table 32.12). Mg^{2+} excess inhibits prejunctional release of acetylcholine and de-

Table 32.12
Clinical Manifestations of Hypomagnesemia

	Serum Mg^{2+} Level (mg/dl)
Normal level	1.7–2.4
Decrease in DTR	4–5
ECG Changes	
e.g., prolonged PR, QRS, ST	4–6
Bradycardia	4–7
Hypotension	5–7
Somnolence	6–8
Respiratory insufficiency	10–12
Heart block	15
Respiratory paralysis	18
Cardiac arrest	15–24

creases motor end plate sensitivity to acetylcholine (104). Excess Mg^{2+} may also cause vasodilation and hypotension. Hypermagnesemia increases neuromuscular sensitivity to the effects of skeletal muscle relaxants and can result in more prolonged and potent effects of these drugs. Hypocalcemia may result from hypermagnesemia-induced parathyroid gland suppression (30).

The neuromuscular and cardiac toxicity of hypermagnesemia can be transiently antagonized by the administration of intravenous Ca^{2+} (5–10 mEq). Definitive therapy to lower the serum Mg^{2+} level consists of stopping all drugs and supplements containing Mg^{2+} and administering saline and furosemide to enhance renal excretion. In patients with renal failure, Mg^{2+} may be removed by dialysis.

PHOSPHORUS

The adult body contains about 700–800 g of PO_4. PO_4 is the major intracellular anion and is essential for a large variety of biochemical processes. It is required in protein, fat, and carbohydrate metabolism and is the source of high-energy bonds in adenosine triphosphate and phosphocreatine. PO_4 high energy bonds provide the energy for maintenance of cellular integrity, muscle contraction, neurologic function, hormonal secretion, and cell division. PO_4 is also a component of 2,3-diphosphoglycerate, which functions as a regulator of oxygen release from hemoglobin. PO_4 is a component of cyclic nucleotides, nicotinamide diphosphate, phospholipids, nucleic acids, and participates in the urinary buffering of acids.

The normal serum PO_4 level is 4.0–7.1 mg/dl in children and 2.7–4.5 mg/dl in adults (29). The average dietary intake of PO_4 ranges from 800–1200 mg/day, with most being absorbed in the small intestine by both passive (50%) and active (vitamin D dependent) transport. Thus, even in vitamin D deficient states the gut is able to absorb enough PO_4 to maintain normal serum levels. PO_4 is excreted in the urine and stool. PO_4 is primarily regulated by the kidneys, with most PO_4 reabsorption occurring in the proximal tubules. Tubular reabsorption increases to a maximum (TmP), with further increases in PO_4 being excreted in the urine. This system is analogous to that which is seen with glucose. The set point for the TmP determines one's fasting serum PO_4 level and is affected by a large number of drugs. It is reduced by aminohippurate sodium, amino acids, dextrose, acetoacetate, sodium bicarbonate, saline, acute hypercapnia, thyroid hormone, estrogen, digoxin, long-term corticosteroids, and renal vasodilation (29, 87). Infusion of dextrose in amounts sufficient to cause glycosuria decrease tubular reabsorption of PO_4 by 20% and both may share a common reabsorptive pathway (87). Extracellular volume expansion is associated with decreases in the proximal tubular reabsorption of both PO_4 and sodium (87), resulting in phosphaturia. Growth hormone increases the TmP and thus decreases the amount of PO_4 excreted in the urine. Higher growth hormone levels in children may explain their higher serum PO_4 concentrations.

The amount of PO_4 in excreted urine also depends upon PTH and its effects upon tubular PO_4 reabsorption. PTH produces phosphaturia by decreasing TmP via the adenyl cyclase system. This phosphaturic effect is important in Ca^{2+} homeostasis. PTH increases bone resorption and releases Ca^{2+} and PO_4. Hyperphosphatemia is avoided by the renal action of PTH. Acute hypercalcemia and hypermagnesemia decrease the renal excretion of PO_4 by inhibiting PTH secretion, whereas hypocalcemia and hypomagnesemia do the reverse. PO_4 has no direct effect upon the parathyoid glands, but rather affects PTH secretion through its affects upon the ionized Ca^{2+} level.

PO_4 affects the 1-hydroxylation of 25-hydroxyvitamin D within the kidney and this effect is independent of PTH. Hypophosphatemia stimulates the 1-hydroxylase, whereas hyperphosphatemia inhibits it. 1,25-Dihydroxyvitamin D can stimulate PO_4 mobilization from bone and enhance absorption from the intestine. It plays a minor role in regulating renal PO_4 reabsorption.

Insulin causes glucose and PO_4 to move into

cells and is responsible for hypophosphatemia seen during insulin administration or high carbohydrate feedings. PO_4 is trapped in the cell when glucose is converted to glucose-6-phosphate.

Hypophosphatemia

CAUSES

Hypophosphatemia results from three primary mechanisms (Table 32.13): intracellular shift of PO_4, increased loss of PO_4 through the kidneys, and decreased gastrointestinal absorption of PO_4.

Carbohydrate loading (e.g., intravenous dextrose solutions and pareneteral nutrition) causes hypophosphatemia by shifting PO_4 into the cell and accounts for about half of the cases of hypophosphatemia seen in hospitalized patients. PO_4 is trapped in the cell when glucose is converted to glucose-6-phosphate (29, 72). Inadequate PO_4 in parenteral nutrition or rapid refeeding of severely starved patients elicits a similar response. Acute respiratory and metabolic alkalosis stimulates intracellular glycolysis, consuming PO_4 in the process (15). Sepsis, central nervous system disorders, and salicylate poisoning cause hyperventilation and respiratory alkalosis. Salicylate poisoning may also stimulate glycolysis directly. Treatment of hypothermia causes a shift of PO_4 into the cell and may also cause hypophosphatemia (81). Hypophosphatemia is common after severe burns and results from a combination of increased metabolism, respiratory alkalosis, sepsis, inappropriate phosphaturia, excess catecholamine and cortisol secretion, and hyperalimentation.

Epinephrine and glucagon, like insulin, can also cause a reduction in the circulating PO_4 level, presumably by stimulating the cellular utilization of glucose and accelerating the formation of intracellular PO_4 esters. The intravenous infusion of epinephrine at a rate of 10 $\mu g/min$ for 10 minutes, results in a 25% fall in the serum PO_4 concentration (86).

Hypomagnesemia augments renal PO_4 excretion; however, hypomagnesemia alone rarely causes hypophosphatemia since it also suppresses parathyroid hormone secretion, causing hypocalcemia and a reduction in PO_4 excretion. The two effects balance out. However, hypophosphatemia may occur in these patients when magnesium is replaced without PO_4, resulting in a surge in parathyroid hormone release and augmented phosphaturia.

Table 32.13
Causes of Hypophosphatemia

Transcellular Shift
 Recovery from malnutrition[a]
 Carbohydrate loading[a]
 Recovery from hypothermia[a]
 Recovery from burns[a]
 Acute alkalosis[a]
 Alcoholism[a]
 Diabetic ketoacidosis[a]
 Sepsis
 Salicylate poisoning
 Hungry bone syndrome
 Anabolic steroids
Gastrointestinal Losses
 Malabsorption
 Emesis
 Diarrhea
 Prolonged NG suction
 PO_4 binding resins
 Vitamin D deficiency
Drug-Induced
 Anabolic steroids
 Antacids[a]
 Calcitonin
 Corticosteroids
 Diuretics
 Epinephrine
 Glucagon
 Insulin[a]
 Sodium bicarbonate
 Saline diuresis
 Salicylates
Renal Losses
 Renal tubular defects e.g., myeloma, heavy metals, RTA, Fanconi syndrome
 Hyperparathyroidism
 Hypomagnesemia
 Hypokalemia
 Acidosis
 Pregnancy
 Vitamin D deficiency or resistance
 Reye's syndrome
 Recovery from ATN
 After renal transplant
 Diuresis
 Oncogenic hypophosphatemia
Miscellaneous
 Hemodialysis
 Inadequate PO_4 in i.v. fluids

[a]Most common causes of severe hypophosphatemia (PO_4 <1 mg/dl).

Diuretic therapy, renal tubular defects (e.g., from myeloma or heavy metals), primary and secondary hyperparathyroidism, vitamin D deficiency, and acidemia are other causes of renal PO_4 wasting and hypophosphatemia. Vitamin D deficiency causes hypophosphatemia via its effects on increasing PTH secretion (induced by hypocalcemia) and reduced intestinal PO_4 absorption. Posttransplantation hypophosphatemia develops in over 50% of patients with a transplanted kidney and results from a combination of renal phosphaturia, persistent hyperparathyroidism, glucocorticoid therapy, 1,25-dihydroxyvitamin D deficiency, and use of antacids (15). Hypophosphatemia has also been associated with a variety of tumors (15). These tumors appear to elaborate substance that interfere with renal PO_4 reabsorption, bone mineralization, and renal 1,25-dihydroxyvitamin D synthesis.

Inadequate PO_4 intake alone rarely causes hypophosphatemia. However, hypophosphatemia may occur in patients on a marginally adequate PO_4 intake when another cause for hypophosphatemia occurs (Table 32.13). A frequently seen clinical situation is that of a chronically ill patient admitted to the hospital and placed on intravenous dextrose solutions (containing little PO_4) or given nonabsorbable PO_4 binding antacids. PO_4 binding antacids, such as aluminum or magnesium hydroxide, are common causes of hypophosphatemia. These antacids bind PO_4 that is found in enteral nutrition as well as PO_4 that is secreted into the gut. Thus, they produce hypophosphatemia even in patients who are not fed enterally. Malabsorption states, such as is seen with pancreatic disease or diarrhea, may also cause hypophosphatemia by impairing PO_4 absorption and increasing gut losses.

Hypophosphatemia is commonly seen during the treatment of diabetic ketoacidosis and hyperglycemic hyperosmolar nonketotic syndromes. Serum PO_4 levels are usually normal at the time the patient is admitted, despite total body depletion of PO_4 (73, 74). After the initiation of insulin therapy, PO_4 shifts into the cells along with glucose and potassium. Plasma levels may decrease to less than 1 mg/dl within 24 hours of initiation of therapy (73, 107). PO_4 deficiency is associated with insulin resistance, decreased levels of 2,3-DPG, and decreased intracellular ATP. Low 2,3-DPG shifts the hemoglobin dissociation curve to the left, decreasing oxygen off-loading to the tissues. This alteration in the oxyhemoglobin dissociation curve may be important clinically in some patients, since elevated levels of glycosylated hemoglobin (found in diabetics) also impairs oxygen off-loading. As acidosis is corrected during the treatment of ketoacidosis, the ability of hemoglobin to release oxygen is even further decreased. PO_4 supplementation can more quickly restore 2,3-DPG levels and intracellular ATP concentrations to normal. Although deleterious effects of hypophosphatemia on the clinical course of diabetic ketoacidosis have not been conclusively shown (69, 130), we have seen a number of patients develop complications believed to be secondary to hypophosphatemia (e.g., seizures and respiratory failure). In addition, if one looks

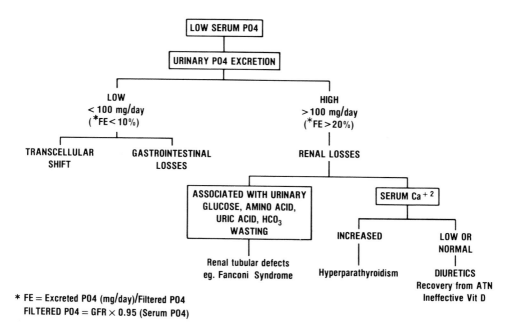

Figure 32.4   Evaluation of hypophosphatemia.

at all patients with hypophosphatemia, diabetic ketoacidosis is a common cause. For the above reasons, we recommend administering PO_4 for the treatment of hyperglycemic states, provided that hyperphosphatemia can be avoided (see Chapter 33).

Hypophosphatemia is common in alcoholics admitted to the hospital (15, 112). These patients are frequently malnourished and suffer from malabsorption processes. When admitted to the hospital, they are given intravenous or oral carbohydrate loads that shift PO_4 into the cells. Respiratory alkalosis may develop, especially during withdrawal, and further exacerbate hypophosphatemia. Hypomagnesemia, hypokalemia, alcohol, and acidosis may lead to impaired renal conservation of PO_4.

Hypophosphatemia (PO_4 <2.4 mg/dl) occurs in approximately 29% of surgical patients (119). Hypophosphatemia develops 24 hours after surgery and results from glucose infusions, increased tissue metabolism, increased catecholamine secretion, and renal PO_4 losses (15, 59, 119). It is not known whether routine PO_4 supplementation in these patients would improve outcome.

The cause of hypophosphatemia can usually be determined from the medical history and clinical setting. When in doubt, measurement of urinary PO_4 excretion may be helpful (Fig. 32.4). Transcelluar shifts of PO_4 and gastrointestinal loss of PO_4 evoke avid renal PO_4 reabsorption, decreasing the fractional excretion of PO_4 in the urine to less than 10%. Renal causes of hypophosphatemia result in PO_4 wasting in the urine and a fractional excretion of PO_4 greater than 20%.

Table 32.14
Clinical Features of Hypophosphatemia

General
  Weakness
  Malaise
Myocardial Insufficiency
Impaired Pressor Responses
Respiratory Insufficiency
Rhabdomyolysis
Hepatocellular Damage
Hematologic
  Hemolysis
  Platelet dysfunction
  Leukocyte dysfunction
Skeletal
  Osteomalacia
  Fractures
  Increased bone resorption
Metabolic
  Impaired glucose tolerance
  Impaired gluconeogenesis
  Impaired phospholipid synthesis
  Hypercalciuria
  Hypermagnesemia
Neurological
  Ataxia
  Confusion
  Obtundation
  Coma
  Delirium
  Dysarthria
  Encephalopathy
  Muscle weakness
  Irritability
  Myopathy
  Paresthesias
  Seizures
  Tremor
Gastrointestinal
  Anorexia
  Nausea
  Vomiting

CLINICAL MANIFESTATIONS

Severe hypophosphatemia is associated with decreased levels of PO_4 containing metabolites (e.g., ATP, 2,3DPG) and membrane phospholipids and may cause a variety of clinical problems (Table 32.14). Patients may develop cardiac insufficiency (15, 37, 46, 100). The cause for cardiac insufficiency is uncertain but may relate to depleted intracellular PO_4 stores (e.g., ATP, creatine phosphate), impaired action of the sodium potassium ATPase pump, decreased calcium flux, or impaired catecholamine action (15, 75).

Patients with serum PO_4 levels of less than 2 mg/dl may complain of muscle weakness, anorexia, or tremor. As PO_4 levels approach 1 mg/dl, respiratory weakness or insufficiency may occur (8, 99, 122). Respiratory failure is more likely to occur in patients with underlying lung disease. In addition, hypophosphatemia may decrease muscle strength and impair weaning from ventilators. PO_4 supplementation in these patients may improve muscle strength (8, 122). We have treated a few patients with advanced pulmonary disease whom we could not wean off the ventilator because of respiratory muscle fatigue. After PO_4 supplementation, these patients were weaned from the ventilator. Hypophosphatemia has been reported to produce a large number of neurologic symptoms that include ataxia, tremor, paresthesias, myopathy, seizures, coma, and death.

Muscle cell integrity depends upon PO_4 and severe hypophosphatemia (< 1 mg/dl) may injure the cell and cause rhabdomyolysis. Severe hypophosphatemia may also affect blood cells and cause hemolysis, platelet dysfunction, and leukocyte dysfunction. Hemolytic anemia is rarely seen unless the plasma PO_4 falls below 0.5 mg/dl. Depressed erythrocyte levels of 2,3DPG shift the oxyhemoglobin dissociation curve to the left (reduces P_{50}), decreasing oxygen delivery to the tissues. Depressed leukocyte chemotaxis, phagocytosis, and bactericidal activity may impair recovery from infection. Metabolic consequences of hypophosphatemia include insulin resistance (38), impaired gluconeogenesis, impaired bone mineralization, and liver dysfunction. Hypercalciuria results from release of Ca^{2+} from bone in an attempt to maintain normal serum PO_4 concentrations (15) and decreased renal absorption of Ca^{2+}. Hypermagnesemia also results from increased mobilization of Mg^{2+} from bone and reduced Mg^{2+} reabsorption in the kidney (15).

PO_4 depletion is associated with three major alterations in renal acid-base regulation: proximal tubular bicarbonate wasting, impaired distal acidification, and decreased buffer excretion (diminished renal ammoniagenesis and hypophosphaturia) (15). Acid-base stability is usually well preserved because of the balance of acidifying and alkalinizing forces (e.g., alkali released from bone). However, prolonged and severe PO_4 depletion may exhaust bone stores of alkali and result in a metabolic acidosis.

THERAPY

The potential consequences of severe hypophosphatemia necessitate prompt recognition and treatment so as to avoid potentially devastating consequences. Serious life-threatening consequences usually do not occur until the serum PO_4 concentration falls below 1 mg/dl. Primary therapy should be oriented towards preventing hypophosphatemia. Serum PO_4 levels, like other primarily intracellular ions, may not adequately reflect body stores. Thus, initial therapy is usually empiric and one must monitor the serum level to avoid hyperphosphatemia.

Initially, one should stop all drugs (if possible) that are contributing to hypophosphatemia. The list of drugs must include PO_4-binding antacids, intravenous glucose, and diuretics.

For immediate correction of profound hypophosphatemia (< 1 mg/dl) or symptomatic hypophosphatemia, intravenous therapy (71, 80, 121) is necessary (Table 32.15), since oral PO_4 preparations when given in large amounts usually cause diarrhea. The rate of administration of PO_4 varies in the literature from 0.3 mg/kg/hour to 4 mg/kg/hour (71, 80, 121).

Based upon our experience we recommend the following: If depletion is recent and uncomplicated give 0.6 mg (0.02 mmol)/kg/hour; if prolonged and multifactorial give 0.9 mg (0.03 mmol)/kg/hour. Check the serum PO_4 level every 6–12 hours until the level has stabilized,

Table 32.15
Phosphate Preparations

Preparation	PO_4 Content[a]	Daily Dose
Enteral		
Whole milk	1 mg/ml	1200 ml
Skim milk	0.9 mg/ml	1330 ml
Neutro-Phos[b]	250 mg/capsule	1–2 t.i.d.
Potassium-PO_4 (K-Phos)	125 mg tablet	3–4 t.i.d.
	250 mg tablet	1–2 t.i.d.
Parenteral		
Potassium-PO_4	93 mg/ml	1000 mg/day
	(4 mEq/ml K^+)	
Sodium-PO_4	93 mg/ml	1000 mg/day
	(4 mEq/ml Na^+)	
Neutral Sodium-PO_4	2.8 mg/ml	1000 mg/day
	(0.16 mEq/ml Na^+)	
Neutral Sodium Potassium-PO_4	3.1 mg/ml	1000 mg/day
	(0.16 mEq/ml Na^+; 0.02 mEq/ml K^+)	

[a] 31 mg PO_4 = 1 mmol PO_4
[b] Also available as a solution.

so as to avoid hyperphosphatemia. Hyperkalemia may result from excessive administration of potassium phosphate, especially in patients with impaired renal function. If the patient is also hypocalcemic or hypercalcemic, PO_4 should be administered at a slower rate and both PO_4 and Ca^{2+} monitored. Risks of treatment include hyperphosphatemia, hypocalcemia, hypotension, hyperkalemia (with potassium PO_4), hypomagnesemia, hyperosmolality, metastatic calcification, and renal failure. Extreme caution must be used when administering PO_4 to patients with renal insufficiency or failure, since these patients have a diminished ability to excrete PO_4. Parenteral solutions of PO_4 are hypertonic and should be diluted before use or given by central line. The addition of calcium to PO_4-containing solutions or administration through the same intravenous line may cause precipitation. Parenteral PO_4 may be discontinued and enteral therapy (Table 32.15) started when the serum PO_4 level exceeds 2 mg/dl. Repletion should be carried out over 5–7 days to replace intracellular stores and then the patient placed on a maintenance dose (e.g., 1200 mg/day orally or 1000 mg/day intravenously in the adult). Additional PO_4 may be required if excess losses are present. Hypomagnesemia is common in patients with PO_4 deficiency and should always be measured and replaced as needed (121).

Hyperphosphatemia

CAUSES

Hyperphosphatemia results from three basic mechanisms (Table 32.16): reduced renal excretion, increased entrance of PO_4 into the extracellular space from the intracellular space, and increased PO_4 or vitamin D intake.

Levels of PO_4 remain within normal ranges until the glomerular filtration rate falls below 20–25 ml/minute. Hyperphosphatemia, as well as renal failure, impair the renal conversion of 25-hydroxyvitamin D to 1,25-dihydroxyvitamin D. Impaired synthesis of 1,25-dihydroxyvitamin D contributes to hypocalcemia and secondary hyperparathyroidism. PO_4 rises in patients with acute renal failure and frequently occurs before the rise in blood urea nitrogen or creatinine. Elevated PO_4 levels are also seen in patients with hypoparathyroidism due to the loss of the phosphaturic action of parathyroid hormone. Hyperphosphatemia and

Table 32.16
Causes of Hyperphosphatemia

Reduced Renal Excretion
  Renal insufficiency
  Hypoparathyroidism
  PTH resistance
  Hyperthyroidism
  Acromegaly
  Diphosphonates
  Tumoral calcinosis
Increased PO_4 or Vitamin D Intake
  Ingestion of PO_4 (e.g., laxatives)
  Intravenous PO_4
  PO_4 enemas
  Vitamin D
Increased PO_4 Entrance into Extracellular Fluid
  Acidosis
  Chemotherapy
  Rhabdomyolysis
  Sepsis
  Malignant hyperpyrexia
  Fulminant hepatitis
  Severe hypothermia
  Hemolysis

hypercalcemia occur in hyperthyroidism as a result of increased bone resorption, parathyroid gland suppression, and increased tubular reabsorption of PO_4. Diphosphonates are used to treat patients with Paget's disease of bone and hypercalcemia. These agents cause hyperphosphatemia by reducing PO_4 excretion and altering its distribution between cellular compartments.

Hyperphosphatemia may occur when PO_4 enters the extracellular space after cellular damage induced by chemotherapy (tumor lysis syndrome), rhabdomyolysis, malignant hyperthermia, hypothermia, sepsis, or hepatic necrosis. The hyperphosphatemia is exaggerated when there is concomitant renal insufficiency. Hyperphosphatemia may also occur from overzealous administration of PO_4-containing compounds (25) or from laxative abuse. PO_4 deficiency is common in patients with diabetic ketoacidosis. However, since potassium deficits are usually twice that of PO_4 deficits, potassium should be replaced with a combination of KCl and K_2PO_4 so that hyperphosphatemia is avoided. Serum PO_4 levels may be artificially increased as a result of hemolysis during blood drawing.

Measurement of glomerular filtration and urinary PO_4 excretion are helpful in evaluating the etiology of hyperphosphatemia (Fig. 32.5). A glomerular filtration rate less than 20–25 ml/minute suggests renal failure as the cause. Relatively normal glomerular filtration with a PO_4 excretion greater than 1500 mg/day sug-

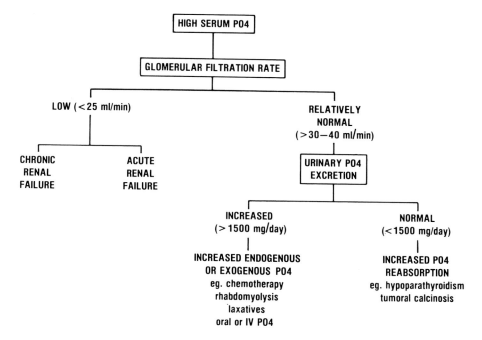

Figure 32.5 Evaluation of hyperphosphatemia.

gests increased PO₄ loading from either endogenous or exogenous sources. Normal renal filtration with a PO₄ excretion less than 1500 mg/day indicates increased PO₄ reabsorption as the cause.

Symptoms of hyperphosphatemia relate primarily to the hypocalcemia that it induces and ectopic calcification. Soft tissue calcification usually occurs when the calcium-phosphate product exceeds 75. In addition, alkalosis favors calcification.

THERAPY

The therapy of hyperphosphatemia is aimed at eliminating the PO₄ source, removing PO₄ from the circulation, and at correcting any associated hypocalcemia. Dietary PO₄ intake should be restricted. PO₄ excretion in the urine can be increased by saline (250–500 ml/hour) and acetazolamide (500 mg every 6 hours) (4). Intestinal PO₄ absorption can be minimized and PO₄ can be removed from the body via the gastrointestinal tract with oral PO₄ binders (e.g., aluminum hydroxide), which are of benefit even if no oral PO₄ is given. If renal insufficiency is not a problem, alternating aluminum hydroxide with magnesium salts can decrease aluminum-induced constipation. If symptomatic hypocalcemia is present the patient

should be given calcium. Hemodialysis or peritoneal dialysis are effective in removing PO₄ in renal failure.

References

1. Abbasi AA, Chemplavil JK, Farah S, et al: Hypercalcemia in active pulmonary tuberculosis. *Ann Intern Med* 90:324–328, 1979.
2. Abraham AS, Rosenmann D, Kramer M, et al: Magnesium in the prevention of lethal arrhythmias in acute myocardial infarction. *Arch Intern Med* 147:753–755, 1987.
3. Aguanno JJ, Ladenson JH: Influence of fatty acids on the binding of calcium to albumin. *J Biol Chem* 257:8745–8748, 1982.
4. Agus ZS, Goldfarb S, Wasserstein A: Disorders of calcium and phosphate balance. In Brenner BM, Rector FC (eds): *The Kidney,* 2nd ed. Philadelphia, WB Saunders 1981, pp 940–1022.
5. Aldinger KA, Samaan NA: Hypokalemia with hypercalcemia. *Ann Intern Med* 85:571–573, 1977.
6. Altura BM, Altura BT, Carella A: Magnesium deficiency induced spasms of umbilical vessels: Relation to preeclampsia, hypertension, growth retardation. *Science* 221:376–378, 1983.
7. Anast CS, Winnacker JL, Forte LR, et al: Impaired release of parathyroid hormone in magnesium deficiency. *J Clin Endocrinol Metal* 42:707–717, 1976.
8. Aubier M, Murciano D, Lecocguic Y, et al: Effect of hypophosphatemia on diaphragmatic contractility in patients with acute respiratory failure. *N Engl J Med* 313:420–424, 1985.
9. Bell NH, Stern PH, Pantzer E, et al: Evidence that increased circulatory 1α, 25-dihydroxyvitamin D is the

probable cause for abnormal calcium metabolism in sarcoidosis. *J Clin Invest* 64:218–225, 1979.

10. Beller GA, Hood WB, Smith TW, Abelmann WH, Wacker WEC: Correlation of serum magnesium levels and digitalis intoxication. *Am J Cardiol* 33:225–229, 1974.

11. Benabe JE, Martinez-Maldonado: Disorders of calcium metabolism. In Maxwell MH, Kleeman CR, Narins RG: *Clinical Disorders of Fluid and Electrolyte Metabolism,* 4th ed. New York, McGraw Hill, 1987, pp 759–788.

12. Benson RC, Riggs BL, Pickard BM, Arnaud DC: Radioimmunoassay of parathyroid hormone in hypercalcemic disease. *Am J Med* 56:821–826, 1974.

13. Berkelhammer C, Bear RA: A clinical approach to common electrolyte problems: hypomagnesemia. *Can Med Assoc J* 132:360–368, 1985.

14. Bohmer T, Mathiesen B: Magnesium deficiency in chronic alcoholic patients uncovered by an intravenous load test. *Scand J Clin Lab Invest* 42:633–636, 1982.

15. Brauthbar N, Kleeman CR: Hypophosphatemia and hyperphosphatemia: clinical and pathophysiologic aspects. In Maxwell MH, Kleeman CR, Narins RG: *Clinical Disorders of Fluid and Electrolyte Metabolism,* 4th ed. New York, McGraw Hill, 1987, pp 789–830.

16. Brautbar N, Massry SG: Hypomagnesemia and hypermagnesemia. In Maxwell MH, Kleeman CR, Narins RG: *Clinical Disorders of Fluid and Electrolyte Metabolism,* 4th ed. New York, McGraw Hill, 1987, pp 831–849.

17. Breslau NA, McGuire JL, Zerwekh JE, et al: Hypercalcemia associated with increased serum calcitriol levels in three patients with lymphoma. *Ann Intern Med* 100:1–7, 1984.

18. Bristow MR, Ginsburg R, Minobe W, et al: Decreased catecholamine sensitivity and beta-adrenergic receptor density in failing human hearts. *N Engl J Med* 307:205–211, 1982.

19. Bristow MR, Schwartz D, Binetti G, Harrison DC, Daniels JR: Ionized calcium and the heart. *Circ Res* 41:565–574, 1977.

20. Buckle R: Ectopic PTH syndrome, pseudohyperparathyroidism, hypercalcemia of malignancy. *J Clin Endocrinol Metab* 3:237–251, 1974.

21. Burch GE, Giles TD: The importance of magnesium deficiency in cardiovascular disease. *Am Heart J* 94:649–657, 1977.

22. Cardella CJ, Birkin BL, Roscoe M, Rapoport A: Role of dialysis in the treatment of severe hypercalcemia: report of two cases successfully treated with hemodialysis and review of the literature. *Clin Nephrol* 12:285–290, 1979.

23. Chaimovitz C, Abinader E, Benderly A, et al: Hypocalcemic hypotension. *J Am Med Assoc* 222:86–87, 1972.

24. Chang J, Abramson EC, Mayer M, et al: The effects of cisplatin on parathyroid hormone and tumor-induced bone resorption. *Clin Res* 33:888A, 1985.

25. Chernow B, Rainey TG, Georges LP, et al: Iatrogenic hyperphosphatemia: a metabolic consideration in critical care medicine. *Crit Care Med* 9:772–774, 1981.

26. Chernow B, Smith J, Rainey TG, et al: Hypomagnesemia: implications for the critical care specialist. *Crit Care Med* 10:193–196, 1982.

27. Chernow B, Zaloga GP: SCCM - ions for society members (sulfate, chloride calcium, magnesium). In *Critical Care - State of the Art.* Fullerton, CA, Society of Critical Care Medicine, 1984, vol 4, pp K1–43.

28. Chernow B, Zaloga GP, Malcolm D, Clapper M, Holaday JW: Glucagon's chronotropic action is calcium dependent. *J Pharmacol Exp Ther* (in press)

29. Chester WL, Zaloga GP, Chernow B: Phosphate metabolism in the critically ill patient. In Geelhoed G, Chernow B (eds): *Endocrine Aspects of Acute Illness: Clin-*

ics in Critical Care Medicine. New York, Churchill Livingstone, 1985, vol 5, pp 205–216.

30. Cholst IN, Steinberg SF, Tropper PJ, et al: The influence of hypermagnesemia on serum calcium and parathyroid hormone levels in human subjects. *N Engl J Med* 310:1221–1225, 1984.

31. Chopra D, Janson P, Sawin CT: Insensitivity to digoxin associated with hypocalcemia. *N Engl J Med* 296:917–918, 1977.

32. Cohen L, Kitzes R: Magnesium sulfate and digitalis-toxic arrhythmias. *JAMA* 249:2808–2810, 1983.

33. Condon JR, Ives D, Knight MJ, Day J: The aetiology of hypocalcemia in acute pancreatitis. *Br J Surg* 62:115–118, 1975.

34. Connor TB, Rosen BL, Bleaustein MP et al: Hypocalcemia precipitating congestive heart failure. *N Engl J Med* 307:869–872, 1982.

35. Cronin RE, Knochel JP: Magnesium deficiency. *Adv Intern Med* 28:509–533, 1983.

36. Cushard WG, Simon AB, Canterbury JM, et al: Parathyroid function in sarcoidosis. *N Engl J Med* 286:395–398, 1972.

37. Darsee JD, Nutter DO: Reversible severe congestive cardiomyopathy in three cases of hypophosphatemia. *Ann Intern Med* 89:867–870, 1978.

38. DeFronzo RA, Lang R: Hypophosphatemia and glucose intolerance. Evidence for tissue insensitivity to insulin. *N Engl J Med* 303:1259, 1980.

39. Denlinger JK, Nahrwold ML, Gibbs PS, et al: Hypocalcemia during rapid blood transfusion in anaesthetized man. *Br J Anaesth* 48:995–999, 1976.

40. Drop LJ: Ionized calcium, the heart and hemodynamic function. *Anesth Analg* 64:432–451, 1985.

41. Dyckner T: Serum magnesium in acute myocardial infarction. Relation to arrhythmias. *Acta Med Scand* 207:59–66, 1980.

42. Dycker T, Weater PO: Relation between potassium, magnesium and cardiac arrhythmias. *Acta Med Scand* (Suppl) 647:163–169, 1981.

43. Ellman H, Dembin H, Seriff N: The rarity of shortening of the QT interval in patients with hypercalcemia. *Crit Care Med* 10:320–322, 1982.

44. Flink EB: Therapy of magnesium deficiency. *Ann NY Acad Sci* 162:901–905, 1969.

45. Forster J, Querusio L, Burchard KW, Gann DS: Hypercalcemia in critically ill surgical Patients. *Ann Surg* 202:512–517, 1985.

46. Fuller TJ, Nichols WW, Brenner BJ, et al: Reversible depression in myocardial performance in dogs with experimental phosphorus deficiency. *J Clin Invest* 62:1194, 1978.

47. Gallagher JC, Wilkinson R: The effect of ethinyloestradiol on calcium and phosphorus metabolism of postmenopausal women with primary hyperparathyroidism. *Clin Sci* 45:785–802, 1973.

48. Ginsburg R, Esserman LJ, Bristow MR: Myocardial performance and extracellular ionized calcium in a severely failing heart. *Ann Intern Med* 98:603–606, 1983.

49. Glover D, Riley L, Carmichael K, et al: Hypocalcemia and inhibition of parathyroid hormone secretion after administration of WR-2721 (a radioprotective and chemoprotective agent). *N Engl J Med* 309:1137–1141, 1983.

50. Glover DJ, Shaw L, Glick JH, et al: Treatment of hypercalcemia in cancer with WR-2721, S-2-(3-aminopropylamino) ethyl-Phosphorothioic Acid. *Ann Intern Med* 103:55–57, 1985.

51. Goldman RH, Kleiger RE, Schweizer E, et al: The effect on myocardial ^{3}H-digoxin in magnesium deficiency. *Proc Soc Exp Biol Med* 136:747–749, 1971.

52. Habener JF, Potts JT: Parathyroid physiology and primary hyperparathyroidism. In Avioli LV, Krane M (eds): *Metabolic Bone Disease,* vol 2. New York, Academic Press, 1978, pp 1–147.

53. Haldimann B, Goldstein DA, Akmal M, Massry SG: Renal function and blood levels of divalent ions in acute pancreatitis. *Mineral Electrolyte Metab* 3:190–199, 1980.

54. Haynes RC, Murad F: Agents affecting calcification: calcium, parathyroid hormone, calcitonin, vitamin D, and other compounds. In Gilman AG, Goodman LS, Rall TW, Murad F (eds): *The Pharmacological Basis of Therapeutics,* New York, Macmillan, 1985, pp 1517–1543.

55. Hauser CJ, Kamrath RO, Sparks J, Shoemaker WC: Calcium homeostasis in patients with acute pancreatitis. *Surgery* 94:830–835, 1983.

56. Heath DA: The emergency management of disorders of calcium and magnesium. *Clin Endocrinol Metab* 9:487–502, 1980.

57. Heckman BA, Walsh JH: Hypernatremia complicating sodium sulfate therapy for hypercalcemic crisis. *N Engl J Med* 276:1082–1083, 1967.

58. Henrich WL, Hunt JM, Nixon JV: Increased ionized calcium and left ventricular contractility during hemodialysis. *N Engl J Med* 310:19–23, 1984.

59. Hessov I, et al: Prevention of hypophosphatemia during post-operative routine glucose administration. *Acta Clin Scand* 146:109, 1980.

60. Horowitz M, Wishart J, Need A, Morris H, Philcox J, Nordin C: Treatment of postmenopausal hyperparathyroidism with norethindrone. *Arch Intern Med* 147:681–685, 1987.

61. Howland WS, Schweizer O, Jascott D, et al: Factors influencing the ionization of calcium during major surgical procedures. *Surg Gynecol Obstet* 143:895–900, 1976.

62. Iseri LT, Chung P, Tobis J: Magnesium therapy for intractable ventricular tachyarrhythmias in normomagnesemic patients. *Western J Med* 138:823–828, 1983.

63. Iseri LT, Freid J, Barnes AR: Magnesium deficiency and cardiac disorders. *Am J Med* 58:837–846, 1975.

64. Jacobs ML, Daggett WM, Civetta JM, et al: Acute pancreatitis: analysis of factors influencing survival. *Ann Surg* 185:43–51, 1977.

65. Jacobs TP, Siris ES, Bilezikian JP, Baquiran DC, Shane E, Canfield RE: Hypercalcemia of malignancy: treatment with intravenous dichloromethylene diphosphonate. *Ann Intern Med* 94:312–316, 1981.

66. Jung A: Comparison of two parenteral diphosphonates in hypercalcemia of malignancy. *Am J Med* 72:221–226, 1982.

67. Kafka H, Langevin L, Armstrong PW: Serum magnesium and potassium in acute myocardial infarction. *Arch Intern Med* 147:465–469, 1987.

68. Kahn RC, Jascott D, Carlon GC, et al: Massive blood replacement: correlation of ionized calcium, citrate, and hydrogen ion concentration. *Anesth Analg* 58:274–278, 1979.

69. Keller V, Berger W: Prevention of hypophosphatemia by phosphate infusion and during treatment of diabetic ketoacidosis and hyperosmolar coma. *Diabetes* 29:87, 1980.

70. Kingston ME, Al-Siba'i MB, Skooge WC: Clinical manifestations of hypomagnesemia. *Crit Care Med* 14:950–954, 1986.

71. Kingston M, Al-Siba'i MB: Treatment of severe hypophosphatemia. *Crit Care Med* 13:16–18, 1985.

72. Fitzgerald FT: Hypophosphatemia. *Adv Internal Med* 23:137, 1978.

73. Knochel JP: The pathophysiology and clinical characteristics of severe hypophosphatemia. *Arch Intern Med* 137:203–220, 1977.

74. Kreisberg RA: Diabetic ketoacidosis. New concepts and trends in pathogenesis and treatment. *Ann Intern Med* 88:681, 1978.

75. Kreusser W, Vetter HO, Mittmann U, Horl WH, Ritz E: Haemodynamics and myocardial metabolism of phosphorus depleted dogs: effect of catecholamines and angiotensin II. *Eur J Clin Invest* 12:219, 1982.

76. Kukla LJ, Abramson EC, McGuire WP, et al: Cis-platinum treatment for malignancy-associated humoral hypercalcemia in an athymic mouse model. *Calcif Tissue Int* 36:559–562, 1984.

77. Lad TE, Mishoulam HM, Shevrin DH, Kukla LJ, Abramson EC, Kukreja SC: Treatment of cancer-associated hypercalcemia with cisplatin. *Arch Intern Med* 147:329–332, 1987.

78. Ladenson JH, Lewis JW, Boyd JC: Failure of total serum calcium corrected for protein, albumin, and pH to correctly assess free calcium status. *J Clin Endocrinol Metab* 46:986–993, 1978.

79. Lee C, Zaloga GP: Magnesium metabolism. *Semin Resp Med* 7:75–80, 1985.

80. Lentz RD, Brown DM, Kjellstrand CM: Treatment of severe hypophosphatemia. *Ann Intern Med* 89:941, 1978.

81. Levy LA: Severe hypophosphatemia as a complication of the treatment of hypothermia. *Arch Intern Med* 140:128, 1980.

82. Loeb HS, Petras RM, Gunrar RM, et al: Paroxysmal ventricular fibrillation in two patients with hypomagnesemia. *Circulation* 37:210–215, 1967.

83. Marcus R, Madvig P, Crim M, et al: Conjugated estrogens in the treatment of postmenopausal women with hyperparathyroidism. *Ann Intern Med* 100:633–640, 1984.

84. Marx SJ, Attie MJ, Levine MA, et al: The hypocalciuric or benign variant of familial hypercalemia: clinical and biochemical features in fifteen kindreds. *Medicine* 60:397–412, 1981.

85. Marx SJ, Bourdeau JE: Calcium metabolism. In Maxwell MH, Kleeman CR, Narins RG: *Clinical Disorders of Fluid and Electrolyte Metabolism,* 4th ed. New York, McGraw Hill, 207–244, 1987.

86. Massara F, Camanni F: Propranolol block of adrenaline-induced hypophosphatemia in man. *Clin Sci Mol Med* 38:245, 1970.

87. Massry SG, Friedler RM, Coburn JW: Excretion of phosphate and calcium. *Arch Intern Med* 131:828, 1973.

88. Massry SG, Silby MS: Hypomagnesemia and hypermagnesemia. *Clin Nephrol* 7:147–153, 1977.

89. Mason RS, Frankel T, Chan YL, et al: Vitamin D conversion by sarcoid lymph node homogenate. *Ann Intern Med* 100:59–61, 1984.

90. Maynard JC, Cruz C, Kleerekoper M, et al: Blood pressure response to changes in serum ionized calcium during hemodialysis. *Ann Intern Med* 104:358–361, 1986.

91. McPherson ML, Prince SR, Atamer ER, Maxwell DB, Ross-Clunis H, Estep HL: Theophylline-induced hypercalcemia. *Ann Intern Med* 105:52–54, 1986.

92. Medalle R, Waterhouse C, Hahn TJ: Vitamin D resistance in magnesium deficiency. *Am J Clin Nutrition* 29:854–858, 1976.

93. Miravet L, Ayigbede O, Carre M, Rayssiguier Y, Larvor P: Lack of vitamin D action on serum calcium in magnesium deficient rats. In Catin M, Seelig MS (eds): *Magnesium in Health and Disease.* New York, SP Medical and Scientific Books, 1980, pp 281–289.

94. Molloy DW, Dhingra S, Solven F, Wilson A, McCarthy DS: Hypomagnesemia and respiratory muscle power. *Am Rev Respir Dis* 129:497–498, 1984.

95. Moore EW. Ionized calcium in normal serum, ultrafiltrates and whole blood determined by ion exchange electrodes. *J Clin Invest* 49:318–334, 1970.

96. Mordes JP, Wacker WE: Excess magnesium. *Pharmacol Rev* 29:273–300, 1978.

97. Mundy GR, Raisz LG, Cooper RH, et al: Evidence for the secretion of an osteoclast stimulating factor in myeloma. *N Engl J Med* 291:1041–1046, 1974.

98. Nagant De Deuxchaisnes C, Krane SM: Hypoparathy-

roidism. In Avioli LV, Krane SM (eds): *Metabolic Bone Disease*. Orlando, FL, Academic Press, 1978, vol 2, pp 217–445.

99. Newman JH, Neff TA, Ziporin P: Acute respiratory failure associated with hypophosphatemia. *N Engl J Med* 296:1101, 1977.

100. O'Connor LR, Wheeler WS, Bethune JR: Effect of hypophosphatemia on myocardial performance in man. *N Engl J Med* 297:901, 1977.

101. Okayama H, Aikawa T, Okayama M, Sasaki H, Mue S, Takishima T: Bronchodilating effect of intravenous magnesium sulfate in bronchial asthma. *J Am Med Assoc* 257:1076–1078, 1987.

102. Orwoll ES: The milk-alkali syndrome: current concepts. *Ann Intern Med* 97:242–248, 1982.

103. Potts M, Doppelt S, Taylor S, Folkman J, Neer R, Potts JT: Protamine: A powerful in-vivo inhibitor of bone resorption. *Calcif Tissue Int* 36:189–193, 1984.

104. Quamme GA, Dirks KJ: Magnesium metabolism. In Maxwell MH, Kleeman CR, Narins RG: *Clinical Disorders of Fluid and Electrolyte Metabolism*, 4th ed. McGraw Hill, New York, 1987, pp 297–316.

105. Rasmussen HS, Aurup P, Hojberg S, Jensen EK, McNair P: Magnesium and acute myocardial infarction. *Arch Intern Med* 146:872–874, 1986.

106. Rasmussen HS, Norregard P, Lindeneg O, et al: Intravenous magnesium in acute myocardial infarction. *Lancet* 1:234–235, 1986.

107. Riley MS, Schade DS, Eaton RP: Effects of insulin infusion on plasma phosphate in diabetic patients. *Metabolism* 28:191, 1979.

108. Robertson GM, Moore EW, Switz DM, Sizemore GW, Estep HL: Inadequate parathyroid response to acute pancreatitis. *N Engl J Med* 294:512–516, 1976.

109. Robertson WG: Measurement of ionized calcium in body fluids - a review. *Ann Clin Biochem* 13:540–548, 1976.

110. Rude RK, Oldham SB, Singer FR: Functional hypoparathyroidism and parathyroid hormone end-organ resistance in human magnesium deficiency. *Clin Endocrinol* 5:209–224, 1976.

111. Rude RK, Singer FR: Magnesium deficiency and excess. *Annu Rev Med* 32:245–259, 1981.

112. Ryback R, Eckardt MJ, Paulter MA: Clinical relationship between serum phosphorus and other blood chemistry values in alcoholics. *Arch Intern Med* 140:673, 1980.

113. Ryzen E, Martodam RR, Troxell M, Benson A, Paterson A, Shepard K, Hicks R: Intravenous etidronate in the management of malignant hypercalcemia. *Arch Intern Med* 145:449–452, 1985.

114. Seller RH, Cangiano J, Kim KE, et al: Digitalis toxicity and hypomagnesemia. *Am Heart J* 79:57–68, 1970.

115. Seyberth HW, Segre GV, Morgan JL, et al: Prostaglandins as mediators of hypercalcemia associated with certain types of cancer. *N Engl J Med* 293:1278–1283, 1975.

116. Silva OL, Becker KL: Calcitonin in the treatment of hypercalcemia. *Arch Intern Med* 132:337–339, 1973.

117. Singer FR, Neer RM, Murray TM, et al: Mithramycin treatment of intractable hypercalcemia due to parathyroid carcinoma. *N Engl J Med* 283:634–636, 1970.

118. Stewart AF, Horst R, Deftos LJ, Cadman EC, Lang R, Broadus PE: Biochemical evaluation of patients with cancer-associated hypercalcemia. *N Engl J Med* 303:1377–1383, 1980.

119. Swaminathan R, et al: Hypophosphatemia in surgical patients. *Surg Gynecol Obstet* 148:448, 1979.

120. Turk J, Morrell L, Avioli L: Ethylene glycol intoxication. *Arch Intern Med* 146:1601–1603, 1986.

121. Vannatta JB, Whang R, Papper S: Efficacy of intrave-

nous phosphorus therapy in the severely hypophosphatemic patient. *Arch Intern Med* 141:885, 1981.

122. Varsano S, Shapiro M, Taragan R, Bruderman I: Hypophosphatemia as a reversible cause of refractory ventilatory failure. *Crit Care Med* 11:908–909, 1983.

123. Wacker WEC, Parisi AF: Magnesium metabolism. *N Engl J Med* 278:658–663, 712–717, 772–776, 1968.

124. Warrell RP, Bockman RS, Coonley CJ, Isaacs M, Staszewski H: Gallium nitrate inhibits calcium resorption from bone and is effective treatment for cancer-related hypercalcemia. *J Clin Invest* 73:1487–1490, 1984.

125. Watson CG, Steed DL, Robinson AG, Deftos LJ: The role of calcitonin and parathyroid hormone in the pathogenesis of post-thyroidectomy hypocalcemia. *Metabolism* 30:588–589, 1981.

126. Webb S, Schade DS: Hypomagnesemia as a cause of persistent hypokalemia. *J Am Med Assoc* 233:23–24, 1975.

127. Whang R, Flink EB, Dyckner T, Wester PO, Aikawa JK, Ryan MP: Magnesium depletion as a cause of refractory potassium repletion. *Arch Intern Med* 145:1686–1689, 1985.

128. Whang R, Morosi HJ, Rodgers D, et al: The influence of continuing magnesium deficiency on muscle K repletion. *J Lab Clin Med* 70:895–902, 1967.

129. Whang R, Oei TO, Watanabe A: Frequency of hypomagnesemia in hospitalized patients receiving digitalis. *Arch Intern Med* 145:655–656, 1985.

130. Wilson R, Kever SP, Lee AS, et al: Phosphate therapy in DKA. *Arch Intern Med* 142:517, 1982.

131. Zaloga GP, Chernow B: Hypocalcemia and rhabdomyolysis. *J Am Med Assoc* 257:626, 1987.

132. Zaloga GP, Chernow B: Hypocalcemia in critical illness. *J Am Med Assoc* 256:1924–1929, 1986.

133. Zaloga GP, Chernow B: Stress-induced changes in calcium metabolism. *Sem Respir Med* 7:52–68, 1985.

134. Zaloga GP, Chernow B: The multifactorial basis for hypocalcemia during sepsis: studies of the PTH-vitamin D axis. *Ann Intern Med* 107:36–41, 1987.

135. Zaloga GP, Chernow B, Cook D, et al: Assessment of calcium homeostasis in the critically ill patient. The diagnostic pitfalls of the McLean Hastings Nomogram. *Ann Surg* 202:587–594, 1985.

136. Zaloga GP, Chernow B, Eil C: Hypercalcemia and disseminated cytomegalovirus infection in the acquired immune deficiency syndrome. *Ann Intern Med* 102:331–333, 1985.

137. Zaloga GP, Chernow B, Hodge J, Eil C: Hypocalcemia and altered vitamin D metabolism in patients with small intestinal disease. *Military Med* 153:34–37, 1988.

138. Zaloga GP, Chernow B, Pock A, et al: Hypomagnesemia is a common complication of aminoglycoside therapy. *Surg Gynecol Obstet* 158:561–565, 1984.

139. Zaloga GP, Eil C, Medberry CA: Humoral hypercalcemia in Hodgkin's disease associated with elevated 1,25(OH)$_2$D levels and subperiosteal bone resorption. *Arch Intern Med* 145:155–157, 1985.

140. Zaloga GP, Eil C, O'Brian JT: Reversible hypocalciuric hypercalcemia associated with hypothyroidism. *Am J Med* 77:1101–1104, 1984.

141. Zaloga GP, Malcolm DS, Holaday J, Chernow B: Verapamil reverses calcium cardiotoxicity. *Ann Emerg Med* 16:637–639, 1987.

142. Zaloga GP, Wilkens R, Tourville J, Wood D, Klymer DM: A simple method for determining physiologically active calcium and magnesium concentrations in critically ill patients. *Crit Care Med* 15:813–816, 1987.

143. Zaloga GP, Willey SC, Chernow B: Free fatty acids alter calcium binding. A cause for misinterpretation of serum calcium values and hypocalcemia in critical illness. *J Clin Endocrinol Metab* 64:1010–1014, 1987.

33

Part 1.
Insulin and Oral Hypoglycemics

Gary P. Zaloga, M.D., F.A.C.P., F.A.C.N.
Bart Chernow, M.D., F.A.C.P., F.C.C.P

Insulin is a polypeptide hormone that is essential for normal metabolic activity. Deficiency of the hormone results in diabetes mellitus. This chapter details the pharmacology of insulin and the application of insulin therapy in the treatment of diabetic ketoacidosis, hyperglycemic nonketotic syndromes, alcoholic ketoacidosis, parenteral nutrition and the diabetic surgical patient.

Insulin, which consists of two polypeptide chains connected by disulfide bridges, is synthesized by the β cells of the islets of Langerhans. The pancreas secretes insulin into the portal vein and the liver removes 50–60% before it reaches the peripheral circulation. The normal fasting venous immunoreactive insulin concentration in healthy individuals is 10–20 μU/ml and represents a basal secretory rate of 0.25–1.5 U/hour.

Glucose is the primary regulator of the β cells and stimulates insulin secretion by a process that involves an increase in intracellular calcium availability (enhanced by cAMP) (36). Glucose-induced insulin release is biphasic. The first phase of insulin secretion is brief (0–5 minutes) and involves release of stored insulin; whereas the second phase of insulin release (which is more gradual, lasting 5–60 minutes) involves the secretion of newly synthesized insulin. The plasma insulin response to an oral glucose load is greater than that after an intravenous glucose load. Part of the reason for the enhanced insulin secretion to oral glucose loads involves the release of gastrointestinal hormones that enhance glucose-stimulated insulin secretion (26). Gastric inhibitory polypeptide (GIP), pancreozymin-cholecystokinin, gut glucagon, and vasoactive intestinal polypeptide have been shown to stimulate insulin secretion (15). Protein, amino acids, and

fatty acids also stimulate insulin secretion, an effect enhanced by gastrointestinal hormones. Adrenergic agents affect insulin release via α- and β-adrenergic receptors involving cAMP (112). α-Adrenergic action is inhibitory and predominates over the β stimulatory effect. As a result, epinephrine and norepinephrine inhibit, whereas isoproterenol stimulates, insulin secretion. Propranolol blocks the isoproterenol effect. Catecholamine effects are responsible for the hypoinsulinemia that accompanies "stress" hyperglycemia (e.g., in severe burns). Such states may occur when the autonomic nervous system is activated during hypoxia, hypothermia, surgery, and burns. Parasympathetic stimulation increases insulin secretion, an effect that is partially antagonized by atropine. Dopamine diminishes insulin release in vitro (79). Prostaglandins are inhibitory to insulin release and may play a role in insulin-dependent diabetes (120). Prostaglandin inhibitors (e.g., acetylsalicylic acid) augment (22, 55, 56), whereas prostaglandin stimulators (e.g., furosemide) reduce, insulin secretion (55). A variety of other hormones effect insulin action. Glucagon, growth hormone, glucocorticoids, estrogens, progestins, and PTH each increase insulin levels. Somatostatin inhibits both insulin and glucagon secretion. Agents that destroy the β cells induce hypoinsulinemic diabetes mellitus (e.g., alloxan and streptozotocin). Some of these agents have been used to treat insulin-secreting tumors.

Insulin controls the storage and metabolism of a variety of metabolic fuels including glucose, fat, and amino acids (Table 33.1). Insulin affects a variety of enzyme systems in the course of its work. In the liver, insulin stimulates glucokinase (phosphorylation of glucose),

Table 33.1
Insulin Action

	Liver	Adipose	Muscle	Periphery
Glucose uptake	+	+	+	+
Glycogen synthesis	+		+	
Fatty acid synthesis	+	+		
Protein synthesis			+	
Glycerol synthesis		+		
Amino acid uptake			+	
Glycogenolysis	−			
Gluconeogenesis	−			
Ketogenesis	−			
Lipolysis		−		
Protein catabolism			−	

Increases (+); decreases (−).

phosphofructokinase (which decreases glycogen breakdown), and glycogen synthetase while inhibiting phosphorylase (which decreases glycogen breakdown) and phosphoenolpyruvate carboxykinase (which decreases gluconeogenesis). Insulin suppresses ketogenesis by inhibiting fatty acid release from adipose tissue and hepatic oxidation of fatty acids to ketones. It accelerates muscle uptake and oxidation of ketone bodies. Insulin effects may cause hypokalemia, hypophosphatemia, and antinatriuresis (36). The antinatriuretic action may account for edema occasionally seen during insulin treatment of patients with diabetic ketoacidosis.

Insulin circulates in plasma predominantly as the free unbound hormone and distributes in the extracellular fluid (78). The pancreas secretes 20 μg of insulin per hour into the portal vein; the concentration in portal blood is 2–4 mg/ml (50–100 μU/ml) and that in the peripheral circulation is 500 pg/ml (12 μU/ml) (78). The plasma half-life of insulin is 5–9 minutes. The major sites of degradation are the liver (40–60%) and kidney (15–20%) (33). Fifty percent of insulin that reaches the liver via the portal vein is destroyed in a single passage.

The decrease in insulin requirements in renal failure is due to decreased renal degradation of insulin.

INSULIN PREPARATIONS

Insulin is available in a variety of forms which differ in onset of action and duration of effects (Table 33.2) (34, 76). Insulin is mixed with solutions containing protamine and zinc to slow absorption and prolong duration of action. The Lente insulins employ different concentrations of zinc while neutral protamine Hagedorn (NPH) and protamine zinc insulin (PZI) employ both zinc and protamine. NPH insulin is formulated by mixing together regular and PZI in proportions to maintain action throughout the day. PZI should not be given with regular insulin since excess zinc slows the time course of the regular insulin. "Single peak" refers to insulin that yields a single peak when gel chromatography is performed. It is 98% pure and contains small amounts of intermediates in the conversion of proinsulin to insulin. "Single component" refers to single-peak insulin that has been further purified

Table 33.2
Insulin Preparations

Type of Insulin	Action	Protein	Peak SQ Action (hr)	Duration SQ (hr)	Route	Dose (U/ml)
Regular (crystalline)[a]	Rapid	None	1–3	5–7	i.v., s.c., i.m.	100, 500
Semilente	Rapid	None	2–4	10–16	s.c.	100
NPH[a]	Intermediate	Protamine	6–14	18–28	s.c.	100
Lente[a]	Intermediate	None	6–14	18–28	s.c.	100
Ultralente	Prolonged	None	18–24	30–40	s.c.	100
PZI	Prolonged	Protamine	18–24	30–40	s.c.	100

[a] Available as human insulin.

using cellulose chromatography. It is over 99% pure and is used in patients with insulin allergy or insulin-induced lipoatrophy. Most insulin today is marketed as U-100 (100 units/ml) insulin although U-500 insulin (500 units/ml) is available for patients resistant to the hormone. Insulin is available as pure beef, pork, beef-pork, fish, or human insulin. Porcine insulin is most similar to that of humans and differs only in the substitution of alanine for threonine at the carboxy-terminus of the β chain. Human insulin is obtained either by synthesis from pork insulin or by recombinant DNA techniques in *Escherichia coli*. Regular insulin in the United States is supplied at neutral pH, which improves its stability. Refrigeration is no longer required, but extremes of temperature and sunlight exposure should be avoided. Regular insulin is the only form approved for intravenous use (Table 33.2). It may also be used intramuscularly, (60, 72) where it has faster and more predictable absorption than subcutaneous injection. Insulin should not be mixed with sodium bicarbonate since insulin is unstable in the presence of alkali (61).

FACTORS THAT INFLUENCE RESPONSE TO INSULIN

There is a marked individual variability in insulin absorption and half-life. Duration of effect and magnitude of hypoglycemic response (at peak action) vary with the dose (16); the larger the dose, the longer the duration of action and the greater the hypoglycemic effect. Rate of absorption varies with the site and depth of injection (47). Absorption is more rapid from the deltoid area and abdomen than from thighs and buttocks. Deep intramuscular injections are more rapidly absorbed than superficial intramuscular injections, and both are absorbed more rapidly than subcutaneous injections. Some patients are insensitive to subcutaneous or intramuscular insulin but sensitive to intravenous insulin (73, 103). This may be related to excessive protease activity in the subcutaneous tissue, resulting in excessive insulin degradation at the injection site (13, 42). The effectiveness of subcutaneously administered insulin can be increased by mixing the insulin with aprotinin, a protease inhibitor (13, 42).

Changes in insulin receptors are important in insulin-resistant states and states of increased insulin sensitivity. In circumstances

of hyperinsulinemia (such as obesity) the insulin receptor concentration (sites/cell) is reduced (down-regulation), while the reverse occurs in hypoinsulinemia.

The most common cause of insulin resistance is obesity (46). In obesity, the defect is at the target cell (decreased number of insulin receptors) and is proportional to the degree of basal hyperinsulinemia (10, 40). Several weeks of a low carbohydrate diet corrects this abnormality. Insulin resistance may be seen in association with acanthosis nigricans because of a decrease in the number of insulin receptors, or with antireceptor antibodies that decrease insulin binding (40). Additional causes of decreased insulin binding include glucocorticoid excess (e.g., Cushing's disease), growth hormone excess (e.g., acromegaly), and lipoatropic diabetes mellitus. Increased insulin binding (augmented sensitivity) is seen in trained athletes, starvation, and in glucocorticoid or growth hormone deficiency. Insulin resistance may also result from postreceptor deficits (e.g., type II diabetes mellitus).

Patients taking insulin develop antibodies to the insulin molecule (46). These antibodies may cause a slower onset and longer duration of insulin action, insulin resistance, or insulin allergy. Resistance occurs when the titer of IgG rises to a level sufficient to necessitate daily insulin doses in excess of 200 U. Initial treatment consists of switching to a less antigenic insulin. Pork is less immunogenic than beef insulin, and single component is less immunogenic than single peak. Lente and protamine (NPH) insulins produce higher antibody titers than does regular insulin (NPH > Lente > regular). Human insulins are least immunogenic. We use only human insulin in our intravenous insulin infusions and in patients in whom short-term insulin therapy is contemplated (e.g., after surgery) so as to avoid antigenicity. If this treatment fails, systemic steroids (prednisone 60–80 mg/day for 10 days) usually results in a marked reduction in insulin requirements (36, 46). Additional therapeutic approaches include the use of sulfated insulins (28), fish insulin (138), immunosuppressants (90), and U-500 regular insulin (95). Insulin allergy results from production of IgE antiinsulin antibodies (87, 102, 136). Local symptoms manifest as induration, pruritus, erythema, or pain at the injection site. Systemic symptoms of insulin allergy include generalized pruritus and urticaria, angioneurotic edema, anaphylaxis, and bronchospasm. Symptoms appear 30 minutes to several hours after injection and usually disappear spontaneously within a few weeks. Many patients exhibit allergic responses following an interval during which insulin therapy had been discontinued and reinstituted (17, 81). The allergy may at times be attributed to exogenous contaminants (from the extraction process) rather than to the insulin (81). If allergic symptoms persist, treatment may be required (Table 33.3) (17, 87). One must first rule out contamination of the insulin. Sources include a dirty bottle, poor injection technique, or reaction to material used in the commercial process of preparing the insulin (e.g., acid, alcohol). Before treating with other agents one should review the requirements for insulin therapy. If insulin is required, switch to a less antigenic form. We recommend using *E. coli* recombinant human insulin. A trial of antihistamines (74) or systemic steroids (25, 97, 126) may decrease adverse reactions. Corticosteroids have been given as oral prednisone (30 mg daily) (97) or as injectable hydrocortisone (10 mg) mixed with the insulin (25). Slow desensitization occurs under corticosteroid coverage and it can be discontinued at a future time. At times desensitization is required (27, 81, 87, 136). Patients should be skin tested against different insulin preparations and the least antigenic form used. Begin intradermally, and if a local reaction occurs, repeat the dose or go to a lower dose before proceeding (Table 33.3). Once desensitization is completed, insulin should be given at frequent intervals (e.g., twice to four times a day). Other factors to be considered in insulin resistance include severe stress, infection, drug antagonism (see "Drug Interactions"), and ketosis.

COMPLICATIONS

The most common complication of insulin therapy is hypoglycemia. Symptoms include neuroglucopenic (e.g., confusion, bizarre behavior, depression, seizures, coma) and hyperadrenergic manifestations (e.g., tachycardia, palpitations, diaphoresis, vasoconstriction, piloerection, anxiety). Localizing neurologic symptoms (e.g., hemiplegia, or visual disturbances) may occur secondary to underlying vascular disease. Hypothermia may be an important clue to hypoglycemia in a comatose patient (21). Symptoms occur with rapid falls in blood glucose, even though the plasma glucose value may be normal (60–120 mg/dl) (29). The most common causes of hypoglycemia are excessive insulin dosage, omission or delay in meals, heavy exercise, and poor injection technique (e.g., failure to mix insulin properly or accidental injection into muscle). When recurrent hypoglycemic episodes develop, one should consider progressive renal insufficiency, failure to reduce dosage after resolution of a stress, onset of adrenal insufficiency, pregnancy, and drug interactions (e.g., with propranolol).

The "Somogyi effect" is the occurrence of posthypoglycemic hyperglycemia and ketonuria after excessive insulin administration. Rebound hyperglycemia results from the release of counterregulatory hormones (e.g., cortisol, catecholamines, glucagon, growth hormone). Widely varying urine glucose values suggest the Somogyi effect. Detection is accomplished by frequent blood glucose monitoring. Treatment consists of decreasing the insulin dose.

An occasional patient will develop edema during insulin therapy. The edema partially results from reduced urinary sodium excretion induced by insulin.

Table 33.3
Treatment of Insulin Allergy

1. Rule out foreign material being injected; switch to new bottle of insulin, review injection technique, and check for sensitivity to solvent.
2. Consider diet and oral hypoglycemics.
3. Switch to a less antigenic insulin:
   Escherichia coli (human) <fish <pork <beef
   Regular < Lente < NPH
   Single component < single peak
4. Antihistamines
5. Corticosteroids
6. Desensitization
   a. Use insulin preparation with least skin test reactivity
   b. Slow desensitization:

Day	Time	Units of Insulin	Route
1	0730 AM	0.00001	i.v.
	1200	0.0001	
	0430 PM	0.001	
2	0730 AM	0.01	i.v.
	1200	0.1	
	0430 PM	1	
3	0730 AM	2	s.c.
	1200	4	
	0430 PM	8	
4	0730 AM	12	s.c.
	1200	16	
	0430 PM	20	
5	0730 AM	25	s.c.
6	0730 AM	30	s.c.

   c. Fast desensitization: double dose every 30–60 minutes and cover with steroids

Insulin deficiency results in the production of diabetes mellitus and can be classified, based upon the cause, into various groups: insulin-dependent diabetes mellitus (type I), non-insulin-dependent diabetes mellitus (type II), secondary diabetes mellitus (e.g., drug induced, pancreatic disease, hormonal), carbohydrate intolerance, and gestational diabetes mellitus. Long-term management of these patients with insulin is discussed elsewhere (130). Major surgery and critical illness are stressful events that stimulate the secretion of "antiinsulin" hormones. Normally, these changes in metabolism are balanced by an increase in insulin secretion. Patients with a diminished ability to secrete insulin may be unable to counterbalance the antiinsulin hormonal effects, and hyperglycemia and ketosis may result. Acute metabolic decompensation in these patients may result in diabetic ketoacidosis or diabetic hyperglycemic nonketotic states.

DIABETIC KETOACIDOSIS

The most severe manifestation of insulin lack is diabetic ketoacidosis (DKA). Mortality in DKA has declined since the advent of insulin therapy; however, it may still be as high as 5–15% (5, 36). Major causes of death include irreversible circulatory shock, myocardial infarction, sepsis, cardiac arrest, stroke, renal failure, pulmonary aspiration, cerebral edema, adult respiratory distress syndrome, thrombosis, pulmonary embolism, gastrointestinal hemorrhage, and electrolyte abnormalities (35).

Hyperglycemia and ketoacidosis result from an imbalance between the actions of anabolic (insulin) and catabolic (glucagon, cortisone, growth hormone, catecholamines) hormones (88, 140). The importance of glucagon in the pathogenesis of DKA forms the basis of the bihormonal theory of diabetes mellitus (114, 115, 130, 131). In this theory glucagon is thought

of as the major agent responsible for the massive production of ketones and glucose. In humans about 75% of hepatic glucose production is mediated by glucagon, whereas only about 40% of glucose utilization occurs in insulin-sensitive tissues. If both glucagon and insulin were lacking glucose, production would decline by 75%, utilization would decline by 40%, and serum glucose levels would most likely decline (130). The major direct effect of insulin on the liver is to oppose the effects of glucagon, and insulin would have minimal influence on hepatic glucose and ketone metabolism unless glucagon is present (130). Diabetic patients fail to normally suppress glucagon during hyperglycemia. The loss of glucose-induced glucagon suppression can be improved by infusion of insulin (130).

A fall in the insulin/glucagon ratio causes increased glucose production by the liver while the absolute decline in insulin levels or action reduces glucose utilization in peripheral tissues.

Glucagon, when unopposed by insulin in the liver, increases glycogenolysis, gluconeogenesis, and ketogenesis (Table 33.4). Insulin deficiency is the mechanism by which substrates for hepatic glucose and ketone production (e.g., amino acids and free fatty acids) are delivered to the liver in increased quantities; glucagon is the switch that activates the production machinery for glucose and ketones (130).

In DKA, hyperglycemia results from decreased utilization of glucose (reduced rate of entrance of glucose into cells) and glucose overproduction by the liver (Table 33.4). Insulin does not influence the rate of glucose transfer across the cell membrane in hepatocytes, brain cells, erythrocytes, leukocytes, and cells of the renal medulla (78). It does affect transfer in muscle and fat cells. Insulin deficiency also impairs the activity of glycogen synthetase, activates lipolysis, accelerates protein catabolism, causes hyperglucagonemia,

Table 33.4
Effect of Insulin and Glucagon on Glucose and Ketone Metabolism in Diabetes

	Insulin Deficiency	Relative Glucagon Excess
Hyperglycemia		
Decreased glucose utilization	+ + + +	0
Hepatic glucose production	+	+ + + +
Ketonemia		
Lipolysis	+ + + +	+
Hepatic ketogenesis	+	+ + + +

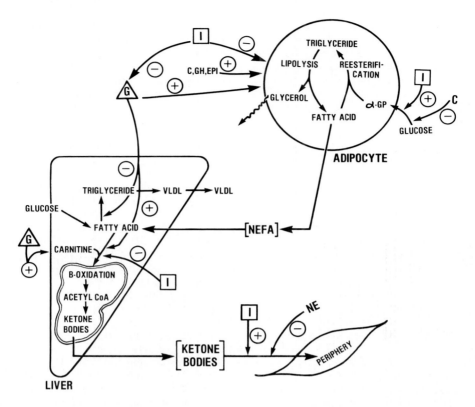

Figure 33.1. Hormonal control of ketogenesis.

intensifies glucagon's effects in the liver, and stimulates hepatic gluconeogenesis. Protein is degraded to amino acids and converted to glucose in the liver. Insulin reverses these effects. Ketones accumulate due to increased lipolysis, decreased fatty acid synthesis in adipose tissue, increased hepatic ketogenesis, and decreased ketone utilization in the periphery. In the absence of insulin, lipolysis, facilitated by various counterregulatory hormones, proceeds unchecked. The liver picks up liberated free fatty acids and converts them to ketones (since insulin deficiency impairs their conversion to triglycerides) (Fig. 33.1) (88, 140). In the absence of glucagon, insulin deficiency leads to only a modest increase in glucose and ketones (114, 115, 131). Suppression of glucagon by somatostatin (50, 52, 54, 116, 130) results in attenuation of hyperglycemia and hyperketonemia in diabetes. Hyperglycemia and ketonemia appear readily when glucagon is infused (130). However, somatostatin offers no advantage over insulin alone in the treatment of established DKA (83). Hyperglycemia in diabetic rats may be decreased by blocking glucagon action with a glucagon receptor antag-

onist (68). Glucagon-suppressing agents may some day provide an additional therapeutic agent in the treatment of diabetes mellitus.

Most cases of DKA are not a result of simple insulin deficiency but result from identifiable precipitating factors that alter antiinsulin hormonal levels (e.g., epinephrine, cortisol, norepinephrine, and growth hormone). These counterregulatory hormones oppose insulin action and stimulate glucagon release and action. Hypovolemia due to glucose-induced diuresis also increases glucagon secretion and release of catecholamines and other stress hormones. The most common precipitating factor for DKA is infection followed by myocardial infarction, cerebrovascular accidents, and trauma (5). Many patients will present with DKA as the initial clinical manifestation of diabetes mellitus.

Signs and symptoms of DKA relate to the presence of hyperglycemia (e.g., osmotic diuresis, dehydration, hyperosmolality, or electrolyte depletion) or ketoacidosis (e.g., acidosis or osmotic diuresis) (140). The major presenting symptoms and signs of DKA include nausea, vomiting, labored (Kussmaul) breathing,

Table 33.5
Clinical Features of Diabetic Ketoacidosis

General
   Malaise, weakness
   Dehydration (dry mucous membranes, decreased
      skin turgor)
   Polyuria, polydipsia
   Muscle aches
Neurological
   Depressed mental function
   Drowsiness, stupor, coma
   Headache
Cardiac
   Tachycardia
   Hypotension
   Heart failure
Gastrointestinal
   Anorexia
   Nausea, vomiting
   Gastric stasis, distention
   Ileus
   Abdominal pain
Respiratory
   Hyperpnea
   Kussmaul breathing
   Fruity odor on breath
Laboratory
   Metabolic acidosis
   Ketonemia, ketonuria
   Hyperglycemia, glucosuria
   Hyperosmolality
   Hypokalemia
   Hypomagnesemia
   Hyponatremia
   Hypophosphatemia
   Leukocytosis
   Elevated serum amylase, CPK, transaminases

polyuria, polydpsia, depressed mental function, dehydration, tachycardia, fruity odor of breath, abdominal pain, and hypotension (Table 33.5). Laboratory examination characteristically shows hyperglycemia, metabolic acidosis with an increased anion gap, ketonemia, glucosuria, ketonuria, hemoconcentration with hyperosmolality, and leukocytosis. Other causes of an anion gap acidosis include alcoholic ketoacidosis, lactic acidosis, renal failure, and certain poisons (e.g., ethylene glycol, or methyl alcohol). Ketoacidosis can be distinguished by the presence of ketonemia. Diabetic ketoacidosis is suggested by the concomitant presence of hyperglycemia.

The cause of the altered consciousness in DKA is uncertain and correlates poorly with blood glucose, ketone bodies, hydrogen ions, or electrolyte levels. Plasma hyperosmolality provides the best correlation to date. The explanation for nausea, vomiting, gastric stasis, and ileus is also unknown. They may be secondary to intracellular potassium and/or mag-

nesium deficiency. Acute abdominal pain occurs in 20–25% of decompensated diabetics (19) and may be the result of intestinal distension. Differentiation from an acute intra-abdominal problem may be difficult. Leukocytosis is common and correlates with the degree of ketosis but not with infection (3). In addition, many DKA patients with infection fail to mount a fever.

An understanding of the nitroprusside reaction (NTPR) (e.g., Acetest) for measuring ketones is essential in the therapy of DKA to avoid inappropriate use of insulin (143). Nitroprusside reacts with acetoacetate (AcAc) and weakly with acetone but not with β-hydroxybutyrate (βOHB). Normally ketones are present in low concentration with a βOHB/AcAc ratio of 3:1. During DKA, total ketones increase and the βOHB/AcAc ratio may approach 30:1. Hence, a negative or trace NTPR may mislead the clinician to underestimate the severity of ketoacidosis when most of the ketones are in the βOHB form. When the NTPR is used to assess response to insulin therapy one can be misled in the opposite direction. With insulin therapy βOHB decreases more rapidly than AcAc. In addition, βOHB is reoxidized to AcAc and the absolute levels of AcAc may rise while total ketones are falling and metabolic status improving. Nitroprusside results may erroneously indicate a worsening of ketosis, and the insulin dosage may be unnecessarily increased. Indirect measures of ketonemia (e.g., anion gap and blood pH) may be useful in these situations.

DKA must be distinguished from other causes of metabolic acidosis and altered mental function (Table 33.6). Hypoglycemia should be quickly ruled out with bedside blood glucose test strips (23). Cerebrovascular accidents may lead to glycosuria and ketonuria, but can usually be distinguished on clinical grounds and by obtaining blood glucose and ketone levels. Nonketotic hyperosmolar syndrome and alcoholic ketoacidosis are discussed in later sections.

Therapy in DKA (Table 33.7) is aimed at correcting fluid and electrolyte abnormalities, correcting the metabolic consequences of insulin lack, and identification of precipitating factors (141). The airway must be protected, and if the patient is obtunded with vomiting, nasogastic suctioning should be undertaken. A comprehensive flow sheet of vital signs, laboratory data, and treatment given aids in proper assessment of therapy. Routine bladder catheterization should not be performed, un-

Table 33.6
Serum Changes in the Differential Diagnosis of Diabetic Ketoacidosis

Diagnosis	Glucose	Ketones	pH	Anion Gap	Sodium	BUN
Diabetic ketoacidosis	3+ (400–800 mg/dl)	3+	3–	2+	N to –	3+ (30–60 mg/dl)
Hyperglycemic hyperosmolar nonketotic syndrome	4+ (>600 mg/dl)	0 to +	–	N	N to 3+	4+ (70–90 mg/dl)
Alcoholic ketoacidosis	– to + (50–250 mg/dl)	+	+ –	+	+	N
Lactic acidosis	N	0 to +	3–	+	N to –	N to 3+
Hypoglycemia	2–	0 to +	N	N	N	N

Increased (+, 2+, 3+, 4+); decreased (–, 2–, 3–); normal (N).

Table 33.7
Treatment of Diabetic Ketoacidosis

Fluids
Give 1 liter isotonic saline on admission followed by 1 liter in 1 hour, 1 liter in 2 hours, then 250–500 ml/hour. If serum sodium rises above 150–155 mEq/liter, switch to 0.5 N saline. When plasma glucose falls below 250 mg/dl, switch to D_5W. Central hemodynamic monitoring may be required in elderly or in patients with cardiac or renal disease.
Insulin
Begin with continuous i.v. infusion of 5–10 U regular insulin per hour (in isotonic saline). Double infusion rate if glucose does not fall by 10%/hour. When plasma glucose drops to 250 mg/dl, decrease i.v. infusion to 1–3 U regular insulin per hour and continue until acidosis is corrected (glucose "clamp").
Alternative:
Use 0.3 U regular insulin per kg i.m. or s.c. initially then 5–10 U regular insulin i.m. or s.c. per hour; when glucose drops to 250 mg/dl, continue i.m. or s.c. injections at 2–4 hour intervals using glucose clamp until acidosis clears. Give injections into deltoids.
Potassium
Give 20 mEq/hour; if oliguric, give 5–10 mEq/hour; if K+ above 6 mEq/liter, stop infusion; if K below 4 mEq/liter, increase infusion. Use continuous ECG monitoring.
Phosphorus
Oral: Neutra-Phos 250 mg every 6 hr
IV: potassium phosphate 0.08–0.16 mmol/kg/6 hours. Measure serum phosphorous levels.
Bicarbonate
If arterial pH <7.1 or bicarbonate <5–7 mEq/liter, give one ampule bicarbonate (44 mEq); if pH <7.0, give two ampules bicarbonate (88 mEq); monitor arterial or venous pH hourly.
Magnesium
If less than 1.2 mg/dl give
Oral: Mg oxide 35 mEq Q6–24 hours
IV: Mg SO_4 or $MgCl_2$ 20–80 mEq/day
Monitor serum glucose (Chemstrip bG), electrolytes, arterial blood gas, anion gap, and hemodynamic and mental status.

less the patient does not void in 3–4 hours or has cardiovascular depression. DKA develops over a number of days and should not be corrected all at once since rapid changes may be harmful by creating harmful osmotic and biochemical gradients (e.g., cerebral edema and pulmonary edema).

Fluid replacement (Table 33.7) is the first step in the therapy (141) of DKA. Dehydration and intravascular volume depletion (average 6–10 liters) result from glucosuria (osmotic diuresis) and vomiting. The circulating volume should be restored with normal saline to promote proper organ function and to assure insulin action. Volume repletion alone can lower plasma glucose levels and decrease counterregulatory hormone concentrations but does not reverse the acidosis. Thus, insulin is also required. Arguments abound regarding the type of fluid replacement. The body is deficient in hypotonic (0.7 N) saline and many centers replace fluid losses with 0.5 N saline or an equivalent hypotonic fluid. We favor the use of isotonic saline. Despite losses of water, plasma sodium concentration is usually normal (25%) or low (67%) (77) and the hypernatremic effect of an isotonic saline infusion is small. Isotonic saline dampens the fall in extracellular osmolality that occurs during fluid and insulin treatment and may lessen the chance of cerebral and pulmonary edema (due to unfavorable osmotic gradients). However, if the plasma sodium rises above 150–155 mEq/liter, hypotonic fluid should be substituted. Large amounts of sodium chloride may contribute to hyperchloremic acidosis during treatment (98). We usually give 1 liter of isotonic saline when the patient is admitted, followed by 1 liter over 1 hour, 1 liter over 2 hours, and finally 250–500 ml/hour depending on the clinical response. When the blood glucose falls below 250 mg/dl, the intravenous infusion is switched to 5% dextrose in water (D_5W), 5% dextrose in 0.5 N saline ($D_5\frac{1}{2}NS$), or 5% dextrose in normal saline (D_5NS), depending on the serum sodium concentration. For example, if the patient is hypernatremic (> 150 mEq/liter) we use D_5W, whereas if the patient is hyponatremic (< 135 mEq/liter) we give D_5NS. When the serum sodium is between 135 and 150 mEq/liter, $D_5\frac{1}{2}NS$ is the best choice. The importance of administering glucose is not only to avoid hypoglycemia but to protect against the development of cerebral edema (discussed later in this section). Hemodynamic monitoring may be required in the elderly and in patients with cardiac or renal disease.

Total body potassium (K^+) and phosphorus (PO_4^{2-}) are depleted in DKA, despite normal or elevated plasma levels on admission (11, 77, 107). K^+ deficits average 3–10 mEq/kg of body weight. In 4–10% of patients with DKA serum K^+ may be decreased on presentation, implying severe K^+ deficiency. The serum K^+ falls with therapy, reaching a nadir at 1–4 hours. The decrease is a result of (a) dilution from rehydration, (b) continued urinary K^+ loss because of volume expansion and hyperaldosteronism, (c) correction of acidosis with reentry of K^+ into the cell, and (d) increased cellular K^+ uptake as a result of insulin therapy (less with low-dose insulin). During treatment of DKA 20–50% of administered K^+ is lost in the urine (77). If bicarbonate is used, K^+ will reenter cells at an accelerated rate in exchange for hydrogen ions. We recommend adding K^+ to bicarbonate therapy (13–20 mEq K^+ per 100 mEq bicarbonate). K^+ requirements are reduced with renal insufficiency. However, these patients still require K^+ because other factors responsible for hypokalemia (discussed earlier in this section) are still operative. We withhold K^+ only when the serum K^+ is elevated. Otherwise, we begin with 20 mEq K^+/hour, as the chloride and/or PO_4^{2-} salt (Table 33.7). If the patient is oliguric we reduce the K^+ dose by 20–50%. Potassium should be given along with insulin, since without insulin potassium cannot enter cells effectively and hyperkalemia may result. Adjustments are made based on serum K^+ measurements at intervals of 2–4 hours. ECG monitoring is also used as an index of hypokalemia or hyperkalemia (86). Hypokalemia is suggested by prominent U waves with apparent Q-T prolongation, T wave inversion, and sagging ST segments. Hyperkalemia produces peaked T waves, P-R prolon-

gation, ST depression, QRS widening, P wave disappearance, and finally a sine wave configuration. PO_4^{2-} deficiency (deficits range from 0.5 to 1.5 mM/kg) results from increased urinary losses, increased tissue catabolism, and impaired tissue uptake due to insulin deficiency. Despite PO_4^{2-} deficiency, only 11% of patients with DKA show hypophosphatemia when admitted to the hospital (94). PO_4^{2-} decreases in the first 4–5 hours of DKA therapy as a result of insulin-induced shifts into cells and may reach levels less than 1 mg/dl (70, 77). PO_4^{2-} deficiency is associated with insulin resistance (30, 64), decreased 2,3-diphosphoglycerate (2,3-DPG) (2, 30, 77), and decreased intracellular ATP. Depletion of 2,3-DPG alters the oxygen-hemoglobin dissociation curve and may produce tissue ischemia. This is important since patients with DKA have elevated hemoglobin A_{1c} levels, a hemoglobin with very high affinity for oxygen. PO_4^{2-} supplementation can restore 2,3-DPG levels to normal within 12–24 hours (62); whereas without supplementation it takes 72–96 hours (2). PO_4 deficiency is also associated with cardiac insufficiency, hemolysis, respirator failure, and rhabdomyolysis (see Chapter 32). Although studies have not clearly demonstrated a benefit of PO_4^{2-} therapy in DKA, some (32, 41) have suggested more prompt recovery. In addition, if one evaluates all patients with severe hypophosphatemia who develop symptoms, insulin treatment of DKA is a common cause of the hypophosphatemia. K^+ deficits (3–10 mEq/kg) exceed PO_4^{2-} deficits (1 mmol/kg), and thus to avoid hyperphosphatemia one should replace K^+ with a combination of KCl and K_2PO_4. We recommend giving PO_4^{2-} orally (Neutra-Phos 250-mg capsule every 6 hours) if possible and if parenteral therapy is required the dosage should be 0.08-0.16 mmol/kg/6 hours as potassium phosphate. Serum PO_4^{2-} and calcium levels should be monitored every 6 hours and the PO_4^{2-} dosage adjusted accordingly. Complications of PO_4^{2-} therapy include hyperphosphatemia, hypocalcemia, hypotension, and metastatic calcification (24, 135). Bicarbonate therapy should be withheld unless the arterial pH is less than 7.1, since acidosis is well tolerated in patients with DKA (93). Acidosis shifts the oxygen-hemoglobin dissociation curve to the right (increases tissue oxygenation) and counteracts the effect of lowered 2,3-DPG levels; therefore, rapid correction of the pH may augment tissue hypoxia. In addition, rapid correction of pH with bicarbonate exaggerates hypokalemia and can lead to a paradoxical fall in CNS pH (99). Upon initiation of insulin, AcAc and βOHB are metablized to bicarbonate and thus the pH will correct on its own. If alkali is given, there may be an overshoot and late alkalosis. On the other hand, severe acidosis (pH < 7.1) should also be prevented since it produces cardiovascular, CNS, and respiratory depression. We suggest treating a pH less than 7.1 or a serum bicarbonate level less than 5–7 mEq/liter. Give one ampule of bicarbonate (44 mEq) for a pH less than 7.1 and two ampules of bicarbonate (88 mEq) for a pH less than 7.0. We also recommend checking serum magnesium since hypomagnesemia is common in DKA (due to renal losses and intracellular shift with insulin) and treating with magnesium if it is low (see Chapter 32).

Low-dose intravenous insulin infusion regimens (3–10 U regular insulin/hour) are as effective as high-dose insulin in reducing blood sugar and correcting acidosis in DKA and are associated with a decreased incidence of hypoglycemia, hypokalemia, hypophosphatemia, and hypomagnesium (1, 4, 12, 39, 65, 72, 77). Insulin suppresses glucagon levels, reestablishing hepatic glycogenesis and preventing glycogenolysis. Insulin causes a rise in fructose 2,6-bisphosphate, which blocks hepatic gluconeogenesis and activates hepatic glycolysis. A rise in malonyl CoA inhibits ketogenesis. In adipocytes, insulin inhibits lipolysis and in the periphery insulin increases glucose uptake (Fig. 33.1). The blood glucose falls at a rate of 70–75 mg/dl/hour in most patients with DKA reaching a level of 250 mg/dl in 4–8 hours. Correction of acidosis usually takes 8–12 hours because of the slower metabolism of ketone bodies.

In the critical care setting regular insulin should be given intravenously in the initial phases of therapy. Intramuscular or subcutaneous insulin injections may be poorly and eratically absorbed in the dehydrated patient and may produce undesirable tissue depots. In addition, in the event of complications (i.e., hypokalemia or hypoglycemia) the intravenous infusion can be stopped, allowing for quick reversal of the insulin effect (plasma half-life of 3–5 minutes). Intravenous insulin should be given as a continuous infusion rather than by bolus injection since bolus administration results in stimulation of counterregulatory hormones (5, 127). A loading dose of insulin is also unnecessary in view of the rapid rate at which insulin values reach a plateau

with an infusion (127). Despite this, there may be a theoretical advantage of a small intravenous bolus (4–6 U regular insulin) to saturate insulin receptors. We recommend starting with a continuous infusion of 5–7 U regular insulin per hour (in isotonic saline). In children, a dose of 0.1 U/kg/hour may be used. If serum glucose does not fall by at least 10% each hour the infusion rate should be doubled and the process repeated. In evaluating the effectiveness of the insulin dose remember that blood glucose falls 35–70 mg/dl in the first hour from hydration alone. Patients with DKA may on rare occasions have insulin resistance and require larger doses of insulin. Failure to respond to 5–7 U/hour, however, should suggest infection. The dosages just discussed apply to DKA; however, insulin infusions are also used to treat non-DKA hyperglycemia in critically ill patients. In this latter group, who may be receiving 50% dextrose (in total parenteral nutrition), corticosteroids, or catecholamines, large insulin infusion dosages (>20 U/hour) may be required (18).

Insulin should be diluted with protein-containing solutions (e.g., plasma or albumin) to minimize loss by absorption to glassware and plastic tubing (75, 132). An alternative is to run 50–100 ml of insulin solution (5 U/dl) through the intravenous tubing before connecting it to the patient (105). This infusion will saturate all "insulin binding" sites on the tubing. If this technique is not used or protein is not added, lesser amounts of insulin may be inadvertently administered for the initial 1–2 hours and may contribute to apparent insulin resistance. Apparent loss of insulin effect would also occur when changing intravenous tubing and glassware. We always add 500 mg of albumin to our insulin infusion bottles, which eliminates any concern of insulin binding to tubing or glassware. This small amount of protein costs less than 5 dollars. Once the plasma glucose level reaches 250 mg/dl, the insulin infusion is decreased to 1–3 U/hour and 5% dextrose is administered to maintain a serum glucose concentration of 200–250 mg/dl. The intravenous insulin infusion should be continued until acidosis is corrected, an effect that usually takes twice as long as normalization of the blood glucose. It is important to maintain blood glucose in the 150–200 mg/dl range for 24–48 hours in order to avoid potential complications of cerebral and pulmonary edema and hypoglycemia.

Cerebral edema (35, 91, 139) is a rare complication of DKA. It becomes clinically apparent 6–10 hours after therapy has begun, at a time when severe acidosis has been partially corrected, the blood glucose level is falling, adequate circulation has been restored, and all indications suggest that the patient is recovering satisfactorily. Cerebral edema is believed to result largely from the development of unfavorable osmotic gradients that favor intracellular movement of water (77). During sustained hyperglycemia the brain makes "idiogenic osmoles" that protect it from continued dehydration (9, 63). Cerebral edema develops when the osmotic gradient between brain and plasma exceeds 35 mosm/kg of water. If blood glucose concentration remains above 200–250 mg/dl (with initial values of 800 mg/dl) and the serum osmolality is not reduced faster than 2–3 mosm/kg/hour, the osmolar gradient usually remains below 30 mosm/kg water (63). Thus, it is recommended that blood glucose not be reduced faster than 100 mg/dl/hour or below 200–250 mg/dl during early therapy. The clinical picture of cerebral edema is characterized by deteriorating mental status, abnormal neurologic signs, progression to coma, papilledema, headache, dilated or unequal pupils, hyperpyrexia, and occasionally diabetes inspidus. Respiratory arrest may occur in association with brainstem herniation. Cerebral edema complicating DKA has a mortality rate of about 90%. Treatment with glucocorticoids or mannitol is recommended, although there is little experience with this approach. Subclinical brain swelling is felt to be common during treatment of DKA (76), even though most patients fail to develop symptoms of cerebral edema.

Pulmonary edema (128) also results from unfavorable osmotic gradients and may cause hypoxia in over 50% of those treated for DKA (59). Supplemental use of oxygen should be administered to these patients. Volume loading with crystalloid produces an acute hypooncotic state and may contribute to the development of pulmonary and cerebral edema (5). Most instances appear to be subclinical.

Stupor and coma in DKA correlate best with osmolality and not acidosis (44, 45). If the plasma osmolality does not exceed 340–350 mosm/liter, other causes of coma should be sought. Plasma osmolality (mosm/liter) may be measured directly or calculated as: $P_{osm} = \{2 \times [Na^+ + K^+ \ mEq/liter]\} + glucose \ (mg/dl)/18 + BUN(mg/dl)/2.8$ (normal = 285–300 mosm/liter).

To minimize wide swings in the blood glucose concentrations during intravenous insulin therapy, the carbohydrate substrate should be fixed at a given rate. To avoid intermittent boluses of dextrose, all intravenous additives should be in saline. By fixing carbohydrate substrate while infusing insulin, one can achieve a glucose "clamp" and avoid hypoglycemia and hyperglycemia.

The endpoint in the therapy of DKA is attainment of a desirable blood glucose level (usually 150–250 mg/dl) and correction of acidosis. A blood glucose in this range offers protection from sudden drops in glucose, which may cause hypoglycemia. Based on the volume of the glucose space (approximately that of extracellular fluid) and rate of glucose decline, it is possible to approximate the rate of glucose administration. For example, in a 70–kg individual (glucose space = 21 liters) with a glucose disappearance rate of 100 mg/dl/hour the rate of glucose administration is 21 g/hour.

If staffing is short or close monitoring of the rate of intravenous insulin infusion cannot be achieved, it can be administered intramuscularly (half-life of 2 hours) or subcutaneously (half-life of 4 hours) (1, 39, 72). However, the initial decline in glucose and ketones will be slower in the first 2 hours when compared with intravenous insulin (39). Both of these routes carry the risk of erratic absorption (especially if dehydrated) and tissue depot accumulation (which can lead to late hypoglycemia). Another potential problem is the injection site. Injections into the buttocks can give variable absorption as a result of underperfusion (especially in supine patients). If intravenous administration is impossible or impractical, we suggest following the practice of Kitabchi et al. (72) and giving injections into the deltoid. We recommend giving 0.3 U regular insulin per kilogram initially, then 5–10 U regular insulin intramuscularly or subcutaneously hourly until the blood glucose level is less than 250 mg/dl. At that point switch fluids to D_5NS, $D_5\frac{1}{2}NS$, or D_5W (glucose clamp) and continue intramuscular or subcutaneous insulin at 2–4 hour intervals until acidosis resolves.

The response to treatment (e.g., normalization of plasma glucose, electrolytes, arterial blood gases, hemodynamic and mental status) must be monitored carefully (at least hourly) and therapy adjusted accordingly. We follow blood glucose at the bedside using Chemstrip bG (Biodynamics) blood glucose test strips (23, 143) and find them to accurately reflect the measured serum glucose levels. Urine glucose

Day	NPH Insulin	Regular Insulin	(Sliding Scale)
1	24 U NPH s.c. at 0600 AM; continue insulin infusion for 4–6 hours following NPH	0600 AM 1200 1800 PM 2400	4 U 0 U 6 U 4 U 14 U/2 = 7 U
2	24 U + 7 U = 31 U NPH s.c. at 0600 AM	0600 AM 1200 1800 PM 2400	4 U 0 U 4 U 0 U 8 U/2 = 4 U
3	31 U + 4 U = 35 U NPH s.c. at 0600 AM	0600 AM 1200 1800 PM 2400	0 U 0 U 0 U 0 U 0 U
4	35 U NPH at 0600 AM		

Figure 33.2. Adjustment of NPH insulin. Patient receiving continuous insulin infusion at 2 U/hour (48 U/day).

is inaccurate in estimating the serum glucose concentration in many patients (142).

As soon as the DKA is under control NPH insulin is begun and is supplemented with regular insulin given subcutaneously according to a sliding scale (Fig. 33.2). The insulin infusion is continued for 4–6 hours after the NPH insulin is given to keep the insulin receptors saturated, thereby preventing rebound hyperglycemia. We begin the subcutaneous NPH insulin by giving half of the patient's previous daily maintenance dose. Supplemental regular insulin is given at 6-hour intervals depending on plasma glucose. We increase the next day's NPH insulin by half the amount of supplemental regular insulin used in the preceding 24 hours (Fig. 33.2). There is a tremendous variability in the total dose of insulin required by any patient, depending on whether one is dealing with a type I or type II diabetic; the presence of insulin-binding antibodies; the patient's diet, activity level, and stress state; and other factors (34). Most newly diagnosed type I diabetics require approximately 0.5 U/kg/day, whereas established type I diabetics usually require 0.6–0.7 U/kg/day. Some patients may be controlled on a single dose of intermediate-acting insulin per day (with or without concomitant short acting insulin); others require twice-daily injections of intermediate/short-acting insulin. Dosage decisions are based upon fasting and postprandial serum or blood glucose concentrations. Patients who eat three meals during the day and who require multiple insulin injections usually require two-thirds of their total insulin dose before breakfast and one-third of their insulin dose before supper (34).

There is usually no need to give less than 3–4 U regular insulin per hour during the initial few hours of DKA therapy. Use of too little insulin may be dangerous by delaying correction of metabolic abnormalities. Doses below 2.4 U regular insulin per hour have not been found to correct metabolic derangements with acceptable rapidity (106, 123) and if insulin resistance is present such doses are insufficient (37). Maximal biologic effect of insulin requires serum insulin concentrations in the 100–200 μU/ml range (124, 127). This level is usually obtained with an insulin infusion rate of approximately 0.1 U/kg/hour.

Treatment of DKA must not be confined to correction of biochemical abnormalities alone. Precipitating factors and complications must be sought and treated. Common precipitating factors include infection, myocardial infarction, pancreatitis, and discontinuance of insulin therapy. Shock may develop as a consequence of hypovolemia and reduced myocardial contractility. Cerebral and pulmonary edema were discussed previously. Diffuse intravascular coagulation is also being increasingly recognized (5).

HYPERGLYCEMIC HYPEROSMOLAR NONKETOTIC SYNDROME

The hyperglycemic hyperosmolar nonketotic-syndrome (HHNS) typically develops in middle-aged and elderly patients in the setting of previously mild, non-insulin-dependent (type II) diabetes mellitus or as the first manifestation of diabetes (8, 53, 71, 108, 129). The syndrome can also occur in nondiabetic patients as a complication of extensive burns, heat stroke, myocardial or cerebral infarction, acute pancreatitis, infections, surgery, thyrotoxicosis, trauma, and acromegaly (71). In addition, it may occur in association with dialysis or intravenous hyperalimentation. Mortality is between 5 and 40%. Most patients experience polydipsia and polyuria during a prodromal phase of several days to a few weeks, culminating in severe dehydration and altered consciousness. The syndrome most frequently occurs in older patients in whom an intercurrent illness increases glucose production (from stress hormones) and impairs the capacity to ingest fluids. Drugs most frequently associated with the syndrome include thiazide diuretics, phenytoin, corticosteroids, cimetidine, furosemide, propranolol, chlorpromazine, and L-asparaginase (see "Drug Interactions"). The pathophysiology involves an imbalance between glucose production and its excretion in the urine. Maximal hepatic production of glucose results in a plateau of plasma glucose in the 400–500 mg/dl range provided urine output is maintained. Severe hyperglycemia results when there is renal impairment (progressive glucose accumulation due to impaired renal glucose excretion) and dehydration (8, 53, 67, 129). The exact mechanism by which ketoacidosis is suppressed despite extreme hyperglycemia is unknown but appears to result from impaired lipolysis and liver ketogenesis. Joffe and associates (66) suggest that the syndrome occurs because the liver is insulinized while the periphery is diabetic. Others have postulated a defect in ketone synthesis within the liver.

Symptoms (Table 33.8) last longer (12 days) than in DKA (3 days) (53, 71). Transient, focal neurologic signs may occur (84) and occasionally the patient is misdiagnosed as having had a stroke. Some patients present with seizures since hyperosmolality may activate epileptogenic foci (71). It is important to recognize the hyperosmolar nature of the etiology since treatment with phenytoin may be hazardous since it impairs insulin release. The depressed sensorium parallels the hyperosmolarity and requires prompt treatment (108). Therapeutic delay is a primary cause of mortality (8). Osmolarity may be measured by the freezing point depression technique or calculated and values above 350 mosm/liter are typically seen. Hy-

Table 33.8
Clinical Features of Hyperglycemic Hyperosmolar Nonketotic Syndrome

General
  Polydipsia, polyuria
  Dehydration
  Gastric distension
  Hyperthermia
  Ileus
Neurological
  Seizures
  Mental obtundation (lethargy to coma)
  Focal neurologic signs (hemiparesis, unilateral
    hyperreflexia, aphasia, hemianopsia)
Cardiovascular
  Hypotension, shock
  Thromboses
Respiratory
  Tachypnea (no Kussmaul breathing)
Laboratory Findings
  Hyperglycemia (>600 mg/dl)
  Hyperosmolality (>350 mosm/l)
  Azotemia (BUN 70–90 mg/dl)
  Absent or mild ketonemia
  Glycosuria (4+)
  Acidosis (lactate)
  Hemoconcentration

perglycemia is usually severe, with levels as high as 4800 mg/dl recorded. Total absence of ketonuria is not essential, but when present it is mild and may result from starvation. Patients are severely dehydrated on presentation despite adequate (> 0.5 ml/kg/hr) urine output due to the glucosuria-induced osmotic diuresis. The serum sodium concentration may be low, normal, or elevated when the patient is admitted. However, one must remember that serum sodium is lowered by about 1.5 mEq/liter for each 100 mg/dl of glucose above normal. The hematocrit is usually elevated as a result of hemoconcentration. Nearly all HHNS patients present with azotemia, which may be of both renal and prerenal origin. A metabolic acidosis is often present with a large anion gap. Unmeasured anions are thought to result from lactate, renal insufficiency, and other unidentified organic acids.

Therapy of HHNS (Table 33.9) is aimed at correction of the volume depletion and metabolic abnormalities (e.g., hyperosmolarity) and detection of precipitating factors. The first priority is immediate restoration of intravascular volume, which is accomplished with 0.9% saline. Once hypotension is abolished, hypotonic saline should be given to replace free water losses. The glucose-induced osmotic diuresis results in large urinary losses of both water and electrolytes.

Table 33.9
Treatment of Hyperglycemic Hyperosmolar
Nonketotic Syndrome

Fluids
 Restore intravascular volume with isotonic saline,
 then

 Give 2–3 liters hypotonic saline (0.45%) in first 2
 hours followed by one-half of the body water deficit
 [0.25 × total body water (kg) + urinary losses]
 over the next 12 hour; give the remainder of the
 body water deficit over the next 24 hour; central
 hemodynamic monitoring may be required in
 elderly or in those with cardiac or renal disease.
Insulin
 Begin with i.v. infusion of 5–7 U regular insulin per
 hour (in hypotonic saline). When serum glucose
 drops to 250 mg/dl switch fluid to D_5W and
 decrease infusion rate of regular insulin to 1–3
 U/hour (glucose clamp technique). Maintain
 infusion for 24–36 hours. Increase infusion rate if
 glucose does not fall by 10%/hour.
Alternative
 5–7 U regular insulin i.m. or s.c. per hour; when
 glucose drops to 250 mg/dl continue i.m. or s.c.
 injections at 2–4 hour intervals using glucose
 clamp.
Potassium
 Give 15–20 mEq/hour; if oliguiric, give 5–10
 mEq/hour; if K^+ above 6 mEq/liter stop infusion of
 K^+; if K^+ below 4 mEq/liter, increase infusion rate.
 Use continuous ECG monitoring.
Phosphorus
 Oral: Neutra-Phos 250 mg every 6 hours
    i.v.: potassium phosphate
 0.08–0.16 mmol/kg/6 hours.
Bicarbonate
 If arterial pH <7.1 or bicarbonate <5–7 mEq/liter,
 give one ampule bicarbonate (44 mEq); if pH
 <7.0, give two ampules bicarbonate (88 mEq);
 monitor arterial or venous pH hourly.
Magnesium
 If less than 1.2 mg/dl give:
    p.o.: Mg oxide 35 meq Q6–24 hour
    i.v.: $MgSO_4$ or $MgCl_2$ 20–80 meq/day
 Monitor serum glucose (Chemstrip bG),
 electrolytes, arterial blood gas, anion gap, and
 hemodynamic and mental status.

Contraction of intravascular volume is partially compensated for by movement of intracellular and interstitial fluid and electrolytes into the intravascular space. The result is a contraction of the intracellular compartment and depletion of sodium, potassium, phosphorus, and magnesium. Balance studies suggest that the fluid lost in HHNS contains about 60 mEq/liter of sodium plus potassium (8), which closely approximates half-normal saline. Use of isotonic saline and isotonic glucose are associated with higher mortality rates (108).

We assume that the patient with HHNS is about 25% total body water depleted on presentation (8). Using the patient's usual weight, we estimate the body water deficit (mean total body water in elderly patients is about 50% of body weight in kilograms). We administer half of the estimated water deficit as 0.45% saline (including urinary losses) in the first 12 hours and the remainder in the next 24 hours. We usually give 2–3 liters of 0.45% saline over the first 2 hours followed by one-half the body water deficit over the next 12 hours. Usual deficits range from 6 to 18 liters of fluid (8, 53, 108). Water can abruptly shift into cells as the plasma glucose concentration falls. Patients must be observed closely and adjustments in the rate of fluid administration made as indicated. Dangers inherent in aggressive fluid therapy (especially in the elderly) can be reduced with central hemodynamic monitoring.

Patients with HHNS are depleted of potassium, phosphorous, and magnesium (see "Diabetic Ketoacidosis"). Hypokalemia in patients who have just been admitted indicates severe depletion and is occasionally associated with acute quadriplegia (85). The potassium requirements in the first 36 hours usually average 200–300 mEq (8, 108). Precipitous falls in serum potassium occur as a result of hemodilution, insulin therapy, correction of acidosis, and continued urinary losses. If the patient is hyperkalemic we withhold potassium therapy until the serum potassium concentration normalizes. Otherwise we give 10–20 mEq of potassium per hour, mostly as the chloride and to a lesser degree as the phosphate salt. The potassium replacement dose is reduced by 50% if the patient is oliguric. Further therapy with phosphorus, magnesium, and bicarbonate are the same as for DKA.

Intravenous regular insulin should be administered by continuous infusion. Patients with HHNS are usually more sensitive to insulin than those with DKA and therefore less total insulin is required. We begin the insulin infusion at 5–7 U/hour (mixed in hypotonic saline) and taper accordingly (see "Diabetic Ketoacidosis"). When the blood glucose concentration reaches 250–300 mg/dl, the intravenous fluid is switched to D_5W and the insulin infusion rate decreased to 1–3 U/hour. A glucose clamp is established and maintained for 24–36 hours to avoid the possibility of cerebral edema. The endpoint of the initial therapy is correction of hyperglycemia, normalization of serum osmolality (to less than 310 mosm/liter), and stabilization of the hemodynamic status (e.g., urine output and blood pressure). The change from intravenous to subcutaneous insulin is similar to that for DKA. Complications of therapy include hypokalemia, hypophosphatemia, hypomagnesemia, hypoglycemia, cerebral edema, pulmonary edema (from aggressive fluid resuscitation and unfavorable osmotic gradients), and rarely intravascular hemolysis. As in DKA, careful monitoring of the plasma glucose and electrolytes, ECG, and hemodynamic status are essential.

ALCOHOLIC KETOACIDOSIS

Alcoholic ketoacidosis is seen in the setting of recently discontinued heavy alcohol use (43, 57, 77, 80, 92). Differentiation from DKA with a low blood glucose may be difficult (especially if it occurs in a known diabetic). Typically, these patients are chronic alcoholics with diminished food intake. There is usually little or no ethanol in the blood at the time of presentation. The mechanism responsible for alcoholic ketoacidosis is only partially understood. Ethanol is metabolized by alcohol dehydrogenase to acetaldehyde which is metabolized to acetly-CoA. The process generates reduced nicotinamide adenine dinucleotide (NADH) from NAD$^+$. Gluconeogenesis is impaired because this process requires NAD$^+$. When glycogen is exhausted, hypoglycemia results. The resultant low insulin state promotes lipolysis and ketogenesis. A "reduced" environment also inhibits the tricarboxylic acid cycle and favors the formation of lactate instead of pyruvate and βOHB instead of AcAc, contributing to acidosis. A variety of lipolytic hormones are released, possibly due to the hypoglycemia that results from inhibited gluconeogenesis and depleted glycogen stores. Released growth hormone, cortisol, glucagon, and catecholamines increase the availability of free fatty acids, which results in the formation of ketones. Low blood insulin levels, as well as alcohol itself, augment the ketotic state. The final result is augmented hepatic ketogenesis and decreased peripheral ketone utilization.

When metabolic acidosis occurs in an alcoholic with high blood alcohol concentrations it is likely to be lactic acidosis. However, when it occurs in the presence of falling, low, or absent blood ethanol concentrations, the acidosis is usually due to alcoholic ketoacidosis (77).

Patients with alcoholic ketoacidosis present with normal or altered mental status, tachycardia, tachypnea, dehydration, and signs of alcohol abuse (e.g., hepatomegaly, jaundice, and portal hypertension). Laboratory studies show a metabolic acidosis (mean anion gap 25 mEq/liter) with ketosis. The arterial pH is usually less than 7.20. The predominant ketone in this condition is βOHB and thus the nitroprusside reaction underestimates the degree of ketosis. Blood glucose concentrations vary from hypoglycemia ($\leq$ 50 mg/dl) to mild hyperglycemia (300 mg/dl). Blood ethanol is usually absent and most patients have azotemia and hemoconcentration due to dehydration. Patients may also have elevated serum transaminases, alkaline phosphatase, bilirubin, and amylase. Management (38, 57, 80, 92) consists of replacement of intravascular volume, in addition to the administration of glucose, electrolytes, and thiamine (100 mg administered intravenously). In diabetics or in patients with hyperglycemia, insulin may also be required (38, 57, 80, 92). Sodium bicarbonate is given only if the pH is less than 7.10. Glucose stimulates phosphorylation of ADP to ATP and reduces lactate production. The intracellular availability of glucose and thiamine produces NADPH via the pentose phosphate shunt. NADPH, in turn, decreases fatty acid metabolism to ketones. During correction of alcoholic ketoacidosis there is a decrease in the serum potassium, phosphate, and magnesium concentrations. Hypophosphatemia (92) results from phosphaturia and phosphate utilization in metabolic processes.

CARE OF THE DIABETIC SURGICAL PATIENT

Preoperative evaluation of the diabetic includes identification of other underlying diseases (58, 134). Such patients frequently have coronary artery disease, a major cause of perioperative mortality, and peripheral vascular disease. Those with renal disease require careful fluid and electrolyte management and adjustment of drug dosages. Some diabetics have autonomic neuropathy that may predispose them to respiratory depression, cardiac arrest, urinary retention, and postural hypotension (101). Diabetics often have an increased risk of infection and poor wound healing.

Cardiac bypass surgery may present special problems for the diabetic (69). The bypass pump may have glucose-containing fluids and as a result patients may receive up to 500 g of extra glucose during surgery. In addition, hypothermia and use of sympathomimetic drugs cause insulin resistance.

The objective of the management of diabetes before, during, and after operations is to prevent excessive hyperglycemia and glycosuria, to prevent ketosis and to prevent hypoglycemia. Prior to surgery the diabetic's blood glucose level should be well controlled (150–200 mg/dl range) and the patient should be free of acidemia (58). The patient should not have symptoms of polydipsia, polyuria, or hypoglycemia. Slight hyperglycemia is desirable to protect against hypoglycemia during surgery. Electrolyte concentrations and volume status should also be normalized.

For minor surgery, in the diet-controlled diabetic in good glycemic control, no insulin therapy is required. Glucose-containing solutions should be avoided and if control deteriorates, insulin can be given. In patients taking oral hypoglycemic agents, stop the medication 3 days prior to surgery. If glycemic control is good on diet alone, no insulin is required for minor surgery. If glucose control becomes poor or major surgery is required, insulin may be needed.

In the diabetic undergoing major surgery or in insulin-dependent diabetics, the combined administration of glucose-insulin-potassium is often effective (84) (Table 33.10). Intravenous glucose is needed to avoid starvation ketosis. Patients are stabilized preoperatively on twice-daily subcutaneous injections of insulin, with only regular insulin (every 6 hours) being given on the day prior to surgery. No subcutaneous insulin is given on the day of surgery. On the morning of surgery, an insulin infusion at 2–

3 U regular insulin per hour with 100 ml/hour of 10% dextrose and 2 mEq potassium chloride per hour is begun and continued until the patient resumes oral feeding and subcutaneous insulin. Glucose, electrolytes, and ketones are monitored at 2–3 hour intervals and intravenous insulin adjusted accordingly. Insulin requirements are increased with infection and decreased in patients undergoing adrenalectomy, hypophysectomy, and postdelivery.

An alternative form of perioperative therapy includes the use of subcutaneous insulin and intravenous glucose. Patients are stabilized on subcutaneous injections of regular insulin (6, 69). On the operative day, oral carbohydrate is replaced with an equivalent amount of 5% or 10% dextrose by intravenous infusion. Insulin therapy (regular) is given by subcutaneous injection every 6 hours. Additional perioperative insulin is given intramuscularly or intravenously as needed, and electrolytes are replaced as required.

Another method for managing the diabetic in the perioperative period is to give one-half of the usual dose of insulin (NPH + Reg) as NPH on the morning of surgery and to cover the patient with a short-acting insulin at frequent intervals. We give regular insulin by the subcutaneous route (every 4–6 hours) or intravenous route (every 1–2 hours). However, one must remember that subcutaneous insulin may be poorly absorbed in the perioperative period. Hypoglycemia is prevented by intravenous administration of dextrose.

The most important factor in managing the diabetic in the perioperative period is careful and frequent monitoring. Blood glucose must be monitored (every 2–3 hours) so as to avoid marked hyperglycemia or hypoglycemia. This step is particularly important in the early perioperative period when counterregulatory hormones are elevated. We use Chemstrip bG blood glucose test strips (23, 143) for rapid evaluation of blood glucose and find them to be more reliable than urine glucose measurements. The renal threshold for glucose may be elevated (due to renal insufficiency) and lead to an underestimation of blood glucose (143). In addition, a number of drugs interfere with urine measurements. For Clinitest, Clinistix, or Diastix these include cephalosporins, chloramphenicol, tetracycline, sulfonamides, and salicylates. Ketones should also be monitored (every 4–6 hours) so as to avoid ketoacidosis. Albumin or blood should be added to insulin infusions to avoid adsorption to glassware and plastic tubing (see "Diabetic Ketoacidosis").

Table 33.10
Glucose-Insulin-Potassium During Surgery

Preoperative
  Switch to twice daily s.c. insulin; give short-acting insulin only on day prior to surgery (every 6 hours).
Operation
  Begin i.v. infusion of 100 ml D_{10} plus 2–3 U regular insulin plus 2–3 mEq K per hour on morning of surgery. Monitor glucose and K^+ at 2–3 hour intervals and readjust as required. Use Chemstrip bG for quick evaluation of blood glucose.
Postoperative
  Continue glucose-insulin-potassium until oral feeding is resumed. Check glucose and electrolytes at 4- to 6-hour intervals. When feeding resumed, return to preoperative s.c. insulin.

Hypoglycemia during surgery is uncommon with these regimens since the stress of surgery leads to hyperglycemia because of the action of counterregulatory hormones.

INSULIN-INFUSION PUMP THERAPY

Two types of insulin-infusion pumps exist for improvement of diabetic control (48, 96, 117, 118): closed loop systems (artificial pancreas), in which the rate of insulin administration is controlled by changes in plasma glucose, and open loop systems, in which predetermined amounts of insulin are administered on the basis of previous estimates of insulin requirement. In the critically ill patient with fluctuating metabolic status a closed loop system would be required. At present, these units are large, bulky, expensive, and have not been shown to be superior to continuous intravenous insulin infusion therapy for short-term diabetic control.

TOTAL PARENTERAL NUTRITION

Serum glucose should not exceed 150–200 mg/dl during total parenteral nutrition (TPN) to allow for maximal cellular glucose utilization. Glucosuria should be prevented since it produces an osmotic diuresis (with loss of fluid and electrolytes) and calorie loss. Glucosuria also prevents the clinician from using urine output as an index of tissue perfusion. As TPN is started, the pancreas responds by increasing insulin secretion. Exogenous insulin is required when the rate of glucose administration exceeds the ability of the pancreas to respond. In some patients, insulin administration may be reduced after 3–6 days as endogenous insulin secretion becomes adequate and insulin resistance (e.g., malnutrition, stress, or infection) decreases (60). Sudden discontinuation of TPN may cause hypoglycemia because of high rates of endogenous insulin secretion, and thus TPN should be tapered as oral intake increases or intravenous dextrose should be administered. To avoid large fluctuations in blood glucose, exogenous insulin should be administered by continuous infusion in the parenteral nutrition fluid. We recommend following the schedule of Grant (60) by adding regular insulin to parenteral nutrition fluid based upon the blood glucose level (Table 33.11). Blood glucose is monitored and additional insulin added as required (see

Table 33.11
Initial Insulin Requirements for Parenteral Nutrition

Blood Glucose (mg/dl)	Regular Insulin (U/250 g dextrose)
<120	0
120–150	6–10
150–200	10–20
>200	21 (or more)

Chapter 44). Insulin requirements may vary from 5 to 40 U/hour and at very high rates of dextrose administration normoglycemia may be unobtainable (due to down-regulation of insulin receptors). Decreasing the infusion rate may allow for return of insulin sensitivity. Insulin, as an anabolic hormone, may also help the severely catabolic patient convert from negative to positive nitrogen balance.

DRUG INTERACTIONS

A number of drugs affect insulin secretion or action (Table 33.12). Prostaglandin E (PgE) inhibits insulin secretion (55, 89, 121). Furosemide, by stimulating PgE, inhibits insulin secretion; whereas tolbutamide, phentolamine, and salicylates stimulate insulin secretion by inhibiting PgE synthesis (22, 55, 56, 89, 121). Thiazides, phenytoin, α-adrenergic receptor agonists (e.g., norepinephrine and epinephrine), verapamil, somatostatin, dopamine, diazoxide, and propranolol decrease insulin secretion (19, 41, 51, 109–113, 122).

A variety of agents interfere with peripheral insulin action (Table 33.12). Corticosteroids decrease hepatic and extrahepatic insulin sensitivity (119) enhancing gluconeogenesis while they decrease peripheral glucose utilization by decreasing the insulin receptor concentration (31). In addition, estrogens, growth hormone, and L-asparaginase (20) also decrease insulin binding to insulin receptors. Sulfonylureas increase insulin secretion and receptor binding (100). Sulfonylureas cross the placenta and stimulate hypersecretion of insulin in neonates. Neonates of mothers receiving these agents require intravenous glucose for 3–4 days after delivery to prevent hypoglycemia.

In hyperthyroidism there is decreased insulin sensitivity (133), whereas in endotoxemia there is increased sensitivity as well as decreased gluconeogenesis (38). These effects of endotoxemia are responsible for the hypoglycemia occasionally seen with sepsis. In sep-

Table 33.12
Insulin-Drug Interactions

Inhibit Insulin Secretion
  Prostaglandin E (furosemide)
  Thiazides
  Phenytoin
  Diazoxide
  α-Adrenergic agonists
  Propranolol
  Verapamil
  Somatostatin
  Dopamine
Suppress Insulin Action or Increase Insulin
    Requirements
  Glucocorticoids
  Oral contraceptives
  L-Asparaginase
  Growth hormone
  Obesity
  Pregnancy
  Infection
  Hyperthyroidism
  Hyperadrenocorticism
Stimulate Insulin Secretion
  Sulfonylureas
  Phentolamine
  Prostaglandin inhibitors
  Glucagon
  β-Adrenergic agonists
Potentiate Insulin Action or Decrease Insulin
    Requirements
  Sulfonylureas
  Clonidine
  Dicumarol
  Terramycin
  Monoamine oxidase inhibitors
  Endotoxin
  Weight loss
  Exercise
  Renal insufficiency
  Hypothyroidism
  Hypoadrenocorticism

sis, antagonism of insulin by dexamethasone and ATP improves survival (38). Ethanol enhances insulin action (137) by impairing gluconeogenesis and secretion of counterregulatory hormones. In renal insufficiency and malnutrition, decreased gluconeogenesis and slowed insulin degradation contribute to enhanced insulin effect (104).

ORAL HYPOGLYCEMIC AGENTS

A variety of oral agents (Table 33.13) are available for the treatment of diabetes mellitus which stimulate insulin secretion and improve insulin action. Sulfonylurea drugs are the only oral agents available in the United States. These agents are well absorbed from the gastrointestinal tract (125) and peak levels occur at 1–4 hours after ingestion.

Sulfonylurea compounds (Table 33.13) acutely stimulate the islet tissue to secrete insulin and are primarily effective in patients who retain the capacity to secrete insulin (e.g., type II diabetes mellitus). However, during chronic therapy a significant portion of their hypoglycemic action results from increases in the number of insulin receptors and postreceptor effects (49, 125). Sulfonylureas act synergistically with insulin to enhance glucose disposal with little effect on glucose production. Sulfonylureas are ineffective in type I insulin-dependent diabetes mellitus and in pancreatectomized animals, suggesting that their major mechanism of action is dependent upon β cell function. The most important differences among the sulfonylureas, for clinical purposes, are their different potencies, duration of action (34, 49, 78, 125, 130), and metabolism.

These drugs are relatively contraindicated in patients with type I diabetes mellitus; in patients during pregnancy or lactation; in patients with hepatic or renal disease, because of the importance of the liver in metabolizing these drugs and kidney in excreting them; in patients with known allergy to sulfa drugs; and during stressful conditions in diabetics (such as during infection, myocardial infarc-

Table 33.13
Sulfonyluria Oral Hypoglycemic Agents

	Tolbutamide	Acetohexamide	Tolazamide	Chlorpropamide	Glipizide	Glyburide
Relative Potency	1	2.5	5	5	100	150
Duration (hr)	6–8	8–12	12–18	24–72	12–18	16–24
Daily dose	0.5–3 g	0.25–1.5 g	0.1–1 g	0.1–0.5 g	2.5–30 mg	1.25–20 mg
Doses per day	2–3	1–2	1–2	1	1–2	1–2
Inactivation	Hepatic	Renal	Hepatic	Hepatic/Renal	Hepatic	Hepatic
Diuretic	Yes	Yes	Yes	No	No	Yes
Antidiuretic	Yes?	No	No	Yes	No	No
Antabuse effect	No	No	No	Yes	No	No
Frequency of hypoglycemia	Rare	<1%	<1%	2–3%	3–5%	4–6%

Table 33.14
Drugs That Alter the Effect of Oral Hypoglycemic Agents

Potentiate	Antagonize
Alcohol	Chronic ethanolism
Anabolic steroids	Corticosteroids
β-Adrenergic blockers	Diazoxide
Bishydroxycoumarin	Estrogens
Chloramphenicol	Furosemide
Clofibrate[a]	Nicotinic acid
Cyclophosphamide	Phenytoin (decreased
Diphenylhydantoin[a]	insulin)
Guanethidine	Rifampin
Halofenate	Thiazides
Methysergide	Thyroid hormone
Monoamine oxidase	
inhibitors	
Oral anticoagulants	
Oxyphenbutazone[a]	
Phenylbutazone[a]	
Salicylates[a]	
Sulfonamides	
Tetracyclines	

[a] Decrease binding to plasma proteins

tion, or surgery, when the ability to increase insulin secretion is diminished).

The major complication from sulfonylurea drugs is hypoglycemia (49, 125). Hypoglycemic episodes may last for several days because of the long duration of action of these drugs, and prolonged or repeated glucose administration may be required. Chlorpropamide and tolbutamide potentiate antidiuretic hormone action in the kidney and may cause water retention and hyponatremia. They may also cause an antabuse-like reaction. Sulfonylurea drugs have also been associated with a small incidence of hematologic (leukopenia, pancytopenia, and bone marrow depression), cutaneous, endocrine (e.g., hypothyroidism) and gastrointestinal (e.g., cholestatic jaundice and nausea) side effects. Drugs that may potentiate the action of sulfonylurea drugs (Table 33.14) are alcohol, β-adrenergic blockers, monoamine oxidase inhibitors, phenylbutazone, oxyphenbutazone, clofibrate, bishydroxycoumarin, sulfonamides, salicylates, and diphenylhydantoin (34, 78, 125). Drugs that may antagonize the action of sulfonylureas are thiazide and loop diuretics, estrogens, and corticosteroids (34).

Most authorities feel that there is little indication for use of sulfonylureas together with insulin. However, some patients may not respond well to insulin because of severe resistance. Such patients may show better glucose regulation using a combination of insulin and

sulfonylureas (7, 82). Allen et al. (7) treated six patients with non-insulin-dependent diabetes mellitus and insulin resistance with combination insulin-glipizide therapy. Four patients had considerable improvement in glycemic control when the sulfonylurea was added to their insulin treatment program. We have used combined sulfonylurea-insulin therapy on occasion to treat severely stressed (e.g., sepsis or trauma) non-insulin-dependent diabetics in the ICU who demonstrated resistance to infusions of insulin and have also noted improvement in their glycemic control.

References

1. Alberti KGMM: Low dose insulin in the treatment of diabetic ketoacidosis. *Arch Intern Med* 137:1367, 1977.
2. Alberti KGMM, Darley JH, Emerson PM, et al: 2,3-Diphosphoglycerate and tissue oxygenation in uncontrolled diabetes mellitus. *Lancet* 2:391, 1972.
3. Alberti KGMM, Hockaday TDR: Diabetic coma, a reappraisal after five years. *Clin Endocrinol Metab* 6:421, 1977.
4. Alberti KGMM, Hockaday TDR, Turner RC: Small doses of intramuscular insulin in the treatment of diabetic "coma." *Lancet* 2:515, 1973.
5. Alberti KGMM, Nattrass M: Severe diabetic ketoacidosis. *Med Clin North Am* 62:799, 1978.
6. Alberti KGMM, Thomas DJB: The management of diabetes during surgery. *Br J Anaesth* 51:663, 1979.
7. Allen BT, Feinglos MN, Lebovitz HE: Treatment of poorly regulated non-insulin-dependent diabetes mellitus with combination insulin-sulfonylurea. *Arch Intern Med* 145:1900, 1985.
8. Arieff AI, Carroll HJ: Nonketotic hyperosmolar coma with hyperglycemia: clinical features, pathophysiology, renal function, acid-base balance, plasma-cerebrospinal fluid equilibria and the effects of therapy in 37 cases. *Medicine* 51:73, 1972.
9. Arieff AI, Kleeman CR: Studies on mechanisms of cerebral edema in diabetic comas. *J Clin Invest* 52:571, 1973.
10. Bar RS, Roth J: Insulin receptor status in disease states in man. *Arch Intern Med* 137:474, 1977.
11. Beigelman PM: Potassium in severe diabetic ketoacidosis. *Am J Med* 54:119, 1973.
12. Bendezu R, Wieland RG, Furst BH, et al: Experience with low-dose insulin infusion in diabetic ketoacidosis and diabetic hyperosmolarity. *Arch Intern Med* 138:60, 1978.
13. Berger M, Cuppers HJ, Halban PA, et al: The effect of aprotinin on the absorption of subcutaneously injected insulin in normal subjects. *Diabetes* 29:81, 1980.
14. Bowman HM, Cowan D, Kovach G, et al: Renal effects of glucagon in rhesus monkeys during hypovolemia. *Surg Gynecol Obstet* 134:937, 1972.
15. Brown JC: Gastrointestinal hormones and the control of insulin secretion. *Diabetes* 27:782, 1977.
16. Brownlee M: Insulin treatment in diabetes. *Hosp Pract* April:85, 1979.
17. Bucholtz HK: Insulin allergy: an approach to therapy. *South Med J* 69:1118, 1976.
18. Byrne WJ, Lippe BM, Strobel CT, et al: Adaptation to increasing loads of total parenteral nutrition: metabolic, endocrine, and insulin responses. *Gastroenterology* 80:947, 1981.
19. Campbell IW, Duncan LJP, Innes JA, et al: Abdominal

pain in diabetic metabolic decompensation. Clinical significance. *JAMA* 233:166,1975.

20. Carpenturi U, Balch MT: Hyperglycemia associated with the therapeutic use of L-asparaginase: possible role of insulin receptors. *J Pediatr* 93:775, 1978.
21. Carter WP: Hypothermia—a sign of hypoglycemia. *JACEP* 5:594, 1976.
22. Chen M, Robertson RP: Restoration of the acute insulin responses by sodium salicylate. *Diabetes* 27:750, 1978.
23. Chernow B, Diaz M, Cruess D, et al: Bedside blood glucose determinations in critical care medicine: a comparative analysis of two techniques. *Crit Care Med* 10:463, 1982.
24. Chernow B, Rainey TG, Georges LP, et al: Iatrogenic hyperphosphatemia: a metabolic consideration in critical care medicine. *Crit Care Med* 9:772, 1981.
25. Cockel R, Mann S: Insulin allergy treated by low-dosage hydrocortisone. *Br Med J* 3:722, 1967.
26. Cruetzfeldt W: The incretin concept. *Diabetologia* 19:74, 1979.
27. Davidson JK, Galloway JA, Peterson BH, et al: The use of purified insulins in insulin allergy. *Diabetes* 23(Suppl 1):352, 1974.
28. Davidson JK, DeBra DW: Immunologic insulin resistance. *Diabetes* 27:307, 1978.
29. DeFronzo RA, Hendler R, Christensen N: Stimulation of counter-regulatory hormonal responses in diabetic man by a fall in glucose concentration. *Diabetes* 29:125, 1980.
30. DeFronzo RA, Lang R: Hypophosphatemia and glucose intolerance: evidence for tissue insensitivity to insulin. *N Engl J Med* 303:1259, 1980.
31. DePirro R, Bertoli A, Fusco A, et al: Effect of dexamethasone and cortisone on insulin receptors in normal human male. *J Clin Endocrinol Metab* 51:503, 1980.
32. Ditzel J: Importance of plasma inorganic phosphate on tissue oxygenation during recovery from diabetic ketoacidosis. *Horm Metab Res* 5:471, 1973.
33. Duckworth WC, Kitabchi AE: Insulin metabolism and degradation. *Endocr Rev* 2:210, 1981.
34. Fajans SS: The adult diabetic patient. In Krieger DT, Bardin CW: *Current Therapy in Endocrinology and Metabolism.* Toronto, BC Decker, 1985, pp 245–254.
35. Fein IA, Rackow EC, Sprung CL, et al: Relation of colloid osmotic pressure to arterial hypoxemia and cerebral edema during crystalloid volume loading of patients with diabetic ketoaciosis. *Ann Intern Med* 96:570, 1982.
36. Felig P: The endocrine pancreas: diabetes mellitus. In Felig P et al: *Endocrinology and Metabolism.* New York, McGraw-Hill, 1981, pp 761–868.
37. Field JB, Johnson P, Herring B: Insulin resistant diabetes associated with increased endogenous plasma insulin followed by complete remission. *J Clin Invest* 40:1672, 1961.
38. Filkins JP, Figlewicz DP: Increased insulin responsiveness in endotoxicosis. *Circ Shock* 6:1, 1979.
39. Fisher JN, Shahshahani N, Kitabchi AE: Diabetic ketoacidosis: low dose insulin therapy by various routes. *N Engl J Med* 297:238, 1977.
40. Flier JS, Kahn CR, Roth J: Receptors, antireceptor antibodies and mechanisms of insulin resistance. *N Engl J Med* 300:413, 1979.
41. Franks M, Berris RF, Kaplan NO, et al: Metabolic studies in diabetic acidosis. II. The effect of the administration of sodium phosphate. *Arch Intern Med* 81:42, 1948.
42. Freidenberg GR, White N, Cataland S, et al: Diabetes responsive to intravenous but not subcutaneous insulin: effectivenss of aprotinin. *N Engl J Med* 305:363, 1981.
43. Fulop M, Hoberman HD: Alcoholic ketosis. *Diabetes* 24:785, 1975.
44. Fulop M, Rosenblatt A, Kreitzer SM, et al: Hyperosmolar nature of diabetic coma. *Diabetes* 24:594, 1975.
45. Fulop M, Tannenbaum H, Dreyer N: Ketotic hyperosmolar coma. *Lancet* 2:635, 1973.
46. Galloway JA, Bressler R: Insulin treatment in diabetes. *Med Clin North Am* 62:663, 1978.
47. Galloway JA, Spradlin CT, Nelson RL, et al: Factors influencing the absorption, serum insulin concentration, and blood glucose responses after injections of regular insulin and various insulin mixtures. *Diabetes Care* 4:366, 1981.
48. Gamblin GT, Chernow B, Clapper M, et al: Insulin infusion pump therapy: a review. *Military Med* 147:747, 1982.
49. Gerich JE: Sulfonylureas in the treatment of diabetes mellitus - 1985. *Mayo Clinic Proc* 60:439, 1985.
50. Gerich JE: Metabolic effects of long term somatostatin infusion in man. *Metabolism* 25 (Suppl 1):1505, 1976.
51. Gerich JE: Somatostatin and diabetes. *Am J Med* 70:619, 1981.
52. Gerich JE, Lorenzi M, Bier DM, et al: Prevention of human diabetic ketoacidosis by somatostatin. Evidence for an essential role of glucagon. *N Engl J Med* 292:985, 1975.
53. Gerich JE, Martin MM, Recant L: Clinical and metabolic characteristics of hyperosmolar non-ketotic coma. *Diabetes* 20:228, 1971.
54. Gerich JE, Raptis S, Rosenthal J: Somatostatin symposium. *Metabolism* 27(Suppl 1):1, 1978.
55. Giugliano D, Torella R, Sgambato S, et al: Acetylsalicyclic acid restores acute insulin response reduced by furosemide in man. *Diabetes* 28:841, 1979.
56. Giugliano D, Torella R, Siniscalchi N, et al: The effect of acetylsalicylic acid on insulin response to glucose and arginine in normal man. *Diabetologia* 14:359, 1978.
57. Goldfrank L, Starke CL: Metabolic acidosis in the alcoholic. *Hosp Physician* 4:34, 1979.
58. Goldman DR: Surgery in patients with endocrine dysfunction. *Med Clin N Am* 71:499, 1987.
59. Goldstein DA, Oh MS, Fein IA, et al: Transient hypoxemia in diabetic ketoacidosis. *Kidney Int* 10:499, 1976.
60. Grant JP: Administration of parenteral nutrition solutions. In Grant JP: *Handbook of Total Parenteral Nutrition.* Philadelphia, WB Saunders, 1980.
61. Grant JP: Preparation of parenteral nutrition solutions. In Grant JP: *Handbook of Total Parenteral Nutrition.* Philadelphia, WB Saunders, 1980.
62. Guest GM, Rapoport S: Electrolytes of blood plasma and cells in diabetic acidosis and during recovery. *Proc Am Diabetes Assoc* 7:97, 1947.
63. Guisado R, Arieff AI: Neurologic manifestations of diabetic comas: correlation with biochemical alterations in the brain. *Metabolism* 24:665, 1975.
64. Harter HR, Santiago JV, Rutherford WE, et al: The relative roles of calcium, phosphorus, and parathyroid hormone in glucose- and tolbutamide-mediated insulin release. *J Clin Invest* 58:359, 1976.
65. Heber D, Molitch ME, Spirling MA: Low dose continuous insulin therapy for diabetic ketoacidosis. *Arch Intern Med* 137:1377, 1977.
66. Joffe BI, Goldberg RB, Krut LH, Seftel HC: Pathogenesis of non-ketotic hyperosmolar diabetic comas. *Lancet* 1:1069, 1975.
67. Joffe BI, Seftel HC, Goldberg R, et al: Factors in the pathogenesis of experimental nonketotic and ketoacidotic diabetic stupor. *Diabetes* 22:653, 1973.
68. Johnson DG, Goebel CV, Hruly VJ, et al: Hyperglycemia of diabetic rat decreased by glucagon receptor antagonist. *Science* 215:1115, 1982.
69. Johnston DG, Alberti KGMM: Diabetic emergencies: practical aspects of the management of diabetic ketoacidosis and diabetes during surgery. *Clin Endocrinol Metab* 4:437, 1980.
70. Keller U, Berger W: Prevention of hypophosphatemia by phosphate infusion during treatment of diabetic

ketoacidosis and hyperosmolar coma. *Diabetes* 29:87, 1980.

71. Khardori R, Soler NG: Hyperosmolar hyperglycemic nonketotic syndrome. *Am J Med* 77:899, 1984.

72. Kitabchi AE, Ayyagari V, Guerra SDM: The efficacy of low-dose versus conventional therapy of insulin treatment of diabetic ketoacidosis. *Ann Intern Med* 84:633, 1976.

73. Kitabchi AE, Stentz FB, Cole C, et al: Accelerated insulin degradation: an alternate mechanism for insulin resistance. *Diabetes Care* 2:414, 1979.

74. Klein SP: Insulin allergy: treatment with the histamine antagonists. *Arch Intern Med* 81:316, 1948.

75. Kraegen EW, Lazarus L, Meler H, et al: Carrier solutions for low level intravenous insulin infusion. *Br Med J* 2:464, 1975.

76. Krane EJ, Rockoff MA, Wallman JK, Wolfsdorf JI: Subclinical brain swelling in children during treatment of diabetic ketoacidosis. *N Engl J Med* 312:1147, 1985.

77. Kreisberg RA: Diabetic ketoacidosis: new concepts and trends in pathogenesis and treatment. *Ann Intern Med* 88:681, 1978.

78. Larner J: Insulin and oral hypoglycemic drugs, glucagon. In Gilman AG, Goodman LS, Rall TW, Murad F: *The Pharmacological Basis of Therapeutics.* New York, Macmillan, 1985, pp 1490–1516.

79. Lebovitz HE, Feldman JM: Pancreatic biogenic amines and insulin secretion in health and disease. *Federation Proc* 32:1797, 1973.

80. Levy LJ, Duga J, Girgis M, et al: Ketoacidosis associated with alcoholism in nondiabetic subjects. *Ann Intern Med* 78:213, 1973.

81. Lieberman P, Patterson R, Metz R, et al: Allergic reactions to insulin. *JAMA* 215:1106, 1971.

82. Longnecker MP, Elsenhans VD, Leiman SM, Owen OE, Boden G: Insulin and a sulfonylurea agent in non-insulin-dependent diabetes mellitus. *Arch Intern Med* 146:673, 1986.

83. Lundbaek K, Hansen A, Orskov H, et al: Failure of somatostatin to correct manifest diabetic ketoacidosis. *Lancet* 1:215, 1976.

84. Maccario M: Neurological dysfunction associated with nonketotic hyperglycemia. *Arch Neurol* 19:525, 1968.

85. Manzano F, Kozak GP: Acute quadriplegia in diabetic hyperosmotic coma with hypokalemia. *JAMA* 207:2278, 1969.

86. Marriott HJL: Miscellaneous conditions. In *Practical Electrocardiology,* ed 6. Baltimore, Williams & Wilkins, 1977, pp 304–310.

87. Mattson JR, Patterson R, Roberts M: Insulin therapy in patients with insulin allergy. *Arch Intern Med* 135:818, 1975.

88. McGarry JD, Foster DW: Regulation of hepatic fatty acid oxidation and ketone body production. *Ann Rev Biochem* 49:395, 1980.

89. McRae JR, Metz SA, Robertson RP: A role for endogenous prostaglandins in defective glucose potentiation of nonglucose insulin secretagogues in diabetes. *Metabolism* 30:1065, 1981.

90. Merimee TJ: Insulin resistance: study of effect of 6-mercaptopurine. *Lancet* 1:69, 1965.

91. Metzger AL, Robenstein AH: Reversible cerebral edema complicating diabetic ketoacidosis. *Br Med J* 3:746, 1970.

92. Miller PD, Heinig RE, Waterhouse C: Treatment of alcoholic acidosis. *Arch Intern Med* 138:67, 1978.

93. Morris LR, Murphy MB, Kitabchi AE: Bicarbonate therapy in severe diabetic ketoacidosis. *Ann Intern Med* 105:836, 1986.

94. Munro JF, Campbell IW, McCuish AC, et al: Euglycaemic diabetic ketoacidosis. *Br Med J* 2:578, 1973.

95. Nathan DM, Axelrod L, Flier JS, et al: U-500 insulin in the treatment of antibody-mediated insulin resistance. *Ann Intern Med* 94:653, 1981.

96. Nathan DM, Lou P, Avruch J: Intensive conventional and insulin pump therapies in adult type I diabetes. *Ann Intern Med* 97:31, 1982.

97. Oakley WG: Insulin resistance. *Br Med J* 2:134, 1967.

98. Oh MS, Carroll HJ, Goldstein DA: Hyperchloremic acidosis during the recovery phase of diabetic ketosis. *Ann Intern Med* 89:925, 1978.

99. Ohman JL, Marliss EB, Aoki TT, et al: The cerebrospinal fluid in diabetic ketoacidosis. *N Engl J Med* 284:283, 1971.

100. Olefsky JM, Reaven GM: Effects of sulfonylurea therapy on insulin binding to mononuclear leukocytes of diabetic patients. *Am J Med* 60:89, 1976.

101. Page MM, Watkins PJ: Cardiorespiratory arrest and diabetic autonomic neuropathy. *Lancet* 1:14, 1978.

102. Patterson R, Mellies CJ, Roberts M: Immunologic reactions against insulin. IgE anti-insulin, insulin allergy and combined IgE and IgG immunologic insulin resistance. *J Immunol* 110:1135, 1973.

103. Paulsen EP, Courtney JW III, Duckworth WC: Insulin resistance caused by massive degradation of subcutaneous insulin. *Diabetes* 28:640, 1979.

104. Peitzman SJ, Agarival BN: Spontaneous hypoglycemia in end-stage renal failure. *Nephron* 19:131, 1977.

105. Peterson L, Caldwell J, Hoffman J: Insulin adsorbance to polyvinylchloride surfaces with implications for constant-infusion therapy. *Diabetes* 25:72, 1976.

106. Piters K, Goodman J, Bessman A: Treatment of diabetic ketoacidosis with continuous low-dose intravenous insulin. *Diabetes* 24(Suppl 2): 396, 1975.

107. Podolsky S, Emerson K: Potassium depletion in diabetic ketoacidosis. *Diabetes* 22:299, 1973.

108. Podolsky S: Hyperosmolar nonketotic coma in the elderly diabetic. *Med Clin North Am* 62:815, 1978.

109. Podolsky S, Pattavina CG: Hyperosmolar nonketotic diabetic coma: a complication of propranolol therapy. *Metabolism* 22:685, 1973.

110. Porte D Jr: A receptor mechanism for the inhibition of insulin release by epinephrine in man. *J Clin Invest* 46:86, 1967.

111. Porte D Jr: Inhibition of insulin release by diazoxide and its relation to catecholamine effects in man. *Ann NY Acad Sci* 150:281, 1968.

112. Porte D, Smith PH, Ensinck JW: Neurohumoral regulation of the pancreatic islet A and B cells. *Metabolism* 25(Suppl 1):1453, 1976.

113. Porte D Jr, Williams RH: Inhibition of insulin release by norepinephrine in man. *Science* 152:1466, 1966.

114. Raskin P, Unger RH: Effects of exogenous hyperglucagonemia in insulin treated diabetes. *Diabetes* 26:1034, 1977.

115. Raskin P, Unger RH: Glucagon and diabetes. *Med Clin North Am* 62:713, 1978.

116. Raskin P, Unger RH: Hyperglucagonemia and its suppression: importance in the metabolic control of diabetes. *N Engl J Med* 299:433, 1978.

117. Rizza RA: Treatment options for insulin-dependent diabetes mellitus: a comparison of the artificial endocrine pancreas, continuous subcutaneous insulin infusion, and multiple daily insulin injections. *Mayo Clin Proc* 61:796, 1986.

118. Rizza RA, Gerich JE, Haymond MW, et al: Control of blood sugar in insulin-dependent diabetes: comparison of an artificial endocrine pancreas, continuous subcutaneous infusion, and intensified conventional therapy. *N Engl J Med* 303:1313, 1980.

119. Rizza RA, Mandarino LJ, Gerich JE: Cortisol-induced insulin resistance in man: impaired suppression of glucose production and stimulation of glucose utilization due to a postreceptor defect of insulin action. *J Clin Endocrinol Metab* 54:131, 1982.

120. Robertson RP, Chem M: A role for prostaglandin E in defective insulin secretion and carbohydrate intolerance in diabetes mellitus. *J Clin Invest* 60:747, 1977.

121. Robertson RP, Metz SA: Prostaglandins, the glucoreceptor, and diabetes. *N Engl J Med* 301:1446, 1979.

122. Seltzer HS, Allen EW: Hyperglycemia and inhibition of insulin secretion during administration of diazoxide and trichlormethiazide in man. *Diabetes* 18:19, 1969.

123. Semple PF, White C, Manderson WG: Continuous intravenous infusion of small doses of insulin in treatment of diabetic ketoacidosis. *Br Med J* 2:694, 1974.

124. Shade DS, Eaton RP: Dose response to insulin in man. Differential effects on glucose and ketone body regulation. *J Clin Endocrinol Metab* 44:1038, 1977.

125. Shen SW, Bressler R: Clinical pharmacology of oral antidiabetic agents. *N Engl J Med* 296:493–496, 787–792, 1977.

126. Shipp JC, Cunningham RW, Russell RD, et al: Insulin resistance. Clinical features, natural course and effects of adrenal steroid treatment. *Medicine* 44:165, 1965.

127. Sonksen PH, Srivastava MC, Tompkins CV, et al: Growth hormone and cortisol responses to insulin infusion in patients with diabetes mellitus. *Lancet* 2:155, 1972.

128. Sprung CL, Rackow EC, Fein IA: Pulmonary edema: a complication of diabetic ketoacidosis. *Chest* 77:687, 1980.

129. Turpin P, Duckworth WC, Solomon SS: Stimulated hyperglycemic hyperosmolar syndrome: impaired insulin and epinephrine effects upon lipolysis in the isolated rat fat cell. *J Clin Invest* 63:403, 1979.

130. Unger RH, Foster DW: Diabetes mellitus. In Wilson JD, Foster DW (eds): *Williams Textbook of Endocrinology*, 7th ed. Philadelphia, WB Saunders, 1985, pp 1018–1080.

131. Unger RH: Role of glucagon in the pathogenesis of diabetes: the status of controversy. *Metabolism* 27:1691, 1978.

132. Weinsenfeld S, Podolsky S, Goldsmith L, et al: Adsorption of insulin to infusion bottles and tubing. *Diabetes* 17:766, 1968.

133. Wennlund A, Arner P, Ostman J: Changes in the effects of insulin on human adipose tissue metabolism in hyperthyroidism. *J Clin Endocrinol Metab* 53:631, 1981.

134. White VA, Kumagai LF: Preoperative endocrine and metabolic considerations. *Med Clin North Am* 63:1321, 1979.

135. Winter RJ, Harris CJ, Phillips LS, et al: Diabetic ketoacidosis: induction of hypocalcemia and hypomagnesemia by phosphate therapy. *Am J Med* 67:897, 1979.

136. Witters LA, Ohman JL, Weir GC, et al: Insulin antibodies in the pathogenesis of insulin allergy and resistance. *Am J Med* 63:703, 1977.

137. Wright J, Marks V: Alcohol-induced hypoglycacemia. *Adv Exp Med Biol* 126:479, 1980.

138. Yalow RS, Berson SA: Reaction of fish insulins with human insulin antiserums. *N Engl J Med* 270:1171, 1964.

139. Young E, Bradley RF: Cerebral edema with irreversible coma in severe diabetic ketoacidosis. *N Engl J Med* 276:665, 1967.

140. Zaloga GP, Chernow B: The use of hormones as therapeutic agents. *Sem Resp Med* 7:39, 1985.

141. Zaloga GP, Chernow B: Diabetes and diabetic coma. In Parrillo JE: *Current Therapy in Critical Care Medicine*. Toronto, BC Decker, 1987, pp 297–299.

142. Zaloga GP, Chernow B, McFadden E, et al: Urine glucose testing in the critically ill—a comparison of two enzymatic test strips. *Crit Care Med* 12:188, 1984.

143. Zaloga GP: Bedside laboratory testing in critical care medicine. *J Crit Illness* (in press).

33

Part 2.
Glucagon

Gary P. Zaloga, M.D., F.A.C.P., F.A.C.N.
Diana S. Malcolm, Ph.D.
John W. Holaday, Ph.D.
Bart Chernow, M.D., F.A.C.P., F.C.C.P.

Glucagon is a polypeptide hormone produced in the α cells of the pancreatic islets of Langerhans. Extrapancreatic sources of glucagon have also been described in the gastrointestinal tract, salivary glands, and central nervous system (74, 86). Physiologically, glucagon is an important hormone in the maintenance of euglycemia. In pharmacologic doses, however, it also has cardiovascular, gastrointestinal, and genitourinary effects. This article reviews the actions of endogenous glucagon and the therapeutic uses of glucagon in critical care and emergency medicine.

ENDOGENOUS FUNCTIONS

Glucagon is a 29–amino acid polypeptide synthesized within the pancreas by proteolytic cleavage from a larger precursor (proglucagon). Glucagon raises blood glucose levels by stimulating hepatic glycogenolysis and gluconeogenesis. It also stimulates lipolysis, proteolysis, and ketogenesis (47, 74, 126).

Glucagon's metabolic effects are initiated by the binding of the hormone to a receptor and activation of adenylate cyclase. Subsequent activation of protein kinase by cyclic AMP mediates most actions of glucagon (74). However, a number of reports (3, 15, 70, 128) suggest that glucagon elicits changes in cellular calcium that lead to increases in cytosolic free calcium. One of its major effects is to increase cellular calcium influx (3, 128). Glucagon's calcium mobilizing effects may be partially mediated through cyclic AMP. Glucagon's metabolic effects are antagonized by insulin excess and potentiated by insulin deficiency.

In fact, the regulation of hepatic glucose production depends upon the insulin/glucagon ratio rather than the absolute concentrations of either hormone (74).

After protein feeding, insulin assures cellular uptake of nutrients and utilization of amino acids, whereas glucagon limits the degree of insulin-induced hypoglycemia. The brain is dependent on glucose for energy. Glucagon maintains hepatic glucose production, and in starvation states it stimulates hepatic ketogenesis. In starvation, ketones substitute for glucose as a cerebral fuel.

Glucagon is important in maintaining plasma glucose levels and preventing hypoglycemia during fasting and stress states. Seventy-five percent of basal hepatic glucose output is mediated by glucagon (17). Glucagon, along with epinephrine, is responsible for the "moment to moment" regulation of circulating glucose concentrations. Growth hormone and cortisol play an important role in long-term control by altering tissue sensitivity to insulin, glucagon, and epinephrine (74).

During starvation, circulating insulin levels decline, resulting in a marked diminution of glucose uptake by peripheral insulin-sensitive tissues (e.g., muscle and adipose tissue) and a shift toward utilization of fatty acids as energy fuels. Glucose consumption, however, continues by non-insulin-dependent tissues (e.g., brain, renal medulla, and blood cells) and the splanchnic bed, so that total glucose uptake occurs at a rate of 2.0–2.5 mg/kg/minute (200–250 g/day). Maintenance of blood glucose homeostasis in this circumstance is achieved by hepatic glucose production. Glucose is resynthesized from lactate and amino acids (74).

Glucose production in the postabsorptive state is primarily derived from glycogenolysis. Endogenous production after prolonged fasting is accounted for by gluconeogenesis. Hypoinsulinemia and hyperglucagonemia act in concert to maximize hepatic gluconeogenesis. Hypoinsulinemia enhances the delivery of substrate amino acids from muscle to liver, where increased quantities of glucose are synthesized under the influence of both the elevation in plasma glucagon and the depression in plasma insulin. Hypoinsulinemia further contributes to glucose homeostasis by reducing extracerebral glucose consumption and by increasing the availability of free fatty acids for oxidative metabolism by muscle and liver.

During stress, glucose utilization may increase from a normal of 4 g/hour to levels as high as 40 g/hour. Energy requirements during stress are provided by circulating glucose (e.g., hepatic glucose output) and free fatty acids. Hepatic glucose output and free fatty acid release are stimulated by increases in circulating catecholamines and glucagon (35, 74, 110). Relative insulinopenia is important for optimal activity of these counterregulatory hormones. Counterregulatory hormones (e.g, epinephrine, growth hormone, cortisol, and endorphins) also stimulate glucagon output (60, 90, 133). The adrenergic influence on the islets perpetuates "stress hyperglycemia" by blocking hyperglycemic suppression of glucagon secretion (138).

The normal pancreatic islets are composed of 60% β cells (insulin synthesis), 30% α cells (glucagon synthesis) and 10% Δ cells (somatostatin synthesis) (139). In type I (insulin-dependent) diabetes mellitus, the islets lose β cells. With the loss of insulin inhibition of glucagon secretion, there is an inappropriate elevation in circulatory glucagon levels and these patients are prone to hyperglycemia and ketoacidosis (48, 123, 124). In type I diabetics, when glucagon is suppressed by a somatostatin infusion, the observed hyperglycemia and ketosis is attenuated (48, 77). Glucagon is also important in preventing hypoglycemia in patients receiving insulin for their diabetes mellitus.

Hyperglucagonemia is seen in patients with cirrhosis, chronic renal failure, myotonic dystrophy, acute pancreatitis (25), starvation, glucagonomas, and shock (61, 89, 96, 138). The increase in the plasma glucagon concentration seen in acute illness and shock results from adrenergic hyperactivity and from the release of catecholamines, growth hormone, cortisol, and β-endorphins (60, 90, 133). Hyperglucagonemia probably contributes to the glucose intolerance found in all these conditions (74).

There have been several case reports of hypoglucagonemia (7, 53, 54). These patients have hypoglycemia that can be controlled with frequent feedings, or with the use of an intravenous glucagon infusion or subcutaneous glucagon injections. The documentation of hypoglucagonemia without insulin excess in these cases is poor, and it remains unclear whether glucagon deficiency alone (e.g., without insulin elevation) causes hypoglycemia. Glucagon deficiency may occur in patients with chronic pancreatitis (25) or after duodenopancreatectomy (74). In these conditions, glucagon deficiency is not associated with persistent hypoglycemia. In addition, somatostatin analogs have been used to suppress growth hormone secretion from pituitary tumors. Hypoglycemia has not been reported with such therapy.

In contrast to the fluctuations in insulin secretion that accompany meals and minor changes in blood glucose, the secretion of glucagon from the pancreas is fairly constant throughout the day. Physiological stimuli of glucagon secretion include protein ingestion, amino acid infusion, exercise, and the administration of epinephrine (or other β-adrenergic receptor agonists), growth hormone, β-endorphin or cortisol (126, 138) (Table 33.15). Glucocorticoids increase glucagon release (147), an effect that partially explains the hyperglycemia observed during glucorticoid adminis-

Table 33.15
Stimulators and Inhibitors of Glucagon Secretion

Stimulate	Inhibit
Amino acids	Atropine
β-Adrenergic agonists	β-Adrenergic blockers
β-Endorphin	Calcitonin
Cholecystokinin	Free fatty acids
Dopamine	Glucose
Epinephrine	Insulin
Exercise	Ketones
Gastric inhibitory peptide	Secretion
Gastrin	Somatostatin
Glucocorticoids	Verapamil
Growth hormone	
Hypoglycemia	
L-Dopa	
Nicotinic acid	
Pancreozymin	
Protein	
Vasoactive intestinal peptide	

tration. In addition, glucocorticoids potentiate the glucagon response to amino acids and protein. This effect may contribute to hyperglycemia in patients receiving parenteral nutrition. Tissue glucopenia stimulates glucagon secretion, an effect blocked by atropine (58). Calcium helps to mediate the release of glucagon from the pancreas into the circulation (137). Verapamil, a calcium channel blocker, may inhibit the secretion of glucagon in response to stimuli such as hypoglycemia or an arginine infusion (73). Somatostatin, insulin, and the ingestion or infusion of glucose (in the presence of insulin) each suppresses glucagon secretion (Table 33.15). Somatostatin's inhibition of pancreatic α-cell function is the basis for its use as an adjunct in the management of insulin-dependent diabetes mellitus (49). Suppression of glucagon secretion minimizes ketosis and helps in the control of hyperglycemia.

CLINICAL USES

Glucagon was discovered in 1923, purified in 1955, and accepted for treatment of hypoglycemia in 1962. Subsequently, it has been found to affect the heart, vascular smooth muscle, and the gut. The metabolic clearance rate (MCR) is the least amount of plasma totally cleared of a substance per unit of time. The MCR for glucagon in humans is approximately 10 ml/kg/minute and is unaffected by insulin and somatostatin (74). The MCR is reduced during starvation, liver disease, and in uremia; it is unchanged in diabetes mellitus. The plasma half-life is dependent on MCR and volume of distribution. Glucagon has a plasma half-life of 3–6 minutes and is degraded primarily in the liver and kidneys (74).

Hypoglycemia

The immediate treatment of hypoglycemia is to administer carbohydrate (e.g., a sweetened drink, food, or intravenous glucose). When glucose is not available or its intravenous injection is not feasible, 1 mg of intramuscular glucagon can increase the serum glucose level (Table 33.16). Because this immediate antihypoglycemic effect of glucagon results from its potent hepatic glycogenolytic properties, glucagon is not effective in states of hepatic gly-

cogen depletion (e.g., starvation, adrenal insufficiency, or chronic hypoglycemia). Glucagon also works poorly in patients with impaired liver function (e.g., those with hepatitis, or severe hepatic congestion from congestive heart failure). The hyperglycemic action of exogenous glucagon is poorly maintained during continuous infusion, because of increased insulin release, which suppresses hepatic glucose release and increases peripheral utilization. Glucagon produces a greater hyperglycemic response in type I than in type II diabetics.

Glucagon works well in insulin excess (38, 39, 105) and has been used to terminate insulin-induced coma in suicidal patients, some of whom had received 2000 U of insulin. It is minimally effective in treating hypoglycemia due to sulfonylureas, insulinoma, nesidioblastosis, glycogen storage disease, and alcohol (74).

Glucagon is effective in raising the blood glucose concentration and improving cerebration in patients unconscious from hypoglycemia caused by extrapancreatic neoplasms, provided the patients are not also malnourished or suffering from liver disease (94). We have also used intramuscular injections of glucagon to prevent symptomatic hypoglycemia in a patient with postprandial hypoglycemia resulting from gastrointestinal ulcer surgery.

Glucagon may be given subcutaneously, intramuscularly, or intravenously in a dose of 1–5 mg (105). Its onset of action is 1 minute after intravenous administration, and 8–10 minutes after intramuscular or subcutaneous administration. Glucagon's hyperglycemic effect lasts only 10–30 minutes, although glucagon-induced gluconeogenesis continues for 30–60 minutes after drug administration. The antihypoglycemic action of glucagon has little use in the hospital critical care setting, where intravenous glucose is available and many hypoglycemic patients may not respond to glucagon (74, 83). However, because it is packaged in a small volume, it is useful in field situations where intravenous glucose is not practical. It may also be administered intramuscularly or subcutaneously by nonmedical personnel (e.g., patients or relatives) and it is useful in the semiconscious or convulsing hypoglycemic patient. If glucagon fails to restore consciousness within 20–30 minutes, intravenous glucose must be given to avoid permanent CNS damage from prolonged hypoglycemia. Recovery of consciousness produced by

Table 33.16
Glucagon Therapy

Indication	Dose (mg)	Time for Response	Duration of Action	Comments[a]
Hypoglycemia	1–5 mg s.c., i.m., or i.v. bolus	<20 minutes	Depends on liver glycogen	Start i.v. glucose; may repeat dose
Cardiogenic shock or heart failure	1–5 mg i.v. bolus every 30–60 minutes or 1–10 mg/hour i.v. infusion	5–10 minutes	20–30 minutes for bolus	Use antiemetic; watch glucose and K+
β-Blocker overdose	1–5 mg i.v. bolus every 30–60 minutes or 1–10 mg/hour i.v. infusion	5–10 minutes	20–30 minutes for bolus	Repeat dose every 30 minutes as needed; watch glucose and K+
Esophageal meat impaction	1 mg i.v. bolus	5 minutes	30 minutes	Repeat every 30 minutes; follow with barium
Diverticular disease	1 mg i.v. bolus every 4 hours	3–12 hours	2–4 hours	Repeat as needed
Renal or biliary calculi	1 mg i.v. bolus every 4 hours	1–2 hours	2–4 hours	Repeat as needed

[a] Administer cautiously to patients with suspected pheochromocytoma or insulinoma.

glucagon should be followed by ingestion of a meal or oral glucose.

Differential Diagnosis of Hypoglycemia

Glucagon causes initial hyperglycemia followed by rebound hypoglycemia (at 90–150 minutes) after its injection in patients with insulinoma. Rebound hypoglycemia results from a stimulation of insulin secretion (74). In contrast, normal subjects rendered hypoglycemic by insulin do not develop rebound hypoglycemia after glucagon injection (e.g., they have a reduced or absent insulinemic response to glucagon). Roughly 70% of insulinoma patients respond with excessive and prolonged insulin release. Thus, the insulinemic response to glucagon can be useful in the differential diagnosis of fasting hypoglycemia since insulinoma alone is associated with an exaggerated response to glucagon. Patients with fasting hypoglycemia due to extrapancreatic neoplasms have an impaired or absent glucagon-induced rise in plasma insulin concentration. Patients with fasting hypoglycemia of endocrine origin or from alcohol have a reduced glycemic and insulinemic response to glucagon.

The glucagon test is useful in the differential diagnosis of fasting hypoglycemia due to inborn errors of metabolism (e.g., glycogen storage disease) (32, 74). These children fail to show a glycemic response to glucagon, whereas hypoglycemia due to hyperinsulinism (e.g., exogenous insulin or nesidiblastosis) does respond (45). Glucagon unresponsiveness may also result from chronic carbohydrate deprivation. This entity can be ruled out by repeating the test after a period of carbohydrate repletion.

CARDIOVASCULAR EFFECTS

Glucagon has both inotropic and chronotropic cardiac effects in animals (42, 74) and humans (41, 67, 74, 81, 82, 111, 127). It is also a peripheral vasodilator (41). Glucagon's inotropic effects are not dependent on catecholamines or adrenergic receptors and they are unaltered by norepinephrine depletion or α- and β-adrenergic receptor blockade (51, 82, 111). They are enhanced by glutathione (134) and glucose administration (29). The cardiotonic effects of glucagon may also be greater in the hypothermic heart than normothermic

heart (91). Glucagon's chronotropic effects are only partially reduced by β-adrenergic blockade. These cardiotonic actions of glucagon are not associated with increased myocardial irritability (81, 111) as seen with isoproterenol.

Glucagon increases intracellular cyclic AMP levels (74, 132) and increases the movement of calcium ions into myocardial cells (107). Its cardiac actions are dependent upon the circulating ionized calcium concentration (16). Glucagon's chronotropic effects are inhibited by both ionized hypocalcemia and hypercalcemia. The overall data suggest that glucagon mediates its cardiotonic actions via both cyclic AMP dependent and independent mechanisms (74). Glucagon may also be of benefit through its opiate antagonistic action (86).

Glucagon decreases atrioventricular conduction time (41, 74, 130) and may improve heart block. It has been shown to increase the ventricular rate during atrial flutter or fibrillation without altering atrial rate (74). Glucagon increases the rate of discharge of the atrioventricular pacemaker and increases the discharge rate in spontaneously beating Purkinje fibers (74). Madan (84) studied idioventricular rhythms in dogs after coronary artery ligation. Glucagon (30–100 µg/kg) reduced the rate of an idioventricular rhythm and in some experiments produced a complete reversal to sinus rhythm. Despite successful defibrillation after cardiac arrest, postcountershock pulseless rhythms may occur. Niemann et al. (108) studied this phenomenon in the canine model of induced-ventricular fibrillation. In 14 of 19 postcountershock episodes, unresponsive to cardiopulmonary resuscitation (CPR) alone, glucagon (1 mg intravenously administered) restored effective spontaneous circulation (e.g., restored cardiac electrical activity and contractile function).

Glucagon's inotropic and chronotropic effects appear to be independent of the β-adrenergic receptor. It can antagonize a propranolol-induced decrease in atrioventricular conduction velocity (74, 144) and has been used effectively to treat hypotension and bradycardia in propranolol overdose (2, 15, 51, 69, 115), even when isoproterenol has failed. Zaloga et al. (149) recently reported the effective use of glucagon in reversing hypotension following anaphylactoid shock in a patient taking propranolol. Madan and Jain (85) also combined glucagon with a β-blocker for the successful treatment of arrhythmias accompanying myocardial infarction. Glucagon has been reported to reverse the cardiotoxic effects of procainamide (120), ouabain (18, 74, 119), verapamil (150), and quinidine (118, 120). Glucagon is more effective in converting ouabain-induced ventricular arrhythmias in hypokalemic versus normokalemic animals (36). There have been no controlled human trials on the efficacy of glucagon in these states.

The observations that glucagon produced positive chronotropic and inotropic responses in animals and that it could act synergistically with β-adrenergic catecholamines (127, 132), prompted a variety of clinical studies in humans. Parmley et al. (111) injected glucagon (3–5 mg intravenously administered) in patients undergoing cardiac catheterization and found an increase in heart rate, cardiac index, and rate of pressure change (dp/dt) with no change in left ventricular end diastolic pressure or systemic vascular resistance. These results have been documented by others (74) in patients with normal and diseased coronary arteries.

Glucagon has been used effectively in heart failure and cardiogenic shock (26, 29, 34, 81, 112). In heart failure, the increase in heart rate is less marked than in normal subjects (74). The results obtained in acute low-output cardiac failure indicate that glucagon causes a dose-dependent increase in cardiac output and heart rate and is not arrhythmogenic (26, 34, 81, 112, 113, 129). Maximal cardiac effects are obtained with 5–10 mg of intravenous glucagon. The chronic forms of heart failure are less responsive to glucagon than the acute types, and variable or sometimes absent responses are reported (74). Armstrong et al. (4) reported that the degree of heart failure determined the response of the heart to glucagon. Patients with class 1 or 2 heart failure had significantly greater increases in cardiac output than those with class 3 or 4 heart failure. Animal experiments show that heart failure due to metabolic failure is less responsive to glucagon than heart failure caused by interference with coupling mechanisms (74). A zinc protamine glucagon formulation has been administered intramuscularly (5 mg twice a day) to patients with heart failure with beneficial results (74). Experimental work using a canine heart-lung preparation suggests that glucagon may increase myocardial efficiency (1). In our experience, however, glucagon is less effective in increasing cardiac output and blood pressure than other inotropic drugs such as dobutamine, dopamine, amrinone, or epinephrine.

Glucagon has improved cardiac function and blood pressure in experimental myocardial infarction (87, 95) and after myocardial infarction in humans (27, 52, 74, 106, 112). Glucagon is less dysrhythmogenic following infarction than β-adrenergic catecholamines (34). Increases in cardiac oxygen consumption result from glucagon-induced increases in heart rate and contractility. Cardiac oxygen consumption is less with glucagon than with adrenergic stimulation (74).

Glucagon improved hemodynamic variables in experimental endotoxin (8, 55, 135) and hypovolemic shock (8, 9, 125, 141). Glucagon transiently increased circulating glucose levels in endotoxin shock (143) and increased survival in swine (143). Glucagon also increased survival in rat hemorrhagic shock (63). On the other hand, Markovitz et al. (92) have reported no improvement in hemodynamic status after glucagon administration to the isolated septic rat heart.

Endogenous glucagon levels increase during shock states (61, 62, 89). The role that this glucagon plays in shock remains uncertain.

Glucagon's cardiac effects begin in 1–5 minutes, peak in 5–15 minutes, and last 20–30 minutes after a single 5-mg bolus (26, 111). Glucagon may be given in 1-mg to 5-mg intermittent boluses every 20–30 minutes or a continuous infusion of 1–10 mg/hour (Table 33.16). Continuous intravenous infusion (140) is effective and may be discontinued if complications develop.

The general conclusions regarding glucagon are that it is a moderately effective inotropic and chronotropic agent in humans and, in contrast to the catecholamine, does not usually produce arrhythmias. Its peripheral dilator properties produce a modest reduction in afterload. It is more effective in acute low-output failure than in chronic heart failure. Cardiac effects of glucagon are not dependent upon β-adrenergic receptors, thus, making it a useful agent in treating cardiodepression resulting from β-blocking agents.

VASCULAR EFFECTS

Glucagon is a potent vasodilator of the splanchnic vascular bed (41, 74). It can increase mesenteric blood flow and survival in experimental models of acute mesenteric ischemia and may be useful in treating nonocclusive mesenteric ischemia (20, 66, 74). Since glucagon is a vasodilator, volume expansion along with glucagon is important so as to maximize tissue perfusion (20).

Glucagon causes renal vasodilation and a resulting diuresis and natriuresis. Its effects are similar to low dose dopamine, but less potent. It may increase renal blood flow in the kidney during ischemic states (76). The combined use of dopamine and glucagon warrants investigation.

GASTROINTESTINAL EFFECTS

Glucagon relaxes smooth muscle in the lower esophageal sphincter (LES), stomach, small and large intestine, gallbladder, and bile ducts (74). Glucagon's enteric and biliary effects do not appear to involve adenylate cyclase (74) or catecholamines. It may work by interfering with ganglionic transmission.

Glucagon reduces LES pressure without decreasing esophageal peristalsis (59), and a 1 mg intravenous dose can relieve esophageal meat impaction (43, 56, 93, 117) (Table 33.16). Glucagon has been found to decrease the elevated resting pressure of the LES of patients suffering from achalasia (74). It can relieve dysphagia, and zinc protamine glucagon may be useful in treating patients with this disorder.

Glucagon decreases LES pressure and suppresses gut motility and gastric secretion. It has been used to aid in the treatment of esophageal perforation by diminishing reflux of esophagogastric contents (116).

Glucagon can be administered to relax gut smooth muscle, allowing better endoscopic visualization of the intestine (13, 121) and bile ducts (44, 52). Glucagon reduces bile duct sphincter pressure and bile duct pressure (12). It has been used to relieve the pain and help the passage of gallstones (28, 74, 131). Glucagon has also been used to relieve narcotic-induced choledochoduodenal sphincter spasm and improve visualization of the bile ducts during operative cholangiography (65).

An intravenous infusion or bolus of glucagon relieves the pain of acute diverticulitis more quickly than conventional therapy with analgesics or antispasmotics (22), and does not block the pain response or alter the abdominal examination. Daniel et al. (22) administered glucagon to 20 patients with attacks of diverticulitis (1 mg intravenously every 4 hours or 1 mg over 4 hours by infusion). Patients were pain free in a mean period of 12 hours compared with 4 days in a control group receiving conventional therapy. Glucagon has been used to relieve intestinal spasm and aid in surgical

end-to-end anastomosis during gastrointestinal surgery (57).

Glucagon inhibits gastric acid (78) and pancreatic juice (30, 31) secretion. It has been used in the treatment of acute pancreatitis (19, 24, 33, 50, 71, 98, 102, 109, 142). It does not alter the severity of pancreatitis, duration of pain, hospital duration, or mortality. However, glucagon may have prophylactic value (99) when given before an insult (e.g., ERCP). Glucagon has been used to decrease pancreatic secretions and accelerate closure of pancreatic fistula (40).

Glucagon is hepatotrophic (23) and has been used in the treatment of advanced liver disease. Baker and colleagues (5) compared insulin and glucagon infusion with dextrose infusion in patients with alcoholic hepatitis and found a tendency (although not significant) toward improved survival in the glucagon group. Jaspan et al. (64) reported an improvement in hepatic function in a patient with liver failure. Animal studies of insulin/glucagon in galactosamine-induced fulminant hepatitis found no benefit (101). Further studies are needed to evaluate hormonal therapy for liver failure.

Glucagon may be useful in differentiating obstructure from nonobstructive jaundice (6, 14). A 1-mg dose of glucagon increases cyclic AMP levels over 40-fold in obstructive jaundice, whereas in nonobstructive jaundice cyclic AMP levels rise less than 20-fold (14). Bernstock et al. (6) were able to differentiate obstructive from hepatocellular jaundice by the glucose response to glucagon injection.

UROLOGIC EFFECTS

Glucagon is filtered and reabsorbed across the luminal membrane of renal tubular cells and degraded, predominantly in the proximal tubule (74). Pharmacologic doses of glucagon increase urinary flow and ion excretion (e.g., sodium, phosphorus, and calcium) (41). These effects result from an increase in glomerular filtration rate due to a selective dilatation of afferent arterioles, a natriuretic effect related to prostaglandin synthesis, and a direct depressant effect on tubular reabsorption (74). Further studies are needed to determine whether physiologic changes in glucagon levels alter renal function during disease states.

Glucagon blocks ureteral peristalsis and has diuretic action within the kidney. It may be useful in relieving ureteral colic due to calculi and may aid in the passage of renal stones (80, 102). Lowman et al. (80) treated 10 patients with glucagon (1 mg administered intravenously) for colic due to ureterolithiasis. Pain was promptly relieved in all patients (lasted 1–3 hours), and calculi passed in 4–8 hours in three cases. Morishima and Ghaed (102) successfully treated five cases of ureteral colic with glucagon and forced diuresis. However, Zobbe et al. (151) found no benefit from glucagon in a randomized trial in patients with ureteral colic from calculi.

RADIOLOGIC EFFECTS

Glucagon-induced gut relaxation and decreased motility help enhance visualization of gastrointestinal lesions (74, 100). This technique is particularly useful for the detection of small occult neoplasms, early Crohn's disease, and Meckel's diverticulum (74). Glucagon has resulted in less discomfort, faster procedures, and better radiologic images during barium enema examination (74). During fluoroscopy, glucagon helps separate functional spasm from organic lesions. Glucagon may also assist in the resolution of intussusception by barium enema (46).

Glucagon is useful in cholangiography (11). The administration of glucagon relieves pain and spasm in the bile ducts and may help in the passage of gallstones and visualization of the gallbladder. Glucagon may also help differentiate functional from organic obstructions.

Glucagon has been used to reverse cornual spasm during hysterosalpingography (146). This technique may reduce the number of artifactual tubal obstructions seen during hysterosalpingography and reduce subsequent laparoscopies. Abdominal digital angiography and selective angiography is used to visualize intestinal blood vessels. Peristalsis-induced artifacts can be reduced or eliminated by 1 mg of intravenous glucagon (122). Glucagon abolishes ureteral peristalsis but does not improve visualization of the ureters during urography (136).

RESPIRATORY EFFECTS

Glucagon relaxes bronchial smooth musculature (37, 74). Lockey et al. (79) reported improvement in airway obstruction in patients with asthma after they received intravenous glucagon. The mechanism for decreased airway obstruction may relate to elevations in intracellular cyclic AMP.

SIDE EFFECTS

Nausea and vomiting, the most common side effects of glucagon administration, are usually associated with large bolus injections (26) and intravenous infusions of greater than 5 mg/hour (81). Antiemetic therapy can minimize these symptoms. Glucagon-induced hypokalemia (26, 81, 107) results from increased insulin secretion with intracellular transfer of glucose and potassium. Both hyperglycemia and hypoglycemia can occur with glucagon therapy. Hyperglycemia is mild and requires no treatment. Hypoglycemia is seen in patients lacking hepatic glycogen (due to unopposed insulin action). Hypoglycemic symptoms can be avoided by carefully monitoring the serum glucose level.

Glucagon is a vasodilator and may lower arterial pressure. Arterial pressure is usually maintained by a concomitant increase in cardiac output. The volume depleted patient is more susceptible to decreases in blood pressure. Glucagon may also cause tachycardia. Glucagon must be given cautiously to hypertensive patients or patients with suspected pheochromocytoma because it stimulates the release of endogenous catecholamines (72, 75, 97, 148). Hypertension usually responds to treatment with phentolamine. Caution is also advised in patients with an insulinoma, since glucagon-stimulated insulin release may cause severe hypoglycemia.

Glucagon is insoluble in saline or water solutions at a pH of between 3 and 9.5 and must be solubilized in the accompanying diluent prior to dilution or administration. The diluent contains phenol (0.2%) and glycerin. Large doses or continuous infusion should be solubilized in the smallest amount of diluent possible and diluted in 5% dextrose solution to avoid the central nervous system and myocardial depression that may be produced by phenol (21). Rarely, a patient may have an allergic reaction to glucagon.

PRESCRIBING INFORMATION AND DRUG INTERACTIONS

Glucagon for clinical use is extracted from beef and pork pancreas. It is relatively insoluble in water unless the pH is less than 3 or greater than 9.5. Glucagon is supplied as a lyophilized powder (1-mg or 10-mg ampules) mixed with lactose and is stable at room temperatures. It is usually solubilized in a phenol diluent and once reconstituted, should be used immediately.

Glucagon may be given subcutaneously, intramuscularly, or intravenously. Boluses of 1–5 mg/hour are usually used in patients with heart failure (Table 33.16) (10, 145). A weight-dependent dose of 50 μg/kg (bolus) of intravenous glucagon (88) is an alternative therapeutic approach. Doses of 1 mg (intravenous bolus) are used for gastrointestinal, urologic, and radiographic studies. One to 5 mg of glucagon is used to treat hypoglycemia (Table 33.16).

Glucagon potentiates the anticoagulant effect of warfarin (68) by depressing vitamin K–sensitive clotting factors and/or increasing warfarin receptor affinity. When glucagon is given to patients receiving warfarin, careful monitoring of the prothrombin time is required to avoid bleeding. Glucagon does not affect the actions of heparin.

References

1. Abel FL: Action of glucagon on canine left ventricular performance and coronary hemodynamics. *Circ Shock* 11:45, 1983.
2. Agura ED, Wexler LF, Witzburg RA: Massive propranolol overdose—successful treatment with high dose isoproterenol and glucagon. *Am J Med* 80:755–757, 1986.
3. Altin JG, Bygrave FL: Ca^{2+} uptake stimulated by the synergistic action of glucagon and Ca^{2+}-mobilizing agents in the perfused rat liver occurs through the activation of a undirectional Ca^{2+} influx pathway. *Biochem Biophy Res Comm* 142:745–753, 1987.
4. Armstrong PW, Gold HB, Daggett WM, Austen WG, Sanders CA: Hemodynamic evaluation of glucagon in symptomatic heart disease. *Circulation* 44:67–73, 1971.
5. Baker AL, Jaspan JB, Haines NW, et al: A randomized clinical trial of insulin and glucagon infusion for treatment of alcoholic hepatitis: Progress report in 50 patients. *Gastroenterology* 80:1410–1414, 1981.
6. Berstock DA, Wood JR, Williams R: The glucagon test in obstructive and hepatocellular jaundice. *Postgrad Med J* 58:485–486, 1982.
7. Bleicher SJ, Levy LJ, Zarowitz H, et al: Glucagon-deficiency hypoglycemia: A new syndrome. *Clin Res* 18:355, 1970.
8. Bower MG, Okude S, Jolley WB, Smith LL: Hemodynamic effects of glucagon following hemorrhage and endotoxic shock in the dog. *Arch Surg* 101:411–415, 1970.
9. Bowman HM, Cowan D, Kovach G, et al: Renal effects of glucagon in rhesus monkeys during hypovolemia. *Surg Gynecol Obstet* 134:937, 1972.
10. Brogan E, Kozonis MC, Overy DC: Glucagon therapy in heart failure. *Lancet* 1:482, 1969.
11. Cannon P, Legge D: Glucagon as a hypotonic agent in cholangiography. *Clin Radiol* 30:49, 1979.
12. Carr-Locke DL, Gregg JA, Aoki TT: Effects of exogenous glucagon on pancreatic and biliary ductal and sphincter pressures in man demonstrated by endoscopic manometry and correlation with plasma glucagon. *Dig Dis Sciences* 28:312–320, 1983.
13. Carsen GM, Finby N: Hypotonic duodenography with glucagon. *Radiology* 118:529, 1976.
14. Carstensen HE, Vrunn E, Hansen OH, et al: Glucagon stimulated plasma cyclic adenosine $-3',5'$-monophosphate in the differential diagnosis of jaundice. *Surg Gynecol Obstet* 149:503, 1979.
15. Chernow B, Reed L, Geelhoed GW, et al: Glucagon: Endocrine effects and calcium involvement in cardiovascular actions in dogs. *Circ Shock* 19:393–407, 1986.
16. Chernow B, Zaloga GP, Malcolm D, Clapper M, Holaday JW: Glucagon's chronotropic action is calcium dependent. *J Pharmacol Exp Ther* 241:833–837, 1987.
17. Cherrington AD, Liljinquist JE: Role of glucagon in regulating glucose production in vivo. In Unger RH, Orce L (eds): *Glucagon*. New York, Elsevier, 1981, pp 221–253.
18. Cohn KE, Agmon J, Gamble OW: The effect of glucagon on arrhythmias due to digitalis toxicity. *Am J Cardiol* 25:683–689, 1970.
19. Condon JR, Knight MJ, Day JL: Glucagon therapy in acute pancreatitis. *Br J Surg* 60:509, 1973.
20. Cronenwett JL, Ayad M, Kazmers A: Effect of intravenous glucagon on the survival of rats after acute occlusive mesenteric ischemia. *J Surg Res* 38:446–452, 1985.
21. Cronk JD: Phenol with glucagon in cardiotherapy. *N Engl J Med* 284:219, 1971.
22. Daniel O, Basu PK, Al-Samarrae HM: Use of glucagon in the treatment of acute diverticulitis. *Br Med J* 3:730, 1974.
23. deDiego JA, Molina LM, Bujan J, Simon P, Gea M, Menchero A, Balibrea JL: Influence of the conjoint administration of insulin and glucagon upon hepatic regeneration. *Surg Gyn Obstet* 163:443–447, 1986.
24. Debas H, Hancock RJ, Soon-Shiong P, Smythe HA, Cassim MM: Glucagon therapy in acute pancreatitis: Prospective randomized double blind study. *Can J Surg* 23:578–580, 1980.
25. Denowitz M, Hendler R, Spiro HM, et al: Glucagon secretion in acute and chronic pancreatitis. *Ann Intern Med* 83:778, 1975.
26. Deraney MF: Glucagon? One answer to cardiogenic shock. *Am J Med Sci* 261:149, 1971.
27. Diamond G, Forrester J, Danzig R, Parmley WW, Swan HJC: Acute myocardial infarction in man. Comparative hemodynamic effects of norepinephrine and glucagon. *Am J Cardiol* 27:612–616, 1971.
28. Doman DB, Ginsberg AL: Glucagon infusion therapy for biliary tree stones. *Gastroenterology* 80:1137, 1981.
29. Drucker MR, Pindyck F, Brown RS, et al: The interaction of glucagon and glucose on cardiorespiratory variables in the critically ill patient. *Surgery* 75:487–495, 1974.
30. Dyck WP, Rudick J, Hoexter B, et al: Influence of glucagon on pancreatic exocrine secretion. *Gastroenterology* 56:531, 1969.
31. Dyck WP, Texter EC, Lasater JM, et al: Influence of glucagon on pancreatic exocrine secretion in man. *Gastroenterology* 58:532, 1970.
32. Dunger DB, Leonard JV: Value of the glucagon test in screening for hepatic glycogen storage diseases. *Arch Dis Child* 57:384, 1982.
33. Durr HK, Maroske D, Zelder O, Bode JCK: Glucagon therapy in acute pancreatitis: Report of a double-blind trial. *Gut* 19:175, 1978.
34. Eddy JD, O'Grien ET, Singh SP: Glucagon and hemodynamics of acute myocardial infarction. *Br Med J* 4:663, 1969.
35. Eigler N, Sacca L, Sherwin RS: Synergistic interactions

of physiologic increments of glucagon, epinephrine and cortisol in the dog. *J Clin Invest* 63:114, 1979.

36. Einzig S, Todd EP, Nicoloff DM, Lucas RV: Glucagon in prevention and abolition of ouabain-induced ventricular tachycardia in normokalemic and hypokalemic dogs. *Circ Res* 29:88–95, 1971.

37. El Naggar M, Collins VJ: Spirometry following glucagon and isoproterenol in chronic obstructive lung disease. *Crit Care Med* 2:82–85, 1974.

38. Elrich H, Witten TA, Arai Y: Glucagon treatment of insulin reactions. *N Engl J Med* 258:476, 1958.

39. Esquibel AJ, Kurland AA, Mendelsohn D: The use of glucagon in terminating insulin coma. *Dis Nerv Syst* 19:485–486, 1958.

40. Fallingborg J, Andersen SP, Laustsen J, Christensen LA: Glucagon treatment of external pancreatic fistula. *Acta Chir Scand* 151:183–184, 1985.

41. Farah AE: Glucagon and the circulation. *Pharmacol Rev* 35:181–217, 1983.

42. Farah A, Tuttle R: Studies on the pharmacology of glucagon. *J Pharmacol Exp Ther* 129:49, 1960.

43. Ferrucci JT, Long JA: Radiologic treatment of esophageal food impaction using intravenous glucagon. *Diag Radiol* 125:25, 1977.

44. Ferrucci JT, Wittenberg J, Stone LB, et al: Hypotonic cholangiography with glucagon. *Radiology* 118:466, 1976.

45. Finegold DN, Stanley CA, Baker L: Glycemic response to glucagon during fasting hypoglycemia: an aid to the diagnosis of hyperinsulinism. *J Pediatr* 96:257–260, 1986.

46. Fisher JK, Germann DR: Glucagon-aided reduction of intussusception. *Radiology* 122:197–198, 1977.

47. Fradkin J, Shamoon H, Felig P, et al: Evidence for an important role of changes in rather than absolute concentrations of glucagon in the regulation of glucose production in man. *J Clin Endocrinol Metab* 50:698, 1980.

48. Gerich JE, Lorenzi M, Bier DM, et al: Prevention of human diabetic ketoacidosis by somatostatin. Evidence for an essential role of glucagon. *N Engl J Med* 292:985, 1975.

49. Gerich JE, Raptis S, Rosenthal J: Somatostatin symposium. *Metabolism* 27(Suppl 1):1, 1978.

50. Gilsanz V, Oteyza CP, Rebollar JL: Glucagon vs anticholinergics in the treatment of acute pancreatitis. A double-blind controlled trial. *Arch Intern Med* 138:535, 1978.

51. Glick G, Parmley WW, Wechsler AS, et al: Glucagon: Its enhancement of cardiac performance in the cat and dog and persistence of its inotropic action despite beta-receptor blockade with propranolol. *Circ Res* 22:789, 1968.

52. Golikov AP, Berestov AA, Maiorov WI: Differential use of glucagon in the acute period of myocardial infarction. *Kardiologia* 19:11–17, 1979.

53. Gotlin RW, Silver HK: Neonatal hypoglycemia, hyperinsulinism and absence of pancreatic alpha-cells. *Lancet* 1:1346, 1970.

54. Grollman A, McCaleb WE, White FN: Glucagon deficiency as a cause of hypoglycemia. *Metabolism* 13:686, 1964.

55. Guillen J, Pappas G: Improved cardiovascular effects of glucagon in dogs with endotoxin shock. *Ann Surg* 175:535, 1972.

56. Handal KA,, Riordan W, Sriae J: The lower esophagus and glucagon. *Ann Emerg Med* 9:577, 1980.

57. Harford FJ: Use of glucagon in conjunction with the end-to-end anastomosis (EEA) stapling device for low anterior anastomoses. *Dis Colon Rectum* 22:452–454, 1979.

58. Hedo JA, Villaneuva ML, Marco J: Stimulation of pancreatic polypeptide and glucagon secretion by 2-deoxy-D-glucose in man: Evidence for cholinergic mediation. *J Clin Endocrinol Metab* 47:366, 1978.

59. Hogan WJ, Dodds WJ, Hoke SE, et al: Effect of glucagon on esophageal motor function. *Gastroenterology* 69:160, 1976.

60. Ipp E, Dobbs R, Unger RH: Morphine and beta-endorphin influence the secretion of the endocrine pancreas. *Nature* 276:190, 1978.

61. Ishida K, Hayasaka H, Hinshaw LB, Williams GR: Release of glucagon in septic patients (abstract). *Circ Shock* 21:293, 1987.

62. Ishida K, Hinshaw LB: Changes of plasma gastrointestinal glucagon concentrations following lethal infusions of E. coli. *Circ Shock* 19:301–308, 1986.

63. Jain KM, Rush BF, Hastings OM, Ghosh A, Slotman G, Abousam S. Glucagon treatment of hemorrhagic shock: improved survival and metabolic parameters in a murine shock model. *Adv Shock Res* 1:149–157, 1979.

64. Jaspan JB, Landau RL, Schneider J: Insulin and glucagon infusion in the treatment of liver failure. *Arch Intern Med* 144:2075–2078, 1984.

65. Jones RM, Fiddian-Green R, Knight PR: Narcotic-induced choledochoduodenal sphincter spasm reversed by glucagon. *Anesth Analg* 59:946–947, 1980.

66. Kazmers A, Zwolak R, Appleman HD, et al: Pharmacologic interventions in acute mesenteric ischemia: improved survival with intravenous glucagon, methylprednisolone, and prostacyclin. *J Vasc Surg* 1:472–481, 1984.

67. Klein SW, March JE, Mahon WA: Cardiovascular effects of glucagon in man. *Can Med Assoc J* 98:1161, 1968.

68. Koch-Weser J: Potentiation by glucagon of the hypoprothrombinemic action of warfarin. *Ann Intern Med* 72:331, 1970.

69. Kosinski EJ, Malendzak GS: Glucagon and isoproterenol in reversing propranolol toxicity. *Arch Intern Med* 132:840, 1973.

70. Kraus-Friedmann N: Effects of glucagon and vasopressin on hepatic CA^{2+} release. *Proc Natl Acad Sci USA* 83:8943–8946, 1986.

71. Kornborg O, Bulow S, Joergensen PW, et al: A randomized double-blind trial of glucagon in treatment of first attack of severe acute pancreatitis without associated biliary disease. *Am J Gastroenterol* 73:423, 1980.

72. Lawrence AM: Glucagon provocation test for pheochromocytoma. *Ann Intern Med* 66:1091, 1967.

73. Leclercq-Meyer V, Malaisse WJ: The role of calcium in glucagon release—studies with verapamil. *Diabetes* 27:996, 1978.

74. Lefelovre PJ (ed): *Glucagon.* Berlin, Springer-Verlag, 1983, vols 1 and 2.

75. Levinson PD, Hamilton BP, Mersey JH, et al: Plasma norepinephrine and epinephrine responses to glucagon in patients with suspected pheochromocytomas. *Metabolism* 32:998, 1983.

76. Levy M: The effect of glucagon on glomerular filtration rate in dogs during reduction of renal blood flow. *Can J Physiol Pharmacol* 53:660–668, 1978.

77. Lickley HLA, Kemmer FW, Doi K, Vranic M: Glucagon suppression improves glucoregulation in moderate but not chronic severe diabetes. *Am J Physiol* 245:E424–429, 1983.

78. Lin TM, Spray GR: Effect of glucagon on gastric HCl secretion. *Gastroenterology* 54:1254, 1968.

79. Lockey SD, Reed CE, Ouellette JJ: Bronchodilatory effect of glucagon in asthma (abstract). *J Allerg* 43:177, 1969.

80. Lowman RM, Belleza NA, Goetsch JB, Finkelstein HI, Berneike RH, Rosenfield AT. Glucagon. *J Urol* 118:128, 1977.

81. Lroff R, Welcken DEL: Glucagon in heart failure and in cardiogenic shock. *Circulation* 45:534, 1972.

82. Lucchese BR: Cardiac actions of glucagon. *Circ Res* 22:777, 1968.

83. MacCuish AC, Munro JF, Duncan LJP: Treatment of

hypoglycemic coma with glucagon, intravenous glucose, and mannitol infusion in a hundred diabetics. *Lancet* 2:946–949, 1970.

84. Madan BR: Effect of glucagon on ventricular arrhythmias after coronary artery occlusion and on ventricular automaticity in the dog. *Br J Pharmacol* 43:279–286, 1971.

85. Madan BR, Jain BK: Combined use of glucagon and beta-adrenoreceptor antagonists in ventricular arrhythmias accompanying myocardial infarction. *Indian J Med Res* 61:1535–1543, 1973.

86. Malcolm DS, Zaloga GP, Chernow B, Holaday JW: Glucagon is a potent antagonist of morphine bradycardia and antinociception. *Life Sci* 39:399–405, 1986.

87. Manchester JH, Parmley WW, Matloff JM, Sonnenblick E: Beneficial effects of glucagon on canine myocardial infarction and shock. *Clin Res* 17:252, 1969.

88. Manchester JH, Parmley WW, Matloff JM, et al: Effects of glucagon on myocardial oxygen consumption and coronary blood flow in man and in dog. *Circulation* 41:579, 1970.

89. Manson NH, Hess ML: Role of angiotensin I and glucagon in canine endotoxin shock. *Circ Shock* 12:177–189, 1984.

90. Marco J, Colle C, Roman D, et al: Hyperglucagonism induced by glucocorticoid treatment in man. *N Engl J Med* 288:128, 1973.

91. Marcus ML, Skelton CL, Prindle KH, Epstein SE: Potentiation of the inotropic effects of glucagon by theophylline. *J Pharm Exp Ther* 179:331–337, 1971.

92. Markovitz LJ, Hasin Y, Freund HR: The effect of insulin and glucagon on systolic properties of the normal and septic isolated rat heart. *Basic Res Cardiol* 80:377–383, 1985.

93. Marks HW, Lousteau RJ: Glucagon and esophageal meat impaction. *Arch Otolaryngol* 106:367, 1979.

94. Marks V, Samols E: Hypoglycaemia of non-endocrine origin (non-islet cell tumours). *Proc R Soc Med* 59:338–340, 1966.

95. Matloff JM, Parmley WW, Manchester JH, Berkovits B, Sonnenblick EH, Harken DE: Hemodynamic effects of glucagon and intra-aortic baloon counterpulsation in canine myocardial infarction. *Am J Cardiol* 25:675–682, 1970.

96. McLeod MK, Carlson DE, Gann DS: Secretory response of glucagon to hemorrhage. *J Trauma* 23:445, 1983.

97. McLoughlin MJ, Langer B, Wilson DR: Life-threatening reaction to glucagon in a patient with pheochromocytoma. *Radiology* 140:841, 1981.

98. Medical Research Council Trial: Morbidity of acute pancreatitis: the effect of aprotinin and glucagon. *Gut* 21:334–339, 1980.

99. Menabe T, Steer ML: Experimental acute pancreatitis in mice—protective effect of glucagon. *Gastroenterology* 76:529, 1979.

100. Miller RE, Chernish SM, Greenman GF, Maglinte DT, Rosenak BD, Brunelle RL: Gastrointestinal response to minute doses of glucagon. *Radiology* 143:317–320, 1982.

101. Minuk GY, Sherman TA, Shaffer EA, Kelly SK: A comparative study of the effects of insulin/glucagon infusions, parenteral amino acids and high dose corticosteroids on survival in a rabbit model of acute fulminant hepatitis. *Hepatology* 6:73–78, 1986.

102. Morishima MS, Ghaed N: Glucagon and diuresis in the treatment of ureteral calculi. *Radiology* 129:807, 1978.

103. Moseson MD, Hoexter B, Labow SB: Glucagon, a useful adjunct in anastomosis with a stapling device. *Dis Colon Rectum* 23:25, 1980.

104. MCR Working Party: Death from acute pancreatitis. MCR multicentre trial of glucagon and aprotinin. *Lancet* 2:632, 1977.

105. Muhlhauser I, Koch J, Berger M: Pharmacokinetics and bioavailability of injected glucagon: differences between intramuscular, subcutaneous, and intravenous administration. *Diabetes Care* 8:39–42, 1985.

106. Murtagh JG, Binnion PF, Lol S, Hutchison KJ, Fletcher E: Hemodynamic effects of glucagon. *Br Heart J* 32:307–315, 1970.

107. Nayler WG, McInnes I, Chipperfield D, et al: The effect of glucagon on calcium exchangeability, coronary blood flow, myocardial function and high energy phosphate stores. *J Pharmacol Exp Ther* 171:265, 1970.

108. Niemann JT, Haynes KS, Garner D, Jagels G, Rennie CJ: Postcountershock pulseless rhythms: Hemodynamic effects of glucagon in a canine model. *Crit Care Med* 15:554–558, 1987.

109. Olazabal O, Fuller R: Failure of glucagon in the treatment of alcoholic pancreatitis. *Gastroenterology* 74:489, 1978.

110. Palmer JP, Porte D Jr: Control of glucagon secretion. The central nervous system. In Unger RH, Orce L (eds): Glucagon. New York, Elsevier, 1981, pp 133–159.

111. Parmley WW, Glick G, Sonnenblick EH: Cardiovascular effects of glucagon in man. *N Engl J Med* 279:12, 1968.

112. Parmley WW, Matloff JM, Sonnenblick EH: Hemodynamic effects of glucagon in patients following prosthetic valve replacement. *Circulation* 39:163–167, 1969.

113. Parmley WW, Sonnenblick EH: A role for glucagon in cardiac therapy. *Am J Med Sci* 258:224–229, 1969.

114. Patel GK, Whalen GE, Soergel KH, Wu WC, Meade RC: Glucagon effects on the human small intestine. *Dig Dis Sciences* 24:501–507, 1979.

115. Peterson CD, Leeder JS, Sterner S: Glucagon therapy for β-blocker overdose. *Drug Intel Clin Pharmacy* 18:394–398, 1984.

116. Pickard R: Glucagon in management of perforated esophagus. *Br Med J* 4:232, 1974.

117. Pillari G, Bank S, Katzka I, et al: Meat bolus impaction of the lower esophagus associated with paraesophageal hernia. *Am J Gastroenterol* 71:287, 1979.

118. Prasod K: Use of glucagon in the treatment of quinidine toxicity in the heart. *Cardiovasc Res* 11:55, 1977.

119. Prasad K, DeSousa HH: Glucagon in the treatment of ouabain-induced cardiac arrhythmias in dogs. *Cardiovasc Res* 6:333, 1972.

120. Prasad K, Wickworth P: Glucagon in procainamide induced cardiac toxicity. *Toxicol Appl Pharmacol* 46:517, 1978.

121. Qvigstad T, Larsen S, Myren J: Comparison of glucagon, atropine, and placebo as premedication for endoscopy of the upper gastrointestinal tract. *Scand J Gastroent* 14:231–235, 1979.

122. Rabe PE, Yune HY, Klatte EC, et al: Efficacy of glucagon for abdominal digital angiography. *Am J Radiol* 139:618, 1982.

123. Raskin P, Unger RH: Glucagon and diabetes. *Med Clin North Am* 62:713, 1978.

124. Raskin P, Unger RH: Hyperglucagonemia and its suppression: Importance in the metabolic control of diabetes. *N Engl J Med* 299:433, 1978.

125. Schumer W, Miller B, Nichols RL, McDonald GO, Nyhus LM: Metabolic and microcirculatory effects of glucagon in hypovolemic shock. *Arch Surg* 107:176–180, 1973.

126. Sherwin RS, Felig P: Glucagon physiology in health and disease. In McCann SM (ed): *International Review of Physiology: Endocrine Physiology*. Baltimore, University Park Press, 1977.

127. Siegel JH, Levine MJ, McConn R, et al: The effect of glucagon infusion on cardiovascular function in the critically ill. *Surg Gynecol Obstet* 131:505, 1970.

128. Sistare FD, Picking RA, Haynes RC: Sensitivity of the response of cytosolic calcium in Quin-2-loaded rat hepatocytes to glucagon, adenine nucleosides, and adenine nucleotides. *J Biol Chem* 260:12744–12747, 1985.

129. Sonnenblick EH, Parmley WW, Matloff J: Hemody-

namic effects of glucagon after prosthetic valve replacement. *Circulation* 37:183, 1968.

130. Steiner C, Wit AL, Damato AB: Effects of glucagon on atrioventricular conduction and ventricular automaticity in dogs. *Circ Res* 24:167–177, 1969.

131. Stower MJ, Foster GE, Hardcastle JD: A trial of glucagon in the treatment of painful biliary tract disease. *Br J Surg* 69:591–592, 1982.

132. Sutherland EW, Robinson GA, Butcher RW: Some aspects of biological role of adenosine 3′,5′-monophosphate (cyclic AMP). *Circulation* 35:279, 1968.

133. Tai TY, Pek S: Direct stimulation by growth hormone of glucagon and insulin release from isolated rat pancreas. *Endocrinology* 99:669, 1976.

134. Talesnik J, Tsoporis J: Enhancement by glutathione of the inotropic actions of catecholamines and glucagon. *J Mol Cell Cardiol* 16:573–576, 1984.

135. Teich S, Malcolm D, Zaloga GP, Holaday J, Chernow B: Beneficial effects of glucagon in endotoxic shock in rats. *Circ Shock* 16:95, 1985.

136. Thomsen HS, Hartelius H, Jensen R, Flindt-Nielsen N, Ohlhues L: Excretory urography with glucagon: a randomized trial. *Radiology* 147:335–338, 1983.

137. Torella R, Giugliano D, Scognamiglio G, et al: Glucagon secretion in patients with hypoparathyroidism: Effect of serum calcium on glucagon release. *J Clin Endo Metab* 54:229, 1982.

138. Unger RH, Orce L: Glucagon and the A cell. *N Engl J Med* 304:1518, 1575, 1981.

139. Unger RH, Orce L: Role of glucagon in diabetes. *Arch Intern Med* 137:482, 1977.

140. Vanderark CR: Clinical evaluation of glucagon by continuous infusion in the treatment of low cardiac output states. *Am Heart J* 79:481, 1970.

141. Vanderwall DA, Stowe NT, Spangenberg R, et al: Effect of glucagon in hemorrhagic stock. *J Surg Oncology* 2:177, 1970.

142. Waterworth NW, Barbezat GO, Hickman R, et al: A controlled trial of glucagon in experimental pancreatitis. *Br J Surg* 63:617, 1976.

143. Weingand KW, Fettman MJ, Phillips RW, Hand MS: Metabolic effects of glucagon in endotoxemic minipigs. *Circ Shock* 18:289–300, 1986.

144. Whitsitt LS, Lucchesi BR: Effects of beta-receptor blockade and glucagon on the atrioventricular transmission system in the dog. *Circ Res* 23:585–595, 1968.

145. Wilcken DEL, Lvoff R: Glucagon in resistant heart-failure and cardiogenic shock. *Lancet* 1:1315, 1970.

146. Winfield AC, Haway DP, Maxson W, et al: Apparent cornual occlusion in hysterosalpingography: Reversal by glucagon. *Am J Radiol* 139:525, 1982.

147. Wise JK, Hendler R, Felig P: Influence of glucocorticoids on glucagon secretion and plasma amino acid concentrations in man. *J Clin Invest* 52:2774, 1973.

148. Yoshimasa T, Nakao K, Li S, et al: Plasma methionine-enkephalin and leucine-enkephalin in normal subjects and patients with phenochromocytoma. *J Clin Endocrinol Metabol* 57:70b, 1983.

149. Zaloga GP, DeLacey W, Holmboe E, Chernow B: Glucagon reverses the hypotension of anaphylactic shock. *Ann Intern Med* 105:65–66, 1986.

150. Zaloga GP, Malcolm D, Holaday J, Chernow B: Glucagon reverses the hypotension and bradycardia of verapamil overdose in rats. *Crit Care Med* 13:273, 1985.

151. Zobbe VB, Rygaard H, Rosmussen D, et al: Glucagon in acute ureteral colic. *Eur Urol* 12:28–31, 1986.

34

Thyroid Hormones

Kenneth D. Burman, M.D., Col., M.C.

In the last several years, our understanding of thyroid physiology and the mechanism of thyroid hormone action has progressed at an unheralded rate. As a result, we can now apply these newly acquired principles to clinical settings and, thus, appropriately alter our approach to patients with thyroid disease. We have accrued an understanding of the pathophysiologic alterations in thyroid metabolism that occur in ambulatory patients. In this chapter, basic thyroid hormone physiology, the laboratory tests available to assess thyroid hormone function, and the therapeutic agents employed to treat patients with altered thyroid hormone function are reviewed. Unfortunately, however, our knowledge of the critically ill individual is still clouded by a lack of understanding of the mechanism for the perturbations in thyroid function tests and by the lack of a definitive tissue marker denoting metabolic hypothyroidism at the cellular level. As a result, I also review in this chapter the findings relative to thyroid function in the critically ill subject and will give my opinion concerning the interpretation of these tests and how to apply them to systemically ill patient. These opinions, of course, are subject to modification as further research and experience evolve. (A very useful aid in understanding the action, kinetics and adverse effects of the drugs mentioned in this chapter is the Rocky Mountain Drug Consultation Center, West 8th and Cherokee, Denver, CO 80204. Much of the data in this chapter were checked with that source.)

THYROID HORMONE PHYSIOLOGY

Although thyroid function tests and clinical examination are extremely useful in ascertaining if an individual is euthyroid, these parameters are less useful and perhaps even misleading when applied to a patient in the intensive care unit (21, 27, 28, 50, 124). The interpretation of the appropriateness of these tests is dependent upon an understanding of the basic physiology of the hypothalamic-pituitary-thyroid axis. Hypothalamic thyrotropin-releasing hormone (thyrotropin, or TRH) stimulates pituitary synthesis and release of thyroid-stimulating hormone (TSH), a hormone that then stimulates thyroidal synthesis and release of $3,5,3',5'$-L-tetraiodothyronine (T_4) and $3,5,3'$-L-triiodothyronine (T_3) (Figs. 34.1 and 34.2). Circulating T_4 is derived entirely from direct thyroidal secretion, whereas only approximately 25% of circulating T_3 is derived from glandular release, the remainder being derived from peripheral conversion of T_4 to T_3 (16, 18, 71, 113). Another metabolite, reverse T_3 (rT_3), is also principally derived from T_4. These conversions of T_4 to T_3 and rT_3 are dependent upon an enzyme(s) that resides in many tissues including brain, liver, and kidney. In normal subjects about 40% of the T_4 secreted is eventually monodeiodinated, resulting in about 80% of all serum T_3 being derived from this extrathyroidal source. Pituitary conversion of T_4 to T_3 probably accounts for approximately 50% of the local pituitary T_3, the remainder being derived from circulating T_3 that is transported to the pituitary (71). In either case, it is probably the local pituitary T_3 content that regulates TSH synthesis and release. Of course, there are other factors, which are capable of stimulating TSH release, e.g., TRH (Fig. 34.3) and hypothermia, whereas inhibitory factors include dopamine, somatostatin, hyperthermia, glucocorticoids, and, of course, T_4/T_3 (47, 66, 82).

In the serum, T_4 and T_3 circulate tightly bound to serum proteins (thyroxine-binding globulin (TBG), thyroxine-binding prealbumin (TBPA), and albumin) and only about 0.3% of T_3 and 0.03% of T_4 are unbound. This unbound fraction is believed to be the major portion of the hormone capable of traversing

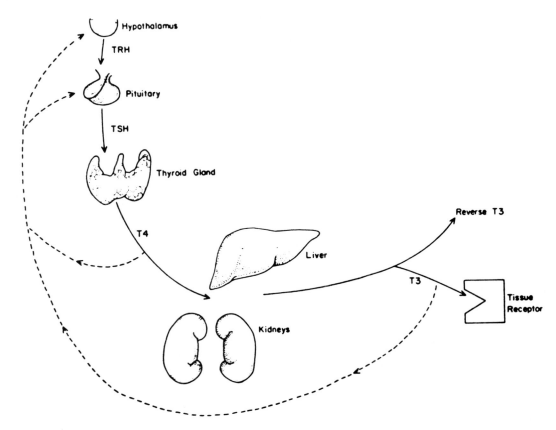

Figure 34.1. Hypothalamic-pituitary-thyroid axis in a euthyroid individual. (From Burman KD: *Thyroid: University Case Reports,* vol 3. Morris Plains, NJ, Parke-Davis, Division of Warner-Lambert, Inc., 1981.)

membranes and exerting its influence upon nuclear receptors (e.g., to increase protein synthesis) (64, 88, 95, 102). Since nuclear receptors have affinities for T_3 about 10 times greater than for T_4 and since T_3 is also less tightly bound to serum proteins than T_4, one can account for most, if not all, of thyroid hormone action by T_3 alone. In selected circumstances T_4 may be active, albeit less than T_3, but in most situations T_4 could be thought of as a prohormone. Understanding these considerations helps us conceptualize why the serum T_4 concentration may not always be an accurate reflection of the tissue effects by thyroid hormones.

Peripheral deiodination proceeds enzymatically (Fig. 34.1) and in some circumstances this conversion is altered, such that less T_3 (active hormone) and more rT_3 (inactive metabolite) is formed (5, 19, 26, 64, 111, 119). This decrease in conversion to T_3 may be homeostatic as it would reduce catabolism, thus

theoretically being beneficial during critical illness. Several of the conditions or agents which decrease T_4-to-T_3 conversion are listed in Table 34.1.

Although a great deal is understood about the physiology of thyroid hormone and its mechanism of action, there are no accurate, reproducible parameters available for assessing the metabolic state of any patient, especially one in the intensive care unit. A physician must depend to a large degree on his or her clinical skills to assess the thyroid status of a systemically ill patient. A complete medical history including family history of thyroid disease, medications ingested, and a physical examination of the neck revealing a surgical scar or enlarged gland are extremely helpful and crucial to the correct interpretation of the thyroid function test results. Of course, exophthalmos or pretibial myxedema are also important findings, reflecting the likelihood of hyperthyroidism (present or past). However,

DEIODINATIVE PATHWAYS OF IODOTHYRONINES

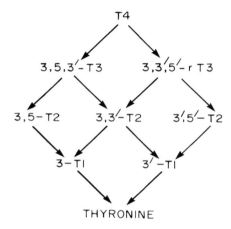

THYROXINE (T4)

T4

3,5,3'-T3   3,3',5'-r T3

3,5-T2   3,3'-T2   3',5'-T2

3-TI   3'-TI

THYRONINE

Figure 34.2. The deiodinative cascade of T_4 to lesser iodinated iodothyronines. (Adapted from Smallridge RC: *Heart and Heart-like Organs.* New York, Academic Press, 1980.)

commonly used parameters such as hand tremor, reflex return phase, and skin condition are nonspecific and difficult to assess in the ambulatory patient, much less in the critically ill subject. There are no laboratory tests available that can accurately assess the action of T_3/T_4 at the cellular level. Indeed, development of such tests is crucial to our understanding, interpretation, and treatment of thyroid function tests in the critically ill patient.

LABORATORY TESTS THAT REFLECT THYROID FUNCTION

T_4 Assay

Most clinical T_4 laboratory tests analyze the serum T_4 concentration by a specific radioimmunoassay (RIA), in which there are few known

factors that may artifactually influence the results (127). The normal range for serum T_4 is approximately 4–12 μg/dl. Although this range is useful as a guideline in the majority of cases, not every patient who has a serum T_4 outside of the normal range has a metabolic derangement in thyroid hormone function and action. In addition, some patients with "normal" T_4 values may actually be hyperthyroid or hypothyroid at a tissue level. Alterations in the serum T_4 level can result from disturbed thyroid function resulting from increases or decreases in serum iodothyronine levels; in addition, changes in serum binding proteins may result in values outside the normal range, despite normal free thyroxine (FT_4) levels and euthyroidism. Situations associated with an acquired increase in TBG, with an elevated serum T_4 and lowered resin T_3 uptake (RT_3U), yet clinical euthyroidism, are summarized in

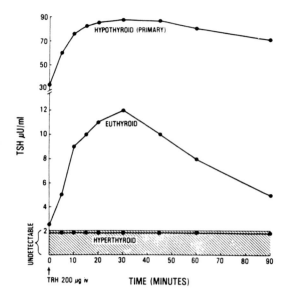

Figure 34.3. Idealized representation of the serum TSH response to the intravenous administration of TRH in a euthyroid, hypothyroid (primary), and hyperthyroid patient.

Table 34.2 (12). Euthyroidism with an elevated serum total T_4 can also occur in conditions (Table 34.3) other than those that have elevated TBG. During the acute phase of any systemic illness serum T_4 may be transiently elevated (12, 35, 58, 79). This increase is seen infrequently and the great majority of patients with systemic illnesses have decreased serum T_4 levels and an elevated RT_3U. Psychiatric illness of any type may also be associated with

Table 34.1
Conditions or Agents Associated with Decreased T_4-to-T_3 Conversion

Systemic illnesses
  Chronic renal failure, malignancy, thermal injury, diabetes mellitus, acute infections, and chronic hepatic disease
Fasting or caloric deprivation
Surgery and the postoperative period
β-Adrenergic blockers
Propylthiouracil
Glucocorticoids
Lithium[a]
Amiodarone
Radiopaque dyes (e.g., ipodate, iopanoic acid)
Neonatal period

[a]Studies indicate lithium may decrease T_4 disappearance and theoretically may decrease T_4-to-T_3 conversion.

Table 34.2
Conditions That Increase or Decrease Serum Thyroxine-Binding Globulin Levels[a]

Increase Serum Thyroxine-Binding Globulin (TBG) Concentrations[a]
  Physiological
    Inherited
    Pregnancy
    Newborn
  Nonthyroidal illness
    Infectious hepatitis
    Chronic active hepatitis
    Primary biliary cirrhosis
    Acute intermittent prophyria
    Estrogen producing tumors
    Hydatidiform mole
    Lymphosarcoma
  Drug-induced
    Exogenous estrogens
    Oral contraceptives
    Heroin and methadone
    Perphenazine
    Clofibrate
    Carbamazepine[b]
Decrease Serum Thyroxine-Binding Globulin Levels or Decrease Binding of T_4 or T_3 to TBG
  Systemic illness (e.g., nephrotic syndrome)
  Glucocorticoids
  Androgens
  Danazol
  L-Asparaginase
  Salicylates
  Phenylbutazone
  Halofenate
  Mitotane

[a]Patients with an elevated TBG concentration would be expected to have an elevated serum T_4, a lowered RT_3U, a normal free T_4, and clinical and biochemical euthyroidism. Similarly, patients with decreased TBG would have a decreased T_4, increased RT_3U, and also a normal free T_4. (Adapted with permission from Borst GC et al: Euthyroid hyperthyroxinemia. *Ann Intern Med* 98:366–378, 1983.)
[b]Carbamazepine may increase TBG, but also most commonly decreases serum T_4 and T_3 (1), possibly because it also enhances extrathyroidal iodothyronine metabolism (1).

elevations in serum T_4; these alterations seem to normalize after several days to weeks.

T_3 Assay

The serum T_3 assay is also performed by RIA and is specific; it measures total serum T_3 and not simply the small unbound fraction. The normal serum T_3 range is about 80–220 ng/dl. Serum T_3 levels are frequently elevated in thyrotoxic subjects but commonly are in the normal range in hypothyroid individuals. As a

Table 34.3
Situations Associated with Elevated Serum Thyroxine Concentrations yet with Clinical and Biochemical Euthyroidism

Acquired or inherited increase in serum thyroxine-binding globulin
Peripheral resistance to thyroid hormones
Transient hyperthyroxinemia of acute medical illness (e.g., hepatitis)
Transient hyperthyroxinemia of acute psychiatric illness
Drug-related hyperthyroxinemia
  Iopanoic acid
  Ipodate
  Amiodarone
  Propranolol

Adapted from Borst GC et al: Euthyroid hyperthyroxinemia. *Ann Intern Med* 98:366–378, 1983.

result, a serum T_3 by RIA would not be expected to aid in the differentiation of hypothyroid and euthyroid patient, but is useful in diagnosing hyperthyroidism.

Resin T_3 Uptake

This test is most appropriately performed as an accompaniment to the T_4 assay. It is not an immunoassay and the test consists of incubating serum with ^{125}I-T_3. The isotope binds to the available hormone binding sites, and then a resin is added which nonspecifically binds the ^{125}I-T_3 that had not been bound in the serum; the number of counts resin bound are then determined. The resin T_3 uptake test does not measure hormone levels directly but simply assesses indirectly the number of serum thyroid hormone binding sites available. This test is elevated in hyperthyroid and decreased in hypothyroid subjects, but in my view, is an insensitive indicator of thyroid hormone levels and action. Indeed, its major utility lies in the simple fact that it reflects the number of available binding sites. Generally, if the RT_3U values are discordant with serum T_4 levels (e.g., serum T_4 elevated and RT_3U decreased) then there probably is a binding abnormality present rather than a true metabolic derangement in thyroxine action. For example, if a patient does have elevated TBG levels secondary to estrogen administration, the T_4 level would be elevated and the RT_3U would be decreased. Of course, a patient with an altered TBG level and a normal free T_4 index is believed to be metabolically euthyroid (1, 124). On the other hand, if the T_4 level and the RT_3U level are altered concordantly (i.e., in the same direction) then one can preliminarily assume altered thyroid function may be present.

Reverse T_3

The serum reverse T_3 level is measured by RIA and has a normal range of 20–40 ng/dl. Reverse T_3 levels are frequently elevated in thyrotoxic and decreased in hypothyroid individuals. In addition, rT_3 concentrations are elevated in euthyroid critically ill subjects, either due to enhanced conversion from T_4 or to decreased rT_3 clearance (64).

Serum-Free T_4

Free T_4 (FT_4) concentrations may be performed by estimating the total T_4 concentration by RIA and then by multiplying this value by the dialyzable percentage of T_4. This dialyzable percentage figure is obtained by placing serum in dialysis tubing along with ^{125}I-T_4. The amount of ^{125}I-T_4 that crosses the membrane is then determined and used to derive the serum-free T_4 value, normally about 1.5–5.0 ng/dl (102, 122). This method of analysis yields excellent discrimination among hypothyroidism, euthyroidism, and hyperthyroidism in the ambulatory patient. Most euthyroid critically ill subjects have a normal or even elevated FT_4 by dialysis, despite low total T_4 levels. The problem is that this method of analysis is relatively expensive, time consuming, and generally is only performed in research or specific reference laboratories and, thus, may have a turn-around time of about 2–5 days. Because of these limitations several newer tests that measure free T_4 directly have been commercially manufactured. There is a controversy as to the validity of each of the marketed kits; the debate centers around their ability to obtain "normal values" in most critically ill subjects (29, 65, 78, 97). Although the argument is somewhat circular, it is reasonable to assume that most critically ill subjects are euthyroid and, thus, the FT_4 should be normal. However, many commercial FT_4 kits obtain low values in this setting, a fact that allows investigators to conclude that such a kit would be inappropriate when applied to critically ill patients. In one or two separate studies (29, 65, 78) the Clinical Assays (Cambridge, MA), Corning (Medfield, MA), or Damon Kits (Needham

Heights, MA) were relatively consistent in obtaining normal FT_4 values in most critically ill subjects. It is expected that these controversies will subside as FT_4 kits are analyzed in more detail and as further studies are performed. Of course, the availability of accurate FT_4 kits with a rapid turn-around time would be extremely useful in the interpretation of thyroid function tests in critically ill subjects. Unfortunately, it is in the critically ill subjects where indirect estimates of FT_4, such as the "FT_4 index", are thought to be misleadingly low (28). Since most conditions associated with altered thyroid hormone binding to their serum binding proteins also have discordantly altered serum T_4 and RT_3U, it seems reasonable that multiplying these two measurements might lead to an accurate estimate of the FT_4. This derived number has been called an "FT_4 index". This index correlates well with the serum FT_4 level by dialysis in most conditions, except in systemically ill patients, where it appears to be inappropriately low, erroneously suggesting hypothyroidism in a presumed euthyroid patient.

Serum-Free T₃

At present, the most accurate method of assessing free T_3 (FT_3) is by equilibrium dialysis (93, 122). Several new kit methods that measure FT_3 (and FT_4) have recently been used to detect low FT_3 levels in the "euthyroid sick syndrome" (122). Further studies with these methods should help determine if they will be useful clinically.

Thyroid-Stimulating Hormone

Within the last several years, highly sensitive commercial thyroid-stimulating hormone (TSH) assay kits have been developed and their use has become routine (73, 90, 101, 110). These methods are generally immunoradiometric (IRMA) or enzyme-linked immunosorbent assays (ELISA) and can measure serum TSH levels as low as $0.04-0.25$ $\mu U/ml$. Normal subjects almost always have detectable TSH levels, and all patients with thyrotoxicosis are expected to have undetectable levels. The normal range varies by each assay, but is usually about $0.5-4.0$ $\mu U/ml$. Primary hypothyroid subjects are expected to have elevated TSH concentrations and euthyroid patients with "nonthyroid" illnesses are expected to have

detectable levels that are usually within the normal range. Some studies suggest that serum TSH may decrease to even undetectable levels in patients with systemic illness, although a summary of reports indicates that usually TSH levels are normal or only slightly low in these patients. TSH can rise during recovery from systemic illness, generally resulting in TSH levels as high as about 15 $\mu U/ml$ that may persist for several days (51). The serum T_4 also increases slightly, suggesting the biologic relevance of this TSH increase, and when such patients are followed, their TSH and T_4 concentrations usually remain normal.

TRH responsiveness, as determined by these highly sensitive TSH assays, are interpreted similarly as with the older assays; thyrotoxic patients do not respond, euthyroid patients have a normal response, and patients with primary hypothyroidism hyperrespond (100). Although further studies are required, it seems that normal subjects have a TSH level at 15 or 30 minutes after TRH administration (usually 500 μg administered intravenously) of between $5-30$ $\mu U/ml$. Each laboratory should assess their own assay, but a hyperresponsive patient has a level greater than 30 or 40 $\mu U/ml$.

Radioiodine Uptake

The radioiodine uptake (RAIU) test is performed by administering radioactive iodine orally and determining how much is accumulated by the thyroid gland. The normal range is about $8-30\%$. The major drawback of this test, as applied to the critically ill subject, is the lack of practicality of measuring thyroidal uptake in the intensive care unit because of the nonmobility of the equipment required to accurately detect the amount of isotope residing in the thyroid gland. Further, there is a large amount of overlap in RAIU values in hypothyroid and euthyroid subjects, although this test is very useful in discriminating hyperthyroid from euthyroid individuals.

HYPERTHYROIDISM

Therapeutic Agents Commonly Used in Hyperthyroidism

The prescribing physician should be very familiar with the mechanisms of action, and patient warnings or adverse effects of these

Table 34.4
Pharmacology of Agents Used to Treat Hyperthyroidism[a]

Agent	Maintenance Dose	Mechanism of Action	Common or Serious Adverse Effects
Commonly Used			
Propylthiouracil (6-propyl-2-thiouracil)	50–300 mg t.i.d., p.o.	Inhibition of thyroid hormone synthesis; inhibits T_4 extrathyroidal conversion to T_3	Skin rash, nausea, epigastric distress, agranulocytosis, granulocytopenia, hepatitis, lupus-like syndrome
Methimazole (1-*methyl*-2-mercapto imidazole)	5–30 mg t.i.d., p.o.	Inhibition of thyroid hormone synthesis	As above
DL-Propranolol or	10–80 mg q.i.d., p.o.	Decreases β-adrenergic mediated activity and helps ameliorate signs and symptoms of thyrotoxicosis	Cardiovascular, bronchospasm, central nervous system, must be used with care in patients with congestive heart failure or asthma
Atenolol[b]	50–100 mg, once daily, p.o.		
Nonroutine Agents[c]			
Lithium carbonate	600 mg t.i.d., p.o. to produce blood levels betwen 0.5 and 1.3 mEq/liter	Probably decreases thyroidal secretion and possibly inhibits extrathyroidal T_4 to T_3 conversion	Hand tremor, polyuria, drowsiness, lack of coordination, ataxia, blurred vision; may cause increased thyroid size and in certain subjects may cause either hypothyroidism or, rarely, hyperthyroidism
Iodides[d]	5 drops SSKI t.i.d., p.o. or 5 drops Lugol's solution t.i.d. p.o.	Decreases thyroidal secretion	Parotitis or skin rash or serum sickness-like reaction; prolonged use may lead to unabated hypersecretion of thyroid hormone
Ipodate sodium[d]	3 g p.o. every 2–3 days or 1 g daily	Decreases thyroidal secretion and extrathyroidal T_4 to T_3 conversion	Skin rash, agranulocytosis, liver disease; should not be used in patient with history of iodide allergy

[a]The prescribing physician should be very knowledgeable with regard to the mechanism of action and potential warnings and potential side effects of these agents and appropriately detailed textbooks or articles should be consulted prior to their use.
[b]Any β-adrenergic blocking agent can be used. DL-propranolol has been utilized for the longest time, and thus, is preferred in some unusual circumstances (e.g., pregnancy). On the other hand, a cardioselective, long-acting blocker (e.g., atenolol) may have advantages in the routine thyrotoxic patient.
[c]None of these agents has been studied adequately in the prolonged treatment of hyperthyroidism. As a general rule these agents should not be utilized for longer than 1 month since the potential complications have not been investigated and the likelihood of causing unabated thyrotoxicosis exists, especially with iodide-containing substances.
[d]SSKI (1 g/ml) contains 76.4% iodine. Five drops t.i.d. (assuming 20 drops/ml) gives about 573 mg iodine. Lugol's solution (125 mg/ml) of total iodine contains in each 100 ml, 5 g iodine, and 10 g potassium iodide. Five drops t.i.d. gives about 94 mg iodine daily. It is assumed at present that the antithyroid action of ipodate is related partly to the release of iodides and partly to the ipodate molecule itself. Contains 61.4% iodine so that one 3-g dose of ipodate has 1842 mg iodine. For purposes of this chapter, iodide and iodine are used interchangeably.

agents prior to their use. Table 34.4 lists several therapeutic agents used in hyperthyroidism.

PROPYLTHIOURACIL

Propylthiouracil (PTU) is an effective inhibitor of thyroidal synthesis of T_4 and/or T_3 (31, 114). This agent is frequently employed either in the short-term situation to decrease thy-roidal secretion, or over the long term to maintain a euthyroid patient with Graves' disease or to induce a remission. PTU also has a peripheral effect in that it decreases extrathyroidal deiodination of T_4, such that serum T_3 levels decrease. PTU (and methimazole) may also have a direct immunological effect in decreasing the synthesis of TSH receptor antibodies (22, 120, 121). This agent is usually administered orally, although the tablets may be crushed and the pills placed down a naso-gastric tube. Alternatively, the drug theoreti-cally can be given rectally [as may methima-zole (84)], although I am unaware of such usage of PTU being reported in the literature. Cooper and his colleagues (34, 36) have re-cently developed a specific sensitive RIA for PTU. A single 150-mg oral dose of PTU is absorbed rapidly, appearing in serum of both normal and thyrotoxic subjects within 5 min-utes and peaking at 65 ± 10 minutes (level 3.3 ± 0.3 $\mu g/ml$) in the former group and at 54 ± 6 minutes (level 4.5 ± 0.6 $\mu g/ml$) in the latter (34). In both groups, detectable PTU was observed to be present in the serum for as long as 6–8 hours after a single dose. In further studies, using various doses of PTU, Cooper et al. (36) noted that comparable serum PTU serum levels were obtained in thyrotoxic and normal subjects after 50- and 200-mg PTU, but after 300 mg of oral PTU the serum PTU concentra-tions were significantly higher in the thyro-toxic subjects. The explanation for this differ-ence possibly relates to enhanced intestinal absorption of PTU in thyrotoxic subjects; this theoretical explanation, however, requires sci-entific validation. Food ingestion did not ap-pear to influence the amount of PTU absorbed although further studies in this area seem war-ranted because of the variable and inconsistent results obtained.

PTU is concentrated within the thyroid gland, and the serum PTU level may correlate with its ability to block thyroidal organification (36). However, the actual duration of effect of PTU within the thyroidal gland or its time of effec-tive residence time within the thyroidal gland is unknown. In contrast, even a single PTU dose can inhibit T_4 conversion such that serum T_3 decreases as early as 1 hour following the dose, reaching its nadir at about 6–10 hours and gradually returning toward basal levels (36). After doses of 50, 200, and 300 mg PTU in euthyroid subjects, the serum T_3 levels after 24 hours were quite close to basal, pretreat-ment levels (36). In the hyperthyroid subjects, 50- and 300-mg doses resulted in a return at or near baseline by 20–24 hours, whereas 200 mg PTU still resulted in significantly de-creased T_3 levels after 24 hours (36). Thus, even though the serum PTU concentration and its effect on thyroidal organification are cor-related with the oral dose given, apparently the influence on extrathyroidal conversion is not dose related since T_3 levels decreased fur-ther after a single dose of 200 mg PTU than after 300 mg PTU. These data obtained by RIA

are similar to those observed by other types of assays. Earlier studies also indicated that PTU absorption was significantly delayed in euthy-roid elderly subjects compared with euthyroid younger individuals. Vesell et al. (118) used a spectrophotometric assay to estimate that the plasma half-life of PTU was 6.7 ± 1.0 hours in normal subjects, 4.3 ± 0.7 hours in thyrotoxics, and 24.7 ± 34.5 hours in hypothyroid subjects. Schuppan et al. (96) and Sitar and Hunning-hake (99) used gas-liquid chromotography techniques to estimate that the plasma half-life of PTU is about 1 hour, an estimate similar to observations of other investigators (60–63, 77). Conceivably, spectrophotometric assays might result in a longer estimated half-life by measuring metabolites; gas-liquid chromotog-raphy and specific RIA techniques should be able to directly measure the parent compound alone. Cooper et al. (34) specifically tested the major metabolites of PTU (propyluracil, S-*methyl* PTU, and PTU-S-glucuronide) and concluded that there was no significant cross-reaction in their PTU assay.

A mildly hyperthyroid subject is generally started on 100–300 mg of PTU daily in three or four divided doses, a moderately thyrotoxic patient on 300–600 mg daily, and a severely hyperthyroid subject should be started on 600–900 mg PTU daily. Serum T_4 is monitored frequently (about every 1–4 weeks) and PTU doses are adjusted to keep the T_4 value in the normal range. Adverse effects of PTU are thought to increase with increasing PTU doses, the most common side effects being skin rash and a metallic taste in the mouth. More severe, and fortunately less common, adverse effects include hepatotoxicity, granulocytopenia, and agranulocytosis (2, 4, 87, 114, 116). PTU and methimazole should be used with caution in nursing women. Tegler and Lindstrom (106) proposed that the estimated dose to the child would be less with PTU; however, recent stud-ies find no evidence of hypothyroidism in nursing infants exposed to low-dose carbima-zole. Cooper et al. (31, 33, 34) concluded that the mean methimazole serum and breast milk levels were both about equal, with about a total of 70 μg excreted in 8 hours after a single 40-mg dose, representing about 0.75% of the ingested amount. Further, they calculated that a 70-μg dose was the equivalent of about 17.5 $\mu g/kg$ in a 4-kg infant and could possibly have antithyroid effects. Since methimazole is 10 times more active than PTU on a milligram basis, and because they believed that breast milk concentrations of PTU were only about

10% of PTU serum levels (61), PTU may be preferred in breast-feeding women (70). The frequency of serious untoward effects from PTU is less than 1%, while skin rashes may occur in 5–10% of patients (32, 129). Some clinicians monitor the hematocrit and white blood count in patients taking PTU; I generally obtain a hemogram and "SMAC-20" prior to and during therapy, although the time of onset of adverse effects (e.g., agranulocytosis or hepatotoxicity) is unpredictable (52). Clinical findings or complaints such as sore throat or infection could indicate agranulocytosis. In those circumstances a hemogram including total white blood cell and differential counts and a peripheral blood smear is indicated, in conjunction with an appropriate history and physical examination. Interestingly, there is one report of a 12-year-old girl who was taking PTU for thyrotoxicosis. She acutely ingested at least 5000 mg PTU prior to admission and she excreted over 90 mg/dl PTU within the first 12 hours after admission (57). Her T_4 level dropped only from 6.5 μg/dl to 4.8 μg/dl and she had no symptoms referable to this dose of PTU.

METHIMAZOLE

Methimazole is an effective inhibitor of thyroidal hormone synthesis and this drug may also be used either for a short term to induce the euthyroid state or long term to attempt to induce a remission in patients with hyperthyroidism. Despite similar effects on the thyroid gland, this drug differs from PTU in that it does not inhibit peripheral T_4 conversion to T_3. Its serum half-life is probably longer than PTU, although it is also concentrated within the thyroid gland, and the duration of its influence upon secretion is unknown. A mildly thyrotoxic subject may require a total of 10–30 mg daily and a severely thyrotoxic individual may require a total of 60–90 mg daily, each in divided doses. Methimazole can also be administered via nasogastric tube or rectally (84).

Methimazole pharmacokinetics have been investigated less thoroughly than those of PTU. In 1969, Alexander and associates (3) administered ^{35}S-labeled methimazole to one patient with thyrotoxicosis and to another patient with inoperable carcinoma of the cervix, renal failure, and a goiter. The distribution space, plasma half-life, and renal clearance were 34.2 liters, 13.8 hours, and 20 ml/minute in the hyperthyroid patient and 35.7 liters, 20.7 hours, and

11.9 ml/min in the euthyroid patient. Cooper et al. (33), using an RIA to document that peak methimazole levels were comparable in normal and thyrotoxic subjects, found the serum half-life to be about 6–7 hours. Cirrhotic patients had a prolonged serum half-life (about 21 hours). In other reports (6, 85, 118), the half-life ranged from 6.4 to 13.6 hours in normal subjects. Obviously, further studies investigating methimazole kinetics with more sensitive and specific techniques (e.g., RIA) are warranted. Methimazole absorption occurs within 30–60 minutes of either oral or rectal administration. Nabil and associates (84) also observed that a 60-mg dose of methimazole resulted in comparable plasma levels whether given orally or rectally to six healthy volunteers.

Although controversial, it is my opinion that PTU and methimazole are essentially interchangeable with regard to their clinical use as they have basically the same mechanism of action and the same types and frequency of adverse reactions. The initial use of PTU or methimazole is arbitrary except if a patient has a known hypersensitivity to one agent or if a woman is pregnant, in which case PTU may be preferred (see below).

Methimazole administration has been associated with the following adverse reactions: skin rash, hepatic toxicity, fever, leukopenia, agranulocytosis, adenopathy, lupus-like syndrome, circulating immune complexes, nausea, vomiting, and hypothyroidism (87).

In a retrospective study, Cooper and associates (37) have given new insight into the likelihood of a patient developing agranulocytosis with PTU or methimazole. They compared the clinical characteristics of hyperthyroid patients who had untoward hematologic reactions and those who did not. The mean age of 14 subjects who had an untoward hematologic reaction was 50.6 ± 16 years, a value significantly higher than that of 35.7 ± 13.7 years in patients who had no reaction. Also, the mean dose of methimazole was higher in the patients who had a reaction (43.8 ± 9.9 mg/day vs. 29.5 ± 10.5 mg/day). They concluded that there was an 8.6-fold increased risk of agranulocytosis with methimazole doses greater than 40 mg/day. The mean doses of PTU, however, were not different in patients who did or did not have a reaction. They suggested that low-dose methimazole (<30 mg/day) may be safer with regard to the development of agranulocytosis than conventional dose PTU. However, agranulocytosis is rare and probably occurs in

0.3–0.6% of hyperthyroid patients ingesting either PTU or methimazole. When agranulocytosis does occur it usually becomes manifest within 2 months of the initiation of therapy (37). If a patient has a mild adverse reaction (e.g., skin rash) to either PTU or methimazole, I recommend immediately switching to the other agent. The frequency of cross allergies to these agents is unknown, but I estimate it to be about 20–30%.

In a pregnant thyrotoxic subject I prefer to use PTU since only methimazole has been associated with a rare scalp condition, in the infant, called "aplasia cutis" (81, 83). A retrospective review, however, questions this effect of methimazole (115). In addition, Momotano et al. (80) studied 643 neonates from mothers with Graves' disease and concluded that the risk of malformation in the infants was 1.7% or less if the mother had received methimazole during pregnancy. Further, it appeared that thyrotoxicosis itself seemed to be more related to the development of malformation than did euthyroidism, even with antithyroid drug administration.

β-ADRENERGIC RECEPTOR BLOCKERS

β-Adrenergic receptor antagonists (β blockers) are very helpful in ameliorating the signs or symptoms of thyroidal hyperthyroidism but they do not alter thyroid hormone synthesis or action (98, 109). The β-blockers, however, result in prompt improvement in tachycardia, fever, sweating, anxiety, and muscle weakness. Propranolol, but probably not other β-blockers, has a slight ability to decrease T_4-to-T_3 conversion so that serum T_3 levels may drop by about 10–20% (42, 43, 53, 59, 117, 130). Although β-blockers are very useful in the treatment of hyperthyroidism, there are reports of individuals developing thyroid storm when only β-blockers and no other agents, such as PTU or methimazole, have been used (40). I believe that, in an ordinary case of thyrotoxicosis, patients should not be treated solely with β-blockers.

Propranolol is the most studied and most commonly employed of the β-blockers and the usual oral dose for a mildly thyrotoxic patient is 20–80 mg daily. A severely thyrotoxic subject may require as much as a total of 160–320 mg daily (in three to four divided doses) (41, 48). Feely and associates (42) noted that propranolol doses of 160 mg/day or greater were required to achieve adequate β-adrenergic blockade. Moreover, they emphasize that resting heart rate alone does not always provide as accurate an estimate of the full effect of β-adrenergic blockade in hyperthyroidism as does its effect upon exercise-induced tachycardia. Plasma propranolol levels appear to depend upon the age of a patient: they were lower in younger subjects. Levels also tend to be lower in smokers than nonsmokers. Rubenfeld et al. (91) noted that after a single oral 80–mg dose there were variable plasma propranolol levels in both normal and thyrotoxic subjects; the former group achieved peak levels between 59 and 226 ng/ml and the latter group had peak levels between 54 and 211 ng/ml. The peak was achieved at 125 ± 16 minutes, with a plasma half-life of 4.5 ± 0.5 hours in the normal subjects; the thyrotoxic patients had peak levels achieved at 108 ± 11 minutes, with a plasma half-life of 3.7 ± 0.4 hours. These values were not significantly different in the two groups. Plasma propranolol concentrations after the 22nd dose of 40 mg propranolol given every 6 hours orally were also studied in thyrotoxic subjects (91). Peak levels varied from 48 to 169 ng/ml, and levels at the end of the interval varied from 16 to 118 ng/ml. Plasma propranolol levels between 50 and 100 ng/ml probably result in adequate β-adrenergic blockade and seem to be associated with a 25–50% reduction in the exercise-induced increase in heart rate. Intravenous doses have a shorter half-life (2.4 hours) than oral doses (3.3 hours). Chronic renal insufficiency was reported to have no effect on half-life in one study, but in another, the half-life increased with decreasing creatinine clearance (14, 72). Hemodialysis does not significantly remove propranolol and thus essentially leaves the half-life unaltered, whereas plasmapheresis in one reported case appeared to remove significant amounts of propranolol, so that the half-life was about 25% of the initial value (105).

In special circumstances, propranolol can be administered intravenously to severely thyrotoxic patients. The dose by this route is 1 mg given slowly with careful monitoring of cardiovascular function (e.g., ECG and CVP). The major side effects of all β-blockers include precipitation or aggravation of congestive heart failure or asthma. Propranolol is contraindicated for use in patients with bronchial asthma, sinus bradycardia, pre-existing heart block greater than first degree, cardiogenic shock, congestive heart failure, right ventricular failure secondary to pulmonary hypertension, or Raynaud's disease. In addition, propranolol should not be given to patients receiving myocardial depressant anesthetics, psychotropic drugs with adrenergic augmenting properties or MAO inhibitors (and during the 2-week withdrawal period of such agents). Propranolol should be used cautiously in patients with renal or hepatic dysfunction, cardiac failure, angina pectoris, Wolff-Parkinson-White syndrome, and during anesthesia or surgery. In general, β-blockers should not be abruptly discontinued but should be gradually decreased since rapid tapering might exacerbate catecholamine-mediated actions (89). I now prefer to use a cardioselective, long-acting agent in the treatment of thyrotoxicosis. β-Blockers, other than propranolol, have not been as extensively studied in the treatment of hyperthyroidism, but they appear to be equally effective in the treatment of thyrotoxicosis (for comparable effect of β-blockade).

OTHER AGENTS

In an unusual or particularly resistant case of hyperthyroidism, one can employ lithium or iodine (11, 25, 69, 107). Both of these agents decrease thyroidal secretion. Lithium may also inhibit adenyl cyclase generation in the thyroid and decrease extrathyroidal conversion of T_4 to T_3. Serum lithium concentrations of 0.5–1.3 mEq/liter appear optimal; if higher levels are achieved adverse reactions such as renal and CNS effects (e.g., tremor, drowsiness, blurred vision, and tinnitus) may be seen (4).

Iodides decrease thyroid hormone synthesis by directly inhibiting the organization of iodide in the thyroid gland (11). This effect occurs rapidly so that a 30–50% decrease in serum T_4 may be observed after only 5–10 days of treatment in a thyrotoxic subject. In a study by Wartofsky et al. (125), after a control period, hyperthyroid patients were administered Lugol's solution 5 drops three times a day for 6–7 days; the mean serum T_4 concentration decreased by about 20–50%. Boehm and associates (11) performed a similar study using the same dose of Lugol's solution; the mean serum T_4 decreased in four thyrotoxic subjects from 26 μg/dl during the control period to 14 μg/dl after about 5 days of Lugol's solution. Unfortunately, in some patients this effect of iodides upon inhibition of T_4 secretion may gradually be overcome by the thyroid gland resulting in subsequent elevated thyroidal synthesis and release (112). This untoward effect may be extremely difficult to control and represents the rationale for why most clinicians recommend that iodides should not be utilized alone

or in the routine management of thyrotoxic subjects. Iodides should not be administered to individuals with a known allergy; other adverse effects may include parotitis and skin rash. Some physicians prefer to administer iodides in the 7–10 day period prior to surgery; this short-term use should not worsen the course of thyrotoxicosis and would likely lower the serum T_4 level. I do not generally prefer this approach, especially in an unreliable subject, because of the possibility that the patient might not return in 10 days but would still continue taking iodide, a circumstance that might lead to unabated thyroidal secretion. I would much prefer to produce euthyroidism by agents that block thyroid gland synthesis, e.g., PTU or methimazole. Radiocontrast agents (e.g., ipodate) have not been studied extensively in the treatment of thyrotoxicosis but may be useful in this regard (17, 44, 67, 103, 104, 131, 132).

Lithium carbonate is an effective second-line agent for the treatment of thyrotoxicosis. Although lithium has not been extensively studied in this role, its major use appears to be limited to the short-term treatment of thyrotoxic subjects who may be allergic to PTU and/or methimazole. However, in one study, Boehm et al. (11) administered lithium carbonate in a total daily dose of 300–3000 mg (average 2100 mg daily) to maintain a total therapeutic serum lithium level in the therapeutic range of 1.0–1.5 mEq/liter (blood samples for lithium determination were drawn 1 hour after the early morning dose). After only about 5 days of lithium carbonate therapy, the mean serum T_4 in four thyrotoxic patients decreased from 22 μg/dl to 13 μg/dl. In this study lithium carbonate appeared to act by decreasing thyroidal secretion and may have also decreased T_4 disappearance. Kristensen et al. (69) observed comparable results as the mean percentage fall in T_4 was 24% after 10 days of lithium carbonate administration to thyrotoxic subjects. All workers also observed a high frequency of adverse reactions to lithium carbonate and strongly urge that the serum lithium level be maintained between 0.5 and 1.3 mEq/liter. Further studies investigating the use of lithium carbonate in the treatment of thyrotoxicosis are warranted, but at present its use is limited to certain specific short-term settings; very careful attention to serum levels and potential adverse effects is necessary. On very rare occasions long-term lithium use may be associated with the development of thyrotoxicosis (76).

Hyperthyroidism in a Critically Ill Subject

Hyperthyroidism, of course, can occur in critically ill subjects, and some of the usual history and physical findings would be similar to those noted in an ambulatory patient (7, 24, 38, 39, 75). However, because of the age of the patient as well as the accompanying systemic illness, hyperthyroidism can be extremely difficult to recognize in an intensive care unit setting. So-called apathetic hyperthyroidism may occur, a situation in which the customary findings of heightened anxiety and nervousness and stare may be subtle or lacking (108). In addition, tachycardia as a discriminating parameter is less helpful than in an ambulatory patient, since there are so many other reasons for there to be an elevated heart rate in a systemically ill subject. The condition of hepatic coma may be difficult to differentiate from thyrotoxicosis or thyroid storm because many of the physical findings (e.g., hand tremor or disorientation) may be similar. In the intensive care setting greater reliance must be placed upon interpretation of the thyroid function tests and the examination of the thyroid gland.

A radioactive iodide uptake test, assessing thyroid gland activity, is a very useful test in discriminating hyperthyroidism from euthyroidism in a critically ill patient. Also, administration of 200–500 μg of TRH (Fig. 34.3) is an excellent indicator of thyrotoxicosis, since a metabolically hyperthyroid subject essentially always demonstrates no rise (compared with baseline) in the serum TSH level when measured at 0, 15, and 30 minutes after TRH injection, whereas a euthyroid individual has an increase in serum TSH from less than 5 μU/ml basally to about 10–25 μU/ml after TRH. The finding of an undetectable TSH concentration basally that remains undetectable after TRH injection is very suggestive of thyrotoxicosis, especially in the presence of physical findings (e.g., enlarged thyroid gland) and historical findings compatible with overproduction of thyroid hormones. In my view, a "blunted" TSH response to TRH injection (e.g., TSH rises from less than 2.5 to 6 μU/ml) does not indicate the presence of thyrotoxicosis, assuming a sensitive TSH assay is used. Also, occasionally, a patient who has had hyperthyroidism in the recent past (1–3 months) but who is clinically and metabolically euthyroid when studied may demonstrate no TSH response to TRH.

It appears that several alterations in thyroid function tests can occur in thyrotoxic systemically ill subjects, but these perturbations per se should not obscure the diagnosis of thyrotoxicosis. The serum FT_4 level by dialysis or kit method and the serum T_4 are usually elevated in a thyrotoxic critically ill subject, although the total T_4 may be less elevated (due to altered binding proteins) than if the patient were healthier. On occasion, the total T_4 may be in the upper part of the normal range in a thyrotoxic critically ill subject. The resin T_3 uptake is expected to be high in most critically ill subjects whether or not they are hyperthyroid; the serum T_3 may not be elevated since critical illness may decrease extrathyroidal T_4 to T_3 conversion. In sum, a hyperthyroid critically ill subject should have appropriate physical findings (e.g., enlarged thyroid gland), elevated RAIU and/or no TSH response to TRH stimulation, and an elevated or high normal T_4 and free T_4. The treatment of a thyrotoxic critically ill subject who is not in impending thyroid storm should probably be as described above. The pharmacological parameters for essentially all drugs or agents mentioned in this chapter have not been studied in critically ill subjects. At present we can only assume the doses, half-lives, and mechanisms of action are comparable in the ambulatory and critically ill subjects. Further, the issue of definitive (surgery or radioactive iodine) therapy may be addressed after the patient has become euthyroid with antithyroid medications (49).

THYROID STORM

A patient with thyroid storm displays an exaggeration of the customary findings of thyrotoxicosis and, in addition, exhibits temperature elevation, diarrhea and central nervous system symptoms (e.g., disorientation) (129). Because of the potentially lethal nature of this disorder, thyroid storm should be anticipated since it can generally be avoided by the early and appropriate diagnosis and treatment of thyrotoxicosis. Frequently, thyroid storm is precipitated by a major stressful event such as surgery or anesthesia. The treatment of thyroid storm depends primarily upon its early diagnosis and is directed at the systemic signs or symptoms (e.g., a cooling blanket and acetaminophen for hyperthermia) and at the thyroid hormone excess. PTU (800–1200 mg daily in 4–6 divided doses) or methimazole (80–100 mg daily in four to six divided doses) is the mainstay of therapy, even though their maximal effects may not be achieved for 7–14 days. Propranolol is given orally (120–400 mg daily in four to six divided doses) but alternatively might be administered intravenously (1–2 mg given slowly with careful monitoring of cardiovascular function). I also administer sodium iodide intravenously (1 g in 1 liter); 3 liters may be given over a 24–hour period, although oral iodide [30 drops of potassium iodide (SSKI) daily] may be given instead. Adequate fluids (3–4 liters daily) are administered and there should be careful monitoring for cardiac or renal decompensation. Most clinicians also give glucocorticoids (hydrocortisone 200 mg three times a day), partly because they decrease T_4 to T_3 conversion and partly because of the theoretical possibility of the precipitation of adrenal insufficiency by the hypermetabolic state. Indeed, the coexistence of Graves' disease and other autoimmune endocrine disease (e.g., Addison's disease) is thought to occur relatively frequently. The best treatment of thyroid storm, however, lies in realizing the circumstances that predispose to it and adequately treating thyrotoxic subjects prior to their having medical or surgical interventions.

HYPOTHYROIDISM

As previously mentioned, the prescribing physician should, once again, be familiar with mechanisms and adverse effects of agents used in treating hypothyroidism (Table 34.5).

Pathophysiology

Hypothyroidism is a disease of inadequate levels of T_4 and/or T_3 characterized by malaise, cold intolerance, dyspnea, bradycardia, constipation, weakness, dry skin, central nervous system findings and occasionally pleural, pericardial, or peritoneal effusions (23, 123, 129). Hypothyroidism can be either primary, that is,

as a consequence of thyroid gland failure, or secondary, as a result of hypothalamic-pituitary gland failure. In all patients with hypothyroidism, pituitary disease must be excluded. Generally, the finding of an elevated serum TSH concentration is adequate for this purpose, but if the patients have either other significant signs or symptoms related to the cranial area (e.g., headache or visual field impairment) or lack of normal secretion of other pituitary hormones, further appropriate laboratory and radiologic studies should be performed to rule out a pituitary or cranial tumor. The most common causes of primary hypothyroidism are either chronic thyroiditis or idiopathic disease. About 10–15% patients with primary hypothyroidism have disease caused by antibodies against the TSH receptor (68). The routine ambulatory patient with primary hypothyroidism should have a complete evaluation including a thorough physical examination and measurement of serum T_4, RT_3U, and TSH levels; RAIU; or thyroid scan and thyroid antibodies. A hemogram and SMAC-20 are also of value. The overall prevalence of overt hypothyroidism is about 1% in females and somewhat less in males. Nevertheless, among elderly patients perhaps 5% of females and 2% of males have serum TSH values between 5 and 10 μU/ml and 2.5% of females and 1.9% of men have TSH values greater than 10 μU/ml (7). In the elderly, many of the symptoms of hypothyroidism may be absent and there must be increased reliance on thyroid function tests. One should initiate therapy gradually using L-thyroxine, starting with oral daily doses of 0.0125–0.050 mg and gradually increasing to maintenance doses of about 0.10–0.15 mg daily (Table 34.5) (23, 54, 123). The average L-thyroxine replacement dose is about 1.7 μg/kg body weight. Clinical findings and serum T_4 and TSH levels are monitored to assess adequacy of treatment. The serum TSH may require as long as several months to normalize but may start to decrease within several days of the initiation of therapy. Although following

Table 34.5
Pharmacology of Agents Used to Treat Hypothyroidism[a]

Medication	Maintenance Dose	Common or Serious Adverse Affects
L-Thyroxine	0.075–0.200 mg daily (75–200 μg)	Precipitation or aggravation of cardiac disease, arrhythmias, angina pectoris; may aggravate diabetes mellitus, and adrenal insufficiency
L-Triiodothyronine	25 μg t.i.d. or q.i.d.	As above

[a] These guidelines refer to the routine ambulatory patient with hypothyroidism; consult the text for the treatment of myxedema coma.

the TSH and T_4 values probably represents the most sensitive laboratory indicators of adequacy of therapy, clinical findings such as heart rate and nervousness and personal history relative to such factors as anxiety or palpitations also represent important parameters to assess whether the therapeutic dose is optimal. The doses recommended are adequate for adults; however, specific texts should be consulted for the treatment of hypothyroid children.

MYXEDEMA COMA

Myxedema coma is a condition that represents an exaggeration of the usual symptoms and signs of hypothyroidism. A patient with myxedema coma may also have the following characteristics: coma or stupor, hypothermia, hypoventilation, hypotension, hypothermia, hyponatremia, or hypoglycemia (23, 128, 134, 135). This condition should be especially suspected in patients with a known history of thyroid abnormalities (regardless of type), a family history or thyroid problems, in a patient with a surgical scar in the lower anterior neck, a patient with proptosis (suggesting a history of Graves' disease that frequently evolves into hypothyroidism) or in a patient who appears to be unusually sensitive to medications or narcotics.

The treatment of myxedema coma involves thyroid replacement, alleviation of any possible precipitating cause, and amelioration of hypotension, hypothermia, hypercapnia or hypoxia (23, 123). Because definitive laboratory diagnosis may require several days, and because these patients are extremely ill, in an appropriate setting, therapy should be instituted immediately based upon clinical, historical and available laboratory data, even though definitive thyroid tests may have been drawn but have not yet returned.

Alleviation of the hypotension should be performed with any conventional regimen, although adrenal steroids probably should be given because of the potential coexistence of adrenal insufficiency and because theoretically, initiation of thyroid hormone treatment may increase the clearance of endogenous steroids. Definitive testing for the presence of adrenal insufficiency can be performed at a later date. In many patients, hyponatremia is observed and may be secondary to inappropriate ADH secretion; this hyponatremia is optimally treated by water restriction. Hypoxia is frequently noted and is treated by conventional means. The treatment of hypothermia is more controversial: some have suggested that warming the patient is unnecessary and potentially dangerous since it may shunt blood to the smaller vessels in the skin.

Thyroid hormone replacement regimens in a patient with myxedema coma are different than in a routine ambulatory hypothyroid patient. Although some thyroidologists may approach such a patient differently, the author begins therapy with 50–75 μg L-thyroxine daily orally or intravenously (23). This medicine can be given orally or crushed and placed into a nasogastric tube. The serum half-life of L-thyroxine in a euthyroid subject is 7 days, and preliminary studies suggest about 50–75% absorption in systemically ill individuals, although this absorption may be decreased with specific gastrointestinal diseases. At present, there is available a parenteral L-thyroxine preparation and this drug can be administered intravenously in a critically ill patient (50–75 μg L-thyroxine daily). Clinical findings and serum T_4 and TSH levels should be followed to assess the adequacy of treatment. As noted earlier, however, a systemically ill patient may have decreased binding of thyroid hormones to serum proteins and the serum T_4 may even be below the usual normal range, yet the dose employed still may represent adequate therapy. Therefore, it becomes a very complicated matter to assess the adequacy of therapy in systemically ill subjects. Since serum T_4 level may be misleading and because serum TSH values may be a better indicator but may require several days or weeks to return to normal, the only practical solution is to pick a dose of L-thyroxine that is reasonable and to continue this dose (which is enough to treat myxedema coma but not enough to cause hypermetabolism) until definitive testing can be achieved. This time, of course, may be only when the patient has significantly improved and is out of the intensive care unit.

Some clinicians prefer to treat myxedema coma with T_3 (12.5–25 μg every 6–8 hours), which has a serum half-life of 24–30 hours in a euthyroid subject. It should also be noted that some clinicians give 300–500 μg L-thyroxine intravenously initially followed by 50–100 μg intravenously daily (55). I do not prefer this approach and feel that it may be dangerous in some patients, possibly due to cardiac arrhythmias. Hylander and Rosenqvist (56) recently retrospectively studied patients with myxedema coma. Patients who died were older (78.9 yrs vs. 66.8 yrs) and had initial heart rates that were lower (43 vs. 50 beats/minute). Although only 11 patients were studied (7 died, 4 survived), it also seemed that the surviving patients had a lower serum T_3 level during treatment compared with those in the nonsurviving patients (1.7 ± 0.6 nmol/liter vs. 3.3 ± 0.4 nmol/liter). There were many contributing factors leading to death, but circulatory failure was frequent. Although larger studies need to be performed, this preliminary study supports using low-dose T_4 treatment for myxedema coma.

Regardless of the treatment plan employed, the physician should be very familiar with the usage and possible complications of thyroid medications and should be current in his or her understanding of the interpretation of thyroid function tests in systemically ill patients. Further, as a general rule, administration of thyroid medications to a patient with cardiac disease (either ambulatory or in myxedema coma) should be instituted gradually and with careful attention to monitoring for the possibility of arrhythmias and increasing angina. Only in life-threatening emergencies should vigorous thyroid hormone replacement be given to a hypothyroid patient with cardiac disease. Lastly, clearances and thus half-lives of other medications may change as the hypothyroid patient becomes euthyroid.

INTERPRETATION OF THYROID FUNCTION TESTS IN EUTHYROID CRITICALLY ILL SUBJECTS: "EUTHYROID SICK SYNDROME"

Interpretation of thyroid function tests in a critically ill subject is very complex (Tables 34.6–34.9) (4, 8–10, 45, 46, 47, 124, 133). The important question the clinician wants answered is, Which patients are hypothyroid and require treatment and which patients are euthyroid? However, these decisions are extremely difficult, largely because normal ranges for thyroid function tests obtained in ambulatory subjects generally are not applicable to the critically ill subject and at present there are no sensitive tissue markers to help determine if there is adequate thyroid hormone at a tissue level. A full discussion of the "euthyroid sick syndrome" is beyond the scope of this chapter and the interested reader is referred to several reviews (124, 128). However, summarized in Tables 34.6–34.9 are the commonly observed changes in thyroid function tests associated with various systemic illnesses or with several drugs known to affect thyroid function tests (124). In addition to those noted, hyperemesis gravidarum may elevate free T_4 and decrease TSH response to TRH (10), and carbamazepine has also been associated with lowered total and free T_4 and T_3 (1).

A special emphasis should be given in the intensive care unit patient to the relationship

Table 34.6
Systemic Illnesses Associated with Commonly Observed Changes in Thyroid Function Tests

	TOTAL T_4	FREE T_4	TOTAL T_3	FREE T_3	REVERSE T_3	BASAL TSH	TSH RESPONSE to TRH
PRIMARY DEPRESSION	↑, N.C.	↑, N.C.	N.C.	N.C.	↑	N.C.	↓
INFECTION	↓	↑	↓	N.C.	↑	N.C., ↓	N.C.
MALIGNANCY	N.C.	↑, N.C.	↓	N.S.	↑	N.C.	N.S.
THERMAL INJURY	↓	↓	↓	↓, N.C.	↑	N.C.	N.C., ↑
CRITICAL ILLNESS	↓	N.C.*	↓	↓*	↑	N.C.	N.S.

Table 34.7
Conditions Associated with Commonly Observed Changes in Thyroid Function Tests

	TOTAL T_4	FREE T_4	TOTAL T_3	FREE T_3	REVERSE T_3	BASAL TSH	TSH RESPONSE to TRH
FASTING	N.C.	N.C., ↑	⬇	⬇	⬆	↓	↓
ANOREXIA NERVOSA	↓	Probably N.C.	⬇	N.S.	↑	N.C.	Late Peak
PROTEIN-CALORIE MALNUTRITION	↓	N.C.	⬇	↓	⬆	N.C., ↑	Exaggerated Delayed
OBESITY	N.C.	N.C.	N.C., ↑	N.C.	N.C.	N.C.	N.C.
DIABETES MELLITUS, CONTROLLED	N.C.	N.C.	N.C., ↑	N.S.	N.C., ↑	N.C.	N.C.
DIABETES MELLITUS, KETOACIDOSIS	↓	N.C., ↑	⬇	N.S.	⬆	N.C.	Blunted

of dopamine to thyroid hormone levels. Endogenous dopamine deceases TSH secretion physiologically. In the intensive care setting, the constant intravenous administration of dopamine (6.5 ± 0.4 μg/kg minute) for 48 hours decreased serum TSH to 0.9 ± 0.04 μU/ml compared with 2.3 ± 0.4 μU/ml in non-dopamine-treated subjects (66, 94). Total and free T_4 indexes were not significantly altered, although both parameters were markedly decreased compared with normal subjects. It also appears that dopamine infusion could even suppress basal serum TSH levels and the TSH response to TRH to within the normal ranges

in hypothyroid subjects, thus obscuring the diagnosis of primary hypothyroidism.

In addition to the effect of dopamine in a "typical euthyroid" critically ill subject there are profound alterations in serum thyroid function tests. Serum T_4 levels are decreased, probably secondary to alterations in binding to serum proteins, and serum T_3 by RIA is low because of decreased extrathyroidal conversion of T_4 to T_3 (30). The alteration in binding of iodothyronine to binding proteins may be related to increased levels of free fatty acids. Serum levels determined by equilibrium dialysis are either normal or even elevated,

Table 34.8
Drugs Known to Affect Thyroid Function Tests

	TOTAL T_4	FREE T_4	TOTAL T_3	FREE T_3	REVERSE T_3	BASAL TSH	TSH RESPONSE to TRH
DOPAMINE	↓	↓	↓	↓	N.C.	↓	↓
GLUCOCORTICOIDS	↓	N.C.	⬇	N.S.	⬆	↓	↓
RADIO-OPAQUE DYES	N.C., ↑	N.C.	⬇	↓	⬆	N.C., ↑	↑, N.C.
PROPRANOLOL	N.C.	N.C.	↓	N.S.	↑	N.C.	N.C.
AMIODARONE	↑	↑	⬇	↓	⬆	↑	↑

Table 34.9
Factors or Conditions That Affect Thyroid-Stimulating Hormone Levels[a]

Decrease
Dopamine agonists
Corticosteroids
Diphenylhydantoin
Low caloric uptake (<500 cal/day)
Somatostatin
Opioids
Serotonin antagonists
Increase
Hypothermic cardiovascular surgery
Recovery from systemic illness
Dopamine antagonists
Iodide
Lithium
Cimetidine
Theophylline
Amphetamines

[a] Artifactual elevation due to the presence of heterophilic antibodies to rabbit or mouse immunoglobulins may also have an effect on TSH levels.

whereas free T_4 calculation estimates are generally decreased. There are now available commercial kits capable of directly measuring free T_4; investigations have demonstrated that some of these kits may be capable of differentiating hypothyroid from euthyroid critically ill subjects (29, 66, 79). However, more studies in this area need to be performed and it appears that some commercial kits are more effective discriminators than others. The question also remains as to the extent to which free T_4 and T_3 in the serum of critically ill subjects is available for uptake into tissues (92). Although

there may be alterations in the regulation of TSH secretion even in euthyroid critically ill subjects, the basal serum TSH concentration still appears to be the best laboratory aid in discriminating hypothyroidism from euthyroidism. In my view, serum TSH values greater than 10 μU/ml represent evidence that there is biochemical hypothyroidism, whereas basal TSH concentrations less than 5 μU/ml are indicative that the patient is euthyroid. In my opinion, values between 5 and 10 μU/ml are in a borderline zone and in a critically ill subject may reflect only mild tissue hypothyroidism. Caloric deprivation, dopamine, and systemic illness itself can lower TSH in hypothyroid subjects (5, 13, 20, 126) (Table 34.10). Recovery from systemic illness could transiently elevate TSH to as high as about 15–20 μU/ml even in euthyroid subjects (51). A TRH stimulation test (Fig. 34.3) (100) is helpful in that a patient with an elevated basal TSH level would probably hyperrespond, i.e., have TSH levels greater than about 30 μU/ml. However, in my opinion, this test is only an aid in helping to diagnose the hypothyroid critically ill subject and a basal TSH is probably more helpful. Practically, if a basal serum TSH is greater than 10 μU/ml a TRH test probably need not be performed in a routine case; if the TSH is between 5 and 10 μU/ml a TRH test may be useful. A serum FT_4 by dialysis that is low may also be helpful in indicating hypothyroidism since in most euthyroid critically ill subjects the FT_4 level is either normal or high; lastly, a serum rT_3 that is low suggests hypothyroidism since most euthyroid criti-

Table 34.10
Symptoms Distinguishing Patients with Primary Hypothyroidism from Those Who are Euthyroid or Hypothyroid

Symptom	Primary Hypothyroidism	Euthyroid Critically Ill	Hypothyroid Critically Ill
Cold intolerance	+	+	+
Dry Skin	+	+	+
Edema	+	+	+
Malaise	+	+	+
Pallor	+	+	+
Anemia	+	+	+
Constipation	+	+	+
Mental slowing	+	+	+
Enlarged thyroid gland	+	−	+/−
Serum T_4	Low	Normal/Low	Low
Serum TSH	Elevated	Normal	Elevated
Serum reverse T_3	Low	Normal/Elevated	Low
Free T_4 (dialysis)	Low	Normal/High	Low
Free T_3 (dialysis)	Low	Normal/Low	Low

From Burman KD: *Thyroid: University Case Reports, vol 3*. Morris Plains, NJ, Parke-Davis, Division of Warner-Lambert, Inc., 1981.

cally ill subjects have a normal or elevated rT_3. Thus, in my view, there are only three thyroid function tests primarily capable of helping to discriminate the hypothyroid from the euthyroid critically ill subject: the serum TSH, free T_4 by dialysis (or specific kit method), and the rT_3 level. If the serum TSH level is greater than 10 μU/ml, the serum FT_4 is low, the rT_3 level is low, and there is a compatible clinical picture, then I would start treatment with exogenous L-thyroxine in a dosage plan detailed herein, which depends on the clinical severity of the patient's illness. If only one or two of these tests are consistent with hypothyroidism, in a proper clinical setting, judicious and gradual therapy with L-thyroxine may be instituted if, in the physician's view, the likelihood of hypothyroidism is great and the circumstances urgent. In the great majority of cases, a serum TSH value can be obtained within several days, and if the TSH is less than 5 μU/ml replacement therapy is not usually indicated (assuming secondary hypothyroidism is not a consideration). If, however, this value is greater than 10 μU/ml most clinicians would institute L-thyroxine therapy as detailed herein, even if the FT_4 and rT_3 values had not returned. TSH regulation may be altered in critically ill subjects (74). My comments regarding TSH depend on the use of a newer highly sensitive TSH assay that has a normal range of about 0.5–3.8 μU/ml.

It does appear that mortality is higher in "euthyroid" critically ill subjects with a decreased serum T_4. Indeed, mortality rates of about 70–80% have been found in those patients with a serum T_4 less than 3 μU/dl. The question of whether T_3 or T_4 treatment might benefit these patients remains largely unanswered. However, oral T_3 given to extensively burned patients did not reduce mortality (8). Further, Brent and Hershman (15) published a randomized prospective study in which critically ill subjects with serum T_4 levels less than 5 μU/dl were assigned either to a control group or to a treatment group that received 1.5 μg/kg L-thyroxine intravenously daily for 2 weeks. Even though the free T_4 index increased in the treatment group, the free T_3 index was comparable in the control and treatment group, as was mortality.

Thyroid function test "abnormalities" observed to occur in euthyroid critically ill subjects may also occur in all hospitalized patients as well as in most ambulatory patients who have systemic illnesses. Further, although I have just outlined the generally observed

alterations in thyroid function tests in systemically ill subjects, there are exceptions based upon the specific illness a patient may have or agents he may be receiving (Tables 34.6–34.9). The reader is referred to appropriate reviews for specific details of specific diseases (124, 128).

Last, I would emphasize that the question of whether a systemically ill patient is hypothyroid and therefore requires therapy arises quite frequently. However, the majority of these patients, when fully evaluated, are deemed euthyroid and do not require therapy. Indeed, the observed changes in thyroid function tests (e.g., decreased serum T_3) are thought to even be beneficial because they probably represent homeostatic alterations for conserving energy by reducing catabolic expenditure. Despite these cautions, a patient who really may be hypothyroid should be diagnosed and treated as rapidly as possible since undue delays may be detrimental, and treatment in these subjects should be instituted without hesitation. There are not ideal methods to help select these patients with a high likelihood of being hypothyroid, but the following findings maybe helpful: a history of thyroid surgery or radioiodine therapy, enlarged thyroid gland, hypothermia, macroglossia, unexplained pleural or peritoneal effusions, and/or presence of other autoimmune endocrine hypofunction (Table 34.10).

Acknowledgments

I am grateful to Dr. Robert C. Smallridge and Dr. Leonard Wartofsky for their assistance in the preparation of this chapter and for their critical reviews. Mrs. Estelle C. Coleman and Mrs. Barbara A. Kuffler provided expert editorial assistance.

References

1. Aanderud S, Myking OL, Strandjord RE: The influence of carbamazepine on thyroid hormones and thyroxine binding globulin in hypothyroid patients substituted with thyroxine. *Clin Endocrinol* 15:247–252, 1981.
2. Aksoy M, Erdem S: Aplastic anemia after propylthiouracil. *Lancet* 1:1379, 1968.
3. Alexander WO, Evans V, MacAulay A, et al: Metabolism of ^{35}S-labeled antithyroid drugs in man. *Br Med J* 2:290–291, 1969.
4. American Medical Association Council on Drugs: *Drug Evaluations*, ed 4. Chicago, American Medical Association, 1980.
5. Azizi F: Effect of dietary composition of fasting-induced changes in serum thyroid hormones and thyrotropin. *Metabolism* 27:935–942, 1978.
6. Balzer J, Lahrtz HG, van Zwieten PA: Serum level and urinary excretion in ^{14}C-thiamol in patients with hyperthyroidism. *Dtsch Med Wochenschr* 100:548–552, 1975.

7. Bastenie PA, Bonnyns M, VanHaelst L: Natural history of primary myxedema. *Am J Med* 79:91–100, 1985.
8. Becker RA, Vaughan GM, Ziegler MG, t al: Hypermetabolic low triiodothyronine syndrome of burn injury. *Crit Care Med* 10:870–875, 1982.
9. Bermudez F, Surks MI, Oppenheimer JH: High incidence of decreased serum triiodothyronine concentration in patients with nonthyroidal disease. *J Clin Endocrinol Metab* 41:27–40, 1975.
10. Bober SA, McGill AC, Tunbridge WMG: Thyroid function in hyperemesis gravidarum. *Acta Endocrinol* 111:404–410, 1986.
11. Boehm TM, Burman KD, Barnes S, et al: Synergism of lithium and iodide in the treatment of thyrotoxicosis. *Acta Endocrinol* 94:174–183, 1980.
12. Borst GC, Eil C, Burman KD. Euthyroid hyperthyroxinemia. *Ann Intern Med* 98:366–378, 1983.
13. Borst GC, Osburne RC, O'Brian JT, George LP, Burman KD: Fasting decreases thyrotropin responsiveness to thyrotropin-releasing hormone: a potential cause of misinterpretation of thyroid function tests in the critically ill. *J Clin Endocrinol Metab* 57:380–383, 1983.
14. Branch RA, Jaes J, Read AE: A study of factors influencing drug disposition in chronic liver disease, using the model drug propranolol. *Br J Clin Pharmacol* 2:243–249, 1976.
15. Brent GA, Hershman JM: Thyroxine therapy in patients with severe nonthyroidal illnesses and low serum thyroxine concentration. *J Clin Endocrinol Metab* 63:1–8, 1986.
16. Brown J, Chopra IJ, Cornell JS, et al: Thyroid physiology in health and disease. *Ann Intern Med* 81:68–81, 1974.
17. Burgi H, Wimpfheimer C, Burger A, et al: Changes of circulating thyroxine, triiodothyronine and reverse triiodothyronine after radiographic contrast agent. *J Clin Endocrinol Metab* 43:1203–1210, 1976.
18. Burman KD: Recent developments in thyroid hormone metabolism: interpretation and significance of measurements of reverse T_3, $3,3'$-T_2, and thyroglobulin. *Metabolism* 27:615–630, 1978.
19. Burman KD, Dimond RC, Harvey GS, et al: Glucose modulation of alterations in serum iodothyronine concentrations induced by fasting. *Metabolism* 28:291–299, 1979.
20. Burman KD, Smallridge RC, Osburne R, et al: Nature of suppressed TSH secretion during undernutrition: effect of fasting and refeeding on TSH responses to prolonged TRH infusion. *Metabolism* 29:46–52, 1980.
21. Burman KD: Interpretation of thyroid function tests in critically ill patients. In Wilber JF: *Thyroid: University Case Reports*, vol 3. Morris Plains, NJ, Parke-Davis, Division of Warner-Lambert, 1981.
22. Burman KD, Baker JR, Jr: Immune mechanisms in Graves' disease. *Endocrine Rev* 6:183, 1985.
23. Burman KD: Hypothyroidism. In Conn HF: *Current Therapy*. Philadelphia, WB Saunders, 1986, pp 521.
24. Burrow GN: The management of thyrotoxicosis in pregnancy. *N Engl J Med* 313:562–565, 1985.
25. Carlson HE, Temple R, Robbins J: Effect of lithium on thyroxine disappearance in man. *J Clin Endocrinol Metab* 36:1251–1254, 1973.
26. Chopra IJ, Solomon DH, Chopra U, et al: Pathways of metabolism of thyroid hormones. *Recent Prog Horm Res* 34:521–567, 1978.
27. Chopra IJ, Solomon DH, Chua Teco GN, et al: An inhibitor of the binding of thyroid hormones to serum proteins is present in extrathyroidal tissues. *Science* 215:407–409, 1982.
28. Chopra IJ, Solomon DH, Hepner GS, et al: Misleadingly low free thyroxine index and usefulness of reverse triiodothyronine measurement in nonthyroidal illnesses. *Ann Intern Med* 90:905–912, 1979.
29. Chopra IJ, Van Herle AJ, Chua Teco GN, et al: Serum free thyroxine in thyroidal and nonthyroidal illnesses: a comparison of measurements by radioimmunoassay, equilibrium dialysis, and free thyroxine index. *J Clin Endocrinol Metab* 51:135–143, 1980.
30. Chopra IJ, Huang T-S, Solomon DH, Chaudhuri G, Chua-Teco GN: The role of thyroxine (T_4)-binding serum proteins in oleic acid-induced increase in free T_4 in nonthyroidal illness. *J Clin Endocrinol Metab* 63:776–779, 1986.
31. Cooper DS: Antithyroid drugs. *N Engl J Med* 311:1353–1362, 1984.
32. Cooper DS, Halpen R, Wood L, Levin AA, Ridgway EC: L-thyroxine therapy in subclinical hypothyroidism: a double-blind placebo-controlled trial. *Ann Intern Med* 101:18–24, 1984.
33. Cooper DS, Bode HH, Nath B, Saxe V, Maloof F, Ridgway EC: Methimazole pharmacology in man: studies using a newly developed radioimmunoassay for methimazole. *J Clin Endocrinol Metab* 58:473, 1984.
34. Cooper DS, Saxe VC, Maloff F, et al: Studies of propylthiouracil using a newly developed radioimmunoassay. *J Clin Endocrinol Metab* 52:204–213, 1981.
35. Cooper DS, Daniels GH, Landenson PW, et al: Hyperthyroxinemia in patients treated with high-dose propranolol. *Am J Med* 73:867–871, 1982.
36. Cooper DS, Saxe VC, Meskell M, et al: Acute effects of propylthiouracil (PTU) on thyroidal iodide organification and peripheral iodothyronine deiodination: correlation with serum PTU levels measured by radioimmunoassay. *J Clin Endocrinol Metab* 54:101–107, 1982.
37. Cooper DS, Goldminz D, Levin AA, et al: Agranulocytosis associated with antithyroid drugs: effects of patient age and drug dose. *Ann Intern Med* 98:26–29, 1983.
38. Davis PJ, Davis FB: Hyperthyroidism in patients over the age of 60 years: clinical features in 85 patients. *Medicine* 53:161–181, 1974.
39. Engler D, Donaldson EB, Stockigt JR, et al: Hyperthyroidism without triiodothyronine excess: an effect of severe non-thyroidal illness. *J Clin Endocrinol Metab* 46:77–82, 1978.
40. Eriksson M, Rubenfeld S, Garber AJ, et al: Propranolol does not prevent thyroid storm. *N Engl J Med* 296:263–24, 1977.
41. Evans GH, Shand DG: Disposition of propranolol. VI. Independent variations steady-state circulating drug concentrations and half-life. *Clin Pharmacol Ther* 14:494–500, 1973.
42. Feely J, Forrest A, Gunn A, et al: Propranolol dosage in thyrotoxicosis. *J Clin Endocrinol Metab* 51:658–661, 1980.
43. Feely J, Isles TE, Ratcliffe WA, et al: Propranolol, triiodothyronine, reverse triiodothyronine and thyroid disease. *Clin Endocrinol* 10:531–538, 1979.
44. Felicetta JV, Green WL, Nelp WB: Inhibition of hepatic binding of thyroxine by cholecystographic agents. *J Clin Invest* 65:1032–1040, 1980.
45. Finucane JF, Griffiths TS: Thyroid function non-thyroidal illness. *Int J Med Sci* 146:103–107, 1977.
46. Gardner DF, Carithers RL, Galen EA, et al: Thyroid function tests in patients with acute and resolved hepatitis B infection. *Ann Intern Med* 96:450–452, 1982.
47. Gavin LA, McMahon FA, Castle JN, et al: Alterations in serum thyroid hormones and thyroxine-binding globulin in patients with nephrosis. *J Clin Endocrinol Metab* 46:125–130, 1978.
48. George CF, et al: Pharmacokinetics of dextro, laevo, and racemic propranolol in man. *Eur J Clin Pharmacol* 4:74–76, 1972.
49. Graham G, Burman KD: Radioiodine treatment of Graves' disease: an assessment of its potential risks. *Ann Intern Med* 105:901–905, 1986.
50. Gregerman RI, Davis PJ: Effects of intrinsic and extrinsic variables on thyroid hormone economy. In Werner

SC, Ingbar SH: *The Thyroid: A Fundamental and Clinical Text.* New York, Harper & Row, 1978, p 223.

51. Hamblin PS, Dyer SA, Mohr VS, LeGrand BA, Lim C-F, Tuxen DV, Topliss DJ, Stockigt JR: Relationship between thyrotropin and thyroxine changes during recovery from severe hypothyroxinemia of critical illness. *J Clin Endocrinol Metab* 62:717–722, 1986.
52. Hanson JS: Propylthiouracil and hepatitis. *Arch Intern Med* 144:994–996, 1984.
53. Harrower ADB, Fyffe JA, Horn DB, et al: Thyroxine and triiodothyronine levels in hyperthyroid patients during treatment with propranolol. *Clin Endocrinol* 7:41–44, 1977.
54. Hennessey JV, Evaul JE, Tseng Y-C, Burman KD, Wartofsky L: L-thyroxine dosage: A reevaluation of therapy with contemporary preparations. *Ann Intern Med* 105:11–15, 1986.
55. Holvey DN, Goodner CJ, Nicoloff JT, et al: Treatment of myxedema coma with intravenous thyroxine. *Arch Intern Med* 113:89–96, 1964.
56. Hylander B, Rosenquist U: Treatment of myxoedema coma factors associated with fatal outcome. *Acta Endocrinol* 108:65, 1985.
57. Jackson GL, Flickinger FW, Wells LW: Massive overdosage of propylthiouracil. *Ann Intern Med* 91:418–419, 1979.
58. Jonckheer MH: Amiodarone and the thyroid gland: a review. *Acta Cardiol* 36:199–205, 1981.
59. Jones MK, John R, Jones GR: The effect of oxprenolol, acebutolol, and propranolol on thyroid hormones in hyperthyroid subjects. *Clin Endocrinol* 13:343–347, 1980.
60. Kampmann JP: Pharmacokinetics of propylthiouracil in man after intravenous infusion. *J Pharmackinet Biopharm* 5:435–443, 1977.
61. Kampmann JP, Johansen K, Molholm Hansen J, Helweg J: Propylthiouracil in human milk. Revision of a dogma. *Lancet* 2:736, 1980.
62. Kampmann P, Skovsted L: The kinetics of propylthiouracil in hyperthyroid subjects. *Acta Pharmacol* 37:201–210, 1975.
63. Kampmann JP, Skovsted L: The pharmacokinetics of propylthiouracil. *Acta Pharmacol Toxicol* 35:361–369, 1974.
64. Kaptein EM, Grieb DA, Spencer C, et al: Thyroxine metabolism in the low thyroxine state of critical nonthyroidal illnesses. *J Clin Endocrinol Metab* 53764–771, 1981.
65. Kaptein EM, MacIntyre SS, Weiner JM, et al: Free thyroxine estimates in nonthyroidal illness: comparison of eight methods. *J Clin Endocrinol Metab* 52:1073–1077, 1981.
66. Kaptein EM, Spencer CA, Kamiel MB, et al: Prolonged dopamine administration and thyroid hormone economy in normal and critically ill subjects. *J Clin Endocrinol Metab* 51:387–393, 1980.
67. Kleinmann RE, Vagenakis AG, Braverman LE: The effect of iopanoic acid on the regulation of thyrotropin secretion in euthyroid subjects. *J Clin Endocrinol Metab* 51:399–403, 1980.
68. Konishi J, Iida Y, Kasagi K, Misaki T, Nakashima T, Endo K, Mori T, Shinpo S, Nohara Y, Matsuura N, Torizuka K: Primary myxedema with thyrotropin-binding inhibitor immunoglobulins: clinical and laboratory findings in 15 patients. *Ann Intern Med* 103:26–31, 1985.
69. Kristensen O, Harrestrup Anderson H, Pallisgaard G: Lithium carbonate in the treatment of thyrotoxicosis: a controlled study. *Lancet* 1:603–605, 1976.
70. Lamberg B-A, Ikonen E, Osterlund K, et al: Antithyroid treatment of maternal hyperthyroidism during lactation. *Clin Endocrinol* 21:81–87, 1984.
71. Larsen PR: Thyroid pituitary interaction: feedback regulation of thyrotropin secretion by thyroid hormones. *N Engl J Med* 30623–32, 1982.

72. Lowenthal DT, et al: Pharmacokinetics of oral propranolol in chronic renal disease. *Clin Pharmacol Ther* 16:761–769, 1974.
73. Martino E, Bambini G, Bartalena L, Mammoli C, Aghini-Lombardi F, Baschieri L, Pinchera A: Human serum thyrotropin measurement by ultrasensitive immunoradiometric assay as a first-line test in the evaluation of thyroid function. *Clin Endocrinol* 24:141–148, 1986.
74. Maturlo SJ, Rosenbaum RL, Pan C, et al: Variable thyrotropin response to thyrotropin-releasing hormone after small decreases in plasma free thyroid hormone concentrations in patients with nonthyroidal disease. *J Clin Invest* 66:451–456, 1980.
75. Mayfield RK, Sagel J, Colwell JA: Thyrotoxicosis without elevated serum triiodothyronine levels during diabetic ketoacidosis. *Arch Intern Med* 140:409–410, 1980.
76. McDermott MD, Burman KD, Hofeldt FD, Kidd GS: Lithium-associated thyrotoxicosis. *Amer J Med* 80:1245–1248, 1986.
77. McMurry JF, Gilliland PF, Ratliff CR, Bourland PD: Pharmacodynamics of propylthiouracil in normal and hyperthyroid subjects after a single dose. *J Clin Endocrinol Metab* 41:362–364, 1975.
78. Melmed S, Geola FL, Reed AW, et al: A comparison of methods for assessing thyroid function in nonthyroidal illness. *J Clin Endocrinol Metab* 54:300–306, 1982.
79. Melmed S, Nademance K, Reed AW, et al: Hyperthyroxinemia with bradycardia and normal thyrotropin secretion after chronic amiodarone administration. *J Clin Endocrinol Metab* 53–997–1001, 1981.
80. Momotani N, Ito K, Hamada N, Ban Y, Nishikawa Y, Mimura T: Maternal hyperthyroidism and congenital malformation in the offspring. *Clin Endocrinol* 20:695–700, 1984.
81. Momotani N, Noh J, Oyanagi H, Ishikawa N, Ito K: Antithyroid drug therapy for Graves' disease during pregnancy: optimal regimen for fetal thyroid status. *N Engl J Med* 315:24–28, 1986.
82. Morley JE: Neuroendocrine control of thyrotropin secretion. *Endocrinol Rev* 2:396–436, 1981.
83. Mujtaba Q, Burrow GN: Treatment of hyperthyroidism in pregnancy with propylthiouracil and methimazole. *Obstet Gynecol* 46:282–286, 1975.
84. Nabil N, Miner DJ, Amatruda JM: Methimazole: an alternative route of administration. *J Clin Endocrinol Metab* 54:180–181, 1982.
85. Pittman JA, Beschi RJ, Smitherman TC: Methimazole: its absorption and excretion in man and tissue distribution in rats. *Endocrinology* 33:182–185, 1971.
86. Reus VI, Gold P, Post R: Lithium-induced thyrotoxicosis. *Am J Psychiatry* 136:191–194, 1974.
87. Reveno WS, Rosenbaum H: Observations on the use of antithyroid drugs. *Ann Intern Med* 60:982–989, 1964.
88. Robbins J, Rall JE: The interaction of thyroid hormones and proteins in biological fluids. *Recent Prog Horm Res* 13:161–208, 1957.
89. Ross TJ, Jones MK, John R: The effect of propranolol withdrawal on thyroid hormones in normal and hyperthyroid subjects. *Clin Endocrinol* 13:27–31, 1980.
90. Ross DS: New sensitive immunoradiometric assays for thyrotropin. *Ann Intern Med* 104:718–720, 1986.
91. Rubenfeld S, Silverman VE, Welch KMA, et al: Variable plasma propranolol levels in thyrotoxicosis. *N Engl J Med* 300:353–354, 1979.
92. Sarne DH, Refetoff S: Measurement of thyroxine uptake from serum by cultured human hepatocytes as an index of thyroid status: reduced thyroxine uptake from serum of patients with nonthyroidal illness. *J Clin Endocrinol Metab* 61:1046–1052, 1985.
93. Sawin CT, Chopra D, Albano J, et al: The free triiodothyronine (T_3) index. *Ann Intern Med* 88:474–477, 1978.

94. Scanlon MF, Weightman DR, Shale DJ, et al: Dopamine is a physiological regulator of thyrotropin (TSH) secretion in normal man. *Clin Endocrinol* 10:7–15, 1979.

95. Schimmel M, Utiger RD: Thyroidal and peripheral production of thyroid hormones. Review of recent findings and their clinical implications. *Ann Intern Med* 87:760–768, 1977.

96. Schuppan D, Et al: Preliminary pharmacokinetic studies of propylthiouracil in humans. *J Pharmacokinet Biopharm* 1:307–318, 1973.

97. Schussler GC: Thyroid function tests in patients with non-thyroidal disease. In *Thyroid Today*, vol 3, no 3. Morton Grove, IL, Flint Laboratories, 1980.

98. Shand DG: Propranolol. *N Engl J Med* 293:280–285, 1976.

99. Sitar DS, Hunninghake DB: Pharmacokinetics of propylthiouracil in man after a single oral dose. *J Clin Endocrinol Metab* 40:26–29, 1975.

100. Snyder PJ, Utiger RD: Response to thyrotropin-releasing hormone (TRH) in normal man. *J Clin Endocrinol Metab* 34:380–385, 1972.

101. Spencer CA, Lai-Rosenfeld AO, Guttler RB, Lopresti J, Marcus AO, Nimalasuriya A, Eigen A, Doss RG, Green BJ, Nicoloff JT: Thyrotropin secretion in thyrotoxic and thyroxine-treated patients: assessment by a sensitive immunoenzymometric assay. *J Clin Endocrinol Metab* 63:349–355, 1986.

102. Sterling K, Brenner MA: Free thyroxine in human serum: simplified measurement with the aid of magnesium precipitation. *J Clin Invest* 45:155–163, 1966.

103. Suzuki H, Kadena N, Taekuchi K, et al: Effects of three-day oral cholecystography on serum iodothyronines and TSH concentrations: comparison of the effects among some cholecystographic agents and the effects of iopanoic acid on the pituitary-thyroid axis. *Acta Endocrinol* 92:477–488, 1979.

104. Suzuki H, Noguchi K, Nakahata M, et al: Effect of iopanoic acid on the pituitary-thyroid axis: time sequence of changes in serum iodothyronines, thyrotropin, and prolactin concentrations and responses to thyroid hormones. *J Clin Endocrinol Metab* 53:779–788, 1981.

105. Talbert RL, Wong YY, Duncan RB: Propranolol plasma concentrations and plasmapheresis. *Drug Intell Clin Pharm* 15:993–995, 1981.

106. Tegler L, Lindstrom B: Antithyroid drugs in milk (letter). *Lancet* 2:591, 1980.

107. Temple R, Berman M, Robbins J, et al: The use of lithium in the treatment of thyrotoxicosis. *J Clin Invest* 51:2746–2756, 1972.

108. Thomas FB, Mazzaferri IL, Skillman G: Apathetic thyrotoxicosis: a distinctive clinical and laboratory entity. *Ann Intern Med* 72:679–685, 1970.

109. Toft AO, Irvine WJ, Sinclair I, et al: Thyroid function after surgical treatment of thyrotoxicosis: A report of 100 cases treated with propranolol before operation. *N Engl J Med* 298:643–647, 1978.

110. Tseng Y-C, Burman KD, Baker JR Jr., Wartofsky L: A rapid, sensitive enzyme-linked immunoassay for human thyrotropin. *Clin Chem* 31:1131–1134, 1985.

111. Utiger RD: Decreased extra thyroidal triiodothyronine production in non-thyroidal illness: Benefit or harm. *Am J Med* 69:807–810, 1980.

112. Vagenakis AF, Braverman LE: Adverse effects of iodine on thyroid function. *Med Clin North Am* 59:1075–1088, 1975.

113. Vagenakis AG, Portnay GI, O'Brian JT, et al: Effect of starvation on the production and metabolism of thyroxine and triiodothyronine in euthyroid obese patients. *J Clin Endocrinol Metab* 45:1205–1309, 1977.

114. Vanderlaan WP: Antithyroid drugs in practice. *Mayo Clin Proc* 47:962–965, 1972.

115. Van Dijke CP, Heydendael RJ, DeKleine MJ: Methimazole, carbimazole and congenital skin defects. *Ann Intern Med* 106:60–61, 1987.

116. Vasily BD, Tyler WB: Propylthiouracil-induced cutaneous vasculitis: case presentation and review of the literature. *JAMA* 243:458–461, 1980.

117. Verhoeen RP, Visser TJ, Docter R, et al: Plasma thyroxine 3,3',5-triiodothyronine during beta-adrenergic blockade in hyperthyroidism. *J Clin Endocrinol Metab* 44:1002–1005, 1977.

118. Vesell ES, Shapiro JR, Passananti GT, et al: Altered plasma half-lives of antipyrine, propylthiouracil and methimazole in thyroid dysfunction. *Clin Pharmacol Ther* 17:48–52, 1975.

119. Visser TJ: A tentative review of recent in vitro observations of the enzymatic deiodination of iodothyronines and its possible physiological implications. *Mol Cell Endocrinol* 35:241, 1978.

120. Volpe R, Karlsson A, Jansson R, Dahlberg P: Evidence that antithyroid drugs induced remissions in Graves' disease by modulating thyroid cellular activity. *Clin Endocrinol* 25:453–462, 1986.

121. Wall JR, Fang SL, Kuroki T, Ingbar SH, Braverman LE: In vitro immunoreactivity to propylthiouracil methimazole, and carbimazole in patients with Graves' disease: A possible cause of antithyroid drug-induced agranulocytosis. *J Clin Endocrinol Metab* 58:868–872, 1984.

122. Wang Y-S, Pekary AE, England MS, Hersaman JM: Comparison of a new ultrafiltration method for serum-free T4 and free T3 with two RIA kits in eight groups of patients. *J Endocrinol Invest* 8:495–500, 1985.

123. Wartofsky L, Burman KD: Hypothyroidism. In Conn HF: *Current Therapy*. Philadelphia, WB Saunders, 1979.

124. Wartofsky L, Burman KD: Alterations in thyroid function in patients with systemic illness: "The euthyroid sick syndrome." *Endocrine Rev* 3:164–217, 1982.

125. Wartofsky L, Ransil BJ, Ingbar SH: Inhibition by iodine of the release of thyroxine from the thyroid glands of patients with thyrotoxicosis. *J Clin Invest* 49:78–86, 1970.

126. Weetman RE, Gregerman RI, Burns WH, Saral R, Santos GW: Suppression of thyrotropin in the low-thyroxine state of severe nonthyroidal illness. *N Engl J Med* 312:546–552, 1985.

127. Wenzel KE: Pharmacological interference with in vitro tests of thyroid function. *Metabolism* 30:7171–732, 1981.

128. Werner SC: Thyroid function tests in non-thyroidal illness are diagnostically and prognostically important. *Ariz Med* 38:356–358, 1981.

129. Werner SC, Ingbar SH: *The Thyroid: A Fundamental and Clinical Text.* Hagerstown, MD, Harper & Row, 1978.

130. Wiersinga WM, Touber JL: The influence of β-adrenoceptor blocking agents on plasma thyroxine and triiodothyronine. *J Clin Endocrinol Metab* 45:293–298, 1977.

131. Wu SY, Chopra IJ, Solomon DH, et al: Changes in circulating iodothyronines in euthyroid and hyperthyroid subjects given ipodate (Oragrafin), an agent for oral cholecystography. *J Clin Endocrinol Metab* 46:691–697, 1978.

132. Wu SY, Shyh TP, Chopra IJ, et al: Comparison of sodium ipodate (Oragrafin) and propylthiouracil in early treatment of hyperthyroidism. *J Clin Endocrinol Metab* 54:630–642, 1982.

133. Zaloga GP, Chernow B, Smallridge RC, Zajtchuk R, Hall-Boyer K, Hargraves R, Lake CR, Burman KD: A longitudinal evaluation of thyroid function in critically ill surgical patients. *Ann Surg* 201:456–464, 1985.

134. Zwillich CW, Pierson DK, Hofeldt FD, et al: Ventilatory control in myxedema and hypothyroidism. *N Engl J Med* 292:662–665, 1975.

135. Zwillich CW, Sahn SA, Weil JV: Effects of hypermetabolism on ventilation and chemosensitivity. *J Clin Invest* 60:900–906, 1977.

35

Antimicrobials

Henry Masur, M.D.

Infection is frequently suspected or documented in critically ill patients either as the primary process that brings the patient to an intensive care unit (ICU) or as a complication of diagnostic procedures, surgical intervention, drug therapy, or nosocomial exposure in patients who originally entered the ICU for other indications. Therapy of suspected infections in critically ill patients must often be more empirical than in other hospitalized patients, because the critically ill patient may be too sick to tolerate diagnostic procedures. Treatment must also be more encompassing since the critically ill patient may not survive if a causative organism is not immediately treated, whereas a less ill patient may be able to tolerate inadequately treated infection for a few days until the specific pathogens are identified.

Another major consideration for treating critically ill patients is the route of drug administration and the dose and interval that are required. Oral and intramuscular routes usually must be avoided because of uncertainty of absorption. Hepatic and renal dysfunction must be carefully monitored and the fluid and colloid status assessed so that drug levels are maintained in therapeutic but nontoxic ranges.

The focus of this chapter is on the antimicrobial agents commonly employed for critically ill patients in the United States. In the late 1980s a plethora of antimicrobial agents has become available, and a major issue is which of these agents really represent an advance in terms of improved efficacy, lower cost, or reduced toxicity (2, 3, 15, 51, 59, 60). These newer drugs vary greatly in their antimicrobial spectrum, toxicity, doses, distribution, half-lives, and routes of elimination. It is probably preferable for intensivists to be very familiar with a limited number of antimicrobial drugs so that these drugs are used correctly rather than attempting the use of numerous costly agents, many of which are quite similar to each other.

SPECIFIC ANTIMICROBIAL AGENTS

Antibacterial Agents

PENICILLINS

The penicillins are a group of natural and semisynthetic compounds that share a basic structure that consists of a thiazolidine ring connected to a β-lactam ring with an attached side chain. The biologic activity of the penicillins is determined by the integrity of the thiazolidine and β-lactam structures. The antibacterial and pharmacologic properties of penicillin are modified by altering the side chain, resulting in a wide variety of available penicillin compounds (Table 35.1). These penicillins are most usefully classified according to their antibacterial spectrum. They all have similar, though not necessarily identical, mechanisms of action, the details of which are currently being elucidated. Penicillins kill bacteria by interfering with synthesis of the peptidoglycan component of the bacterial cell wall (28). Without effective cell walls the bacteria either fail to divide or swell and rupture.

Penicillins do not kill or inhibit all bacteria. Bacteria may be intrinsically resistant or may acquire resistance to the penicillins (72, 73). Differential permeability to penicillins and differential binding of a specific penicillin to receptor proteins account for different activity of various penicillin compounds against specific bacteria. Other bacteria contain enzymes that inactivate the drugs (72). In Gram-positive bacteria, for instance, the peptidoglycan polymer is near the cell surface and is thus readily acted upon. In Gram-negative bacteria, however, the cell wall is protected from the hydrophilic penicillins by a complex surface structure. While some microorganisms are inherently resistant to the penicillins, other microorganisms produce enzymes that can inactivate various β-lactam drugs. Gram-positive organisms generally secrete extracellular enzymes, whereas Gram-negative organisms produce small quantities of enzymes that remain in the periplasmic space between the inner and outer cell membranes. Each bacterial species produces a somewhat different β-lactamase, and each specific penicillin, or cephalosporin, varies in its susceptibility to the particular enzyme produced. The information for penicillinase is encoded on a plasmid that can be transferred by phages to other organisms. Ability to produce the enzyme is often inducible by exposure to the appropriate substrate. Some of the β-lactamases secreted by Gram-negative bacteria are inducible while others are constitutive.

Penicillins are most readily classified for clinical purposes on the basis of their antimicrobial spectrum. Table 35.1 lists the most commonly used penicillins, and their major routes of excretion. Table 35.2 indicates organisms for which penicillin drugs are effective therapy.

Distribution and Elimination

Most penicillins are widely distributed throughout the body though local concentrations may vary substantially. In CSF, levels are generally well below serum concentrations, though the presence of fever or meningeal inflammation usually augments penetration such that subarachnoid concentrations are therapeutic for the most common community acquired organisms that cause meningitis. Concentrations in obstructed bile and in prostatic tissue are often subtherapeutic for the most likely pathogens.

Adverse Reactions

The most common adverse reactions to the penicillins are hypersensitivity reactions. All of the penicillin compounds have potential to cause allergic phenomena (66). In order of decreasing frequency, these reactions are maculopapular rash, urticaria, fever, bronchospasm, vasculitis, serum sickness, exfoliative dermatitis, and anaphylaxis. The true incidence of such reactions is probably between 0.5% and 10%, although some hypersensitivity

reactions may occur particularly frequently with one penicillin compound. A hypersensitivity response after one administration of a drug does not guarantee a similar response for each of its subsequent administrations. It is not safe clinical practice to give a patient a penicillin compound if the patient has a reliable history of immediate hypersensitivity response to any drug in the penicillin group (41, 66). Whether or not desensitization of the patient to the penicillin compound decreases the likelihood of a subsequent allergic response is uncertain, but desensitization in a controlled medical setting, such as an ICU, is a standard practice for patients who have no therapeutic alternative to penicillin. Skin testing with both major and minor determinants of penicillin is useful for predicting which patients are most likely to have a hypersensitivity response. Reliable preparations of antigens should be used for skin testing. Both major and minor determinants must be employed.

Serious toxic reactions to the penicillins are unusual events. The drugs provoke an inflammatory response that appears to be concentration dependent; inflammation at injection sites and thrombophlebitis occasionally occur. Very high serum concentrations are associated with confusion, lethargy, and seizures, especially in those patients with pre-existing cerebral disorders. Intrathecal administration of penicillins can cause arachnoiditis, but such administration is almost never warranted. Other toxic reactions reported include nephritis (especially with methicillin) (34), bone marrow depression (especially with methicilin or nafcillin) (35), hepatitis (especially with oxacillin) (54), and impaired platelet aggregation (especially with carbenicillin and ticarcillin) (12, 67).

Because of their proven clinical efficacy and their safety, penicillins are commonly used in critically ill patients. Table 35.1 indicates the recommended doses for the commonly used penicillin drugs.

Numerous new penicillin compounds have appeared in recent years. The acylamino penicillins, for example (azlocillin, mezlocillin, piperacillin) are broad-spectrum penicillins with activity against many enterobacteriaceae and *Pseudomonas aeruginosa* (22). Piperacillin is widely used because of its excellent in vitro activity against *P. aeruginosa*, but the major determinant of the drug of choice among these acylamino penicillins is probably cost rather than efficacy or safety, because the effi-

Table 35.1
Antimicrobial Agents for Bacterial, Fungal, and Viral Infections in Critically III Patients

Drug	Usual Adult Daily Dose (Recommended Dose Interval)	Route of Administration	Peak Serum (μg/ml) Concentration (i.v. Dose)	Hepatic Metabolism/ Excretion	Dose Alteration with Renal Dysfunction	Serum Concentration Altered by: Hemodialysis	Peritoneal Dialysis
Penicillins							
Aqueous crystalline penicillin G	0.6–20 million units/day (continuous-q4h)	i.v., i.m.	18 (1×10^6 U/hr)	No	Major	No	No
Ampicillin	4–12 g/day (q4–6h)	i.v., i.m.	6 (0.5 g)	Yes	Major	Yes	No
Carbenicillin	0.5 g/kg/day (q4h)	i.v., i.m.	150 (2 g)	Yes	Major	Yes	Yes
Ticarcillin	0.25 g/kg/day (q4h)	i.v., i.m.	140 (3g)	Yes	Major	Yes	Yes
Timentin	18.6 g/day (q4–6h)	i.v., i.m.		Yes	Major	Yes	Yes
Piperacillin	0.2–0.5 g/kg/day (q4h)	i.v., i.m.	320 (4 g)	Yes	Minor	Yes	Yes
Oxacillin	4–8 g/day (q4–6h)	i.v., i.m.	50 (0.5 g)	No	Minor	No	No
Nafcillin	4–8 g/day (q4h)	i.v., i.m.	11 (0.5 g)	Yes	Minor	No	No
Methicillin	6–12 g/day (q4–6h)	i.v., i.m.	72 (2.0 g)	No	Minor	No	No
Cephalosporins and Cephamycins							
Cephalothin	4–12 g/day (q4–6h)	i.v., i.m.	100 (2 g)	Yes	Minor	Yes	Yes
Cefazolin	2–6 g/day (q6–8h)	i.v., i.m.	188 (1 g)	Yes	Major	Yes	No
Cefoxitin	4–12 g/day (q4–6h)	i.v., i.m.	110 (1 g)	Yes	Major	Yes	
Cefamandole	4–12 g/day (q4–6h)	i.v., i.m.	80 (1 g)	Yes	Major	No	No
Cefotaxime	4–12 g/day (q6–8h)	i.v., i.m.	214 (2 g)	Yes	Minor	No	No
Ceftazidime	4–6 g/day (q6–8h)	i.v., i.m.	130 (2 g)	No	Major	Yes	Yes
Ceftriaxone	2–4 g/day (q12h)	i.v., i.m.	250 (2 g)	Yes	Minor	No	No
Other β-Lactams							
Imipenem/Cilastatin	3 g/day (q6–8h)	i.v., i.m.	70 (1 g)	No	Major	Yes	
Aztreonam	8 g/day (q8–12h)	i.v., i.m.	125 (1 g)	Yes	Major	Yes	Yes
Aminoglycosides							
Gentamicin	3–6 mg/kg/day (q6–8h)	i.v., i.m.	3–6 (1 mg/kg)	No	Major	Yes	Yes
Tobramycin	3–6 mg/kg/day (q6–8h)	i.v., i.m.	4–10 (1 mg/kg)	No	Major	Yes	Yes
Amikacin	15 mg/kg/day (q12h)	i.v., i.m.	20 (1.0 g)	No	Major	Yes	Yes

Agent	Dose	Route					
Antimycobacterial Agents							
Isoniazid	300 mg/day (q24h)	p.o.	1.0 (10 mg/kg)	Yes	Minor	Yes	No
Rifampin	600 mg/day (q24h)	p.o.	7 (600 mg)	Yes	Minor	No	No
Ethambutol	15 mg/kg/day (q24h)	p.o.		No	Major	Yes	No
Other Antibacterial Agents							
Trimethoprim/sulfamethoxazole	320–960 mg trimethoprim/day	i.v.	100–150 S (25 mg/kg)	Yes	Major	Yes	Yes
Vancomycin	2 g/day (q6h or q12h)	i.v.	20–40 (0.5 g)	No	Major	No	No
Erythromycin lactobionate	2 g/day (q6h)	i.v.	9.9 (0.50g)	Yes	No	No	No
Clindamycin	2.4 g/day (q6h)	i.v.	14 (0.6 g)	Yes	Minor	No	No
Chloramphenicol	2–6 g/day (q6h)	i.v.	11 (1.0 g)	Yes	Minor	No	No
Metronidazole	2.25 g/day (q6–8h)	i.v.	26 (0.5 g)	Yes	Major	Yes	No
Tetracycline	2 g/day (q6h)	i.v.	8.5 (0.5 g)	Yes	Avoid	Yes	No
Antiprotozoal Agents							
Pentamidine	4 mg/kg/day (q24h)	i.v.	0.612 (4 mg/kg)	?	No	No	No
Trimethoprim/sulfamethoxazole	20 mg/kg/day (T) and 100 mg/kg/day (S) (q6h)	i.v., p.o.	100–150 S (25 mg/kg)	Yes	Major	Yes	Yes
Sulfadiazine	4–8 g/day (q6h)	i.v.		Yes	Yes	Yes	Yes
Pyrimethamine	25 mg/day (q24h)	p.o.		No		No	
Antifungal Agents							
Amphotericin B	0.6 mg/kg/day (q24h)	i.v.		No	Minor	No	No
Flucytosine	150 mg/kg/day (q6h)	p.o.	75 (2.0 g)	No	Yes	Yes	Yes
Ketoconazole	400 mg/day	p.o.	3.5 (200 mg)	No	Yes	No	No
Antiviral Agents							
Acyclovir	15–30 mg/kg/day (q8h)	i.v.	20 (10 mg/kg)	No	Yes	Yes	Yes
Amantadine	100–200 mg/day (q24h)	p.o.	0.3 (100 mg)	No	Yes	Yes	No
Azidothymidine	1000 mg/day (q4h)	p.o.		Yes			
Ribavirin	aerosol	aerosol		No			
DHPG	10 mg/kg/day (q12h)	i.v.		No	Yes		

cacy and safety profiles of these drugs are so similar. Ticarcillin has been marketed as a combination with potassium clavulanate, a noncompetitive inhibitor of many β-lactamases. The combination is available as Timentin, and has increased in vitro activity against a variety of organisms (55, 77). This drug combination may be useful against certain aerobic Gram-negative bacilli, anerobes, and *Staphylococcus aureus* that produce β-lactamase, but it has no clear advantage over older drugs or drug combinations.

CEPHALOSPORINS

Cephalosporins are a group of natural and semisynthetic compounds with broad antibacterial activity. They are structurally similar to penicillins and inhibit bacterial cell wall synthesis in much the same manner as the penicillins. Cephamycins are structurally similar to cephalosporins and act in a similar manner, and thus are also considered in this section.

A large and expanding number of cephalosporin and cephamycin compounds are avail-

Table 35.2
Antimicrobial Drugs of Choice for the Treatment of Specific Infectious Agents in Critically Ill Patients

Organism	Antimicrobial Agent of Choice	Alternative Agents
BACTERIA		
Gram-positive cocci (aerobic)		
Staphylococcus aureus		
Non-penicillinase-producing	Penicillin	Vancomycin, cephalosporin
Penicillinase producing	Nafcillin, oxacillin	Vancomycin, cephalosporin
α-Streptococci (viridans streptococcus	Penicillin	Erythromycin, clindamycin, cephalosporin
β-Streptococci (A,B,C,G)	Penicillin	Cephalosporin, erythromycin
Streptococcus fecalis		
Serious infection	Ampicillin + aminoglycoside	Vancomycin + aminoglycoside
Uncomplicated urinary infection	Ampicillin	Vancomycin
Streptococcus bovis	Penicillin	Cephalosporin, vancomycin
Streptococcus pneumoniae	Penicillin	Erythromycin, vancomycin, cephalosporin
Gram-negative cocci (aerobic)		
Neisseria meningitidis	Penicillin	Cefotaxime, chloramphenicol
Neisseria gonorrheae	Penicillin	Spectinomycin, ceftriaxone
Gram-positive bacilli (aerobic)		
Corynebacterium JK	Vancomycin	
Gram-negative bacilli (aerobic)		
Acinetobacter sp.	Aminoglycoside + carbenicillin	Trimethoprim-sulfamethoxazole
Campylobacter sp.	Erythromycin	Tetracycline
Enterobacter sp.	Aminoglycoside	Third generation cephalosporin
Escherichia coli	Ampicillin	Cephalosporin, aminoglycoside
Haemophilus influenza	Second- or third-generation cephalosporin	Trimethoprim-sulfamethoxazole
Klebsiella pneumoniae	Aminoglycoside	Cephalosporin, aztreonam
Legionella sp.	Erythromycin + rifampin	Rifampin, quinolones
Proteus mirabilis	Ampicillin	Aminoglycoside, cephalosporin
Other proteus species	Aminoglycoside	Cephalosporin, aztreonam
Providencia sp.	Aminoglycoside (amikacin)	Cephalosporin, aztreonam
Pseudomonas aeruginosa	Aminoglycoside + carbenicillin	Third-generation cephalosporin, aztreonam
Salmonella sp.	Trimethoprim-sulfamethoxazole	Ampicillin, chloramphenicol, third-generation cephalosporins
Serratia marcescens	Aminoglycoside	Third generation cephalosporin
Shigella sp.	Ampicillin	Chloramphenicol
Anaerobes		
Anaerobic streptococci	Penicillin	Clindamycin, metronidazole
Bacteroides sp.		
Oropharyngeal strains	Penicillin	Clindamycin
Gastrointestinal strains	Clindamycin	Metronidazole, cefoxitin
Clostridium sp. (except C. difficile)	Penicillin	Clindamycin, metronidazole

Organism	Antimicrobial Agent of Choice	Alternative Agents
Clostridium difficile	Vancomycin	Metronidazole
Other Bacteria		
Actinomyces and *Arachnia*	Penicillin G	Tetracycline
Nocardia sp.	Trimethoprim-sulfamethoxazole	Minocycline
Mycobacterium tuberculosis	INH + rifampin	Ethambutol, streptomycin
FUNGI		
Aspergillus sp.	Amphotericin B	
Elastomyces dermatitidis	Amphotericin B	
Candida sp.	Amphotericin B	Ketoconazole
Coccidioides immitis	Amphotericin B	
Cryptococcus neoformans	Amphotericin B + flucytosine	
Histoplasma capsulatum	Amphotericin B	Ketoconazole
Mucor-Absidia-Rhizopus	Amphotericin	
PROTOZOA		
Pneumocystis carinii	Trimethoprim-sulfamethoxazole	Pentamidine
Toxoplasma gondii	Sulfadiazine + pyrimethamine	
VIRUSES		
Herpes simplex	Acyclovir	
Influenza A	Amantadine	
Herpes zoster	Acyclovir	
OTHER ORGANISMS		
Mycoplasma pneumoniae	Erythromycin	Tectracycline
Chlamydia psittaci	Tetracycline	Chloramphenicol
Chlamydia trachomatis	Erythromycin	Tetracycline
Leptospira sp.	Penicillin G	Tetracycline
Rickettsia sp.	Tetracycline	Chloramphenicol

able, which vary considerably in antibacterial spectrum, pharmacokinetics, and cost (3, 50). For most clinicians it is necessary to be knowledgeable about only a few of these many compounds but to be aware that if the cephalosporin they are accustomed to using does not have the desired antimicrobial spectrum or tissue penetration, other cephalosporin compounds should be considered. The availability of new, extended-spectrum cephalosporins often makes it possible now to use a relatively nontoxic cephalosporin drug as a single agent rather than a multiple-drug regimen that includes an aminoglycoside. The relative role of newer cephalosporins compared with imipenem, timentin, aztreonam, or the quinolones is currently a matter of great debate (2, 3, 15, 51, 59).

Cephalothin and cefazolin are the prototype compounds against which subsequent cephalosporins should be judged. They have wide activity against almost all aerobic cocci including *Staphylococcus aureus* (but not *Streptococcus faecalis*) and against many enteric Gram-negative bacilli (but not against *P. aeruginosa*). Cefazolin is less phlebogenic than cephalothin, and can be given either intramuscularly or intravenously as opposed to cephalothin, which should not be given intramuscularly.

Cefoxitin offers the advantage, compared with cephalothin or cefazolin, of outstanding activity against almost all anaerobic organisms including *Bacteroides fragilis*, and more activity for indole positive proteus and serratia. Thus it can be of particular use for purulent pulmonary infections such as empyemas and abscesses and for mixed abdominal infections. Cefamandole has excellent activity against *Haemophilus influenzae* as well as aerobic Gram-positive cocci and an extended spectrum of enteric bacilli. Cefuroxime, however, probably has more activity than cefamandole and is preferred over cefamandole by some experts. Its usefulness is primarily for mixed upper and lower respiratory infections that are likely to involve Gram-positive cocci and *H. influenzae*.

The extended-spectrum cephalosporins (the so called third generation) offer improved in vitro activity compared with second-generation cephalosporins for aerobic Gram-negative bacilli (3, 23, 49, 50, 51, 52, 58, 59). As a group these drugs are active against most aerobic Gram-positive cocci (but not *S. faecalis*, methicillin resistant *S. aureus*, or many *Staphylococcus epidermidis*), *Neisseria meningitidis*, and *Neisseria gonorrheae*, many anaerobic organisms (but not *B. fragilis*), and aerobic Gram-negative bacilli including, for a few cephalosporins, *P. aeruginosa*. Cefotaxime, ceftizoxime, and ceftriaxone are the most commonly used third-generation cephalosporins that have broad spectrum activity which does not include *P. aeruginosa*. Ceftriaxone has the advantage of a longer half-life (49). Ceftazidime has a similar (but not identical) spectrum of activity to these latter drugs but is also active against *P. aeruginosa* (58, 59). All the third-generation cephalosporins mentioned above cross inflamed meninges (17, 40). The emergence of resistance during therapy has been reported for third-generation cephalosporins (62). The major advantage of this group of cephalosporins is their low toxicity compared with aminoglycosides, activity against certain unusual multiple-drug-resistant bacilli, and the opportunity in many situations to administer a single drug rather than multiple agents. These drugs are clearly effective clinically, but their relative efficacy compared with older antibiotic combinations has not been clearly established, particularly when these agents are used as monotherapy for immunologically abnormal patients (e.g., the efficacy of ceftazidime compared with combination regimens for therapy of fever and neutropenia or sepsis and neutropenia has not been unequivocally established) (58, 59, 77).

Distribution and Elimination

Therapeutic cephalosporin levels can be found in most body sites including bile, synovial fluid, and pericardial fluid. Cephalothin, cefazolin, cefoxitin, and cefamandole penetrate the subarachnoid space poorly, but several of the third-generation cephalosporins appear to penetrate sufficiently to have therapeutic potential (17). These include cefotaxime, ceftriaxone, ceftizoxime, and ceftazidime. The elimination of cephalosporins varies with the specific agent (Table 35.1).

Adverse Effects

Hypersensitivity reactions are the most common adverse effects for the cephalosporins and cephamycins (66). No one cephalosporin or cephamycin seems to cause dramatically more hypersensitivity responses than the others. Clinical manifestations of hypersensitivity are similar to those described with the penicillins. Clinically, about 5–10% of patients with a penicillin allergy demonstrate an allergic response when challenged with a cephalosporin (57). Skin test antigen is not available to assess cephalosporin hypersensitivity. It is imprudent to administer a cephalosporin to any patient with a history of immediate hypersensitivity reactions to a penicillin drug.

Other serious adverse effects are uncommon. They include positive Coombs test, hemolytic anemia, nephrotoxicity (especially when cephalosporins are used in combination with aminoglycosides), thrombocytopenia, and granulocytopenia.

OTHER β-LACTAM DRUGS

Imipenem is a β-lactam antibiotic that is sold in a fixed combination with cilastatin (Primaxin) (15, 53). Cilastatin inhibits the renal metabolism of imipenem and is included to decrease the production of potentially nephrotoxic compounds. Imipenem has the broadest activity of any β-lactam drug including extended-spectrum cephalosporins: its spectrum includes Gram-positive cocci (except some *Streptococcus fecium*, *S. epidermis*, and some methicillin-resistant staphylococci), most aerobic Gram-negative bacilli including *P. aeruginosa*, (but excluding *Pseudomonas capacia* and *Pseudomonas maltophilia*), and many anaerobic bacteria including *B. fragilis*; it does not cover *Corynebacterium JK*. Emergence of resistance during therapy, particularly for *P. aeruginosa*, is a concern, as is superinfection and the induction of β-lactamases, which would make Gram-negative bacilli more resistant to other β-lactam drugs. The role for imipenem is similar to that for extended-spectrum cephalosporins, but imipenem should not be used as a single agent for *P. aeruginosa* infections because of the possible emergence of resistance (61, 64). Patients allergic to other β-lactam drugs are likely to be allergic to imipenem. Imipenem should be avoided in patients with seizures.

Aztreonam is a synthetic β-lactam antibiotic that is structurally different from cephalosporins and penicillins (2). It is the first monobactam approved for clinical use. Aztreonam has broad activity against aerobic Gram-negative organisms including *N. gonorrheae*, most enteric Gram-negative rods, and *P. aeruginosa*. It has no activity against Gram-positive organisms or anerobes. Aztreonam is clinically effective against a broad range of Gram-negative organisms, although its efficacy for meningitis has not been established. Adverse effects are similar to other β-lactam drugs. There appears to be little cross allergenicity with penicillins and cephalosporins. The major advantage of aztreonam is that it has potent activity against Gram-negative bacilli without the toxicity of aminoglycosides. It remains to be determined whether for therapy of Gram-negative bacillus infections there is any advantage of aztreonam over imipenem or cephalosporins for patients who are not allergic to these β-lactam drugs.

AMINOGLYCOSIDES

The aminoglycosides are a group of natural and semisynthetic compounds that have broad activity against Gram-negative bacilli. The clinically useful drugs are gentamicin, tobramycin, amikacin, and netilmicin (5, 60). The group also includes streptomycin, neomycin, and kanamycin, which are infrequently used in the 1980s. Because aminoglycosides have broad activity against Gram-negative bacilli and because they are proven to be clinically efficacious, they are a major component of the antimicrobial armamentarium for the critically ill. They are widely used as part of multiple-drug empiric therapy and as specific therapy for infections caused by organisms not susceptible to less toxic drugs.

Gentamicin, tobramycin, netilmicin, and amikacin have excellent activity against aerobic Gram-negative bacilli including most *Pseudomonas* species. These drugs have no activity against anaerobic organisms and limited activity against aerobic Gram-positive cocci. *S. faecalis* are susceptible to aminoglycosides in the presence of penicillins. Aminoglycosides have excellent activity against most *P. aeruginosa*: they act synergistically against these organisms and against some enterobacteriaceae when used in combination with carbenicillin or ticarcillin or piperacillin (22, 39). Aminoglycosides are active in vitro against most *S. aureus* and *S. epidermidis*, but clinical efficacy against staphylococci has never been proved, and staphylococci rapidly become resistant when treated with aminoglycosides alone. The aminoglycosides act at the 30S bacterial ribosomal unit, where they inhibit protein synthesis and interfere with the translation of mRNA. These mechanisms do not, however, explain the bactericidal effects of these drugs. Bacterial resistance to aminoglycosides is usually caused by elaboration of enzymes that inactivate the drugs, though failure to penetrate into the bacteria

and low affinity of the drug for ribosomes are also factors (21, 46). These enzymes are located in the bacterial membrane. They adenylate, acetylate, and phosphorylate the aminoglycosides at numerous sites. Aminoglycosides that are poor substrates for these enzymes are active against more organisms. Thus amikacin, a compound that is a substrate for only one of the common enzymes, an acetylase, is active against more Gram-negative bacilli than the other aminoglycosides. However, it is not clear whether clinicians should use this semisynthetic compound in preference to the other aminoglycosides since resistance to amikacin could spread if this drug were used more commonly. Many consultants prefer to withhold amikacin for the treatment of microorganisms that are suspected or documented to be resistant to other aminoglycosides.

Distribution and Elimination

Aminoglycoside concentrations are high in the renal cortex. Levels are low in other tissues, and aminoglycosides do not reliably penetrate into the subarachnoid space. Concentrations in bile are about 30% of serum levels unless the biliary system is obstructed, in which case levels are even lower. Aminoglycosides are eliminated by glomerular filtration. Some tubular reabsorption of these agents probably occurs.

Adverse Effects

Aminoglycosides are toxic to renal, auditory, and cochlear function (4, 5, 48). Toxicity is concentration dependent and the predilection for site of toxicity varies with each specific drug. Ototoxicity occurs due to progressive destruction of vestibular or cochlear sensory cells when the aminoglycoside is concentrated in the perilymph of the inner ear. Ototoxicity can occur abruptly or gradually. Gentamicin and streptomycin primarily affect auditory function, and tobramycin affects both equally. All the aminoglycosides are nephrotoxic (4). The frequency of clinical nephrotoxicity is influenced by the frequency and severity of concurrent nephrotoxic insults and by preexisting renal pathology. Nephrotoxicity characteristically occurs after 5–7 days of therapy: proteinuria and tubular casts initially occur, followed by a reduction in glomerular filtration. The process is usually reversible. Tobramycin is slightly less nephrotoxic than gentamicin; the difference is probably not clinically important. In patients who are seriously ill it is important to measure serum levels of aminoglycosides in order to avoid drug accumulation and toxicity, and conversely to avoid inappropriately low levels and ineffectiveness. Peak serum levels of 2–3 μg/ml are usually needed to produce concentrations greater than the minimum inhibitory concentration of most *Pseudomonas* and many *Enterobacteriaceae* (47). Gentamicin or tobramycin levels greater than 12 mg/ml are associated with toxicity. There is controversy concerning the optimal peak and trough levels to maximize efficacy but avoid toxicity. It seems reasonable to try to maintain peak gentamicin or tobramycin levels of 6–12 μg/ml, and trough levels of 1–2 μg/ml. Peak amikacin levels should be maintained at 25–30 μg/ml. Serum aminoglycoside levels (peak and trough) should be measured at least two or three times weekly in seriously ill patients regardless of renal function. Many factors affect serum level, including the underlying disease and fever. Although nomograms and formulas are available, measurement of serum levels is the only accurate method of assuring the desired range. Either the total daily dose or the interval between doses can be altered. A useful method of estimating the appropriate interval between 1-mg/kg doses of gentamicin or tobramycin while awaiting laboratory results is to estimate the interval in hours to be equal to the product of eight times the serum creatinine. Thus, if the serum creatinine is 3 mg/dl, 1 mg/kg of gentamicin should be given every 24 hours (8 × 3). Peak and trough levels should then be measured, and the dose readjusted as indicated by the levels.

MACROLIDE ANTIBIOTICS

The macrolide antibiotics are a group of compounds that contain a lactone ring to which are attached one or more deoxy sugars. Because of their excellent gastrointestinal absorption, erythromycin and clindamycin are widely used antibiotics in ambulatory medicine. In critically ill patients, their use as intravenous preparations relates primarily to their excellent activity against agents causing atypical pneumonia and anaerobic infections, respectively.

Erythromycin

Erythromycin is either bacteriostatic or bacteriocidal depending on the microorganism and the serum concentration. The drug is effective in vitro for almost all *Streptococcus pyogenes*, *Streptococcus pneumoniae*, and *Viridans streptococcus*, though a few strains of these organisms may be resistant, particularly if the patient has recently been exposed to a macrolide antibiotic. The antibiotic is also useful against all *Mycoplasma pneumoniae*, *Legionella pneumophila*, and *N. gonorrheae*. Erythromycin is active against only some *S. aureus* and *H. influenzae*, and thus is not recommended as first-line therapy for infections involving these organisms. Erythromycin has little activity against most Gram-negative bacilli with the exception of *Campylobacter* species. In critically ill patients the major role for erythromycin is to treat suspected *legionella* or *mycoplasma* pneumonias.

Erythromycin binds to the 50S subunit of bacterial ribosomes and thus interferes with protein synthesis.

Distribution and Elimination. Erythromycin diffuses into intracellular fluids and adequate concentration is attained in almost all tissues except the brain and CSF. It penetrates the prostate well, though its antimicrobial spectrum renders it of little utility in prostatic infections.

Erythromycin is concentrated in the liver and excreted in the bile. About 15% of the intravenous form is excreted in the urine.

Adverse Effects. Serious adverse effects due to erythromycin are rare. The drug is irritating in its intravenous form and frequently causes phlebitis. Fever, eosinophilia, and rashes occasionally occur. Cholestatic hepatitis rarely occurs with the intravenous preparations. This complication is more often observed with the oral estalate.

Clindamycin

Clindamycin is a macrolide antibiotic that, like erythromycin, has excellent activity against *S. pyogenes*, *S. pneumoniae*, and *V. streptococcus*. It is active against many but not all *S. aureus*. Because clindamycin is only bacteriostatic against *S. aureus*, and because resistance develops during experimental infection, clindamycin is not first-line antistaphylococcal therapy. Clindamycin differs from erythromycin in that it has excellent activity against almost all anaerobic bacteria except for a few peptococci, a few *Clostridium perfringens*, a few *B. fragilis*, and many nonperfringens clostridia. The major role for clindamycin in the treatment of critically ill patients is to provide therapy for anaerobic infections (6).

Clindamycin inhibits protein synthesis by binding to the 50S subunit of bacterial ribosome.

Distribution and Elimination. Clindamycin penetrates most body sites well, particularly bone. It does not reliably enter the CSF. Only about 10% of clindamycin is excreted unchanged in the urine. The rest of the drug is metabolized in the liver and excreted in the bile and urine.

Adverse Effects. The most prominently described adverse effect of clindamycin is pseudomembranous colitis, which is a serious inflammatory process caused by the toxin of *Clostridium difficile*, a normal bowel organism (7, 8). This syndrome presents as persistent copious watery stool or sudden bloody stool associated with fever and abdominal pain. The frequency of its occurrence differs sharply in various series from 0.2% to 20% of patients. It must be recognized, however, that pseudomembranous colitis has been reported with almost every currently used antibiotic, not just clindamycin, and concern about this potential complication should not be an important factor in deciding whether or not to include clindamycin in an antibiotic regimen.

Skin rashes, transaminasemia, and bone marrow suppression have occasionally been associated with clindamycin administration. Diarrhea without pseudomembrane formations is quite common. This form of diarrhea is probably due to alteration of bowel flora. It usually resolves when antimicrobial therapy is stopped.

CHLORAMPHENICOL

Chloramphenicol is a natural compound with a unique structure unrelated to other antimicrobials. Like the macrolide antibiotics, chloramphenicol binds to the 50S ribosomal subunit, preventing formation of peptide bonds. Chloramphenicol also inhibits mitrochondrial protein synthesis in mammalian cells, especially those in the erythropoietic system. This drug can be useful in critically ill patients because of its antibacterial spectrum and distribution; its marrow toxicity, however, is a major drawback that results in this drug being used with decreasing frequency, now that clindamycin, metronidazole, and extended spectrum β-lactam drugs are available as less toxic alternatives.

Chloramphenicol is bacteriostatic for a wide variety of Gram-positive and Gram-negative organisms including almost all nonenterococ-

cal streptococci, *Neisseria meningitidis*, *N. gonorrhoae*, *Salmonella* species, most anaerobes, *H. influenzae* and many enteric Gram-negative bacilli. *P. aeruginosa* is not inhibited. High concentrations inhibit many *S. aureus*. Resistance of Gram-negative bacilli is spread by a R factor.

Distribution and Elimination

Chloramphenicol penetrates all body tissue including the brain and CSF. Only about 5–10% of biologically active chloramphenicol is excreted in the urine. The rest of the drug is metabolized in the liver. The half-life of the drug correlates with the plasma bilirubin concentration. The dosage must therefore be reduced for patients with hepatic insufficiency but not for patients with renal insufficiency.

Adverse Effects

There are two separate and distinct types of bone marrow toxicity that are the major toxicities. The idiopathic type of marrow aplasia is usually irreversible especially if the onset occurs more than 2 months after the last dose. Aplastic anemia is the most common manifestation. This form occurs only once per 25,000 treated patients, and almost exclusively in young women receiving oral therapy who had previous exposure to the drug.

A dose-related hematologic toxicity also occurs, producing increased serum iron levels, cytoplasmic vacuolization of granulocyte and erythroid precursors, and anemia, often with leukopenia and thrombocytopenia. This syndrome regularly occurs when the serum level is greater than $25\mu g/ml$. It should be watched for by monitoring the serum iron level and the percent saturation of the total iron binding capacity and the platelet count. This type of marrow toxicity is reversible when the drug is stopped. Blurred vision, digital paresthesias, and allergic phenomena are observed rarely.

VANCOMYCIN

Vancomycin is a natural compound that is structurally unlike the other antimicrobial compounds (19, 24). It is bactericidal against essentially all staphylococci (both *S. aureus* and *S. epidermidis*), all *S. pneumoniae*, *S. pyogenes*, and *V. streptococci*. It is bacteriostatic against all *S. faecalis* and most *Corynebacterium* species. A few anaerobes are susceptible, but virtually no Gram-negative organisms are susceptible to vancomycin. Vancomycin has a prominent role in therapy of critically ill patients (19, 24). To an increasing extent critically ill patients have temporary or permanent foreign bodies implanted as pacemakers, vascular access, valves, or shunts. These devices are especially predisposed to infection by staphylococci including S. aureus, and S. epidermidis, an increasing fraction of which are methecillin resistant. In addition, the importance of S. epidermidis and diphtheroid species in patients with prosthetic valves or malignant tumors and the emergence of drug-resistant S. pneumoniae has made vancomycin a particularly useful bactericidal antibiotic. Vancomycin is also useful for patients with Gram-positive infection and a history of serious penicillin allergy (24).

Distribution and Elimination

Vancomycin penetrates most body tissues well, including the brain and inflamed meninges. It is excreted almost unchanged by the kidneys.

Adverse Effects

Nephrotoxicity and ototoxicity are uncommon with the modern drug preparation if peak serum levels are maintained below 50 μg/ml. Phlebitis is common with intravenous vancomycin. Flushing, tingling, and erythema ("red neck syndrome") are usually associated with rapid infusion, especially if 1-g doses are used. Leukopenia occasionally occurs.

SULFONAMIDES, TRIMETHOPRIM, AND PYRIMETHAMINE

Sulfonamides are a large group of compounds that were the first chemotherapeutic agents employed systematically for the prevention and treatment of bacterial infection in humans. They have a wide antibacterial spectrum that includes Gram-positive cocci, Gram-negative rods, chlamydia, nocardia, neisseria, and protozoa (toxoplasma, pneumocystis, malaria). More effective drugs have taken the place of sulfonamides for the treatment of most bacterial processes. They have an important role for treating uncomplicated urinary tract infections. They are also first-line therapy for nocardia, pneumocystis, and toxoplasma infections, particularly when combined with trimethoprim and pyrimethamine (33, 71).

The sulfonamides are structural analogs and competitive antagonists of para-aminobenzoic acid, and thus interfere with the production of folic acid. Sulfonamides exert a synergistic effect when they are combined with agents such as trimethoprim or pyrimethamine that act at sequential steps in folic acid synthesis. For this reason a fixed combination preparation of two of these sequential blockers, trimethoprim-sulfamethoxazole (in a ratio of 1:5), has proven to be an effective and widely used therapeutic product (71). It is the drug of choice for pneumocystosis. Sulfadiazine or sulfasoxazole are still preferred for nocardiosis. Pyrimethamine is the preferred choice in combination with sulfadiazine for toxoplasmosis.

Distribution and Elimination

Sulfonamides are widely distributed throughout the body including the CSF. They are metabolized in the liver to varying degrees depending on the compound involved. The parent drug and the metabolites are excreted in the urine.

Adverse Effects

For most patient groups, about 5% of recipients have adverse reactions to sulfonamides. Hypersensitivity reactions, especially skin, mucous membrane, and vasculitic lesions can be life threatening. Acute hemolytic anemia, often associated with glucose-6-phosphate dehydrogenase deficiency, and agranulocytosis, thrombocytopenia, aplastic anemia, crystalluria, and hepatic necrosis are also seen. For AIDS patients, up to 70% can have fever, leukopenia, hepatitis, nephritis, or rash when treated with trimethoprim-sulfamethoxazole: these reactions appear to be related to the sulfamethoxazole rather than the trimethoprim, and often necessitate cessation of therapy.

METRONIDAZOLE

Metronidazole is a synthetic nitroimidazole that has an increasingly important role in the treatment of serious anaerobic infections as well as in the treatment of certain protozoal infections (27). Metronidazole is active against almost all anaerobes; some cocci and a few non-spore-forming Gram-positive bacilli are resistant. Ameba, giardia, and trichomonas are generally susceptible. Because metronidazole is the only bactericidal drug available for most anaerobic organisms, it has a potentially important role for critically ill patients with anaerobic infections. Its role compared to clindamycin or chloramphenicol is currently being defined. With regard to mechanism of action, the nitro group of metronidazole is reduced by electron transport proteins with low redox potentials. The cell is thus deprived of reducing equivalents, and the reduced form of metronidazole is able to alter the helical structure of DNA.

Although metronidazole is well absorbed after oral administration, it should be given intravenously to seriously ill patients.

Distribution and Elimination

Good drug levels are attained in most tissues; particularly high levels are found in the CSF. Both metabolized and unmetabolized metronidazole are excreted in the urine.

Adverse Effects

Metronidazole causes considerable headache and gastrointestinal symptoms including anorexia, nausea, vomiting, diarrhea, epigastric pain, and cramps. Neurotoxic effects such as dizziness, vertigo, and ataxia and peripheral neuropathy may occur. Reversible neutropenia may be noted during therapy.

PENTAMIDINE

Pentamidine is a diamidine compound that is effective for the therapy of pneumocystis pneumonia (33, 56). Formerly available only from the Centers for Disease Control, this drug is now available commercially. For protozoa the mechanism of action of pentamidine is unclear; it may inhibit replication of protozoan kinetoplast DNA.

Pentamidine isethionate should be reconstituted in sterile water and administered by slow intravenous infusion (30–60 minutes). Clinically important hypotension is not frequently associated with slow intravenous infusion despite older reports to the contrary (42). Intramuscular administration often causes painful sterile abscesses and is no longer recommended. Aerosolized pentamidine appears to be well tolerated and effective as either therapy or prophylaxis for pneumocystis pneumonia in preliminary studies, but further studies concerning dose, delivery devices, schedules, efficacy, and safety are needed.

Distribution and Elimination

Concentrations of drug are detectable for at least 24 hours after a 4 mg/kg dose. The half-

life after intravenous administration is about 6.5 hours (18). The routes of metabolism and elimination are not well worked out.

Adverse Effects

Parenteral pentamidine is associated with renal failure in a high percent of patients, as well as dysglycemia (hypoglycemia followed by hyperglycemia, both of which can be clinically severe) and pancreatitis. AIDS patients appear to be particularly predisposed to leukopenia, which is usually quickly reversed when drug is discontinued.

ANTIMYCOBACTERIAL THERAPY

Although many antituberculous drugs are available, the most important drugs for therapy of critically ill patients are isoniazid, rifampin, streptomycin, and ethambutol (69). The first three of these drugs are available for intramuscular administration.

Isoniazid (INH) is the hydrazide of isonicotinic acid. It is bactericidal against dividing typical mycobacteria *(Mycobacterium tuberculosis)* and some atypical mycobacteria. It appears to work by inhibiting synthesis of the cell wall. About one in 10^6 *M. tuberculosis* are genetically impermeable to INH.

Isoniazid is readily absorbed orally. The drug penetrates all body tissues including the CSF. The drug is acetylated and hydrolyzed, and then excreted in the urine. The rate of acetylation is racially dependent. The serum INH concentration of rapid acetylators is 50–80% less than that of slow acetylators.

About 5% of patients develop INH-induced untoward reactions including rash, jaundice, peripheral neuritis, fever, seizures, bone marrow depression, hypersensitivity reactions and arthritis. The peripheral neuritis is quite common if pyridoxine is not given concurrently (30). The most common concern with isoniazid therapy is hepatic injury. Mild transaminasemia (SGOT and SGPT two to three times normal) is a common occurrence that does not predict more serious injury. Bridging necrosis can be caused by isoniazid. The drug should immediately be stopped in patients with symptoms of hepatitis (anorexia, nausea, malaise, and jaundice) and transaminases that are more than three times normal. Older patients are more likely to have substantial hepatic damage than are younger patients.

Rifampin is a zwitterion that inhibits many

Gram-positive and Gram-negative organisms by inhibiting DNA-dependent RNA polymerase, leading to suppression of the initiation of RNA chain synthesis. *In vitro* and *in vivo* resistance develops rapidly.

The drug is well absorbed orally; the parenteral form is available only as an investigational drug. Rifampin is metabolized in the liver via an active deacetylation and ultimately excreted via bile in the gastrointestinal tract. Rifampin is widely distributed in body tissue, including the CSF.

Less than 4% of patients suffer fever, rash, jaundice, various gastrointestinal complaints, and hypersensitivity reactions.

Ethambutol is an oral compound with excellent tuberculostatic activity. The drug is widely distributed. About 50% is excreted unchanged in the urine. Optic retinitis occurs only rarely in patients who are receiving 15 mg/kg or less of the drug. Other adverse effects are rare.

Streptomycin is tuberculocidal. Vestibular toxicity, auditory toxicity, and nephrotoxicity are not uncommon.

A variety of other antimycobacterial drugs are available for the therapy of *M. tuberculosis* or atypical mycobacteria such as *M. avium intracellulare*. Clofzimine and ansamycin are investigational agents that have been used in AIDS patients to treat *M. avium intracellulare*, but their efficacy or the efficacy of any other agents for the treatment of this organism has not been shown yet.

Antifungal Agents

AMPHOTERICIN B

Amphotericin B is a polyene antibiotic that is fungistatic or fungicidal for a wide variety of fungi but has no activity against bacteria or viruses (11, 14, 44). Amphotericin B is active against most *Candida* species, *Cryptococcus neoformans*, and *Torulopsis glabrata* as well as some *Aspergillus* and *Rhizopus* species, and most *Histoplasma capsulatum*, *Coccidioides immitis*, *Blastomyces dermatiditis*, and *Sporotichum schenkii*. Amphotericin B binds to the sterol component of fungal membranes, creating channels that increase the permeability of the membrane. Amphotericin B does not bind to the membranes of resistant organisms. Fungi do not become resistant to amphotericin B *in vivo*.

Amphotericin B must be administered by slow intravenous infusion after the amphotericin B has been dissolved in 5% dextrose in water. The drug precipitates in solutions containing acids, preservatives, or electrolytes. Because of the serious adverse effects, a 1-mg test dose is usually given in 20 ml of 5% dextrose solution over 1 hour. The next dose can be given immediately if there are no adverse effects. Although some experts suggest a gradual increase in dosage by 5-mg steps, it is prudent in critically ill patients to proceed directly to 0.6 mg/kg/day, administered in 500 ml of 5% dextrose solution over 2–6 hours. Few patients tolerate higher daily doses. Alternate-day therapy may be useful for some critically ill patients, especially after their fungal disease is clearly controlled. Hypersensitivity effects can be diminished by premedication with meperidine (50 mg intravenously administered) and diphenhydramine HCL (50 mg intravenously administered), and heparin (1000 units) added to the infusion. Premedication with hydrocortisone (10–100 mg intravenously administered) may be necessary to reduce the adverse effects, but this immunosuppressive agent should not be automatically given unless the other premedications are not effective. Amphotericin B can be administered intrathecally though there are few cases where this is warranted. Coccidioidomycosis meningitis may be one such indication.

Amphotericin B is a highly tissue bound drug that penetrates most body compartments, though concentrations in CSF and vitreous humor are low. Its metabolic pathways are incompletely understood. Very little of the drug is excreted in the urine, though the drug can be detected in the urine for 6–8 weeks after the last dose is given. Altered renal function or hemodialysis do not necessitate changes in drug dosage.

Adverse Effects

Amphotericin B is associated with a substantial number of adverse reactions such as flushing, chills, fever, anorexia, and headache. When severe, these untoward effects can be associated with tachypnea, hypoxemia, and hypotension. Slowing the infusion and premedicating the patient can diminish or eliminate these untoward effects.

Renal function is impaired by long courses of amphotericin B in over half of patients (13). Renal dysfunction can be reduced in severity and frequency by maintaining good hydration for the patient. Often the patient's serum creatinine, initially normal, will plateau in the 2–3 mg/dl range. In most cases, the renal dysfunction is largely but not completely reversible. If the serum creatinine rises about 3.0 mg/dl, the amphotericin B should be discontinued or the dose should be reduced if the danger of uremia outweighs the acute danger of the fungal process. Renal tubular function is often impaired by amphotericin B, resulting in hypokalemia, hypomagnesemia, and renal tubular acidosis that may be permanent. Anemia is also reported as a consequence of amphotericin B therapy, but leukopenia and thrombocytopenia are rare.

FLUCYTOSINE

Flucytosine, or 5-fluorocytosine, is a fluorinated pyrimidine that has activity against *C. neoformans*, some *Candida* species, and occasional isolates of other fungal species. Because 30% of cryptococci develop resistance during therapy, and resistance has also been observed to develop during therapy of *Candida* infection, flucytosine has no role as a single agent except perhaps in the treatment of chronic blastomyeosis. Its primary use is in combination with amphotericin B for cryptococcal infections and some candida infections (10).

Flucytosine is converted to fluorouracil by fungal cells, but not by host cells. The fluorouracil ultimately inhibits hymidylate synthetase.

Flucytosine is well absorbed orally and is widely distributed in body tissues, penetrating CSF and aqueous humor quite well. About 80% of the drug is excreted unchanged in the urine.

Adverse Effects

Bone marrow depression is a common occurrence in patients receiving flucytosine, especially those whose marrows have been previously compromised by malignancy, radiation, or myelosuppressive drugs. Bone marrow suppression can be minimized by maintaining peak serum levels below 100–125 μg/ml. Hepatomegaly, transaminasemia, nausea, rash, emesis, diarrhea, and enterocolitis are also seen occasionally.

KETOCONAZOLE

Ketoconazole is an oral agent that is effective against mucosal candidiasis as well as less common fungal diseases such as histoplas-

mosis, coccidiomycosis, and blastomycosis. For patients with life-threatening fungal disease, ketoconazole has no role as a single agent. Nausea is the major adverse effect; numerous endocrinologic effects have also been described although their clinical importance when conventional doses are used is unclear. Ketoconazole is not absorbed unless there is gastric acidity.

MICONAZOLE

The indications to use miconazole in an intensive care setting are extremely rare although this imidazole does have activity against yeasts and filamentous fungi (70).

Antiviral Agents

RIBAVIRIN

Aerosolized ribavirin is effective therapy for severe respiratory syncytial virus (RSV) infections in children. Precipitation of the aerosolized drug on the valves and tubing of mechanical ventilators can lead to potentially hazardous malfunctions, especially if prefilters are not used. Other adverse effects associated with its use include anemia. There is no clear role for ribavirin in adults.

ACYCLOVIR

Acyclovir is a purine nucleoside analogue that has excellent activity against herpes simplex and herpes zoster but not against cytomegalovirus or Epstein-Barr virus (32, 37). The drug acts by inhibiting viral DNA synthesis. Some herpesviruses are resistant by virtue of thymidine kinase deficiency as well as by other mechanisms. Resistance developing during therapy has been described (20). Intravenous acyclovir is the drug of choice for life-threatening herpes simplex or herpes zoster infections such as disseminated disease or Herpes simplex encephalitis. Because herpes zoster is less sensitive to acyclovir than is herpes simplex, serious herpes zoster disease requires higher doses of acyclovir than serious herpes simplex. Acyclovir is excreted largely unchanged by the kidney, so dose adjustments must be made in the presence of renal dysfunction.

Adverse Effects

Intravenous acyclovir is well tolerated: phlebitis, rash, hypotension, nausea, headache, and encephalopathic changes can occur, as can reversible renal dysfunction.

9-1,3 DIHYDROXY-2-PROPOXYMETHYL-GUANINE

9-1,3 Dihydroxy-2-propoxymethyl-guanine (DHPG) inhibits the replication of all herpes viruses in vitro including cytomegalovirus, herpes zoster, and herpes simplex (16, 43, 68). DHPG is highly bone marrow suppressive in the doses employed clinically, so it is less desirable than acyclovir for therapy of Herpes simplex and herpes zoster infections. Its major clinical role is for therapy of cytomegalovirus disease. In AIDS patients it has been used to successfully treat cases of cytomegalovirus retinitis, pneumonia, esophagitis, and colitis. As of 1987 the specific indications for its use and the optimal treatment regimens are being delineated.

AZIDOTHYMIDINE

Azidothymidine (AZT, zidovudine) is a synthetic thymidine analog that has activity against human immunodeficiency virus (HIV). It is the first drug that has been shown to clearly prolong the life of patients with acquired immunodeficiency syndrome (AIDS). It is currently available commercially only in oral form. There is no evidence that therapy during life-threatening illness improves short-term survival. Major adverse effects including neutropenia, anemia, and headache. Little data are available about its interactions with other marrow suppressive drugs.

VIDARABINE

Vidarabine (adenosine arabinoside) is a derivative of adenosine. It is effective for herpes simplex encephalitis and keratoconjunctivitis, but there is almost no occasion to use it since intravenous acyclovir has become available (32, 75, 76). Acyclovir is at least as effective and considerably less toxic. The vidarabine must be administered intravenously in large volumes of fluid (15 mg/kg dissolved in 2.5 liters) given over 12–24 hours. This fluid bolus presents a management problem for patients with increased intracranial pressure, or with renal failure.

Adverse Effects

Thrombophlebitis occasionally occurs at the site of administration. Nausea, emesis, diarrhea, and malaise can also occur. Ataxia, tremor, seizures, and psychiatric disturbances can occur, particularly when serum levels are high.

CLINICAL USE OF ANTIMICROBIAL AGENTS IN CRITICALLY ILL PATIENTS

General Considerations

The successful use of antimicrobial therapy in the critically ill depends on an understanding of the pharmacology of the agents employed. For optimal therapy of an infectious process the drug must have good activity against the suspected or documented pathogen, it must be administered in such a way that active forms of the drug reach the site of infection at concentrations greater than the minimum inhibitory concentration (MIC) of the organism, and adverse effects must be avoided (9, 25). The activity of the drug against the presumed pathogens must be based on both in vitro susceptibility testing and clinical trials. Certain antibiotics have excellent in vitro activity but poor clinical efficacy. For example, polymixins may be quite active against Gram-negative bacilli, yet clinical response is unimpressive. Salmonella species may be susceptible to cephalothin, and S. aureus may be susceptible to chloramphenicol, yet patients do not have dramatic clinical response to these drugs compared with ampicillin and methicillin, respectively. Similarly, drugs may fail because organisms quickly develop resistance such as rifampin and S. aureus or carbenicillin and P. aeruginosa.

The mechanism of antimicrobial action is frequently considered in the choice of an antimicrobial agent. Common sense deems it preferable to use an agent that is bactericidal rather than bacteriostatic, especially if the patient's immune function is abnormal. In bacterial endocarditis, bactericidal agents are much more efficacious than bacteriostatic compounds (36, 45, 65, 74). For the treatment of other infections the importance of microbicidal as opposed to microbistatic drugs is unconvincing (38). Thus, the optimal antibiotic is probably best chosen on the basis of activity against the pathogen, distribution, and toxicity rather than mechanism of action.

Additive or synergistic drug combinations are popular approaches to the treatment of infectious processes (1, 36, 45, 63, 65). For bacterial endocarditis the addition of an aminoglycoside to a penicillin enhances serum bactericidal activity and the likelihood of clinical cure. These observations have been applied to other clinical situations where *in vitro* testing shows synergy for the offending microbe. In fact, there are little data, except for endocarditis, that document the clinical usefulness of these drug combinations, and in many situations, toxicity of the second drug can outweigh its usefulness (36, 45, 63). In some situations, however, the addition of a second drug may provide sufficient synergy that the dose of the first drug can be reduced, thus decreasing the toxicity. This is the case when flucytosine is added to amphotericin B for the treatment of cryptococcal meningitis (10).

Antagonism between bactericidal and bacteriostatic drugs is another in vitro phenomenon that is frequently applied to clinical situations (1, 63). With the exception of a trial of penicillin plus tetracycline for the treatment of pneumococcal meningitis, however, there is little documentation that antibiotic antagonism should be an important consideration in the choice of antibiotics. To ascertain that adequate antibiotic concentration reaches the site of infection is an essential consideration. An antibiotic must be present at a concentration equal to or greater than the MIC of the organism. Measuring antibiotic levels or measuring bacteriostatic activity in joint fluid, CSF, or bone may help determine the adequacy of drug dose (38). For anesthetic agents or for pressors, augmented clinical responses can be obtained by augmenting drug concentrations. With antibiotics, however, increased drug concentrations over the MIC for the pathogen do not correlate with enhanced clinical response in any predictable manner. The clinician often takes solace in attaining serum or body fluid drug levels that are much higher than the MIC of the causative organism. Attaining very high serum levels at peak and trough periods may in fact be useful: They ensure the clinician that sufficient antibiotic will be available if renal or hepatic drug excretion suddenly increases or if the infection occurs at a site where drug diffusion is poor. Only in bacterial endocarditis, however, does a specific measurement of serum killing activity correlate with clinical efficacy.

Measuring serum levels of antibiotics is important for ensuring adequate dosing and for preventing toxicity. In critically ill patients, renal and hepatic function may be difficult to assess and may fluctuate rapidly. Formulas and nomograms may help to estimate proper drug dose. Drug levels should be measured on a regular basis, particularly if the drug is potentially toxic, such as an aminoglycoside or vancomycin. Measuring drug levels several times weekly may be expensive on an absolute basis, yet such measurements represent a small fraction of total patient cost and prevent distressing and expensive complications.

Empirical Therapy

When patients are critically ill their survival is often dependent on the prompt initiation of appropriate antimicrobial therapy. If the identity of the etiologic microorganism(s) is uncertain, empirical therapy that covers the full range of likely pathogens pending the outcome of diagnostic procedures must be initiated. For many critically ill patients, however, the optimal diagnostic procedure cannot be performed because the patient is too hypoxic for a bronchoscopy, too thrombocytopenic for a biopsy, or too hemodynamically unstable to be transported to radiology or the operating suite. This scenario is especially common when dealing with immunosuppressed patients.

Traditionally, empirical antimicrobial regimens were likely to include multiple drugs, since no one agent has broad coverage that included aerobic and anaerobic organisms, Gram-positive and Gram-negative bacteria, rods, and cocci. The past few years have been characterized by the appearance of third-generation cephalosporins, thienamycin, quinolones, and β-lactam/β-lactamase inhibitor combinations that can provide broad coverage. Single agents have the advantage of being less time consuming to administer. Moreover, several of these drugs are considerably less toxic than the aminoglycosides that were previously included in most multiple-drug empirical regimens, particularly those used for neutropenic patients. In the middle 1980s a major unresolved issue was whether single agents such as ceftazidine, or imipenem, or timentin would be as effective as multiple-drug regimens, thus allowing clinicians the ease of monotherapy and the diminution in direct toxicity (15, 51, 53, 58, 59). Whether these benefits will outweigh the high absolute cost of many of these newer drugs remains to be determined.

Epidemiological and Other Factors

The epidemiology of highly pathogenic or multiple antibiotic resistant organisms is an important consideration in the choice of antimicrobial agents in critically ill patients. Many patients who are critically ill have been exposed to hospital flora during previous hospitalization. Many critically ill patients are hospitalized in an ICU where they can acquire resistant organisms and become superinfected. Substantial antibiotic pressure on these patients can also select out endogenous flora that are multiply antibiotic resistant (26). These organisms can cause serious disease in the infected patient and they can be transmitted to other patients. A physician caring for a critically ill patient is obligated to use the most efficacious antimicrobial therapy available. The physician must also, however, introduce antibiotics appropriately so that resistance to newer antibiotics is delayed, thus saving these drugs for unusual situations where they are uniquely useful. For instance, amikacin has decided advantages over gentamicin and tobramycin because it is often more active against more Gram-negative bacilli. Gram-negative bacilli that are resistant to gentamicin and tobramycin will sometimes be susceptible to amikacin, yet the more frequently this latter drug is used, the more amikacin resistant organisms will likely appear. Thus, amikacin should probably be used only if the organism is known to be resistant to other therapeutic agents, or if there is some reason to strongly suspect such resistance. Similarly, some third-generation cephalosporins appear to be useful, nontoxic agents for the treatment of organisms that previously required toxic agents such as the aminoglycosides. If they are used indiscriminately to treat organisms susceptible to more conventional agents, however, resistance may rapidly develop, thus decreasing their usefulness and the usefulness of other β-lactam drugs.

The cost of newer antibiotics should also influence the drug selected. Newer drugs are often much more expensive than older, generically available agents, and their routine use can dramatically increase a hospital's pharmacy expenditure.

Finally, the choice of antimicrobial agent must be influenced by a physician's familiarity with the drug. The rapid explosion of penicillin, cephalosporin and quinolone agents makes it impossible for physicians to be familiar with the doses, pharmacokinetics, and adverse effects of all agents. Errors in selection and administration are more frequent if the physician attempts to use too large an armamentarium of drugs, especially when dealing with critically ill patients with changing hepatic and renal function and when considering the interaction of the drug with other medications. It seems preferable for the physician to be very familiar with the pharmacology of a limited antibiotic armamentarium and to select other agents or newer agents only when clearly indicated.

References

1. Acar JF, Sabath JP, Ruch PA: Antagonism of the antibacterial action of some penicillins by other penicillins and cephalosporins. *J Clin Invest* 55:446–453, 1975.
2. Acar JF, Neu HC (eds): Gram-negative aerobic bacterial infections: a focus on directed therapy, with special reference to aztreonam. *Rev Infect Dis* 7(Suppl 4):5537–5840, 1985.
3. Allan JD, Eliopoulos GN, Moellering RC: The expanding spectrum of beta-lactam antibiotics. *Adv Intern Med* 00:119–146, 1986.
4. Appel GB, Neu HC: The nephrotoxicity of antimicrobial agents. *N Engl J Med* 296:663, 676, 1977.
5. Appel GB, Neu HC: Gentamicin in 1978. *Ann Intern Med* 89:528, 538, 1978.
6. Bartlett JG, Gorbach SL: Penicillin or clindamycin for primary lung abscess? An Editorial. *Ann Intern Med* 98:546, 1983.
7. Bartlett JG, Chang TW, Gurwith M, et al: Antibiotic associated psuedomembranous colitis due to toxic producing clostridia. *N Engl J Med* 298:531, 534, 1978.
8. Bartlett JG, Onderdonk AB, Cisneros RL: Clindamycin. Associated colitis due to a toxin producing species of clostridia in hamsters. *J Infect Dis* 136:701–707, 1977.
9. Bauer AW, Kirby WMM, Sherris JC, et al: Antibiotic susceptibility testing by a standardized single disc method. *Am J Clin Pathol* 45:493–496, 1966.
10. Bennett JE, Dismukes NE, Duma RJ, et al: A comparison of amphotericin B alone and combined with flucytosine in the treatment of cryptococcal meningitis. *N Engl J Med* 301:126–131, 1979.
11. Bennett JE: Antifungal agents. In Mandell GL et al: *Principles and Practices of Infectious Diseases.* New York, John Wiley & Sons, 1985, pp 263–269.
12. Brown CH, Natelson EA, Bradshaw E, et al: The hemostatic defect produced by carbenicillin. *N Engl J Med* 291:265–270, 1974.
13. Burgess JL, Birchall R: Nephrotoxicity of amphotericin B with emphasis on changes in tubular function. *Am J Med* 53:77–84, 1972.
14. Carrizosa J, Kaye D: Antibiotic concentrations in serum, serum bactericidal activity and results of therapy of streptococcal endocarditis in rabbits. *Antimicrob Agents Chemother* 12:479–483, 1977.
15. Clissold SP, Todd PA, Campoli-Richards DM: Imipenem/Cilastin—A review of its antibacterial activity, pharmacokinetic properties, and therapeutic efficacy. *Drugs* 33:183–241, 1987.
16. Collaborative DHPG Treatment Study Group. Treatment of serious cytomegalovirus infections with 9-(1,3-dihydroxy-2-propoxymethyl) guanine in patients with AIDS and other immunodeficiencies. *N Engl J Med* 314:801–805, 1986.
17. Congeni BL: Comparison of ceftriaxone and traditional therapy of bacterial meningitis. *Antimicrob Agents Chemother* 25:40–44, 1984.
18. Conte JE, Upton RA, Phelps RT, et al: Use of a specific and sensitive assay to determine pentamidine pharma-

cokinetics in patients with AIDS. *J Infect Dis* 154:923–929, 1986.

19. Cook RV, Farrar WE Jr: Vancomycin revisited. *Ann Intern Med* 88:318–321, 1978.

20. Crupacker CS, Schnipper LE, Marlowe SI, et al: Resistance to antiviral drugs of Herpes simplex virus isolated from patients treated with acyclovir. *N Engl J Med* 306:343, 1982.

21. Davies J, Courvalin P: Mechanisms of resistance to aminoglycosides. *Am J Med* 62:868–877, 1977.

22. Elipoulos GM, Moellering RC: Azlocillin, mezlocillin, piperacillin: new broad spectrum penicillins. *Ann Intern Med* 97:755–760, 1982.

23. Farrar WE Jr, O'Dell NM: Comparative beta-lactamase resistance and antistaphylococcal activities of parenterally and orally administered cephalosporins. *J Infect Dis* 137:490–493, 1978.

24. Geraci JE, Hermans PE: Vancomycin. *Mayo Clin Proc* 58:88–91, 1983.

25. Fekety FR Jr, Norman PS, Cluff LE: Treatment of Gram-negative bacillary infections with colistin. *Ann Intern Med* 57:214–227, 1962.

26. Finland M: Emergence of antibiotic resistance in hospitals, 1935–1975. *Rev Infect Dis* 1:4, 1979.

27. Galgiani JN, Busch DF, Brass C, et al: *Bacteriodes fragilis* endocarditis bacteremia and other infections treated with oral or intravenous metronidazoles. *Am J Med* 65:284–289, 1978.

28. Ghysen JM: Penicillin-sensitive enzymes of peptidoglycon metabolism. In Schlessinger D: *Microbiology-1977*. Washington, DC, American Society for Microbiology, 1977, p 195.

29. Gilman AG, Goodman LS, Gilson: *The Pharmacologic Basis of Therapeutics*, ed 8. New York, Macmillian, 1980.

30. Gronhagen-Riska C, Hellstrom PE, Froseth B: Predisposing factors in hepatitis induced by isoniazide-rifampin treatment of tuberculosis. *Am Rev Respir Dis* 105:292–295, 1978.

31. Handbook on antimicrobial therapy: *Med Lett Drugs Ther* 1986.

32. Hirsch MS, Schwartz ML: Antiviral agents. *N Engl J Med* 302:903–907, 949–953, 1980.

33. Hughes WT, Feldman S, Chaudhary SC, et al: Comparison of pentamidine isethionate and trimethoprim-sulfamethoxazole in the treatment of *Pneumocystis carinii* pneumonia. *J Pediatr* 92:285–291, 1978.

34. Kancir LM, Tuazon CU, Cardella TA, et al: Adverse reactions to methicillin and Naficillin during treatment of serious *Staphylococcus aureus* infections. *Arch Intern Med* 138:909–911, 1978.

35. Kaufman C, Frame PT: Bone marrow toxicity associated with 5-fluorocytosine therapy. *Antimicrob Agents Chemother* 11:244–247, 1977.

36. Kaye D: *Infective Endocarditis*. Baltimore, University Park Press, 1976.

37. King DHJ, Galasso G (ed): Proceedings of a symposium on acyclovir. *Am J Med* July 20, 1982.

38. Klastersky J, Daneau D, Weerts D: Antibacterial activity in serum and urine as a therapy guide to bacterial infection. *J Infect Dis* 129:187–193, 1974.

39. Kluge RM, et al: Carbenicillin-gentamicin combination against *Pseudomonas aeruginosa*. *Ann Intern Med* 81:584, 1974.

40. Landesman SH, Corrado ML, Shah PM, et al: Past and current roles for cephalosporin antibiotics in treatment of meningitis. Emphasis on use in gram-negative bacillary meningitis. *Am J Med* 71:693, 1981.

41. Levine BB: Skin rashes with penicillin therapy: current management. *N Engl J Med* 286:42–43, 1972.

42. Mallory DL, Parrillo JE, Lane HC, et al: The hemodynamic effects and safety of intravenous pentamidine. *Critical Care Med* 15:503–505, 1987.

43. Masur H, Lane HC, Palestine A, et al: Effect of 9-(1,3-dihydroxy-2-propoxymethyl) guanine on serious cytomegalovirus disease in eight immunosuppressed homosexual men. *Ann Intern Med* 104:41–44, 1986.

44. Medoff G, Kobayashi GS: Strategies in the treatment of systemic fungal infections. *N Engl J Med* 302:145–148, 1980.

45. Moellering RC Jr, Wennersten C, Weinberg AN: Synergy of penicillin and gentamicin against enterococci. *J Infect Dis* 124:5207, 1971.

46. Moellering RC Jr, Wennersten C, Kung LJ, et al: Resistance to gentamicin, tobramycin, and amikacin among clinical isolates of bacteria. *Am J Med* 62:873–877, 1977.

47. Moore RD, Smith CR, Lietman PS: The association of aminoglycoside plasma levels with mortality in patients with gram-negative bacteremia. *J Infect Dis* 149:443, 1984.

48. Moore RD, Smith CR, Lipsky JJ, et al: Risk factors for renal dysfunction in patients treated with aminoglycosides. *Ann Intern Med* 100:352, 1984.

49. Nahata MC, Barson WJ: Ceftriaxone: A third generation cephalosporin. *Drug Intell Clin Pharm* 19:900–906, 1985.

50. Neu HC: The new β-lactamase stable cephalosporins. *Ann Intern Med* 97:408–413, 1982.

51. Neu HC: Antibiotics in the second half of the 1980's—Areas of future development and the effect of new agents on aminoglycoside use. *Am J Med* 80(Suppl 6B):195–203, 1986.

52. Neu HC, Turck M, Phillips I: Ceftizoxime: A broad spectrum beta-lactamase stable cephalosporin. *J Antimicrob Agents Chemother* 10(Suppl C):1, 1982.

53. Neu HC: Beta-lactamase inhibitors. In Mandel GL, Douglas RG, Bennett JE (eds): *Principles and Practice of Infectious Diseases*, ed 2, New York, John Wiley & Sons, 1985, pp 190–192.

54. Onorato IM, Axelrod JL: Hepatitis from intravenous high dose oxacillin therapy. Findings in an adult inpatient population. *Ann Intern Med* 89:497–500, 1978.

55. Parter RH, Eggleston M: Beta-lactamase inhibitors: Another approach to overcoming antimicrobial resistance. *Inf Control* 8:36–40, 1987.

56. Pearson RD, Hewlett EL: Pentamidine for the treatment of pneumocystis pneumonia and other protozoal disease. *Ann Intern Med* 103:783–786, 1985.

57. Petz LD: Immunologic cross reactivity between penicillins and cephalosporins: a review. *J Infect Dis* 137:574–579, 1978.

58. Pizzo PA, Hathorn JW, Hiemenz J, et al: A randomized trial comparing ceftazidime alone with combination antibiotic therapy in cancer patients with fever and neutropenia. *N Engl J Med* 315:552–558, 1986.

59. Pizzo PA, Thaler M, Hathorn JW, et al: New Beta-lactam antibiotics in granulocytopenic patients: new options and new questions. *Am J Med* 79(Suppl 2A):75–82, 1985.

60. Pratt WB, Fekety R: *The Antimicrobial Drugs*. New York, Oxford University Press, 1986.

61. Quinn JP, Dudek EG, Divincenzo CA, et al: Emergence of resistance to imipenem during therapy for *Pseudomonas aeruginosa* infections. *J Infect Dis* 154:289, 1986.

62. Quinn JP, Divincenzo CA, Foster J: Emergence of resistance to ceftazidime during therapy for Enterobacter-cloacal infections. *J Infect Dis* 155:942–947, 1987.

63. Rahall JJ Jr: Antibiotic combinations: clinical relevance of synergy and antagonisms. *Medicine* 570:179–183, 1978.

64. Rouveix E, Bure AM, Regnier B, et al: Experience with imipenem/cilastatin in the intensive care unit. *J Antimicrob Agents Chemother* 18(Suppl):153–180, 1986.

65. Sande MA, Courtney KB: Nafcillin-gentamicin synergism in experimental staphylococcal endocarditis. *J Lab Clin Med* 88:118, 1976.

66. Saxon A: Immediate hypersensitivity reactions to Beta-lactam antibiotics. *Rev Infect Dis* 5(Suppl 2):5368, 1983.

67. Shattil JS, Bennett JS, McDonough M, et al: Carbenicillin and penicillin inhibit platelet functions in vitro by impairing the interactions of agonists with the platelet surface. *J Clin Invest* 65:329–337, 1980.

68. Shepp DH, Dandliker PS, Myers JD: Treatment of *Varicella zoster* virus infection in severely immunocompromised patients: a randomized comparison of acyclovir and vidarabine. *N Engl J Med* 314:208–212, 1986.

69. Snider DE, Cohn CL, Davidson PT, et al: Standard therapy for tuberculosis. *Chest 1985* 87(supp):1175–1245, 1985.

70. Stevens DA: Miconazole in the treatment of systemic fungal infection. *Am Reve Respir Dis* 116:801–806, 1977.

71. Symposium. Trimethoprim-sulfamethoxazole. *J Infect Dis* 128(Suppl):425–816, 1973.

72. Tomasz A: The mechanism of the irreversible effects of penicillins. How the β-lactam antibiotics kill and lyse bacteria. *Ann Rev Microbiol* 33:113, 1979.

73. Weinstein L, Dalton AC: Host determinants of response to antimicrobial agents. *N Engl J Med* 279:467, 1968.

74. Weinstein L: Experimental staphylococcal endocarditis. *J Lab Clin Med* 88:118, 1976.

75. Whitley RJ, Alford CA, Hirsch MS, et al: Vidarabine versus acyclovir therapy in Herpes simplex encephalitis. *N Engl J Med* 314:144–149, 1986.

76. Whiteley RJ, Ch'ien LT, Dolin R, et al: Adenosine arabinoside therapy of Herpes zoster in the immunosuppressed. *N Engl J Med* 297:289–294, 1977.

77. Williams ME, Harman C, Scheld M, et al: A controlled study: Ticarcillin plus clavulanic acid versus piperacillin as empiric therapy for fever in the immunosuppressed host. *Am J Med* 79(Suppl 5B):67, 1985.

36

Topical Therapy

H.D. Peterson, D.D.S., M.D.

Topical therapy is probably best defined as a manipulation on the surface of a patient to correct, or prevent, a problem arising on that surface. These manipulations may be pharmacological, such as the application of an antimicrobial agent to a burn, or physical, as in the management of a patient on a pressure equalizing bed. The manipulation may be therapeutic as in the cleansing and debridment of an established decubital ulcer, or prophylactic, as in topical care of a central line in an effort to avoid catheter sepsis. The problems addressed with topical therapy can be divided into life threatening, such as a large burn or severe toxic epidermal necrolysis, and non-life-threatening, such as in a skin slough from an intravenous infiltration. In the former, mortality is the prime consideration, in the latter morbidity is the primary concern. The final division as to type of topical therapy is patients that are critically ill as the result of the cutaneous problem. The large burn is an example of this. The other group are those patients whose cutaneous problem is the result of another disease process making them critically ill. The immunosuppressed chemotherapy patient with generalized Herpes is an expression of this group.

Before addressing individual topical therapy problems, I shall review several general principles. The first premise is that the natural course of a wound is to heal and that many of the things that we do may delay this healing. As an example, the application of hydrogen peroxide to a clean granulating would is common, yet it slows the healing in a normal wound and can prevent healing in a compromised wound such as a radiation ulcer. A brilliant man in 1783 said "We must be careful what unctions we put on a small burn, or wound, because it is going to heal anyway, and if we do something several times and

healing results, we will begin to ascribe healing qualities to that maneuver, whatever it might be" (11). This statement not only holds true for burns but for all wounds in general.

The second premise is that surface cultures of an open wound are usually without value. There are exceptions, such as recovering acid fast organisms from a draining neck node. The surface of decubital ulcers, open wounds, healing burns, and draining sinuses are rich in bacteria. Literally tons of systemic antibiotics have been given in a misguided reaction to surface cultures. Thus, the presence of bacteria on the surface of a wound does not constitute proof of systemic infection, nor, for that matter, local infection. Pseudomonas, an omnipresent organism in our daily lives can grow on the surface of a wound or in a neglected dressing, without harming the patient. Conversely, it can cause fatal cutaneous infection, such as Psuedomonas burn wound sepsis. It is incumbent upon the physician to understand the difference.

The third premise is that granulation tissue in a healthy or relatively healthy patient cannot be infected, but granulation tissue in an immunocompromised patient, such as a large burn, can be rapidly invaded. Finally, the last premise is that cleanliness is second to godliness except in wounds where it is ahead of godliness. A clean wound is a healing wound, and many wound problems result from neglect of local care. The local care may vary from washing with soap and water to surgical debridement under general anesthesia, but cleanliness must always accompany topical therapeutic efforts. There is no magic potion that we can spread on or give by mouth or vein that will substitute for good wound care. The search for this potion has enriched a great many manufacturers and proved deleterious to a great many patients.

BURNS

In order to understand the proper use of topical therapy for burns, the reader must possess a working knowledge of burn care. This is beyond the scope of this chapter and one should seek the appropriate text to understand the modern principles of burn wound care (1, 2, 13). Briefly, the general principles of burn would care are to avoid dessication, mechanical trauma, and infection. The two topical modalities that are used to prevent infection are topical antimicrobial agents and covering membranes, either biologic or synthetic.

Since humans first discovered fire they have looked for something to put on their burns. This has run the gamut of soot from the inside of the cave, through picric acid, to modern antimicrobial agents. Topical therapies were ineffective in preventing bacterial growth in the eschar, or more importantly, at the interface of eschar and the unburned tissue, until the advent in the early 1960s, of 0.5% silver nitrate ($AgNO_3$) soaks and mafenide hydrocloride. The latter is now marketed as mafenide acetate under the tradename Sulfamylon. Prior to the 1960s, the course of a patient with a large burn was to survive the period of resuscitation, only to succumb to sepsis, originating in the burn wound at 4–5 weeks postinjury. Only large burns became septic, the smaller ones had their dead tissue invaded by bacteria, and as a result bacterial lysis separated the burn eschar from the living tissue, without developing systemic sepsis. The clean wound then either healed or was grafted.

Carl Moyer introduced 0.5% $AgNO_3$ soaks and John A Moncrief introduced Sulfamylon at approximately the same time in the early 1960s (3, 12). Both of these topical agents significantly increase the LD_{50} size of burns in all age groups. Silver sulfadiazine appeared in the early 1970s and is also an efficacious agent. All the other topical agents that have come and gone in the past 15 years have never been demonstrated to be of any therapeutic efficacy. Therefore, we will just consider the efficacious agents.

SILVER NITRATE

Silver nitrate ($AgNO_3$), used in the form of a 0.5% solution applied to the wound, is an efficacious treatment to prevent infection in the burn wound. It is placed on the affected area in several layers of gauze and must be kept wet at all times with distilled water. It has several advantages: (a) it is easy to apply, (b) the bulky dressings maintain the patient's body heat and make heat loss from the patient less of a problem, (c) there are essentially no organisms resistant to silver nitrate, and (d) it is relatively inexpensive.

There are several major disadvantages. The first is that the silver nitrate solution is very hypotonic, and when placed in contact with the burn wound over a large surface area of the body it promotes electrolyte loss from the patient. The most critical of these is sodium, and a marked hyponatremia will occur very rapidly if this problem is not appreciated. This is especially true in children; silver nitrate soaks must be used with great care in all patients, but especially in children. The second disadvantage is that it does not penetrate the eschar. It will not affect bacterial growth below the surface. Therefore it is a topical agent that must be applied to the burn wound early on, before significant seeding of the wound occurs. It is not useful in heavily contaminated burn wounds. A third and major disadvantage is that $AgNO_3$ is damaging to the surroundings of the patients. It stains everything that comes in contact including the hospital linens, furniture, floors, and attendant's clothing and skin. Lastly, it is the most misused of the topical applications to burn wounds. As stated earlier, it is very hypotonic and will deplete electrolytes from the patient. It also cannot be allowed to dry out. If 0.5% $AgNO_3$ is allowed to dry in dressings, it quickly becomes 1,2, or 3% $AgNO_3$ which is very caustic. The dessication of silver nitrate dressings will convert open wounds to neoeschar and kill freshly grafted skin. Because of these disadvantages 0.5% $AgNO_3$ probably should not be used for wound care in ICU patients with multiple problems, but should be relegated to burn care under the supervision of individuals familiar with its use (17).

Mafenide

Mafenide, either hydrochloride or acetate, in an 11% cream, is the first efficacious topical burn cream. As a cream it is much easier to use than 0.5% $AgNO_3$ soaks, and it has several advantages in use on the burn wound. It has a very broad spectrum of antimicrobial activity, although some Gram-negative organisms have developed resistance. It also has no antifungal activity. Unlike $AgNO_3$, mafenide penetrates the eschar, where there is often a heavy growth of organisms. Despite those advantages, mafenide has several severe disadvantages, making it an agent that should be used only for specific indications. It is extremely painful during application and for approximately one-half hour after application. It is also a potent carbonic anhydrase inhibitor and can produce metabolic acidosis since it is rapidly absorbed through the eschar. Complete absorption from the vehicle occurs in 2–3 hours, and clinically important blood levels are achieved rapidly. When applied to a 30% total body surface burn mafenide concentrations of 3 mg/dl of the active drug are achieved and the paracarboxy benzenesulfonamide metabolite will exceed 6 mg/dl. These levels are in patients with normal renal function. With renal failure, paracarboxy benzenesulfonamide levels of 200 mg/100 ml are observed (9).

The active drug is rapidly broken down upon entering the systemic circulation (2, 21). The acid salt that is formed is excreted in the urine and this represents a large osmotic load, causing an osmotic diureses. More importantly the carbonic anhydrase inhibition of the active drug and its paracarboxy benzene metabolite prevents bicarbonate reabsorption in the renal tubule. As a result, an alkaline urine is excreted and the serum bicarbonate decreases. The loss of bicarbonate combines with the increased acid load resulting from mafenide metabolism to produce a metabolic acidosis. The metabolic acidosis is initially compensated by increased respiratory rate. In addition, mafenide may increase ventilatory rate by a central mechanism.

Application of mafenide to a burn patient without pulmonary problems increases the minute ventilation 2- to 3-fold. As long as there is adequate respiratory function, the metabolic acidosis may remain compensated. However, this delicate balance may be upset by either an increased acid load such as from poor perfusion or sepsis, or from failure of CO_2 elimination because of pulmonary problems such as pneumonitis or interstitial edema. When a patient demonstrates increasing ventilatory rate and minute volume while being treated with mafenide, the agent must be discontinued at once.

Mafenide must not be used under occlusive dressings, since it is rapidly absorbed from the vehicle and leaves the wound unprotected. For example, using a 12-hour dressing change regimen of mafenide provides 2–3 hours of protection and 9–10 hours of ideal growth con-

ditions for the eschar bacteria. Thus, Sulfamylon must be used in an open fashion of burn treatment, which results in additional problems such as loss of body heat and the rubbing off of the agent, which removes antimicrobial protection.

Mafenide has a broad antibacterial spectrum, but because of its deleterious actions on large burns and the pain of application, it should be reserved for use in infected burn wounds, or where bacterial control has been lost with another agent. Mafenide, like $AgNO_3$, is best used by experienced personnel (2, 16).

SILVER SULFADIAZINE

In the late 1960s, Charles Fox amalgamated sulfadiazine and silver into an insoluble complex of silver sulfadiazine (4). This drug has been suspended in a vehicle to make a burn treatment cream (Silvadene) that has a narrower antibacterial spectrum than mafenide, but is a relatively benign agent that provides bacterial control of the burn wound. Most importantly, it is very difficult to produce serious toxicity with this agent. It has several advantages: (a) it offers fairly wide antibacterial activity, probably controlling Gram-positive somewhat better than Gram-negative organisms; (b) it has some antifungal and anti-*Candida* properties; (c) it is soothing upon application to the wound; and (d) it may be used with both open and closed techniques of burn care.

There are also a number of disadvantages of silver sulfadiazine. The antimicrobial spectrum is narrower than either mafenide or 0.5% $AgNO_3$. There is less eschar penetration than mafenide, but more than $AgNO_3$ soaks. There are also allergic reactions, which are usually urticarial in nature and respond to antihistamines. These reactions are far less frequent than to mafenide, but more common than allergy to silver nitrate soaks. Prolonged use of silver sulfadiazine can result in hyponatremia. The mechanism of hyponatremia is not well understood, but it is a common clinical observation. One only needs to be aware of this and be sure that there is adequate sodium replacement throughout the burn course if the wounds are being treated with silver sulfadiazine. Perhaps the most worrisome, and yet not clinically significant disadvantage is that silver sulfadiazine may cause a circulating leukopenia in the early postburn course. This problem is manifested within 24 to 36 hours and lasts usually throughout the course of the use of this medication. The total white blood cell count may go as low as 500 to 700 mm³, but concomitant bone marrow examination is either normocellular or hypocellular (6). There is no adequate explanation for the leukopenia. Early after the introduction of silver sulfadiazine, marked leukopenia was considered an indication for discontinuing the medication and changing topical agents. In the last several years, however, it has been common practice to treat the patients through their leukopenia since it resolves within a few days. The author reviewed three groups of 100 patients, each matched for burn size and age. The groups were treated with silver nitrate, mafenide, or silver sulfadiazine. Circulating white blood cell count was significantly lower at each day of the first 14 days of burn therapy in patients treated with silver sulfadiazine. There was no correlation between white blood cell count and morbidity and mortality; indeed, the silver sulfadiazine group had a higher burn area LD$_{50}$ than the other two groups.

The European and Oriental burn community uses chlorhexidine with silver sulfidiazine. When critically examined, however, chlorhexidine fails to demonstrate any improvement in survival and fails to alter the bacterial milieu of the burn wound. Of interest, Dr. William Monafo in the mid-1970s added cerium, a rare earth, to silver sulfidiazine and reported truly outstanding burn wound bacterial flora control; however, these results were not duplicatable at several other centers. In reality this probably represents a tribute to Dr. Monafo's excellent wound care and nursing care, rather than an endorsement of cerium (19).

The mode of action of silver sulfadiazine is not clearly delineated. It bears no relationship to the activity of sulfadiazine on the burn wound flora, since sulfadiazine alone is ineffective in clinical treatment of the burn wound and in the rat burn model. It is most likely that the insoluble molecule of sulfadiazine releases silver in an ionized form when it is in contact with the wound, having less toxicity than silver nitrate soaks (15).

Numerous topical agents have been advocated for burn wound care. These include Furicin; Gentamycin cream and ointment; Neomycin cream, ointment, and soaks; Povidine Iodine; acetic acid; and DAPS solution (a triple antibiotic applied by dabbing it on the burn wound). None of these have proven efficacy in either altering the morbidity or mortality of age-matched and size-matched burns.

WOUND COVERAGE MEMBRANES

Membranes used to cover burn wounds can be divided into two basic types: biological membranes, such as homograft and xenograft, and artificial membranes manufactured from various materials. The artificial membranes fall in two categories: those that are bilaminate and those that are unilaminate. Many of the artificial membranes have specific uses in burn care and will be covered briefly.

Modern burn care only employs two biological wound dressings: those that are homograft (14), and xenograft (22). Homograft is partial-thickness skin graft obtained either from cadavers or living donors. Xenograft is a split-thickness skin graft from another species; in the case of clinical burn care, only pig skin is used. Experimentally dog skin, chicken skin, and bovine skin have been found to adhere to fresh burn wounds but have never been of practical use. Amnion is another biological dressing used at some burn centers (8). However, because of preparation problems, lack of sterility, and rapid drying and cracking, it should not be considered for occasional use.

The role of a biological dressing in burn care is to prevent dessication, and in so doing prevent deepening of the wound. When biological dressings are applied to superficial, moist, sensitive, partial-thickness injuries, they adhere and permit the wound to heal under the dressings. Another use of biological dressings is to place them as temporary coverage over areas that are excised to fascia, or excised to viable tissue, if autograft is not available or autograft is not a wise choice of coverage at the time. Although the U.S. Army Institute of Surgical Research recommends the use of homograft to clean up dirty wounds, other centers find it no better than course mesh gauze changed from wet to dry (20). Other than the use of biological dressings for the treatment of superficial, partial-thickness injuries, its other indications relate to the use of biological dressing with surgical excision of the burn wound, which are topics that are best addressed in a burn care text.

Artificial dressings that are bilaminate have two separate layers. An outer lamina provides a seal for the wound, allowing only the egress of water vapor and preventing the entrance of bacteria; a second layer, such as nylon mesh, permits fibroplastic ingrowth to attach the dressing to a freshly excised burn wound (11). The unilaminate artificial dressing is a single-layer dressing, which is usually a film of some type, such as polyurethane, that is coated with an adhesive that sticks to the dry skin. The problem with these unilaminate dressings is that they will not adhere to a wet burn wound. The monolayer artificial dressings are useful only for treating very small burns and for isolating intravenous sites or for covering small surgical incisions. The bilaminate artificial dressings are useful in various forms of superficial burn wound excision and coverage, for which the reader is referred to a burn care text (78).

WOUND CARE

Armed with topical agents, available membrane covers, soap and water, and a pair of pickups and a sharp scalpel, the critical care physician is ready to care for the cutaneous problems of his or her patients.

Small burns in either multiple trauma patients or critical medical patients are best treated by daily cleansing with a soap, and daily or twice-daily application of silver sulfadiazine. The wound should then be covered with a light dressing. A superficial burn treated in this fashion will heal in 10–21 days. A deeper burn will either take longer to heal, or the eschar will separate and leave granulating tissue that requires grafting. Daily debridement of small burns is to be discouraged. There is no benefit to picking off portions of necrotic tissue. It hurts the patient, it traumatizes the wound, and unless the debrider cuts down into viable tissue, it does not speed healing or readiness for graft, since the clinically important biologic invasion of the wound is at the interface of the viable and nonviable tissue. Burns of less than 10% can be managed in the above fashion and will almost never cause systemic complications even in the compromised patient.

Small necrotic skin areas, such as those caused by infiltration of caustic substances like potassium, or cytotoxic substances like adriamycin, are treated as small burns. There is a given amount of tissue necrosis that will form an eschar and the necrotic area should be kept clean, moist, and allowed to separate. Early excision and grafting probably do well in infiltrations that did not need to be excised, but fail with more serious ulcerations. Excision and grafting almost always result in the sacrifice of tissue that would have survived if not

removed. Injection of either steroids or specific antagonists have had occasional anecdotal successes, but these are impossible to evaluate.

The best policy with an intravenous infiltration is to keep the area clean, moist, lightly dressed, and protected with a topical agent, and to keep the limb elevated and at rest. It is also critically important to monitor the distal pulses. If peripheral pulses are lost it is most likely due to fascial compartment swelling and the fascia needs to be surgically opened. Intraarterial vasodilators rarely, if ever, are efficacious.

Multiple abrasions and small lacerations are treated like small burns, except that they need to be thoroughly cleaned when first seen. In multiple-trauma patients this task is done in the operating room while other procedures are being done. Failure to clean deep abrasions will result in tattooing that is almost impossible to remove at a later date. Once the wounds are cleaned, they are kept clean, moist, and protected with some form of topical antibacterial agent.

A major ICU problem is the development of decubital ulcers. The ulcers are caused by pressure between an external source and a boney pressure point. When cutaneous pressure exceeds the capillary perfusion pressure of the tissue in question and the ischemia lasts for over 2 hours, tissue death results. A commonly quoted critical pressure is 70 mm Hg (18), but this is only true for the normotensive patient. Much less pressure will cause ischemia in a hypotensive patient. This realization is critical in an ICU, where many patients spend prolonged periods with hypotension or poor peripheral perfusion. Once tissue necrosis has occured, the eschar that will form is no different from that of a burn, except there is more deep tissue necrosis relative to the surface area involved.

Prevention is the key to decubital ulcer treatment. All the admonitions for the nursing home patient are valid: provision of adequate nutrition, avoidance of maceration, and good skin care. In addition, in the acutely ill ICU patient unremitting pressure must be avoided. Decubitus ulcers can often be avoided by positioning and by routine turning and supporting with pillows, but this therapy must be compulsively done and not just ordered and neglected. A single night of neglect will result in 6 weeks of decubitus care. Unfortunately, there are critically ill patients who must be kept supine. Some form of pressure relief should be considered in all comatose or paralyzed patients, and in these patients early use of a pressure equalization bed is helpful. The air fluidized bed is an effective pressure equalizer but creates nursing care difficulty. Some form of pressure relief should be considered in all comatose or paralyzed patients; sheepskins, egg crates, and other local measures provide temporary protection, but there is no substitute for a pressure equalizing bed.

Despite all efforts, some decubital problems develop. The decubiti in a surviving patient who has intact sensation and regains consciousness are best treated conservatively. They are completely different from decubiti in chronically ill patients or in paraplegics and quadraplegics without sensation. An acute decubital ulcer in a patient with normal sensation is best treated by cleansing with soap and water, protection with a topical agent, and relief of the pressure either by positioning or a pressure equalizing bed. If the patient improves and is ambulatory, the wound can be treated by showering with soap and water, and even very large acute decubital ulcers will heal rapidly. If the patient's condition is stable and the patient is not ambulatory, large acute decubital ulcers will heal rapidly on a pressure equalizing bed. If the ulcer is cleansed daily with soap and water, has minimal debridement, and has the pressure removed, it will heal in a period of weeks.

Chronic undermined bed sores with exposed boney prominences are not usually a problem in ICUs. They are generally seen in the nursing home setting or with paraplegics and quadraplegics. The care of these sores represents a surgical problem; as a temporizing measure they only need to be cleaned with soap and water, debrided, packed loosely, and the pressure removed from the area.

SUMMARY

In a text on the therapeutic management of ICU patients, it may seem rather mundane to repeatedly emphasize keeping a wound clean, moist, and free of excess bacterial growth. It would seem that in an era when we can judge the rejection of a heart by an endocardial biopsy, determine the status of the left ventricle by placing a tiny balloon in a terminal branch of the pulmonary artery, and do countless other wonderful things, that there should be some miraculous way to take care of a wound and avoid wound sepsis and necrosis.

It is seeking this modality that has given rise to a score of covering membranes, and half a score of topical agents, all developed in an effort to skirt the need for routine meticulous wound care. We must never lose sight of the fact that the natural course of a wound, even in a compromised patient, is to heal. It is always easier to smear something on a wound, or to cover it with a membrane, than to really clean it, debride it, and make sure that it remains moist. In this era of modern medicine we need to stop looking for magical treatments for any type of wound and practice good debridement, meticulous wound care and maintenance of an environment that will encourage healing, that environment being low bacterial count and moisture. We will be rewarded with a well-healed wound that is simply tended.

References

1. Achauer Bruce M: *Management of the Burned Patient.* Appleton & Lange, 1987.
2. Boswick John A: *The Art and Science of Burn Care.* Aspen Publishers, 1987.
3. Brentano L, Moyer CA, Gravens D, et al: Bacteriology of large human burns treated with silver nitrate. *Arch Surg* 93:456, 1966.
4. Constable JD: Silver nitrate in the treatment of burns. *Symposium on the Treatment of Burns.* St. Louis, CV Mosby Co, 1973, p 113.
5. Dimsdale SM: Decubital ulcers: role of pressure and friction in causation. *Arch Phys Med Rehabil* 55:147, 1974.
6. Fox CL: Clinical experience with silver sulfadiazine: a new topical agent for control of pseudomonas infections in burns. *J Trauma* 9:377, 1969.
7. Frank DH, Wachtel T, Frank HA, et al: Comparison of biobrane, porcine, and human allograft as biological dressings for burn wounds. *J Burn Care Rehab* 4:186, 1983.
8. German JC, Wolley TE, Achauer B, et al: Porcine xenograft burn dressings: a critical reappraisal. *Arch Surg* 104:806, 1972.
9. Harrison HN, Blackmore WP, Bales HW, et al: The absorption of C-14 labeled sulfamylon acetate through burned skin. 1. Experimental methods and initial observation. *J Trauma* 12:986, 1972.
10. Kentish E: *Essay On Burns.* London, Longman, Hurst, Rees, Orme and Brown, 1817.
11. Levine N, Linberg R, Salisbury R, et al: Comparison of course mesh gauze with biologic dressings on granulating wounds. *Am J Surg* 131:727, 1979.
12. Lindberg RB, Moncrief JA, Mason AD: Control of experimental and clinical burn wound sepsis by topical application of sulfamylon compounds. *Ann NY Acad Sci* 150:950, 1968.
13. McDougal WS, Slade CL, Pruitt BA: *Manual of Burn Care.* Berlin, Springer-Verlag, 1978.
14. McManus AT, Denton CL, Mason AD: Mechanisms of in vitro sensitivity of silver sulfadiazine. *Arch Surg* 118:161, 1983.
15. Monafo WW, Tandon SN, Ayvazian VH, Tuchschmidt J, Skinner AM: Cerium nitrate: a new topical antiseptic for extensive burn surgery. 80:465, 1976.
16. Moncrief JA: Topical therapy of the burn wound: present status. *Clin Pharmacol Ther* 10:439, 1969.

17. Moyer CA, Brentano L, Gravens DL, et al: Treatment of large human burns with 0.5% silver nitrate solution. *Arch Surg* 90:812, 1965.
18. Nahas LF, Swartz BL: Use of semipermeable polyurethane for skin graft dressing. *Plastic Surg* 67:791, 1981.
19. Peterson HD: Report presented at ISBI Meeting, Stockholm Sweden, 1978.
20. Quinby WC, Hoover HC, Scheflan M, et al: Clinical trials of amniotic membranes in burn wound care. *Plast Reconstruct Surg* 70:711, 1982.
21. Schaner P, Shuck JM, Ritchey CR: A possible ventilatory effect of carbonic anhydrase inhibition following topical sulfamylon in burn patients. *Anesthesiology* 29:207, 1968.
22. Shuck J: The use of homograft in burn therapy. *Surg Clin North Am* 50:1325, 1970.

Special Considerations in Critical Care Pharmacology

37

Endogenous Opioids and Other Peptides: Evidence for Their Clinical Relevance in Shock and CNS Injury[a]

John W. Holaday, Ph.D.
Diana S. Malcolm, Ph.D.

Over the past decade, research defining the physiological, pharmacological, and behavioral importance of peptides and their receptors has opened new areas of investigation to define their role in the etiology and treatment of disease. The enormous diversity of information contained in the various amino acid sequences of these small proteins is reflected in their equally diverse biological actions. Peptides have clasically been defined on a basis of their initially described functions and localizations. However, peptides, like most drugs, do not subserve a single, specific biological role. These biological messengers are found in virtually all tissues, such as the gut, skin, kidney, immunological tissues (i.e., spleen, lymphocytes), endocrine systems, and the nervous system. They may function as endocrine substances, paracrine substances, neurotransmitters, or all three. Indeed, recent evidence indicates that certain "neuropeptides" function simultaneously as neurotransmitters in the brain, in digestive processes within the gut, and as modulators of the immune system. Thus, categories assigned on the basis of initially described peptide functions unnecessarily limit perceptions about the full scope of their biological actions.

This chapter focuses on peptides initially described as "neurotransmitters" or "gut peptides", and emphasizes those for which a role in the etiology or treatment of critical illnesses has been defined. Among the neuropeptide systems that have been investigated, the endogenous opioids and their receptors, collectively referred to as "endogenous opioid systems", have played a pivotal role. These endogenous opioid systems are described, and their role in autonomic function is emphasized. Specifically, extensive basic and clinical evidence is reviewed in order to address the

[a] The opinions or assertions contained herein are the private views of the authors and should not be construed as offical or as necessarily reflecting the views of the U.S. Army Medical Research Development and Command, Uniformed Services University of the Health Sciences, or the Department of Defense. There is no objection to its presentation and/or publication.

pathophysiological role of endogenous opioids in the etiology of circulatory shock, spinal injury and CNS ischemia. The therapeutic effects of thyrotropin releasing hormone (TRH) and glucagon in experimental models of critical illnesses are also described.

ENDOGENOUS OPIOIDS AND THEIR RECEPTORS

There are three general categories of endogenous opioid peptides—enkephalins, B-endorphin and dynorphins—each of which derives from a distinctly different larger peptide precursor. Enkephalins, including methionine (Met-) enkephalin, and leucine (Leu-) enkephalin fragments, derive from proenkephalin A; B-endorphin [along with adrenocorticotropic hormone (ACTH) and various melanocyte stimulating hormones] derives from proopiomelanocortin (POMC); and dynorphins derive from prodynorphin (65). These related peptides share an initial amino acid sequence [Tyr-Gly-Gly-Phe-Met (or Leu)], followed by distinctively different numbers and types of amino acids that impart their unique biological profiles. These different "profiles" are mediated by the different opiate receptor types upon which opioid peptides act (Table 37.1).

At least five types of opiate receptors have been defined on the basis of the unique pharmacological effects of various synthetic and natural opioid ligands. These include the μ, δ, κ, ϵ, and σ receptors. Enkephalin peptides predominantly act upon δ receptors, β-endorphin acts upon δ and μ receptors (or possibly on its own ϵ receptor) and dynorphins act primarily on κ receptors. However, these ligands are not absolutely selective for these receptor types, and evidence is accumulating to indicate that the various opiate "receptor" subtypes may instead be different binding surfaces on a common macromolecular complex (77). Nonetheless, depending upon the receptor type involved, the binding of opioid ligands to their receptors may result in ion fluxes, alterations in guanine nucleotide coupling proteins, and/or the inhibition of cyclic adenosine monophosphate (cAMP) that serves as a second messenger to carry information into the cell.

In many ways, the pharmacological effects of injected opioid alkaloid and peptide agonists mimic the actions of endogenously released opioid substances (25). For example, the injection of opioid peptides into the CNS can result in an elevation of nociceptive latencies (analgesia), catalepsy, electroencephalographic changes and associated anticonvulsant responses, changes in body temperature, hypoventilation, and an alteration of heart rate and arterial pressure. Although pharmacological studies using opioid agonists confirm the existence of functional receptor and effector mechanisms, they do not necesarily mimic the integrated interactions of the many endogenous opioids released as part of the orchestrated responses of the intact organism. Differences in doses required (relative to physiological concentrations), routes of injection, sites of injection, the use of anesthetics, and other variables can result in opposing biological re-

Table 37.1
Opioid Receptor Subtypes and Ligands

Receptor Subtype	Endogenous Agonists	Prototype Agonist	Representative Agonists	Representative Antagonists
μ	β-endorphin Met-enkephalin	morphine	morphiceptin [Tyr-D-Ala-Gly-N Me -Phe-Gly-ol](DAGO)	naloxazonazine β-funaltrexamine naloxone
δ	Leu-enkephalin	Leu-enkephalin	[D-Ala^2-D-Leu^5 enkephalin](DADLE) [D-Pen^2-D-Pen^5 enkephalin]	ICI 154,129 ICI 174,864 16-Me-Cyprenorphine Naloxone
κ	dynorphin 1-17	ketocyclazocine	U 50,488 dynorphin 1-17	WIN-44,441-3 MR 2266 binaltorphamine Naloxone
ϵ	β-endorphin	β-endorphin	β-endorphin	Naloxone
σ	Unsequenced peptides	SKF 10047 (N-allylnormetazocine)	Phencyclidine?	?

sponses, thus further compromising the value of many pharmacological studies using opioid injections as predictors of their endogenous function.

Much of the information defining the various functions of endogenous opioid systems has been derived from the use of the opioid antagonist, naloxone. Naloxone has provided an important inferential tool in establishing the many physiological and behavioral effects of endogenous opioid systems. Since endogenous opioid systems are usually quiescent during homeostasis, naloxone injections have relatively little effect in resting organisms. However, the occurrence of stress, disease, or injury activates the release of endogenous opioids that, in turn, act upon their receptors to result in profound alterations of behavioral, autonomic, or immune function. In these situations, naloxone displaces endogenous opioids from their different receptor types, thereby antagonizing their many effects and allowing us to infer an etiological role of endogenous opioids. Since opioids are generally inhibitory in their actions, injections of naloxone usually result in stimulatory responses when administered after disruption of behavioral or physiological homeostasis.

Largely through the use of naloxone and related substances, investigations at a biochemical, cellular, and whole-organism level have demonstrated the importance of both the central nervous system and peripheral autonomic effector sites in mediating the many therapeutic actions of opioid antagonists in models of critical illnesses. However, the use of opioid antagonists for the treatment of shock and CNS injury has prompted concerns about the management of pain after naloxone treatment. These concerns have resulted in further studies defining the opiate receptor subtypes that may be involved in shock, trauma, and pain relief. Various antagonist molecules have recently become available that act with greater selectivity upon δ, μ, and κ opiate receptors. With the use of these molecules, it is possible to define the particular receptor subtypes responsible for the many biological effects of endogenous opioids (82). Furthermore, such knowledge serves to stimulate the development of more selective drugs in order to optimize therapeutic effects.

There are two important consideratons regarding the use of opioid antagonists. Although naloxone readily displaces morphine or synthetic opioid analgesics (e.g., fentanyl and meperidine) from μ opiate receptors and reverses their actions, endogenous peptide ligands bind much more avidly to their receptors and therefore require much higher doses of naloxone to reverse their effects. Additionally, naloxone is not equally selective for the different opiate receptor types, being a far better μ antagonist than δ or κ antagonist. Both of these reasons point to the need for far greater doses of naloxone to reverse the actions of endogenously released opioids than one would conventionally use to reverse the effects of administered morphine or its congeners.

OTHER SELECTED PEPTIDES

Thyrotropin-Releasing Hormone

Although originally discovered as the hypothalamic substance responsible for the release of thyrotropin from the pituitary gland, thyrotropin-releasing hormone (TRH) has numerous biological actions in the CNS and periphery that do not depend on this endocrine role (67). TRH, like most other neuropeptides, is also a product of ribosomal biosynthesis in the mammalian CNS, and this tripeptide derives from its own precursor, a decapeptide termed pro-TRH-SH (90).

The injection of TRH as a drug produces a spectrum of pharmacological effects that are generally opposite to those resulting from opioid injections (10, 67, 83, 85). Whereas opioid substances usually are inhibitory, TRH exerts stimulatory (analeptic) effects that counteract opioid inhibition. Although some evidence indicates that high doses of TRH may interact with certain opiate receptor types (9), the actions of TRH appear to be predominantly mediated by its own receptors distributed throughout the CNS and possibly at peripheral sites (43, 109). Unlike the opioid systems, presently there are no antagonists for TRH that would allow for an inference that TRH subserves *physiological* roles opposite to those defined for the endogenous opioid sytems.

We were concerned that the use of opioid antagonists such as naloxone to treat critical illness or injury would potentially enhance pain by blocking opioid analgesia. Importantly, TRH does not antagonize opioid analgesia, and in fact it may even potentiate the pain-relieving effects of morphine or endogenous opioids (12, 75, 83). Since TRH does not alter opioid analgesia (while opposing many of the other actions of opioids), we tested the effects of TRH in various forms of shock and CNS ischemia (see below).

Glucagon

Glucagon is a large peptide molecule that is best known for its actions in stimulating glucose release. As with the other peptide substances described in the preceding section, the prohormone for glucagon has been characterized (44). In addition to its location in the pancreas, glucagon and its receptors have recently been defined in the brain (84). Thus, glucagon joins many other peptides that are known to be localized in the CNS and peripheral tissues. This distribution indicates that glucagon may function in many other biological roles beyond its known metabolic effects. Unfortunately, as with TRH, no receptor antagonists for glucagon are available to assist in defining those functions.

Glucagon is kown to activate adenylate cyclase, and its effects are dependent upon calcium flux (17, 20). Pharmacologically, glucagon injections result in increased heart rate, improved cardiac contractility, as well as elevated blood glucose levels. Perhaps these biological responses account for some reports indicating that glucagon has therapeutic effects in clinical cardiogenic shock (106). Because of these stimulatory properties of glucagon, we tested glucagon to determine its potential as yet another physiological antagonist of opioid systems (see next section).

CIRCULATORY SHOCK

From a simplistic perspective, there are many similarities between the signs of opioid (narcotic) overdose and those of circulatory shock. Inasmuch as stress activates endogenous opioids, it seemed possible that endogenous opioid systems were in part responsible for the pathophysiologic effects of some forms of shock. Could the organism "overdose" itself with endogenous opioids activated by the stress of shock or trauma? To confirm this hypothesis, it was demonstrated that the opioid antagonist naloxone blocked or reversed the hypotensive effects of endotoxin injections in rats (74), dogs, cats, horses, pigs, and other species (118, 120, 129). These results encouraged the use of naloxone in other forms of shock, including models of anaphylaxis, hemorrhagic shock, and neurogenic shock following acute spinal cord transection or injury (8, 64, 65). From these observations, we extended our work to include an evaluation of the effects of TRH and glucagon in experimental models of endotoxic, hemorrhagic, and anaphylactic shock as well as CNS ischemia.

There are many in-depth reviews available to provide historical evidence and detailed information regarding sites and mechanisms of opioid antagonist actions in shock and trauma (8, 28, 29, 64–67, 77, 82). The following emphasizes more recent and controversial research findings and their potential clinical importance.

Endotoxic Shock

The cell wall of Gram-negative bacteria contain lipopolysaccharides that are released into the bloodstream upon destruction of these bacteria. It is believed that these bacterial endotoxins may account for many of the pathophysiological effects of Gram-negative sepsis. For this reason, endotoxin injections have been used in experimental models of septic shock to assess etiological and therapeutic strategies.

After endotoxin administration in mammals there is a precipitous fall in arterial pressure, usually followed by a spontaneous recovery prior to a second hypotensive interval. Early experiments established that the opioid antagonist naloxone either blocked or rapidly reversed this hypotension in rats (74) and other species (for review, see 64–67). These observations have been extended in several recent reports. Although Hinshaw and colleagues (62) have reported excellent success with naloxone in live *Escherichia coli* sepsis in dogs, they found no apparent effect of naloxone in baboons injected with *E. coli*. In other canine studies by Reynolds and colleagues, naloxone specifically improved left ventricular contractility without affecting calculated total peripheral vascular resistance (118). Thus, from a hemodynamic perspective, naloxone appears to improve arterial pressure and tissue perfusion by increasing cardiac contractility and not by increasing total peripheral vascular resistance.

In rat studies, these pressor effects of naloxone in endotoxic shock are dose-related, with maximum effects observed at naloxone doses ≥ 1.0 mg/kg. The specific involvement of opiate receptors was demonstrated by the use of stereoisomers of naloxone. Only the $(-)$-isomer of naloxone [and not the $(+)$-isomer] demonstrated biochemical and biological activity at opiate receptors, and only this isomer reversed endotoxic hypotension (32).

More recent studies have used antagonists with selective actions at μ and δ binding sites. The μ antagonists, β-funaltrexamine (β-FNA) and naloxazone, failed to block or reverse endotoxic hypotension, whereas the δ-antagonists ICI-154,129 and ICI-174,864 improved arterial presssure in endotoxemic rats whether administered intracerebroventricularly into the brain at low doses or intravenously at high doses (22, 70, 76, 79, 81, 103). From these studies, it was concluded that δ (not μ) receptors mediate the pathophysiological actions of endogenous opioids in endotoxic shock. Furthermore, these actions are, at least in part, mediated within the brain since intravenous doses of these antagonists that failed to improve arterial pressure, were effective when injected into the ventricles of the brain. Many subsequent studies have further established that endogenous opioids, possibly localized in the hypothalamic autonomic centers of the brain, are released during endotoxemia to act upon δ opioid receptors, thereby inhibiting sympathomedullary outflow and exacerbating the hypodynamic state. Opioid antagonists block this action, presumably resulting in improved sympathetic function and arterial pressure (see below).

As an alternative therapeutic strategy to opiate receptor antagonists, we investigated the effects of TRH in the rat endotoxic shock model (71, 80). Unlike naloxone and other opioid antagonists, TRH exerts direct pressor effects. In mild endotoxemia, TRH improves arterial pressure and survival (80). However, in severe endotoxic shock, although TRH improves arterial pressure, survival is diminished (101). This pressor effect of TRH is mediated in part by CNS actions (increased sympathomedullary outflow) as well as direct peripheral effects (75, 101, 110). Perhaps because of its early hyperactivation of compensatory mechanisms during endotoxic shock (including increased catecholamine and glucose release), fewer resources are available during the later stages of shock to maintain vital functions. In addition to these considerations, different responses to TRH may be obtained in different species. Although TRH improved hemodynamic status in primate endotoxic shock, it was less effective in dogs receiving similar treatment (54). On

the basis of these experimental observations, we recommend *against* TRH for the clinical treatment of endotoxemia or sepsis. However, in other forms of circulatory shock or CNS injury, TRH or its structrual analogs may be of greater therapeutic value than opioid receptor antagonists.

Glucagon is another peptide that may provide yet another rational therapeutic strategy for the treatment of shock and trauma. In addition to elevating serum glucose, glucagon is known to increase heart rate and contractility (18, 19). We found that glucagon also improves survival in endotoxemic rats, although it failed to demonstrate pronounced effects on the early hypodynamic stages of endotoxic shock (124). Since many compounds that reverse shock can also function as opioid antagonists, we evaluated the effects of glucagon as an antagonist of morphine-induced analgesia and bradycardia (108). Indeed, glucagon potently blocks these actions of morphine in rats, indicating its possible physiological function as an opioid antagonist. Recent studies have extended these observations to the mouse (107), where it was shown that centrally administered glucagon antagonized morphine and "stress induced" antinociception resulting from endogenous opioid release. As with TRH, glucagon does not displace opioid ligands from their receptors, indicating that the antiopioid properties of glucagon are through opposing biochemical or physiological systems (108).

Anaphylactic Shock

Over 25 years ago, Spink and Vick (122) noted that there are many characteristics of endotoxic shock that resemble anaphylaxis. Not only do these include the early hypodynamic effects, but also changes in hematological variables (51, 89). In both situations, activation of the complement system plays an important role. The generation of the anaphylatoxins C3a, C4a and C5a following complement activation by anaphylactic reactions or by endotoxin exposure may serve as one common denominator linking the pathophysiology of anaphylactic and endotoxic shock.

In addition to the anaphylatoxins, many of the other mediators of anaphylaxis are known. These include histamine, platelet activating factor (PAF), slow reactive substance (SRS, now known to be leukotrienes C4, D4, and E4), and chemotactic factors. The anaphylatoxins, particularly C5a, are potent stimuli that promote mast cell degranulation, resulting in the release of these substances. Moreover, anaphylatoxins are hypotensive (89), as are histamine, PAF, and leukotriene D4 (47, 104), and the hypotension resulting from these substances is reversed by antagonists of opioid systems (30). It is possible that anaphylatoxins produce hypotension by their release of these secondary mediators.

Although not equally effective in all species or models (106), the opioid antagonist naloxone improves survival in mouse anaphylactic shock produced by sensitization to bovine serum albumin (2) and improves hemodynamic variables in rats sensitized to *B. pertussis* (115). Similar to endotoxic shock, an intact sympathomedullary system is required for the therapeutic actions of naloxone and TRH to be manifested (3–5). Endogenous opioids may also be involved in the disruption of glucose homeostasis in anaphylaxis, since both naloxone and TRH attenuated the hyperglycemic effects of anaphylactic shock in mice (6). As a further indication of the role of endogenous opioids in anaphylactic shock, naloxone partially reverses the hypotension produced by other mediators of anaphylactic responses, including PAF (47) and histamine, although it is without effect in reversing leukotriene D4-induced hypotension (104). Collectively, the cascade of events produced during anaphylactic shock must also include the activation of endogenous opioid systems as well as the release of these other mediators.

To test the primary hypothesis that activation of anaphylatoxins (e.g., C3a or C5a) either directly or indirectly accounts for the subsequent hypotension in both anaphylaxis and endotoxemia, we used cobra venom factor (CVF) derived from *Naja naja* (unpublished data). CVF injections acutely activate both C3a and C5a, and these anaphylatoxins have an extremely short half-life. Thus, 18-24 hours following CVF treatment, the complement system is depleted (89). For this reason, pretreatment with CVF prevents the acute hypotensive response to re-challenge with CVF or endotoxin 18 hours later.

In support of the hypothesis that the initial hypotension produced by endotoxin injection is mediated by anaphylatoxins, we found that chronic pretreatment of rats with CVF prevented the initial hypotension produced by endotoxin or rechallenge with CVF (unpublished data). Furthermore, the initial hypotension produced by acute CVF is partially reversed by naloxone and completely reversed

by TRH treatment. preliminary results indicate that glucagon is also effective in treating anaphylactic shock in mice (Amir, personal communication) and humans (20). Thus, anaphylatoxins may account for the similarities between anaphylactic and endotoxic shock, including the ability of opioid receptor antagonists or stimulatory peptides (e.g., TRH or glucagon) to reverse their effects.

Hemorrhagic Shock

Naloxone and nalbuphine (a mixed opioid agonist-antagonist) are also quite effective in reversing hemorrhagic shock in mammals (21, 31, 55, 111–113, 125). Early studies with rats (31, 78) and dogs (126) demonstrated that naloxone reverses hemorrhagic shock in a dose-related manner even without re-infusion of shed blood (56) (Fig. 37.1). Although there is one negative report from a study that used the rat hemorrhagic shock model (48), observations from many other laboratories in numerous species indicate that naloxone may be of value in stabilizing hemorrhagic hypotension in patients before classic volume loading or other resuscitative measures can be implemented (64).

Important advances have been made in defining a peripheral site and mechanism of action for naloxone in dogs subjected to hemorrhagic shock (97–99). As with endotoxemia, naloxone injections after hemorrhagic shock in dogs increase cardiac performance, resulting in improved tissue perfusion (98). Similar to endotoxic shock studies, an intact sympathomedullary system was required for naloxone's therapeutic effects (next section). Although naloxone does not alter the usual pattern of increased catecholamine secretion produced by acute hemorrhage in dogs (97,99) and cats (45), others have reported that increased circulating catecholamines accompany the pressor effects of naloxone in rabbits (120) and baboons (111). As with endotoxic shock, an intact sympathomedullary system is required for naloxone's therapeutic actions (next section).

Thyrotropin releasing hormone has also been demonstrated to improve hemodynamic status in rats (71) and monkeys (54) when administered after hemorrhagic shock. In monkeys, TRH also significantly improved survival. However, dogs appear to be resistant to TRH since TRH was without effect on hemodynamics or survival when administered after

CANINE HYPOVOLEMIC SHOCK, DOSE RESPONSE
SYSTEMIC MEAN ARTERIAL PRESSURE

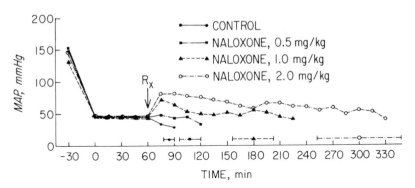

Figure 37.1.   Mean arterial pressure (MAP) in millimeters of mercury (mmHg) following naloxone injection in a canine model of hemorrhagic shock. In this model, shed blood was *not* reinfused after 1 hour of sustained hemorrhagic hypotension (45 mmHg). Naloxone treatment produced dose-dependent increases in MAP and survival time, shown along abscissa as means ±S.E.M. Saline control (●——●); naloxone (●••••●) 0.5 mg/kg; naloxone (▲ – – – – ▲) 1.0 mg/kg; naloxone (○—•—○) 2.0 mg/kg. For details, see Gurll et al. (56). (From Gurll NJ, Reynolds DG, Vargish T, et al: Naloxone without transfusion prolongs survival and enhances cardiovascular function in hypovolemic shock. *J Pharmacol Exp Ther* 220:621–624, 1982.

hemorrhagic shock in this species (54). Thus, additional evidence is required to delimit the potential therapeutic effects of TRH in hemorrhagic shock.

Spinal Injury and Stroke

In an initial test of the effects of opioid antagonists in neurogenic shock, we demonstrated that naloxone acts within the CNS to rapidly reverse the hypotension that follows acute cervical spinal transection (73). Cervical transection at C5-C6 results in a disruption of supraspinal control of sympathetic outflow by severing the pathways between the brain and sympathetic ganglia. Since naloxone injected into the brain ventricles improved arterial pressure following cervical transection, the remaining parasympathetic pathways had to have been involved (35). This conclusion was confirmed by demonstrations that vagotomy blocked the pressor actions of naloxone in spinally transected rats and cats (35).

Both complete spinal transection and spinal trauma result in a loss of autoregulatory control of spinal cord blood flow, and perfusion of the injured area becomes dependent upon peripheral arterial pressure. Since naloxone and TRH improved hemodynamics in spinally transected rats and cats, the potential therapeutic effects of these substances in animal models of spinal trauma were investigated (36–40). We and others (50) have shown that naloxone improves neurological function as well as spinal cord perfusion following injury produced by the classic Allen technique (calibrated weight drop, 400–600 gm-cm, on the exposed spinal cord). Indeed, TRH was even more effective than naloxone in improving neurological function and survival, whereas standard dexamethasone therapy was without therapeutic benefit (29, 38–40). Importantly, these drugs produced an improvement in function when administered 1–24 hours *after* the injury was produced (29). This is a clinically reasonable time frame relative to elapsed time following injury and before treatment can be initiated.

As with all new research areas, there are reports that extend information about naloxone's efficacy (50, 130), and reports that failed to demonstrate improved neurologic function following naloxone treatment after spinal injury (127, 128). These latter studies used an extradural clip compression injury in rats, a species in which we have also demonstrated a lack of effect of naloxone following percussion spinal injury in rats that have not been subjected to laminectomy (102). In one additional report using the Allen technique in cats, naloxone was without effect on somatosensory evoked potentials (SEP) (57). However, in that study, an impact force of only 120 gm-cm was used; this force was insufficient to demonstrate a significant change in SEP by itself, even without naloxone injections.

There has been considerable interest and debate about the therapeutic use of opioid antagonists in the treatment of stroke and cerebral ischemia (7, 27, 59, 64, 68, 69, 87, 92). The impetus for these investigations evolved from the observed therapeutic benefit of naloxone in treating spinal injuries (36). One model of stroke that does respond well to opioid antagonists is spinal ischemia produced by cross clamping the distal aorta in the rabbit (27, 41, 92). This model not only applies to the paralysis following certain forms of stroke, but is also directly pertinent as a model of paralysis resulting from aortic cross-clamping during the surgical repair of aneurysms.

Recent research investigating the role of endogenous opioids and their receptors in acute spinal injury or stroke has sparked further controversy. Although naloxone is efficacious in certain animal models of stroke as described above, this opioid antagonist acts upon all types of opioid receptors if adequate concentrations are administered. Research has focused upon which receptors are involved in these situations (34, 41, 94). Evidence indicates that δ receptor antagonists (with proven therapeutic effects in endotoxic shock) (22, 81, 103) appear to be relatively ineffective as therapeutic agents in spinal injury (41). However, Faden and Jacobs (34) report that WIN 44,441, an opioid antagonist with both κ and μ antagonist properties, has potent, stereospecific effects in improving neurologic function following spinal injuries in cats or spinal stroke in rabbits. Additionally, several reports indicate that the endogenous κ agonist, dynorphin, induces paralysis upon intrathecal injection into the spinal cord (33, 60, 102, 116) and that dynorphin concentrations increase in proximity to the spinal lesion (42). Of the multiple opiate receptor subtypes, only κ receptors increase in proximity to the spinal injury site (26, 29).

From this work with κ antagonists, agonists, and receptors, Faden and colleagues have posed the hypothesis that endogenous dynorphin in the spinal cord, released in response to neuronal ischemia, acts upon κ receptors to mediate the endogenous opioid-induced paralysis following spinal injury or stroke (34, 40). Our studies and those of others indicate that this may be an overly simplistic hypothesis (102). In agreement with other laboratories (33, 60, 116), we find that the paralysis induced by

intrathecal dynorphin injections is *not* reversed by naloxone or the more κ-selective antagonist, WIN 44,441 (100, 102). Moreover, partial removal of the N-terminal amino acids of dynorphin, which are responsible for κ opioid receptor binding, still results in a compound that induces paralysis. Lastly, when several other opioid and nonopioid peptides (including the δ antagonist ICI 174,864, substance P antagonists, vasopressin and somatostatin) are administered intrathecally, they produce identical paralytic effects (102). Thus, the pharmacological link between dynorphin-induced paralysis and the potential physiological events that characterize the opioid component of spinal ischemia do not agree. Opiate antagonists such as naloxone or WIN 44,441 fail to antagonize dynorphin-induced paralysis, while effectively reversing paralysis following spinal injury or ischemia. By contrast with the observed effects of opioid antagonists, κ agonists (7,123) also improve outcome following experimental cerebral ischemia. The precise mechanisms of therapeutic action of opioid antagonists in spinal injury and stroke require further investigation (102).

SITES AND MECHANISMS OF ACTION OF OPIOID RECEPTOR ANTAGONISTS

Endotoxic shock models helped to provide the initial evidence that the site of action where endogenous opioids (or therapeutic effects of opioid antagonists) contributed to shock pathophysiology is in the brain. In endotoxemic rats, naloxone improves hemodynamics following direct intracerebroventricular brain injections at a dose that when administered intravenously fails to produce a pressor response. Furthermore, Jansen and Lutherer (91) demonstrated that ventriculocisternal perfusion of naloxone in endotoxemic dogs results in an improvement in hemodynamic status. In other forms of shock and trauma, the importance of the CNS has also been demonstrated. For example, in rats rendered hypotensive by acute hemorrhage or spinal transection, low doses of naloxone administered intracerebroventricularly improve arterial pressure (32, 73, 78). Thus, in these models of circulatory shock, evidence is provided for an involvement of opioid receptors within the CNS.

Since the heart possesses opioid ligands and receptors, a direct myocardial action of naloxone can be possible as well. Lechner et al. (96) addressed this issue by infusing naloxone into the coronary artery in hemorrhaged dogs. They reported that naloxone improved mean arterial pressure (MAP), cardiac contractility, and cardiac output at a dose that when administered intravenously was without effect on hemodynamics. Furthermore, they were able to show that naloxone's effects were stereospecific. Thus, at least in this canine model of hemorrhagic shock, endogenous opioids and their antagonists appear to be acting upon stereospecific opioid receptors directly at the myocardium to improve cardiac function in the shock state. Several in vitro studies also confirm a myocardial site of action for naloxone (11, 13, 15, 21, 24, 95, 96, 119).

Additional studies of the sources and types of opioids involved in the pathophysiology of shock and trauma have yielded complex and sometimes paradoxical results. Circulating endorphins and enkephalins both increase dramatically during endotoxic and hemorrhagic shock (16, 58), however these observations alone are insufficient to implicate circulating opioids as the causative factors in the naloxone-reversible pathogenesis of circulatory shock. It is possible that the increases of circulating opioid peptides during shock could merely reflect a generalized endocrine response to stress, without immediate consequences for circulatory homeostasis. It is also possible that the surgical interventions (hypophysectomy and adrenalectomy) used to manipulate endogenous opioid release could compromise other essential compensatory responses that may or may not involve endogenous opioids. For example, the lack of adrenal function sensitizes

animals and humans (e.g., Addisons' disease) to circulatory shock. We have demonstrated that hypophysectomy or adrenal demedullation sensitized rats to the hypotensive effects of acute hemorrhage or endotoxin administration (65, 78, 101). These findings argue against a direct causative role of circulating pituitary and/or adrenal opioids in the hemodynamic responses of circulatory shock and have led to further investigations on the role of pituitary-sympathoadrenal function in the pressor response to naloxone in endotoxic shock.

As noted above, adrenalectomy and adrenal demedullation (or deafferentation) in rats and dogs not only enhances sensitivity to endotoxin-induced hypotension, but also abolishes the usual pressor response to centrally or intravenously administered naloxone during hemorrhagic or endotoxic shock (65, 99). In support of the importance of sympathoadrenal function to naloxone's actions, it was shown that the pressor response to naloxone occurred simultaneously with an increase in the firing rate of the splanchnic nerve; denervation of the adrenal medulla by cutting this nerve greatly attenuated these effects of naloxone (93).

These observations indicate that endogenous opioids within the CNS act during endotoxic shock to inhibit sympathoadrenomedullary outflow. Indeed, the adrenal medulla releases vasoactive catecholamines in response to stress, including shock. Since naloxone requires an intact adrenal medulla to exert pressor actions, one might expect that naloxone would further enhance the release of adrenomedullary catecholamines. Although some

Table 37.2
Effects of Endotexemia and Treatment with Naloxone on Plasma Catecholamines in Endotoxin-Treated Rats[a]

No. Rats	Treatment	Pre-endotoxin	Postendotoxin	15 Min Post-treatment
		Epinephrine (pg/ml)		
9	Saline[b]	91.0 ± 28.0	2665.0 ± 582.0	6187.0 ± 153.0
8	Naloxone[c]	86.0 ± 30.0	3126.0 ± 598.0	4624.0 ± 677.0
		Norepinephrine (pg/ml)		
9	Saline	316.4 ± 34.5	1336.1 ± 34.5	2771.4 ± 404.6
8	Naloxone	361.6 ± 38.6	1513.0 ± 202.5	2536.0 ± 275.0
		Dopamine (pg/ml)		
9	Saline	34.0 ± 10.0	139.0 ± 33.0	358.0 ± 60.0
8	Naloxone	46.0 ± 9.0	150.0 ± 17.0	328.0 ± 52.0

[a]When a 20 mmHg drop in mean arterial pressure was recorded following endotoxin administration (20 mg/kg, i.v.), venous blood samples were withdrawn through external jugular catheters, and rats were immediately treated with [b] saline (0.1 ml/kg, i.v.) or [c] naloxone (3 mg/kg, i.v.) in an equal volume. Further samples were withdrawn 15 minutes after drug treatment. Immediately after withdrawal of blood samples, rats were reinfused with an equal volume of blood taken from a common pool to alleviate the hypovolemia accompanying repeated blood sampling. Saline alone did not alter circulating catecholamine content across samples. For details, see Long et al. (101).

investigations have shown increases in catecholamines following naloxone administration in hemorrhagic shock (46, 112), we were unable to demonstrate this in our endotoxemic rat model (Table 37.2). Nonetheless, since catecholamine antagonists block the effects of naloxone in various forms of shock, this suggests that catecholamine receptors are somehow ultimately involved (6, 8, 14, 97, 120). Thus, it appears likely that opioids and their antagonists potentiate the actions of catecholamines at the receptor or postreceptor level.

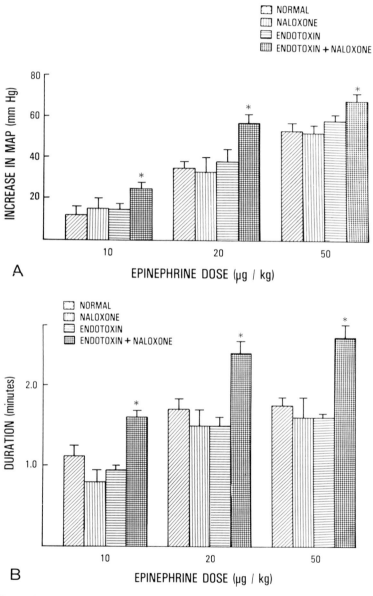

Figure 37.2. Effects of naloxone on the magnitude *(A)* and duration *(B)* of epinephrine-induced increases in mean arterial pressure (MAP) in normal and endotoxemic rats. Rats *(n = 8)* were injected with either saline (1 mg/kg, i.v.) or *E. coli* endotoxin (5 mg/kg, i.v.). Sixty minutes later, rats were infused with saline (1 ml/hr, i.v.) or naloxone HCl (3mg/hr, i.v.) following a bolus loading dose of 1 ml/kg and 33 mg/kg, respectively. Each animal received three doses of epinephrine (10, 20, and 50 µg/kg) with a 15 minute delay between injections. Naloxone potentiated the magnitude *(A)* and duration *(B)* of epinephrine's pressor effect in endotoxemic, but not normal rats. Endotoxin alone had no effect on epinephrine-induced increases in MAP.

To address this possibility, we determined whether naloxone potentiated the pharmacological actions of epinephrine in animals subjected to endotoxic shock. Dose-response curves to intravenous epinephrine (10-, 20-, and 50-μg/kg bolus doses) were constructed prior to and after naloxone injections in control and endotoxemic rats. The magnitude and duration of the pressor responses produced by epinephrine are shown in Figure 37.2.

Since endogenous opioid systems are not tonically involved in cardiovascular function during homeostasis, it was not surprising that naloxone failed to alter the hemodynamic effects of epinephrine in control animals (Fig. 37.2). Also, in hypotensive-endotoxemic animals, the absolute magnitude and the duration of the pressor actions of epinephrine injections were unaltered. This finding was surprising in view of the enormous elevation of endogenous epinephrine produced by endotoxin administration (Table 37.2). In endotoxemic rats receiving naloxone, however, the magnitude and duration of epinephrine's pressor effects were elevated by approximately 40%. From these data, we conclude that the pathophysiological actions of endogenous opioids activated by endotoxemia prevent the full expression of the cardiovascular actions of epinephrine. Naloxone, by antagonizing endogenous opioids, therefore potentiates the epinephrine response. Thus, although naloxone does not further augment the release of catecholamines in endotoxemia (Table 37.2), it may facilitate their effects through interactions with catecholamine receptors or postreceptor systems (Fig. 37.2).

Data supporting these observations were independently derived by Lechner et al. (97). In dogs subjected to hemorrhagic shock, both ganglionic blockade with chlorisondamine and adrenal denervation were required to prevent the therapeutic effects of naloxone. In these animals, naloxone's pressor actions were fully resorted if minimal pressor doses of isoproterenol and phenylephrine were previously administered. Once again, catecholamines were required for naloxone to improve hemodynamic status in animals subjected to circulatory shock.

Although these investigations reinforce the importance of opioid-catecholamine interactions in cardiovascular function, the precise role of the sympathoadrenomedullary system in shock remains to be firmly resolved. The role of parasympathetic outflow in circulatory shock is also controversial. As reviewed previously (64, 66), naloxone effectively improves arterial pressure after spinal transection (where only parasympathetic pathways remain intact), and vagotomy or atropine abolish this effect (35). Also, bilateral vagotomy abolishes the pressor effect of naloxone in the mouse anaphylactic shock model (6). In the rodent, the preganglionic vagal motor nuclei contain populations of leucine-enkephalin-containing neuronal cell bodies; opioid antagonists could be acting here to modify vagal activity. However, in other shock models, atropine and vagotomy have not significantly modified the response to naloxone (64, 99).

CLINICAL PERSPECTIVES

The studies reviewed in the preceding sections emphasize the potential importance of peptides such as opioids, TRH, glucagon and others in the pathophysiology or therapy of shock and ischemic disorders. Without doubt, of the various peptides yet investigated, evidence that endogenous opioids are involved in shock and trauma is the best established. Over the past few years, many great strides have been made in defining the sites and mechanisms of endogenous opioid involvement in experimental studies of shock and trauma. From these studies, it is clear that the vast majority of experimental results support the observation that opioid antagonists significantly improve hemodynamic, metabolic and neurologic function as well as survival in many models of circulatory shock, trauma, and CNS ischemia. Additionally, the critical importance of opioid antagonists in facilitating the expression of catecholamine effects is firmly established.

Despite these initial inroads into defining the mechanisms of opioid involvement in ischemic disorders, there are many opioid interactions with other systems (e.g, biogenic amines, cellular and noncellular components of immune responses, or eicosanoids) that must be determined (66, 114). For example, recent evidence indicates that endogenous opioids can promote neutrophil and monocyte chemotaxis, enhance or diminish immune responses, and modify eicosanoid effects (for review, see reference 66). These are all important mediators of ischemic disorders. Furthermore, it is far too simplistic to suppose that opioid antagonists by themselves can reverse all forms of ischemic insult. Like most drugs, there are many conditions that severely limit their therapeutic effects (e.g., acidosis, hypothermia, altered endocrine status) (66, 86, 125). Clearly, different stages of these progressive disorders require different therapeutic strategies, and opioid antagonists may provide one component of therapeutic cocktails devised for the future treatment of shock and trauma.

There are many anecdotal reports in the literature regarding the therapeutic effects of naloxone in the clinical setting (for review, see reference 52). These include reports of the successful treatment of cardiogenic, septic, anaphylactic and hemorrhagic shock as well as therapeutic effects of naloxone in spinal injury or stroke. Putterman and colleagues (117) demonstrated therapeutic effects of very low doses of naloxone administered early in human septic and cardiogenic shock, and similar findings were obtained in other studies (61, 88), using repeated naloxone doses. Perhaps because naloxone potentiates the actions of catecholamines in pathophysiological states (see preceding section), there is a clinical rationale for using naloxone in weaning patients from catecholamine drips (61, 97). The therapeutic effects of naloxone after CNS injury/ischemia have been demonstrated by Adams et al. (1), who provided preliminary evidence for improved neurologic function following human stroke, and Flamm and colleagues (49), who reported that naloxone improved function when administered following acute human spinal cord injury. Both of these studies used high doses of naloxone similar to those required in animal studies (> 1 mg/kg) without adverse effects.

Recently, reports have also been presented to indicate that naloxone may not have therapeutic effects in certain forms of clinical shock. Research by DeMaria et al. (23) failed to observe therapeutic responses with very low (0.005 mg/kg) doses of naloxone in human sepsis. However, they correctly concluded that insufficient doses of naloxone were used in their studies. Despite the tremendous safety of high doses of naloxone in humans, as noted by Groeger (52), large, prospective, double-blind studies evaluating the effects of naloxone on the morbidity and mortality of shock must be performed before its routine use is recommended. Based on the theoretical and experimental evidence reviewed above, such studies must be conducted with large doses of naloxone. Although other neuropeptides reviewed above have been defined as potential therapeutic agents in these pathologial conditions, they also require rigorous clinical trials before hu-

man efficacy is confirmed or refuted. Regardless of the therapeutic strategies that may evolve from studies with peptides, it is highly unlikely that there is a single mechanism of action or "magic bullet" therapy that will be universally efficacious in treating these critical illnesses. Despite these caveats, research with peptides has opened new areas of investigation that may ultimately recommend the use of peptides or their antagonists as adjunctive therapy to alleviate circulatory shock, CNS trauma, or stroke.

References

1. Adams HP Jr, Olinger CP, Barsan WG, et al: A dose-escalation study of large doses of naloxone for treatment of patients with acute cerebral ischemia. *Stroke* 17(3):404–409, 1986.
2. Amir S: Opiate antagonists improve survival in anaphylactic shock. *Eur J Pharmacol* 80: 161–162, 1982.
3. Amir S: Antianaphylactic effect of naloxone in mice is mediated by increased central sympathetic outflow to sympathetic nerve endings and adrenal medulla. *Brain Res* 274:180–183, 1983.
4. Amir S: Beneficial effects of icv naloxone in anaphylactic shock is mediated through peripheral beta-adrenoceptive mechanisms. *Brain Res* 290:191–194, 1984.
5. Amir S: Anti-anaphylactic action in the mouse of thyrotropin-releasing hormone is mediated through beta-1-adrenoceptive effectors. *Neurosci Lett* 46:127–130, 1984.
6. Amir S: Endorphins contribute to the loss of glucose homeostasis in anaphylactic shock. In *Progress in Opioid Research:* Proceedings of the International Narcotics Research Conference. NIDA Research Monograph Series Vol H 75, 1986, pp 539–542.
7. Baskin DS, Hosobuchi Y, Loh HH, et al: Dynorphin (1–13) improves survival in cats with focal cerebral ischaemia. *Nature* 312:551–552, 1984.
8. Bernton EW, Long JB, Holaday JW: Opioids and neuropeptides: mechanisms in circulatory shock. *Federation Proc* 44:290–299, 1985.
9. Bhargava HN, Das S: Evidence for opiate action at the brain receptors for thyrotropin-releasing hormone. *Brain Res* 368:262–267, 1986.
10. Bhargava HN, Yousif DJ, Matwyshyn GA: Interactions of thyrotropin releasing hormone, its metabolites and analogues with endogenous and exogenous opiates. *Gen Pharmacology* 14(6):565–570, 1983.
11. Brasch H: Influence of the optical isomers (+)- and (−)-naloxone on beating frequency, contractile force and action potentials of guinea-pig isolated cardiac preparations. *Br J Pharmacol* 88:733–740, 1986.
12. Butler PD, Bodnar RJ: Potentiation of foot shock analgesia by thyrotropin releasing hormone. *Peptides* 5:635–639, 1984.
13. Caffrey JL, Gaugl JF, Jones CE: Local endogenous opiate activity in dog myocardium: receptor blockade with naloxone. *Am J Physiol* 248 (*Heart Circ Physiol* 17):H382–H388, 1985.
14. Caffrey JL, Wooldridge B, Gaugl JF: The interaction of endogenous opiates with autonomic circulatory control in the dog. *Circ Shock* 17:233–242, 1985.
15. Caffrey JL, Wooldridge B, Gaugl JF: Naloxone enhances myocardial responses to isoproterenol in dog isolated heart-lung. *Am J Physiol* 250 (*Heart Circ Physiol* 19):H749–H754, 1986.

16. Chernow B, Lake CR, Teich S, et al: Hemorrhagic hypotension increases plasma beta-endorphin concentrations in the nonhuman primate. *Crit Care Med* 14(5):505–507, 1986.

17. Chernow B, Reed L, Geelhoed GW, et al: Glucagon: endocrine effects and calcium involvement in cardiovascular actions in dogs. *Circ Shock* 19:393–407, 1986.

18. Chernow B, Roth B: Pharmacologic manipulation of the vasculature in shock states: clinical and experimental approaches. *Circ Shock* 18:141–155, 1986.

19. Chernow B, Zaloga GP, Malcom DS, et al: Glucagon-calcium interactions: implications for treatment of verapamil and calcium overdoses. *Ann Emerg Med* (in press).

20. Chernow B, Zaloga GP, Malcolm DS, et al: Glucagon's chronotropic action is calcium dependent. *J Pharm Exp Ther* 241(3):833–837, 1987.

21. Curtis MT, Lefer AM: Protective actions of naloxone in hemorrhagic shock. *Am J Physiol* 239:H416–H421, 1980.

22. D'Amato RJ, Holaday JW: Multiple opiate receptors in endotoxic shock: evidence for δ involvement and μ - δ interactions in vivo. *Proc Natl Acad Sci* 81:2898–2901, 1984.

23. DeMaria A, Heffeman JJ, Grindlinger GA, et al: Naloxone versus placebo in treatment of septic shock. *Lancet* June 15:1363–1365, 1985.

24. Eiden LE, Ruth JA: Enkephalins modulate the responsiveness of rat atria in vitro to norepinephrine. *Peptides* 3(3):475–478, 1982.

25. Evans AGJ, Nasmyth PA, Steward HC: The fall of blood pressure caused by intravenous morphine in the rat and cat. *Br J Pharmacol* 7:542–552, 1952.

26. Faden AI: Recent pharmacological advances in experimental spinal injury: theoretical and methodological considerations. *Trends Neurosci* 6:375–377, 1983.

27. Faden AI: Opiate antagonists in the treatment of stroke. *Stroke* 8:27–31, 1983.

28. Faden AI: Opiate antagonists and thyrotropin-releasing hormone: Potential role in the treatment of shock. *JAMA* 252(9):1177–1180, 1984.

29. Faden AI: Opiate antagonists and thyrotropin-releasing hormone: Potential role in the treatment of central nervous system injury. *JAMA* 252(11):1452–1454, 1984.

30. Faden AI, Feuerstein G, Hayes E, et al: Leukotrienes and anaphylactic shock: a therapeutic role for thyrotropin-releasing hormone. *Circ Shock* 10:246, 1983.

31. Faden AI, Holaday JW: Opiate antagonists: a role in the treatment of hypovolemic shock. *Science* 205:317–318, 1979.

32. Faden AI, Holaday JW: Naloxone treatment of endotoxin shock: stereospecificity of physiologic and pharmacologic effects in the rat. *J Pharm Exp Ther* 212:441–447, 1980.

33. Faden AI, Jacobs TP: Dynorpin-related peptides cause motor dysfunction in the rat through a non-opiate action. *Br J Pharmacol* 81:271–276, 1984.

34. Faden AI, Jacobs TP: Opiate antagonist WIN 44,441-3 stereospecifically improves neurologic recovery after ischemic spinal injury. *Neurology* 35:1311–1315, 1985.

35. Faden AI, Jacobs TP, Holaday JW: Endorphin-parasympathetic interaction in spinal shock. *J Autonom Nerv Sys* 2:295–304, 1980.

36. Faden AI, Jacobs TP, Holaday JW: Opiate antagonist improves neurologic recovery after spinal injury. *Science* 211:493–494, 1981.

37. Faden AI, Jacobs TP, Holaday JW: Comparison of early and late naloxone treatment in experimental spinal injury. *Neurology* 32:677–681, 1982.

38. Faden AI, Jacobs TP, Holaday JW: Thyrotropin-releasing hormone improves neurologic recovery after spinal trauma in cats. *N Engl J Med* 305:1063–1067, 1981.

39. Faden AI, Jacobs TP, Mougey EH, et al: Endorphins in experimental spinal injury: therapeutic effect of naloxone. *Ann Neurol* 10:326–332, 1981.

40. Faden AI, Jacos TP, Smith GP, et al: Neuropeptides in spinal cord injury: comparative experimental models. *Peptides* 4:631–634, 1983.

41. Faden AI, Jacobs TP, Zivin JA: Comparison of naloxone and a delta-selective antagonist in experimental spinal "stroke." *Life Sci* 33:707–710, 1983.

42. Faden AI, Molineaux CJ, Rosenberger JG, et al: Endogenous opioid immunoreactivity in rat spinal cord following traumatic injury. *Ann Neurol* 17:386–390, 1985.

43. Faden AI, Pilotte NS, Burt DR: Experimental spinal cord injury: effects of trauma or ischemia on TRH and muscarinic receptors. *Neurology* 36:723–726, 1986.

44. Farah AE: Glucagon and the circulation. *Pharmacol Rev* 35:181–217, 1983.

45. Feuerstein G, Ailam R, Bergman F: Reversal by naloxone of hemorrhagic hypotension in anephric cats. *Eur J Pharmacol* 65:93–96, 1980.

46. Feuerstein G, Chiueh CC, Kopin IJ: Effects of naloxone on the cardiovascular and sympathetic response to hypovolemic hypotension in the rat. *Eur J Pharmacol* 75:65–69, 1981.

47. Feuerstein G, Lux WE Jr., Snyder F, et al: Hypotension produced by platelet-activating factor is reversed by thyrotropin-releasing hormone. *Circ Shock* 13:255–260, 1984.

48. Feuerstein G, Siren AL: Effect of naloxone and morphine on survival of conscious rats after hemorrhage. *Circ Shock* 19:293–300, 1986.

49. Flamm ES, Young W, Collins WF, et al: A phase 1 trial of naloxone treatment in acute spinal cord injury. *J Neurosurg* 63:390–397, 1985.

50. Flamm ES, Young W, Demopoulos HB, et al: Experimental spinal cord injury: treatment with naloxone. *Neurosurgery* 10(2):227–231, 1982.

51. Garner R, Chater BV, Brown DL: Role of complement in endotoxin-shock and disseminated intravascular coagulation—experimental observations in dogs. *Br J Haem* 28(3):393–401, 1974.

52. Groeger JS: Opioid antagonists in circulatory shock. *Crit Care Med* 14(2):170–171, 1986.

53. Gurll NJ, Ganes E, Reynolds DG: Central nervous system is involved in the cardiovascular responses to naloxone in canine endotoxic but not hemorrhagic shock. *Circ Shock* 22:115–125, 1987.

54. Gurll NJ, Holaday JW, Reynolds DG et al: Thyrotropin releasing hormone: effects in monkeys and dogs subjected to experimental circulatory shock. *Crit Care Med* 15(6):574–581, 1987.

55. Gurll NJ, Reynolds DG, Vargish T, et al: Primate hemorrhagic shock responds to naloxone. *Circ Shock* 9:189, 1982.

56. Gurll NJ, Reynolds DG, Vargish T, et al: Naloxone without transfusion prolongs survival and enhances cardiovascular function in hypovolemic shock. *J Pharmacol Exp Ther* 220(3):621–624, 1982.

57. Haghighi SS, Cherhrazi B: Effect of naloxone in experimental acute spinal cord injury. *Neurosurgery* 20(3):384–388, 1987.

58. Hamilton AJ, Carr DB, LaRovere JM, et al: Endotoxic shock elicits greater endorphin secretion than hemorrhage. *Circ Shock* 19:47–54, 1986.

59. Hariri RJ, Supra EL, Roberts JP, et al: Effect of naloxone on cerebral perfusion and cardiac performance during experimental cerebral ischemia. *J Neurosurg* 64:780–786, 1986.

60. Herman BH, Goldstein A: Antinociception and paralysis induced by intrathecal dynorphin A. *J Pharmacol Exper Ther* 232(1):27–32, 1985.

61. Higgins TL, Sivak ED, O'Neil DM, et al: Reversal of hypotension by continuous naloxone infusion in a ventilator-dependent patient. *Ann Intern Med* 98(1):47–48, 1983.

62. Hinshaw LB, Beller BK, Chang AC, et al: Evaluation of naloxone for therapy of Escherichia coli shock *Arch Surg* 119:1410–1418, 1984.

63. Hock CE, Lefer AM: Lack of effect of thyrotropin releasing hormone (TRH) in circulatory shock. *Peptides* 6(3):547–554, 1985.

64. Holaday JW: Cardiovascular effects of the endogenous opiate system. *Ann Rev Pharmacol* 23:541–594, 1983.

65. Holaday JW: Neuropeptides in shock and trauma injury: sites and mechanisms of action. *Neuroendo Persp* 3:161–199, 1984.

66. Holaday JW: Endogenous opioids and their receptors. In *Current Concepts.* Kalamazoo MI, Scope Publications, Upjohn, 1985.

67. Holaday JW, Bernton EW: Thyrotropin releasing hormone: a potent neuromodulator with therapeutic potential. *Arch Int Med* 144:1138–1140, 1984.

68. Holaday JW, D'Amato RJ: Naloxone and ischemic neurologic deficits in the gerbil: is there an effect? *Science* 218:592–593, 1982.

69. Holaday JW, D'Amato RJ: Naloxone or TRH fails to improve neurologic deficits in gerbil models of "stroke". *Life Sci* 31:385–392, 1982.

70. Holaday JW, D'Amato RJ: Multiple opioid receptors: evidence for μ - δ binding site interactions in endotoxic shock. *Life Sci* 33:703–706, 1983.

71. Holaday JW, D'Amato RJ, Faden AI: Thyrotropin releasing hormone improves cardiovascular function in experimental endotoxic and hemorrhagic shock. *Science* 213:216–218, 1981.

72. Holaday JW, D'Amato RJ, Ruvio BA, et al: Adrenalectomy blocks pressor responses to naloxone in endotoxic shock: evidence for sympathomedulary involvement. *Circ Shock* 11:201–210, 1983.

73. Holaday JW, Faden AI: Naloxone acts at central opiate receptors to reverse hypotension, hypothermia, and hypoventilation in spinal shock. *Brain Res* 189:295–299, 1980.

74. Holaday JW, Faden AI: Naloxone reversal of endotoxin hypotension suggests role of endorphins in shock. *Nature* 275:450–451, 1978.

75. Holaday JW, Faden AI: TRH: Autonomic effects upon cardiorespiratory function in endotoxic shock. *Reg Peptides* 7:111–125, 1983.

76. Holaday JW, Kenner JR, Glatt CE, et al: Dynorphin: cardiovascular consequences of opioid receptor interactions in normal and endotoxemic rats. *Proc West Pharmacol Soc* 27:429–433, 1984.

77. Holaday JW, Long JB, Tortella FC: Evidence for kappa, mu, and delta opioid binding site interactions in vivo. *Federation* Proc. 44:2860–2862, 1985.

78. Holaday JW, O'Hara M, Faden AI: Hypophysectomy alters cardiorespiratory variables: central effects of pituitary endorphins in shock. *Am J Physiol* 241 *(Heart Circ Physiol)* 10:H479–H495, 1981.

79. Holaday JW, Pasternak GW, D'Amato RJ, et al: Naloxazone lacks therapeutic effects in endotoxic shock yet blocks the effects of naloxone. *Eur J Pharmacol* 89:293–296, 1983.

80. Holaday JW, Ruvio BA, Faden AI: Thyrotropin releasing hormone improves blood pressure and survival in endotoxic shock. *Eur J Pharmacol* 74:101–105, 1981.

81. Holaday JW, Ruvio BA, Robles LE, et al: ICI M154,129, A putative delta antagonist, reverses endotoxic shock without altering morphine analgesia. *Life Sci* 31:2209–2212, 1982.

82. Holaday JW, Tortella FC: Multiple opioid receptors: Possible physiological functions of μ and δ binding sites in vivo. In Mueller EE, Genazzani AR: *Central and peripheral Endorphins.* New York, Raven, 1984, pp 237–250.

83. Holaday JW, Tseng LF, Loh HH, et al: Thyrotropin releasing hormone antagonizes β-endorphin hypothermia and catalepsy. *Life Sci* 22:1537–1544, 1978.

84. Hoosein NM, Gurd RS: Identification of glucagon receptors in rat brain. *Proc Natl Acad Sci USA* 81:4368–4372, 1984.

85. Horita A, Carino MA, Lai H: Pharmacology of thyrotropin-releasing hormone. *Ann Rev Pharmacol Toxicol* 26:311–332, 1986.

86. Horton JW, Tuggle DW, Kiser RS: Effect of temperature on naloxone treatment in canine hemorrhagic shock. *Circ Shock* 14:251–265, 1984.

87. Hosobuchi Y, Baskin DS, Woo SK: Reversal of induced ischemic neurologic deficit in gerbils by the opiate antagonist naloxone. *Science* 215:69–71, 1982.

88. Hughes GS: Naloxone and methylprednisolone sodium succinate enhance sympathomedullary discharge in patients with septic shock. *Life Sci* 35(23):2319–2326, 1984.

89. Hugli TE: The structural basis for anaphylatoxin and chemotactic functions of C3a, C4a, and C5a. *CRC Crit Rev Immunol* 1(4):321–366, 1981.

90. Jackson IMD, Wu P, Lechan RM: Immunohistochemical localization in the rat brain of the precursor for thyrotropin-releasing hormone. *Science* 229:1097–1098, 1985.

91. Jansen HF, Lutherer LO: Ventriculocisternal administration of naloxone protects against severe hypotension during endotoxin shock. *Brain Res* 194:608–612, 1980.

92. Kinney RC, Holaday JW, Harmon JW: Naloxone decreases neurologic deficits in experimental aortic cross-clamping ischemia. *Surg Forum* 36:460–461, 1985.

93. Koyama S, Santiesteban HL, Ammons WS, et al: The effects of naloxone on the peripheral sympathetics in cat endotoxin shock. *Circ Shock* 10:7–13, 1983.

94. Krumins SA, Faden AI: Traumatic injury alters opiate receptor binding in rat spinal cord. *Ann Neurol* 19(5):498–501, 1986.

95. Krumins SA, Faden AI, Feuerstein G: Opiate binding in rat hearts: modulation of binding after hemorrhagic shock. *Biochem Biophys Res Comm* 127(1):120–128, 1985.

96. Lechner RB, Gurll NJ, Reynolds DG: Intercoronary naloxone in hemorrhagic shock: dose-dependent stereospecific effects. *Am J Physiol* 249:H272–277, 1985.

97. Lechner RB, Gurll NJ, Reynolds DG: Naloxone potentiates the cardiovascular effects of catecholamines in canine hemorrhagic shock. *Circ Shock* 16:347–361, 1985.

98. Lechner RB, Gurll NJ, Reynolds DG: Effects of naloxone on regional blood flow distribution in canine hemorrhagic shock. *Proc Soc Exper Biol Med* 178:227–233, 1985.

99. Lechner RB, Gurll NJ, Reynolds DG: Role of the autonomic nervous system in mediating the response to naloxone in canine hemorrhagic shock. *Circ Shock* 16:279–295, 1985.

100. Long JB, Echevarria EE, Mobley WC, et al: Non-opioid hindlimb paralytic actions of intrathecally administered ICI 174864 and dynorphin A-related peptides. INRC, Alcohol and Substance Actions/Misuse 1985.

101. Long JB, Lake CR, Reid AA, et al: Effects of naloxone and thyrotropin releasing hormone on plasma catecholamines, corticosterone, and arterial pressure in normal and endotoxemic rats. *Circ Shock* 18:1–10, 1986.

102. Long JB, Martinez-Arizala A, Petras JM, et al: Endogenous opioids in spinal cord injury: a critical evaluation. *CNS trauma* 3(4):295–315, 1986.

103. Long JB, Ruvio BA, Glatt CE, et al: ICI 174864, a putative δ opioid antagonist, reverses endotoxemic hypotension: pretreatment with dynorphin 1-13, a k agonist, blocks this action. *Neuropeptides* 5:291–294, 1984.

104. Lux WE Jr, Feuerstein G, Faden AI: Alteration of leukotriene D4 hypotension by thyrotropin releasing hormone. *Nature* 302:822–824, 1983.

105. Lux WE Jr, Feuerstein G, Faden AI: Thyrotropin-releasing hormone reverses experimental anaphylactic shock through non-endorphin-related mechanisms. *Eur J Pharmacol* 90:301–302, 1983.

106. Lvoff R, Wilcken DEL: Glucagon in heart failure and in cardiogenic shock. *Circulation* 45:534–542, 1972.
107. Malcolm DS, Amir S, Holaday JW: Central glucagon antagonizes morphine- and stress induced antinociception in the mouse. Presented at Progress in Opioid Research: Proceedings of the International Narcotics Research Conference. NIDA Research Monograph Series, vol 75, 1986, pp 539–542.
108. Malcolm DS, Zaloga GP, Chernow B, et al: Glucagon antagonizes morphine-induced bradycardia at a site within the central nervous system. *Life Sci* 39:399–405, 1986.
109. Manaker S, Winokur A, Rhodes CH, et al: Autoradiographic localization of thyrotropin-releasing hormone (TRH) receptors in human spinal cord. *Neurology* 35:328–332, 1985.
110. McIntosh TK, Faden AI: Thyrotorpin-releasing hormone (TRH) and circulatory shock. *Circ Shock* 18:241–258, 1986.
111. McIntosh TK, Palter M, Grasberger R, et al: Endorphins in primate hemorrhagic shock: beneficial action of opiate antagonists. *J Surg Res* 40:265–275, 1986.
112. McIntosh TK, Palter M, Grasberger R, et al: Effect of an opiate antagonist (naloxone) and an agonist/antagonist (nalbuphine) in primate hemorrhagic shock. *Circ Shock* 17:313–325, 1985.
113. McKenzie JE, Anselmo DM, Muldoon SM: Nalbuphine's reversal of hypovolemic shock in the anesthetized rat. *Circ Shock* 17:21–33, 1985.
114. McMenamin DV, Smith EM, Blalock JE: Endotoxin induction of leukocyte-derived proopiomelanocortin-related peptides. *Infect Immunol* 48:813–817, 1985.
115. Paciorek P, Todd MH: Comparison of the cardiovascular effects of meptazinol and naloxone following anaphylactic shock in anesthetized rats. *Br J Pharmacol* 76 (Suppl):245P, 1982.
116. Przewlocki R, Shearman GT, Herz A: Mixed opioid/nonopioid effects of dynorphin and dynorphin related peptides after their intrathecal injection in rats. *Neuropeptides* 3:233–240, 1983.
117. Putterman C, Halpern P, Leykin Y, et al: Early use of naloxone in shock—a clinical trial. *Resuscitation* 13:185–190, 1986.
118. Reynolds DG, Gurll NJ, Vargish T, et al: Blockade of opiate receptors with naloxone improves survival and cardiac performance in canine endotoxic shock. *Circ Shock* 7:39–48, 1980.
119. Riggs TR, Yano Y, Vargish T: Morphine depression of myocardial function. *Circ Shock* 19:31–38, 1986.
120. Schadt JC, York DH: The reversal of hemorrhagic hypotension by naloxone in conscious rabbits. *Can J Physiol Pharmacol* 59:1208–1213, 1981.
121. Sharif NA: Diverse roles of thyrotropin-releasing hormone in brain, pituitary and spinal function. *TIPS* 3:119–122, 1985.
122. Spink WW, Vick J: A labile serum factor in experimental endotoxin shock: cross-transfusion studies in dogs. *J Exp Med* 114:501–510, 1961.
123. Tang AH: Protection from cerebral ischemia by U-50,488E, a specific kappa opioid analgesic agent. *Life Sci* 37:1475–1482, 1985.
124. Teich S, Malcolm D, Zaloga G, et al: Beneficial effects of glucagon in endotoxic shock in rats. *Circ Shock* 16:95, 1985.
125. Van DeMeer K, Valkenburg PW, Bastiaans AC, et al: Effect of naloxone on blood pressure and survival in different shock models in rats. *Eur J Pharmacol* 124:299–308, 1986.
126. Vargish T, Reynolds DG, Gurll NJ, et al: Naloxone reversal of hypovolemic shock in dog. *Circ Shock* 7:31–38, 1980.
127. Wallace MC, Tator CH: Failure of naloxone to improve spinal cord blood flow and cardiac output after spinal cord injury. *Neurosurgery* 18(4):428–432, 1986.
128. Wallace MC, Tator CH: Failure of blood transfusion or naloxone to improve clinical recovery after experimental spinal cord injury. *Neurosurgery* 19(4):489–494, 1986.
129. Weld JM, Kamerling SG, Combie JD, et al: The effects of naloxone on endotoxic and hemorrhagic shock in horses. *Res Comm in Chem Pathol Pharmacol* 44(2):227–238, 1984.
130. Young WE, Flamm ES, Demopoulos HB, et al: Effect of naloxone on posttraumatic ischemia in experimental spinal contusion. *J Neurosurg* 55:209–219, 1981.

38

Arachidonic Acid Metabolites

H. David Reines, M.D.
James A. Cook, Ph.D.

Eicosanoids are a group of fatty acid metabolites derived from arachidonic acid, a component of cell membrane phospholipids. A variety of stimuli mediated via specific receptors or nonspecifically can activate enzymes capable of cleaving membrane phospholipids with the release of the constituent fatty acid. Arachidonic acid is stored and released from specific phospholipid pools. The release of arachidonic acid from phospholipids is catalyzed by phospholipase A_2 or phospholipase C (103).

Once released, arachidonic acid is oxidatively processed (dependent upon cell origin) to a variety of metabolites by specific enzyme pathways. Cyclooxygenase catalyzes conversion of arachidonic acid to the cyclized endoperoxide metabolites PGG_2 and PGH_2 (Fig. 38.1). These unstable intermediates are in turn converted to a cascade of metabolites including thromboxane (Tx)A_2 and prostaglandins, PGE_2, PGD_2, PGF_2, and prostacyclin (PGI_2).

Synthesis of TXA_2 and PGI_2 requires thromboxane and prostacyclin synthetase enzymes, respectively. The presence of those enzymes vary with the cell type. For example, platelets synthesize large quantities of TXA_2 but not PGI_2 (71), whereas endothelial cells generate mainly PGI_2 (70). Thromboxane A_2 and PGI_2 have opposing actions on platelet aggregation and vasoactivity and are potentially important factors in the regulation of vascular homeostasis and hemastasis (71). Thromboxane A_2 induces platelet aggregation and is an extremely potent vasoconstrictor (40, 97). Thromboxane A_2 has a short half-life (approximately 30 seconds) and is quickly hydrolyzed to the stable and inactive metabolite, TxB_2 (70, 97). PGI_2, a potent endogenous inhibitor of platelet aggregation and a vasodilator, has a half-life of approximately 2 minutes and hydrolyzes to its stable and inactive metabolite, 6-keto-PGF_1 (13, 71). Measurement (by radioimmunoassay) of the stable products TXB_2 and 6-keto-PGF, in plasma thus serves as markers for TxA_2 and PGI_2 production.

Another oxidative pathway of arachidonic acid metabolism is via 5-, 12-, or 15-lipoxygenase enzymes. The 5-lipoxygenase pathway leads to the biosynthesis of leukotrienes through an ordered cascade of enzymes (88). Two classes of leukotrienes (LT) are produced from the enzymatic conversion of the LTA_4 precursor: the sulfidopeptide leukotrienes (LTC_4, LTD_4, and LTE_4) and the nonpeptide metabolite, LTB_4. These lipoxygenase products have a variety of proinflammatory properties and hemodynamic effects. LTB_4 stimulates neutrophil and eosinophil chemotaxis, leukostasis, lysosomal enzyme release, superoxide generation, and the expression of C3b receptors (35, 36, 73, 76). The sulfidopeptide leukotrienes, which together constitute the "slow reacting substance of anaphylaxis" (62), augment microvascular permeability changes in response to a variety of injuries (29, 57). These latter leukotrienes also can induce bronchoconstriction and are potent vasoconstrictors in coronary, mesenteric, renal, and pulmonary vascular beds in certain species [Table 38.1] (27, 48, 57, 66, 86). Leukotrienes are quickly eliminated from the circulation. LTC_4, for example, has a plasma clearance half-time of approximately 30 seconds from the vascular compartment (41, 50). Cell surface bound enzymes, glutamyl transferase, and dipeptidase, located in the kidney, lung, and liver are responsible for the rapid uptake and metabolism of leukotrienes. The liver has a higher affinity for LTE_4 where there is partial metabolism of LTE_4 by an acetyltransferase to N-acetyl LTE_4 (100). The latter appears as a major bile metabolite in the rat (23). Because of their rapid catabolism, leukotriene metabolites are measured in bile (23), urine (22), or lung lavage fluid (2) as an index of endogenous production.

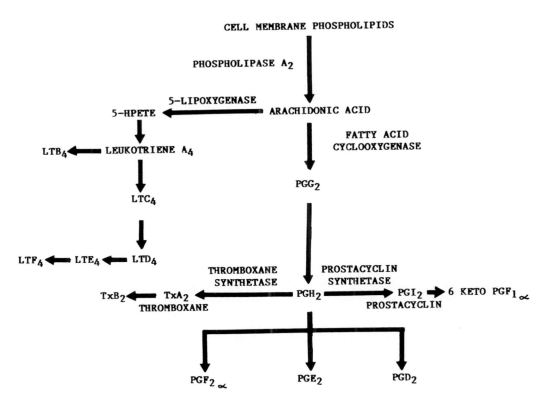

Figure 38.1. Archidonic acid cascade.

EICOSANOIDS IN SEPSIS AND ADULT RESPIRATORY DISTRESS SYNDROME

The clinical entity of septic shock (frequently associated with Gram-negative bacteremia) is a dramatic complication in patients. The incidence of this entity has steadily risen during the past two decades (56). It is esti-mated that 15 per 1,000 hospital admissions may develop gram-negative sepsis amounting to as many as 71,000 to 330,000 cases annually in the United States (4, 65, 105). Circulatory shock occurs in 20% of these septic patients and produces a complex sequence of pathophysiological changes frequently culminating in multiple organ system failure and death.

Table 38.1
Biological Activity of Arachidonic Acid Metabolites

Product	Hemodynamic Effect	Action
Cyclooxygenase		
PGE$_2$	Vasodilation	Inhibits immunoregulatory mechanisms
PGI$_2$	Vasodilation	Inhibits platelet aggregation
PGF$_{2\alpha}$	Vasoconstriction	
TxA$_2$	Vasoconstriction	Stimulates platelet aggregation
Lipoxygenase		
LTB$_4$		Increased adhesiveness and chemotaxis of leukocytes
LTC$_4$		
LTD$_4$	Vasoconstriction	Increased microvascular permeabilities
LTE$_4$		

Despite the use of specific antibiotics, surgical intervention, and careful monitoring, the mortality rate from septic shock still remains between 30 to 80% (4, 56, 65, 85, 105).

A frequent concomitant complication of septic shock is the adult respiratory distress syndrome (ARDS), an acute form of respiratory failure presenting as noncardiogenic pulmonary edema. Alveolar edema produced by increased permeability of the alveolar-capillary membrane and decreased compliance associated with the development of refractory arterial hypoxemia are the major clinical hallmarks (58, 65). As with septic shock, the mortality rate from ARDS remains high (25, 30, 69).

The activation of systemic inflammatory mediators that normally serve a protective function against microbes and toxins contributes to the pathophysiologic events leading to metabolic and vascular deterioration in sepsis and ARDS. There is considerable experimental evidence that eicosanoids are important inflammatory mediators in Gram-negative bacteremia and other forms of acute lung injury (3). Although there have been few clinical investigations examining the potential role of eicosanoids in sepsis and ARDS, several studies have now demonstrated abnormal prostanoid, thromboxane, and leukotriene production associated with these clinical disorders.

Reines et al. (81) measured central venous plasma $iTxB_2$ levels in patients diagnosed as septic based upon positive blood or peritoneal cultures, hypotension without pressor drugs, febrile response, and abnormal white blood cell count. All patients received standard therapy with the exception of nonsteroidal antiinflammatory drugs. In six patients with no evidence of septicemia, mean plasma $iTxB_2$ concentrations (91 ± 18 pg/ml) were similar to four surviving septic patients (92 ± 25 pg/ml). However, in eight nonsurviving septic patients plasma $iTxB_2$ levels were increased 10-fold (912 ± 250 pg/ml). Intrapulmonary shunting (as determined by alveolar-arterial oxygen gradients), and prothrombin and partial thromboplastin time were significantly worse in septic non-survivors. These studies thus suggested that increased thromboxane production in severe sepsis may be involved in respiratory distress and hematologic disorders (81).

Increased thromboxane also has been demonstrated in patients with septic and nonseptic burns (44). Patients in the acute phase of injury (less than 3 days postburn) exhibited increased mean plasma $iTxB_2$ concentrations relative to nonburn controls (2.6 ± 0.85 vs.<0.03 pmol/ml $N = 5$). Levels were lower (0.24 ± 0.03 pmol/ml) in a group of patients at 7–14 days postburn injury, but were markedly raised (3.47 ± 0.61 pmol/ml) in nine burn patients that developed septic complications. Plasma i6-keto-$PGF_1\alpha$ levels were not above detectable limits in this study regardless of the clinical course.

In contrast to the above studies, Rie et al. (83) found no consistent change in plasma $iTxB_2$ taken from eight septic patients with positive blood cultures compared with nine critically ill patients with negative blood cultures. Mean $\pm$ SEM plasma levels of i6-keto-$PGF_1\alpha$ however, were increased in septic patients relative to the control group (721 ± 41 pg/ml vs. 65 ± 12 pg/ml, respectively). Plasma i6-keto-$PGF_1\alpha$ levels have also been measured in septic patients employing gas chromatography/mass spectrometry techniques (39), a more sensitive measurement tool of prostacyclin than radioimmunoassay. This study demonstrated that mean central venous plasma 6-keto-$PGF_2\alpha$ levels in control patients were less than 4 pg/ml, whereas six septic survivors exhibited a median level of 30 pg/ml (range 22 to 194). Plasma 6-keto-$PGF_1\alpha$ levels, however, in eight septic nonsurvivors were raised to a median level of 229 pg/ml (range 31 to 21,998). A potential role of prostacyclin in septic shock is further supported by the studies of Slotman et al. (92), who assessed the interaction of thromboxane, prostacyclin, and activated complement in clinical sepsis and hypotension. Forty-eight critically ill patients were divided into four groups: nonseptic normotensive, hypovolemic shock, normotensive severe sepsis, and septic shock. Mean plasma $iTxB_2$ levels were significantly increased (approximately 200 pg/ml) in hypotensive, normotensive septic, and septic shock groups relative to normal controls (<50 pg/ml). There were, however, no significant differences in $iTxB_2$ among these latter critically ill patients. On the other hand, plasma i6-keto-$PGF_1\alpha$ levels were greatly increased in septic shock patients (856 ± 439 pg/ml vs.<82 pg/ml in normal controls) as were the levels of complement component C3a in plasma. Since PaO_2/F_1O_2 ratios correlated directly with PGI_2 and inversely with plasma TxB_2/PGI_2 ratios or plasma C3a, these investigators concluded that imbalances in these agents were involved in the pathogenesis of hypovolemic and septic shock (92).

Oettinger et al. (75) assessed endogenous prostaglandin $F_2\alpha$ production in the hyperdynamic stage of severe sepsis in patients. Their results indicated pulmonary net release of PGF_2 since mean $\pm$ SEM arterial plasma levels $(1252 \pm 119$ pg/ml) were elevated more than those in mixed venous plasma $(824 \pm 89$ pg/ml, $N = 9$). In contrast to studies with prostacyclin however, plasma $PGF_2\alpha$ concentrations did not correlate individually with hemodynamic and respiratory changes.

Altered eicosanoid production has also been demonstrated in patients with ARDS. Deby-Dupont et al. (21) measured arterial plasma $iTxB_2$ in 38 patients during the course of ARDS. Plasma $iTxB_2$ concentrations in 79% of the group were greater than 100 pg/ml, which was the maximum value found in normal subjects. In 17% of the patients with ARDS, plasma TxB_2 levels were greater than 2000 pg/ml. These investigators also examined the correlation between plasma $iTxB_2$ levels and plasma trypsin-like activity in 117 patients at risk of developing ARDS (20). Increased plasma levels of immunoreactive trypsin (IRT) were associated with high mortality. Plasma TxB_2 increased simultaneously with increases in plasma IRT activity or within 24 hours of IRT release. Plasma values of $iTxB_2$ above 2000 pg/ml were measured in patients when IRT values increased above 500 ng/ml (20). These studies suggested that plasma $iTxB_2$ concentrations parallel protease release from the gastrointestinal tract or ischemic pancreas during the development of ARDS.

In addition to thromboxane, there is evidence that lipoxygenase metabolism is increased in ARDS. Matthay et al. (64) demonstrated significant increases in LTD_4 in pulmonary edema fluid of patients with ARDS, compared with five patients with cardiogenic pulmonary edema $(18.5 \pm 6.8$ vs. 4.4 ± 1.1 pmol/ml). Other eicosanoid products in lung edema fluid (TxB_2, PGE_2, LTB_4, and LTC_2) were not significantly different between these two patient groups. These investigators (98) also observed increased LTD_4 and LTB_4 concentrations in pulmonary edema fluid of a patient that developed pulmonary congestion after cardiopulmonary bypass. Stenmark et al. (96) reported increased lung lavage LTC_4 and LTD_4 levels in five infants exhibiting persistent pulmonary hypertension, bronchoconstriction, and pulmonary edema, compared with 14 infants without a diagnosis of persistent pulmonary hypertension. These studies suggest that leukotrienes may function as local pathogenic mediators in these forms of pulmonary dysfunction.

There have been limited clinical trials assessing the effect of therapeutic agents on eicosanoid metabolism in sepsis and ARDS. Since phospholipase A_2 is inhibited by corticosteroids (6), the possibility that steroids may inhibit the release of arachidonic acid and its metabolism to TxB_2 in sepsis was investigated. Reines et al. (80) measured $iTxB_2$ in central venous plasma obtained from septic patients within 1–4 hours after administration of a single dose of methylprednisolone (15–30 mg/kg, $N = 9$). Despite marked increases in plasma $iTxB_2$ in patients dying of sepsis (>700 pg/ml), $iTxB_2$ levels did not vary significantly from those patients not receiving steroids ($N = 12$). Mortality and hematologic and respiratory parameters also were not significantly different between the two groups. Mean plasma levels of $iTxB_2$, however, were significantly reduced in four septic patients given aspirin $(444 \pm 159$ pg/ml to 174 ± 33 pg/ml).

Selective thromboxane synthetase inhibitors have been assessed in both sepsis and ARDS. The thromboxane synthetase inhibitor, dazoxiben, significantly inhibited increases in plasma TxB_2 in septic patients (82). However, changes in mean arterial pressure, peripheral vascular resistance, intrapulmonary shunting, extravascular lung water, and hematologic parameters were not improved. Leeman et al (59) demonstrated that dazoxiben administration in patients with ARDS did not affect pulmonary hemodynamics even though platelet thromboxane production was largely inhibited. The only effect seen with this compound was a slight increase in arterial oxygenation and decrease in venous admixture. Therefore, these data suggest that selective thromboxane synthetase inhibitors are not beneficial in the management of patients with established septic shock and ARDS. However, such compounds might be potentially useful as adjunctive therapy in patients at risk of developing these clinical disorders. Slotman et al. (93) gave ketocanozole (an antibiotic and imidazole-based thromboxane synthetase inhibitor) prophylactically in 71 critically ill patients at risk of developing ARDS. Eighteen percent of these patients developed ARDS with a high mortality (nine of 13). However, the incidence of ARDS was significantly less among ketocanozole-treated patients compared with the placebo group (2/35 v. 11/36). Whether this beneficial effect is derived from antimicrobial and/or thromboxane synthetase inhibitor properties of the drug merits further investigation.

Potentially beneficial prostanoids rather than

eicosanoid inhibitors have provided alternative approaches to the treatment of ARDS. Prostaglandin E_1 has properties that make it attractive as a therapeutic agent since this prostanoid has anti-inflammatory functions and is largely degraded by the lung (94). The infusion of PGE_1 proximal to the lung has the advantage of maximizing anti-inflammatory effects in ARDS while minimizing systemic effects because of rapid pulmonary metabolism. Holcroft et al. (46) examined the effect of 7-day infusion of PGE_1 or placebo in 41 ARDS patients. Thirty-day survival was significantly improved in PGE_1 patients (15 of 21 alive) compared with seven of 20 placebo patients. Shoemaker et al. (90) also demonstrated beneficial effects of PGE_1 infusion in 15 severely ill patients with ARDS. Prostaglandin E_1 reduced pulmonary artery pressure, pulmonary systemic vascular resistance and increased cardiac output, arterial PO_2 and oxygen consumption when compared with preinfusion values or with placebo-treated patients. A recent multicenter study of PGE_1, however, has not verified these early results (Upjohn Co, personal communication).

Since there have been no published clinical trials employing nonsteroidal anti-inflammatory drugs or lipoxygenase inhibitors in sepsis and ARDS, the potential pathophysiologic significance of eicosanoids (e.g., PGI_2 or leukotrienes) is currently unknown. At least one limitation of the use of nonsteroidal anti-inflammatory drugs in sepsis is their potential adverse effect upon renal function through inhibition of beneficial vasodilating prostaglandins (12, 28). It thus remains to be determined if the potential deleterious effect of these drugs in septic patients will outweigh their potential beneficial actions. The therapeutic efficacy of glucocorticoids in these clinical disorders, however, remains controversial (26, 95). Because of the continued high mortality rate in sepsis and ARDS, further clinical trials with drugs that alter eicosanoid metabolism and further testing of beneficial prostanoids appears warranted.

EICOSANOIDS IN OTHER CARDIOPULMONARY CONDITIONS

Transmural myocardial infarction is generally associated with thrombotic occlusion of the diseased coronary artery. Platelet adhesion and aggregation are essential to thrombosis. Platelet release of TXA_2 may also contribute to coronary artery spasms. This relationship has been experimentally (17, 89) and clinically demonstrated by the observation that patients with Prinzmetal's angina have increased plasma TXA_2 levels (85).

A randomized prospective study of 555 patients with unstable angina treated with aspirin, resulted in an 8.6% death and nonfatal MI rate vs. 17% in controls. This study provides strong evidence that antiplatelet therapy with a cyclooxygenase inhibitor is effective in the prevention of coronary occlusion (9). Antiplatelet therapy using aspirin has also proved useful in other manifestations of peripheral vascular disease. Low-dose aspirin given to patients undergoing aorta-coronary bypass significantly lowers the generation of venous plasma TXA_2 and can inhibit platelet aggregation (104). This therapy appears to increase coronary artery bypass patency without increasing bleeding complications. The impact of this approach to peripheral vascular surgery awaits confirmation. PGI_2 has also been utilized when heparin is contraindicated in cardiopulmonary bypass, hemodialysis, and transplanted livers (38).

Another area of interest has been the role of eicosanoids in pulmonary emboli. Experimentally it has been demonstrated that a significant rise in plasma TXB_2 and 6-keto-$PGF_{1}\alpha$ follows pulmonary emboli in the dog (101). The intravenous infusion of prostacyclin can decrease pulmonary resistance and increase cardiac output in the same model (99). Pretreatment with imidazole, a thromboxane synthetase inhibitor, does not lower pulmonary artery pressure and results in an increase mortality (51).

PGE_1 has been used to increase cardiac index and lower systemic vascular resistance in patients with acute myocardial infarction with left ventricular failure (78). Intravenous pulmonary arterial infusions of PGE_1 given simultaneously with left atrial injection of norepinephrine have been used to successfully treat five patients with refractory heart failure following mitral valve replacement (19). All five survived with significant improvement in cardiac performance.

EICOSANOIDS IN CENTRAL NERVOUS SYSTEM DISEASE

Eicosanoids are ubiquitous within the central nervous system and are produced in response to numerous stimuli. The role of eicosanoids in the pathophysiology of central nervous system injury have not been defined, although early experimental results demonstrate an interrelation of eicosanoid production and cerebral ischemia. A possible role for leukotrienes in the formation of cerebral edema accompanying reperfusion following stroke and vasospasm following subarachnoid hemorrhage has been proposed. Leukotrienes C_4 and D_4 are synthesized in gerbil forebrains following ischemia (72) and also increase water accumulation in ischemic baboon cortical preparation (43). Further work in subarachnoid hemorrhage in a concussive brain injury model also produces elevations in LT C_4 and D_4 (52).

There are no clinical data supporting the role of eicosanoid blockade in the prevention of ischemic stroke associated with transient ischemic attacks (TIA). The Canadian Cooperative Study has demonstrated the efficacy of aspirin and aspirin plus sulfinpyrazone in reducing the frequency of stroke and mortality with TIA (10, 11). Results with other cyclooxygenase inhibitors, however, have not been as promising (42).

Prostacyclin is a potent cerebral vasodilator that may have a role in the reperfusion of ischemic areas. Prostacyclin has been successfully used in models of reversible global ischemia in dogs (37). It may be that other arachidonic acid metabolites and free oxygen radicals released during ischemia inhibit the vasodilating effects of PGI_2 and increase ischemic damage. Several clinical trials with PGI_2 have been performed in patients with acute cerebral infarct, and there was some neurological improvement although no change in computerized tomographic findings was demonstrated. (68). Prostacyclin has also been utilized in the treatment of acute vasospasm following subarachnoid hemorrhage in animals and humans (61). In spinal cord injuries, an imbalance of TXA_2 - PGI_2 synthesis is thought to be responsible for ischemic changes, whereas leukotrienes are thought to contribute to the edema and disruption of tissue ion homeostasis (47).

Further studies in cats have demonstrated a decrease an infarct size and neurological deficit in cats fed fish oil compound compared with those receiving a regular diet (5). Fish oil is a source of PGI_3, which is a potent vasodilator and inhibitor of platelet aggregaters.

PROSTAGLANDINS AND NEONATES

One of the first clinical applications of prostaglandin research was in the treatment of diseases in infants involving the ductus arteriosus. This large channel between the pulmonary trunk and descending aorta bypasses the lung in the fetus and normally closes completely within hours of birth to divert blood flow normally to the lung of the breathing infant. Ductal closure occurs in two stages. Initially, smooth muscles constrict in the wall of the vessel; this event is followed by permanent closure, secondary to the destruction of endothelial and connective tissue formation, to seal the lumen (15). In the presence of congenital heart disease, the ductus may close, creating serious problems for children with cardiac lesions associated with decreased pulmonary blood flow such as pulmonary atresia. These infants are dependent upon ductal flow to maintain pulmonary flow and thereby increase oxygenation of systemic blood flow. Without ductal flow, hypoxemia and acidosis quickly insure progress and maintenance of a patent ductus (PDA), therefore becomes a lifesaving measure in these infants. As neonatal intensive care became more successful in the resuscitation of small babies, another group of children with a problem opposite from the congenital heart group appeared. These were premature infants in whom the ductus did not close normally, creating congestive heart failure from their large left to right shunt. Closure of the shunt in these babies usually required surgery.

Attempts to modulate the response of the ductus with vasoactive drugs were unsuccessful until Coceani and Olley (16) discovered that isolated strips of sheep ductus arteriosus were relaxed by E-type prostaglandins (PGE_1 and PGE_2) in a dose-dependent fashion. Rudolph and Hymen (87) studied fetal lambs to test this hypothesis in vivo. Acetylsalicylic acid (aspirin) was injected to inhibit prostaglandin synthesis and cause closure of the ductus while injection of PGE_1, reversed these changes (87).

Arachidonic acid relaxes the oxygen-constricted ductus arteriosus, and indomethacin completely blocks this reaction (15). Although thromboxane A_2 and PGF_2a have been implicated in this reaction, the most potent relaxant in the ductus is PGE_2. PGE_2 is formed intramurally and exerts its effect on the muscle cells. PGI_2 is also produced in quantity by the ductus arteriosus; however, PGE_2 is three orders of magnitude more potent than PGI_2 in relaxing the ductus arteriosus (15). Utilizing these concepts, clinical trials involving manipulation of prostaglandins were implemented.

In children with cyanotic heart disease,

maintenance of a PDA became a palliative procedure until more definitive therapy could be instituted. Infusion of PGE_1 and PGE_2 were given to 11 infants with congenital heart disease secondary to pulmonary stenosis of the great vessels, resulting in an increase in oxygen saturation secondary to ductal dilation in 10 of 11 patients (74). The use of PGE_1 infusion is now an accepted procedure in the palliation of congenital heart disease requiring maintenance of the patent ductus. Therapy is maintained for several days until corrective surgery can be performed.

Another application of prostaglandins in neonates is to promote nonsurgical closure of PDA with nonsteroidal anti-inflammatory compounds. Two simultaneous studies published in 1976 demonstrated the usefulness of indomethacin in premature neonates with respiratory distress syndrome and congestive heart failure unresponsive to digitalis and diuretics (31, 45). Prior to the institution of prostaglandin blockade, the only alternative in these children was surgical closure of the ductus. Pharmacologic closure of the ductus was demonstrated in all children with marked improvement in symptoms of congestive heart failure. Indomethacin was chosen over aspirin because the latter displaces bilirubin from binding sites and irreversibly inhibits platelet aggregation (31, 45).

Further studies have confirmed the usefulness of indomethacin to close PDA; however, failures have been reported. One reason proposed for this lack of response may be the existence of a subset of patients with alterations in indomethacin metabolism (7). The majority of children with PDA and respiratory distress, however, can be treated medically without surgical closure.

PROSTAGLANDINS AND GASTRIC ACID SECRETIONS

Aspirin and nonsteroidal anti-inflammatory drugs (NSAIDS) have an irritating effect on gastric mucosa that results in gastritis, bleeding, and even perforation. These lesions resemble those of stress ulceration seen in critically ill patients. Both aspirin and indomethacin significantly decrease total gastric mucosa blood flow, while simultaneously potentiating stimulated acid production (34). Numerous prostaglandins are synthesized in the submucosa of the gastrointestinal tract and inhibit gastric acid secretion (54, 67). This inhibition has been confirmed in humans (55). The exact mechanisms by which prostaglandins inhibit gastric acid secretion in humans are unknown, although direct inhibition of parietal cell function is possible (53).

Topical prostaglandins E_1 and E_2 prevent gross gastric mucosal lesions induced by chemical irritation (84). Cytoprotection from sucralfate is, in part, related to the ability of the drug to enhance prostaglandin production (63). Furthermore, H_2 blockers can increase PGE_2 in normal and in peptic ulcer disease patients (77). Direct application of PGI_2 experimentally increased gastric mucosal blood flow and yielded a cytoprotective effect in the absence of vasopressors (33). However instillation of PGE_2 did not offer significant protection in two studies in patients (91, 102).

Recently a new synthetic analog of PGE_1, misoprostol has been undergoing extensive testing in the prevention of stress ulceration. This drug has been efficacious in decreasing acid secretion in normal volunteers (1). Misoprostol was compared with antacids in a randomized prospective study that demonstrated excellent cytoprotection from PGE_1 instillation (G. D. Searle, Inc., personal communication).

It appears, therefore, that eicosanoids may be important in the pathophysiology of acute ulceration, and modulation of these effects yields hope for new preventive therapies in the future.

PROSTAGLANDINS AND RENAL COMPLICATIONS

Administration of nonsteroidal anti-inflammatory agents was observed to lead to retention of sodium and water and a decrease in glomerular filtration rate (GFR). As early as 1976, these changes were felt to be prostaglandin mediated (24). Arachidonic acid metabolites are produced throughout the kidney, in the medullary interstitial cells, distal tubules, endothelial cells, and collecting tubes (18, 79). Numerous clinical renal disorders have been reported secondary to NSAID, which block cyclooxygenase products. NSAIDs can interfere with urine output and sodium excretion and impair diuretic action. They have also been associated with renal failure due to papillary necrosis, acute interstitial nephritis, and vasculitis (32). PGE_2, PGI_2, and PGF_2 tend to promote an increase in renal blood flow and increase GFR to augment the filtered load of sodium. Blood flow is preferentially increased to the inner cortex and medullary regions. Renin release is enhanced by PGE_2, while PGE_2 blocks the effects of ADH on collecting tubules to reduce water reabsorption (12).

A review of NSAID by Carmichael et al. (12) revealed 274 cases of acute renal disease caused by NSAIDs, including 34 cases of nephrotic syndrome associated with fenoprofen. A number of cases documenting acute renal insufficiency after NSAID was administered are reported (32). Renal failure occurred from 1 to 21 days and was heralded by a decrease in urine output, increasing creatinine, and a fractional excretion of sodium $<1\%$. Most of these patients were hospitalized with other problems, especially collagen vascular disease. Only three of 27 patients required dialysis. The remaining 24 recovered normal function after discontinuation of the drug. One patient had permanent severe disease requiring permanent dialysis (32). On the other hand, Sulindac, a newer agent, appears to have less effect on renal function (14).

Although prostaglandins appear to have little influence on renal hemodynamics among normal controls (79), a decrease in renal perfusion results in an increase in PGI_2 production to maintain renal blood flow (49). Renal ischemia in dogs has been associated with a rise in TxB_2 and shift of blood flow to the medulla (8). The opposing action of prostacyclin may be a clinical determinant of the extent of renal damage in ischemia (60). Using specific Tx synthetase inhibitors, these authors demonstrated a decrease in postischemic renal damage by shifting metabolism cyclooxygenase metabolism prostacyclin. These preliminary studies thus suggest that manipulation of eicosanoid metabolisms may be effective in preventing postperfusion injury in ischemic renal failure.

References

1. Akdamur K, Agrawal N, Ertan A: Inhibition of nocturnal gastric secretion in normal human volunteers by misoprostol: a synthetic prostaglandin E_1 methyester analog. *Am J Gastroenterol* 77:902, 1982.
2. Ball HA, Cook JA, Spicer KM, Halushka PV: LY171883, a leukotriene D_4/E_4 antagonist, attenuates leak in oleic acid induced pulmonary injury. *Circ Shock* 12:106, 1985.
3. Ball HA, Cook JA, Wise WC, Halushka: Role of thromboxane, prostaglandins and leukotrienes in endotoxic and septic shock. *Intensive Care Med* 12(3):116, 1986.
4. Berringer R, Hardwood-Nuss AL: Septic shock (part I). *Emer Med Rev* 3:75, 1985.
5. Black KL, Culp B, Madison P, et al: The protective effects of dietary fish oil on focal cerebral infarction. *Prostag Med* 3:257, 1979.
6. Blackwell GJ, Carnuccio F, DiRosa M, et al: Metal glucocorticoids induce the formation and release of antiinflammatory and anti-phospholipase proteins into the peritoneal cavity of the rat. *Br J Pharmacol* 76:185, 1982.
7. Brash AR Hickey DE, Graham TP, et al: *Pharmacokinetics of indomethacin in the neonate: relation of plasma indomethacin levels to response of the ductus arteriosus. N Engl J Med* 305(2):67, 1981.
8. Bretton PR, Tempel G, Rajagopalan PR et al: Effects of hemodilution on renal cortical blood flow following ischemic renal failure. *Surg Forum* 35:640, 1984.
9. Cairns JA, Gent M, Singer J, et al: Aspirin, sulfinpyrazone or both in unstable angina. Results of a Canadian multicenter trial. *N Engl J Med* 313(22):1369, 1985.
10. Canadian Cooperative Study Group: A randomized trial of aspirin and sulfinpyrazone in threatened stroke. *N Engl J Med* 299:53, 1978.
11. Candelise L, Landi G, Perrone P, et al: A randomized trial of aspirin and sulfinpyrazone in patients with TIA. *Stroke* 13:175, 1982.
12. Carmichael J. Shankel SW: Effects of nonsteroidal and antiinflammatory drugs on prostaglandins and renal function. *Am J Med* 78:992, 1985.
13. Cho MG, Allen MA: Chemical stability of prostacyclin (PGI_2) in aqueous solution. *Prostaglandin* 15:943, 1978.
14. Ciabattoni G, Cinotti GA, Pierucci A, et al: effects of sulindac and ibuprofen in patients with chronic glomerular disease. *N Engl J Med* 310(5):279, 1984.
15. Clyman RI: Ontogeny of the ductus arteriosus response to prostaglandins and inhibitors of their synthesis. *Semin Perinatol* 4(2):115, 1980.
16. Coceani F, Olley PM, Bodach E: Lamb ductus arteriosus: effect of prostaglandin synthesis inhibitors on muscle tone and the response to prostaglandin E_2. *Prostaglandins* 9:299, 1975.
17. Coker SJ, Paratt JR, Ledingham IM, et al: Thromboxane and prostacyclin release from ischemic myocardium in relation to arrhythmias. *Nature* 291:323, 1981.
18. Currie MG, Needleman P: Renal arachidonic acid metabolism. *Ann Rev Physiol* 46:327, 1984.
19. D'Ambra MN, LaRaia PJ, Philbin DM, et al: Prostaglandin E_1: a new therapy for refractory right heart failure and pulmonary hypertension after mitral valve replacement. *J Thoracic Cardiovas Surg* 89:567, 1985.
20. Deby-Dupont G, Pincemail J, Faymonville ME, Braun M, Deby C, Goutier R, Lamy M, and Franchimont P: Trypsin-like activity and thromboxane release in adult respiratory distress syndrome. *Prostaglandins* 32:106, 1986.
21. Deby-Dupont G, Rodoux L, Mass M, Larbuisson R, Noell FX, Lamy M: Release of thromboxane B_2 during adult respiratory distress syndrome and its inhibition by nonsteroidal antiinflammatory substance in man. *Arch Int Pharmacodyn* 259:317, 1982.
22. Denzlinger C, Guhlmann A, Scheuber PH, Wilker D, Hammer DK, and Keppler D: Metabolism and analysis of cysteine leukotrienes in the monkey. *J Biol Chem* 261:15601, 1986.
23. Denzlinger C, Rapp S, Hagmann W, Keppler D: Leukotrienes as mediators in tissue trauma. *Science* 230:330, 1985.
24. Donker AJM, Arisz L, Brentjens JRH, et al: The effect of indomethacin on kidney function and plasma renal activity in man. *Nephron* 17:288, 1976.
25. Douglas ME, Downs JB: Pulmonary function following severe acute respiratory failure and high levels of positive end expiratory pressure. *Chest* 71:18, 1977.
26. DuToit HG, Erasmus FR, Macfarlane CM: Methylprednisolone and adult respiratory distress syndrome. *South Afr Med J* 65:1049, 1985.
27. Feuerstein G, Zukowska-Grojec Z, Kopin IJ: Cardiovascular effects of leukotriene D_4 in SHR and WKY rats. *Eur J Pharmacol* 76-107-110, 1981.
28. Fink MP, MacVittie TJ, Casey LC: Effects of nonstero-

idal antiinflammatory drugs on renal function in septic dogs. *J Surg Res* 36:516, 1984.

29. Ford-Hutchinson AW, Rackman A: Leukotrienes as mediators of skin inflammation. *Br J Dermatol* 109:26, 1983.

30. Fowler AA, Hamman RF, Good JT, et al: Adult respiratory distress syndrome: Risk with common predisposition. *Ann Int Med* 98:593, 1983.

31. Friedman WF, Hirschklau J, Printz M, et al: Pharmacologic closure of patent ductus arteriosus in the premature infant. *N Engl J Med* 295(10):526, 1976.

32. Garella S, Matarese RA: Renal effects of prostaglandins and clinical adverse effects of nonsteroidal antiinflammatory agents. *Medicine* 63(3):165, 1984.

33. Gaskill HV, Sirinek KR, Levine BA: Prostacyclin-mediated gastric cyto-protection is dependent on mucosal blood flow. *Surgery* 92(2):221, 1982.

34. Gerkens JF, Shand DG, Flexner C, et al: Effect of indomethacin and aspirin on gastric blood flow and acid secretion. *J Pharmacol Exp Ther* 203(3):646, 1977.

35. Goetzl EJ, Brindley LL, Goldman DW: Enhancement of human neutrophil adherence by synthetic leukotriene constituents of the slow-reacting substance of anaphylaxis. *Immunology* 50:35, 1983.

36. Goetzl EJ, Pickett WC: Novel structural determinants of the human neutrophil chemotactic activity of leukotriene B₂. *J Exp Med* 153:482, 1981.

37. Hallenbeck JM, Furlow TW: Prostaglandins influence nutrient perfusion in brain during the post ischemic period. *Prostacyclin* 299; 1979.

38. Halushka PV, Dollery CT, MacDermot J, et al: Thromboxane and prostacyclin in disease: a review. *Q J Med* 52:461, 1983.

39. Halushka PV, Reines HD, Barrow SE, Blair IA, Dollery CT, Rambo W, Cook JA, Wise WC: Elevated plasma 6-keto-prostaglandin F₁ in patients in septic shock. *Crit Care Med* 13:451, 1985.

40. Hamberg M, Svenson J, Samuelson B: Thromboxanes: a new group of biologically active compounds derived from prostaglandin endoperoxides. *Proc Natl Acad Sci USA* 72:2994, 1975.

41. Hammerstrom S, Ornig L, Bernstrom K, Gistafsson B, Norin E, Kaijser L: Metbolism of leukotriene C₄ in rat and man. *Ad Prost Thromb Leuk Res* 15:185, 1985.

42. Harris RJ, Bayhan M, Branston NM et al: Modulation of the pathophysiology of primate focal cerebral ischaemia by indomethacin. *Stroke* 13:17, 1982.

43. Harris RJ, Lindquist C, Kaniya K, et al: The effect of LTC₄ and its antagonist FPL 55712 on the formation of cerebral ischemic edema in the primate. *Stroke* (in press).

44. Herndon DN, Abston S, Stein MD: Increased thromboxane B₂ levels in the plasma of burned and septic burned patients. *Surg Gynecol Obstet* 159:210, 1984.

45. Heymann MA, Rudolph AM, Silverman NH: Closure of the ductus arteriosus in premature infants by inhibition of prostaglandin synthesis. *N Engl J Med* 295(10):530, 1976.

46. Holcroft JW, Vassar MJ, Weber CJ: Prostaglandin E/₁ and survival in patients with the adult respiratory distress syndrome: A prospective trial. *Ann Surg* 203:371, 1986.

47. Hsu CY, Halushka PV, Hogan EL, et al: Alteration of thromboxane and prostacyclin levels in experimental spinal cord injury. *Neurology* 35:1003, 1985.

48. Iacopina VJ, Fitzpatrick TM, Ramwell RW, Rose JC, Kot PA: Cardiovascular response to leukotriene C₄ in the rat. *J Pharmacol Exp Ther* 227:224, 1983.

49. Johnston HH, Herzog JP, Lauler DP: Effect of prostaglandin E₁ on renal hemodynamics, sodium and water excretion. *Am J Physiol* 213:939, 1967.

50. Keppler D, Hagmann W, Rapp S, Denzlinger C, Koch H: The relation of leukotrienes to liver injury. *Hepatology* 5:883, 1985.

51. Kapsch DN, Metzler M, Silver D: Contributions of

prostaglandin F and Thromboxane A₂ to the acute cardiopulmonary changes of pulmonary embolism. *J Surg Res* 30(5):522, 1981.

52. Kiwak KJ, Moskowitz MA, Levine L: Leukotriene production in gerbil brain after ischemic insult, subarachnoid hemorrhage, and concussive injury. *J Neurosurg* 62:865, 1985.

53. Konturek SJ, Pawlik, MD: Physiology and pharmacology of prostaglandins. *Digestive Dis Sci* 31(2):65, 1986.

54. Konturek SJ, Robert A, Haucher AJ, et al: Comparison of prostacyclin and prostaglandins E₂ on gastric secretions, gastric release, and mucosal flow in dogs. *Digestive Dis Sci* 25:673, 1980.

55. Konturek SJ, Tasler J, Kwiecien N, et al: Mechanism of inhibitory action of prostaglandin on mean induced gastric secretions. *Digestion* 17:281, 1978.

56. Kreger BE, Craveb DE, Carling PC, et al: Gram-negative bacteremia III. Reassessment of etiology, epidemiology and ecology in 612 patients. *Am J Med* 68:332, 1980.

57. Kreutner W, Siegal MI: Biology of leukotrienes. *Ann Rep Med Chem* 19:241, 1984.

58. Lee CT, Fein AM, Lippmann ML, Holzmann H, Kimbel P, Weinbaum G: Elastolytic activity in pulmonary lavage fluid from patients with adult respiratory distress syndrome. *N Engl J Med* 304:192, 1981.

59. Leeman M, Boeynaems J, Degaute J, Vincent J, Kahn RJ: Administration of dazoxiben, a selective thromboxane synthetase inhibitor, in the adult respiratory distress syndrome. *Chest* 87:726, 1985.

60. Lelcuk S, Alexander F, Kobbzik L, et al: Prostacyclin and thromboxane A₂ moderate post-ischemic renal failure. *Surgery* 98:207, 1985.

61. Leslie JB, Watkins WD: Eicosanoids in the central nervous system. *J Neurosurg* 63:659, 1985.

62. Lewis RA, Drazen JM, Austen KF, et al: Identification of the C(6)-S-conjugate of leukotriene A with cysteine as a naturally-occurring slow reaction substance of anaphylaxis (SRS-A): Importance of the 11-*cis*-geometry of biological activity. *Biochem Biophs Commun* 95:271, 1980.

63. Ligumsky M, Karmel R, Rachmilewitz D: Sucralfate stimulation of gastric PGE₂ synthesis. *Gastroenterology* 86:1164, 1984.

64. Matthay MA, Eschenbacker WL, Goetzel EJ: Elevated concentrations of leukotriene D₄ in pulmonary edema fluid of patients with the adult respiratory distress syndrome. *J Clin Immunol* 4:479, 1984.

65. McCabe WR: Gram-negative bacteremia. *Adv Intern Med* 19:135, 1974.

66. Michalassi F, Landa L, Hill RD, Lowenstein E, Watkins WD, Petkau AJ, Zapol WM: Leukotriene D₄: A potent coronary artery vasoconstrictor associated with impaired ventricular contraction. *Science* 217:841, 1982.

67. Miller TA, Jacobsen ED: Gastrointestinal cyto-protection by prostaglandins. *Gut* 20:75, 1979.

68. Miller VT, Coull BM, Tatso SM, et al: Prostacyclin infusion in acute cerebral infarction. *Neurology* 34:1431, 1984.

69. Modig J: Adult respiratory distress syndrome pathogenesis and treatment. *Acta Chir Scand* 152:241, 1986.

70. Moncada S. Higgs GA, Vane JR: Human arterial and venous tissues generate prostacyclin (glandin x), a potent inhibitor of platelet aggregation. *Lancet* 1:18, 1977.

71. Moncada S, Vane JR: Pharmacology and endogenous roles of prostaglandin, endoperoxides, thromboxane A₂ and prostacyclin. *Pharmacol Rev* 30:293, 1979.

72. Moskowitz MA, Kiwak KJ, Hekimian K, et al: Synthesis of compounds with properties of leukotrienes C₄ and D₄ in gerbil brains after ischemia and reperfusion. *Science* 224:886, 1984.

73. Nagy L, Lee TH, Goetzl EJ, Pickett WC, Kay AB: Compliment receptor enhancement and chemotaxis of human neutrophils and eosinophils by leukotrienes and

other lipoxygenase products. *Clin Exp Immunol* 47:541, 1982.

74. Neutze JM, Starling MB, Elliott RB, et al: Palliation of cyanotic congenital heart disease in infancy with E-type prostaglandins. *Circulation* 55(2):238, 1977.

75. Oettinger WKE, Walker GO, Jensen UM, Beyer A, Peskar A: Endogenous prostaglandin F_2 in the hyperdynamic state of severe sepsis in man. *Br J Surg* 70:237, 1983.

76. O'Flaherty JT, Hammett MJ, Shewmake TB, Wykl RL, Love SH, McCall CE, Thomas MJ: Evidence of 5,12-dihydroxy-6,819,14-eicostatetraenoate as a mediator of human neutrophil aggregation. *Biochem Biophy Res Commun* 103:552, 1981.

77. Okada M, Nagao S, Imai S: Effects of cimetidine on prostaglandin level and blood flow of gastric mucosa. Presented at the 12th International Congress of Gastroenterology, Lisbon, Portugal, September 1984.

78. Popat KD, Pitt B: Hemodynamic effects of prostaglandin E_1 infusion in patients with acute myocardial infarction and left ventricular failure. *Am Heart J* 103:485, 1982.

79. Pugliese F, Ciabattoni G: The role of prostaglandins in the control of renal function: renal effects of nonsteroidal anti-inflammatory drugs. *Clin Exp Rheumatol* 2:345, 1984.

80. Reines HD, Halushka PV, Cook JA, Loadholt CB: Lack of effect of glucocorticoids upon plasma thromboxane in patients in a state of shock. *Surg Gynecol Obstet* 160:320, 1985.

81. Reines HD, Halushka PV, Cook JA, Wise WC, Rambo W: Plasma thromboxane concentrations are raised in patients dying with septic shock. *Lancet* 24: 174, 1982.

82. Reines HD, Halushka PV, Olanoff LS, Hunt PS: Dazoxiben in human sepsis and adult respiratory distress syndrome. *Clin Pharmacol Ther* 37:391, 1985.

83. Rie M, Peterson M, Kong D, Quinn D, Watkins D: Plasma prostacyclin increases during acute human sepsis. *Circ Shock* 10:232, 1983.

84. Robert A: Cyto-protection by prostaglandins. *Gastroenterology* 77:761, 1979.

85. Robertson RM, Robertson D, Roberts LJ, et al: Thromboxane A_2 in vasotonic angina pectoris. *N Engl J Med* 304(17):998, 1981.

86. Roth DM, Lefer AM: Mechanism of the constrictor action of leukotrienes in cat coronary arteries. *Pharmacologist* 24:142, 1983.

87. Rudolph AM, Heymann MA: Medical treatment of the ductus arteriosus. *Hosp Prac* 57, 1977.

88. Samuelson B: Leukotrienes: mediators of immediate hypersensitivity reactions and inflammation. *Science* 220:568, 1983.

89. Schror K, Smith EF III, Bickerton M, et al: Preservation of ischemic myocardium by pinane thromboxane A_2. *Am J Physiol* 238:H87, 1980.

90. Shoemaker WC, Appel PL: Effects of prostaglandin E_1 in adult respiratory distress syndrome. *Surgery* 90:279, 1986.

91. Skillman JJ, Lisbon A, Long PC, et al: 15(R)-15 methyl prostaglandin E_2 does not prevent gastrointestinal bleeding in seriously ill patients. *Am J Surg* 147:451, 1984.

92. Slotman GJ, Burchard KW, Williams J, D'Arezzo A, Yellin SA: Interaction of prostaglandins, activated compliment and granulocytes in clinical sepsis and hypotension. *Surgery* 99:744, 1986.

93. Slotman GJ, D'Arezzo A, Burchard KW, Gann DS: Ketoconazole prevents acute respiratory failure in critically ill surgical patients. *J Trauma* 26:684, 1986 (abstract).

94. Slotman GJ, Machiedo GW, Casey KF, et al: The hemodynamic effects of prostaglandin E_1 (PGE_1) in acute hypoxic respiratory failure. *Adv Shock Res* 3:283, 1980.

95. Sprung CL, Caralis PV and, Marical EH, et al: The effects of high-dose corticosteroids in patients with septic shock: a prospective, controlled study. *N Engl J Med* 311:1137, 1984.

96. Stenmark KR, James SL, Voelkel NF, Toews WH, Reeves JT, Murphy RC: Leukotriene C_4 and D_4 in neonates with hypoxemia and pulmonary hypertension. *N Engl J Med* 309:77, 1983.

97. Svenson J, Fredholm BB: Vasoconstriction effect of thromboxane A_2. *Acta Physiol Scand* 101:366, 1977.

98. Swerdlow BN, Mihm FG, Goetzl EJ, Matthay MA: Leukotrienes in pulmonary edema fluid after cardiopulmonary bypass. *Anesth Analog* 65:306, 1986.

99. Takajoth U, Kraus M, Valeri CR, et al: Treatment of pulmonary embolism with prostacyclin. *Surgery* 88:25, 1980.

100. Uiehara N, Ormastaf K, Ornig L, Hammerstrom S: Characteristics of the uptake of cysteine-containing leukotrienes by isolated hepatocytes. *Biochem Biophys Acta* 732:69.

101. Utsunomiya T, Krausz MU, Levine L, et al: Thromboxane mediation of cardiopulmonary effects of embolism. *J Clin Invest* 70:361, 1982.

102. Van Essen HA, van Blankenstein M, Wilson HP, et al: Intragastric prostaglandin E_2 and the prevention of gastrointestinal hemorrhage in ICU patients. *Crit Care Med* 13(11):957, 1985.

103. Waite M: Approaches to the study of mammalian cellular phospholipases. *J Lipid Res* 26:1379.

104. Weksler BB, Pett SB, Alonso D, et al: Differential inhibition by aspirin of vascular and platelet prostaglandin synthesis in atherosclerotic patients. *N Engl J Med* 308(14):800, 1983.

105. Wolff SM, Bennet JV: Gram-negative bacteremia (editorial). *N Engl J Med* 291:733, 1974.

39

Poisoning

Glenn C. Freas, M.D., F.A.C.E.P.

Mortality from poisoning ranges from 5,000 to 12,000 deaths per year (20, 67). Accidents are the leading cause of death in Americans up to age 40. In this category, poisoning is outranked only by motor vehicle fatalities. Suicide from poisoning is the second leading cause of death among adolescents and young adults (46). Current estimates attribute 1% to 10% of all emergency room visits to poisoning (46). Roughly 15% of all ICU admissions are for acute poisoning (8). Only a minority of poisoned patients presenting to a hospital are cared for in a critical care setting since less than 15% of self-poisonings result in changes in level of consciousness (21). The overall mortality rate from poisoning in hospitalized patients is low, less than 1% of admitted patients (28). Preschoolers (children less than 5 years of age) tend to be victims of accidental, nontoxic ingestions or exposures. Ingestion in older patients is more likely to be purposeful and toxic. Data from the National Clearinghouse for Poison Control Centers in 1978 revealed that only 2% of poisoned preschoolers required hospitalization, and preschoolers were involved in only 9% of fatal poisonings. The 1978 NCPCC data show that the mode of poisoning was accidental in only 36% of cases involving the older population, as opposed to essentially 100% of cases in preschoolers (46).

Carbon monoxide, alcohols, acetaminophen, opioids, salicylates, sedative-hypnotics, psychotherapeutic agents, cardiac glycosides, β-blockers, and anticonvulsants account for the large majority of poisoning deaths and ICU admissions in this country (20, 90). Carbon monoxide is the most common cause of death by poisoning.

PHARMACOLOGY

Poisons may be inhaled, injected, absorbed through the skin and mucous membranes, and ingested. Many drugs can be used and abused via all four routes. The pharmacokinetics of drugs or toxins taken in toxic doses may be much different than when taken in therapeutic dosages. Absorption, distribution, metabolism, and excretion may all be altered by an overdose (137).

Many poisons can alter absorption rates by delaying gastric emptying; this is especially true of drugs that possess anticholinergic properties. Delayed absorption may have some indirect benefit in the poisoned patient because most drugs are not absorbed in the stomach but in the small intestine. Many authors advocate inducing emesis or gastric lavage even several hours after ingestion because of this delay in gastric emptying (19).

This concept of gastric emptying as one of the determinants of intestinal absorption rates is important when considering the use of dilutents, with or without syrup of ipecac. When copious fluids are given in an effort to dilute a poison or to follow a dose of ipecac, gastric emptying may be increased because of gastric distention. Animal studies demonstrate that the oral lethal dose of a variety of drugs is decreased as the volume of diluent is increased (48). These considerations make judicious use of fluids (limited to 8–10 oz in adults or 5 ml/kg of body weight in children) imperative when used as a diluent or "chaser" for ipecac.

Enterohepatic circulation plays a major role in drug overdoses. Recent reports indicate that repeated doses of orally administered activated charcoal increase clearance of certain agents from the systemic circulation. The proposed mechanism is adsorption of drug that has passively diffused or has been actively secreted from the systemic circulation into the gastrointestinal tract. This mode of therapy is called "gastrointestinal dialysis" (95).

Many drugs are eliminated by first-order kinetics in which the amount of drug eliminated is directly proportional to the concentration of that drug. Zero-order kinetics (e.g., the amount of drug eliminated is constant and independent of drug concentration) may result if enzyme systems are saturated. Methanol, ethanol, salicylates, and phenytoin exhibit zero order or saturation kinetics at all clinically important blood concentrations (4).

The reader is referred to other sources for a more indepth discussion of the pharmacology of poisoning (6). Concepts such as solubility, volume of distribution, protein binding, and active metabolites have important implications for the clinician. The choice of interventional means such as hemodialysis or hemoperfusion is based on these concepts. Later in this chapter, in the discussion of specific poisons, significant pharmacologic characteristics will be addressed as they relate to management of each toxin.

RESUSCITATION AND STABILIZATION

In most cases the intensivist assumes care for the poisoned patient when the patient is transferred from the emergency room to the intensive care setting. It is imperative that all prior therapy, intervention, and perhaps aborted attempts at intervention be carefully reviewed once the patient is admitted to the ICU. In the vast majority of poisoned patients nonspecific supportive therapy is all that is necessary to assure complete recovery. Some basic points about resuscitation bear re-emphasizing.

Airway

Poisoned patients may lose their ability to protect their airway rather rapidly. Obtundation, hypoventilation, a weak or absent gag reflex, signs of airway obstruction, or associated maxillofacial injuries all warrant immediate management with nasotracheal or orotracheal intubation. Aspiration of gastric contents is the most frequent complication of poisoning (127). Nasotracheal intubation, if possible, is preferable because it is better tolerated by the semiconscious patient and it allows easier access for eventual placement of a large-bore orogastric tube.

A question often arises regarding airway protection for the patient who is not a candidate for ipecac (and who consequently requires gastric lavage), yet who is responsive enough to fight insertion of a nasotracheal tube.

Although some might consider paralysis with succinylcholine prior to intubation and lavage, this approach may be hazardous. Succinylcholine may affect the ingested toxin; for example, succinylcholine may produce cardiac arrhythmias and obscure the clinical picture in tricyclic antidepressant overdose (69). A safer approach would be to attempt nasotracheal intubation without the use of succinylcholine. Should patients be so combative as to inflict harm on themselves or the staff, one can cease attempts at intubation and observe the patient carefully during insertion of the orogastric tube and subsequent lavage.

Breathing

Proper oxygenation is required to meet metabolic needs (often increased by seizures, hyperpyrexia, etc.) and is specifically therapeutic in the treatment of toxins such as carbon monoxide, which interferes with the transport of oxygen. In paraquat poisoning tissue damage is mediated by superoxide ions. In this type of poisoning, supplemental oxygen should be avoided (47). Supplementing a hypoventilating patient's respirations with a bag-valve-mask for prolonged periods is to be discouraged because it may overdistend the stomach and result in vomiting and aspiration. Respiratory rate, effort, and breath sounds must be constantly reassessed. Noncardiogenic pulmonary edema or direct gaseous toxins may complicate pulmonary function.

Circulation

Maintenance of adequate end organ perfusion requires that intravascular volume, cardiac function, and systemic vascular resistance be controlled. Hypotension on admission is the most important prognostic factor for mortality in severe poisoning (3). Even if normotensive initially, at least one large-bore intravenous line should be inserted to provide venous access should hypotension later develop. Direct arterial monitoring and measurements of pulmonary capillary wedge pressures may need to be initiated in the patient whose fluid management is complex. Use of pressor agents should be reserved until failure of fluid resuscitation is clearly demonstrated; toxins that cause hypotension by venous pooling far outnumber the agents, such as propranolol, that might cause myocardial depression (46).

Other Stabilizing Measures

All patients with a depressed sensorium or in coma should receive naloxone hydrochloride in an initial intravenously administered dosage of at least 0.8 mg (two ampules). This specific narcotic antagonist will reverse the central nervous system depression associated with the overdose of opiates as well as other drugs. Larger doses and repeated doses may be necessary to achieve or maintain the desired response. All patients with a depressed sensorium should also receive 50 g of dextrose intravenously if indicated by a spot, bedside glucose determination. Thiamine 100 mg, intravenous or intramuscular, should be given prior to or concomitant with dextrose to prevent the development of Wernicke-Korsakoff syndrome in the patient who may be severely thiamine depleted (67).

DIAGNOSIS

The history may be unreliable in the poisoned patient as a result of drug induced confusion, amnesia, misinformation (particularly important in recreational drug overdoses), and deliberate attempts at deception (68). Despite these handicaps the physician must elicit as much information from as many sources as possible. Family, friends, emergency department personnel, pre-hospital-care providers, pharmacists, bystanders, and police can be contacted and significant historical clues can emerge, even when the patient is comatose. It is incumbent upon the physician to determine what toxin (or toxins) is involved, the mode of exposure, the amount ingested, the time since ingestion, and the circumstances surrounding the overdose. One should also attempt to determine coexisting medical, surgical, or psychiatric conditions, current medications, and any drug allergies. If applicable, an occupational and vocational history should be obtained.

The aim of the physical examination is to detect signs that may lead to a determination of the type and severity of poisoning, as well as evidence of underlying systemic disease or trauma. Additionally, the intensivist must look for complications of therapy that may have occurred in the pre-hospital-care setting or the emergency room.

Particular attention should be paid to vital signs, the integument, the cardiopulmonary system, the abdomen, the neurologic examination, and products of secretion and excretion. Patients may be profoundly hypothermic due to prolonged periods of exposure and inactivity as well as prolonged resuscitation and stabilization. Temperature elevation may be due to specific poisons (salicylates or anticholinergics) or related to coexistent medical problems producing a fever.

Many severely poisoned patients will have alterations in blood pressure, heart rate, and respiratory rate. These must be followed closely and appropriate therapy initiated when indicated by the clinical picture.

Along with a general description of the patient and vital signs, the examiner should note any characteristic odors on the patient's breath. The breath may smell like alcohol (e.g., ethanol, methanol, ethylene glycol), gasoline (hydrocarbons),or fruit (diabetic ketoacidosis or alcoholic ketoacidosis).

Fresh or old, scarred needle puncture or "tracks" suggest intravenous drug abuse. Cutaneous bullae may be seen in barbiturate, glutethamide, and carbon monoxide poisoning (69). Diaphoresis may be due to salicylates or organophosphates. Hot, dry skin may be characteristic of anticholinergic poisoning, as well as severe heat stroke. Cyanosis may be due to oxidizing agents that cause methemaglobinemia.

A whole host of poisons may cause noncardiogenic pulmonary edema and a wide variety of toxins can cause alterations in cardiac function. In the intravenous drug abuser with a cardiac murmur, the examiner should think of endocarditis with embolic phenomenon as a source for persistent neurologic signs. In hydrocarbon ingestion, the onset of wheezing or rales may precede the development of chest x-ray findings.

The abdominal examination should focus on the presence or absence of bowel sounds, presence of involuntary guarding, evidence of urinary retention, and the presence of signs such as hepatomegaly and/or splenomegaly that may signify chronic alcohol abuse or other medical conditions. In the poisoned trauma victim with changes in mental status the abdominal examination can be unreliable as an indicator of a potential surgical problem. In most cases further investigation by peritoneal lavage or abdominal imaging techniques will be necessary.

A careful neurological examination is mandatory. Serial determinations of level of consciousness by a standardized evaluation system or by the same examiner is invaluable.

Changes in level of consciousness not consistent with the suspected ingestion should lead the examiner to further investigate other possible etiologies. Pinpoint pupils suggest either a pontine lesion or use of opiates, organophosphates, phenothiazines, or chloral hydrate. Midpoint or dilated pupils are less specific. Extraocular movements and the presence of nystagmus should be examined and noted. Ingestion of PCP may cause nystagmus. Testing the cranial nerves and checking the gag reflex are mandatory. The presence of focal neurological findings is highly suggestive of a structural lesion and further investigation is warranted, it is re-emphasized that repeated neurological examinations may detect expanding masses (e.g., hemorrhage) or evolving metabolic abnormalities.

Finally, attention to secretory and excretory products may yield characteristic findings. Salivation, lacrimation, urination, and defecation (SLUD) are characteristic of muscarinic signs of anticholinesterase poisoning (63). On the other hand, anticholinergic agents can cause dry mouth, urinary retention, and decreased gastrointestinal motility.

Careful and selective use of laboratory tests can be extremely valuable. An indiscriminate "shotgun" approach or delaying therapy while awaiting results can be disastrous. In general, any severely poisoned patient should have blood collected for hemoglobin, hematocrit, blood counts, serum electrolytes, blood urea nitrogen, creatinine, glucose, prothrombin time, and arterial blood gases. A urine analysis should also be obtained. Depending on the clinical scenario, other commonly needed studies include a carboxyhemaglobin, serum ketones, serum osmolality, and liver function studies. Specific laboratory abnormalities will be discussed in the sections dealing with individual poisons.

Judicious use of the toxicology lab can help confirm a suspected diagnosis. In most cases a qualitative urine screen is sufficient for the poisoned patient. If positive, it confirms the suspected diagnosis and may add additional unsuspected information. If negative, it suggests the presence of another etiology.

Quantitative drug concentrations are essential in the management of some toxins. These include acetaminophen, digoxin, ethanol, methanol, ethylene glycol, carbon monoxide, salicylates, iron, lead, and lithium. If a toxic blood level is reported by the laboratory but is not supported by the clinical picture, the level should be repeated before instituting specific treatment based on that result.

Tablets that are radiopaque on x-ray flat plate of the abdomen include chloral-hydrate, heavy metals (arsenic, lead, iron), iodides, psychotropics (phenothiazines and tricyclics), and enteric-coated tablets. ECGs, while nonspecific, can have some important therapeutic considerations in certain overdoses such as tricyclic antidepressants. Since many poisons can complicate pulmonary function (e.g., cause pulmonary edema or aspiration pneumonitis) a chest x-ray is a valuable adjunct as well.

DRUG REMOVAL

Once the patient is stabilized and diagnostic measures have been undertaken the focus of therapy shifts to removal of the offending agent(s). This goal can be accomplished by decreasing absorption of the poison and hastening its elimination.

While the vast majority of poisons are ingested and absorbed via the gastrointestinal tract, it bears emphasizing that some toxins are absorbed in other ways and it is necessary to decontaminate any portal of entry. When the portal of entry is dermal, it is imperative that all clothing be removed and the skin washed so as to prevent continued absorption.

Measures to Decrease Absorption

Spontaneous emesis often occurs with such substances as theophylline, iron, and salicylates. This is probably not an efficacious way of decontaminating the gastrointestinal tract, and the clinician should not let an episode of spontaneous emesis deter further attempts to empty the upper part of the gastrointestinal tract (44). Mechanically induced emesis (e.g., tongue blade, finger) is likewise ineffective in emptying the stomach (35).

Induced emesis is most frequently accomplished with either ipecac syrup or apomorphine. Ipecac is the agent of choice for most clinicians. The best candidate for induced emesis is the awake, alert, cooperative patient who demonstrates an intact gag reflex. Contraindications to induced emesis include coma, manifest or incipient seizures, loss of a gag reflex, ingestion of a caustic agent, or ingestion of a hydrocarbon where the risk of aspiration outweighs the risk of systemic toxicity if intestinal absorption is permitted (46).

Syrup of ipecac is derived from the dried root of *Cephaelis ipecacuanha*. The principle alkaloids producing emesis are emetine and cephaline. Both agents exert central effects on the medulla's chemoreceptor trigger zone, as well as a local irritant effect on the gastric mucosa. Fluid extract of ipecac is no longer used. It is 14 times more concentrated than syrup of ipecac, and it caused a variety of cardiovascular complications.

Recommended doses of ipecac are 10 ml for children under 1 year of age, 15 ml for children 1–12 years of age, and 30 ml for those over 12 years of age. This dose should be followed by 8–12 oz of water in adults or 5 ml of water per kilogram of body weight in children (165). In more than 90% of cases, emesis will ensue within 30 minutes (98). If emesis has not occurred within 30 minutes the dose of ipecac may be repeated. A recent prospective study showed that the use of syrup of ipecac in the 9- to 12-month-old child appears to be safe and effective (57).

Most authorities caution against the simultaneous use of ipecac and activated charcoal. The proposed reasoning is that activated charcoal significantly absorbs the ipecac and thus decreases its efficacy. In a recent, small prospective study, administration of activated charcoal 10 minutes after ipecac (and prior to emesis) found no significant decrease in the ability of ipecac to produce emesis. After emesis subsided, a repeat dose of charcoal was given (53). These results take on significant implications when one considers the recent recommendations that activated charcoal be given as rapidly as possible (discussed below). Ipecac is effective when administered to patients who have ingested an overdose of antiemetics (161).

Apomorphine is a morphine congener that acts by stimulating the medullary chemoreceptor trigger zone. It is unstable in solution and only effective when used parenterally. Thus, a tablet must be crushed and dissolved to create a fresh, stable solution. Apomorphine causes respiratory depression and CNS sedation, which can be reversed with naloxone (39). Because of the inconvenience in preparation and its CNS sedation and respiratory depression, apormorphine is not used extensively.

Gastric lavage is an alternate method for preventing absorption of toxin from the gastrointestinal tract. It is commonly employed when the need to empty the stomach is present but the patient does not meet the criteria for induced emesis or in the rare case where ipecac (two doses) has not produced emesis. Contraindications to gastric lavage include caustic ingestions, hydrocarbon poisoning, and lack of ability to protect the airway (46).

A large-bore gastric tube of at least 36-F diameter should be used and the stomach lavaged with 4 ml/kg/cycle to a maximum of 200 ml/cycle of fluid. The patient should be on the left side to pool gastric contents in the fundus, tilted head down to deter aspiration, and turned slightly on the stomach. Lavage should be continued until the gastric return is "clear" but this approach does not guarantee removal of dissolved toxin (138). Protection of the airway is important during lavage. Repeated assessments of the level of consciousness and the presence of a gag reflex are mandatory.

The use of tap water is advocated by many. It is just as efficacious as saline solutions, can be warmed easily, causes no demonstrable electrolyte imbalances in adults, and is much less expensive (138). Use of saline when lavaging children is advocated by some because it is less likely than tap water to produce electrolyte imbalances. In selected cases it may be advantageous to modify the lavage fluid. In cases of oxalate poisoning it is useful to add calcium to the lavage fluid to precipitate these ions. In poisoning with enteric-coated tablets or with iron it is useful to use a bicarbonate solution (152). In glutethamide overdose it is recommended that a lavage solution of castor oil and water be used.

An age-old debate in clinical toxicology is the question of the comparative efficacy of gastric lavage and induced emesis in gastrointestinal decontamination. This question is still unresolved. The clinician must tailor his approach to the clinical setting. Effective results from induced emesis or gastric lavage might take anywhere from 30 minutes to 2 hours. One prospective study showed that gastric-emptying procedures in the emergency room were not of benefit unless gastric lavage was performed within 1 hour of ingestion in obtunded patients (90).

Large pill concretions, which are resistant to easy removal via traditional gastric emptying methods, can form in the stomach. Successful removal of tablets of meprobamate, ferrous sulfate, and aspirin has been accomplished by endoscopy or removal of the mass via gastrotomy (100). These techniques should be reserved for the patient in whom ongoing absorption of the poison from the concretion is deleterious and cannot be prevented by repeated doses of activated charcoal.

Activated charcoal is formed by burning such substances as wood, bone, starch, and other organic substances. The residue is "activated" by treatment with superheated steam or with other chemicals to remove any adsorbed substances and to increase the surface area available for adsorption. When charcoal is used in poisoning, the quantity of drug adsorbed at equilibrium is proportional to the amount of internal surface area. There is a wide variety of commercially available activated charcoal preparations, and they vary in their adsorption capacity. Activated Charcoal Merck, Norit A, and Nuchar C are the most efficient commercial preparations (89).

Activated charcoal is administered orally as a suspension, or alternately the suspension can be instilled via an orogastric tube (after lavage) or via a nasogastric tube (after induced emesis). The desired ratio of activated charcoal to ingested toxin is 10:1. However, the amount of poison is frequently unknown. For most adults, 50–100 g in 8 oz of water creates the desired slurry. For children, 20–50 g is recommended, depending on age and habitus. Activated charcoal is nontoxic and completely inert if aspirated. The sooner charcoal is administered, the more efficacious it is for preventing absorption of toxin (96). Activated charcoal is poorly tolerated orally, and it may be necessary to insert a small-bore nasogastric tube (which is left in place when repeated doses are necessary) for installation of the slurry. This method saves precious time and nursing efforts.

Activated charcoal should be withheld when N-acetylcysteine is going to be administered for the treatment of acetaminophen overdose. This approach is based on the assumption that activated charcoal will adsorb this antidote. Although a recent study has challenged this assumption, the recommendation to withhold charcoal in this situation should stand until further in vivo studies are completed (138).

Repeated doses of activated charcoal are advised for those toxins that undergo enterogastric or enterohepatic recirculation. This method of enhancing gastrointestinal clearance by activated charcoal has been termed "gastrointestinal dialysis" (95). Drugs amenable to this form of treatment include phenobarbital and cyclic antidepressants and related compounds, phenylbutazone, digitoxin, theophylline, glutethimide, and meprobamate (32, 50, 73). Rec-

ommended doses for this purpose are 50 g every 2–6 hours for four doses. Charcoal is not efficacius in treatment of poisoning with cyanide, lithium, iron, alkalies, or mineral acids.

Measures to Enhance Elimination

The administration of cathartics to hasten elimination of both adsorbed toxin and free toxin has traditionally been advocated. Commonly used agents are sodium sulfate, magnesium sulfate, or magnesium citrate. However, there have been no clinical studies confirming that catharsis decreases the total adsorption of an ingested toxin (44). On the other hand, there are many reports of complications related to cathartic therapy, including a case report of profound cathartic-induced magnesium toxicity (86).

Clinical studies on cathartics have examined only immediate-release dosage forms of potential poisons. Studies need to be done which evaluate the effect of rapid catharsis on the bioavailability of sustained-release preparations such as theophylline or delayed-release, enteric-coated products. Recommended doses of cathartics in these situations is 15–30 g of magnesium citrate in adults and 250 mg/kg in pediatric patients. Cathartics should not be used in the very young, the patient who may have an ileus, the patient in renal failure, or the patient in whom fluid and electrolyte balance is problematic.

Fluid loading and forced diuresis may help eliminate toxic agents from the body but may also lead to complications that include electrolyte disturbance, acid-base disorders, cerebral edema, and pulmonary edema.

The following general criteria should be considered before instituting forced diuresis: (a) renal excretion of the unchanged drug is the major route of elimination, (b) the drug is extensively reabsorbed in the renal tubules, and (c) the drug is distributed mainly in the extracellular fluid compartment and is minimally protein bound.

Cell membranes are relatively impermeable to ionized (polar) molecules, whereas nonionized (nonpolar) molecules can easily cross cell membranes. By increasing the ratio of ionized to nonionized drug by altering urine pH, less drug is available for absorption through cell membranes.

Alkalinization of urine is achieved with sodium bicarbonate, 1 to 2 mEg/kg intravenously every 3–4 hours. Maintenance of a urinary pH of 7.5–8.5 is desired and the amount of bicarbonate administered is guided by this endpoint. A urine flow of 5 ml/kg/hour is desired. Toxins amenable to alkaline diuresis are salicylates and barbiturates (156, 97). Cyclic antidepressant poisoning is treated with systemic alkalinization (but not forced diuresis).

Acid diuresis is usually accomplished with ammonium chloride (either orally or intravenously). Hydration is maintained with 5% dextrose in saline. Ammonium chloride, 4 g every 2 hours orally or a 1–2% solution in normal saline intravenously, should be given to maintain a urinary pH of 5.5–6 (171). Forced acid diuresis can increase the excretion of phencyclidine, amphetamines, quinine, fenfluramine, and quinidine (171, 128).

Hemoperfusion or hemodialysis is indicated (171, 128) when (a) progressive deterioration of the patient occurs despite careful and intensive supportive care, (b) severe clinical intoxication occurs with abnormal vital signs signifying depression of midbrain functioning, (c) the compound ingested has been absorbed or ingested in a potentially lethal dose, (d) a blood or plasma concentration of the compound is in the lethal range, (e) there is impairment of the patient's normal excretory capacity for eliminating the ingested poison, or (f) the drug ingested can be removed at a rate that exceeds the endogenous elimination by the liver or kidneys.

Drugs that can effectively be removed by hemodialysis include ethylene glycol (124), methanol (102), lithium (171), salicylates (77), and ethanol (171). Drugs in which hemoperfusion plays a role in active removal include quinine (109); isopropyl alcohol (9); diquat (171); barbiturates (195); digitalis glycosides; tricyclic antidepressants (188); other lipid soluble drugs (171); and nonbarbiturate hypnotics, sedatives, and tranquilizers (171).

SPECIFIC TOXINS

Acetaminophen

Acetaminophen is currently available in more than 250 pharmaceutical products in the United States (25). Cases of acute hepatocellular necrosis in association with paracetamol (acetaminophen) overdoses were reported in 1966 (38). Two-hundred patients die every year from acetaminophen overdose in the United Kingdom, where the drug is the leading cause of acute hepatic necrosis (75). In the United States

the incidence of poisoning from acetaminophen overdose is rising, and in some areas may constitute 10–12% of patients who are admitted for poisoning (141).

Acetaminophen is primarily metabolized to glucuronide and sulfate conjugates, which are nontoxic. A small proportion of the parent compound (about 4%) is metabolized by the cytochrome P-450 dependent, mixed function oxidase enzymes to a poorly described reactive intermediate (105). With therapeutic doses of acetaminophen this intermediate is detoxified by conjugation with glutathione and excreted by the kidney as cysteine and mercapturate metabolites of acetaminophen (79). However, when acetaminophen is given in toxic doses, glutathione becomes depleted and the hepatotoxic metabolite cannot be adequately detoxified. The metabolite binds to sulfhydryl groups in hepatic intracellular proteins and causes acute, widespread hepatocyte death (19). Acetylcysteine can prevent this process. N-acetylcysteine is metabolized to cysteine, a glutathione precursor, thereby providing additional glutathione for use in the detoxification of acetaminophen metabolite (139).

Toxic ingestion of acetaminophen is characterized by four clinical stages (139). Stage 1 occurs 12–24 hours after ingestion and is typified by nausea, vomiting, diaphoresis, and anorexia. There may be some patients with few symptoms in this stage, even after ingesting large amounts. Stage 2 occurs 1–2 days after ingestion. Typically the previous stage's symptoms abate, however, liver enzymes and prothrombin time begin to rise. Some right upper quadrant pain and tenderness may develop at the end of this stage. Stage 3 develops 3 days postingestion and correlates with peak hepatotoxicity. This phase is characterized by jaundice, coagulopathy, hypoglycemia, encephalophathy, and occasionally renal failure and cardiomyopathy. The SGOT may reach 20,000 IU or more, and in one case the SGOT reached 321,900 IU (145). Stage 4 occurs 7–8 days after ingestion and is the recovery stage for patients who survive.

Treatment of acetaminophen overdose is centered around N-acetylcysteine. Treatment is most effective with N-acetylcysteine when it is administered within 16 hours after acetaminophen ingestion. Current recommendations are to institute treatment if the ingestion occurred within 24 hours. Use of a nomogram (Fig. 39.1) to guide therapy requires that plasma levels be drawn at least 4 hours after ingestion. It is important to note that nonspecific colori-

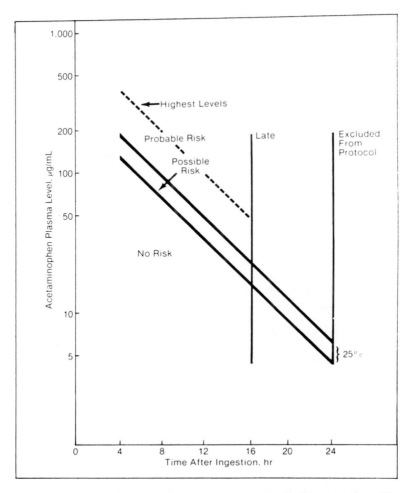

Figure 39.1. Revised nomogram for estimating toxicity from acetaminophen overdose. (From Rumack BH, Peterson RG, Koch GG, Amara IA: Acetaminophen overdose: 662 cases with evaluation of oral acetylcysteine treatment. *Arch Intern Med* 141:380, 1981. Copyright 1981, American Medical Association.)

metric assays may underestimate acetaminophen levels by as much as 700% (123). If levels are not readily available, starting treatment with N-acetylcysteine is advised until a plasma level can be obtained. If a pretreatment plasma level is in the nontoxic range then treatment can be stopped. If a previously toxic plasma level becomes nontoxic during therapy, treatment should continue for the full course of therapy. Most authorities agree that 7.5 g of acetaminophen represents a toxic dose in adults and 150 mg/kg represents a toxic dose in children. Because of inaccuracies in some patient's histories, it is best to draw a level (at least 4 hours postingestion), start therapy, and continue or stop treatment based on the pretreatment serum acetaminophen level.

N-acetylcysteine should be given after appropriate stabilizing measures have been accomplished. If activated charcoal has been instilled, it is recommended that the stomach be lavaged clear of charcoal prior to the first dose of N-acetylcysteine. An initial loading dose of 140 mg/kg is given orally. The solution is prepared by mixing one part (20%) N-acetylcysteine with three parts soda, or water, or grapefruit juice. This yields a 5% solution. Maintenance doses are 70 mg/kg administered every 4 hours for a total of 68 hours (17 doses). Intravenous N-acetylcysteine is used in the United Kingdom with good success. Currently, this is not available in the United States. Palatability of N-acetylcysteine is its major drawback. If the patient vomits less than 1 hour after ingestion of any dose of N-acetylcysteine, it should be repeated. An occasional patient will require placement of a duodenal tube for administration of the antidote.

Salicylates

Children make up the largest group of patients who present with salicylate poisoning (20, 156, 159). The most commonly encountered salicylates are acetylsalicylic acid (aspirin), sodium salicylate, and salicylic acid. A less common yet very concentrated form of salicylate is methyl salicylate (oil of wintergreen), which is a component of Ben-Gay. Oral ingestion of a little as 5 ml of oil of wintergreen is equivalent to 21 325-mg tablets of aspirin, a lethal dose in young children (22).

Salicylates follow zero-order kinetics; thus an increase in dose does not result in a linear increase in serum level. Rather, at saturation an increase in dose causes a higher than expected serum level. In addition, children's metabolic pathways are more rapidly saturated than adults (156).

The two major modes of presentation of severe salicylism are metabolic alterations and CNS manifestations. The biochemical actions responsible for the metabolic derangements include direct stimulation of the medullary respiratory center (respiratory alkalosis), uncoupling of oxidative phosphorylation, inhibition of amino acid metabolism, inhibition of Krebs Cycle enzymes, stimulation of gluconeogenesis, and inhibition of glycolysis (149). Metabolis acidosis predominates in young children (less than 4 yours of age) while respiratory alkalosis is more common in older children and in adults (130).

Neurologic disturbances such as confusion, delirium, and coma are the best clinical indications of severe intoxication (129). CNS toxicity is most frequently demonstrated in those patients in whom a picture of metabolic acidosis dominates (130). The acidosis is thought to favor a shift of salicylates from extracellular fluid into cells, particularly the brain (78). Additionally it is postulated that some CNS effects may be caused or exacerbated by a relatively hypoglycemic environment in the brain despite normal serum glucose levels.

Patients with mild toxicity typically show nausea and vomiting, tinnitus and other hearing disturbances, hyperpnea, respiratory alkalosis, and slight restlessness or lethargy. Those with moderate toxicity have more pronounced hyperpnea, fever, varying degrees of dehydration, metabolic acidosis, and marked lethargy and/or excitability. Severe toxicity can manifest as stupor, coma, seizures, severe metabolic acidosis, noncardiogenic pulmonary edema, renal failure, and hepatic failure (156, 159).

Severity of salicylate poisoning can be determined from a serum salicylate level (Fig. 39.2). The Done nomogram is only useful in estimating severity of acute poisoning. The serum level should be drawn at least 6 hours postingestion. Peak levels correlate best with toxicity (41). With ingestion of large amounts, or with ingestion of enteric-coated preparations, there may be prolonged absorption and levels may continue to rise for 24 hours after ingestion. Salicylate ingestion is also sug-

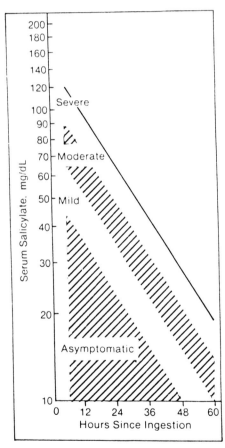

Figure 39.2. Nomogram for estimating the severity of poisoning form the serum salicylate level at varying intervals after ingestion of a single dose. (From Done AK: Salicylate intoxication. Significance of measurements of salicylate in blood in cases of acute ingestion. *Pediatrics* 26:800, 1960. Reproduced with permission of the publisher.)

gested by positive results on several qualitative screening tests. These include an increased anion gap, a positive urine Clinitest with a negative glucose oxidase strip test, and a positive ferric chloride test on a boiled sample of urine. Prior to return of the serum salicylate level, the severity of toxicity can be estimated as follows: (a) no toxic reaction if ingested dose is 150 mg/kg, (b) mild to moderate toxicity if ingested dose is 150 –300 mg/kg, (c) serious toxicity if ingested dose is 300–500 mg/kg, and (d) potentially lethal reaction if ingested dose is 500 mg/kg.

The diagnosis of chronic salicylism may be very difficult since typically symptoms are minimal and nonspecific. Many elderly patients undergo a neurologic workup for altered mental status before the diagnosis of chronic salicylism is entertained. Delayed diagnosis is associated with a higher morbidity and mortality (5).

Treatment of salicylate poisoning is aimed at correcting fluid, electrolyte, and acid-base disturbances and enhancing elimination of the salicylate. Initial measures include hydration, administration of dextrose for hypoglycemia, correction of acidemia with sodium bicarbonate, and administration of vitamin K (2–5 mg/kg administered intravenously) if the patient manifests any evidence of a bleeding disorder secondary to hypoprothrombinemia. Gastrointestinal decontamination with lavage and activated charcoal is important, particularly when large amounts or enteric-coated preparations are ingested. Elimination of salicylates is enhanced by alkaline diuresis (107), as previously described.

Hemodialysis can be used in the severely poisoned patient. It is usually reserved for the patient who is likely to develop fluid overload and pulmonary edema with forced diuresis (as in cardiac or renal failure). Other indications for hemodialysis are a plasma salicylate level of greater than 100 mg/dl and acidemia with neurotoxicity, refractory to bicarbonate administration.

Cyclic Antidepressants

Tricyclic antidepressants are used by over 25 million people annually (99) and are the fourth most common cause of drug overdose in the United States (26). There is an associated 3% mortality (26). The narrow and sometimes overlapping margin of safety between thera-

peutic and toxic effects mandates close follow-up of all patients taking these medications.

The active agents responsible for both therapeutic and toxic effects are the parent tertiary amine compound (e.g., imipramine, amitryptyline, doxepin) and their metabolites (desipramine, nortriptyline, desmethyldoxepin). It should be noted that cyclobenzaprine (Flexeril) and carbamazepine (Tegretol) are similar to the cyclic antidepressants in their presentation and management of overdose.

Cyclic antidepressants undergo rapid absorption from the gastrointestinal tract. Metabolism takes place mainly via N-demethylation, N-oxidation, and hydroxylation reactions in the liver. They all possess a large volume of distribution, signifying extensive tissue binding (81). Because of the extensive protein binding of these compounds and the large volume of distribution, forced diuresis, hemoperfusion, and hemodialysis have no role in the management of these overdoses (33).

Additionally, because of their wide volume of distribution, serum levels of these compounds are not reflective of potential toxicity. Tissue levels may be 10 times serum levels (51). Cyclic antidepressant medications also undergo an enterohepatic circulation that makes repeated doses of activated charcoal advisable in treatment of overdoses (33).

Cyclic antidepressants and related compounds exert four pharmacological actions that can result in both therapeutic and toxic effects. They sedate, exert both central and peripheral anticholinergic effects, block presynaptic uptake of amine neurotransmitters (norepinephrine, serotonin, and dopamine), and exert a quinidine-like effect on the cardiac conduction system.

As a result of these pharmacological effects there are three major manifestations of toxicity: CNS signs, anticholinergic signs, and cardiopulmonary signs. CNS effects may occur with both toxic and therapeutic doses. In a typical overdose, an initial phase of excitement and restlessness is followed by sedation, which may progress to coma, seizures, and autonomic changes (132). Amoxapine and maprotiline are associated with a higher incidence of seizures compared with older tricyclic antidepressants and trazodone (167). Typical anticholinergic signs include fever, fixed dilated pupils, dry mouth, flushed hot skin, excitement, hallucinations, and coma. Cardiopulmonary toxicity is manifested by supraventricular and ventricular dysrhythmias, conduction disturbances, hypotension, and pulmonary edema.

Cardiac toxicity is the major concern in tricyclic overdose. There have been various attempts to establish criteria for predicting the likelihood of cardiac toxicity from an overdose. In the absence of an atrioventricular conduction disturbance it is reasonable to assume that the absence of a tachycardia means there is a low probability of significant cardiac toxicity (80). A QRS duration greater than 100 ms signifies cardiac toxicity and is usually associated with serum levels of greater than 1000 mg/dl (18). Others have found that a prolonged corrected QT interval and a terminal QRS vector of 130° to 270° indicate significant cardiac toxicity. It was also found that a QRS duration of 100 ms or more was associated with a higher incidence of seizures, whereas a QRS duration of greater than 160 ms was associated with a higher incidence of ventricular dysrhythmias (18). Despite these guidelines, there is still a paucity of data predicting the likelihood of cardiac disturbances from cyclic antidepressant overdose, as well as predicting when a patient is "out of the woods" and can be transferred to an unmonitored setting.

Treatment for the patient with a cyclic antidepressant overdose is based on general supportive measures and liberal criteria for admitting the patient to the intensive care setting. Early airway control cannot be overemphasized. Patients with a significant overdose may initially present awake, alert, and with an intact gag reflex. Within minutes they can become obtunded and lose their gag reflex. Because of the delayed gastric emptying associated with these medications, measures to empty the upper gastrointestinal tract (lavage or induced emesis) should be attempted within 4–6 hours of ingestion. Repeated doses of activated charcoal may help remove the drug because of its enterohepatic circulation. Because of the possibility of pulmonary edema, intravenous fluids should be kept at maintenance infusion rates unless hypotension is present.

The use of physostigmine salicylate in the management of cyclic antidepressant overdose remains controversial. In this setting, physostigmine can arouse a comatose patient, stop seizures, and terminate tachydysrhythmias. However, arousal after physostigmine administration is not diagnostic of poisoning with anticholinergics because it can arouse victims of other poisonings (117). Physostigmine can aggravate conduction abnormalities and pro-

duce asystole in patients with severe tricyclic poisoning (125). Physostigmine may also precipitate seizures (115). Thus, physostigmine should be used only when other measures have failed. The usual dose in adults is 0.2 mg/minute intravenously over 10 minutes.

Diazepam is the agent of choice for treating seizures (82). Intractable seizures can be treated with phenytoin or other anticonvulsants. Sodium bicarbonate administration to achieve a pH of 7.5 has been shown to suppress dysrhythmias, narrow the QRS complex, and significantly improve hypotension (24). When bicarbonate is unsuccessful in terminating ventricular dysrhythmias in adults, phenytoin is recommended (59, 103). In children, propranolol is recommended for dysrhythmias unresponsive to bicarbonate (134). In the patient with hypotension resistant to bicarbonate therapy, fluid and pressor therapy is indicated. Logical pressors to choose are norepinephrine or dopamine since they are two of the amine neurotransmitters that cyclic antidepressants affect.

Several patients have died from dysrhythmias as late as 6 days postingestion despite apparent hemodynamic stability (54). However, absence of tachycardia, absence of QRS, PR, and QT prolongation, absence of ventricular dysrhythmias, and absence of anticholinergic and CNS signs for at least 24 hours suggest that the patient can be safely discharged from a monitored bed.

Carbon Monoxide

Carbon monoxide (CO) poisoning accounts for one-half of all poisoning deaths in the United States (120) and may contribute to many others (116). CO is a tasteless, odorless, and colorless gas that is the product of incomplete combustion of carbon-containing substances. Some common sources include combustion engine exhaust fumes, defective heating systems, smoke, fires, faulty gas and kerosene space heaters, and improperly ventilated charcoal briquette or Sterno fires. Methylene chloride is a volatile solvent used in many home and industrial preparations. Accidental exposure or purposeful inhalation of this solvent may result in CO poisoning (155). The resting carboxyhemoglobin level in normal nonsmokers is about 0.8–1.0% while the level in normal smokers is about 4–6.8% (30, 112).

The effects of acute CO poisoning vary

depending on the inspired concentration of CO, the activity level of the victim, and the duration of the exposure. The nonspecific nature of the initial presentation forces the clinician to have a high index of suspicion, if the condition is to be correctly and promptly diagnosed. Over-reliance on carboxyhemoglobin levels and inadequate attention to clinical signs and symptoms may lead to incomplete treatment with subsequent permanent neurological sequelae.

CO has two major actions as a poison. It crosses the alveolar-capillary membrane and binds to hemoglobin with an affinity 200–250 times greater than that of oxygen. CO also causes the oxyhemoglobin dissociation curve to shift to the left. These effects dramatically reduce the blood's oxygen carrying capacity. In addition, CO is a direct cellular toxin for the cytochrome A3 oxidase system, preventing aerobic cellular metabolism (29).

These toxic effects primarily impact on the tissues with the highest oxygen consumption, such as the myocardium and the brain. The principal initial clinical manifestations of CO poisoning are neurological. The symptoms are nonspecific and are easily confused with those caused by ingestion of other substances, particularly alcohol. The diagnosis may further be confused by the fact that up to 60% of CO poisoning victims also ingest alcohol in varying amounts (173). Some of the presenting symptoms and signs include headache, nausea, confusion, poor judgment, visual disturbances, shortness of breath, fatigability, memory deficits, somnolence, coma, and seizures. Dermatologic manifestations include erythema, bullae, and edema. Cherry red discoloration of the lips or skin is usually a postmortem finding and rarely seen as a presenting sign in the alive patient. Rhabdomyolysis may occur from pressure necrosis of muscle or as a direct toxic effect (166). Fever and leukocytosis may also be present. An ECG should be obtained to rule out evidence of myocardial ischemia from hypoxia.

The intensivist is cautioned against over-reliance on carboxyhemoglobin levels. Past attempts to correlate these blood levels with severity of symptoms have been unsuccessful. Carboxyhemoglobin levels obtained in the ICU do not reflect peak levels that may have been partially treated by EMS personnel or emergency room physicians. A normal carboxyhemoglobin level does not rule out CO poisoning (113). Levels between 10 and 70% may be associated with the entire spectrum of clinical

CO poisoning. In general, brief exposures to high levels of CO will have much less clinical toxicity than prolonged exposures to lower levels (166).

The mainstay of treatment for victims of CO poisoning is oxygen. The half-life of CO in a patient breathing room air is about 5 hours. With 100% oxygen administration, the half-life is reduced to about 1½ hours. Hyperbaric oxygen at 3 atm reduces the half-life to 23 minutes (113). The mode of oxygen therapy depends on the clinical condition, the carboxyhemoglobin level, and the availability and proximity of a hyperbaric chamber. In suspected cases of CO poisoning, immediate applications of 100% oxygen should precede any other therapy while awaiting a laboratory report on carboxyhemoglobin levels. Since CO is eliminated by adequate ventilation, patients demonstrating inadequate ventilation should be intubated and mechanically ventilated. Treatment of other medical or surgical conditions should be instituted simultaneously. Arterial pH should be monitored and corrected as necessary.

Current recommendations for the use of hyperbaric oxygen therapy following CO exposure include (120) (a) any patient with a carboxyhemoglobin level of 25% or more; (b) any patient exhibiting neurological symptoms other than a mild headache and nausea, regardless of carboxyhemoglobin level; (c) a patient with a history of unconsciousness; and (d) a patient with new cardiac abnormalities such as arrhythmias or ischemic changes.

Oxygen therapy should continue until the patient clinically improves. Clinical recovery usually lags hours to days behind normalization of carboxyhemoglobin levels.

Cyanide

Cyanide poisoning, although relatively rare, represents one of the most severe poisonings a clinician can encounter. More importantly, cyanide is one of the few poisons that can be successfully treated with a specific antidote. The intensivist must be able to rapidly recognize a victim of cyanide poisoning, initiate resuscitative efforts promptly, and administer the antidote in the proper sequences and dosages.

Cyanide can exist in several forms. Hydrocyanic acid is the highly volatile acid that liberates the deadly gas hydrogen cyanide. The gas has the distinctive smell of bitter almonds.

Cyanide also exists as the sodium and potassium salts of hydrocyanic acid. Derivations of hydrogen cyanide include acrylonitrile, cyanamide, cyanogen chloride, and nitroprusside (31). Industrial sources for cyanide compounds include fumigation, ore extraction, electroplating, synthetic ruber production, fertilizers, silver polishes, and rodenticides. Natural sources of cyanide include amygdalin, which is found in the seeds of many fruits such as cherries, plums, peaches, pears, and apricots. Amygdalin is harmless unless the seed that contains it is crushed and moistened, which allows the enzyme emulsin to drive the chemical reaction that produces cyanide. Laetrile is a synthetic agent, allegedly antineoplastic, that contains amygdalin usually from apricot or peach pits. There have been several cases of cyanide poisoning from Laetrile, at least one resulting in death (43). Recently, there have been several tragic deaths from apparently purposeful contamination of over-the-counter medications with cyanide salts.

Cyanide causes hypoxia by binding to the ferric (Fe+3) iron of mitochondrial cytochrome oxidase. This results in an almost total inhibition of cytochrome oxidase activity and thus inhibition of cellular respiration. This leads to anaerobic metabolism and an accumulation of lactic acid (71).

The clinical presentation depends on the amount inhaled or absorbed and the duration of exposure. Symptoms begin within minutes to an hour after oral ingestion; skin absorption usually produces symptoms in minutes; and inhalation may produce symptoms and even death within seconds. The symptoms occur in rapid succession and include giddiness, palpitations, headache, dyspnea, and unconsciousness. Usually, gastrointestinal symptoms from ingestion of the salts do not occur because of the rapidity of the onset of CNS depression. Seizures and dysrhythmias result from profound hypoxia. Lactic acidosis occurs because of anaerobic metabolism and hypoxia.

Diagnosis rests on a history of potential exposure and rapidly progressive clinical signs, as described above. Lactic acidosis is helpful but nonspecific. Other clinical clues include equally red arteries and veins on funduscopic examination and signs and symptoms of severe hypoxia in patients who do not appear cyanotic (71). Cyanide levels are not usually available in the acute setting. Plasma thiocyanate (an indication of the amount of endogenous detoxification of cyanide by the naturally occurring enzyme rhodanase) may be measured and followed to detect cyanide poisoning in patients on nitroprusside therapy.

Successful treatment involves simultaneous resuscitation and stabilization efforts, and administration of the appropriately sequenced and dosed antidotes. All emergency rooms and intensive care units should have the Lilly Cyanide Antidote kit. This contains instructions, pediatric dose tables, and prepackaged forms of amyl nitrite "perles," 10% sodium nitrite, and 25% sodium thiosulfate.

Inhalation of amyl nitrite and intravenous injection of sodium nitrite causes a methemoglobinemia (Fe+3) which has a greater affinity for cyanide than does the ferric iron (Fe+3) of cytochrome oxidase. Methemoglobin remove cyanide from the respiratory enzyme, allowing normal cellular respiration to resume. Sodium thiosulfate is given intravenously to enhance the metabolism of cyanide to thiocyanate, a relatively nontoxic substance that is excreted by the kidneys. In adults, amyl nitrite "perles" should be broken in a gauze pad and inhaled by the patient while the sodium nitrite solution is being prepared. Usually 10 ml of the sodium nitrite (330 mg) is given intravenously (slowly to prevent hypotension). Subsequently 50 ml (12.5 g) of sodium thiosulfate is given intravenously. Repeat doses may be necessary as clinically indicated.

Theophylline

The incidence of theophylline poisoning is on the rise (45). Some cases are a result of intentional overdoses, but many others are the result of physician-prescribing errors (110). The availability of slow-release preparations has also contributed to the increased incidence of theophylline poisonings. Available forms of theophylline include aminophylline, oxtriphylline, dyphylline, slow-release theophylline, and slow-release aminophylline. Theophylline is a methylxanthine similar in structure to caffeine. Short-acting preparations are rapidly absorbed from the gastrointestinal tract, and peak blood levels occur within 2 hours. Slow-release preparations have delayed absorption and peak serum levels may not occur for 8–12 hours depending on the preparation. Once absorbed, approximately 60% of theophylline is protein bound. Only free theophylline is pharmacologically active. Serum levels measure both bound and unbound theophylline. Theophylline is metabolized in the liver, and diseases or drugs affecting the liver's ability to metabolize theophylline may result in higher blood levels.

At therapeutic levels, theophylline is metabolized by first-order kinetics. However, at blood levels of 10 μg/ml or above, metabolizing enzymes become saturated and zero-order kinetics ensues. Thus, patients with therapeutic blood levels of theophylline, may become toxic if doses are increased or liver function is decreased. Medical conditions that may predispose patients to theophylline toxicity include age over 60 years, liver disease (cirrhosis, hepatitis, cholestasis), COPD, cor pulmonale, congestive heart failure, viral illnesses, febrile illnesses, and influenza vaccine. Medications that can predispose to toxicity include cimetidine, erythromycin, and noncardioselective β-blockers (103).

Serum theophylline levels are best determined by high-pressure liquid chromotography. Both symptoms of toxicity and clinical response to therapy correlate well with peak serum levels. Therapeutic serum concentrations range from 10 to 20 μg/ml. Acute single ingestions (in a patient not on maintenance therapy) of less than 10 mg/kg are unlikely to produce symptoms of toxicity. Acutely toxic patients can tolerate much higher theophylline levels than patients on chronic therapy who become toxic (121).

Mild manifestations of toxicity usually occur with serum levels between 20 and 35 μg/ml. These signs and symptoms include nausea and vomiting, tremors, irritability, polyuria, tachycardia, tachypnea, and headaches. Severe toxic manifestations occur above serum levels of 80 μg/ml in acute toxicity and above 50 μg/ml in chronic toxicity. Severe toxicity includes supraventricular arrhythmias, ventricular arrhythmias, hypotension, seizures, coma, and cardiopulmonary arrest. Metabolic abnormalities of toxicity include hypokalemia, hyperglycemia, leukocytosis, respiratory alkalosis, metabolic acidosis, hypomagnesemia, and hypophosphatemia (72). The presence of seizures carries up to a 50% mortality in some series (179).

The hypotension seen in severe toxicity is usually mediated by a decrease in systemic vascular resistance. It is proposed that this decrease in systemic vascular resistance is secondary to an increase in β-adrenergic activity causing vasodilation in skeletal muscle (36). This has led some authorities to advocate the use of β-blockers or pure α-agonists (methox-amine) for the treatment of hypotension. In one limited series, β-blockers did indeed raise blood pressure (17). Many of the metabolic abnormalities may also result from a hyperadrenergic state (17).

Treatment includes general supportive measures, institution of gastrointestinal dialysis with repeated doses of activated charcoal, and careful selection of patients for charcoal or resin hemoperfusion. Theophylline levels should be drawn every 2 hours until a trend is established and efficacy of therapeutic measures is proven. Once theophylline toxicity is established, anticipation of life-threatening dysrhythmias or seizures is paramount.

Early and repeated doses of activated charcoal can decrease ongoing absorption of theophylline and increase elimination, because of theophylline's enterohepatic circulation (144, 96). Initial doses of activated charcoal range from 50–100 g and are followed by 30–50 g every 2–4 hours until levels are below the toxic range. Sorbitol (100 ml of 70% solution) may be given as a cathartic along with the charcoal (160).

Treatment of arrhythmias from theophylline toxicity follows conventional guidelines. Seizures associated with theophylline overdose may be prolonged and intractable. They carry a high mortality and survivors may show permanent neurologic sequelae. Diazepam should be used as a first-line drug. If diazepam (or one of its benzodiazepine analogues) is given to a total dose of 20–30 mg and the seizures persist beyond 15–20 minutes, phenobarbital should be added. Phenobarbital can be given at a dose of 10 mg/kg intravenously. A repeat dose of 10 mg/kg may be given in 15 minutes. If seizure activity persists beyond 45 minutes, thiopental general anesthesia is recommended (103).

Hemoperfusion may be useful in removing theophylline and minimizing life-threatening complications of toxicity. Criteria for selecting patients for hemoperfusion are poorly defined. Some recommend hemoperfusion in the setting of a rising serum concentration greater than 60 μg/ml (17). Others recommend it when levels exceed 80 μg/ml (61). In chronic toxicity, hemoperfusion may be instituted when levels exceed 50 μg/ml in a patient who is over 60 years of age and has heart or liver failure. Hemoperfusion may also be useful in the elderly patient who is unable to tolerate oral activated charcoal. While decisions are being made about hemoperfusion, all patients should have oral charcoal therapy started.

Alcohols

An osmolal gap of greater than 10 suggests the presence of osmotically active substances such as the alcohols, mannitol, or glycerol. The most commonly ingested alcohols are ethanol, methanol, ethylene glycol, and isopropyl alcohol.

ETHANOL

Ethyl alcohol is the most common drug consumed (49). It is oxidized in the liver to carbon dioxide and water by the alcohol dehydrogenase system. This is a nicotinamide adenine dinucleotide (NAD) dependent enzyme. Other enzyme systems may play a role in ethanol metabolism, but alcohol dehydrogenase is the major route by which ethanol is detoxified. Hepatic ethanol metabolism follows zero-order kinetics, with 7–10 g of ethanol metabolized each hour in the adult. Chronic alcoholics and children metabolize alcohol more rapidly than the average adult (131).

Whisky and wine are involved in most reported serious ethanol poisonings in children. Mouthwashes and colognes may also be involved. In the very small child, a potentially lethal dose is provided by just 5–10 oz of mouthwash or 1–2 ounces of cologne (170). Ethanol serum concentrations of 338–575 mg/dl have been associated with coma and subsequent survival without sequelae in toddlers (131). The occurrence of concomitant hypoglycemia in children is of major concern.

Although serum ethanol levels may be helpful in establishing a diagnosis, they frequently do not correlate well with the level of intoxication because of tolerance. For the novice drinker, or the person never exposed to alcohol, death from medullary failure may occur at serum ethanol levels of 500 mg/dl. However, there is one anecdotal report of a patient with an ethanol level of 999 mg/dl, who was treated and discharged from an emergency room (162).

The clinical features of ethanol intoxication range from mild mental impairment to coma and death. The degree of intoxification depends upon the rapidity of the rise of the blood ethanol level, the level reached, and the length of time high levels are maintained. With severe toxicity, hypotension, hypoventilation, hypothermia, and coma may develop. Tachycardia is commonly seen, even without hypotension. Patients must be examined for evidence of complications of the acute intoxication (such

as aspiration, gastrointestinal bleeding, or core hypothermia) as well as coexistent medical or surgical conditions (such as multiple trauma, diabetes, or other ingestions).

Treatment of the acutely poisoned patient is supportive. Early airway protection is paramount. Alcohol is a gastric irritant and carries high risk of aspiration in the obtunded patient. Lavage and instillation of charcoal are indicated if the ingestion is acute (e.g., within 2 hours of presentation). After blood is drawn for a glucose determination, administer 50 g of dextrose intravenously and 100 mg of thiamine intravenously or intramuscularly. Hypotension usually responds to fluid therapy. The Wernicke-Korsakoff Syndrome (ataxia, dysarthria, and sixth-nerve palsy or oculomotor paralysis) requires the administration of 500–1000 mg of thiamine intravenously.

Some have tried the administration of naloxone in order to reverse the CNS and respiratory depression associated with ethanol poisoning. There are some data to indicate that naloxone reverses the ethanol-induced depression of the hypercapnic drive. There are also anecdotal reports of boluses of naloxone dramatically improving the mental status of the acutely intoxicated patient. However, this same effect reportedly is not operative in the acutely intoxicated chronic alcoholic (104). Further studies are needed to determine its place, if any, in the treatment of acute ethanol intoxication. Hemodialysis can be employed when ethanol levels are high and the patient exhibits profound midbrain and medullary dysfunction despite supportive measures.

The intensivist must also be aware of the potential for alcohol withdrawal syndromes in their poisoned patients. Alcohol withdrawal seizures ("rum fits") are major motor seizures that may manifest before the onset of other withdrawal symptoms. They occur typically in burst of two to three seizures and begin 8–12 hours after cessation of drinking. Prior to the onset of full-blown delirium tremens, the patient may show tremors, tachycardia, insomnia, and irritability. These symptoms may occur even in the presence of elevated blood ethanol levels. The full spectrum of delirium tremens usually manifests 36–96 hours after cessation of drinking. Symptoms and signs include marked tachycardia, diaphoresis, hypertension, visual hallucinations, psychosis, and uncontrollable tremors. Intravenous diazepam or easily titratable short-acting benzodiazepines are effective in controlling delirium tremens. Huge doses may be necessary, mandating careful monitoring of the patient's airway and respiratory status. Withdrawal seizures rarely require treatment because status epilepticus is unusual. Use of phenothiazines is contraindicated because they decrease the seizure threshold. Those patients with underlying seizure disorders should receive phenytoin intravenously both therapeutically and prophylactically.

METHANOL

Methyl alcohol (methanol) in its distilled form is a nearly odorless and palatable alcohol. Crude wood alcohol (methanol) has many impurities that give it a very disagreeable odor and taste. Methanol is obtained from the destructive distillation of wood and is found in antifreeze fluid, windshield de-icers, varnishes, and shellacs. "Bootleg" whiskey may contain significant amounts of methanol. Methanol is not taxed, and because of its low cost has led the occasional unwary alcoholic to imbibe it in lieu of more expensive ethanol.

Methanol is rapidly absorbed from the gastrointestinal tract, with peak levels occurring 30–60 minutes after ingestion. Toxicity can also result from inhalation and skin absorption. Methanol, being water soluble, distributes in total body water.

The primary route of elimination of methanol is oxidation to formaldehyde, formic acid, and carbon dioxide. The rate limiting step in methanol metabolism is its conversion by alcohol dehydrogenase to formaldehyde. Formaldehyde is then rapidly converted to formic acid. Formic acid, in turn, is metabolized by a folate-dependent enzyme to carbon dioxide and water. Formaldehyde and formic acid are much more toxic than methanol, and it is now believed that formic acid is the major toxin. Formic acid levels correlate with the degree of acidosis and magnitude of the anion gap (143). Clinically, mortality rates and severity of visual symptoms also correlate with the degree of acidosis (12). There is an enormous variability in the reported doses necessary to cause acidosis, blindness, or death. This variability is partially due to the total amount of methanol ingested, the extent of concomitant ethanol ingestion, and the folate levels present at the time of ingestion. The generally accepted lethal dose of methanol is 30 ml.

Typically there is a lag time of 8–72 hours from ingestion to onset of symptoms. The onset of symptoms correlates with the appearance of metabolic acidosis (162). The most important initial symptom is altered visual perception, which may be described as blurred vision or photophobia. Permanent and complete blindness may eventually develop. Initially, optic disc hyperemia and papillary edema are evident. With permanent visual sequelae, optic atrophy and attenuation of blood vessels occur. No patient with normally reactive pupils has suffered permanent visual loss (14). Conversely, decreased pupillary function may occur in patients who recover completely. Other signs and symptoms of methanol poisoning are abdominal pain, vomiting, dyspnea with Kussmaul respirations, headache, nuchal rigidity, weakness, confusion, seizures, and coma. The most striking laboratory finding is a high anion gap metabolic acidosis. Serum bicarbonate levels may reach zero. Other characteristic laboratory values include increased osmolal gap, increased amylase, increased serum glucose, and lactic acidemia. The finding of a profound metabolic acidosis in a patient with visual disturbances should lead the clinician to consider methanol poisoning.

After initial resuscitation and gastric decontamination, treatment of suspected methanol poisoning centers on (a) prompt correction of metabolic acidosis, (b) prompt initiation of ethanol therapy, (c) administration of folate, and (d) selection of patients for hemodialysis. Large doses of sodium bicarbonate may be necessary to correct the metabolic acidosis. Arterial blood gases and serum bicarbonate determinations should be used to guide therapy.

Ethanol competitively inhibits alcohol dehydrogenase from converting methanol to formaldehyde because ethanol has a ninefold higher affinity for this enzyme. Ethanol therapy should be instituted in all cases of suspected or confirmed methanol poisoning. Therapy should precede the return of blood methanol determinations. Ethanol therapy is given to maintain a serum ethanol concentration of 100 mg/dl. McCoy (102) suggests the following regimen: (a) a loading dose of 0.6 g/kg, (b) a maintenance dose for nondrinkers of 66 mg/kg/hr, and (c) a maintenance dose for drinkers of 153 mg/kg/hour. If hemodialysis is instituted, the ethanol infusion will need to be increased because ethanol is removed by dialysis. McCoy suggests increasing the infusion rate in adults to 7.2 g/hour (102). Folate doses of 1 mg/kg (up to 50 mg/dose) intravenously every 4 hours for a total of six doses is given to replete folate stores.

Patients with a serum methanol level of 50 mg/dl should undergo hemodialysis. Ethanol therapy increases methanol's half-life from 8 hours to 30 or more hours. Hemodialysis will decrease the half-life to about 2.5 hours and thus shorten the length of time intensive care management is necessary (67). Hemodialysis will remove both methanol and formic acid. Other indications for hemodialysis include a history of ingestion of more than 30 ml of methanol, intractable acidosis, and deterioration of vision or CNS function (64). Hemodialysis should be continued until the serum methanol level is reduced to 20 mg/dl or below.

ETHYLENE GLYCOL

Ethylene glycol is a colorless, and sweet-tasting liquid. It is a common component of antifreeze, lacquer, polish, and de-icers. Approximately 1.4–1.6 ml/kg constitutes a minimum lethal dose, about 100 ml in adults (23).

Unmetabolized ethylene glycol has about the same CNS toxicity as ethanol. Once ingested it is rapidly absorbed and peak serum levels occur in 1–4 hours. Like methanol, it is distributed evenly throughout the body tissues. Although the parent compound is relatively nontoxic, the metabolic by-products are extremely toxic. Metabolism takes place mainly in the liver and, like methanol, the major converting enzyme is alcohol dehydrogenase. Toxic by-products are aldehydes, glycolate, oxalate, and lactate. Ethanol, with its higher enzyme affinity, prevents the metabolism of ethylene glycol into its more toxic by-products.

Toxic manifestations are due primarily to the development of metabolic acidosis and tissue destruction due to the deposition of oxalate crystals. Hypocalcemia may result from calcium chelation with oxalate. The onset of symptoms may be delayed up to 12 hours or more depending on the amount of ethylene glycol ingested and the extent of coingestion of ethanol. Berman (15) described three stages of intoxication: stage 1 (occurring 20 minutes to 12 hours after ingestion) consists of symptoms of intoxication such as nausea, vomiting, seizures, and coma; stage 2 (12–24 hours post-ingestion) is manifest by tachypnea, tachycardia, congestive heart failure, or pulmonary edema; and stage 3 (24–72 hours after ingestion) is characterized by renal failure secondary to acute tubular necrosis. In reality, the distinction between the phases is not clear cut, particularly between the CNS manifestations (stage 1) and the cardiovascular manifestations (stage 2). Other prominent CNS signs include nystagmus, myoclonus, and ophthalmoplegia. Pulmonary edema may result from both congestive heart failure and the adult respiratory distress syndrome (ARDS) (27). Laboratory findings include a high anion gap metabolic acidosis, hypocalcemia, and calcium oxalate crystals in the urine. With the onset of renal failure, there will be an elevation in BUN and creatinine. Hematuria and proteinuria may also be seen.

Ethylene glycol intoxication is suggested by the presentation of a patient who appears markedly intoxicated but does not have the smell of ethanol on the breath, the presence of coma with a large anion gap acidosis and an osmolal gap, and the presence of calcium oxalate crystals in the urine.

After initial resuscitation measures and gastrointestinal decontamination, therapy consists of maintenance of a high urine flow, administration of ethanol, administration of thiamine and pyridoxine supplements, correction of acidosis, correction of hypocalcemia, and hemodialysis. Some authorities advocate maintaining a high urine output until crystalluria disappears (164). Urine output may need to be augmented by furosemide or mannitol. If congestive heart failure or ARDS ensues, fluid therapy should be appropriately altered.

Ethanol should be administered to maintain a blood level of 100 mg/dl. Peterson suggests a loading dose of 0.6 to 0.8 g/kg, followed by a maintenance dose of 110–130 mg/kg/hour. If dialysis is performed the maintenance dose must be increased to 250–350 mg/kg/hour (126).

Correction of acidemia may require large amounts of sodium bicarbonate. To correct hypocalcemia the intensivist may use calcium chloride or calcium gluconate. Thiamine and pyridoxine are administered to prevent depletion of these cofactors, which are necessary for ethylene glycol detoxification. Thiamine (100 mg) and pyridoxine (100 mg) are given intramuscularly or intravenously every 6 hours for the first 24 hours (62).

Hemodialysis is recommended in ethylene glycol poisoning when ethylene glycol levels are above 50 mg/dl or if severe toxicity occurs. With ethanol blocking therapy, the half-life of ethylene glycol increases from 3 hours to 17 hours or more (126). In a small series, patients who had hemodialysis instituted prior to the onset of renal failure did better clinically than those in whom it was instituted after renal failure developed (9). Both ethylene glycol and intermediate toxic aldehydes are dialyzable. For these reasons, early and aggressive use of hemodialysis is recommended, rather than waiting for symptoms and signs of severe toxicity to develop. An exception to early hemodialysis would be rapid clinical improvement and/or rapidly falling ethylene glycol levels associated with ethanol therapy. All treatment should continue until ethylene glycol is undetectable in serum.

ISOPROPANOL

Isopropanol (isopropyl alcohol) is a clear, colorless, volatile liquid with a characteristic odor and a slightly bitter taste. Ingestion is common in young children and in suicidal or derelict adults. It is commonly found in the home as rubbing alcohol. It is also found in disinfectants, solvents, cleaning agents, and cosmetics.

Absorption from the stomach is rapid, occurring within 30 minutes, and peak blood levels are achieved within 1–1½ hours. It is more toxic than ethanol; its clinical effects last two to four times longer; and CNS depression is more pronounced. Dermal absorption is insignificant yet inhalation can be a significant route of exposure, particularly in children who are being sponged down with isopropanol for treatment of fever. Serious toxicity has been reported with this type of exposure (56).

Approximately 80% of isopropyl alcohol is metabolized by the liver to acetone, which is excreted by the kidneys (primarily) and the lungs. A small amount of unchanged isopropanol is resecreted into the stomach and saliva. Isopropanol appears to follow first-order kinetics, with a half-life of 2.5–3 hours (37). Acetone elimination occurs much more slowly. A lethal dose of isopropanol in adults is about 3 ml/kg.

Symptoms of acute intoxication, including abdominal pain, vomiting, and CNS effects usually occur within 30 minutes of ingestion. The CNS manifestations are similar to those of ethanol except they are more pronounced and they last longer. The acetone probably contributes to the more prolonged symptoms. Deep coma may develop rapidly and respiratory arrest may ensue. Gastrointestinal symptoms are more severe than with ethanol, and hemorrhagic gastritis has been reported (94). With severe toxicity (serum concentrations above 300–400 mg/dl) myocardial depression and severe hypotension can result. Less common ef-

fects include renal tubular necrosis, hypothermia, acute myopathy, and hemolytic anemia (91). The most characteristic and specific laboratory findings are an elevated anion gap, elevated osmolal gap, acetonemia, and acetonuria. Acidosis is less common, and when present, it is not as severe as that associated with methanol or ethylene glycol. Acidosis with isopropanol poisoning is likely due to lactic acidosis associated with hypotension and hypoxia. Hypotension is a poor prognostic indicator. In one series, the presence of hypotension carried a 45% mortality, while those patients in grade III or IV coma without hypotension had a 25% mortality (92).

Treatment involves gastric emptying, lavage, and activated charcoal if the ingestion was within 2 hours, and continuous nasogastric suction to remove re-secreted isopropanol. The clinician should be alert to the possibility of significant gastrointestinal bleeding and intervene appropriately.

Hemodialysis is effective in removing both isopropanol and acetone. Some investigators have reported beneficial clinical outcomes with the early institution of hemodialysis (171). No widely accepted guidelines are available for the use of dialysis. In view of the mortality figures associated with deep coma and hypotension, hemodialysis is appropriate in these settings as well as with blood levels in excess of 400 mg/dl. As is the trend with treatment of other alcohol poisonings, early institution of dialysis before severe complications set in may decrease mortality. Controlled studies comparing this approach with supportive treatment alone are not yet available.

Opiates

The term *opiates* generally refers to all drugs with pharmacological effects similar to the parent drug opium. For the purpose of this chapter opiates include medications derived from opium (morphine and codeine), drugs that are semisynthetic derivatives of opium (heroin, oxycodone, hydromorphone, etc.), and drugs that are synthetic compounds with opiate-like properties (meperidine, methadone, propoxyphene, and newer generation synthetics). The intensivist will most frequently face opiate overdoses in the setting of intravenous drug abuse (e.g., heroin, methadone), childhood ingestions of diphenoxylate or propoxyphene, or adolescent or adult oral overdoses of prescribed pain medications or antitussives.

Opiates are readily absorbed from the gastrointestinal tract, nasal mucosa, pulmonary mucosa, and parenterally (subcutaneous, intravenous, and intramuscular). When orally ingested, a significant percentage of the dose undergoes first-pass hepatic metabolism. Thus, there is less effect from an oral dose than an intravenous dose. Opiates are well distributed throughout the body. Blood levels may not correlate with the clinical picture nor reflect the ingested dose. Hemodialysis does not remove significant amounts of opiates from the body (2). Hepatic metabolism is relatively rapid, and major metabolic pathways differ with each opiate. Metabolism and toxic effects can be prolonged in hepatic disease and with delayed gastric emptying (2). About 90% of an ingested or injected drug is excreted in the urine, making this the fluid of choice for toxicology screening.

Opiates have their most pronounced effects on the central nervous system and the respiratory system. CNS effects include analgesia, euphoria, sedation, suppression of the cough reflex, dysphoria, nausea and vomiting, respiratory depression, fixed miotic pupils, and seizures. Seizures are due to a brief excitatory effect early after ingestion. The respiratory depression is secondary to a blunted medullary response to hypercarbia. In addition, patients may develop noncardiogenic pulmonary edema (13, 154). Other clinical effects include peripheral vasodilation with orthostatic hypotension, flushed skin, pruritis, diminished peristalsis, delayed gastric emptying, and urinary retention. A clue to diagnosis may be the presence of fresh or sclerotic needle puncture marks overlying blood vessels. Laboratory tests are not helpful in making the diagnosis of opiate overdose, with the exception of qualitative urine toxicology screens. A significant percentage of the time, other drugs or toxins are coingested with opiates. Opiates may mask manifestations of other drugs and vice versa.

Supportive measures are the mainstay of therapy. Once the airway is secured and respirations controlled or supplemented, the remainder of the resuscitation can take place in a controlled orderly fashion. Intravenous access should be established, blood and urine collected for routine laboratory tests, and toxicology screens and glucose and thiamine should be given. Naloxone is then administered. Once aroused with naloxone, the patients may be quite agitated and uncooperative with further procedures. Some clinicians favor

application of therapeutic restraints prior to reversing the CNS depression of opiates.

Naloxone is a superior antidote. It has no agonist properties and there are no contraindications to its use. Naloxone is a competitive antagonist at all three proposed opiate receptor subtypes (87). Naloxone restores pulmonary ventilation, reverses postural hypotension, and improves the patient's level of consciousness. It can also reverse the delay in gastric emptying caused by opiates. An initial dose of 0.8–2.0 mg may be given intravenously. If no response is elicited, repeat doses are given every 3–5 minutes to a total of 4 mg. If no improvement is noted, the clinician should suspect another cause for the patient's clinical status. With a child, initial doses can be given in the range of 0.01–0.02 mg/kg. Repeated doses up to 0.05 mg/kg should produce the desired response (85). Subsequent administration is titrated to the desired clinical response. Naloxone has a half-life of 12–20 minutes (a fraction of the half-life of the ingested opiate), and frequent repeat doses or initiation of a naloxone drip (0.4–0.8 mg/hr) may be necessary. Naloxone has also been successfully administered via the endotracheal tube (158).

Delayed gastric emptying occurs following oral ingestion and may be a reason to institute a gastric lavage. As mentioned above, administration of naloxone can speed gastrointestinal transit. Naloxone should not be administered to awaken a comatose patient so that ipecac syrup can be administered.

Organophosphates

Insecticides come under two general classes, organophosphates and carbamates. The organophosphate compounds are the type of insecticide most commonly associated with serious toxicity, accounting for more than 80% of pesticide-related hospitalizations (157). The popularity of these agents for commercial use has been growing because after application, they are rapidly hydrolyzed in the environment and little long-term accumulation occurs. Poisoning usually occurs in children who accidentally ingest the substance, in farmworkers who are accidentally exposed, and in victims of suicide attempts. Organophosphates sold for household use are usually made of more dilute formulations, about 1–2%, in contrast to the 40–50% concentrations in agricultural compounds (65). Just a few drops of the agricultural compounds can be fatal in children (42). Organophosphate poisoning can be rapidly fatal. One study (157) revealed that in hospitalized patients the fatality rate was 50% in children and 10% in adults.

Organophosphate poisoning can be successfully treated with chemical and physiological antidotes. However, recognizing a victim or organophosphate poisoning can be difficult. Organophosphate toxicity results from the disruption of normal cholinergic neurotransmission at multiple sites in the body (11). The organophosphates gain entrance to the body via gastrointestinal absorption, dermal absorption, and absorption through the ocular and respiratory mucosa. Acetylcholine is the neurotransmitter at the affected synaptic junctions. Normally acetylcholine is broken down into acetic acid and choline by the enzyme acetylcholinesterase. Acetylcholinesterase (true cholinesterase) is found primarily in erythrocytes and nervous tissue. Another cholinesterase, pseudocholinesterase, is found in the serum and in the liver. Organophosphates are powerful inhibitors of both cholinesterases, irreversibly binding to them within 24–48 hours (147).

The clinical effects depend on the site and type of acetylcholine synapse affected. The anatomic sites are muscarinic synapses (autonomic effector cells), nicotinic synapses (autonomic ganglia and the adrenal medulla), and central nervous system synapses. Excessive amounts of acetylcholine initially excite and subsequently paralyze normal function of these synapses producing the characteristic effects (11).

The onset of muscarinic effects depends on the route of exposure. In a case of inhalation of fumes or vapors, the ocular and respiratory effects may appear first. These include miosis, eye pain, blurred vision, excessive lacrimation and salivation, wheezing and tightness in the chest (bronchoconstriction and increased tracheobronchial secretions), and dyspnea. Following ingestion, gastrointestinal symptoms may predominate or appear earliest. These include diarrhea, abdominal cramps, nausea, vomiting, and fecal incontinence. Other muscarinic signs and symptoms are bradycardia, diaphoresis, and urinary incontinence.

Nicotinic effects of organophosphates manifest in striated muscle and sympathetic ganglia. These effects include muscle fasciculations, fatigability, weakness, cramps, paralysis (with apnea), tachycardia, hypertension, and, rarely, mydriasis. Central nervous system effects manifest as confusion, slurred speech, ataxia, anxiety, fatigue, psychosis, seizures, coma, and central respiratory paralysis.

A history, if available, should attempt to determine what was taken, how much, and when. The physical examination should search for the muscarinic, nicotinic, and CNS signs just described. Laboratory tests are of limited usefulness. A red cell cholinesterase level is most specific but not readily available in most institutions (115). The serum cholinesterase level is usually more readily available. This is more sensitive but less specific than a red cell cholinesterase. Other conditions that may depress serum cholinesterase levels include hepatitis, cirrhosis, hepatic congestion, metastatic carcinoma, malnutrition, acute infections, anemia, myocardial infarction, and dermatomyositis.

A trial with atropine may be useful in aiding the diagnosis. In organophosphate poisoning, intravenous administration of atropine in doses of 1–2 mg does not result in flushing, dry mouth, tachycardia, or mydriasis. In fact, the ability to administer large doses of atropine without observable adverse effects is virtually diagnostic of organophosphate poisoning.

Treatment of organophosphate poisoning must be individualized. Administration of the antidote atropine prior to stabilization and oxygenation can be catastrophic. Seriously poisoned patients must have their airway controlled. Seizures, aspiration, increased tracheobronchial secretions, and bronchospasm can be managed more easily with adequate airway protection and control. Once the airway is controlled, maximum oxygenation should be accomplished. Suctioning and administration of atropine can lessen the effects of increased secretions. Diazepam can be used to control seizures.

Decontamination of the portal of entry is imperative. Continuous absorption from the clothing and/or skin must be prevented by completely stripping all clothes off and thoroughly washing skin, hair, and under nails. Copious irrigation of eyes should take places in cases of ocular exposure. Even when the vehicle for an ingested organophosphate is a hydrocarbon, gastric lavage or induced emesis should take place. Initial and repeated doses of charcoal are indicated.

Once the patient is stabilized and properly oxygenated, pharmacological treatment can ensue. The use of morphine, aminophylline, phenothiazines, and reserpine are contraindicated (108). Hypoxia and a direct toxic effect of organophosphates often results in a hyper-irritable myocardium, and epinephrine may cause irreversible ventricular fibrillation in such cases (135). Pharmacological treatment is based on the use of atropine and the cholinesterase "activator" pralidoxime. Atropine counters the muscarinic and CNS manifestations of organophosphate poisoning, whereas pralidoxime reverses both the muscarinic and the nicotinic effects.

Atropine may need to be given in large and repeated doses. The most common cause of treatment failure is inadequate atropinization (108). The therapeutic endpoint is evidence of atropinization as manifested by mydriasis, tachycardia, flushing, xerostomia, or anhydrosis. Two milligrams of atropine should be administered intravenously every 15 minutes until atropinization is apparent. The pediatric dose is 0.05 mg/kg every 15 minutes. The severely poisoned patient may require a continuous atropine infusion. Atropine should be tapered slowly during its discontinuation.

Pralidoxime (2-PAM chloride) has three major biochemical effects that are beneficial to the patient poisoned with organophosphates (11). It cleaves the organophosphate bond from cholinesterases, which reactivates the cholinesterase enzyme. It directly reacts with and detoxifies the organophosphate molecule, and it has an anticholinergic atropine-like effect. Pralidoxime should be used in the presence of muscle fasciculations or muscle weakness. For optimum effects, pralidoxime must be administered immediately after poisoning. Early administration may lessen the need for large doses of atropine. Reactivation of cholinesterases may not occur in patients administered the drug more than 36 hours after exposure (11).

The dosage of pralidoxime for adults is 1 g administered intravenously, with a maximum infusion rate of 0.5 g/minute and 20–50 mg/kg with a maximum infusion of one-half the total dose per minute for children (108). Repeat doses depend upon the clinical response. Reversal of muscle weakness and fasciculations usually begins within 10–40 minutes of administration (115).

The major complications of organophosphate poisoning are pulmonary and include aspiration pneumonitis, pulmonary edema, ARDS, and respiratory paralysis. Untreated patients usually die within 24 hours of exposure. In all other cases, provided cerebral hypoxia has been successfully prevented or treated, clinicians can expect total symptomatic recovery within 7–10 days (115).

Digitalis

Digitalis preparations have been used in contemporary medicine for over 200 years and are among the top 10 drugs prescribed in the United States. Iatrogenic digitalis intoxication is one of the most common toxic reactions in clinical medicine and is the most common cause of unintentional poisoning deaths in the elderly (176). Digitalis intoxication causes a morbidity of 8–35% and a mortality of 3–21% (148). Single, massive overdoses of digitalis are a relatively uncommon but significant mode of suicide. Deliberate digoxin overdose is fatal in 50% of patients (122).

Digitalis exerts its action at the cellular level by altering the activity of the sodium-potassium-ATPase membrane transport system. Digitalis preparations come in the form of digoxin (half-life of about 33 hours) and digitoxin (half-life of 6–7 days). Drug action depends on tissue concentration, which is relatively constant in relation to serum levels. The major human depot is skeletal muscle (40). Digoxin is excreted primarily via the kidneys; digitoxin is eliminated after being metabolically inactivated in the body. Both substances undergo enterohepatic circulation. Children are believed to be less sensitive to digoxin and require higher doses (89). Digitalis preparations possess a relatively narrow therapeutic index, with 40–60 percent of the lethal dose being required to achieve maximal therapeutic effect.

Digitalis cardiotoxicity is caused by its effects on cardiac conduction and automaticity, coexistent cardiac disease (both myocardial and conduction system disease), and other noncardiac disease states or medications. Almost any rhythm or conduction disturbance can result from this complex interaction of factors. More characteristic disturbances associated with digitalis toxicity include profound bradycardias with or without associated atrioventricular conduction disturbances, atrial tachycardias with atrioventricular block, and ventricular ectopy and tachydysrhythmias. Ventricular dysrhythmias are associated with a higher mortality, up to 50% in some series (111).

Gastrointestinal manifestations of digitalis toxicity include nausea, vomiting, and anorexia. Hypokalemia appears to be a consistent finding with chronic toxicity (106), while hyperkalemia is a prominent finding in acute, massive overdose (40). Neurologic symptoms include blurred and altered color vision, headache, fatigue, depression, confusion, hallucinations, and delirium. These latter symptoms are not a consistent finding with acute ingestions (142).

Diagnosis of digitalis toxicity is based on a history of ingestion of a digitalis preparation, a history of nausea, vomiting, and anorexia, an ECG demonstrating "digitalis effects" (prolonged PR interval, AV block, ST depression), the presence of arrhythmias, and confirmation with serum levels. The magnitude of the serum level, and its correlation with the degree of toxicity, depend upon the presence or absence of other host disease states or medications. In one study, a significant increase in mortality was correlated with an increasing digoxin level, with a 50% mortality occurring with digoxin levels of above 6 ng/ml. Quinidine causes an increase in serum digoxin in up to 90% of patients. This finding is best explained by the displacement of digoxin from tissue binding sites (70).

Therapy of digitalis intoxication is aimed at intensive cardiovascular support and hastening digitalis removal from the body. Gastric emptying and administration of activated charcoal are indicated. Repeat doses of charcoal may be useful in view of the presence of an enterohepatic circulation. Conduction disturbances of arrhythmias require treatment only if hemodynamic compromise is manifest. Bradydysrhythmias can be treated with atropine and/or placement of a temporary pacemaker. Correction of hypoxia and hypokalemia is imperative for successful treatment of ventricular ectopy and arrhythmias. Lidocaine and phenytoin are the most efficacious agents. Phenytoin doses are similar to those used for anticonvulsant treatment (e.g., 50–100 mg can be given slowly every 5 minutes to a total dose of 600 mg). Direct-current countershock is to be withheld unless all other therapy fails.

Immunotherapy with Fab fragments from digoxin antibodies has recently been reported to dramatically reverse signs of profound digoxin poisoning. Use of these antibodies can terminate life-threatening arrhythmias, lower serum digoxin levels, terminate gastrointestinal side effects, and reverse life-threatening hyperkalemia, all within 1–2 hours of administration (153). Use of immunotherapy is limited mostly to tertiary care institutions.

Sporadic cases of the successful use of hemoperfusion for treating digitalis intoxication are reported in recent literature (93). It is said to cause a more rapid fall in plasma digoxin levels than supportive treatment alone. It is a good therapeutic alternative in digoxin poisoning when adverse factors, such as hyperkalemia, pre-existing heart disease, and chronic renal failure are present. Hemodialysis may be necessary for recalcitrant, life-threatening hyperkalemia; however, it will not eliminate digoxin because of high protein binding.

Benzodiazepines

The popularity of the benzodiazepines needs little re-emphasis here. They are among the most widely prescribed drugs every year. Between 1964 and 1973 the number of prescriptions nearly tripled. In the last 10 years, the number of available benzodiazepine compounds has increased. The popularity of these medications is based on their relative safety as compared with their predecessor sedative, hypnotic-type medications and barbiturates. Indeed, despite sometimes massive doses (2 g of diazepam in one ingestion), patients who ingest benzodiazepines alone seldom suffer any serious medical complications (66). It is their ingestion as part of a polydrug overdose that may result in death or serious consequences. The potentiating effect of alcohol on benzodiazepines is well known.

Benzodiazepines are all derived from a common nucleus. Alterations of this basic nucleus produce the variety of compounds available today. The pharmacokinetics of these compounds can vary widely. Although these pharmacokinetic differences may suggest therapeutic differences, currently there are no data clearly demonstrating the clinical superiority of one compound over another when based solely upon pharmacokinetic properties. In general, the benzodiazepines are rapidly and completely absorbed after oral ingestion. Once into the systemic circulation, all benzodiazepines bind to plasma albumin and are then distributed to tissues at rates dependent upon their lipid solubility. Essentially all benzodiazepines are hepatically biotransformed via oxidation and/or conjugation pathways. Oxidation frequently results in the production of multiple metabolites, some of which are pharmacologically active. Certain benzodiazepines, including diazepam, undergo enterohepatic circulation. These agents primarily affect the CNS. They potentiate the effects of the neurotransmitter GABA without themselves being GABA-mimetic compounds.

Benzodiazepine overdose is characterized by sedation without cardiovascular compromise.

Drowsiness, ataxia, dizziness, and weakness are usual symptoms. Severe CNS depression (deep coma) is unusual and should suggest other coingestants. Patients may take 2 g or more of diazepam and still be oriented and conversant (66). The diagnosis is made by history and qualitative toxicological examination. Since polysubstance ingestion is found in over 80% of hospitalized patients, the intensivist should search carefully for clues revealing other more dangerous toxins (16). In one study, almost 40% of patients who were hospitalized for polydrug ingestion involving benzodiazepines required ventilatory support (3).

Treatment is purely supportive. Ingestion of alcohol or other toxins may depress the patient's ability to protect their airway. In pure benzodiazepine overdoses, the efficacy of gastric emptying is minimal. Repeated doses of activated charcoal may be helpful; but again, given the excellent prognosis for even massive single ingestions of benzodiazepines alone, the indication for even this relatively benign form of therapy is questioned. Observation is usually all that is necessary. Specific therapy is directed at other more toxic agents that may have been ingested. Hemodialysis, hemoperfusion, forced diuresis, physostigmine, and naloxone are not of any proven clinical utility. Recovery from huge, single-dose ingestions is rapid and complete, usually within 24–48 hours.

Calcium Channel Blockers

As the use of calcium channel blockers increases, so has the incidence of both accidental and purposeful poisoning with these agents. Presently, therapeutic modalities are derived mainly from case reports of overdoses and the rational assumption that parenteral calcium administration should and does reverse some of the toxic effects in an overdose scenario. Three preparations of calcium channel blockers are currently in use: verapamil, nifedipine, and diltiazem. These agents are used for the treatment of dysrhythmias, coronary artery spasm, hypertensive emergencies, heart failure, and angina pectoris.

The mechanism of action of these compounds rests on their ability to inhibit the slow calcium channel current. These drugs may cause (106) myocardial depression (negative inotropism), bradycardia, decrease in atrioventricular conduction, inhibition of vascular tone with peripheral and coronary vasodilation, CNS depression, nausea and vomiting, and disordered glucose metabolism and mild acidosis.

Data regarding the pharmacokinetics and toxic effects of calcium channel blockers in a massive overdose scenario are lacking. Most comparisons are limited to side effects or therapeutic effects with therapeutic doses. Documented adverse cardiovascular manifestations with overdoses of diltiazem and verapamil include hypotension, bradycardia, sinus arrest, and cardiogenic shock (151). There are also documented case reports of verapamil causing terminal ventricular fibrillation after being administered to patients with Wolff-Parkinson-White syndrome and atrial tachyarrhythmias (83).

Treatment is aimed at reversing these life-threatening cardiovascular manifestations. Intravenous calcium administration should follow initial resuscitative measures if the patient is not responding to general supportive measures alone. Ten percent calcium chloride can be given in doses of 10 ml for adults and 0.1–0.2 ml/kg in pediatric patients (174). Repeat doses with careful monitoring of the serum calcium concentration may be necessary. Gastrointestinal decontamination should be accomplished. Dopamine or dobutamine can be used for persistent hypotension. For symptomatic persistent bradycardias or sinus arrest, glucagon (177), atropine, or isoproterenol can be tried. A temporary pacemaker may be necessary in some cases. There is one case report of a patient who ingested large quantities of diltiazem and metoprolol who responded well to charcoal hemoperfusion (7). No controlled data are available regarding the use of hemoperfusion in calcium channel blocker overdoses.

β-Blockers

Propranolol is the best known of the β-blocking drugs. Other drugs in this class include metoprolol, nadolol, timolol, atenolol, pindolol, and oxyprenolol. β-blockers are used widely in the treatment of hypertension, arrhythmias, glaucoma, angina, migraine disease, and prophylaxis against sudden death in the postmyocardial infarction period. The rise in β-blocker popularity for treatment of these various disorders has also been accompanied by a rise in the incidence of overdoses with these agents (168). Massive overdoses with β-blockers can pose a significant challenge for the intensivist because frequently, traditional pharmacologic management of decreased cardiac output with catecholamines has been unsuccessful.

β-blocking agents differ in their pharmacologic properties. Metoprolol and atenolol are "cardioselective" (β_1 only) in therapeutic doses. Propranolol exhibits the most pronounced membrane depression (168). Membrane-active drugs are more likely to cause CNS effects (e.g., sedation, coma, and convulsions). Pindolol and oxyprenolol possess partial adrenergic receptor agonist activity, leading to tachycardia and hypertension in overdose situations. The more lipophilic drugs tend to be extensively distributed in body tissues and rapidly metabolized by the liver. They are well absorbed but undergo extensive first-pass metabolism. Less lipophilic drugs are distributed less extensively to tissues and are excreted mostly unmetabolized by the kidneys. Half-lives of the metabolized drugs tend to be shorter than those of the drugs excreted by the kidney (34).

β-blockers function at the β-adrenergic receptors in the body. β-1 stimulation increases sinoatrial rate, myocardial contractility, and conduction velocity. β-2 stimulation dilates bronchial smooth muscle and arterioles in skeletal muscle, stimulates insulin secretion, and increases lactic acid production, lipolysis, and glycogenolysis. β-blockade reverses these adrenergic effects.

β-blocker overdose is manifested by bradycardia (72%), hypotension (76%), seizures (28%), peripheral cyanosis (23%), and coma (26%) (168). Heart failure and/or bronchoconstriction can appear in patients with pre-existing heart or lung disease. Hyperglycemia is uncommon but may be a more prominent problem in children and diabetics (76). Cardiogenic shock, intraventricular conduction delays, and asystole due to direct myocardial depression can occur in previously healthy people (146). As mentioned previously, β-blockers with partial adrenergic agonist activity can produce mild to moderate degrees of tachycardia and hypertension.

Diagnosis rests on the suspicion of β-blocker ingestion coupled with profound hypotension and bradycardia resistant to standard therapy. Patients may initially be ambulatory and conversant and within minutes deteriorate to seizures and severe hemodynamic compromise (169). Blood levels are not necessary to management, yet a qualitative toxicology screen may be helpful in the unknown ingestion. Close monitoring of blood glucose may be necessary, particularly during treatment with glucagon. Serum electrolytes, electrocardiograms, and chest x-rays may be helpful but are not diagnostic.

Management of patients with overdoses of β-blockers primarily focuses on reversal of life-threatening hypotension and bradycardia. Standard resuscitative and decontamination measures should be employed. In a patient with a history of a massive ingestion, anticipation of rapid clinical deterioration should include withholding ipecac, achieving early airway control, and keeping diazepam readily available to treat seizures. When treating ventricular arrhythmias, lidocaine is the agent of choice. Use of quinidine, procainamide, and disopyramide is contraindicated because of their myocardial depressant effects.

Although there are no prospective human studies comparing the efficacy of glucagon alone with β-agonists, atropine, and vasopressors, retrospective studies and case reports clearly point out the superiority of glucagon in reversing hypotension and bradycardia associated with massive β-blocker overdose in patients with low cardiac output and normal capillary wedge pressures (168, 169, 178). Glucagon is the agent of choice in this clinical situation. Glucagon produces a positive inotropic and chronotropic effect on the heart via stimulation of glucagon specific receptors in the myocardium that are not blocked by even massive doses of β-blockers (88). Glucagon can have salutary effects within 5−10 minutes after intravenous administration. The optimal dose is not precisely known, but an initial dose of 2−5 mg is advised. Repeat doses may be administered as necessary. Alternately a continuous intravenous infusion of about 1−5 mg/hour, titrated to desired response, can be employed (See chapter 33 B).

While not proven to be more effective than glucagon, atropine, β-agonists, and fluid treatment in the treatment of bradycardia and hypotension have been recommended by most authors. This author favors maximizing treatment with glucagon (after establishing adequate hydration) prior to initiating other therapy. Glucagon can cause persistent vomiting and hyperglycemia. Airway protection and monitoring of the serum glucose are imperative. Bradydysrhythmias resistant to pharmacological management should be treated with a transvenous pacemaker.

Iron

The accidental ingestion of iron-containing compounds by children less than 5 years old continues to be a very common problem. Most iron preparations are over-the-counter vitamins or vitamin supplements that are available in large quantities. Some vitamins are brightly colored, which makes them appealing to children; many parents still do not recognize the potential danger of these compounds to their children. While the majority of iron ingestions can be managed easily without hospital admission, a small percentage of patients will present after significant and sometimes massive ingestion and present a complex management problem for the intensivist. Despite the widespread experience with iron poisoning over the years, several important aspects of treatment remain controversial, including the techniques of gastric lavage, the route of administration of the complexing agent deferoxamine, and the use of the clinical laboratory in management of iron overdose.

The common ferrous salts are sulfates, fumarates, and gluconates. Iron toxicity is related to the total amount of elemental iron ingested. In ferrous sulfate tables, iron content is 20%. Ferrous fumarate preparations contain 33% elemental iron. Ferrous gluconate tablets are 12% iron. A generally accepted lethal dose is 200–250 mg/kg, although fatal ingestions have been recorded with smaller quantities (136).

Iron content of the body is controlled by alterations in absorption. There is no specific mechanism for excretion. Iron is absorbed in the duodenum and jejunum. After oxidation to the ferric state, iron is complexed to a storage protein called ferritin. When iron is released to plasma from ferritin it is transported by binding to the protein transferrin. When transferrin's capacity to bind iron is exceeded, free iron circulates unbound and exerts its toxic effects by depositing into tissues, particularly cells in the liver.

Iron poisoning has classically been divided into stages. Perhaps the most useful approach is that of Lovejoy and Lecoutre (91), which looks at clinical changes in relation to time after ingestion. Early changes occur from 30 minutes to 6 hours after ingestion. Prominent amongst these early changes are gastrointestinal effects. Vomiting and diarrhea occur; frequently they are severe and complicated by gastrointestinal bleeding. Fever and leukocy-tosis may also be present. Shock may ensue from various mechanisms including gastrointestinal blood loss, venous pooling, and increased capillary permeability, all of which lead to a decrease in cardiac output. Acidosis and hyperglycemia may also occur. Intermediate changes occur between 6 and 48 hours postingestion. A brief period of quiescence is followed by profound shock and vascular collapse (84). Hepatic failure may occur with jaundice, elevated liver enzymes, and bleeding disorders. Hypoglycemia may manifest during this phase, secondary to hepatic damage (60). Late changes manifest from 3 days to 3 weeks after ingestion. Characteristic changes include strictures of the stomach, small bowel infarction, liver cirrhosis, and fatty degeneration of the liver.

Diagnosis and therapy in part depend upon timely and selective use of ancillary studies. Specifically, serum iron levels, total iron binding capacity (TIBC), and flat plate abdominal radiographs can be most helpful. Normal serum iron levels range from 100 to 125 ug/dl. Levels above 300 ug/dl should be treated with chelation therapy until the TIBC becomes available. Iron concentrations measured between 4 and 6 hours after ingestion are the most reliable. Iron levels above 1000 μg/dl carry a large increase in mortality (60). If the serum iron exceeds the TIBC, chelation therapy is recommended. Others caution against over-reliance on the TIBC (10). The abdominal flat plate can be helpful in assessing the adequacy of gastric lavage since iron is radiopaque. A positive flat plate is usually associated with a serum iron level above 300 μg/dl (74).

Treatment of iron overdose centers on gastric decontamination and chelation therapy with deferoxamine. Deferoxamine is a highly specific chelator of ferric (Fe+3) iron and has affinity for iron that is 10 times greater than any other known chelator of iron (136). Iron in the gut can be bound by orally administered deferoxamine. Parenterally administered deferoxamine enhances iron elimination through the formation of the water-soluble, renally excreted ferrioxamine.

Gastric emptying is extremely important because of the direct corrosive effect that iron has on the gastric mucosa. Iron preparations tend to form concretions in the stomach with large ingestions (52). Copious gastric lavage should be performed. Although some recommend addition of bicarbonate or deferoxamine to the lavage solution, this is not proven to be more efficacious than saline or tap water alone. In large ingestions, flat plate abdominal radiographs can demonstrate the efficacy of lavage attempts. Large pill concretions resistant to voluminous lavage may need to be removed endoscopically or surgically (52). After lavage is complete, instillation of 100 ml of a 1% sodium bicarbonate solution is recommended. Bicarbonate promotes formation of a ferrous carbonate salt that is less irritating and poorly absorbed. Others recommend instillation of deferoxamine (10 g in 50 ml of water) at the completion of lavage to chelate any iron remaining in the stomach (74). Activated charcoal is not indicated.

Any patient with a serum iron level greater than 300 ug/dl should undergo parenteral chelation therapy. However, a level below 300 ug/dl does not rule out serious toxicity. Because of this, patients exhibiting clinical signs or symptoms of toxicity should also undergo chelation therapy. Other indications for parenteral chelation are a positive deferoxamine challenge test (appearance of vin rosé urine after a single intramuscular dose of deferoxamine) and evidence of radiopaque densities after gastric lavage. Any patient with a history of significant iron ingestion should receive 2 g of deferoxamine intramuscularly (after serum studies are drawn) until further decisions can be made about indications for continuing chelation therapy.

For normotensive patients, deferoxamine can be given intramuscularly. Doses are 50–100 mg/kg, up to 2 g, every 6–8 hours to a maximum of 6 g/24 hours. For hypotensive patients, a continuous infusion of 15 mg/kg/hour is given (10). Chelation therapy should continue until the disappearance of the vin rosé color from the urine, signifying disappearance of the iron-deferoxamine complex. Others recommend continuing chelation therapy for an additional 24 hours after the urine has cleared in patients with initial serum iron levels above 500 $\mu g/dl$ (58).

Because of the high incidence of shock and acidosis in severe poisoning aggressive supportive therapy is mandatory. Fluid and pressor therapy should be guided by hemodynamic monitoring and clinical response. Blood therapy for gastrointestinal bleeding should be anticipated. Administration of sodium bicarbonate for acidosis may be necessary on repeated occasions. Intensive supportive therapy, combined with aggressive decontamination and chelation therapy, can successfully treat even the most severe overdoses.

References

1. Abramowitz M (ed): Acute drug abuse reactions. *Med Letter* 696:77–80, 1985.
2. Achong MR: Clinical pharmacology of analgesic drugs. *Can Fam Physician* 25:179, 1979.
3. Afife AA, Sacks ST, Liu VY, et al: Accumulative prognostic index for patients with barbiturate glutethamide, and meprobamate intoxication. *N Engl J Med* 285:1497–1502, 1971.
4. Ambre J: Principles of pharmacology for the clinician. Winchester, Haddad (eds): *Clinical Management of Poisoning and Drug Overdose*, Philadelphia, WB Saunders, 1983.
5. Anderson RJ, Potts DE, et al: Unrecognized adult salicylate intoxication. *Ann Intern Med* 85:745, 1976.
6. Anonymous: Carbon monoxide, an old enemy forgot. *Lancet* 2:75–76, 1981.
7. Anthony T, Jastremski M, et al: Charcoal hemoperfusion for the treatment of combined diltiazem and metaprolol overdose. *Ann Emerg Med* 15:1344–1348, 1986.
8. Aquilonius SN, Hedstrand V: The use of physostgimine as an antidote in tricyclic antidepressant intoxication. *Acta Anaesthiol Scand* 22:40–45, 1978.
9. Baker MD: Theophylline toxicity in children. *J Pediatr* 109:538–542, 1986.
10. Banner W, Tong TG: Iron Poisoning. *Pediatr Clin North Am* 33:393–409, 1986.
11. Becker C, Sullivan JB: Prompt recognition and vigorous therapy for organophosphate poisoning. *Emerg Med Rep* 7:33–40, 1986.
12. Bennet IL, Cary FH, Mitchell GL: Acute methyl alcohol poisoning: review based on experiences in outreach of 323 cases. *Medicine* 32:431–463, 1953.
13. Benowitz NL, Rosenberg J, Becker CE: Cardiopulmonary catastrophes in drug overdose patients. *Med Clin North Am* 63:267, 1979.
14. Benton CD, Calhoun FP: The ocular effects of methyl alcohol poisoning: report of a catastrophe involving 320 persons. *Am J Ophthalmol* 36:1677–1685, 1952.
15. Berman LB, Schreiner GE, Feys J: The nephrotoxic lesion of ethylene glycol. *Ann Intern Med* 46:611–619, 1957.
16. Bertino JS, Reed MD: Barbiturate and nonbarbiturate sedative hypnotic intoxication in children. *Pediatr Clinics North Am* 33:703–720, 1986.
17. Biberstein MP, Ziegler MG, Ward DM: Use of beta-blockade and hemoperfusion for acute theophylline poisoning. *West J Med* 141:485–490, 1984.
18. Biggs JT, Spiker DG, et al: Tricyclic antidepressant overdose: incidence of symptoms. *JAMA* 238:135, 1977.
19. Black M: Acetaminophen hepatotoxicity. *Ann Rev Med* 35:377, 1984.
20. Brancato JC, Fow MI: Poisoning. Poisoning mortality in the United States, 1978. *Natl Clearingh Poison Control Cent Bull* 25:11–15, 1981.
21. Brandwin MA: Drug overdose emergency room admissions. *Am J Drug Alcohol Abuse* 3:605–619, 1976.
22. Brenner BE, Simon RR: Management of salicylate intoxication. *Drugs* 24:355, 1982.
23. Brown CG, Trumbull D, et al: Ethylene glycol poisoning. *Ann Emerg Med* 12:501–506, 1983.
24. Brown TC: Tricyclic antidepressant overdosage: experimental studies on the management of circulatory complications. *Clin Toxicol* 9:55, 1976.
25. Byers AJ, Traylor TR, Semmer JR: Acetaminophen overdose in the third trimester of pregnancy. *JAMA* 247:3114–3115, 1982.
26. Callaham M: Epidemiology of fatal tricyclics: antidepressant ingestion: management. *Ann Emerg Med* 14:1–9, 1985.
27. Catchings TT, Beane LC, et al: Adult respiratory distress syndrome secondary to ethylene glycol ingestion. *Ann Emerg Med* 14:594–596, 1985.

28. Clemmensen C, Nilsson E: Therapeutic trends in the treatment of barbiturate poisoning: The Scandanavian method. *Clin Pharmacol Ther* 2:220, 1961.

29. Coburn RF: Mechanisms of carbon monoxide poisoning toxicity. *Prev Med* 8:310–322, 1979.

30. Coburn RF, Danielson GK, et al: Carbon monoxide in blood: analytical method and sources of error. *J Appl Physiol* 19:510, 1964.

31. Cotrell JE, Casthel P, et al: Prevention of nitroprusside induced cyanide toxicity with hydroxycolbalamin. *N Engl J Med* 298:809–811, 1978.

32. Crome P, Dawling S, et al: Effect of activated charcoal on nortriptyline. *Lancet* 2:1203, 1977.

33. Crome P, Braithwaite G, et al: Hemoperfusion in clinical and experimental poisoning. Chang (ed): *Hemoperfusion: Kidney and Liver Support and Detoxification.* Washington, Hemisphere Pub, 1980.

34. Cruickshank JM: The clinical importance of cardioselectivity and lipophilicity in beta blockers. *Am Heart J* 100:160, 1980.

35. Cupit GC, Temple AR: Gastrointestinal decontamination in the management of the poisoned patient. *Emerg Med Clin North Am* 1:3–14, 1984.

36. Curry SC, Vance MV, et al: Cardiovascular effects of toxic concentrations of theophylline in the dog. *Ann Emerg Med* 14:547–553, 1985.

37. Daniel DR, McAnalley BH, Garriot JC: Isopropyl alcohol metabolism after acute intoxication in humans. *J Anal Toxicol* 5:110–112, 1981.

38. Davidson DGD: Acute liver necrosis following overdose of paracetamol. *Br Med J* 2:497–499, 1966.

39. deCastro FJ, Jaeger RW, et al: Apomorphine: clinical trial of a stable solution. *Clin Toxicol* 12:65–68, 1978.

40. Doherty JE, deSoyza N, et al: Clinical pharmacokinetics of digitalis glycosides. *Prog Cardiovas Dis* 21:141, 1978.

41. Done AK: Salicylate intoxication: significance of measurements of salicylate in blood in cases of acute ingestion. *Pediatrics* 26:800–807, 1960.

42. Done AK: The toxic emergency. The great equalizer? Anticholinesterases. *Emerg Med* 11:167, 1979.

43. Dorr RT, Paxinos J: The current status of laetrile. *Ann Intern Med* 89:387–389, 1978.

44. Easom JM, Lovejoy FH: Efficacy and safety of gastrointestinal decontamination in the treatment of oral poisoning. *Pediatr Clin North Am* 2:827, 1979.

45. Ellis EF: Theophylline toxicity. *J Allergy Clin Immunol* 76:297, 1985.

46. Epstein FB, Eilers MA: Rosen, et al (eds): Poisoning. Emergency Medicine. *Concepts and Clinical Practice* St. Louis, CV Mosby, 1983.

47. Fairshter RD, Wilson AF: Paraquat poisoning, manifestations and therapy. *Am J Med* 59:751–753, 1975.

48. Ferguson HC: Dilution of dose and acute oral toxicity. *Toxicol Appl Pharmacol* 4:759, 1962.

49. Fifth Special Report to the US Congress on Alcohol and Health. Washington, DC, US Govt Printing Office, 1983.

50. Fiser RH, Maetz HM, et al: Activated charcoal in barbiturate and glutethamide poisoning. *J Pediatrics* 78:1045, 1971.

51. Food and Drug Administration, Bureau of Drugs: Minutes of Ad Hoc Panel on *Toxicity of the Tricyclic Antidepressants* of the Psychopharmacological Agents Advisory Committee, Rockville, MD, September 10, 1975.

52. Foxford R, Goldfrank L: Gastrotomy—A surgical approach to iron overdose. *Ann Emerg Med* 14:1123–1126, 1985.

53. Freedman GE, et al: A clinical trial using syrup of ipecac and activated charcoal concurrently. *Ann Emerg Med* 2:164–166, 1987.

54. Freeman JW, Mundy GR, et al: Cardiac abnormalities in poisoning with tricyclic antidepressants. *Br Med J* 2:610, 1969.

55. Frejaville JP, Nicaise AM, et al: Etude statistique d'une seconde certaine d'intoxications aiques par les derive de l'iminobenzle. *Bul Soc Med Hop Paris* 117:1151, 1966.

56. Garrison RF: Acute poisoning from use of isopropyl alcohol in tepid sponging. *JAMA* 152:317–318, 1953.

57. Gaudreault P, McCormick MA, et al: Poisoning exposures and use of ipecac in children less than one year old. *Ann Emerg Med* 7:808–810, 1986.

58. Ghandi R, Roberts F: Hourglass stricture of the stomach and pyloric stenosis due to ferrous sulfate poisoning. *Br J Surg* 49:613–617, 1962.

59. Glassman AH: Cardiovascular effects of tricyclic antidepressants. *Annual Rev Med* 35:503–511, 1984.

60. Gleason WA, deMello, et al: Acute hepatic failure in severe iron poisoning. *J Pediatr* 95:138–140, 1979.

61. Goldberg MJ, Park GP, Berlinger WG: Treatment of theophylline intoxication. *J Allerg Clin Immunol* 78: 811–817, 1986.

62. Goldfrank L, Flomenbaum N, et al: The liquid time bomb. *Hospital Physician* 18:38–60, 1982.

63. Goldfrank LR, Kirstein R: *Toxicologic Emergencies: A Comprehensive Handbook in Problem Solving.* New York, Appleton-Century-Crofts, 1981.

64. Gonda A, Gault H, et al: Hemodialysis for methanol intoxication. *Am J Med* 64:749–758, 1978.

65. Gosselin RE, Smith RP, Hodge HC: *Clinical Toxicology of Commercial Products,* ed 5. Baltimore, Williams & Wilkins, 1984.

66. Greenblatt DJ, Allen MD, et al: Acute overdosage with benzodiazepine derivatives. *Clin Pharmacol Ther* 21:497–514, 1977.

67. Gross PL, Schwartz HS: Toxicology emergencies. In Wilkens EW (ed): *MGH Textbook of Emergency Medicine.* Baltimore, Williams & Wilkins, 1982.

68. Guzzardi LJ: Role of the emergency physician in the management of the poisoned patient. *Emerg Med Clinics North Am* 1:3–14, 1984.

69. Haddad L: A general approach to the emergency management of poisoning. In Winchester, Haddad (eds): *Clinical Management of Poisoning and Drug Overdose.* Philadelphia, WB Saunders, 1983.

70. Hager WD, Fenster P, et al: Digoxin-quinidine interaction: Pharmacokinetics evaluation. *N Engl J Med* 300:1238, 1979.

71. Hall AH, Rumack BH: Clinical toxicity of cyanide. *Ann Emerg Med* 15:1067–1074, 1986.

72. Hall KW, Dobson KE, et al: Metabolic abnormalities associated with intentional theophylline overdose. *Arch Intern Med* 101:457–462, 1984.

73. Hassan E: Treatment of meprobamate overdose with repeated oral doses of activated charcoal. *Ann Emerg Med* 15:73–76, 1986.

74. Henretig FN, Karl SR, Weintraub WH: Severe iron poisoning treated with enteral and intravenous deferoxamine. *Ann Emerg Med* 12:306–309, 1983.

75. Henry J, Volans G: ABC of poisoning. Analgesics: II paracetamol. *Br Med J* 289:907, 1984.

76. Heese B, Pederson JT: Hypoglycemia after propanolol in children. *Acta Med Scand* 193:551, 1973.

77. Hill JB: Salicylate intoxication. *N Engl J Med* 292:250, 1975.

78. Hill JB: Experimental salicylate poisoning: Observations on the effects of altering blood pH on tissue and plasma salicylate concentrations. *Pediatrics* 47:658, 1971.

79. Hinson J, Pohl K, et al: Acetaminophen—induced hepatotoxicity. *Life Sci* 29:107, 1981.

80. Hornback KD: Overdoing the anticholinergics. *Emerg Med* 13:45–53, 1981.

81. Jackson JE, Bressler R: Prescribing tricyclic antidepressants, Part I. General considerations. *Drug Ther* 11:87–96, 1981.

82. Jackson JE, Bressler R: Prescribing tricyclic antide-

pressants. Part III. Management of overdose. *Drug Ther* 12:49–63, 1982.

83. Jacob AS, Nielsen DH, Gianelly RE: Fatal ventricular fibrillation following verapamil in Wolff-Parkinson-White syndrome with atrial fibrillation. *Ann Emerg Med* 14:159–160, 1985.

84. Jacobs J, Greens H, Gendel BR: Acute iron intoxication. *N Engl J Med* 273:1124, 1965.

85. Jaffe JH, Martin WR: Opioid analgesics and antagonists. In Goodman, Gilman (eds): *The Pharmacologic Basis of Therapeutics.* ed. 6. New York, MacMillian, 1980.

86. Jones J, Heiselman D, et al: Cathartic-induced magnesium toxicity during overdose management. *Ann Emerg Med* 15:1214–1218, 1986.

87. Kallos T, Smith TG: Naloxone reversal of pentazocine-induced respiratory depression. *JAMA* 204:932, 1968.

88. Kazmers A, Whitehouse W, et al: Dissociation of glucagon's central and peripheral hemodynamic effects: Mechanism of reduction and redistribution on canine hindlimb blood flow. *J Surg Res* 30:384–390, 1981.

89. Kearin M, Kelly JG, O'Malley K: Digoxin "receptors" in neonates an explanation of less sensitivity to digoxin than in adults. *Clin Pharmacol Ther* 28:346–349, 1980.

90. Kulig K, et al: Management of acutely poisoned patients without gastric emptying. *Ann Emerg Med* 14:562–567, 1985.

91. Lacouture PG, Lovejoy FH: Iron. Haddad, Winchester (eds): *Clinical Management of Poisoning and Drug Overdose.* Philadelphia, WB Saunders, 1983.

92. Lacouture PG, Wason S, et al: Acute isopropyl alcohol ingestion: diagnosis and management. *Am J Med* 75:680–686, 1983.

93. Lai KN, Swaminathan R, et al: Hemofiltration in digoxin overdose. *Arch Intern Med* 146:1219–1220, 1986.

94. Lehman AJ, Chase HF: The acute and chronic toxicity of isopropyl alcohol. *J Lab Clin Med* 29:561, 1944.

95. Levy G: Gastrointestinal clearance of drugs with activated charcoal. *N Engl J Med* 307:676–678, 1982.

96. Lim DT, Singh P: Absorption inhibition and enhancement of elimination of sustained-release theophylline tablets by oral activated charcoal. *Ann Emerg Med* 15:1303–1307, 1986.

97. Linton AL, Luke RG, Briggs JD: Methods of forced diuresis and its application in barbiturate poisoning. *Lancet* 2:7512, 1967.

98. Manno BR, Manno JE: Toxicology of ipecac: A review. *Clin Toxicol* 10:221, 1977.

99. Marshall JB, Forker AD: Cardiovascular effects of tricyclic antidepressant drugs: therapeutic usage, overdosage, and management of complications. *Am Heart J* 103:401–414, 1982.

100. Marstellar H, Gugler R: Endoscopic management of toxic masses in the stomach. *N Engl J Med* 196:1003, 1977.

101. McCarthy LG, Speth CP: Diquat intoxication. *Ann Emerg Med* 12:394–396, 1983.

102. McCoy HG, Cipolle RJ, et al: Severe methanol poisoning: application of a pharmacokinetic model for ethanol therapy and hemodialysis. *Am J Med* 67:804, 1979.

103. McGuigan MA: Planning an effective strategy for theophylline poisoning in adults. *Emerg Med Rep* 8:41–48, 1987.

104. Michiels TM, Light RW, Mahutte CK: Naloxone reverses ethanol-induced depression of hypercapnic drive. *Am Rev Respir Dis* 128:823–826, 1983.

105. Mitchell JR, Jollow DT, et al: Acetaminophen-induced hepatic necrosis, role of drug metabolism. *J Pharmacol Exp Ther* 187:184–194, 1973.

106. Mofenson HC, Caraccio TR, Schauber J: Poisoning by antidysrhythmic drugs. *Ped Clinics North Am* 33:723–738, 1986.

107. Morgan AG, Polak A: The excretion of salicylate in salicylate poisoning. *Clin Sci* 41:475–484, 1971.

108. Morgan DP: *Recognition and Management of Pesticide Poisonings,* 3rd ed. Wash DC, US Environmental Protection Agency, 1982.

109. Morgan MD, Pusey CD, et al: Treatment of quinine poisoning with charcoal hemoperfusion, *Post Med J* 59:365–367, 1983.

110. Mountain RD, Neff TA: Oral theophylline intoxication: a serious error of patient and physician understanding. *Arch Intern Med* 144:724–727, 1984.

111. Murphy DJ, Bremer WF, Haber E: Massive digoxin overdose treated with FAB: fragment of digoxin specific antibodies. *Pediatrics* 70:;472, 1982.

112. Myers RAM, Linberg SE, Crowley RA: Carbon monoxide poisoning, the injury and its treatment. *JACEP* 8:479–484, 1979.

113. Myers RAM, Synder SK, et al: Value of hyperbaric oxygen in suspected carbon monoxide poisoning. *JAMA* 246:2478–2480, 1981.

114. Namba T: Diagnosis and treatment of organophosphate insecticide poisoning. *Med Times* 100:100–126, 1972.

115. Namba T, Nolte C, et al: Poisoning due to organophosphate insecticides. *Am J Med* 50:475–492, 1975.

116. National Safety Council: Accident Facts. Chicago, National Safety Council, 1982.

117. Nattel S, Bayne L, Ruedy J: Physostigmine in coma due to drug overdose. *Clin Pharmacol Ther* 25:96–102, 1979.

118. Newton RW: Physostigmine in the treatment of tricyclic antidepressant overdose. *JAMA* 231:941–943, 1975.

119. Niemann JT, Besser HA, et al: Electrocardiographic criteria for tricyclic antidepressant cardiotoxicity. *Am J Cardiol* 57:1154–1159, 1986.

120. Norkool DM, Kirkpatrick JN: Treatment of acute carbon monoxide poisoning with hyperbaric oxygen: a review of 115 cases. *Ann Emerg Med* 14:1168–1171, 1985.

121. Olson KR, Benowitz NC, et al: Theophylline overdose: acute single ingestion versus chronic repeated overmedication. *Am J Emerg Med* 3:408, 1985.

122. Ordog GI, Benaron S, et al: Serum digoxin levels and motality in 5,100 patients. *Ann Emerg Med* 16:32–39, 1987.

123. Osterpoh J: Limitations of acetaminophen assays. *J Toxicol Clin Toxicol* 20:19, 1983.

124. Parry MF, Wallack R: Ethylene glycol poisoning. *Am J Med* 57:143, 1974.

125. Pentel P, Peterson CD: Asystole complicating physostigmine treatment of tricyclic antidepressant overdose. *Ann Emerg Med* 9:588–590, 1980.

126. Peterson C, Collins A, et al: Ethylene glycol poisoning: pharmacokinetics during therapy with ethanol and hemodialysis. *N Engl J Med* 304:21–23, 1981.

127. Piper KW, Griner PF: Suicide attempts with drug overdose. *Arch Intern Med* 134:703–706, 1974.

128. Pond SN: Diuresis, dialysis, and hemoperfusion. *Emerg Med Clin North Am* 2:29–45, 1984.

129. Proudfoot AT: Toxicity of salicylates. *Am J Med* 75:99–103, 1983.

130. Proudfoot AT, Brown SS: Acidemia and salicylate poisoning in adults. *Br Med J* 2:547–550, 1969.

131. Ragan FA, Samuels MS, Hite SA: Ethanol in children. *JAMA* 242:2787–2788, 1979.

132. Reed K: Tricyclic antidepressant blood levels—eight practical questions. *Postgrad Med* 70:81–88, 1981.

133. Renzi FP, Donovan JW, et al: Concomitant use of activated charcoal and N-acetylcysteine. *Ann Emerg Med* 4:568–572, 1985.

134. Roberts RJ, Mueller S, Lauer RM: Propanolol in the treatment of cardiac arrythmias associated with amitryptiline intoxication. *J Pediatr* 82:65, 1973.

135. Roberts RJ, Morgan DP: Organophosphate and N-methyl

carbamate insecticides. Edlick and Spyker (eds): *Current Emergency Therapy*. Rockville, Aspen Systems, 1985.

136. Robotham JL, Lietman PS: Acute iron poisoning. *Am J Dis Child* 134:875–878, 1980.

137. Rosenberg J, Benowitz NL, Pond S: Pharmacokinetics of drug overdose. *Clin Pharmacokinet* 6:161–192, 1981.

138. Rudolph JP: Automated gastric lavage and a comparison of 0.9% normal saline solution and tap water irrigant. *Ann Emerg Med* 14:1156–1159, 1985.

139. Rumack BH: Acetaminophen overdose. *Am J Med* 76:104–111, 1983.

140. Rumack BH, Matthew H: Acetaminophen poisoning and toxicity. *Pediatrics* 55:871–876, 1975.

141. Rumack BH, Peterson RG: Acetaminophen overdose: incidence, diagnosis, and management in 416 patients. *Pediatrics* 62:898–903, 1978.

142. Rumack BH, Wolfe RR, Gilfrick H: Phenytoin treatment of massive digoxin overdose. *Br Heart J* 36:405–408, 1974.

143. Sejersted OM, Jacobson D, et al: Formate concentrations in plasma in patients poisoned with methanol. *Acta Med Scand* 213:105–110, 1983.

144. Sessler CN, Glauser FL, Cooper KR: Treatment of theophylline toxicity with oral activated charcoal. *Chest* 87:325–329, 1985.

145. Severance H: Vomiting and abdominal pain. *Case Stud Emerg Med* 12:4–6, 1986.

146. Shore ET, Cepin D, Davidson MJ: Metoprolol overdose. *Ann Emerg Med* 10:524–526, 1981.

147. Smith PW: Bulletin: Medical problems in aerial applications. Office of Aviation Medicine, Federal Aviation Administration, Department of Transportation, Washington DC, 1977.

148. Smith TW, Haber E: Digitalis IV. *N Engl J Med* 289:1125, 1973.

149. Snodgras WR: Salicylate toxicity. *Ped Clin North Am* 33:381–391, 1986.

150. Snodgras WR, Rumack BH, et al: Salicylate toxicity following therapeutic doses in young children. *Clin Toxicol* 18:247–259, 1981.

151. Snover SW, Bocchino V: Massive diltiazem overdose. *Ann Emerg Med* 15:1221–1224, 1986.

152. Sogge MR, Griffith JL, et al: Lavage to remove enteric coated aspirin and gastric outlet obstruction. *Ann Int Med* 87:721, 1977.

153. Spiegel A, Marchlinski FE: Time course for reversal of digoxin toxicity with digoxin—specific antibody fragments. *Am Heart J* 109:1397, 1985.

154. Steinberg AD, Karliner JS: The clinical spectrum of heroin pulmonary edema. *Arch Intern Med* 122:122, 1968.

155. Sturman K, Mofenson H, Carracio T: Methylene chloride inhalation: an unusual form of drug abuse. *Ann Emerg Med* 14:903–905, 1985.

156. Sullivan JB, Lander DH: Planning an effective therapeutic strategy in salicylate poisoning. *Emerg Med Rep* 7:89–96, 1986.

157. Tafuri J, Roberts J: Organophosphate poisoning. *Ann Emerg Med* 16:193–202, 1987.

158. Tandberg D, Abercrombie R: Treatment of heroin overdose with endotracheal naloxone. *Ann Emerg Med* 11:443–445, 1982.

159. Temple AR: Acute and chronic effects of aspirin toxicity and their treatment. *Arch Intern Med* 141:364, 1981.

160. Tenenbein M: Multiple dose charcoal therapy. *Curr Probl Pediatr* 7:214, 1986.

161. Thompson ME, Verhulst HL: Ipecac syrup in antiemetic ingestion. *JAMA* 196:433, 1966.

162. Tintinalli JE: The alcohols. In Tintinalli, et al (eds): *Emergency Medicine: A Comprehensive Study Guide*. New York, McGraw-Hill, 1985.

163. Uhl JA: Phenytoin: The drug of choice in tricyclic overdose? *Ann Emerg Med* 10:270–274, 1984.

164. Underwood E, Bennet W: Ethylene glycol intoxication. *JAMA* 226:1453–1454, 1978.

165. Veltri JC, Temple AR: Telephone management of poisonings using syrup of ipecac. *Clin Toxicol* 9:407, 1976.

166. Walls RM, Sloan MB: Coma in a fire victim. *Case Stud Emerg Med* 11:10–12, 1985.

167. Weden GP, Oderda GM, et al: Relative toxicity of cyclic antidepressants. *Ann Emerg Med* 15:797–804, 1986.

168. Weinstein RS: Recognition and management of poisoning with beta-adrenergic blocking agents. *Ann Emerg Med* 13:1123–1131, 1984.

169. Weinstein RS, Cole S, et al: Beta blocker overdose with propanolol and atenolol. *Ann Emerg Med* 14:161–163, 1985.

170. Weller-Fahy ER, Berger LR, Troutman WG: Mouthwash: A source of acute ethanol intoxication. *Pediatrics* 66:302–304, 1980.

171. Winchester JF: Active methods for detoxification: oral sorbents, forced diuresi hemoperfusion, and hemodialysis. In Winchester, Haddad (eds): *Clinical Management of Poisoning and Drug Overdose*. Philadelphia, WB Saunders, 1983.

172. Winchester JF, Gelfand MC, et al: Dialysis and hemoperfusion of poisons and drugs. *Trans Am Soc Artif Organs* 23:762, 1977.

173. Winter PM, Miller JN: Carbon monoxide poisoning. *JAMA* 236:1502–1504, 1976.

174. Worthley LIG: Treating the adverse effects of verapamil. *JAMA* 252:1129, 1984.

175. Yatzides H, Voudiclari S, et al: Treatment of severe barbiturate poisoning. *Lancet* 2:216, 1965.

176. Yearly Report. Washington, DC, National Center for Health Statistics, 1977.

177. Zaloga GP, Malcolm D, Holaday J, Chernow B: Glucagon reverses the hypotension and bradycardia of verapamil overdose in rats. *Crit Care Med* 13:273, 1985.

178. Zaloga GP, Delacey W, Holmebae E, Chernow B: Glucagon reverses the hypotension of anaphylactic shock. *Ann Intern Med* 105:65–66, 1986.

179. Zwillich CW, Sutton FD, et al: Theophylline-induced seizures in adults: correlation with serum concentration. *Ann Intern Med* 82:784–787, 1975.

40

Glucocorticoids in Sepsis

John N. Sheagren, M.D.

Glucocorticoids ("steroids") are being used with increasing frequency in medical practice (29). In most situations, steroids are primarily used for their anti-inflammatory effects in an effort to reduce the contribution of the host's inflammatory response to destructive disease processes. In the case of infection, glucocorticoids reduce inflammation just as they do in other situations; however, the downside is that inflammation may be inhibiting progression of the underlying infectious agent. Thus, glucocorticoids, by their anti-inflammatory action, may enhance the proliferation and spread of a number of infectious agents and in the end cause more severe infections than if glucocorticoids were not present. Obviously, if the infectious agent is otherwise harmless, then glucocorticoids can be an excellent, primary therapeutic modality. In most cases, however, proliferation of the causative microbe must be halted, usually by an antimicrobial agent, at the time of glucocorticoid administration; otherwise disastrous results may occur.

In medical practice, the types of diseases treated with glucocorticoids are generally those in which inflammation is a major contributor to the disease process (19). Prime examples are many of the collagen vascular diseases, many "allergic" reactions, and a variety of situations in which nonspecific, inflammatory irritants produce either tissue or organ malfunction. Different dosages of glucocorticoids, produce a variety of different effects, and an understanding of the varying effects of glucocorticoids at different dose levels is crucial to the understanding of their potential use in septic conditions (28).

DOSE-RESPONSE EFFECTS

Physiological Dose

Physiological glucocorticoid doses are 20–100 mg/day of hydrocortisone, 5–20 mg/day of prednisone, or their equivalents. The term "physiological" is used to describe the preceding doses because such doses are at the lower end of the dosage range of the therapeutic use of glucocorticoids. In normal individuals who are not in a stress situation, the amount of hydrocortisone typically secreted by the adrenal cortex in a 24-hour period is approximately 20–30 mg/day (38). Under stress conditions, the adrenal output of cortisol may increase to 100 mg/day or more (38). At these physiological levels, glucocorticoids primarily support the metabolic processes required to meet the energy demands both at basal and stress conditions. There is little evidence that at physiological doses, even up to 100 mg/day of hydrocortisone given briefly (a few days to 1–2 weeks), there is any effect on host defenses. More prolonged exposure to levels of 100 mg/day of hydrocortisone (approximately 20–25 mg/day of prednisone) results in some immunosuppressive and/or anti-inflammatory sequelae. Glucocorticoids produce their anti-inflammatory effect primarily by impairing access of the polymorphonuclear (PMN) leukocyte to foci of inflammation; in addition, some reduction in T cell function also occurs (29). Whether all such immunosuppressive effects are due solely to glucocorticoids or also result from secondary impacts of metabolic and/or nutritional alterations are not known and need to be studied.

Pharmacological Dose

Pharmacological glucocorticoid doses are 40–200 mg or 1–3 mg/kg daily of prednisone or its equivalent. Glucocorticoids used in the preceding doses cause many alterations in the immune system when given daily, especially when administered in divided doses (8). Less effect on immunity (and on metabolic processes) is achieved when the entire dose is given once daily in the morning, and such effects are almost eliminated if such doses are given once every other morning (the so-called alternate-day steroid dosing regimen) (29).

Daily dosing schedules of glucocorticoids, typically at the outset given in divided daily doses (for example, 80 mg of prednisone is usually given as 20 mg four times a day), are highly effective in treating inflammatory and allergic conditions. Such doses substantially suppress acute inflammation under almost all experimental and clinical situations. Such doses almost uniformly impair PMN responses to chemotactic stimuli in peripheral inflammatory sources. Also, PMNs marginate less well and egress from the microvasculature into areas of inflammation very poorly. Thus, such doses of glucocorticoids impair inflammatory cell accumulation in inflammatory exudates, and persons on such doses are known to be especially prone to infections with acute pyogenic bacteria. Not only are pyogenic infections more frequent in patients on pharmacological doses of glucocorticoids, but particularly devastating to the clinician is the fact that signs and symptoms accompanying progression of underlying infection are reduced. Patients on pharmacological doses of glucocorticoids have a delay in the development of fever, and the site of the initial infection does not show the normal inflammatory signs of pain, redness, swelling, and edema (8).

For these reasons, patients on pharmacological doses of glucocorticoids usually have had an infection progress much more extensively when recognized by the clinician than a similar infection in a patient not receiving glucocorticoids. Thus, bacterial infections may become overwhelming, often with bacteremia. Such infections certainly occur more frequently in patients on high doses of glucocorticoids; however, data on the actual frequency of infection in such patients are not now available (28).

It is clear that initiation of pharmacological doses of glucocorticoids does not immediately predispose to infection, and it is not clear how long a patient needs to be on such doses before the risk of infection becomes substantial. It is likely that 2–4 weeks of therapy are required before the risk of serious pyogenic infection is substantially increased (28). For example, it is known that previously healthy young adults with severe head injuries do not develop an increased incidence of pulmonary infections during a 14-day period of ventilation whether or not they received low, moderate, or high doses of the glucocorticoid, dexamethasone (6).

Pharmacological doses of glucocorticoids also impair the cell-mediated and humoral immune systems (8, 29). Again, suppression of these two limbs of the specific immune system are not immediately produced by large doses of glucocorticoids but also evolve progressively over time. The humoral immune system is least affected and requires higher and more prolonged glucocorticoid doses to decrease both numbers and function of B lymphocytes and plasma cells. Patients receiving pharmacological doses of glucocorticoids for prolonged periods of time gradually decrease B cell function and therefore antibody production; however, clinically there does not seem to be a particularly high incidence of infections with encapsulated pyogenic bacteria, agents against which the host depends primarily on the production of opsonizing antibody (6). As noted earlier, it becomes very hard to know whether an increased rate of infection is due solely to the inhibition of the nonspecific inflammatory response in general or to decreased B cell/antibody function in specific.

T cell numbers and functions are substantially altered by pharmacological doses of glucocorticoids (29). Interestingly, some animal species are much more susceptible to the anti-T cell effects of glucocorticoids than others, and humans are relatively steroid-resistant species. In steroid-susceptible species (mice, rats, rabbits, etc), the administration of pharmacological doses of glucocorticoids leads to the breakdown of T cells. In humans, T cells are much more resistant to destruction by glucocorticoids, but measurements of T cell/macrophage (MP) functions reveal impairment (8). For example, patients on pharmacological doses of glucocorticoids gradually lose delayed hypersensitivity-type skin responses to antigens with which they have been previously immunized. In a remarkable study of the effect of prednisone on the tuberculin response, Bovornkitti et al. (5) showed that within 30 days of starting 40 mg/day of prednisone, almost all patients had lost their skin test responses to tuberculin. Those investigators also showed that after glucocorticoids were discontinued, delayed hypersensitivity skin reactions to tuberculin reappeared in 7–14 days. Such observations correlate very well with the demonstrated increase in the incidence and severity of infections with facultative intracellular microbes, the tubercle bacillus being the prime example of such an infectious agent in humans.

Alternate-day dosing schedules of glucocorticoids leave intact inflammatory cell function (9) and permit maintenance of normal delayed hypersensitivity skin responses (21). In long-term follow-up of large numbers of patients maintained on alternate-day glucocorticoid regimens even at very high doses (up to 120 mg of prednisone four times a day), infections have been well tolerated and no reports of more numerous or severe infections have been forthcoming (21, 28). Over the last decade, the principle has emerged that every patient who needs pharmacologic doses of glucocorticoids in order to control an underlying inflammatory or allergic disease should have regular attempts made to switch to an alternate-day glucocorticoid regimen (29).

Suprapharmacological Dose

Suprapharmacological glucocorticoid doses are 30 mg/kg of methylprednisolone sodium succinate (MPSS) or its equivalent. The usefulness of extremely large doses of glucocorticoids has been increasingly documented over the last several years (29); indeed, such doses, usually infused over a 15–30 minute period, may produce dramatic reductions in both acute and chronic inflammatory responses and, if given for a short term, are quite safe. Conditions for which such doses are presently being used include acute transplant rejection, flaring collagen vascular diseases and systemic inflammatory responses generated by drug reactions, or, until recently found to be ineffective, severe bacterial septic episodes with impending septic shock.

Exactly how these high glucocorticoid doses produce their acute anti-inflammatory and immunosuppressive effects are not entirely known. A number of investigators have shown, however, that within minutes after administering such a dose (30 mg/kg of MPSS, for example) there is relatively complete inhibition of the activation of the PMN and its accumulation in inflammatory stimuli (17). Also there is decreased PMN aggregation and adherence, and intravascularly activated PMNs that tend to clump and form leukostatic plugs can be disaggregated, at least in vitro (34). Not only is the PMN physically less involved in the inflammatory response, but biochemically the production of many of its toxic inflammatory substances is impaired (34). In addition, many

humoral inflammatory mediator systems resulting in the production of a variety of pro-inflammatory materials are inhibited by such doses of glucocorticoids. The activation of the complement system is directly impaired (23), as is, probably, activation of the kallikrein-kinin system. Also, the massive release of endorphins, occurring during all stress situations (16), is inhibited by large doses of glucocorticoids via the same negative feedback loop as that which inhibits the release of ACTH. Thus, suprapharmacological doses of glucocorticoids have been suggested as valuable in treating acute systemic inflammatory reactions as well as isolated organ-threatening inflammatory processes (for example, acutely progressive glomerulonephritis in systemic lupus erythematosus).

TREATMENT OF INFECTIOUS SITUATIONS

Glucocorticoids may be helpful in a variety of infectious situations. First, a variety of specific, localized infections have been treated with steroids (28). The primary objective in such situations is to reduce the local inflammatory response that has produced, or may result in organ malfunction or in other ways has threatened to impair host homeostasis. A second situation in which glucocorticoids have been used in infection is during "severe sepsis" (31). Severe sepsis is defined as the presence of signs and symptoms indicating that an individual is likely to be septic and may rapidly deteriorate. The most life-threatening complication of infection is the hemodynamic deterioration resulting in septic shock with or without the syndrome of multiple organ system failure.

In this section, I review the rationale for the use of glucocorticoids in infectious situations, focusing first on their use in specific, isolated infections and then on their use in the septic shock syndrome.

Treatment of Specific Infections: Pathogenetic Aspects

As outlined earlier, as a microbe begins to proliferate during the establishment of a peripheral infection, damage can either be caused directly by the microbe (usually via the production of toxic substances and/or tissue damaging enzymes) or by the reaction of the host to organism proliferation which results in inflammation. Antimicrobial agents (antibiotics) are directed at halting organism proliferation and, of course, are required successfully to treat more serious infections. It is to reduce the potential additional damaging effect of the host's inflammatory response that pharmacological or suprapharmacological doses of glucocorticoids are administered in some specific infections.

High doses of glucocorticoids have been used for many years to reduce the symptoms of acute inflammation and to lessen subsequent fibrotic sequelae caused by certain types of infections. As noted earlier, high doses of glucocorticoids reduce fever as well as the local signs and symptoms of inflammation especially pain, redness, swelling, and warmth (19, 28). Thus, if the symptoms of inflammation are impairing patient well-being or threatening function of a vital organ, high doses of glucocorticoids may be lifesaving and may produce dramatic symptomatic relief. Examples of the use of glucocorticoids in specific infections are described next.

First, steroids may suppress inflammation and/or fibrosis in "critical" closed-space infections such as pericarditis (especially tuberculous) (24), meningoencephalitis and brain abscess (25) (to counteract brain edema), epiglottitis (11) and other soft tissue infections of the neck and upper airway.

Second, some of the distressing local and systemic manifestations of certain viral infections are promptly alleviated by pharmacological doses of glucocorticoids. Best studied have been infectious mononucleosis (30) and varicella zoster infections (20). Glucocorticoids have been used in mumps infections, especially when complicated by orchitis or pancreatitis, although there are no studies of efficacy. It is not known how glucocorticoids are able to limit the symptoms of these viral infections and do so without permitting spread of the agent with potentially calamatous results.

Third, a variety of allergic or hypersensitivity complications of infections can be controlled with high-dose glucocorticoid treatment (28). The asthmatic symptoms accompanying bronchopulmonary aspergillosis rapidly resolve. Patients may develop diffuse dermal hypersensitivity reactions to mycoplasma infections (i.e., the Stevens-Johnson syndrome) which promptly responds to steroids (28). Certain infections caused by streptococci and systemic fungal infections may be associated with erythema nodosum (EN), which may produce substantial disability; EN is rapidly controlled by glucocorticoids. Finally, patients who are receiving lifesaving antibiotics for which there are no alternatives and who have developed hypersensitivity reactions to them may have the drugs continued with the addition of glucocorticoids (28).

Treatment of Septic Shock Syndrome: Rationale

In almost every experimental model of septic shock produced either by administered live bacteria or by an infusion of endotoxin, pretreatment with glucocorticoids dramatically decreases mortality (31). Such favorable results of glucocorticoids in experimental shock models have been described in mice, rats, rabbits, dogs and a variety of primates; the best model has been the baboon during a systemic infusion of *Escherichia coli* (13).

In the baboon model, utilized by Hinshaw et al. (13), complete protection was provided by the simultaneous infusion of 30 mg/kg of methylprednisolone sodium succinate (MPSS) followed by a 15 mg/kg infusion over the next several hours. If the infusion was delayed for 2 hours after the start of the infusion of the E. coli, approximately a 20% mortality rate occurred (14), and if the infusion was delayed for 4 hours, approximately a 40% mortality was observed (12). Thus, in the baboon model, concomitant infusion of suprapharmacological glucocorticoid doses essentially eliminated mortality.

PATHOGENETIC BASIS FOR HIGH-DOSE THERAPY

The following sections touch on each pathogenetic point in which glucocorticoids could have a lifesaving effect during serious systemic infection. Focused upon in this discussion are the anti-inflammatory effects noted previously, the effect of glucocorticoids in countering the output of endorphins, their anti-mast-cell effect, and their ability to reduce the production of cachectin output by macrophages.

Anti-inflammatory Effects

As noted earlier in this chapter, glucocorticoids substantially alter the nonspecific limb of the immune system involving the accumulation and activation of the PMN by inflammatory stimuli (28). As happens locally, systemic activation of a variety of inflammatory mediator systems occurs during the infusion of high-molecular-weight bacterial polysaccharides (31, 32). Endotoxin has been best studied. Endotoxin activates the complement system via the alternative pathway (23), resulting in the production both of anaphylatoxic substances and chemotactic substances. Of the anaphylatoxins, C_{5a} has been best studied, and that small peptide directly causes mast cell degranulation, an effect that is discussed in more detail below. C_{5a} is the major chemotactic substance generated by the complement pathway although other complement components may also play roles in attracting and activating PMNs to inflammatory foci. C_{5a}, as do almost all chemotactic peptide substances, initiates movement of the PMN into the focus of inflammation and activates in a variety of ways the PMNs internal killing systems (40, 7). When infused systemically, C_{5a} causes intravascular activation of PMNs, resulting in aggregation and the formation of small "leukostatic plugs" of aggregated PMNs (40). The activated PMNs also adhere avidly to endothelial cells, releasing their destructive substances in the process (7). Both in vivo and in vitro (34) massive doses of glucocorticoids halt these processes dramatically, reducing the ability of activated PMNs to damage the cells and tissues with which they are in contact (28). Thus, high doses of glucocorticoids predictably should decrease both endothelial cell damage and the capillary leak syndrome (28, 33) that develops rapidly during systemic sepsis.

Anti-Mast-Cell Effects

As noted previously, high doses of glucocorticoids halt the generation of complement components by directly interfering with complement system activation. Further, when present in the medium in which mast cells are incubating, steroids interfere with mast cell activation by a variety of activating substances including complement-generated anaphylatoxic components (1). As with all other granulocytes, glucocorticoids stabilize mast cell cellular components and prevent degranulation, resulting in decreased histamine release.

Antimacrophage Effects

Just as glucocorticoids halt the activation of the macrophage (8) (partially explaining why

glucocorticoids enhance the development of facultative intracellular microbial infections such as tuberculosis), so do high-dose glucocorticoids affect the production of a large number of "monokines" released from the activated macrophage. Of recent interest have been data showing that cachectin (also known as "tumor necrosis factor") participates in (or even mediates) the metabolic deterioration occurring during endotoxemia and Gram-negative sepsis (2). While many immunologic stimuli cause cachectin to be produced, one of the strongest stimuli to cachectin production is bacterial lipopolysaccharide (endotoxin), and an important series of recent studies from the Rockefeller University have shown the following:

1. Glucocorticoids, if given before endotoxin infusion, stop the production of cachectin by macrophages (3). If cachectin production has already been initiated, glucocorticoids do not help (3).
2. Cachectin infusion in experimental animals mimics almost completely the septic shock syndrome (37).
3. An antiserum neutralizing cachectin can, during recombinant cachectin infusion (37), protect animals from organ failure and death.
4. Preliminary experiments (4) show that anticachectin antiserum may protect animals against lethal endotoxin infusion, almost certainly implicating cachectin as a primary mediator of cell and organ system damage during endotoxemia.

In summary, cachectin probably plays a central role in the septic shock syndrome and associated failure of multiple organ system. Cachectin probably explains the heretofore unexplained rapid shutdown of cellular metabolic processes during severe sepsis (22). Therapeutic modalities directed at neutralizing the acute effect of cachectin during systemic sepsis will probably be of major benefit in treatment of septic patients. Glucocorticoids are of theoretical value, but need to be infused before, at, or no later than very shortly after the entry of endotoxin or live bacteria into the bloodstream in order to have a protective effect.

Antiendorphin Effects

The precursor molecule that produces adrenocorticotropic hormone (ACTH) during systemic stress also results in the production of β-lipotropin, which then forms a variety of the endorphins and enkephalins (16). To grossly state what happens during stress: the same stimuli that result in the production of ACTH (which provides metabolic, electrolyte, and volume support during stress) also result in the massive release of a variety of endorphins and enkephalins (16, 32). The latter substances are powerful opiate-like substances that provide pain relief and reduce anxiety during severe stress and trauma. These substances, however, have the same adverse effects as synthetic opiates (like morphine and meperidine) in that they contribute to vasodilation (16) and enhance capillary leakage.

Interestingly, there were no adverse effects of glucocorticoid administration despite the theoretical concern about dissemination of the viral infection. Also, the effect seemed to be much greater in elderly patients. Thus, in patients past midlife who present with particularly painful onset of varicella-zoster infection, a "burst" dose of glucocorticoids seems indicated to reduce postherpetic neuralgia.

In an anecdotal report, patients with infectious mononucleosis with severe pharyngitis interfering with nutrition and with continued high spiking fevers responded, within hours, to pharmacological doses of glucocorticoids (30). Sixty to 80 mg of prednisone daily for several days followed by rapid tapering results in clearing of the clinical symptomatology. The patient becomes afebrile and the severe sore throat rapidly resolves. Again, while not done in a controlled prospective fashion, adverse sequela seem minimal.

As regards bacterial infections, rapid stabilization of airway obstruction has been repeatedly observed in infants and children suffering acute bacterial epiglottis, and many pediatricians use short-term, high-dose glucocorticoid therapy along with broad-spectrum antibiotic coverage in infants who exhibit impending airway obstruction (11).

Finally, in a study that again was not fully controlled, the use of glucocorticoids in tuberculous pericarditis resulted in better outcome than in patients not treated with steroids (24).

Glucocorticoids inhibit the release of ACTH through the classical negative feedback loop (16), and the output of endorphins is also suppressed by glucocorticoids (32). Thus, glucocorticoid infusion early in systemic stress should decrease the contribution of the endorphins to hemodynamic instability and capillary leakage. The rationale for the use of naloxone and other opiate antagonists in the periphery operate on the same principle (16).

High-dose glucocorticoids given early enough in severe sepsis should have the same salutary effect.

CLINICAL CONSIDERATIONS

The preceding sections have outlined the rationale for the use of glucocorticoids in a variety of infectious situations. This section attempts to provide specific clinical data supporting the use of glucocorticoids in sepsis.

Use of Glucocorticoids in Specific Infections

Few controlled studies have been carried out defining unequivocally the beneficial effect of glucocorticoids in specific infections. The best study to date is the prospective randomized administration of glucocorticoids to patients suffering varicellar zoster infections (shingles) (20, 18). In that study, glucocorticoid-treated patients had fewer adverse postherpetic sequelae, especially chronic postherpetic neuralgia.

Use of Glucocorticoids in Severe Sepsis (Impending Septic Shock and/or Multiple Organ System Failure)

Several studies over the last decade have suggested that glucocorticoids might, as expected from experimental and in vitro studies, be beneficial in patients suffering systemic bacteremia and impending septic shock. Schumer (27) published a study in 1976 in which controlled administration of suprapharmacological doses of glucocorticoids reduced mortality. That study was controversial and did not convince the Food and Drug Administration (FDA) to permit septic shock to be an indication for high-dose glucocorticoid administration. Hoffman et al. (15) have convincingly demonstrated that high-dose glucocorticoid treatment reduced mortality in "severe typhoid fever." Typhoid fever is, however, an aberrant type of Gram-negative infection: It is a better tolerated form of Gram-negative bacteremia, and the host depends on the T cell/ macrophage system far more for defense than with acute pyogenic septic episodes and Gram-negative bacteremia. Thus, the data generated by that study are seen directly applicable to the kind of patients treated in most clinical situations. Sprung and his colleagues (36) demonstrated no reduction in mortality of patients administered high-dose glucocorticoids who were in full-blown septic shock. In his studies, patients were randomized after having experienced an average of 18 hours of frank shock: high mortality (70% or greater) was seen in each group. Glucocorticoids did, however, somewhat delay death.

Because of the continued controversy, two multicenter studies of early glucocorticoid treatment of patients suffering the syndrome of severe sepsis were initiated in the early 1980s. Both of those studies have now been terminated. Each study used well-defined entry criteria highly predictive of the patients being bacteremic and at high risk of developing septic shock. In fact, in both studies, approximately half of the patients had positive blood cultures. The studies were planned so that high-dose glucocorticoid administration was initiated within 2–4 hours of the recognition of the septic event. Both studies showed no beneficial effects of high-dose glucocorticoid administration. Further, one of the two studies, the one using higher doses of glucocorticoids for a more prolonged period of time, showed a trend toward *increased* mortality in the glucocorticoid cohort, especially those entering the study with serum creatinine levels in excess of 2 mg/dl. The Upjohn Company, sponsor of the larger of the two studies (19 centers with an enrollment of 382 patients), felt it appropriate to issue a letter to all practicing physicians noting the lack of efficacy of glucocorticoids in severe sepsis and warning that some subgroups of patients could, in fact, suffer increased mortality. In the other study sponsored by the Veterans Administration (VA) (10 centers with an enrollment of 223 patients), no difference was demonstrated in mortality between the glucocorticoid and control patient groups. The VA study showed, however, no adverse glucocorticoid effects. The VA study used lower drug doses for a shorter period of time than did the Upjohn study, making the point that the downside of glucocorticoid use in critically ill, seriously septic patients may be enhanced mortality due primarily to secondary infection.

A variety of studies have failed to show that glucocorticoids are helpful in sepsis-induced ARDS (10, 39). Again, at least one study showed an increased mortality in glucocorticoid-treated patients with ARDS in the intensive care unit. One study of ARDS induced by multiple fractures (bone marrow embolism–induced ARDS), however, showed that prophylactic administration of MPSS did reduce the severity of the bone marrow embolism syndrome (26).

SUMMARY

This chapter has outlined the rationale for, and the current status of, the use of the glucocorticoids in sepsis. There are a variety of isolated, specific, potentially life-threatening infections in which glucocorticoids seem to be helpful: especially acute bacterial infections occurring in critical closed spaces, tuberculous pericarditis and infections in and around the larynx and upper airway. Several severely symptomatic viral infections are also helped by steroid therapy. Despite theoretical indications supporting the use of suprapharmacological doses of glucocorticoids in serious systemic bacterial infection, recent multicenter, prospective, randomized trials have not shown any benefit, and one has shown potential deleterious effects. Thus, the uses of glucocorticoids in sepsis can be summarized as follows:

1. Physiological doses of glucocorticoids are indicated in patients who may be suffering adrenal cortical insufficiency from any type of infection. In this situation, glucocorticoids provide metabolic and electrolyte support, maximizing hemodynamic functioning during septic stress.
2. Pharmacological doses of glucocorticoids can be used briefly to suppress inflammation and theoretically to reduce damaging fibrotic sequelae of selected acute infections in critical closed spaces and to produce symptomatic improvement in several viral infections.
3. Suprapharmacological doses of glucocorticoids at the present time are of no benefit in patients with severe systemic sepsis, septic shock, and/or any of the end organ sequelae thereof, especially ARDS.

Acknowledgment

The excellent secretarial assistance of Mrs. Wendy S. Bottke is very much appreciated.

References

1. Benhamou M, Ninio E, Salem P, et al: Decrease in IgE Fc receptor expression on mouse bone marrow-derived mast cells and inhibition of PAF-Acether formation and of B-Hexosaminidase release by dexamethasone. *J Immunol* 136:1385, 1986.
2. Beutler B, Cerami A: Cachectin: More than a tumor necrosis factor. *N Engl J Med* 316:379, 1987.

3. Beutler B, Krochin N, Milsark IW, et al: Control of cachectin (tumor necrosis factor) synthesis: mechanisms of endotoxin resistance. *Science* 232:977, 1986.

4. Beutler B, Milsark IW, Cerami AC: Passive immunization against cachectin/tumor necrosis factor protects mice from lethal effect of endotoxin. *Science* 229:864, 1985.

5. Bovornkitti S, Kangsadol P, Sathirapat P, and Oonsombatti P: Reversion and reconversion rate of tuberculin skin test reactions in correlation with the use of prednisone. *Dis Chest* 38:51, 1960.

6. Braun SR, Levin AB, and Clark KL: Role of corticosteroids in the development of pneumonia in mechanically ventilated head trauma victims. *Crit Care Med* 14:198, 1986.

7. Craddock PR, Hammerschmidt DE, White JG, et al: Complement (C5a)-induced granulocyte aggregation in vitro: a possible mechanism of complement-mediated leukostasis and leukopenia. *J Clin Invest* 60:260, 1977.

8. Cupps TR, Fauci AS: Corticosteroid-mediated immunoregulation in man. *Immunol Rev* 65:133, 1982.

9. Fauci AS, Dale DC and Balow JE: Glucocorticosteroid therapy: mechanisms of action and clinical considerations. *Ann Int Med* 84:304, 1976.

10. Flick MR, Murray JF: High-dose corticosteroid therapy in the adult respiratory distress syndrome. *JAMA* 251:1054, 1984.

11. Hall CB, Douglas RG: Infections of the upper respiratory tract, trachea and bronchi: epiglottitis. In Reese RF, Douglas RG (eds): *A Practical Approach to Infectious Diseases*. Boston, MA, Little, Brown and Co., 1986, pp 194.

12. Hinshaw LB, Archer LT, Beller-Todd BK, et al: Survival of primates in lethal septic shock following delayed treatment with steroid. *Circ Shock* 8:291, 1981.

13. Hinshaw LB, Archer LT, Beller-Todd BK, et al: Survival of primates in LD_{100} septic shock following steroid/antibiotic therapy. *J Surg Res* 18:100, 1980.

14. Hinshaw LB, Beller-Todd BK, Archer LT, et al: Effectiveness of steroid/antibiotic treatment in primates administered LD_{100} *Echericia coli*. *Ann Surg* 194:51, 1981.

15. Hoffman SL, Punjabi NH, Kumala S, et al: Reduction of mortality in chloramphenicol-treated severe typhoid fever by high-dose dexamethasone. *N Engl J Med* 310:82, 1984.

16. Holaday JW: Opioid antagonists in septic shock. In Sande M, Root R (eds): *Septic Shock: Newer Concepts of Pathophysiology and Treatment*. New York, Churchill Livingston, 1985, pp 201.

17. Jacob HS, Craddock PR, Hammerschmidt DE, et al: Complement induced granulocyte aggregation: an unsuspected mechanism of disease. *N Engl J Med* 302:789, 1980.

18. Keczkes K and Basheer AM: Do corticosteroids prevent postherapeutic neuralgia? *J Dermatol* 102:551, 1980.

19. Kehrl JH, Fauci AS: The clinical use of glucocorticoids. *Ann Allergy* 50:2, 1983.

20. Kilbrich S: Varicella and herpes zoster. In Wyngaarden JB & Smith LH, Jr (eds): *Cecil Textbook of Medicine*, 17th ed. Philadelphia, WB Saunders, 1985, pp 1721.

21. MacGregor RR, Sheagren JN, Lipsett MB, et al: Alternate-day prednisone therapy: evaluation of delayed hypersensitivity responses, control of disease and steroid side effects. *N Engl J Med* 280:1427, 1969.

22. Mela L, Miller LD: Efficacy of glucocorticoids in preventing mitochondrial metabolic failure in endotoxemia. *Circ Shock* 10:371, 1983.

23. Packard BD, Weiler JM: Steroids inhibit activation of the alternative-amplification pathway of complement. *Infect Immun* 40:1011, 1983.

24. Rooney JJ, Crocco JA, Lyons HA: Tuberculous pericarditis. *Ann Int Med* 72, 1970.

25. Scheld WM, Winn MR: Brain abscess. In Mandel GL, Douglas RG, Bennett JE (eds): *Principles and Practice of Infectious Diseases*. New York, John Wiley and Sons, 1985, pp 585.

26. Schonfeld SA, Polysongsang Y, DiLisio R, et al: Fat embolism prophylaxis with corticosteroids: a prospective study in high risk patients. *Ann Int Med* 99:438, 1983.

27. Schumer W: Steroids in the treatment of clinical septic shock. *Ann Surg* 184:333, 1976.

28. Sheagren JN: Antiinflammatory steroid action: infectious diseases. In Lichtenstein LM, Claman HN, Oronsky A, Schleimer RP (eds): *Antiinflammatory Steroids: Basic and Clinical Aspects*. Orlando, FL, Academic Press, 1987.

29. Sheagren JN, Young MK: Glucocorticoids. In Parillo J (ed): *The Critically Ill Immunosuppressed Patient: Diagnosis and Management*. Rockville, MD, Aspen Systems Corp., 1987, in press.

30. Sheagren JN: Glucocorticoid therapy of infectious mononucleosis and aphthous stomatitis. *JAMA* 256:1051, 1986.

31. Sheagren JN: Glucocorticoid therapy in the management of severe sepsis. In Sande M, Root R (eds): *Septic Shock: Newer Concepts of Pathophysiology and Treatment*. New York, Churchill Livingston, 1985, pp 201.

32. Sheagren JN: The pathogenesis and therapy of the complications of severe sepsis. In Chernow B, Schoemaker WC (eds): *Critical Care: State of the Art*. Fullerton, CA, Society of Critical Care Medicine, 1986, pp 465.

33. Sibbald WJ, Anderson RR, Reid B, et al: Alveolocapillary permeability in human septic ARDS. *Chest* 79:133, 1981.

34. Skubitz KM, Craddock PR, Hammerschmidt DE, et al: Corticosteroids block binding of chemotactic peptide to its receptor on granulocytes and cause disaggregation of granulocyte aggregates in vitro. *J Clin Invest* 68:13, 1981.

35. Spriggs DR: Cachexia and Septic Shock: What's in a Name? *J Infect Dis* 154:734, 1986.

36. Sprung CL, Caralis PV, Marcial EH, et al: The effects of high-dose corticosteroids in patients with septic shock: a prospective controlled study. *N Engl J Med* 311:1137, 1984.

37. Tracey KJ, Beutler B, Lowry SF, et al: Shock and tissue injury induced by recombinant human cachectin. *Science* 234:470–474, 1986.

38. Tyrrel JB, Baxter JD: Disorders of the adrenal cortex. In Wyngaarden JB, Smith LH Jr (eds): *Cecil Textbook of Medicine*, ed 17. Philadelphia, WB Saunders, 1985, pp 1300.

39. Weigelt JA, Norcross JF, Borman KR, Snyder WH: Early steroid therapy for respiratory failure. *Arch Surg* 120:536, 1985.

40. Weissman G, Smolen JE, Dorchak HM: Release of inflammatory mediators from stimulated neutrophils. *N Engl J Med* 303:27, 1980.

41

Plasma Fibronectin: Its Potential Therapeutic Value to the Critically Ill Patient

Thomas M. Saba, Ph.D.
Larry F. Cohler, M.D.
Imbesat Daudi, M.D.

ORGAN AND HOST DEFENSE FAILURE IN THE CRITICALLY ILL PATIENT

Multiple organ failure in the critically ill surgical, trauma, and burn patient is of major clinical importance and is associated with a high mortality rate (49). Reticuloendothelial (RE) phagocytic failure has been demonstrated in both experimental models of injury and sepsis as well as in critically ill patients (7, 25, 55) with multiple organ failure. In patients, this impairment of RES function has been correlated with a deficiency of a humoral opsonic factor in plasma that mediates phagocytosis of nonbacterial particulates (47, 49, 54, 55). This humoral component is identical to plasma fibronectin or cold-insoluble globulin (3, 49), which is immunologically similar to cell surface or tissue fibronectin (45) believed to play a role in cell-cell interaction and cell adhesion to a collagenous basement membrane (32, 44). The plasma concentration of fibronectin may have prognostic value in the critically ill surgical or trauma patient (7, 28). Its plasma concentration not only modulates phagocytic function but may influence vascular permeability, tissue repair, and wound healing in view of its ability to become incorporated into the tissue pool of fibronectin (11, 36).

This chapter focuses on the relationship of plasma fibronectin to multiple organ failure in the critically ill, septic, injured patient from the standpoint of its potential prognostic and therapeutic value. Emphasis is placed on host defense failure and alterations in vascular permeability.

FIBRONECTIN AS A UNIQUE MOLECULE

Fibronectin (from Latin *fibra* fiber, *nectere* to bind) is a large-molecular-weight (440,000) glycoprotein that has both "opsonic" and "adhesive" biological functions (49). A soluble form of fibronectin is found in blood, lymph and other tissue fluids, while an insoluble form (cellular or tissue fibronectin) is found in connective tissues and is associated with basement membranes, especially in the vascular system. Fibronectin is a complex molecule with domains that have a high affinity for collagen, gelatin, fibrin, DNA, actin, *Staphylococcus aureus*, and heparin (24, 32). Plasma fibronectin is identical to opsonic α_2 surface binding (SB) glycoprotein (3), which appears to modulate RE or macrophage phagocytic removal (2, 4, 46, 47, 50) of denatured collagen-coated particles, cytoskeletal debris, fibrin-fibrinogen complexes, connective tissue fragments, and intracellular membranous debris. Fibronectin augments clearance of such particulates from the blood, lymph, peritoneal cavity, and tissue spaces. Indeed, the vascular entrance of denatured collagen (gelatin) coated particles (4, 50), gelatin itself, *Staphylococcus aureus*, denatured actin, as well as cellular membranous debris can deplete plasma fibronectin. Opsonic fibronectin deficiency decreases resistance to trauma, while the infusion of opsonically active plasma fibronectin after surgery can prevent the typical postoperative hepatic Kupffer cell phagocytic depression. Typically, rapid removal of blood-borne particulates by the hepatic Kupffer

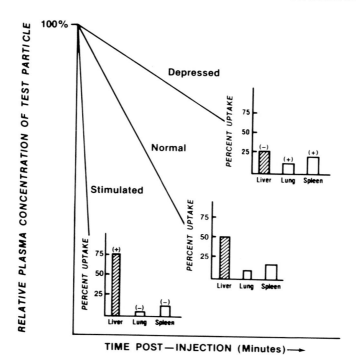

Figure 41.1. Graphic presentation of foreign particulate clearance from the blood and the relationship between rate of particle removal and organ deposition. In most species (rats, dogs, humans), for particles removed by the RES, the level of extrahepatic localization (lung) increases with decreased hepatic phagocytic clearance. Semi-log of plasma concentration is plotted as a function of time. Organ uptake is measured at the end of a defined period of particle removal. Organ deposition is expressed as percent of total bloodborne particles (injected dose) removed per organ. (From Saba TM, Holman JM, Jr: Fibronectin and phagocytic host defense mechanisms. *Surgical Care II.* Philadelphia, Lea & Febiger, 1985, pp 271–282.)

cells results in less localization in the lung (Fig. 41.1).

Cellular or tissue fibronectin is antigenically related to plasma fibronectin, but differences appear to exist between these two forms of fibronectin in terms of adhesive properties as well as solubility. However, both appear to have very similar secondary and tertiary poly-peptide structures and both can bind to col-lagen (15), a connective tissue matrix protein. Fibronectin is localized between lung endo-thelial cells and their collagenous subendo-thelium, in liver sinusoids, on the surface of fibroblasts and selected phagocytic cells, and at the sites of injury (12) and/or wound repair (20). Fibronectin is also found in the provi-sional fibrin matrix during wound healing (20). Endothelial cells, macrophages, fibroblasts, and hepatocytes as well as other cell types such as smooth muscle cells actively synthesize fibro-nectin in culture, but hepatocytes are sus-pected to be the primary site for the production of the soluble fibronectin in plasma. Indeed,

patients with fulminant hepatic failure (19) have very low fibronectin levels, and the syn-thetic rate of fibronectin by the liver is consis-tent with that required to maintain the plasma level, considering estimates of its half-life in plasma (11).

Plasma fibronectin can incorporate into tis-sues (11, 36). Its incorporation into the insol-uble extracellular matrix with the subsequent formation of fibronectin multimers may be due to disulfide exchange in the amino-terminal portion of fibronectin. Factor XIII may also modulate this tissue incorporation. In the fetus or newborn the fibronectin in tissues is most likely locally synthesized; in the adult the plasma pool of fibronectin may contribute sig-nificantly to the fibronectin detected in many tissues by immunofluorescence. Thus, the plasma pool of fibronectin may serve as a res-ervoir for fibronectin in tissues, where it may influence wound repair after injury, as well as vascular and tissue structural integrity.

A fibronectin monomer consists of at least

four globular domains, separated by flexible protease sensitive areas of polypeptide chain (24, 31, 44). The N-terminal domain (molecular weight of 25,000–30,000) binds to fibrin, S. aureus, heparin, and actin. A second domain (molecular weight of 30,000–40,000) contains the collagen and gelatin binding site. The polypeptide chain between these two domains is very sensitive to proteases such as thrombin, plasmin, trypsin, and leukocyte elastase. A third domain (molecular weight of 140,000–160,000), which is actually two subunits, contains the fibroblast or cell adhesion site and can also bind heparin. A fourth domain (molecular weight of 6,000–10,000), which binds to fibrin and contains the C-terminus, is where the two fibronectin monomers are linked by interchain disulfide bond(s). Proteases can also cleave this portion of fibronectin. Thus, fibronectin is an adhesive modular glycoprotein with an affinity for entities, which can be endocytosed by macrophages. Its multiple binding sites, its distribution, and its documented functions suggest that the insoluble tissue fibronectin is an "adhesive or structural" glycoprotein, whereas the soluble fibronectin in plasma or lymph is an "opsonic glycoprotein" that can also incorporate into tissues (49).

PLASMA FIBRONECTIN LEVELS IN INJURED PATIENTS AND CRYOPRECIPITATE INFUSION

Low plasma fibronectin levels have been documented in a variety of clinical situations, especially septic trauma, burn, and surgical patients (7, 39, 40, 47, 51, 54, 56); newborns with sepsis and respiratory distress syndrome (61); patients with acute hepatic failure (19); premature newborns (62); and during periods of malnutrition (13, 23, 52). Our laboratory first documented opsonic deficiency after surgery or trauma in animals and its relationship to phagocytic function as reviewed (49). Subsequently, Scovill et al. (55, 56) and Saba et al. (47) demonstrated a deficit of plasma opsonic activity in patients following trauma or burn. Clinically defined sepsis was preceded by a fall in plasma opsonic activity (28). Furthermore, depression of opsonic activity in nonsurvivors was prolonged, while survivors demonstrated an early restoration of opsonic activity after trauma (55). This plasma factor called "opsonic α_2 surface binding (SB) glycoprotein" was cryoprecipitable, especially in

the presence of heparin (39) and shown to be identical to cold-insoluble globulin or plasma fibronectin (3, 49). Preparation of antibody to fibronectin (2) allowed for its measurement by immunoassay, which correlated with opsonic activity (2, 4, 50). In addition, infusion of fibronectin-rich, fresh plasma cryoprecipitate (usually less than 2 months old) reversed this opsonic deficit in septic surgical and trauma patients (47). Plasma cryoprecipitate that is stored in excess of 3–4 months may not be as biologically active in terms of fibronectin-mediated opsonic activity, since a rapid loss of this function has recently been observed by Blumenstock et al. (5).

In preliminary clinical longitudinal studies, a reduction in the positive end-expiratory pressure needed to maintain arterial PO_2 was observed after elevation of the plasma fibronectin levels in trauma patients (47, 54, 56). Robbins et al. (40) subsequently demonstrated a drop in plasma fibronectin and a sequestration of fibronectin in the drainage fluid of patients following mastectomy. In fact, the relative amount of fibronectin in the drainage fluid at 2, 4, and 8 hours following operation was higher than serum levels. In studying a group of 98 intensive care patients, Rubli et al. (43) observed that fibronectin as well as antithrombin III, transferrin, and prealbumin were low in septic as compared with nonseptic patients, reflecting a pattern of general protein depletion in septic patients. A significant difference in mortality as related to fibronectin levels was noted, in that the mortality was 86% for those patients with plasma fibronectin levels less than 200 ug/ml. If the levels were greater than 200 ug/ml, there was a lower mortality rate.

Richards et al. (39) observed a postoperative drop in plasma fibronectin in patients undergoing surgery, which normalized by 3 days after surgery. They also observed that patients with pre-existing intra-abdominal infections had significantly lower plasma fibronectin levels preoperatively as compared with elective surgery patients with no infections (39). Of the 16 surgical patients with intra-abdominal sepsis, eight developed multiple organ failure, which was temporally associated with a sustained deficiency of plasma fibronectin after surgery. Patients with plasma fibronectin levels that normalized by the fifth postoperative day did not manifest multiple organ failure and had a mortality rate of 12.5%; whereas patients with sustained depression of plasma fibronectin beyond the fifth postoperative day exhibited organ failure and a mortality of 62%. Thus, normalization of plasma fibronectin levels was associated with a better clinical course. This observation is consistent with the data of Brodin et al. (7), who showed that burn patients who manifest a persistently low level of plasma fibronectin, usually in association with sepsis postburn, have a lower survival rate. Indeed, they suggested that sustained plasma fibronectin deficiency may be an indicator of pending septicemia in burn patients, which correlates with a higher risk of organ failure.

Snyder et al. (57) demonstrated a significant decline in fibronectin levels following coronary artery bypass surgery. Plasma fibronectin levels were the lowest in bypass patients with the most severe postoperative complications. In recent studies on nine cardiac bypass patients, we have also observed an acute decline in fibronectin levels during cardiac bypass surgery, which then normalize by 5–6 days postsurgery (Saba et al., unpublished data). Similar to the studies of Richards et al. (39), the data by Snyder et al. (57) also emphasized that the persistently low levels of plasma fibronectin were associated with the development of postsurgical complications in cardiac bypass patients. It would appear that the magnitude of the acute fall in plasma fibronectin in patients undergoing coronary bypass surgery cannot be accounted for by dilution itself. Factors such as opsonic consumption in the process of RES clearance, binding of plasma fibronectin to foreign surfaces when the patients are on the pump, complexing of plasma fibronectin with the anticoagulant heparin, as well as dilution are all contributing variables.

Patients sustaining severe thermal injury often require large amounts of volume support to maintain hemodynamic stability, especially if they become septic. This volume requirement may be due to both loss of fluid and proteins into the area of injury, as well as a generalized increase in vascular permeability. There is an acute depletion of plasma fibronectin following thermal injury, which is often maximal 6–12 hours postburn with restoration of normal levels by 1–3 days (28). A similar acute depletion of plasma fibronectin, as well as the rapid normalization of fibronectin levels, has been reported (12) in animals after sublethal burn injury. In addition to the acute decline of fibronectin after burn injury, a second phase of fibronectin deficiency, can often be observed 5–7 days postburn in patients even before the development of a septic episode (7, 14, 16, 28).

Resolution of the septic episode is associated with normalization of plasma fibronectin. Yoder et al. (61) documented plasma fibronectin deficiency in septic newborn infants with respiratory distress and perinatal asphyxia. An elevation of the fibronectin levels was observed with resolution of the septic episode. Ekindjian et al. (14) have also documented a correlation of low fibronectin levels with the presence of sepsis in burn patients. Others (16) also demonstrated a decrease in fibronectin following excision and grafting of the burn area. A fall in plasma fibronectin preceded by 2–3 days the development of positive blood cultures in one study (16). Thus, as suggested by Saba and Jaffe (49) as well as Brodin et al. (7), plasma fibronectin levels may be of prognostic value with respect to sepsis in patients with thermal injury. Moreover, the magnitude of the acute drop of plasma fibronectin may be a very sensitive index of the severity of burn injury or trauma. However, caution must be noted in that (a) there tends to be a wide range for normal plasma fibronectin values in adults; (b) males tend to have higher levels than females; (c) fibronectin levels are normally lower in infants than adults; (d) plasma concentrations are higher than serum concentrations; and (e) nutritional state can influence the plasma fibronectin concentration.

FIBRONECTIN DEFICIENCY UNRELATED TO TRAUMA

Perturbations in plasma fibronectin levels have been documented in nontrauma disorders, especially disseminated intravascular coagulation (8, 33), fulminant liver failure (18, 19), and starvation (13, 23, 52). A major factor in the fibronectin deficit observed with some forms of hepatic failure may be decreased liver synthesis of fibronectin. Portal insulin concentrations may be one factor that can influence the rate of hepatic fibronectin synthesis. Gonzalez-Calvin et al. (19), studying a group of patients with fulminant hepatic failure secondary to paracetamol overdose, documented a very low plasma fibronectin concentration (117.9 ± 19.4 μg/ml) in these patients. Fibronectin values were even lower in patients that also developed renal failure. The authors postulated that the low prevailing level of plasma fibronectin was due to its opsonic role in the clearance of hepatocyte debris. However, since fibronectin is synthesized by isolated hepatocytes, a synthetic deficit by the liver may also have existed in these patients. Plasma fibronectin levels have been shown to normalize in patients with severe liver disease who undergo successful liver transplantation (38).

Plasma fibronectin levels are depressed in patients with disseminated intravascular coagulation. Cembrowski and Mosher (8) also observed depression of plasma fibronectin in patients with the syndrome of defibrinogenation. They were able to show an association between low plasma fibronectin levels and low levels of antithrombin III and plasminogen. In one of the more complete clinical studies on fibronectin and coagulation, Mosher and Williams (33) documented severe fibronectin deficiency in patients with intravascular coagulation that was associated with a high incidence of organ failure. Experimentally induced intravascular coagulation in rabbits can also lower the plasma fibronectin concentration and alter its rate of removal from the blood. Whether the decline with Gram-negative postoperative septicemia (10, 35, 36) is due, in part, to an endotoxin activation of intravascular coagulation remains to be determined.

The plasma level of any specific protein is obviously influenced by both its rate of synthesis and its rate of utilization/degradation. Thus, low plasma fibronectin levels seen in critically ill, septic, surgical or trauma patients may also be a function of decreased fibronectin synthesis. Dillon et al. (13) documented a rapid decline in immunoreactive fibronectin in blood and associated opsonic activity in rats by 2 days poststarvation with rapid recovery upon feeding. Howard et al. (23) demonstrated a rapid reduction in plasma fibronectin in normal volunteers after starvation prior to any decrease in serum albumin or total iron binding capacity. Because many critically ill patients often become malnourished, this may contribute to the low levels of plasma fibronectin. In fact, fibronectin may be a useful indicator of the nutritional status of a patient, because of its rapid turnover. Compared with albumin, prealbumin, transferrin, and haptoglobin, Sanstedt et al. (52) observed that fibronectin was the only protein which rose significantly following a period of total parenteral nutrition. This finding agrees with the initial report from our laboratory (23) on the rapid restoration of plasma fibronectin after total parenteral nutrition in malnourished patients. It is possible that some specific inhibitor mechanism may exist in septic injured pa-

tients, but not in experimental sepsis in rodents, which limits the synthesis of plasma fibronectin. Indeed, mild postoperative sepsis in rats can actually increase the rate of fibronectin synthesis to a level capable of maintaining the plasma fibronectin concentration even in conjunction with increased fibronectin clearance (26). The exact stimulatory mechanism to account for this response in rats remains undetermined.

ORGAN DYSFUNCTION AND LOW FIBRONECTIN LEVELS

Although numerous studies have documented that persistent depression of plasma fibronectin points to a poor prognosis in the critically ill patient, very few studies have documented a significant correlation of depressed plasma fibronectin levels with dysfunction of a specific organ system, other than RE phagocytic depression and perhaps increased lung vascular permeability with postoperative sepsis. Early findings (1, 47, 54, 56), in a limited number of patients reported low plasma fibronectin levels in trauma and burn patients with severe sepsis that were temporally associated with a ventilation-perfusion mismatch, blunted peripheral vascular response to ischemia, and decreased endogenous creatinine clearance. Following infusion of fresh plasma cryoprecipitate, which is rich in plasma fibronectin, a reduction in the positive end-expiratory pressure necessary to maintain arterial PO_2 was observed. Fourrier et al. (17), studying patients with adult respiratory distress syndrome (ARDS), showed that low angiotensin converting enzyme (ACE) levels, perhaps reflecting pulmonary endothelial injury or dysfunction, were of substantial value in predicting the presence of ARDS. Additionally, they showed that although a low plasma fibronectin level was not predictive of the presence of ARDS, it was correlated with severity of ARDS in such patients. In contrast, Maunder et al. (30) showed low plasma fibronectin levels in septic patients but found no correlation between the development of ARDS and a low plasma fibronectin level.

In a longitudinal study, Scovill et al. (54) reported improvement in peripheral vascular and pulmonary function in surgical and trauma patients after cryoprecipitate infusion. Robbins et al. (41) showed that a burn patient with sepsis and coexistent pulmonary infiltrates who was refractory to antibiotic therapy responded very positively to the infusion of fresh fibronectin-rich cryoprecipitate. In addition to an improvement of the pulmonary status, there was a return of blood lactic acid levels to normal (36). Annest et al. (1) reported an increase in endogenous creatinine clearance independent of an increase in cardiac index following cryoprecipitate infusion in septic surgical and trauma patients. Rogers and Heymach (42) documented a beneficial effect of cryoprecipitate infusion in a postpartum patient with ARDS secondary to amniotic fluid embolism, which they attributed to the fibronectin in the plasma cryoprecipitate. Todd et al. (59) in completing a randomized clinical trial of plasma cryoprecipitate in 93 ICU patients concluded that administration of cryoprecipitate to correct the fibronectin deficiency in septic critically ill patients improved survival. Newman et al. (34) also provided recent data emphasizing the positive therapeutic value of fibronectin rich cryoprecipitate in septic shock patients. Several studies investigating plasma fibronectin deficiency in patients with acute leukemia, also infused cryoprecipitate in an attempt to correct this deficiency. However, they were unable to raise the plasma fibronectin level more than 50% of the level predicted on the basis of body weight and the immunoreactive fibronectin concentration in the cryoprecipitate. This result is in agreement with the findings by Ragni et al. (38), who also recovered less fibronectin than anticipated in patients after cryoprecipitate infusion. Whether there are tissue debris and/or abnormal ligands in the plasma of critically ill patients that acutely deplete the infused fibronectin or alter its detection is not known. There is also a rapid early drop in plasma fibronectin after its initial intravenous infusion (11) as it distributes between vascular and extravascular sites that needs to be considered in quantitating blood recovery. This rapid biphasic loss from plasma has also been observed with purified human plasma fibronectin after its intravenous infusion (46). We have previously estimated that the plasma half-life of fibronectin is 20–24 hours (49). This estimate agrees with the fractional clearance rate studies performed in septic injured patients with the use of radiolabeled fibronectin (37).

The age of the cryoprecipitate infused into patients is important (5). Hellsevik (21) was unable to demonstrate improved organ function in patients using cryoprecipitate that had been stored for 4–12 months, even though its fibronectin antigen content was high and it displayed gelatin binding activity. In contrast, others who used fresh plasma cryoprecipitate (1, 54, 55), most often less than 1–2 months of age, have noted improved organ function in patients entered into a longitudinally designed protocol without a control-placebo solution. Increased duration of survival (29) as well as decreased mortality (59) have also been suggested after elevation of the fibronectin level in septic surgical or injured patients. One explanation for this difference in observations may reside in the recent observation (5) that after 3–4 months of storage, the fibronectin in cryoprecipitate apparently begins to lose its opsonic activity as tested by standard liver slice phagocytic bioassay, whether stored at $-20°C$ or $-80°C$. The basis for this decline in activity may be due to fibronectin fragmentation. Thus, opsonically active, purified plasma fibronectin that has been pasteurized (46) may be more appropriate than plasma cryoprecipitate, since the fibronectin content of cryoprecipitate varies considerably even when prepared at the same blood center (5) and its opsonic activity appears to decline with prolonged storage. Clinical studies that use plasma cryoprecipitate older than 1–2 months (21) may have limited experimental value in testing the therapeutic potential of fibronectin-rich plasma cryoprecipitate in view of the potential lability of its fibronectin-mediated opsonic activity (5). Indeed, its fibronectin antigen content can be normal and its gelatin binding activity can be normal, yet it can lose its opsonic activity with respect to stimulating macrophage phagocytosis of gelatin-coated test particles. Thus, gelatin adherence may not be a reliable index of opsonic activity.

LUNG VASCULAR INJURY AND ADULT RESPIRATORY DISTRESS SYNDROME

Adult respiratory distress syndrome (ARDS) is a common manifestation of the organ failure syndrome in septic trauma patients. Burn patients with mainly cutaneous injury also manifest pulmonary edema and respiratory distress with sepsis. While hydrostatic and oncotic pressures are important to lung fluid balance, studies have emphasized that capillary leaking in the lung can contribute to pulmonary edema and post-traumatic pulmonary insufficiency. Increased lung vascular permeability exists during postoperative bacteremia and/or intravascular coagulation (35) as shown in Figure

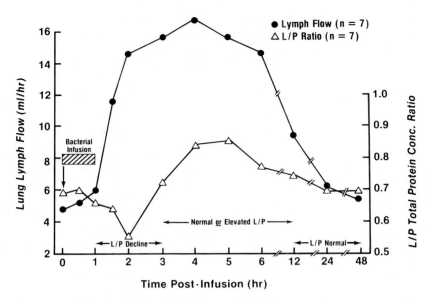

Figure 41.2. Effect of postoperative bacterial challenge on lung lymph flow and the lymph to plasma (L/P) total protein concentration ratio in sheep. Sheep ($n = 7$) underwent sterile thoracotomy for cannulation of the efferent duct of the caudal mediastinal lymph node, and studied 2 days after operative intervention. Sheep were injected intravenously with 5×10^8 live *Pseudomonas aeruginosa* over a 60-minute infusion interval. The early phase associated with a rise in lymph flow and a decline in L/P is mainly due to an elevation of pulmonary microvascular pressure. The second phase of increased lymph flow with elevated L/P ratios reflects an increase in lung vascular permeability and the flux of a protein-rich fluid into the lung interstitial space.

41.2, which depicts the lung lymph flow and lymph-to-plasma (L/P) total protein concentration ratio in sheep after *Pseudomonas* challenge during the postoperative period. The initial increase in lymph flow is hemodynamically mediated and associated with a decline in L/P (washdown). The second phase of rising L/P and elevated lymph flow most likely reflects an increased lung vascular permeability. This acute injury to the lung vascular bed may be functionally mediated by pulmonary microembolization, activation of complement, or the release of proteases and oxygen metabolites from activated leukocytes or macrophages in the lung. Granulocytopenia minimizes the lung vascular injury, which may be due to the fact that proteases released from activated leukocytes and macrophages may degrade the "adhesive" tissue fibronectin in the lung. Such fragmentation of lung tissue fibronectin may contribute to altered integrity of the lung vascular barrier. Oxidant-induced lung injury can also alter the fibronectin content of the lung and may trigger the release of lung tissue fibronectin into both the blood and alveolar spaces.

While the exact relationship between the plasma concentration of fibronectin and lung vascular integrity remains to be defined, the increase in lung vascular permeability with postoperative septicemia in sheep (Fig. 41.2) can be amplified by plasma fibronectin deficiency (10, 35). Moreover, the direct intravenous infusion of a proteolytic enzyme, such as trypsin, depletes plasma fibronectin as well as increases lung vascular permeability (9). Thus, a balance may exist between plasma fibronectin–mediated RES function and the level of bloodborne abnormal particulates that, if disturbed after surgery or trauma, could contribute to inefficient clearance of tissue debris by the RES, resulting in lung vascular injury via microembolism. Plasma fibronectin may also serve as a "temporary reservoir" for fibronectin in vascular beds, where it may influence endothelial integrity (49). This may be another mechanism by which low plasma fibronectin levels potentiate the increase in lung vascular permeability with postoperative sepsis.

Although the etiology of ARDS is unclear, it is generally accepted that alterations in pulmonary microvascular permeability contribute to the increased fluid and protein flux in the lung. Fibronectin may be important to this aspect of the pathophysiology of pulmonary failure. Saba et al. (51) and Niehaus et al. (35), utilizing the lung lymph fistula model, showed an increase in lung transvascular protein clearance following infusion of live *Pseudomonas* especially into fibronectin-deficient sheep. The administration of fibronectin-rich cryoprecipitate resulted in a decrease in the lung transvascular protein clearance (51). Cryoprecipitate depleted of plasma fibronectin by the technique of affinity chromatography was unable to minimize the increase in transvascular protein clearance in the septic sheep (51). More recently, the elevation of plasma fibronectin levels to a state of hyperfibronectinemia by infusion of purified human plasma fibronectin into postoperative septic sheep was also able to blunt the delayed increase in lung vascular permeability (10). Indeed, rebound elevation of plasma fibronectin levels (Fig. 41.3) that can be seen by 48 hours and last for several days, after the early postoperative sepsis-induced decline, appears to limit the typical increase in lung vascular permeability that develops if these sheep are given a second Gram-negative bacterial challenge (10). This action appears not to be mediated by the development of antibodies to the initial bacterial challenge. This protection can be reproduced in normal sheep by treating sheep with infusions of pur-

ified plasma fibronectin (10) to elevate their level by 70–80%.

By immunofluorescence, fibronectin has been localized between lung endothelial cells and their collagenous basement membrane as well as between lung epithelial cells and their basement membranes. Its ability to bind cells to collagen suggests that the "adhesive" fibronectin may play a role in maintaining microvascular integrity. Sequestration of activated leukocytes in the lung (22) with sepsis or disseminated intravascular coagulation (DIC) may result in the local release of proteases, (cathepsin G or leukocyte elastase), which can fragment tissue fibronectin and thus alter vascular integrity. In support of this concept is our documentation of the increased content of fibronectin fragments in lung lymph after intravenous challenge of sheep with human α-thrombin to induce low-grade intravascular coagulation (Daudi et al., unpublished data). The presence of such fragments temporally correlates with a sustained increase in lung protein clearance at a time that the mean pulmonary artery and pulmonary wedge pressures have returned to normal, i.e., during the phase of elevated vascular permeability. The plasma fibronectin pool may be a reservoir for fibro-

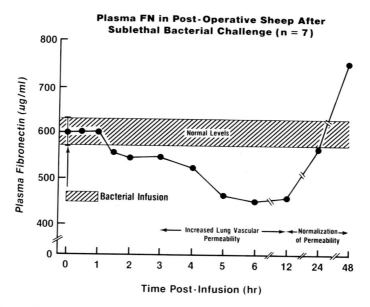

Figure 41.3. Plasma fibronectin levels following the postoperative intravenous infusion of the *Pseudomonas* bacteria. Sheep (*n* = 7) underwent sterile thoracotomy for cannulation of the efferent duct of the caudal mediastinal lymph node, and studied 2 days after operative intervention. Sheep were injected intravenously with 5x10⁸ live *Pseudomonas aeruginosa* over a 60-minute infusion interval. Levels are ug/ml plasma as determined by electroimmunoassay. Restoration of fibronectin levels with rebound hyperfibronectinemia was temporally associated with normalization of both lymph flow and L/P ratios as shown in Figure 41.2.

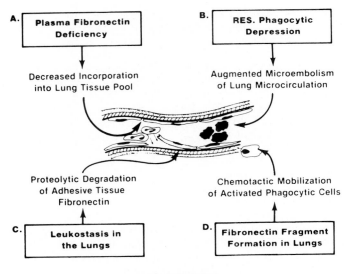

CONSQUENCES

A. Altered Matrix Formation.

B. Impaired Perfusion.

C. Endothelial Detachment.

D. Destruction of Interstitium

Figure 41.4. Mechanisms by which disturbances in fibronectin can contribute to lung vascular injury and altered vascular permeability. Microvascular embolization due to inefficient RES particulate removal; altered gradient for incorporation of plasma fibronectin into tissue pool; proteolytic fragmentation of lung tissue fibronectin by enzymes released from marginated leukocytes and/or activated macrophages with abnormal cell-out contact or endothelial cell adhesion to collagenous substratum; and chemotactic attraction of active monocytes, leukocytes, and other cells by fibronectin fragments. Oxygen metabolites, such as superoxide anion (O_2^-), hydrogen peroxide (H_2O_2), and the hydroxyl radical ($OH°$), released from these activated cells could further injure endothelial and nonendothelial cells. Proteolytic enzyme release can disrupt the interstitial and extracellular matrix. (From Saba TM: Plasma and tissue fibronectin: its role in pathophysiology of the critically ill septic patient. In *Critical Care: State of the Art*, vol 7. Fullerton, CA, The Society of Critical Care Medicine, 1986, pp 437–464.)

nectin that enters injured areas of the microcirculation to serve in a reparative process. As such, plasma fibronectin may influence vascular permeability. Figure 41.4 graphically portrays several mechanisms by which disturbances in either plasma or tissue fibronectin may develop in septic injured or surgical patients as related to the etiology of increased lung vascular endothelial permeability.

BASIS FOR DEFICIENCY OF PLASMA FIBRONECTIN LEVELS

Low plasma fibronectin levels in septic trauma and burn patients have been documented, but the responsible mechanisms have yet to be clearly elucidated. The method of measuring plasma fibronectin may by itself produce inaccuracies and thus contribute to some of the disparate observations in the literature. Electroimmunoassay (4) is commonly used, and we know that a significant alteration in the charge of the molecule and/or its size (if complexed with another molecule in plasma) can affect its measurement by this assay. In fact, Deno et al. (12) demonstrated the appearance of a gelatin-like ligand in the plasma following burn injury to the skin that complexed to plasma fibronectin and inhibited its migration. The gelatin-like ligand in the blood after thermal injury to the skin appears to come from the site of injury. Using crossed immunoelectrophoresis, they observed that the addition of extracts of burned skin or denatured collagen to samples of plasma fibronectin yielded a similar abnormal electrophoretic pattern for fibronectin as that seen with burn plasma (12). Such binding may limit its full detection by electroimmunoassay as well as its opsonic activity.

Another factor that may influence plasma fibronectin levels is the volume or nature of the fluids used in resuscitation. The evidence to date would argue against hemodilution as the major etiological factor in the early decline of fibronectin in most patients, except for cardiac bypass patients where it obviously is an important factor, along with depletion due to binding to the pump oxygenator membrane. Rubli et al. (43) as well as Richards et al. (39) were unable to correlate volumes of fluid infused with the degree of fibronectin depletion observed in surgical or trauma patients. However, specific colloidal solutions used for resuscitation depress RES function (53). For example, Hemaccel, a 3.5% gelatin-based colloid, acutely depletes fibronectin when administered to normal volunteers, whereas plasma fibronectin levels are not depleted when Macrodex (Dextran 70) is infused (6). Blood components by themselves, especially if abnormal upon prolonged storage, may affect plasma fibronectin levels. Snyder et al. (58) demonstrated that infusion of old, packed red cells dropped the plasma fibronectin, whereas the use of filters with great selectivity limited this depletion. Indeed, cryoprecipitate itself, by virtue of its factor XIII content, may influence the prevailing levels of endogenous plasma fibronectin (27) by modulating its incorporation into the insoluble tissue pool of fibronectin.

The plasma level of fibronectin is obviously a reflection of both its synthetic rate and utilization rate. Fibronectin levels fall in patients after fasting and repletion to normal levels can often be accomplished in some patients by total parenteral nutrition. Since low fibronectin levels also limit RES function (43), one might speculate that nutritional support that also provides substrate for fibronectin synthesis may exert a therapeutic value indirectly by way of its influence on fibronectin synthesis. The correlation of malnutrition to poor wound healing after surgery or tissue trauma is most likely mediated, in part, by its influence on fibronectin, which we know has a major regulatory role in wound repair. The association of fibronectin with fibrin may enhance cell adhesion to clots and thus exert a positive influence on wound healing (20). With post-trauma bloodborne particulates, the low levels of plasma fibronectin acutely may be related to consumption following the entrance into the vascular compartment of connective tissue

and cytoskeletal debris (4, 50, 60). Plasma fibronectin binds actin, collagen, and fibrin, and thus may function as an opsonin in the clearance of these products of tissue destruction (15, 49). Whether or not plasma fibronectin is an important opsonin mediating directly the clearance of bacteria in vivo is yet to be determined, but it appears not to be a direct bacterial opsonin (except for selected bacteria) acting independently of other proteins. However, plasma fibronectin binds S. aureus and it can influence complement-mediated phagocytic clearance of Staphylococcus by neutrophils. Fibronectin may also influence the expression of receptors on macrophages as well as the clearance of immune complexes. Certainly, it binds to Clq, which may be relevant to clearance of immune complexes. Since bacteria secrete a variety of substances including collagenase, elastase, and hyaluronidase, that by themselves are capable of eliciting tissue destruction, the depression of plasma fibronectin coincident with sepsis may again be a reflection of the entrance into the vascular compartment of components of tissue debris secondary to bacterial-mediated tissue destruction.

In the case of low fibronectin levels with DIC, one likely explanation may be that plasma fibronectin is covalently linked to fibrin via activated plasma factor XIII during the process of coagulation. In fact, infusion of activated plasma factor XIII results in an acute depletion of plasma fibronectin in animals with experimentally induced hyperfibronectinemia (27). Another likely mechanism may be the proteolytic effect of thrombin on the plasma fibronectin molecule. Depressed levels of antithrombin III are a sensitive indicator of DIC and thus indirectly an index of the presence of activated thrombin. As previously noted, a correlation with depressed antithrombin III levels and depressed plasma fibronectin has been documented (8). The concept of proteolytic degradation being responsible for altered plasma fibronectin levels may be extended to other observations. For example, Cohler et al. (9) demonstrated an acute depletion of plasma fibronectin in sheep following the intravenous infusion of trypsin, which is known to degrade plasma fibronectin. Thus, fibronectin fragments with an altered biological half-life may be formed and rapidly cleared.

Deposition of plasma fibronectin into an area of injury may also contribute to low blood levels in critically ill injured patients, especially patients with a focus of tissue trauma. Deno et al. (12) showed that isotopically labeled plasma fibronectin localizes in the area of burn. Increased vessel permeability coupled with high affinity for collagen and fibrin are undoubtedly factors mediating its sequestration at sites of tissue damage. Indeed, part of its localization may be due to its ability to bind to C-reactive protein which also deposits at sites of tissue injury. Its rapid uptake at sites of injury may also relate to its nonspecific role as an opsonic probe for the clearance of tissue and cellular debris by infiltrating monocytes or macrophages. In this respect, the subsequent release of proteases by neutrophils at sites of tissue injury may, in turn, generate cleavage products of fibronectin that can chemotactically influence fibroblast and macrophage infiltration into sites of injury, thus influencing the process of tissue repair and wound healing.

Thus, the depression of plasma fibronectin in the critically ill, injured patient with or without sepsis could be due to a multitude of factors, including (a) consumption as an opsonic factor in the clearance of bloodborne microparticulate and soluble debris; (b) increased sequestration at sites of tissue injury; (c) altered flux into normal tissues; (d) degradation by proteases; (e) limited synthesis; (f) depletion by transfusion of stored blood containing microparticulates ; (g) dilution due to excessive fluid support; and (h) the presence of bloodborne ligands that bind the molecule and limit its detection. The use of stable-isotope infusion techniques (i.e., ^{15}N-glycine enrichment into fibronectin) to study its synthesis and turnover in patients will provide more specific data on which conclusions regarding the etiology of low plasma fibronectin levels in various disease states can be firmly made.

BENEFICIAL EFFECT AND MECHANISMS

No large scale "randomized and blinded" clinical trial has yet been reported in which fresh (less than 1 month old) fibronectin-rich plasma cryoprecipitate as well as purified opsonically active (documented by phagocytic bioassay) plasma fibronectin is compared with an appropriate control solution in terms of its influence on both organ function and survival. Infusion of fresh cryoprecipitate (47, 48, 54, 56) or purified opsonically active fibronectin (46) corrects both an immunoreactive and opsonic fibronectin deficiency; however, its effect on organ function needs to be fully quan-

tified, with an emphasis on ventilation-perfusion ratios, lung vascular permeability, fluid requirements needed for hemodynamic support, and phagocytic function. Its therapeutic influence, when applied topically, to the treatment of ulcerations or persistent wounds that fail to heal is also worthy of consideration and merits extensive investigation. Plasma cryoprecipitate older than 2–3 months, even when stored at −80°C, may not be adequate (5). If anything, it may have a suppressive effect because of the potential existence of fibronectin fragments, which can be documented by immunoblot analysis. Conversely, before purified plasma fibronectin is used, it must be tested for opsonic activity by phagocytic assay using gelatin-coated test particles. It is not adequate to assume that it has opsonic activity to promote phagocytosis because it has gelatin adherence, because it can be partially fragmented and still retain the 40,000 gelatin binding domain with this property. By facilitating clearance of soluble and microparticulate tissue debris from the vascular compartment, plasma fibronectin may minimize pulmonary and renal microembolization. However, because of its role in mediating cell-cell and cell-matrix interaction, fibronectin may modulate vascular permeability and wound healing. The physiologic role of plasma fibronectin in the healthy state and the consequences of severe injury and/or sepsis is depicted in Figure 41.5.

SUMMARY

In summary, deficiency of plasma fibronectin has now been documented in a variety of clinical entities. Persistently low plasma fibronectin levels may have prognostic value, and infusion of fresh fibronectin-rich cryoprecipitate (48, 49) or purified opsonically active dimeric human plasma fibronectin (46) may have therapeutic value. However, a well-controlled, randomized, multi-institutional clinical trial must now be completed before firm conclusions can be made. If the infusion of plasma fibronectin does provide a valuable therapeutic modality to the critically ill patient, we would speculate that it will be especially valuable in septic surgical, trauma, or burn patients who manifest increased lung vascular permeability, impaired wound healing, and phagocytic dysfunction. Its infusion may increase duration of organ stability, which can provide a more extended time frame to allow other

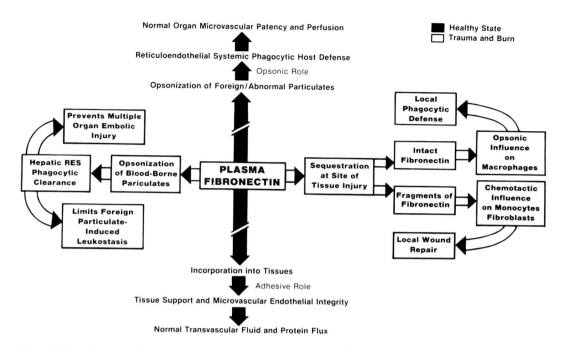

Figure 41.5.   Speculated roles for plasma fibronectin as related to both phagocytic host defense function as well as vascular integrity. Consequences of severe trauma and burn with associated presence of bloodborne microaggregates and tissue debris are depicted as they may alter the kinetics and distribution of plasma fibronectin. Most prominent after injury is the acute depletion of plasma fibronectin due to its consumption as an opsonin, its sequestration at sites of tissue injury, and its complexing with ligands released into the plasma. This would limit the availability of plasma fibronectin for normal hepatic phagocytic function and alter its plasma-tissue concentration gradient, potentially influencing its normal incorporation into tissues. True incorporation into tissues most likely reflects transition from a soluble to insoluble pool of fibronectin. Thus, the balance during a healthy state is disturbed with severe trauma, burn, DIC, or septic shock, leading to increased potential for systemic phagocytic depression, increased vascular permeability, and multiple organ failure.

existing standard therapeutic modalities as well as natural homeostatic mechanisms to have their positive influence on patient survival.

Acknowledgment

Experimental studies presented in this review were supported by grant GM-21447 from the National Institutes of Health. Larry F. Cohler, M.D. and Imbesat Daudi, M.D. are NIH Trauma and Burn postdoctoral research fellows and Ph.D. trainees, supported by grant T32-GM-07033.

References

1. Annest SJ, Scovill WA, Blumenstock FA, Stratton HH, Newell JC, Paloski WH, Saba TM, Powers SR: Increased creatinine clearance following cryoprecipitate infusion in trauma and surgical patients with decreased renal function. *J Trauma* 20(9):726, 1980.
2. Blumenstock FA, Saba TM, Roccario E, Cho E, Kaplan JE: Opsonic fibronectin after trauma and particle injection as determined by a peritoneal macrophage monolayer assay. *J Reticuloendothelial Soc* 30:61–71, 1981.
3. Blumenstock FA, Saba TM, Weber P, Laffin R: Biochemical and immunological characterization of human op-

sonic α_2-SB glycoprotein: Its identity with cold-insoluble globin. *J Biol Chem* 253:4287–4291, 1978.
4. Blumenstock FA, Weber P, Saba TM, Laffin R: Electroimmunoassay of alpha-2-opsonic protein during reticuloendothelial blockade. *Am J Physiol* 232:R80–R87, 1977.
5. Blumenstock FA, Valeri CR, Saba T, Cho E: Progressive loss of fibronectin medicated opsonic activity in plasma cryoprecipitate with storage (abstract). *Fed Proc* 45:707, 1986.
6. Brodin B, Hesselvik F, von Schenck H: Decrease of plasma fibronectin concentration following infusion of a gelatin-based plasma substitute in man. *Scand J Clin Lab Invest* 44:529–533, 1984.
7. Brodin B, von Schenck H, Schildt B, Liljedahl S-O: Low plasma fibronectin indicates septicaemia in major burns. *Acta Chir Scand* 150:5–11, 1984.
8. Cembrowski GS, Mosher DF: Plasma fibronectin concentration in patients with acquired consumptive coagulopathies. *Thrombosis Res* 36:437–445, 1984.
9. Cohler LF, Saba TM, Lewis EP: Lung vascular injury with protease infusion: Relationship to plasma fibronectin. *Ann Surg* 202:240–247, 1985.
10. Cohler LF, Saba TM, Lewis E, Vincent PA, Charash WE: Plasma fibronectin therapy and lung protein clearance with bacteremia after surgery. *J Appl Physiol* 63:623–633, 1987.
11. Deno, DC, Saba TM, Lewis EP: Kinetics of endogenously labelled plasma fibronectin: incorporation into tissues. *Am J Physiol* 245:R564–R575, 1983.

12. Deno DC, McCafferty MH, Saba TM, Blumenstock FA: Mechanism of acute depletion of plasma fibronectin following thermal injury in rats: Appearance of a gelatin-like ligand in plasma. *J Clin Invest* 73:20–34, 1984.

13. Dillon BC, Saba TM, Cho E, Lewis E: Opsonic deficiency in the etiology of starvation-induced reticuloendothelial phagocytic dysfunction. *Exp Molec Pathol* 36:177–192, 1982.

14. Ekindjian OG, Marien M, Wassermann D, Bruxelle J, Cazalet C, Konter E, Younger J: Plasma fibronectin time course in burned patients: Influence of sepsis. *J Trauma* 24(3):214–219, 1984.

15. Engvall E, Ruoslahti E: Binding of soluble form of fibroblast surface protein, fibronectin, to collagen. *Int J Cancer* 20:1–5, 1977.

16. Eriksen HO, Kalaja E, Jensen BA, Clemmensen I: Plasma fibronectin concentrations in patients with severe burn injury. *Burns* 10:422–426, 1984.

17. Fourrier F, Chopin C, Wallaert B, Mazurier C, Mangalaboyi J, Durocher A: Compared evolution of plasma fibronectin and angiotensin-converting enzyme levels in septic ARDS. *Chest* 87:191–195, 1985.

18. Gluud C, Dejgaard A, Clemmensen I: Plasma fibronectin concentrations in patients with liver diseases. *Scand J Clin Lab Invest* 43:533–537, 1983.

19. Gonzalez-Calvin J, Scully MF, Sanger Y, Fok J, Kakkar VV, Hughes RD, Gimson AES, Williams R: Fibronectin in fulminant hepatic failure. *Br Med J* 285:1231–1232, 1982.

20. Grinnell F: Fibronectin and wound healing. *J Cell Biochem* 20:107–116, 1984.

21. Hesselvik F, Brodin B, Carlsson C, Cedergren B, Jorfeldt L, Lieden G: Cyoprecipitate infusion fails to improve organ function in septic shock. A blinded, randomized trial of fibronectin therapy. *Crit Care Med* (in press).

22. Harlan JM, Killen PD, Hanker LA, Striker GE, Wright DG: Neutrophil-mediated endothelial injury in vitro. Mechanisms of cell detachment. *J Clin Invest* 68:1394–1403, 1981.

23. Howard L, Dillon B, Saba TM, Hofmann S, Cho E: Decreased plasma fibronectin during starvation in man. *J Parent Enter Nutri* 8(3):237–244, 1984.

24. Hynes RO, Yamada KM: Fibronectins: multifunctional modular glycoproteins. *J Cell Biol* 95:369–377, 1982.

25. Kaplan JE, Saba TM: Humoral deficiency and reticuloendothelial function after traumatic shock. *Am J Physiol* 230:7–14, 1976.

26. Kiener J, Saba TM, Cho E, Blumenstock FA: Clearance and distribution of plasma fibronectin in septic rats: relationship to synthetic rate. *Am J Physiol* 251:R724–R734, 1986.

27. Kiener JL, Cho E, Saba TM: Factor XIII$_a$ as a modulator of plasma fibronectin alterations during experimental bacteremia. *J Trauma* 26:1013–1023, 1986.

28. Lanser ME, Saba TM, Scovill WA: Opsonic glycoprotein (plasma fibronectin) levels after burn injury: relationship to extent of burn and development of sepsis. *Ann Surg* 192(6):776–782, 1980.

29. Lungsgaard-Hansen P, Doran JE, Rubli E, Papp E, Morgenthaler J-J, Spath P: Purified fibronectin administration to patients with severe abdominal infections: a controlled clinical trial. *Ann Surg* 202:745–759, 1985.

30. Maunder RJ, Harlan JM, Pepe PE, Paskell S, Carrico CJ, Hudson LD: Measurement of plasma fibronectin in patients who develop the adult respiratory distress syndrome. *J Lab Clin Med* 104(4):583–590, 1984.

31. Moseson MW, Amrani DL: The structure and biologic activities of plasma fibronectin. *Blood* 56(2):145–158, 1980.

32. Mosher, DF: Physiology of fibronectin. *Ann Rev Med* 35:561–575, 1984.

33. Mosher DF, William EM: Fibronectin concentration is decreased in plasma of severely ill patients with disseminated intravascular coagulation. *J Lab Clin Med* 91:729–735, 1978.

34. Newman PM, Ramsay G, Ledingham I McA: Cryoprecipitate replacement of fibronectin in septic shock. *Int Care Med* 12:188, 1986.

35. Niehaus GD, Schumacker PT, Saba TM: Influence of opsonic fibronectin deficiency on lung fluid balance during bacterial sepsis. *J Appl Physiol* 49:693–699, 1980.

36. Oh E, Pierschbacher M, Ruoslahti E: Deposition of plasma fibronectin in tissues. *Proc Acad Sci USA* 78:3218–3221, 1981.

37. Pussel BA, Peake PW, Brown MA, Charlesworth JA: Human fibronectin metabolism. *J Clin Invest* 76:143–148, 1985.

38. Ragni MV, Lewis JH, Spero JA, Bontempo FA: Plasma fibronectin levels in clinical disease states after cryoprecipitate infusion. *Thromb Haemostasis* 52:321–324, 1984.

39. Richards WO, Scovill WA, Shin B: Opsonic fibronectin deficiency in patients with intra-abdominal infection. *Surgery* 94(2):210, 1983.

40. Robbins AB, Doran JE, Reese AC, Mansberger AR, Jr: Cold insoluble globulin levels in operative trauma: Serum depletion, wound sequestration, and biological activity: An experimental and clinical study. *Am Surgeon* 46:663–672, 1980.

41. Robbins AB, Doran JE, Reese AC, Mansberger AR, Jr: Clinical response to cold insoluble globulin replacement in a patient with sepsis and thermal injury. *Am J Surg* 142:636–638, 1981.

42. Rodgers GP, Heymach GJ: Cryoprecipitate therapy in amniotic fluid embolization. *Am J Med* 76:916–920, 1984.

43. Rubli E, Bussard S, Frei E, Lundsgaard-Hansen P, Pappova E: Plasma fibronectin and associated variables in surgical intensive care patients. *Ann Surg* 197(3):310–317, 1983.

44. Ruoslahti E, Engvall E, Hayman EG: Fibronectin: current concepts of its structure and function. *Collagen Res* 1:95–128, 1981.

45. Ruoslahti E, Vaheri A: Interaction of soluble fibroblast surface antigen with fibrinogen and fibrin. Identity with cold-insoluble globulin of human plasma. *J Exp Med* 141:497–501, 1975.

45a. Saba TM: Plasma and tissue fibronectin: its role in the pathophysiology of critically ill septic patient. In *Critical Care: State of the Art*, vol 7. Fullerton, CA, The Society of Critical Care Medicine, 1986, pp 437–464.

46. Saba TM, Blumenstock FA, Shah DM, Landaburu RH, Hrinda ME, Deno DC, Holman JM, Cho E, Dayton C, Cardarelli PM: Reversal of opsonic deficiency in surgical, trauma, and burn patients by infusion of purified human plasma fibronectin. *Am J Med* 80:229–240, 1986.

47. Saba TM, Blumenstock FA, Scovill WA, Bernard H: Cryoprecipitate reversal of opsonic α_2-surface binding glycoprotein deficiency in septic surgical and trauma patients. *Science* 201:622–624, 1978.

48. Saba TM, Blumenstock FA, Shah DM, Kaplan JE, Cho E, Scovill W, Stratton H, Newell J, Gottlieb M, Sedransk N, Rahm R: Reversal of fibronectin and opsonic deficiency in patients: a controlled study. *Ann Surg* 199(1):87–96, 1984.

48a. Saba TM, Holman JM, Jr: Fibronectin and phagocytic host defense mechanisms. In Condon RE, DeCosse J (eds): *Surgical Care II*. Philadelphia, Lea & Febiger, 1985, p 273.

49. Saba TM, Jaffe E: Plasma fibronectin (opsonic glycoprotein): Its synthesis by vascular endothelial cells and role in cardiopulmonary integrity after trauma as related to reticuloendothelial function. *Am J Med* 68:577–594, 1980.

50. Saba TM, Di Luzio NR: Reticuloendothelial blockade and recovery as a function of opsonic activity. *Am J Physiol* 216:197–205, 1969.

51. Saba TM, Niehaus GD, Scovill WA, Blumenstock FA, Newell JC, Holman J Jr, Powers SR, Jr: Lung vascular

permeability after reversal of fibronectin deficiency in septic sheep. *Ann Surg* 198(5):654–662, 1983.

52. Sandstedt S, Cederblad G, Larsson J, Schildt B, Symreng T: Influence of total parenteral nutrition on plasma fibronectin in malnourished subjects with or without inflammatory response. *J Parent Ent Nutr* 8(5):493–496, 1984.

53. Schildt B, Bouveng R, Sollenberg M: Plasma substitute induced impairment of the reticuloendothelial system function. *Acta Chir Scand* 141:7–13, 1975.

54. Scovill WA, Annest SJ, Saba TM, Blumenstock FA, Newell JC, Stratton HH, Powers SR: Cardiovascular hemodynamics after opsonic α_2 surface binding glyco-protein therapy in injured patients. *Surgery* 86:284–293, 1979.

55. Scovill WA, Saba TM, Kaplan JE, Bernard H, Powers SR, Jr: Deficits in reticuloendothelial humoral control mechanisms in patients after trauma. *J Trauma* 16(11):898–904, 1976.

56. Scovill WA, Saba TM, Blumenstock FA, Bernard HR, Powers SR, Jr: Opsonic α_2 surface binding glycoprotein therapy during sepsis. *Ann Surg* 188:521–529, 1978.

57. Snyder EL, Barash PG, Mosher DF, Walter SD: Plasma fibronectin level and clinical status in cardiac surgery patients. *J Lab Clin Med* 102(6):881–889, 1983.

58. Snyder EL, Mosher DF, Hezzey A, Golenwsky G: Effect of blood transfusion on in vivo levels of plasma fibronectin. *J Lab Clin Med* 98(3):336–341, 1981.

59. Todd TR, Glynn MFX, Silver E, Redmond MD: A randomized trial of cryoprecipitate replacement of fibronectin deficiencies in the critically ill. *Am Rev Resp Dis* 129:A102, 1984.

60. Walton KW, Almond TJ, Robinson M, Scott DL: An experimental model for the study of the opsonic activity of fibronectin in the clearance of intravascular complexes. *Br J Exp Path* 65:191–200, 1984.

61. Yoder MC, Douglas SD, Gerdes J, Kline J, Polin RA: Plasma fibronectin in healthy newborn infants: Respiratory distress syndrome and perinatal asphyxia *J Pediatr* 102:777–780, 1983.

42

Radiation Injury[a]

Karl F. Hubner, M.D.

Radiation accidents and incidents continue to be of great interest and concern to the public. Issues such as the threat of nuclear war, the Chernobyl reactor accident, or reports of sporadic incidences of accidental radiation exposure keep this interest up and maintain a high level of fear among the public. In this climate of real concern and radiation phobia, physicians should not only be prepared to answer questions about acute or late effects of ionizing radiation, but also be able to participate in the initial assessment and management of individuals who have been exposed to ionizing radiation or contaminated with radioactive material. Some of the key facts about radiation injury and its medical treatment are discussed in this chapter.

SOURCES OF IONIZING RADIATION

Of all radiation exposure, 78% comes from natural sources; 20% from the use of x-rays, accelerators, and radiopharmaceuticals in diagnostic and therapeutic medicine; and the remaining 2% from nuclear energy production and other occupational environments.

For the purpose of discussing the medical consequences of ionizing radiation, it should suffice to distinguish between penetrating radiation (x-rays, γ rays, neutrons) and radiation with less penetrating power (α-particles, β-particles).

X-rays or γ-rays are electromagnetic waves that can easily enter the body. Depending on the amount of energy deposited within the body (absorbed dose) and the radiosensitivity of the irradiated organ or tissue, the resulting "immediate" effect may be clinically evident within minutes or hours or could take days or weeks to manifest itself. Late effects from high or low doses may not become recognizable for many years. On the other hand, α- and β-particles, because of their physical mass, travel only short distances in air and are rapidly slowed down within matter. They loose their kinetic energy within the first few micrometers or millimeters of tissue.

X-rays are produced in x-ray tubes by bombarding a metal target with electrons in a vacuum, while γ-rays are emitted directly from a nuclear fission process or during the radioactive decay of fission products. In addition, some natural radionuclides reach a stable state by decay. Energy is also associated with fast-moving, charged (α and β) or electrically neutral (neutrons) particles. Neutrons produce damage through collision in matter, and charged particles induce electrical instability within cells, causing damage through ionization. α-Particles are released during the radioactive decay of certain radionuclides and occur also as cosmic rays. β-Particles are the product of the decay of a number of radionuclides or can be produced by particle accelerators. Neutrons are typically released in the fission process but can also be produced in cyclotrons and linear accelerators or occur as cosmic rays. The α- and β-emitters in general are not a hazard with regard to external total body irritation; however, they present a serious problem when they enter the body through wounds, or the respiratory or gastrointestinal tracts. Depending on their chemical form, solubility, etc., radionuclides may end up in certain target sites, either destroying the target organ (e.g., ^{131}I destroys thyroid tissue and ^{32}P destroys bone marrow) or inducing neoplasms that appear after long latency periods.

[a]The original version of this chapter is based on work performed under contract no. DE-AC05-760R00033 between the U.S. Department of Energy, Office of Health and Environmental Research, and Oak Ridge Associated Universities. Accordingly, the U.S. government retains a nonexclusive, royalty-free license to publish or reproduce the published form of this contribution, or to allow others to do so for U.S. government purposes.

EFFECTS OF IONIZING RADIATION

Early Somatic Effects

The clinical responses to ionizing radiation are dose-related (Table 42.1), and the symptoms and signs that occur following this exposure are called the "acute radiation syndrome" (ARS).

ARS can be divided into four phases: (a) the prodromal phase (duration 1–2 days, possibly up to 4 days in some cases); (b) the latent phase (duration 2–3 weeks, less with high doses); (c) the bone marrow depression phase, excluding the gastrointestinal and cerebrovascular syndromes (duration 2–6 weeks); and (d) the recovery phase (duration about 3–4 weeks).

During the latent phase the patient may be asymptomatic. However, close clinical observation and laboratory tests should continue in order to detect the onset of manifestations of the ARS. Depending on the dose, the ARS may express itself as a cerebrovascular syndrome, gastrointestinal syndrome, or hematopoietic syndrome (Table 42.2). For more details and in-depth discussions of radiation injury in general and ARS in particular, the reader is referred to several publications released primarily under the auspices of the International Atomic Energy Agency and the World Health Organization (WHO) (2, 4, 6, 13).

Table 42.1
Clinical Response to Radiation Exposure

Dose (rad)	Effect
50	No symptoms
100	Anorexia, nausea
280	Vomiting in 50% of cases
450	Bone marrow suppression, fatal in 50% of cases; survival probable with adequate medical treatment
600–700	Fatal bone marrow suppression; survival possible only with maximum treatment
1000	Severe acute radiation syndrome with gastrointestinal complications; survival possible with bone marrow transplant
1000–2000	Gastrointestinal syndrome; fatal within 2 weeks
5,000–10,000	Cerebrovascular syndrome; fatal within 48 hours
10,000	Probably immediately fatal

Our experience with serious radiation accidents is limited. Sixty-two fatalities (acute effects) have occurred worldwide since 1945 (9). A review of all major radiation accidents (≥25 rad total body dose), including the Chernobyl data, reveals a total of 289 accidents involving approximately 136,363 persons (135,000 at Chernobyl alone), of whom 828 received significant exposures (ORAU/REAC/TS, Oak Ridge, TN; personal communication). Persons who develop the cerebrovascular or gastrointestinal syndromes cannot be saved by medical treatment. Even if death from the cerebrovascular effects of ionizing radiation could be prevented, the problems associated with the gastrointestinal syndrome would still have to be dealt with. It is conceivable that the gastrointestinal syndrome might be controllable by the correction of water and electrolyte imbalances, total parenteral alimentation, and selective treatment with antibiotics. However, even successful treatment of the gastrointestinal syndrome would not eliminate the serious problems of infection and hemorrhage resulting from bone marrow suppression (hematopoietic syndrome). The hematopoietic syndrome, then, remains the real challenge in treating patients having ARS.

Late Somatic Effects

Aside from the prevention of further radiation exposure and the removal of contaminating radioactive material from the skin or body after incorporation, late effects of ionizing radiation are of a minor concern in the immediate treatment of persons injured by radiation. A few general statements about late somatic and possible genetic effects are, however, in order. [For more extensive information, the reader is referred to the report of the United Nations Scientific Committee on the Effects of Atomic Radiation(15).]

CARCINOGENESIS

Radiation-induced changes in tissue may lead to somatic mutation and thus may be carcinogenic. After acute doses of ≥ 100 rad, the frequency of certain types of leukemia increases among the exposed population, with its "peak" occurring about 10 years after the exposure. For solid tumors linked to radiation exposure (thyroid, breast, lung, and bone), the latency period is longer. It is believed that approximately one-half of all radiation-in-

Table 42.2
Acute Radiation Syndrome (ARS)

	Signs and Symptoms	Clinical Course	Cause of Death	Exposure
Cerebrovascular syndrome	Ataxia, disorientation, CNS blackout, quick recovery, projectile vomiting, hemorrhagic diarrhea, shock	Severe hypotension, shock, increasing peripheral edema, coma, death	Irreversible shock; survival time: 6–48 hr	>3,000 R promptly
Gastrointestinal syndrome	Prompt vomiting, short latent phase, abdominal pain, abdominal distention, early diarrhea and dehydration, weight loss, prostration, early pancytopenia	Ulcerative enteritis associated with hemorrhage, infection, malnutrition and toxemia	Electrolyte imbalance with overwhelming septicemia (saprophytes); survival time: 5–15 days	>1,500 R (?) to <3,000 rad (?)[a]
Hematopoietic syndrome	Prodromal phase; latent phase; agranulocyte angina and thrombocytopenia	Granulocytopenia and thrombocytopenia reaching nadir at about 28 days postexposure; bone marrow depression phase: approximately day 20–40 postexposure	Infection and/or hemorrhage	Prodromal response, ED_{50}[b] Anorexia 180 R Nausea 260 R Fatigability 280 R Vomiting 320 R Diarrhea 360 R $LD_{50/60}$[c], 400–450 R $LD_{50/60}$ with medical treatment 600–700 R $LD_{50/60}$ with bone marrow graft 1000 R

[a] The uncertainties regarding the exposure required to produce this syndrome in man stem from the fact that there is only one well-documented case that fits into this category of the ARS, a man involved in the 1946 Los Alamos II radiation accident. His total body exposure was 1900 rad, and he died 8 days postexposure.
[b] Estimated response for 50% of exposed people (12). In order to convert exposure (roentgen, R) to rad (midline dose, rad = radiation absorbed dose), multiply by ⅔.
[c] $LD_{50/60}$: A dose lethal to 50% of a population within 60 days postexposure.

duced tumors will have occurred by 20 years after radiation. A statistically significant increase in cancer risk is demonstrable only for total body doses of ≥ 100 rad. Tumor induction through lower doses is probable, but it is clinically impossible to distinguish between radiation-induced and spontaneous cancers in the population, and any extrapolation from high to lower exposures (x-ray diagnosis, for instance) remains highly problematic.

RADIODERMATITIS

Radiation doses exceeding 1000 rad (fatal if given to the whole body) cause late effects of the skin such as chronic radiodermatitis (dry, atrophic, hairless skin) with a tendency to develop squamous cell or basal cell carcinoma. However, skin cancer induction probably requires thousands of rad.

STERILITY

Spermatogonia are quite radiosensitive. Doses of only 15 rad can lead to temporary oligospermia 45–60 days after exposure. Permanent, radiation-induced sterility is not likely to occur below doses of 500–700 rad (a dose well within the $LD_{50/60}$ range if received by the whole body). Full recovery of fertility is expected after total body doses in the range of 300 rad. In fertile women, doses of less than 400–500 rad causes transient sterility; doses of 500–1000 rad produce permanent sterility.

TERATOGENETIC EFFECTS

Another radiation effect—although not strictly a late effect—is the teratogenetic effect of radiation on the fetus. The specific effect depends primarily on the dose received and the phase of gestation. During the preimplantation (up to 10 days postconception), doses of 10 rad or more are likely to induce abortion rather than produce malformation. During organogenesis (up to the end of the ninth week of gestation), there is only a slight probability of malformation. At the present time, there is no scientific basis for the assumption that doses of <50 rad cause malformations in human fetuses if the exposure occurs during the first 9 weeks of gestation. However, in view of all the uncertainties associated with such assumptions or deductions, it is probably safest to assume that teratogenetic effects on the fetus may be possible after doses as low as 10 rad. Radiation exposure after 9 weeks of gestation

is not expected to cause malformation, but reduced growth and damage to the central nervous system may occur. There is, however, an increased incidence of leukemia during the first few years of life in children exposed to radiation in utero.

CATARACTS

Cataracts require fairly high doses, >600 rad of x-rays or γ-rays or 70 rads of neutrons, and the latency period before opacities may be detected can extend from several months up to 7–10 years. Certainly, if the cataract-inducing dose is "part" of a whole-body exposure, cataracts are of secondary concern since total body dose is already in the lethal range.

GENETIC EFFECTS

The effect of ionizing radiation on germ cells results in an increase in frequency of somatic mutations. Whether or not this effect becomes a deleterious and possibly inheritable health trait in the offspring of exposed persons remains to be documented. The information available from mutation experiments in animals indicates a doubling dose of 30 rad from acute exposure to x-rays. No quantitative data are available for human populations; however, no genetic consequences have been observed in the first- and second-generation offspring of the A-bomb survivors.

CLINICAL STAGING OF EFFECTS OF IONIZING RADIATION

Staging for radiation overexposure should be based primarily on clinical findings and laboratory tests. During the prodromal phase, various signs and symptoms are forerunners of the subsequent clinical course; early gastrointestinal symptoms, for example, allow a broad exposure classification, as indicated in the "prodromal response" section of Table 42.2.

Based on the frequency of nausea and vomiting in a large population following various levels of exposures, a dose-incidence-time pattern has been established (3) to assist in staging radiation overexposure. For example, a dose of 100 rad produces nausea and vomiting in less than 10% of the exposed population (Fig. 42.1). On the other hand, the entire population is expected to have nausea and vomiting 5–8 hours after a dose ≥ 300 rad. The specific time of the onset of nausea and vomiting is also dose related.

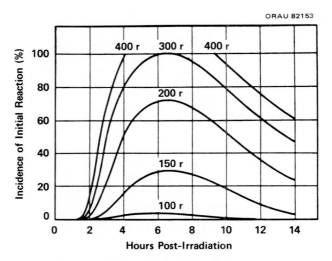

Figure 42.1 Estimation of incidence and duration of severe nausea, with vomiting in most cases, among a large population exposed to various air doses of penetrating ionizing radiation. (From Gerstner HB: Reaction to short-term radiation in man. *Ann Rev Med* 11:289–302, 1960, ©1960 by Annual Reviews, Inc., Palo Alto, CA.)

This simple staging procedure allows a quick assessment of the overall situation. However, continued observation of each overexposure patient is indicated since the clinical picture and stage of the ARS may evolve rather slowly.

Several laboratory tests are extremely helpful in staging radiation injury more accurately. One of the most useful and inexpensive biological dosimeters is the absolute lymphocyte count. Experience has shown that an absolute lymphocyte count taken during the first 48 hours postexposure permits a remarkably reliable classification of the severity of radiation injury (Table 42.3).

Biological dose estimation can also be obtained from chromosome analysis, the most sensitive method (15–10 rad) for providing evidence of radiation exposure (8). Obviously, this method is not very practical for the immediate evaluation of radiation accident vic-

tims because it takes several days before the results of such an analysis are available.

THERAPEUTIC OBJECTIVES AND MEANS FOR THEIR ATTAINMENT

Treatment of the Acute Radiation Syndrome

Every person involved in a radiation accident is likely to require treatment if he or she develops prodromal signs and symptoms and a lymphopenia of $<1,000/mm^3$ during the first 24 hours. Admission or planning for admission to a hospital should include some provision for effective isolation. A final decision about the kind and possible extent of treatment for such a person can be made within the first week after radiation exposure.

There is no question about the need for admission and treatment of persons who have nausea, vomiting, weakness, fatigue, erythema, and signs of cardiovascular involvement or a lymphopenia of $<500/mm^3$ within the first 24–48 hours postexposure. These more severe cases need prompt treatment with intense efforts to avoid serious consequences from cardiovascular or gastrointestinal tract involvement. It is obvious that the physician, when confronted with this type of problem, should observe the patient, categorize the symptoms, and plan treatment. Close laboratory surveillance should

Table 42.3
Prognostic Value of Absolute Lymphocyte Count in Total Body Irradiation

Lymphocytes (mm³) (48-hr postexposure)	Severity of Exposure	Prognosis
1500–3000	No exposure	(Normal range)
1000–1500	Mild exposure	Favorable
500–1000	Serious injury	Fair
100–500	Very serious injury	Poor
<100	Hopeless level of injury	Hopeless

include frequent routine blood counts and differentials, as well as bacteriological surveys from different regions of the body to detect infection or hemorrhage, the most serious complications of the hematopoietic syndrome.

ISOLATION

The clinical management of the hematopoietic syndrome consists of measures aimed at controlling infection and bleeding (1). Although it is most likely that infections in a radiation accident patient are caused by endogenous microorganisms, some sort of isolation is warranted to provide protection against exogenous infections. Protection may be provided by simple reverse isolation or more effective isolation methods such as "life islands" or laminar airflow rooms (this type of isolation is not likely to be available under austere conditions of nuclear warfare or other major nuclear catastrophes).

ANTIBIOTICS

Since increased susceptibility to infection in the hematopoietic syndrome does not develop until about 2–3 weeks postexposure, there is enough time to establish baseline cultures and to treat any existing minor infections using antibiotics chosen on the basis of cultures and sensitivity tests. In severe granulocytopenia ($<750/mm^3$), the prophylactic use of antibiotics is indicated because normally nonpathogenic organisms can cause serious, rapidly developing infections in the neutropenic host and because the typical response to infection (redness, pus formation, exudate, regional lymphadenopathy) are often absent. The choice of antibiotics should be based on the assumption that Gram-negative bacilli constitute the most likely initial risk. A combination of two or three antibiotics, a third-generation cephalosporin, carbenicillin (or ticarcillin), and an aminoglycoside (tobramycin or amikacin) should be effective in over 90% of the cases (16). Toxicity from long-term use of antibiotics is not likely to present a major problem since the period of severe neutropenia lasts only for 3–4 weeks before hematopoietic recovery starts. If recovery does not occur, concerns about toxicity of antibiotics become irrelevant.

GRANULOCYTE TRANSFUSIONS

With the development of filtration techniques and mechanical cell separators, normal granulocytes are becoming more and more available for clinical applications. Granulocyte transfusions are effective in neutropenic patients who have bacterial infections that do not respond to antibacterial agents (5). However, in order to have a chance of being effective, large numbers of granulocytes (10^{10}/day) have to be transfused daily for periods of 5–10 days.

PLATELET TRANSFUSIONS

Patients suffering from radiation-induced thrombocytopenia benefit from platelet transfusions during the thrombocytopenic phase (3–4 weeks). If the platelet count decreases to levels below 10,000 mm^3, platelet transfusions should be given even in the absence of bleeding. If bleeding exists, platelet transfusions are indicated even if the platelet count is as high as 60,000/mm^3. Since platelet transfusions are only required for periods of 2–3 weeks, alloimmunization is not of too much concern in this situation.

BONE MARROW TRANSPLANTATION

If bone marrow transplantation is considered, it has to be done at least 14 days before the recipient's bone marrow becomes totally aplastic, as it takes about 2 weeks before a successful bone marrow graft can provide sufficient numbers of platelets and granulocytes to the host. If possible, the bone marrow transplantation should be done within 7 days of radiation exposure. This potentially lifesaving procedure may be an option for an individual having a compatible bone marrow donor, but in radiation accidents or nuclear warfare involving multiple victims, this form of treatment is not likely to be available for all patients who might benefit from an allogeneic bone marrow transplant.

The reactor accident at Chernobyl in 1986 has clearly demonstrated the magnitude of the problems the medical community would have to address if a truly major radiation accident were to occur. At Chernobyl 135,000 people had to be evacuated (only 60,000 have been allowed to return to their homes as of this writing). Of those, 2000 were evaluated for significant radiation exposure, and 500 were hospitalized. Thirteen fire fighters and nuclear power plant workers, estimated to have received radiation doses in excess of 500 rad, were given bone marrow transplants from siblings. Six other victims, who had also sustained serious and extensive thermal burns, were given human fetal liver cells. The outcome of these transplants is discouraging. Only one of the bone marrow transplant recipients is alive at this time, and the six who received fetal liver cells have died (7).

These results emphasize the fact that even an HLA identical match neither assures a "take" nor excludes a potentially fatal graft-versus-host reaction. The timing of the bone marrow graft is critical; the Chernobyl accident victims received their bone marrow transplants 4–16 days after the accident. These results, presumably obtained with HLA-identical donors, also indicate that bone marrow transplants using random donors are doomed to fail, or to do more harm than good (among 100,000 persons selected at random, only two are likely to be HLA compatible). A possible solution to this problem is the collection and deep-freeze storage of the autologous bone marrow of nuclear power plant workers, who could then receive their own bone marrow in case of serious radiation exposure. This is a monumental task, considering that approximately 120,000 persons are currently employed in nuclear power plants worldwide. Considering the low probability of the recurrence of a serious reactor accident such as the one at Chernobyl, the cost of such measures would not seem justifiable. On the other hand, under "controlled conditions" an allogeneic bone marrow transplant may well be lifesaving in an individual case if dose estimation, clinical response and availability of an HLA-identical, MLC (mixed lymphocyte culture) nonreactive donor warrant this therapeutic approach.

OTHER THERAPEUTIC MEASURES

As indicated above, intensive care directed toward correcting cardiovascular abnormalities or problems associated with the gastrointestinal syndrome is indicated even though the overall prognosis may be poor. The pharmacological basis and principles to be applied in those situations are treatment of shock, management of water and electrolyte imbalances, alleviation of nausea and vomiting, and relief of pain. Under austere conditions, treatment for those victims whose survival is virtually impossible has to be restricted to sedation, analgesics and provision for general patient comfort.

TREATMENT OF RADIATION BURNS

Radiation accidents resulting in partial-body irradiation and potential radiation burns are much more common than those involving serious total-body exposures (10). The skin is extremely vulnerable to radiation, and damage is common following radiotherapy or industrial exposure involving x-ray and gamma sources. The determining factor is the total dose received.

The first noticeable effect is a transient erythema, which appears within 2–3 hours after exposure. This may be associated with a sensation of warmth or, if the dose is high, with severe pain and the sensation of fire in the affected part. Moderate doses will result in an immediate but transient erythema, followed by a more persistent erythema 2 or 3 weeks later. The length of the latent period between the "immediate" and the "fixed" erythema is dose dependent. In contrast to thermal burns, radiation burns deposit their energy much deeper in the skin, which results in damage to subcutaneous tissue, i.e. nerve endings, hair follicles, sweat glands, and, most importantly, the endothelium of the blood vessels. The result of "deep damage" is a progressive, obliterating endarteritis, leading to ischemic pain and irreversible tissue necrosis.

Since the result of such damage is progressive, the evolving effects continue over many weeks or months. The final degree of damage depends on the dose and dose rate. If the dose is 5000 rad or higher, necrosis of bone, muscle, and other internal structures may occur. Doses in excess of 300–400 rad will cause epilation at about 16 days postexposure. Epilation is likely to be permanent after doses above 700 rad.

Medical management of radiation burns during the erythema stage consists of frequent observation of the area in question, perhaps repeated color photographs, and protection of the skin against further thermal, chemical, or mechanical injury. The initial erythema and dry, itchy skin require little treatment other than a bland lotion.

At first, bland lotions are prescribed, and, in the later stages when dry desquamation of the skin develops, 1% aqueous solution of gentian violet may be applied. Cortisone cream may be of value at any stage of the burn. Pain, ischemic in character, may be severe and even require narcotics. Since the control of pain is likely to be required for a long period of time, narcotics should only be used only if ordinary analgesics fail.

Serious radiation burn may progress to blistering (wet desquamation) and, deep tissue necrosis. At this stage, the radiation burn is usually further complicated by infections. The combined problems of ischemia, tissue necrosis, pain, and infection usually require some kind of surgical intervention. The type and extent of surgical procedures such as skin grafting, simple excision or amputation, as well as the timing of such procedures, vary from patient to patient. The decision of surgical intervention should be made by a physician or a medical team experienced in treating radiation burns and only with the aid of additional diagnostic information on the microcirculation (nuclear medicine perfusion scintigraphy and thermography) of the damaged area.

CONTAMINATION BY RADIOACTIVE MATERIALS AND DECONTAMINATION AND DECORPORATION

If radioactive materials have been released into the environment during a radiation accident or the detonation of a nuclear device, external surface skin contamination and internal contamination with eventual deposition at specific target sites (incorporation) may occur. Accidents involving contamination with radioactive materials require immediate attention, and decontamination and decorporation (removal of radioactivity from the body by chelation or other medical treatment) have to be instituted as soon as possible in order to reduce deposition of radionuclides in specific organs, thereby avoiding potential late effects (carcinogenesis).

The most important rule in dealing with external and internal contamination is that any emergency medical care has absolute priority. The problem of contamination can be dealt with effectively only if the patient's condition is stable. Taking into consideration some basic radiation protection rules, the patient should be surveyed for contamination. Removal of clothing followed by decontamination of the skin (shower or localized cleansing) should be done as soon as the patient's condition and other circumstances permit. Contaminated wounds should be decontaminated first and covered with sterile dressings. Decontamination should be done at the site, if at all possible; otherwise at a first-aid station or a hospital

with a radiation emergency treatment area. Useful procedures and instructions as to how to handle a contaminated patient have been published in two manuals: National Council on Radiation Protection and Measurements Report No. 65 (11) and recommendations by the International Atomic Energy Agency in Vienna (12).

Incorporation of radionuclides can occur by absorption from contaminated wounds, by ingestion or by inhalation. The objective of medical treatment of this condition is to reduce incorporation by nonspecific measures such as irrigation of a wound, displacement therapy or chelation therapy. Chelating agents such as Ca- or Zn-diethylenetriaminepentaacetic acid (Ca-DTPA or Zn-DTPA) remove toxic metals by exchanging their cations for metals that form more stable complexes with DTPA. These chelating agents are particularly effective in removing long-lived, highly radiotoxic agents such as the transuranic elements (plutonium, americium, californium, and neptunium) from the body. Typically, Na_3-Ca-DTPA is given intravenously (1 g in 250 ml of 5% dextrose in water) as soon as possible after the incorporation of a transuranic element. If whole-body counts and bioassay data indicate that internal contamination did not exceed maximum permissible body or organ burdens, further chelation therapy is not indicated. In cases of excessive (multiple body burdens) incorporation of transuranic elements, chelation may have to be carried on for several months or perhaps even years. For longer periods of treatment, the Zn- form of DTPA is recommended because of its low toxicity as compared with that of Ca-DTPA.

There are also excellent sources for information on internal contamination and its medical management (5, 11). Both of these books (5, 11) were written by a panel of experts as practical manuals containing a wealth of information on decontamination and decorporation, not only of the transuranic elements but also of all other important radionuclides.

SUMMARY

In attempting to summarize the management of a patient who has sustained radiation injury by external sources or contamination, the following points should be kept in mind:

1. Deal with first-aid emergency care, surgical, and toxicologic problems before addressing

decontamination/decorporation and dosimetry problems.

2. Obtain history and do physical examination.

3. Plan laboratory studies: hematological, bacteriological, cytogenetics, tissue typing.

4. Follow platelet counts, look for evidence of bleeding, arrange for supportive transfusions as required.

5. Follow white blood cell count, isolate patient, watch for evidence of infection. Provide antimicrobial treatment and granulocyte transfusion, as indicated.

Treating radiation accident victims is not unique and does not really differ from treating patients who, for other reasons, have depressed bone marrow with the potential for infection and bleeding. Also the management of patients with the cardiovascular and gastrointestinal syndrome is not an unusual clinical task; unfortunately, there is not adequate treatment that could improve the prognosis of these radiation-induced problems. Finally, handling a radioactively contaminated patient is not an insurmountable problem and can be done quite safely.

References

1. Andrews GA: Medical management of accidental total-body irradiation. In Hubner KF, Fry SA: *The Medical Basis for Radiation Accident Preparedness.* Proceedings of the REAC/TS International Conference, 1979, Oak Ridge, Tn. New York, Elsevier/North Holland, 1980, pp 297–310.
2. Diagnosis and treatment of acute radiation injury: Proceedings of a scientific meeting. International Atomic Energy Agency and World Health Organization, Geneva, 1960, International Documents Service. New York, Columbia University Press, 1961.
3. Gerstner HB: Reaction to short-term radiation in man. *Annu Rev Med* 11:289–302, 1960.
4. Handling of radiation accidents: Proceedings of a Symposium, IAEA and World Health Organization, Vienna, 1969. International Atomic Energy Agency, Vienna, 1969 (SII/PUB/299).
5. Higby DJ, Burnett D: Granulocyte transfusions: current status. *Blood* 55:2–8, 1980.
6. Hubner KF, Fry SA: *The Medical Basis for Radiation Accident Preparedness.* Proceedings of the REAC/TS International Conference, 1979, Oak Ridge, TN. New York, Elsevier/North Holland, 1980.
7. Linnemann RE: Soviet medical response to the Chernobyl nuclear accident. *JAMA* 258:637–643, 1987.
8. Littlefield LG, Joiner EE, DuFrain RJ et al: Cytogenetic dose estimates from in vivo samples from persons involved in renal or suspected radiation exposures. In Hubner KF, Fry SA: *The Medical Basis for Radiation Accident Preparedness.* Proceedings of the REAC/TS International Conference, 1979. New York, Elsevier/North Holland, 1980, pp 375–390.
9. Lushbaugh CC, Fry SA, Hubner KF et al: Total body irradiation: an historical review and follow-up. In Hubner KF, Fry SA: *The Medical Basis for Radiation Accident Preparedness,* Proceedings of the REAC/TS International Conference, 1979, Oak Ridge, Tennessee. New York, Elsevier/North Holland, 1980, pp 3–15.
10. Lushbaugh CC, Fry SA, Ricks RC, Hubner KF, Burr WW: Historical update of past and recent skin damage radiation accidents. *Br J Radiol* (Suppl)19:7–12, 1987.
11. Management of persons accidentally contaminated with radionuclides: National Council on Radiation Protection and Measurements, Washington, DC, 1979 (NRCP Report 65).
12. Manual on early medical treatment of possible radiation injury: International Atomic Energy Agency; Vienna, 1978 (IAEA Safety Series No. 47).
13. Manual on radiation haematology: International Atomic Energy Agency, Vienna, 1971 (IAEA Technical Report Series No. 123).
14. Radiological factors affecting decision-making in a nuclear attack: National Council on Radiation Protection and Measurements, Washington, DC, 1974 (NCRP Report 42).
15. United Nations Scientific Committee on the Effects of Atomic Radiation: Sources and effects of ionizing radiation, United Nations Publication No. E.77.XI.1, 1977.
16. Young LS: fever and septicemia. In Rubin RH, Young LS: *Clinical Approach to Infection in the Compromised Host.* New York, Plenum Medical Book Corp, 1981, pp 75–122.

43

Electrolyte and Acid-Base Disorders

Man S. Oh, M.D.
Hugh J. Carroll, M.D.

Electrolyte and acid-base disorders are common problems in clinical medicine. This chapter reviews some of these disorders with particular reference to those problems that occur frequently in critically ill patients. Discussions stress pathophysiology, diagnosis, and pharmacological aspects of management.

HYPONATREMIA

Hyponatremia, which is defined as a reduced plasma sodium concentration, is the most common electrolyte disorder. The term *pseudohyponatremia* is applied to a spurious reduction in serum sodium concentrations due to a measurement error caused by hyperlipidemia, hyperproteinemia, or increased viscosity of the plasma. Although the sodium concentration in plasma water is normal in pseudohyponatremia, the dilution of the sample causes an error in measurement (33). When measurement is made with an ion-specific electrode without dilution of the sample (direct method), the concentration is normal. However, the error occurs when serum sodium is measured with a flame photometer, because the sample is always diluted before flame-photometric measurement. The error also occurs even when an ion-specific electrode is used, if an indirect method (dilution of the sample) is used (15, 23). In pseudohyponatremia, plasma osmolality, which is customarily measured without dilution, is normal (33). A low plasma sodium concentration with a normal plasma osmolality does not always indicate the presence of pseudohyponatremia; true hyponatremia may be accompanied by a normal plasma osmolality because of hyperglycemia, azotemia, mannitol, or alcohol (31).

Hyponatremia usually signifies a proportionate reduction in plasma osmolality, which causes cellular overhydration by the shift of water into the cells. Cell overhydration, especially when it occurs abruptly, can cause neuromuscular dysfunction, convulsions, and death. Cellular overhydration in hyponatremia is independent of extracellular volume, since the shift of water across the cell membrane depends solely on the osmotic gradient. Accumulation of a substance such as mannitol or glucose that is restricted to the extracellular fluid can cause hyponatremia by increasing extracellular (effective) osmolality and hence causing the shift of water from the intracellular space to the extracellular space. In such situations, despite hyponatremia, cells are dehydrated rather than swollen. Some authors extend the definition of pseudohyponatremia to those hyponatremic states accompanied by increased effective osmolality. However, since the sodium concentration in mannitol- or hyperglycemia-induced hyponatremia is truly low, such an extended definition of pseudohyponatremia is inappropriate and also confusing.

Glucose, sodium, and mannitol are effective osmols, whereas urea and alcohol are ineffective osmols because the former can effectively cause the shift of water across the cell membrane, whereas the latter diffuse freely into the cell and therefore do not cause the water shift (12). Thus, the clinical importance of hyponatremia must be judged in the context of the effective plasma osmolality, which may be determined in two ways. It can be measured by summation of all effective osmols in plasma:

Effective osmolality = Plasma Na (mEq/liter)

$$\times 2 + \frac{glucose\ (mg/dl)}{18} + \frac{mannitol\ (mg/dl)}{18} +$$

Alternatively, the total osmolality can be measured and the osmolality due to ineffective osmols subtracted. Table 43.1 lists the cate-

Table 43.1
Hyponatremia According to Effective Osmolality

Normal effective osmolality-pseudohyponatremia:
hyperlipidemia, hyperproteinemia, increased
viscosity
Increased effective osmolality: hyperglycemia,
mannitol infusion
Low effective osmolality: usual hyponatremia

Table 43.2
**Causes of Hyponatremia According to
Mechanism of Maintenance**

Increased water intake, e.g., primary polydipsia
Reduced water excretion
Reduced delivery of fluid to the distal nephron
because of low effective arterial volume (ADH
is usually present as well)
Heart failure
Nephrotic syndrome
Cirrhosis of the liver
Gastrointestinal sodium loss
Sweating
Diuretic therapy or renal salt wasting
Adrenal insufficiency
Hypothyroidism
Advanced renal failure
Inappropriate secretion of ADH (SIADH)
Tumors
Pulmonary diseases
Central nervous system disorders
Drugs, e.g., chlorpropamide, barbiturates,
morphine, indomethacin
Physical and emotional stress, nausea
Glucocorticoid deficiency
Myxedema
Idiopathic
Reset osmostat

gories of hyponatremia associated with increased, normal, and low effective plasma osmolality.

Causes and Pathogenesis of True Hyponatremia

The initiating mechanism of hyponatremia will be one of the following: (a) shift of water from the cell caused by accumulation of extracellular solutes other than sodium salts; (b) retention of excess water in the body; (c) loss of sodium; and (d) shift of sodium into the cells.

The appropriate physiological response to hyponatremia is suppression of antidiuretic hormone (ADH) release, leading to rapid excretion of excess water and correction of hyponatremia. Persistence of hyponatremia indicates the failure of this compensatory mechanism. In most instances hyponatremia is maintained because the kidney fails to produce water diuresis, but sometimes excessive ingestion of water is responsible.

Among the reasons for the inability of the kidney to excrete water and therefore correct hyponatremia are renal failure, reduced delivery of glomerular filtrate to the distal nephron, and the presence of ADH. The mechanism for impaired water excretion in renal failure is obvious and needs no further explanation. Reduced distal delivery of filtrate results from the low glomerular filtration rate and enhanced proximal tubular reabsorption that characterize volume-depletion states. The normal dilution of urine requires delivery of adequate amounts of fluid to the diluting segment and the reabsorption of solute without water at that segment. ADH impairs urine dilution by reabsorption of water in the collecting duct. The presence of normal amounts of ADH despite hyponatremia would be considered inappropriate, but the release of ADH caused by reduced effective arterial volume is not considered inappropriate. The term "the syndrome of inappropriate ADH secretion" (SIADH) is therefore reserved for hyponatremia with a

normal or increased effective arterial volume. There are many causes of SIADH: tumors, pulmonary diseases including tuberculosis and pneumonias, central nervous system diseases, drugs, etc. (Table 43.2).

Hyponatremia in clinical states associated with reduced effective arterial volume such as congestive heart failure and cirrhosis of the liver is caused by a combination of reduced delivery of fluid to the distal nephron and elaboration of ADH (74). The same appears to be true of myxedema and glucocorticoid deficiency states (24, 34, 67).

Finally, mild hyponatremia may be caused by "resetting of the osmostat" at an osmolality lower than the usual level. In such cases urine dilution occurs normally when the plasma osmolality is brought down below the reset level. Resetting of the osmostat would be considered a form of SIADH, since ADH secretion occurs inappropriately at hyponatremic levels. Patients with chronic debilitating diseases such as pulmonary tuberculosis often manifest this phenomenon (17).

Diagnosis

The presence of a low plasma sodium and normal osmolality suggests pseudohyponatremia, but does not confirm it; hyponatremia accompanied by a high concentration of urea or alcohol might give a normal osmolality. More direct proof is the demonstration of a normal sodium concentration using a sodium-specific electrode or demonstration of reduced water content of plasma. Pseudohyponatremia due to hyperlipidemia is caused by accumulation of chylomicrons, which consist mostly of triglycerides (33), and is obvious from the milky appearance of serum or plasma. Substantial hyponatremia due to hyperlipidemia requires accumulation of more than 5–6 g/dl of lipids, and that degree of hyperlipidemia does not occur with hypercholesterolemia alone. Pseudohyponatremia due to hyperproteinemia can be confirmed by measurement of plasma proteins. Hyponatremia caused by mannitol or glucose is easily detected from the history and simultaneous measurements of plasma sodium, osmolality, and glucose.

In evaluating hyponatremia associated with hypoosmolality, the main concern is to distinguish between SIADH and hyponatremia due to other causes, for the most part volume-depletion states and edematous states. The major distinction between SIADH and other causes of hyponatremia lies in the status of effective arterial volume (EAV); EAV is normal or increased in the former, whereas the latter are associated with reduced EAV. However, there is no diagnostic test that measures effective arterial volume with certainty. A convenient and thus widely practiced technique for estimating EAV consists of measurement of urinary sodium and serum urea nitrogen (SUN), creatinine, and uric acid. Urinary sodium excretion > 20 mEq/liter, SUN < 10 mg/dl (16), serum creatinine < 1 mg/dl, and serum urate < 4.0 mg/dl (5) are suggestive of normal or increased effective arterial volume. In contrast, the measurement of urine osmolality has virtually no diagnostic value, and often misleads physicians. Contrary to common belief, SIADH may be associated with urine osmolality less than plasma osmolality (4). Similarly, other causes of hyponatremia can also be accompanied by urine osmolality higher than plasma osmolality, and a high urine osmolality in hyponatremia does not necessarily favor the diagnosis of SIADH.

The only situation in which urine osmolality may be appropriately low in the presence of hyponatremia is the hyponatremia caused by primary polydipsia, and this is usually apparent when a careful history reveals polyuria (53). In all other disorders that cause hypona-

tremia urine osmolality is inappropriately increased, i.e., greater than 100 mOsm/liter.

Management and Pharmacology

Hyponatremia is treated either by the addition of sodium or by removal of water. Salt is given to patients with hyponatremia due to salt depletion, and water is to be removed in hyponatremic states with normal or increased sodium content. The speed of correction of hyponatremia is very important and should depend on the speed of development of hyponatremia and the patient's symptoms. Clearly, severe symptomatic hyponatremia is a life-threatening condition (2), but there are considerable dangers associated with treatment of hyponatremia. In addition to the danger of volume overload that may occur with administration of a large quantity of salt-containing solution, the possibility of central pontine myelinolysis is now considered a major danger associated with rapid correction of hyponatremia (40, 73). This demyelinating disease of the central pons, which is characterized by motor nerve dysfunction including quadriplegia, may develop following rapid correction of hyponatremia. The complication tends to occur more with chronic hyponatremia in a malnourished and debilitated patient than with acute hyponatremia, and may be avoided by slow correction of hyponatremia (at a speed < 0.5 mEq/liter/hour). Since there is less danger of central pontine myelinolysis with acute hyponatremia than with chronic hyponatremia, and chronic hyponatremia is usually asymptomatic, rapid correction (at a rate of 1–2 mEq/liter/hour) should be restricted to those with acute symptomatic hyponatremia. Even then, there is no advantage in rapidly increasing serum sodium above levels of 125–130 mEq/liter. For patients admitted with hypotonic dehydration and chronic asymptomatic hyponatremia who suffer mainly from volume depletion, the traditional recommendation has been administration of isotonic saline. However, sometimes rapid excretion of water following isotonic saline administration in these patients may leave them particularly vulnerable to the development of central pontine myelinolysis. For those patients, the use of 0.45% sodium chloride solution may be safer (43).

RAPID TREATMENT

For hyponatremia with sodium depletion, intravenous administration of sodium as hypertonic saline will correct hyposmolality effectively. The amount of sodium necessary to increase the sodium to a desired level of serum sodium is calculated as follows:

$$\text{Sodium requirement (in mEq)} =$$
$$\text{TBW X (the desired serum sodium} -$$
$$\text{actual serum sodium)}$$

Sodium may be administered as a 3% or 5% NaCl solution. If the main purpose of treatment is correction of volume depletion rather than of hyponatremia, normal saline may be administered instead. As the ADH release caused by low EAV is suppressed with the volume expansion, excess water is excreted in the urine, resulting in correction of hyponatremia. This approach is feasible, of course, only if there is sufficient renal function for water excretion.

When accumulation of excess water is primarily responsible for hyponatremia, as in SIADH, water may be rapidly removed by administration of intravenous osmotic diuretics such as mannitol. An easier technique to use is to administer a loop diuretic (e.g., furosemide, which causes sodium and water diuresis) and simultaneously to administer hypertonic saline; the net result is removal of water (27). The usual adult dose of furosemide for this purpose is 40 mg. The same dose can be repeated at 2 to 4-hour intervals while hypertonic saline is being given. The response to this regimen cannot be predicted with precision, and frequent follow-up measurements of serum sodium level must be made. There is no theoretical advantage of replacing exactly the amount of sodium lost in urine with hypertonic saline. Administration of hypertonic saline alone usually causes a salt and water diuresis, but addition of a loop diuretic makes the correction of hyponatremia easier by preventing excretion of concentrated urine. Another advantage of adding a diuretic is prevention of fluid overload that may result from the administration of hypertonic saline. Potassium supplements are usually needed with this therapy.

CHRONIC THERAPY

Chronic hyponatremia may be treated by a reduction of water intake or by an increase in renal water excretion. Reduction of water intake is preferable but is not always feasible. If water restriction is difficult or unsuccessful, the latter approach may be used. Increased renal water excretion can be achieved by the use of pharmacological agents that interfere

with urine concentration. Lithium and demeclocycline increase urine output by reducing the production of cyclic AMP and also by interfering with its action (18, 65, 66). Demeclocycline is more effective and has fewer side effects (19), but it may cause nephrotoxicity in patients with liver diseases (11). The usual dose of lithium for this purpose is 300 mg twice or three times a day, and the usual dose of demeclocycline is 300 mg twice to three times a day.

Administration of a loop diuretic such as furosemide in conjunction with increased salt and potassium intake is a safer method of treating chronic hyponatremia than the above methods. The mechanism of action of the diuretic is prevention of high medullary interstitial osmolality by limiting the reabsorption of salt in Henle's loop and hence prevention of urine concentration. The increased salt and potassium intake leads to increased delivery of solutes and hence to increased water output (61). There is evidence that ethacrynic acid may impair ADH-stimulated water movement across the collecting duct, and furosemide may have the same effect. The usual dose of furosemide is 40 mg twice to three times a day.

Finally, the recently discovered vasopressin antagonists, which are not yet commercially available, may become an important addition to the chronic as well as acute treatment of hyponatremia in the future (60). The vascular effect as well as the antidiuretic effect of vasopressin is antagonized by the vasopressin antagonists.

HYPERNATREMIA

Hypernatremia is defined as an increased sodium concentration in plasma water. Whereas hyponatremia may not be accompanied by hyposmolality, e.g., hyponatremia due to hyperglycemia, hypernatremia is always associated with an increased effective plasma osmolality and hence with a reduced cell volume. However, the extracellular volume may be normal, decreased, or increased, depending on the pathogenesis of the hypernatremia.

Pathogenesis

Hypernatremia is caused by either loss of water or gain of sodium (Table 43.3). Loss of water could be due to increased loss or reduced intake, and gain of sodium is due either

Table 43.3
Pathogentic Mechanism of Hypernatremia

Loss of Water
  Reduced water intake
    Defective thirst
    Unconsciousness
    Inability to drink water
    Lack of access to water
  Increased water loss
    Gastrointestinal loss; vomiting, osmotic diarrhea
    Cutaneous loss; sweating and fever
    Respiratory loss; hyperventilation
    Renal loss, diabetes insipidus, osmotic diuresis
Gain of Sodium
  Increased intake
    Hypertonic saline infusion
    Ingestion of sea water
    Hypertonic sodium bicarbonate
  Renal salt retention
    Usually in response to primary water deficit

to increased intake or to reduced renal excretion. Increased loss of water can occur through the kidney (e.g., in diabetes insipidus or osmotic diuresis), the gastrointestinal tract (e.g., gastric suction or osmotic diarrhea), or the skin. Reduced water intake occurs most commonly in comatose patients or in those with a defective thirst mechanism. Less frequent causes of reduced water intake include continuous vomiting, lack of access to water, and mechanical obstruction such as esophageal tumor. The excess gain of sodium leading to hypernatremia is usually iatrogenic, e.g., from hypertonic saline infusion, abortion with hypertonic saline, or administration of hypertonic sodium bicarbonate during cardiopulmonary resuscitation or treatment of lactic acidosis (35). Reduced renal sodium excretion leading to sodium gain and hypernatremia is most commonly observed in patients who are water depleted.

Water depletion due to diabetes insipidus, osmotic diuresis, or insufficient water intake commonly leads to secondary renal sodium retention in those who continue to ingest or are given sodium. Often, hypernatremia observed in such cases is due more to sodium retention than to water loss (Table 43.3). Whether hypernatremia is due to sodium retention or water loss can be determined by examination of the patient's volume status. For example, if a patient with a serum sodium of 170 mEq/liter is normotensive and does not have obvious evidence of dehydration, hypernatremia cannot be caused entirely by water loss. In order to increase a serum sodium to 170 mEq/liter by water deficit alone, one would have to lose more than 20% of total body water.

Whereas the most effective defense against hyponatremia is increased renal water excretion, the most effective defense against hypernatremia is increased water drinking in response to thirst. Because thirst is such an effective and sensitive defense mechanism against hypernatremia, it is virtually impossible to increase serum sodium by more than a few milliequivalents per liter if the water drinking mechanism is intact. Therefore, in a patient with hypernatremia, there will always be a reason for reduced water intake (Table 43.3).

Management

ACUTE TREATMENT

Hypernatremia is treated either by the addition of water or the removal of sodium. The choice depends on the status of the body sodium and water content. If water depletion is the cause of hypernatremia, water is added. If sodium excess is the cause, sodium needs to be removed. When the water deficit is substantial, circulatory disturbances may result from extracellular volume depletion. In this situation, isotonic (0.9%) NaCl or 0.45% NaCl may be given initially to stabilize circulatory dynamics, with subsequent administration of more hypotonic solutions to normalize the tonicity. Administration of 5% dextrose solution would also correct the extracellular volume depletion, but a larger volume than isotonic saline is needed to expand the extracellular volume by the same extent and too rapid reduction of the plasma osmolality may result in cerebral edema. In acute symptomatic hypernatremia, serum sodium may be reduced by 6–8 mEq/liter in the first 3–4 hours, but thereafter the rate of decline should not exceed 1 mEq/liter/hour. As with hyponatremia, chronic hypernatremia usually does not cause CNS symptoms, and therefore does not require rapid correction. The amount of water needed to correct hypernatremia can be estimated with the following equation:

$$\text{Water deficit (in liters)} = \text{TBW}\left(\frac{\text{Na2}}{\text{Na1}} - 1\right)$$

where Na1 is the desired serum sodium level, Na2 the observed serum sodium, and TBW is total body water. Total body water (in liters) can be estimated using the following formula:

$$\text{TBW} = \text{body weight in lb}/4.$$

In hypernatremia with excess sodium, the restoration of a normal volume usually initiates natriuresis, but if natriuresis does not occur promptly, sodium may be removed with diuretics. Furosemide plus 5% dextrose solution might be an appropriate regimen to treat hypernatremia associated with excess sodium, but care must be taken not to allow serum sodium concentration to decline too rapidly. Furosemide can be given at 40–60 mg intravenously at 2–4 hour intervals while 5% dextrose solution is being infused. If the patient has renal failure, salt can be removed by dialysis.

CHRONIC TREATMENT

Hypernatremic disorders that require chronic preventive therapy include diabetes insipidus and primary hypodipsia. If diabetes insipidus is the primary cause of hypernatremia, the distinction should first be made between nephrogenic and neurogenic (pituitary) diabetes insipidus. Administration of pitressin or stimulation of endogenous ADH secretion is helpful only for pituitary diabetes insipidus. Exogenous pitressin is available in three forms: pitressin tannate in oil, which is administered intramuscularly; I, desmopressin (dDAVP), a synthetic analog of ADH, which is administered through a plastic nasal tube (56); and a synthetic lysine vasopressin (lypressin, Diapid), which is administered as a nasal spray. The usual dose of dDAVP is 0.2 ml twice a day, and the usual dose for Diapid is 1–2 sprays in each nostril four times a day.

Some patients may prefer oral agents, and the two that have been used extensively with relatively few side effects are chlorpropamide and thiazide diuretics. Chlorpropamide (100–250 mg/day) stimulates the secretion of endogenous ADH and may also enhance the effect of ADH. Thiazide diuretics produce vascular volume depletion and enhanced reabsorption of fluid in the proximal tubule. Thus, they increase urine concentration by reducing the delivery of fluid to the distal diluting segment of the nephron. Addition of a thiazide diuretic to chlorpropamide may prevent the hypoglycemia that may occur if the latter is used alone. Two other drugs that have been used for the treatment of neurogenic diabetes insipidus are clofibrate (the usual dose, 2 g/day) (38) and carbamazepine (600 mg/day) (52). Since both drugs are less effective than chlorpropamide and have serious side effects, they should be the last resources in the treatment of diabetes

insipidus. Nephrogenic diabetes insipidus cannot be treated with ADH preparations or an agent that stimulates ADH release, but measures to reduce the distal delivery of salt and water, i.e., low salt diet and thiazide diuretics, have been used successfully. Subjects with primary hyodipsia should be educated to drink on schedule. In some instances, stimulation of the thirst center with chlorpropamide has met with success (8).

POTASSIUM METABOLISM

Although most of the body potassium is intracellular, the plasma potassium concentrations usually reflect the total body store of potassium. However, in conditions such as periodic paralysis or acid-base disorders, where abnormal shifts in potassium take place across the cell membrane, the plasma potassium concentration may not accurately reflect body stores. In both hyperkalemic and hypokalemic types of periodic paralysis, abnormal plasma potassium concentrations are explained by transmembrane potassium shifts. Similarly, in acute acidosis hyperkalemia may occur because of the shift of potassium from the cell, while acute alkalosis leads to hypokalemia because of potassium shift into the cells. Catecholamines and respiratory alkalosis are often responsible for hypokalemia in critical care units.

HYPOKALEMIA

Hypokalemia refers to a reduction in the plasma potassium concentration. Except for the situations where hypokalemia is caused by intracellular shift, it usually represents depletion of cellular potassium.

Pathogenesis

There are three basic mechanisms for hypokalemia: (a) intracellular shift, (b) reduced intake, and (c) increased loss (Table 43.4). An intracellular shift of potassium occurs with an increase in blood pH (62). This shift may occur when a patient develops alkalosis or when acidosis is being corrected. Administration of glucose and insulin also causes an intracellular shift of potassium, in part by stimulation

Table 43.4
Causes and Mechanism of Hypokalemia

Shift into the cell
  Correction of acidosis
  Administration of insulin and glucose
  Alkalosis
  Hypokalemic periodic paralysis
  Barium poisoning
  Increased catecholamines due to acute stress
Reduced intake
Increased loss
  Renal loss
    Primary hyperaldosteronism
    Secondary hyperaldosteronism, e.g., diuretic
      therapy, malignant hypertension, Bartter's
      syndrome, renal artery stenosis
    Mineralocorticoids other than aldosterone, e.g.,
      licorice, fluoro-prednisolone ointment,
      carbenoxolone
    Miscellaneous, e.g., hypercalcemia, Liddle's
      syndrome, magnesium deficiency, L-DOPA,
      RTA, acute myelocytic and monocytic
      leukemia, poorly reabsorbable anions
  Gastrointestinal loss
    Vomiting or nasogastric suction
    Diarrhea or fistula drainage

of glucose metabolism, but also by a direct effect of insulin on the cellular uptake of potassium (32, 58). The mechanism of intracellular shift of potassium in familial periodic paralysis is not clearly known.

The ingestion of absorbable barium salts, e.g., carbonate or chloride, causes a prompt reduction in the plasma potassium concentration by an intracellular shift (57). The intracellular shift is due to a decrease in passive outward diffusion of potassium because of decreased conductance of potassium (69).

The major routes of potassium loss are the kidneys and the gastrointestinal tract. There are numerous causes for renal potassium loss, but the two most constant factors are increased sodium delivery to the distal nephron and increased mineralocorticoid activity. Increased sodium delivery with reduced mineralocorticoid activity (e.g., high salt diet), or increased mineralocorticoid activity with reduced renal sodium excretion (e.g., extrarenal salt loss) does not lead to increased renal potassium excretion. Conditions such as primary hyperaldosteronism or chronic diuretic therapy are associated with increased sodium delivery to the distal nephron, even though sodium intake and urinary excretion may be normal. In primary hyperaldosteronism the proximal tubular sodium reabsorption is reduced because of volume expansion, resulting in greater sodium delivery to the distal ne-

phron. Enhanced sodium reabsorption at the Na-K exchange site allows normal amounts of sodium to come out in the urine despite increased delivery of sodium to the distal nephron.

A similar mechanism is responsible for the maintenance of increased sodium delivery to the Na-K exchange site during chronic diuretic therapy even when sodium excretion equals the intake. Hypercalcemia causes hypokalemia through increased renal potassium loss, but the exact mechanism is unknown. Increased urinary sodium excretion, which occurs with calcium infusion, is suggested as a possible mechanism (3). The degree of hypokalemia appears to be positively correlated with the serum calcium concentration. Hypokalemia caused by magnesium deficiency is due to increased renal loss of potassium, perhaps caused by increased production of aldosterone (21). PRA in magnesium deficiency is normal, and the mechanism of increased aldosterone is not known. Although the causal relationship is not entirely clear, the prevalence of hypokalemia in familial hypomagnesemia suggests that they are related (68). L-Dopa also occasionally causes hypokalemia possibly through increased aldosterone secretion (25). Kaliuresis and hypokalemia in renal tubular acidosis are commonly attributed to secondary hyperaldosteronism caused by renal salt wasting. Although renal salt wasting occurs in chronic metabolic acidosis, there is little convincing evidence for secondary hyperaldosteronism. There may be a specific tubular defect causing increased potassium loss in renal tubular acidosis (63). The mechanism of hypokalemia in acute mylelocytic and acute monocytic leukemias is increased renal loss of potassium, but the mechanism of this loss is controversial (36). Delivery to the distal nephron of poorly reabsorbable anions such as penicillin and carbenicillin, leads to increased urinary loss of potassium because increased luminal negativity enhances potassium secretion (29). Vomiting and nasogastric suction cause hypokalemia, in part, because of direct loss of potassium from the stomach, but to a larger extent because of renal loss attributable to the renal bicarbonate wasting that occurs with metabolic alkalosis. Excretion of large amounts of bicarbonate causes renal potassium loss because bicarbonate acts as a poorly reabsorbable anion. Secondary hyperaldosteronism due to volume depletion is an additional factor involved in the pathogenesis of hypokalemia in this setting.

Management

Hypokalemia is usually treated either by potassium administration or by prevention of the renal loss of potassium. Renal loss of potassium is prevented either by treating its cause (e.g., removal of aldosterone-producing adenoma or by discontinuation of diuretics) or by the administration of potassium-sparing diuretics. The potassium-sparing diuretics in current use are aldosterone antagonists (e.g., spironolactone), triamterene, and amiloride. Aldosterone antagonists are effective in preventing renal potassium loss only if an increased mineralocorticoid concentration is responsible for hypokalemia. In disorders such as Liddle's syndrome, spironolactone is ineffective because plasma aldosterone is reduced, whereas triamterene and amiloride are effective regardless of the plasma aldosterone concentration. The daily dose of spironolactone ranges from 25 to 400 mg. The usual doses of triamterene range from 50 to 150 mg twice a day, whereas amiloride is administered at 5 mg/day, and can be slowly increased up to 20 mg/day. Amiloride should be administered with food to avoid gastric irritation. Because reduced delivery of sodium to the distal nephron always reduces potassium secretion, a low salt diet may be effective in reducing renal potassium loss of any cause, independent of the plasma aldosterone concentration.

HYPERKALEMIA

Hyperkalemia may be caused by one of three mechanisms: (a) shift of potassium from the cells to the extracellular space, (b) increased potassium intake, and (c) reduced renal potassium excretion (Table 43.5). Hyperkalemic familial periodic paralysis, use of succinylcholine in paralyzed patients (14), use of cationic amino acids such as epsilon-aminocaproic acid, arginine or lysine (13, 28), rhabdomyolysis or hemolysis, and acute acidosis all cause hyperkalemia by extracellular potassium shift. Rhabdomyolysis and hemolysis cause hyperkalemia only in the presence of renal failure. Acute acidosis has long been regarded as a cause of extracellular potassium shift, irrespective of the type of acidosis, but recent evidence suggests that hyperkalemia is not as predictable with organic acidosis as with inorganic acidosis (46). Furthermore, there is little change in serum potassium concentration with either respiratory acidosis or alkalosis.

Table 43.5
Causes of Hyperkalemia

Pseudohyperkalemia
  Thrombocytosis, massive leucocytosis, use of tourniquet with fist exercise, in vitro hemolysis
True hyperkalemia
  Due to extracellular shift
    Severe acidosis (especially inorganic acidosis)
    Catabolic states
    Periodic paralysis
    Succinylcholine
    Cationic amino acids
  Due to excessive ingestion: rare if renal excretion is normal
  Decreased renal excretion
    Hypoaldosteronism; Addison's disease; selective hypoaldosteronism (hyporeninemic hypoaldosteronism, heparin, congenital adrenal enzyme deficiencies, angiotensin converting enzyme inhibitors)
    Tubular unresponsiveness to aldosterone: congenital, salt-losing nephropathy
    Potassium-sparing diuretics
    Severe dehydration

However, hyperkalemia is common in diabetic ketoacidosis and phenformin-induced lactic acidosis (1). The more frequent occurrence of hyperkalemia in clinical organic acidosis than in experimental organic acidosis may be explained by the longer duration of acidosis and the presence of other factors such as dehydration and renal failure in organic acidosis. Hyperkalemia can also occur in severe digitalis intoxication by extracellular shift of potassium as digitalis inhabits the Na^+-K^+ pump (6).

The kidney's ability to excrete potassium is so great that hyperkalemia rarely occurs solely on the basis of increased intake of potassium. However, increased intake can lead to hyperkalemia when renal excretion of potassium is reduced. There are three major mechanisms of diminished renal potassium excretion: reduced aldosterone or aldosterone responsiveness, renal failure, and reduced distal delivery of sodium.

Aldosterone deficiency may be part of a generalized deficiency of adrenal hormones (e.g., Addison's disease) or it may represent a selective process (e.g., hyporeninemic hypoaldosteronism). Hyporeninemic hypoaldosteronism is not only the most common cause of selective hypoaldosteronism, but also the most common cause of all aldosterone deficiency states (48). Selective hypoaldosteronism with normal glucocorticoid function can also occur with heparin therapy (49). Renal tubular unresponsiveness to aldosterone (pseudohypoaldosteronism) may be congenital, but it is more often an acquired defect. This defect may involve only potassium secretion (pseudohypoaldosteronism type II) (59) or sodium reabsorption as well as potassium secretion. Most cases of so-called salt-losing nephritis appear to represent the latter defect (76). Severe dehydration may cause hyperkalemia despite secondary hyperaldosteronism because delivery of sodium to the distal nephron is markedly reduced (41). Pseudohyperkalemia is defined as an increase in potassium concentration only in the local blood vessel or in vitro, and has no physiological consequences. Prolonged use of a tourniquet with fist exercises can increase the serum potassium level by as much as 1 mEq/liter (10). Thrombocytosis and severe leucocytosis cause pseudohyperkalemia through potassium release from the platelets and white blood cells respectively during blood clotting (9, 26).

Management

Hyperkalemia may be treated by removal of potassium from the body, relocation of extracellular potassium into the cells, and by antagonism of potassium action on the membrane of the cardiac conduction system. Removal of potassium may be accomplished by several routes: through the gastrointestinal tract with a potassium exchange resin given orally or by enema; through the kidney by diuretics, mineralocorticoids, and increased salt intake; or by hemodialysis or peritoneal dialysis. A potassium exchange resin, sodium polystyrene sulfonate (kayexalate), is more effective when it is given with agents that cause osmotic diarrhea such as sorbitol or mannitol. One tablespoon of Kayexalate mixed with 100 ml of 10% sorbitol or mannitol can be given by mouth two to four times a day. When it is given as an enema, a larger quantity is given more frequently. Shift of potassium into cells can be accomplished with glucose and insulin or by increasing the blood pH with sodium bicarbonate. Antagonism of the action of potassium on the heart with intravenous calcium salts or hypertonic sodium solution is the quickest method of treating hyperkalemia, and is used in cases of life-threatening hyperkalemia. Reduced intake is often important in the long-term management of hyperkalemia. Prolonged administration of diuretics and a high salt diet is an effective treatment for hyporeninemic hypoaldosteronism, the most common cause of chronic hyperkalemia. This regimen ensures

the delivery of an adequate amount of sodium to the distal nephron without causing further volume expansion. Mineralocorticoid may be required as an adjunct therapy for hyporeninemic hypoaldosteronism, and the agent most commonly used is a synthetic mineralocorticoid, fludrocortisone (Florinef), 0.1 mg once or twice daily. Since renal salt retention may be an important mechanism in the pathogenesis of hyporeninemic hypoaldosteronism (48), mineralocorticoid replacement may lead to salt retention and worsening hypertension.

METABOLIC ACIDOSIS

Metabolic acidosis is defined as a reduction in extracellular pH resulting from a primary decrease in the bicarbonate concentration. The kidney plays a major role in maintaining the extracellular bicarbonate concentration, and the failure of the kidney in this function results in metabolic acidosis referred to as renal acidosis (Table 43.6). The term "extrarenal acidosis" is used when factors other than defective renal acid-excretory function are responsible. Renal acidosis may occur because of specific defects of tubular function in acid excretion or bicarbonate reabsorption (renal tubular acidosis) (64) or because of reduced nephron mass due to renal parenchymal disease (uremic acidosis). Three types of metabolic acidosis occur most frequently in critically ill patients: lactic acidosis (Table 43.7), ketoacidosis, and uremic acidosis.

When lactic acidosis results from tissue hypoxia, it is called type A lactic acidosis (the most common type). The most common cause

Table 43.6
Causes of Metabolic Acidosis

Renal acidosis
  Uremic acidosis
  Renal tubular acidosis
    Distal renal tubular acidosis (type I)
    Proximal renal tubular acidosis (type II)
    Aldosterone deficiency (type IV)
Extrarenal acidosis
  Gastrointestinal loss of bicarbonate
  Ingestion of acids: ammonium chloride, sulfur
  Acid precursors or toxins
    Salicylate
    Ethylene glycol
    Methanol
    Paraldehyde
  Organic acidosis
    Lactic acidosis (D- and L-)
    Ketoacidosis

Table 43.7
Causes of Lactic Acidosis

Tissue hypoxia, e.g., circulatory shock, severe
  hypoxemia, severe heart failure, severe anemia
Acute alcoholism
Drugs and toxins, e.g., phenformin, isoniazid
Diabetes mellitus
Leukemia
Idiopathic
Short bowel syndrome (D-lactic acidosis)

of tissue hypoxia leading to lactic acidosis is circulatory shock, which may be due to sepsis, hypovolemia, or cardiac failure. Generalized convulsion is also a fairly common cause, but the resulting acidosis is transient. Less commonly, tissue hypoxia may result from severe hypoxemia due to respiratory failure, carbon monoxide poisoning, or severe anemia. In type B lactic acidosis, the less common variety, there is no apparent tissue hypoxia, but the possibility of subtle tissue hypoxia must be considered. The causes of type B lactic acidosis include alcoholic intoxication, various drugs (phenformin, isoniazid), leukemia, and diabetes (47, 54). The prognosis of both types of lactic acidosis is dismal.

Ketoacidosis occurs most frequently in diabetes mellitus, but it occasionally occurs in vomiting, binge-drinking chronic alcoholics. When ketoacidosis occurs in the presence of poor mitochondrial oxidation (e.g., ethanol intoxication, septic shock in the diabetic, use of phenformin) the ratio of the reduced form of ketoacid, β-hydroxybutyrate, to the oxidized form, acetoacetate, increases. The usual ratio of β-hydroxybutyrate to acetoacetate in typical diabetic ketoacidosis is about 2.5–3, and the ratio increases to 8 or higher in β-hydroxybutyric acidosis. Since acetoacetate is the only form measured by the nitroprusside reagent (Acetest), the patient with β-hydroxybutyric acidosis may present with a large unexplained anion gap. Lactic acidosis often coexists with β-hydroxybutyric acidosis, because the abnormal redox state of mitochondria leads to increased production of lactic acidosis. Uremic acidosis is most often a result of chronic end-stage renal failure, but in critically ill patients acute renal failure is a common cause. Lactic acidosis also commonly coexists in this setting.

MANAGEMENT

Restoration of normal blood pH and bicarbonate concentration is the ultimate aim of therapy for metabolic acidosis. Rapid restoration of normal pH is usually unnecessary and may be undesirable for several reasons. When the pH is increased acutely, there may be insufficient time for restoration of a normal concentration of the red blood cell 2,3-DPG (37). In addition, a sudden increase in extracellular pH may cause a paradoxical CSF acidosis (51). Rapid restoration of a normal serum bicarbonate level in metabolic acidosis would be undesirable, because persistent hyperventilation produces a very high blood pH, simulating respiratory alkalosis (50).

The initial aim in the treatment of severe metabolic acidosis should be to increase the blood pH to a level at which adverse cardiovascular effects of severe acidemia can be avoided. Although the risk of acidosis varies with the agent and the cardiovascular status of patients, it is considered prudent, at least in older subjects, to keep blood pH above 7.1–7.2. The blood pH may be increased by the administration of alkali or by allowing alkali to be produced endogenously by metabolism of retained organic anions (OA^-):

$$OA^- + H_2CO_3 \longrightarrow OAH + HCO_3^-$$
$$\downarrow$$
$$CO_2 + H_2O$$

Successful treatment of the cause of organic acidosis increases the serum bicarbonate concentration by the latter mechanisms. When ketoacidosis is treated with insulin and fluid, the outcome is usually predictable: a substantial increase in the plasma bicarbonate concentration with a concomitant increase in arterial pH. Exogenous alkali is rarely necessary in ketoacidosis.

In contrast to the favorable outcome in ketoacidosis, response to treatment in lactic acidosis is usually poor. In lactic acidosis induced by hypoxia (type A), the prognosis depends on the cause of tissue hypoxia. In most cases of circulatory shock, the prognosis is extremely poor, but with seizure-induced lactic acidosis, recovery is usually complete within hours after the control of the seizure (45). Improvement in the microcirculation with the infusion of sodium nitroprusside may be effective in a patient with idiopathic lactic acidosis (75).

Rapid recovery is the rule with alcohol-induced lactic acidosis, but the prognosis of other type B lactic acidosis is usually bad. Treatment for type B lactic acidosis has consisted of the administration of alkali in the hope of spontaneous recovery, but administration of bicarbonate tends to be self-defeating because it may also lead to increased production of lactic acid (20).

Discouraged by the poor results of bicarbonate therapy and offering theoretical arguments against alkali therapy as discussed above, some authors have recommended against the use of bicarbonate in the treatment of all types of lactic acidosis (70). In contrast, others feel that the judicious use of bicarbonate is still beneficial to patients with severe metabolic acidosis (39). Dichloroacetate, an experimental drug, offers some hope in the treatment of type B lactic acidosis (55, 71). Its main action is stimulation by pyruvate dehydrogenase, the enzyme responsible for conversion of pyruvate to acetyl CoA. Increased conversion of pyruvate to acetyl CoA results in a decrease in pyruvate concentration, which in turn increases utilization of lactate as well as alanine. Despite the theoretical prediction that lactic acidosis due to hypoxia should respond only to the supply of sufficient oxygen, dichloroacetate also causes a striking increase in serum bicarbonate concentration in patients with type A lactic acidosis. A major drawback of the drug appears to be the frequent occurrence of CNS side effects when it is used chronically (72).

D-Lactic acidosis is a disorder that occurs in patients with the short bowel syndrome. The acidosis is caused by production of D- and L-lactic acids by the colonic bacteria; L-lactic acid that is absorbed is rapidly metabolized and there is no accumulation, but D-lactate accumulates in the body fluids. Accumulation of D-lactate has been attributed to its slow metabolism, but a recent study showed that the rate of D-lactate metabolism in humans is quite fast, suggesting that there may be an additional defect in the mechanism of D-lactate in those who develop D-lactate acidosis (44). A neurological syndrome characterized by mental confusion, disorientation, and staggering gait commonly accompanies the disease. Treatment consists of sterilization of the gut with an antibiotic (42).

The response to the administration of alkali depends on the type of metabolic acidosis. In nonorganic acidosis, the alkali requirement can be estimated with reasonable accuracy. In organic acidosis, in contrast, the alkali requirement is usually much more than predicted in lactic acidosis, whereas it is much less than predicted in ketoacidosis. In lactic acidosis, almost continuous administration of bicarbonate may be needed to maintain serum bicarbonate at a reasonable level, whereas in ketoacidosis administration of insulin and fluid usually suffices.

There are three types of alkali that can be used for the treatment of metabolic acidosis: bicarbonate, salts of organic acids, and tromethamine (THAM). Organic salts used as a bicarbonate substitute include lactate, acetate, and citrate. Each milliequivalent of the organic salts produces 1 mEq of bicarbonate. Thus, the milliequivalent doses of organic salts are the same as those of bicarbonate. However, because they require metabolism, an increase in bicarbonate concentration is delayed. Furthermore, when metabolism is impaired (e.g., in lactic acidosis) administration of an organic salt may have no effect on the serum bicarbonate concentration. The amount and speed of administration of bicarbonate and organic salts vary widely depending on the severity of acidosis. Shohl's solution (citric acid and sodium citrate) contains 1 mEq of alkali (as citrate) per milliliter and is tkaen orally.

In contrast to the delayed and sometimes uncertain responses to organic salts, THAM increases serum bicarbonate concentration promptly and predictably in the following reaction:

$$THAM + H_2CO_3 \longrightarrow THAM\text{-}H^+ + HCO_3^-$$
$$\downarrow$$
$$CO_2 + H_2O$$

Because formation of bicarbonate by THAM occurs at the expense of carbonic acid, rapid infusion of THAM results in a marked reduction in PCO_2, and therefore it should be given slowly, not exceeding the rate of 2 mmol/minute.

For a given quantity of bicarbonate administration, the rise in serum bicarbonate is less in severe than in mild metabolic acidosis (i.e., the apparent volume of distribution of bicarbonate is greater in severe than in mild metabolic acidosis). However, the absolute increase in pH for a given dose of bicarbonate administered is greater in more severe metabolic acidosis than in mild acidosis, because the proportionate increase in serum bicarbonate is greater with severe acidosis. In practice, however, there is no need to estimate the bicarbonate requirements to achieve a certain specific level. Since pH is determined by the ratio of bicarbonate/PCO_2 and a change in ventilation and PCO_2 following acute increase in serum bicarbonate cannot be accurately predicted, it is difficult to predict what the pH will be, even if the increase in bicarbonate concentration were accurately predicted. The best approach is to administer two to three ampules of sodium bicarbonate (44.5 or 50 mEq/ampule) by direct intravenous bolus injection, and then repeat the blood-gas measurement 20–30 minutes after bicarbonate injection to determine the need for further bicarbonate administration.

For treatment of chronic acidosis, citrate is more palatable than bicarbonate and citrate is available as Shohl's solution. For treatment of uremic acidosis, sodium acetate is the most commonly used alkali in hemodialysis fluids, and sodium lactate in peritoneal dialysis fluids. Administration of THAM probably has no advantage in treatment of metabolic acidosis in most situations (7), but would be more advantageous than bicarbonate in treating metabolic acidosis complicated by respiratory acidosis. THAM is available as a 0.3 M solution, and the rate of infusion of THAM should not exceed 30 ml/minute.

METABOLIC ALKALOSIS

Metabolic alkalosis is defined as an increase in extracellular pH caused by an increase in the serum bicarbonate concentration. Normally, the kidney's ability to excrete the excess bicarbonate when the serum bicarbonate is high is so great that it is virtually impossible to maintain metabolic alkalosis by a mechanism that simply causes increased generation of bicarbonate; another mechanism must coexist that prevents the rapid renal loss of bicarbonate. Hence, there are always two abnormalities for sustained metabolic alkalosis: an abnormality that increases the extracellular bicarbonate concentration and an abnormality that causes increased renal bicarbonate threshold.

Mechanisms for Increase in Serum Bicarbonate

There are several mechanisms for increasing the extracellular bicarbonate concentration. These include: loss of HCl (from the stomach or, rarely, in the stool), administration of bicarbonate or bicarbonate precursors, metabolism of bicarbonate precursors, shift of $H+$ into the cell, contraction of extracellular volume by loss of sodium chloride and water, and increased renal excretion of acid (Table 43.8).

Table 43.8
Mechanisms and Causes of Increasing Extracellular Bicarbonate Concentration

Loss of HCl from the stomach, e.g., gastric suction, vomiting

Administration of bicarbonate or bicarbonate precursors, e.g., sodium lactate, sodium acetate, sodium citrate

Shift of H^+ into the cell, e.g., K^+ depletion

Rapid contraction of extracellular volume by loop diuretics

Increased renal excretion of acid, e.g., diuretic therapy, hypermineralocorticoid state, potassium depletion, high PCO_2, secondary hypoparathyroidism

Of these, the two most frequent causes of metabolic alkalosis are increased renal generation of bicarbonate and loss of HCl from the stomach.

Gastric suction is a particularly frequent cause of metabolic alkalosis in critically ill patients, because acid secretion is often markedly stimulated in these patients owing to the stress of severe illness. Considerable loss of acid may still occur in these patients even when gastric acid secretion is inhibited by cimetidine or ranitidine. Diuretic therapy with complicating hypokalemia is also a common cause of metabolic alkalosis in critically ill patients. Sometimes, metabolic alkalosis is a complication of the treatment of metabolic acidosis; administration of bicarbonate to a patient with lactic acidosis increases the production of lactic acid, which is retained as lactate following titration by bicarbonate. The subsequent metabolism of the lactate can lead to a rapid increase in the serum bicarbonate concentration.

Mechanisms for Maintaining High Serum Bicarbonate

Since the kidney is the organ responsible for excreting the excess bicarbonate when the concentration is abnormally high (77), renal failure would be the most effective mechanism for maintaining excess bicarbonate. However, in mild to moderate renal failure, the ability to excrete bicarbonate is still well preserved (30). Other mechanisms of maintaining a high serum bicarbonate concentrate include contraction of EAV, potassium deficiency, high PCO_2, and secondary hypoparathyroidism. Chloride deficiency is usually listed among the causes of increased renal bicarbonate threshold, but chloride deficiency without reduced

Table 43.9
Mechanisms and Causes of Maintaining High Serum Bicarbonate Concentration

Reduced effective arterial volume, e.g., diuretic therapy, vomiting, heart failure and other edema forming states
Potassium deficiency
Chloride deficiency accompanied by low effective arterial volume, e.g., vomiting
High PCO_2
Secondary hypoparathyroidism, e.g., milk-alkali syndrome, certain malignancy-induced hypercalcemia
Severe renal failure

EAV does not increase the bicarbonate threshold (Table 43.9). For example, in severe hyponatremia due to SIADH, total-body chloride content might be reduced, but renal bicarbonate threshold is not increased because EAV is not reduced.

The commonest causes of increased renal bicarbonate threshold encountered clinically are low EAV and potassium deficiency. These two and severe renal failure are probably the mechanisms responsible for maintenance of over 95% of cases of metabolic alkalosis. In most patients who develop metabolic alkalosis due to gastric suction or vomiting, the high renal bicarbonate threshold is caused by low EAV and hypokalemia. Thus if the renal threshold of bicarbonate is maintained normal by prevention of volume depletion and potassium depletion, large losses of gastric fluid will not lead to metabolic alkalosis.

Management

Since the increased renal bicarbonate threshold in metabolic alkalosis is most often caused by reduced EAV and hypokalemia, correction of these abnormalities leads to rapid restoration of bicarbonate concentration in most patients. Correction of low EAV is accomplished by administration of normal saline or half-normal saline. Sometimes discontinuation of an offending agent (e.g., a diuretic) and restoration of normal salt intake is sufficient. If volume depletion is to be avoided, chloride must be given to replace the excreted bicarbonate; it can be given as either sodium chloride or potassium chloride. In certain clinical situations such as edema-forming states, treatment of reduced EAV with salt solution may not be feasible. A logical and effective choice in such situations is acetazolamide (Diamox),

a carbonic anhydrase inhibitor, which will treat metabolic alkalosis as well as edema. Diamox can be given either intravenously or orally. The starting dose is 250 or 500 mg and can be repeated at 6–hour intervals until a desired serum bicarbonate concentration is achieved. Acetazolamide administration usually reduces the renal bicarbonate threshold to a subnormal level, but when it is administered to patients with severe volume depletion, it may not be able to reduce bicarbonate threshold to even a normal level.

Correction of metabolic alkalosis by renal excretion of bicarbonate requires adequate renal function. In renal failure, metabolic alkalosis can be treated by administration of dilute HCl or acidifying salts or by dialysis; the latter has an advantage in that it treats uremia as well as alkalosis. HCl can be administered in 0.1 or 0.05 N solution into a central vein (78). Acidifying salts include ammonium chloride, arginine chloride, and lysine chloride. Metabolism of these salts results in release of HCl, which then titrates bicarbonate. The amount of acidifying salts to be administered depends on the severity of metabolic acidosis. When they are given by intravenous infusion, the optimal rate is about 1 mEq/minute. If continuous acid loss from the stomach is the cause of metabolic alkalosis, an inhibitor of acid secretion such as cimetidine or ranitidine may be useful. Considerable acid secretion, however, may still occur in some patients even with the maximal dose of these drugs.

References

1. Adrogue HJ, Wilson H, Boyd AE, et al: Plasma acid-base patterns in diabetic ketoacidosis. N Engl J Med 307:1603, 1982.
2. Arieff AL: Hyponatremia, convulsions, respiratory arrest, and permanent brain damage after elective surgery in healthy women. N Engl J Med 314:1529, 1986.
3. Adlinger KA, Samaan NA: Hypokalemia with hypercalcemia. Prevalence and significance in treatment. Ann Intern Med 87:571, 1977.
4. Bartter FC, Schwartz WB: The syndrome of inappropriate secretion of antidiuretic hormone. Am J Med 42:651, 1967.
5. Beck LH: Hypouricemia in the syndrome of inappropriate secretion of antidiuretic hormone. N Engl J Med 301:528, 1979.
6. Bismuth C, Gaultier M, Conso F, et al: Hyperkalemia in acute digitalis poisoning: prognostic significance and therapeutic implications. Clin Toxicol 6:153, 1973.
7. Bleich HL, Schwartz WB: Tris buffer (THAM). An appraisal of its physiological effects and clinical usefulness. N Engl J Med 274:782, 1966.
8. Bode HH, Harley BM, Crawford JD: Restoration of normal drinking behavior by chlorpropamide in patients

with hypodipsia and diabetes insipidus. *Am J Med* 51:304, 1971.

9. Bronson WR: Pseudohyperkalemia due to release of potassium from white blood cells during clotting. *N Engl J Med* 274:369, 1966.

10. Brown JJ, Chin RR, David DL, et al: Falsely high serum potassium levels in patients with hyperaldosteronism. *Br Med J* 2:18, 1970.

11. Carrilho F, Bosch J, Arroyo V, et al: Renal failure associated with demeclocycline in cirrhosis. *Ann Intern Med* 87:195–197, 1977.

12. Carroll HJ, Oh MS: Electrolyte physiology and body composition in *Water, Electrolyte and Acid-Base Metabolism*. Philadelphia, JB Lippincott, 1978, p 1.

13. Carroll HJ, Tice DA: The effects of epsilon aminocaproic acid upon potassium metabolism in the dog. *Metabolism* 15:499, 1966.

14. Cooperman LH: Succinylcholine-induced hyperkalemia in neuromuscular disease. *JAMA* 213:1867, 1970.

15. Cowell DC, McGrady PM: Direct-measurement ion-selective electrodes. Analytical error in hyponatremia. *Clin Chem* 31:2009, 1985.

16. Decaux, Genette F, Mockel J: Hypouremia in the syndrome of inappropriate secretion of antidiuretic hormone. *Ann Intern Med* 93:716, 1980.

17. DeFronzo RA, Goldberg M, Agus ZS: Normal diluting capacity in hyponatremic patients. *Ann Intern Med* 84:538, 1976.

18. Forrest JN, Cohen AD, Torretti J, et al: On the mechanism of lithium-induced diabetes insipidus in man and rat. *J Clin Invest* 53:1115–1123, 1974.

19. Forrest JN, Cox M, Hong C, et al: Superiority of demeclocycline over lithium in the treatment of chronic syndrome of inappropriate secretion of antidiuretic hormone. *N Engl J Med* 298:173–177, 1978.

20. Fraley DS, Adler S, Bruns FJ, et al: Stimulation of lactate production by administration of bicarbonate in a patient with a solid neoplasma and lactic acidosis. *N Engl J Med* 303:1100–1102, 1980.

21. Francisco LL, Sawin LL, DiBona GF: Mechanism of negative potassium balance in the magnesium deficient rat *Proc Soc Exp Biol Med* 168:382, 1981.

22. Frick PG, Schmid JR, Kistler HJ, et al: Hyponatremia associated with hyperproteinemia in multiple myeloma. *Helv Med Acta* 33:317–329, 1967.

23. Furhman SA, Eckfeldt JH: Hyponatremia and ion-selective electrodes. *Ann Intern Med* 102:872, 1985.

24. Graettinge JS, Muenster JJ, Checchia CS, et al: A correlation of clinical and hemodynamic studies in patients with hypothyroidism. *J Clin Invest* 37:502, 1958.

25. Granerus AK, Jagenburg R, Svanborg A: Kaliuretic effect of L-dopa treatment in Parkinsonian patients. *Acta Med Scand* 201-291-297, 1977.

26. Hartman RC, Auditore JC, Jackson DP: Studies in thrombocytosis. I. hyperkalemia due to release of potassium from platelets during coagulation. *J Clin Invest* 37:699, 1958.

27. Hantman D, Rossier B, Zohlman R, et al: Rapid correction of hyponatremia in the syndrome of inappropriate secretion of antidiuretic hormone. *Ann Intern Med* 78:870, 1973.

28. Hertz P, Richardson JA: Arginine-induced hyperkalemia in renal failure patients. *Arch Intern Med* 130:778, 1972.

29. Hoffbrand BI, Steward JD: Carbenecillin and hypokalemia. *Br Med J* 4:746, 1970.

30. Husted FC, Nolph KD, Maher JF: NaHCO₃ and NaCl tolerance in chronic renal failure. *J Clin Invest* 56:414, 1975.

31. Gennari FJ: Current concepts: Uses and limitations. *N Engl J Med* 310:102, 1984.

32. Kestens PJ, et al: The effect of insulin on the uptake of potassium and phosphate by the isolated perfused canine liver. *Metabolism* 12:941, 1963.

33. Ladenson JK, Apple FS, Koch DD: Misleading hyponatremia due to hyperlipemia: A method-dependent error. *Ann Intern Med* 95:707, 1981.

34. Linas SL, Berl T, Robertson GL, et al: Role of vasopressin in the impaired water excretion of glucocorticoid deficiency. *Kidney Int* 18:58–67, 1980.

35. Mattar JA, et al: Cardiac arrest in the critically ill. Hyperosmolar states following cardiac arrest. *Am J Med* 56:162, 1974.

36. Mir MA, Brabin B, Tinag OT, et al: Hypokalemia in acute myeloid leukemia. *Ann Intern Med* 82:54–57, 1972.

37. Mitchell JH, Sildenthal K, Johnson RL: The effects of acid-base disturbances on cardiovascular and pulmonary function. *Kidney Int* 1:375, 1972.

38. Moses AM, Howanitz J, vanGemert M, et al: Clofibrate-induced antidiuresis. *J Clin Invest* 52:535, 1973.

39. Narins RG, Cohen JJ: Bicarbonate therapy for organic acidosis: the case for its continued use. *Ann Intern Med* 106:615, 1987.

40. Norenberg MD, Leslie KO, Robertson AS: Association between rise in serum sodium and central pontine myelinolysis. *Ann Neurol* 11:128, 1982.

41. Oh MS: Selective hypoaldosteronism. *Resident Staff Physician* 28:46S–62S, 1982.

42. Oh MS, Phelps K, Traube M, et al: D-Lactic acidosis in a man with the short bowel syndrome. *N Engl J Med* 301:249, 1979.

43. Oh MS, Uribarri J, Barrido D, et al: Central pontine myelinolysis following isotonic saline infusion: is 0.5 NS better than NS in treating hypotonic dehydration? *Kidney Int* 31:212, 1987.

44. Oh MS, Uribarri J, Alveranga D, et al: Metabolic utilization and renal handling of D-lactate in man. *Metabolism* 34:621, 1985.

45. Orlinger CE, Estace JC, Wunsch CD, et al: Natural history of lactic acidosis after grand mal seizures. *N Engl J Med* 297:796–799, 1977.

46. Olster JR, Perez GO, Vaamonde CA: Relationship between blood pH and phosphorus during acute metabolic alkalosis. *Am J Physiol* 235:F345–F351, 1978.

47. Park R, Arieff AL: lactic acidosis. *Adv Intern Med* 25:33, 1980.

48. Phelps KR, Lieberman RL, Oh MS, et al: The syndrome of hyporeninemic hypoaldosteronism. *Metabolism* 29:186, 1980.

49. Phelps KR, Oh MS, Carroll HJ: Heparin-induced hyperkalemia: report of a case. *Nephron* 25:254–258, 1980.

50. Pierce NF, et al: The ventilatory response to acute base deficit in humans. Time course during development and correction of metabolic alkalosis. *Ann Intern Med* 172:633, 1970.

51. Posner JB, Plum E: Spinal fluid and pH and neurological symptoms in acidosis. *N Engl J Med* 277:605, 1967.

52. Rado JP: Combination of carbamezepine and chloropropamide in the treatment of "hyporesponder" pituitary diabetes insipidus. *J Clin Endo Metab* 38:1, 1974.

53. Raskind M, Burns RF: Water metabolism in psychiatric disorders. *Semin Nephrol* 4:316, 1984.

54. Relman AS: lactic acidosis. In Brenner BM, Stein JH: *Contemporary Issues in Nephrology. Acid-Base and Potassium Homeostasis*. New York, Churchill Livingstone, 1978, vol 2, p 65.

55. Relman ASD: Lactic acidosis and a possible new treatment. *N Engl J Med* 298:564–565, 1978.

56. Robinson AG: DSDAVP in the treatment of central diabetes insipidus. *N Engl J Med* 294–507, 1976.

57. Roza O, Berman LB: The pathophysiology of barium: hypokalemic and cardiovascular effects. *J Pharmacol Exp Ther* 177:433–439, 1971.

58. Santensanio F, et al: Evidence for a role of endogenous insulin and glucagon in the regulation of potassium homeostasis. *J Lab Clin Med* 81:809, 1973.

59. Schambelan M, Sebastian A, Rector FC Jr: Mineralocortcoid-resistant renal hyperkalemia without salt wast-

ing (type II pseudohypoaldosteronism): role of increased renal chloride reabsorption. *Kidney Int* 19:716, 1981.

60. Schrier RW: Treatment of hyponatremia: Editorial. *N Engl J Med* 312:1121, 1985.

61. Schrier RW, Lehman D, Zacherle B, et al: Effect of furosemide on free water excretion in edematous patients with hyponatremia. *Kidney Int* 3:30, 1973.

62. Scribner BH, Burnell JM: Interpretation of serum potassium concentration. *Metabolism* 5:468, 1956.

63. Sebastian A, McSherry E, Morris RC: Renal potassium wasting in renal tubulatr acidosis (RTA). Its occurrence in types I and II RTA despite sustained correction of systemic acidosis. *J Clin Invest* 50:667, 1971.

64. Sebastian A, McSherry Z, Morris RC: Metabolic acidosis with special reference to the renal acidosis. In Brenner BM, Rector FC: *The Kidney.* Philadelphia, WB Saunders, 1976, p 615.

65. Singer I, Rotenberg D, Puschett JB: Lithium-induced nephrogenic diabetes insipidus. *J Clin Invest* 51:1081, 1972.

66. Singer I, Rotenberg D: Demeclocyline-induced nephrogenic diabetes insipidus. In vivo and in vitro studies. *Ann Intern Med* 79:679, 1973.

67. Skowsky WR, Kikuchi TA: The role of vasopresin in the impaired water excretion of myxedema. *Am J Med* 64:613, 1978.

68. Spencer PW, Voyce MA: Familial hypomagnesemia and hypokalemia. *Acta Paediatr Scand* 65:505, 1976.

69. Sperlakis N, Schneider MF, Harris EJ: Decreased K^+ conductance produced by Ba^{++} in frog sartorius fibers. *J Gen Physiol* 50:1565–1583, 1967.

70. Stacpoole PW: The lactic acidosis: the case against bicarbonate therapy (editorial). *Ann Intern Med* 105:276, 1986.

71. Stacpoole PW, Moore GW, Korhauser DM: Metabolic effects of dichloroacetate in patients with diabetes mellitus and hyperlipoproteinemia. *N Engl J Med* 298:526–530, 1978.

72. Stacpoole PW, Harman EM, Curry SH, et al: Treatment of lactic acidosis with dichloroacetate. *N Engl J Med* 309:390, 1983.

73. Sterns RH, Riggs JE, Schochet SS, Jr: Osmotic demyelinating syndrome following correction of hyponatremia. *N Engl J Med* 314:1535, 1986.

74. Szatalowicz VL, Arnold PE, Chaimovitz L, et al: Radioimmunoassay of plasma arginine vasopressin in hyponatremic patients with congestive heart failure. *N Engl J Med* 305:203, 1981.

75. Taradash MR, Jacobson LB: Vasiodilatory therapy of idiopathic lactic acidosis. *N Engl J Med* 293:468, 1975.

76. Uribarri J, Oh MS, Carroll HJ: Salt-losing nephritis. *Am J Nephrol* 3:193, 1983.

77. Van Goidsenhoven GMT, et al: The effect of prolonged administration of large doses of sodium bicarbonate in man. *Clin Sci* 13:383, 1954.

78. Wilson RF, Gibson D, Percivel AK: Severe alkalosis in critically ill surgical patients. *Arch Surg* 105:197, 1972.

44

Parenteral Nutrition

Laurence H. Ross, M.D.
John P. Grant, M.D.

The healthy adult is in a state of nitrogen equilibrium where daily dietary nitrogen intake equals nitrogen loss. When dietary intake is limited or interrupted, the human adapts by reducing physical activity and lowering core body temperature with a reduction in metabolic rate. The term "basal metabolic rate" (BMR) describes the minimal energy expenditure of a trained subject at rest after an overnight fast. In chronic uncomplicated starvation, the body reduces energy expenditure by up to 5–10% below the BMR. If starvation is complicated by stress or sepsis, however, energy expenditure markedly increases and may approach 200% BMR. When dietary intake does not meet an individual's energy requirement, the human resorts to catabolism of body mass to generate energy. Proteins are broken down for gluconeogenesis and lipids are mobilized for lipid oxidation. This catabolic state is not without serious consequences and cannot be sustained indefinitely. The fat mass is relatively expendable. However, there are no known protein reserves in the body; each protein molecule serves some biological function. During acute and chronic starvation, protein is derived from all parts of the body with preservation only perhaps of the brain. Seven-day fasting in rats produces a 30% body weight loss with 30–40% decrease in liver, kidney, lung, gastrointestinal tract, and heart masses with similar losses of organ protein content (2, 79). Similar data are reported in humans (101). Associated with the loss of organ mass and protein content is an impairment of organ function (47). In particular, skeletal muscle function is decreased as starvation progresses as demonstrated by the Minnesota Experiment in 1944 (89). More acute starvation in hospitalized patients also decreases muscle function independent of measured muscle mass (113a). Respiratory muscle function is also impaired in chronic malnutrition as measured by pulmonary function tests (90). Acute starvation decreases maximal inspiratory vacuum and maximal expiratory pressures in hospitalized patients (129). Doekel et al. (33) demonstrated that a short period of semistarvation in normal volunteers impaired the ventilatory response to hypoxia. Likewise Weissman et al. demonstrated loss of chemoreceptor sensitivity to hypercarbic gas mixtures following short periods of protein-free diets in normal volunteers (203). Catabolism of the gastrointestinal tract leads to loss of villous height and absorptive surface with depletion of brush border enzymes and malabsorption (118). Loss of normal gastric acid secretion is associated with bacterial overgrowth of the upper gastrointestinal tract contributing to diarrhea (45). Delayed gastric emptying with small bowel hypermotility also occurs. Hepatic function is markedly impaired with undernutrition both with respect to the microsomal enzyme system as well as the protein synthetic pathways (98, 163). On the other hand, some enzyme systems, including the gluconeogenic series, increase in activity with progressive starvation. Changes in renal function during starvation include loss of concentrating ability with progressive diuresis in the face of dehydration and impaired ability to excrete titrable acid leading to metabolic acidosis (99, 100). In children, impaired clearance of aminoglycosides may occur due to altered glomerular and tubular function with severe protein depletion (16). Cardiac reserves and function are depressed (1, 68). Immune system function becomes impaired as starvation progresses, causing loss of chemotactic and phagocytic activity of the lymphocyte, anergy to common skin test antigens, and impairment of the humoral response (10, 175).

Because of these alterations in organ function, as well as other complex interactions, undernourished patients have an increased incidence of morbidity and mortality. Prognostic relationships exist between morbidity and mortality and serum albumin and transferrin concentrations, delayed-type hypersensitivity skin test reactions, percent weight loss from usual weight, and various combinations of these parameters (27, 62a, 104a, 131, 156a, 159). Surveys of infectious complications in patients undergoing clean surgical procedures demonstrate malnutrition (defined as weight loss and a low serum albumin concentration) to be as important a factor as old age, obesity, diabetes, and infections in other parts of the body (22, 27). It therefore behooves the physician in the critical care unit to consider the patient's nutritional status in the initial patient evaluation. The need for immediate and intensive nutritional support must be considered whenever a patient's nutritional status is threatened by disease or when significant preillness malnutrition is present. Whenever possible the enteral route should be utilized to reduce costs and risks. If the enteral route cannot or should not be utilized for nutritional support, there should be no hesitancy in providing intravenous nutrition. At no time should nutritional support be withheld until some parameter indicates the presence of malnutrition. Instead, emphasis should be placed on prophylactic nutritional support to avoid the occurrence of malnutrition and its complications. As a rule, patients admitted to critical care units for evaluation and treatment should be receiving adequate nutritional support within the first 36 hours of admission.

ENDOCRINE RESPONSE TO STRESS

The endocrine response to stress is a complex feedback system that is intimately related to the metabolic response to stress. In this section only a brief discussion of the endocrine response is presented, and for simplification a division is made between the hormones of catabolism, anabolism, and fluid-electrolyte balance.

Catabolic Hormones

GLUCOCORTICOIDS

Immediately after injury there is a rapid increase in cortisol secretion lasting for 24–48 hours (39). However, even with minor injuries, up to two to five times normal excretion of urinary hydroxycorticoids is found for 7–10 days (77, 124, 125). With severe or prolonged stress, elevations of urinary hydroxycorticoids are detected for weeks to months and may be associated with hypertrophy of the adrenal cortex. Cortisol acts in concert with the catecholamines to stimulate lipolysis (109), to inhibit protein synthesis, to facilitate amino acid mobilization from muscle (21), to induce the enzymes of gluconeogenesis (170, 204), to enhance secretion of glucagon while inhibiting insulin secretion (117, 151), and to stimulate conversion of lactic acid to glycogen (137).

CATECHOLAMINES

Epinephrine and norepinephrine are secreted within seconds of injury (22). Although their biologic half-lives are short, their continued secretion for several days and, in severe stress, several weeks, results in a prolonged metabolic effect (52, 123). Epinephrine induces the enzymes of hepatic glycogenolysis and gluconeogenesis, stimulates glucagon secretion, inhibits insulin secretion, stimulates lipolysis, enhances amino acid release from skeletal muscle, and inhibits the uptake of glucose by peripheral tissues (93, 154). In addition, epinephrine leads to the secretion of pituitary ACTH, which stimulates glucocorticoid secretion (39).

GLUCAGON

Glucagon is a potent catabolic hormone secreted by the pancreatic cells in response to trauma, and is in part mediated by cortisol and catecholamine secretion. It acts predominately on the hepatocyte to prevent hypoglycemia by stimulating gluconeogenesis and glycogenolysis. In the periphery it may enhance lipolysis and proteolysis (192).

Anabolic Hormones

INSULIN

Insulin is a potent anabolic hormone secreted by pancreatic β cells. It plays a central role in the regulation of glucose metabolism by inhibiting gluconeogenesis and glycogenolysis in the hepatic cells through the stimulation of glucokinase and UDPG-glycosyl transferase, and the inhibition of pyruvate carboxylase and phosphorylase. Insulin also promotes glucose and potassium uptake by peripheral tissues, inhibits lipolysis, and favors protein synthesis (125). The stress reaction (largely catecholamine mediated) leads to a marked depression in insulin production and secretion that results in a disproportionately and persistently low serum insulin level (121, 154). With the increase in serum glucagon, the molar insulin:glucagon ratio is depressed resulting in an increase in gluconeogenesis and glycogenolysis.

GROWTH HORMONE

Stress is a strong stimulant of growth hormone secretion (208). Growth hormone stimulates nitrogen, phosphorus and potassium retention, fatty acid oxidation, and ketogenesis. It also inhibits insulin action and promotes amino acid uptake with protein synthesis (108).

ANDROGENS

Testosterone, in addition to its other roles, is a potent anabolic hormone. It stimulates protein synthesis and decreases amino acid catabolism. Retention of nitrogen, potassium, phosphorus, and calcium are manifestations of its anabolic effect. Stress and catecholamines suppress testosterone production (125).

Fluid and Electrolyte Hormones

ANTIDIURETIC HORMONE

Antidiuretic hormone (ADH) is a powerful hormone responsible for maintaining a proper solute/solvent ratio in the serum. Hypovolemia and hypertonicity during stress are strong stimulants for ADH release from the posterior pituitary gland (125). Its primary site of action is the kidney where it promotes water reabsorption.

ALDOSTERONE

Aldosterone hormone promotes reabsorption of sodium bicarbonate while increasing potassium and hydrogen losses. Aldosterone secretion in stress is augmented by catecholamines and hyponatremia. In addition, isotonic hypovolemia, by increasing renin production, leads to angiotensin release that in turn stimulates aldosterone secretion (180). The endocrine response to stress can be graphically displayed as in Figure 44.1.

METABOLIC RESPONSE TO STRESS

The metabolic response to stress and injury as first described by Cuthbertson (29) in the

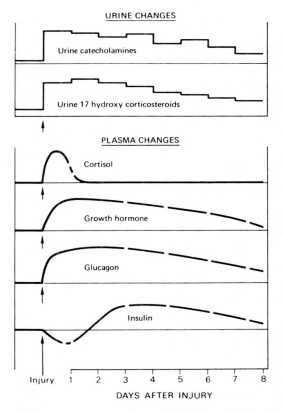

Figure 44.1. Hormone changes after injury. (Reprinted with permission. From Fleck A: Metabolic response to injury. Ledingham IM, Mackay G: *Jamieson and Kay's Textbook of Surgical Physiology*. New York, Churchill Livingstone, 1978, pp 45.)

1930s can be divided into several phases that do not have sharp demarcations but rather gradual transitions.

The acute phase begins immediately following injury and lasts for 12–36 hours. It is characterized by a rapid secretion of the stress hormones (catecholamines, glucocorticoids, glucagon, growth hormones, etc.), marked fluid shifts, acid-base imbalances, and a decrease in energy expenditure, oxygen consumption, and core temperature (94). Therapeutic priorities are to provide hemostasis, cardiovascular stability, and electrolyte balance. If the injury is severe there is an accompanying metabolic acidosis from anaerobic carbohydrate metabolism, development of oxygen deficit, a rise in the acute phase proteins, hyperglycemia due to insulin resistance, and an elevation in serum free fatty acids (39). Vigorous nutritional support during this initial phase in not indicated due to other priorities.

After the first 12–36 hours, the acutely stressed patient enters the catabolic phase when aggressive nutritional support is needed. During this phase there is an increase in urea production and urinary urea nitrogen excretion due to protein catabolism. Uncomplicated starvation does not increase urinary urea nitrogen excretion, instead it is associated with normal or decreased excretion (5–7 g/day) (126). With stress, however, the urinary urea nitrogen excretion may increase to 7–40 g/day depending upon the degree of stress (20 g nitrogen/day = 175 g protein/day = 0.5 kg lean tissue/day) (127). Other potential sources of nitrogen loss during stress include blood, transudates, exudates, and wound drainage. Protein catabolism supplies the carbon skeletons for gluconeogenesis not obtainable from fat oxidation and also provides substrates acutely needed for the synthesis of blood, structural proteins, and enzymes. Prior to the development of intravenous feeding, it was felt that net nitrogen loss was mandatory and irreversible during this phase (29). However, the advent of nonvolitional tube feeding and total parenteral nutrition (TPN) has shown that although the catabolic response cannot be suppressed, the negative nitrogen balance and subsequent body wasting can be reduced and at times overcome by infusion of specially formulated intravenous solutions (19b, 88a, 116a, 165).

The catabolic phase is associated with marked increases in daily caloric expenditure and nitrogen excretion. The two tend to parallel each other with increasing degrees of stress except in severe stress, where the caloric expenditure increases more than nitrogen excretion (111). An equation for estimation of BMR in healthy individuals was first developed by Harris and Benedict in 1919 (62). This equation is still valid but must be adjusted by a factor of approximately 10% to obtain the clinically more useful value of resting metabolic expenditure (RME). In stress the energy expenditure is markedly increased above the predicted RME (Fig. 44.2). After extensive metabolic studies, Long et al. (111) modified the original Harris-Benedict equation to better estimate daily caloric expenditure by adding a stress and activity factor (Table 44.1).

In times of stress, when an individual is usually unable or unwilling to eat, the body adapts by converting from exogenous to endogenous sources of carbohydrate, fat, and protein. Carbohydrates are stored mainly as glycogen (500 g) (126). Mobilization by glycogenolysis can provide only about 1700 kcal, which is exhausted after 8 hours. Certain organs require glucose as their caloric source early in starvation (CNS, heart, renal medulla, leukocytes, fibroblasts). To provide glucose, the body converts protein into glucose in the liver and kidney by gluconeogenesis. The conversion of body protein is an inefficient and

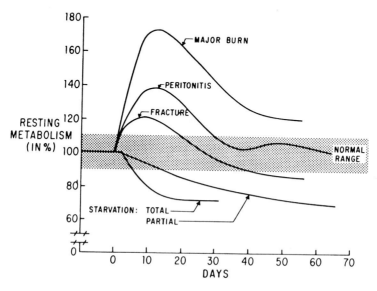

Figure 44.2. Changes in resting metabolic expenditure (RME) in six patient groups with time. (Reprinted with permission. From Long CL et al.: Metabolic response to illness and injury: estimation of energy and protein needs from indirect calorimetry and nitrogen balance. *J Paren Enter Nutr* 3:452–456, 1979.)

Table 44.1
Calculation of Actual Energy Expenditure (AEE)[a]

AEE (men)	$= (66.47 + 13.75W + 5.011 - 6.76A) \times$ (activity factor) $\times$ (injury factor)
AEE (women)	$= (6.55.10 + 9.56W + 4.8511 - 4.68A) \times$ (activity factor) $\times$ (injury factor)

Where AEE = actual energy expenditure, W = weight in kg, 11 = height in cm, A = age in years

Activity factor	Use	Injury factor	Use
Confined to bed	1.2	Minor operation	1.20
Out of bed	1.3	Skeletal trauma	1.35
		Major sepsis	1.60
		Severe thermal burn	2.10

[a] Modified from Long CL et al. Metabolic response to injury and illness: estimation of energy and protein needs from indirect calorimetry and nitrogen balance. *J Paren Enter Nutr* 3:452–456, 1979.

expensive process as it yields few calories (20 kcal gained for each gram of nitrogen excreted = 6.25 g of protein = 30 g of wet muscle tissue) (126). Other tissues can use fatty acids for energy, which are a rich and expendible source. Up to 300–500 g/day of fat may be oxidized, providing 2700–4500 kcal/day (126). Even by providing large amounts of exogenous glucose through TPN, the stressed body prefers to convert excess glucose to glycogen while the endogenous fat stores continue to be oxidized (6). In the unstressed depleted patient, however, extra glucose is converted into fat, and fat oxidation is suppressed. When excess glucose is given to the hypermetabolic, stressed patient, gluconeogenesis is not suppressed and protein catabolism continues (112).

The electrolyte and acid-base derangements that occur during the catabolic phase are largely due to losses from, or shifts between, compartments and reflect cellular destruction, proteolysis, and the body's effort to maintain an effective circulating blood volume. In the urine, excretion of potassium, phosphorus, sulfate, magnesium, creatinine, creatine, and uric acid are elevated (128). Bicarbonate and sodium are retained by the kidney through the effect of aldosterone, which results in kaluresis, acidic urine, and mild metabolic alkalosis that can be aggravated by blood transfusions (citrate metabolized to bicarbonate) and nasogastric suction (hydrogen ion loss).

If the clinical course progresses without complications, the catabolic phase gradually gives way to an anabolic phase (126). There is a decrease in urinary nitrogen excretion that reflects a decrease in protein catabolism, a diuresis of salt and water, a normalization of serum potassium and sodium, and a change in the endocrine pattern from the stress hormones (catecholamine, glucocorticoids, and glucagon) to the growth hormones (insulin, androgens, and growth hormone). The state of

convalescence may continue for weeks to months depending on the body protein and fat lost during catabolism. During recovery, essential amino acids, total protein, and caloric requirements are greater than normal, but less than during the stressed period, and appropriate adjustments must be made. Nutritional support is very important during this period, but since the patient is no longer critically ill, an oral diet is usually resumed and intensive intravenous or enteral nutritional support is usually not necessary.

SUBSTRATE REQUIREMENTS FOR NUTRITIONAL SUPPORT

Fluid Requirements

Fluid requirements for patients on total nutritional support are somewhat greater than for patients on 5% dextrose solutions. The standard formulas used to calculate fluid requirements based either on body weight or body surface area assume a catabolic state with release of 300–500 ml of water a day from oxidation of fat and release of intracellular water. When a patient is converted to an anabolic state with nutritional support, the released intracellular water is no longer available and indeed, in the anabolic state, new cells are being formed and requirements for new intracellular water can be marked. The standard formulas therefore underestimate fluid requirements by 500–800 ml/day. To assure adequate fluid supplementation, one must give consideration to basic fluid requirements, requirements of an anabolic state, the replacement of measured losses, and replacement of estimated insensible and third-space fluid losses. Insensible fluid loss estimates must be increased by 360 ml/°C/day in febrile patients. fluid administration must also be appropriately adjusted in patients with congestive heart failure, renal failure, pulmonary edema, and those receiving humidified air.

Caloric Requirements

An interaction exists between calorie and nitrogen substrates (133, 206). If one increases caloric support to a patient, less nitrogen is required to achieve nitrogen balance. On the other hand, if one increases nitrogen intake, fewer calories are required to achieve nitrogen balance. The optimal ratio of calories-to-nitrogen in the patient requiring intensive care remains to be determined. Usually an estimate of optimal nitrogen supplementation is made and then caloric supplementation is given to assure nitrogen balance. This often results in a calorie-to-nitrogen ratio between 100:1 and 200:1. The caloric source is typically 25–50% glucose providing 0.86–1.72 kcal/ml. Other sugars have been utilized with no improvement in clinical effect.

Recent studies utilizing insulin and glucose clamp techniques show reduced glucose utilization in stressed patients ($6.23 \pm .87$ mg/kg/minute) compared with normals ($9.46 \pm .79$ mg/kg/minute) (11). Furthermore, increases in glucose infusions above 5.0 mg/kg/minute fail to improve protein synthesis and are not associated with increased glucose oxidation (16a).

With limitation on glucose utilization during stress, attention has been given to the use of alternate fuels during stress including lipid, branched chain amino acids, and ketone bodies. In mild stress, clearance of lipids from the blood is increased (56b). One cannot assume, however, that uptake and clearance documents utilization. Goodenough et al. (44a) found only about 8% of infused lipids to be immediately oxidized, with the remainder stored as neutral fats for later use. In addition, Long et al. (113) found less nitrogen-sparing effect with substitution of carbohydrate in a stressed animal model. With severe stress, Lindholm and Rossner (110a) found significant impairment of lipid clearance, especially when multiple organ failure was present.

Difficulty with lipid utilization during stress may in part be related to its dependence on carnitine for transport into the mitochondria for β oxidation. Carnitine deficiency, although rare, has been reported in patients with renal failure, liver disease, cardiac or skeletal muscle disease, patients with stress, and in clinical settings of inadequate intake of carnitine or its

precursors (13a, 184a). A new lipid emulsion, the so-called structured lipid emulsion, which is composed of both long-chain fatty acids and medium-chain fatty acids, has been found by Maiz et al. to be more effective in sparing nitrogen in the stressed animal model (116a). The product they used contained 60% medium-chain fatty acids. These fatty acids can be readily metabolized even in the absence of carnitine and may be of great use in the future as commercial products become available.

Some early investigations with ketone bodies have also been promising. These intermediates of fat metabolism enter the energy cycle more easily than either long-chain fatty acids or medium-chain fatty acids. Sherwin et al. (176a) have demonstrated reasonable tolerance of a conjugated solution in monkeys and some nitrogen-sparing capabilities, however the product is far from being clinically useful.

Another alternate fuel that has attracted much interest recently is branched-cain amino acids. These three amino acids are unique in that they appear to be the preferred fuel of skeletal muscle during stress and are not metabolized by the liver. Infusions of branched chain amino acid–enriched solutions to patients in varying degrees of stress suggest their greatest benefit to be in selected patients with marked stress mainly early during the first week or so (11a, 19b, 88a, 133a). These products are currently available both for enteral and parenteral infusion.

A final alternate fuel of perhaps great importance is the amino acid glutamine. This amino acid is the preferred fuel of the gastrointestinal tract, especially during stress. Currently available amino acid solutions for intravenous use do not contain glutamine, and concern has been raised that the lack of this fuel may result in wasting of the gastrointestinal tract with breakdown of the mucosal barrier and increase risks of sepsis and multiple organ failure. Grant and Snyder (48a) have recently shown preservation of the rat intestine when 1 or 2% glutamine is added to intravenous nutrition solutions compared with wasting when it was not.

Current practice is to attempt to provide stressed patients with their estimated, or preferably measured, caloric needs. Caloric needs can be estimated from the Harris-Benedict equation as in Table 44.1 (95, 111, 207). Roughly, mild stress is associated with a 35–37 kcal/kg/day caloric requirement, moderate stress with 37/42 kcal/kg/day, and severe stress with 42–50 kcal/kg/day. Activity such as vigorous exercise increases requirements by up to 5 kcal/kg/day. Actual measurement of caloric expenditure can be accomplished with one or several metabolic carts available that measure oxygen consumption and carbon dioxide production. An onboard computer calculates energy expenditure, along with several other useful parameters such as respiratory quotient and substrate utilization. Up to 1500–1800 kcal are given daily as carbohydrate with the rest being given as long-chain fatty acids, while one watches carefully to assure lipid clearance from the blood. If the stress is moderate to severe, branched-chain enriched amino acid solutions are used as the protein source. It is hoped that structured lipid emulsions and glutamine supplements will be available soon.

Attempts to improve glucose tolerance with insulin infusion during stress has met with limited success (207). When used, only monocomponent, and preferable recombinant insulin should be given. Although insulin can increase uptake of glucose by peripheral tissues and therefore lower blood glucose concentrations in stress, studies have failed to demonstrate increase in glucose oxidation or nitrogen sparing. Potential adverse effects of insulin must be considered. It has been proposed that increased serum insulin and free fatty acids associated with the neuroendocrine response to stress inhibit and activity or pyruvate dehydroginase, thereby limiting the entry of glucose into the Krebs cycle for oxidative metabolism (194a). The increase in pyruvate favors fat synthesis, which requires energy and produces carbon dioxide. In general, use of insulin beyond 50–75 U/day is not recommended. If intolerance persists, an alternate fuel source should be sought and carbohydrate infusion reduced to 5 mg/kg/day or less.

Nitrogen Requirements

Minimal nitrogen supplementation to maintain nitrogen balance with adequate caloric support is estimated to be between 0.5 and 0.75 g/kg/day. However, to achieve optimal nitrogen utilization and preserve lean body mass, it is recommended that between 1.0 and 1.5 g/kg be administered to the unstressed patient (4). During mild to moderate stress up to 2 g/kg/day should be given, and with severe stress 2.5 g/kg/day may be required. Patients with protein-losing enteropathies or nephropathies, those with exudative wound losses,

or those undergoing hemodialysis or peritoneal dialysis may have markedly increased requirements due to excessive loss of nitrogen. In practice, a level of nitrogen supplementation is selected along with adequate caloric support, and if in doubt, patients are then monitored for nitrogen balance by comparing total nitrogen input to total losses. Either caloric or nitrogen support is increased until the appropriate nitrogen balance is achieved (0.0 for maintenance of body cell mass, ± 0.04–0.07 g/kg/day for body cell mass repletion). Use of amino acid solutions enriched with branched-chain amino acids may have some advantage in the stressed patient and their use is under investigation (11a, 19b, 88a, 133a).

Electrolyte Requirements

Requirements for electrolytes are markedly different in the anabolic state compared with the catabolic state. In particular, those electrolytes in high concentrations within cells are required to a greater extent during total nutritional support than during administration of 5% dextrose solutions. Therefore, supplementation with adequate potassium, phosphorus and magnesium (the anabolic electrolytes) is critical for safe and effective total nutritional support. Rudman et al. (164) demonstrate that not only must all the electrolytes be given, but they must be given in appropriate amounts to establish optimal nitrogen repletion. Requirements occur in three phases. Phase I is during the first 12–24 hours, when anabolic electrolyte deficits must be replaced. Patients who are severely malnourished often have normal serum concentrations of anabolic electrolytes. The true total body deficiency is not apparent until feeding is initiated. Phase II occurs between 12 and 40 hours and follows conversion to an anabolic state. In this phase, increased anabolic electrolyte requirements are due to formation of new intracellular water and the loss of release due to breakdown of body cell mass. Phase III of anabolic electrolyte requirements occurs when patients become stable after repletion of deficits and establishment of the anabolic state. In this phase, anabolic electrolyte shifts are uncommon and requirements are fairly constant. The requirements for other electrolytes, including sodium, chloride, and calcium are not changed from routine 5% dextrose solutions as these are predominantly extracellular ions.

Vitamin Requirement

Requirements for vitamins during intravenous feeding in patients requiring intensive support are not adequately determined. The American Medical Association (AMA) has established guidelines for infusion of vitamins to nonstressed patients receiving intravenous support (Table 44.2) (132). Both B-complex and fat-soluble vitamin deficiencies occur during both short-term and extended periods of nutritional support and must be considered.

Mineral Requirements

The need to provide calcium, phosphorus, and magnesium during total nutritional support is well recognized. Phosphorus is an important component in normal immune function as well as oxygen transport. Routine supplementation with 20 mM phosphorus per 1000 kcal should be modified based on serum concentrations. Deficiency of magnesium is associated with a syndrome similar to hypocalcemia with tetany and muscle fasiculations as well as altered mental status. Routine supplementation ranges between 0.3 and 0.45 mEq/kg/day. Adequate calcium supplementation ranges between 0.2 and 0.3 mEq/kg/day.

Trace Element Requirements

There is controversy over requirements for various trace elements during TPN. Recent AMA guidelines suggest administration of zinc, copper, manganese, and chromium to the unstressed patient (Table 44.3) but offer no advice as to requirements of the critical care patient (55). Deficiency syndromes are identified in patients receiving TPN for zinc, chromium, copper, manganese, selenium, iron and iodine. Preparation and stability of these elements in the TPN solution presents a major challenge to the pharmaceutical industry. However, single components as well as combination solutions are now available. Interactions between various trace elements are well known. Further discussion of calcium, phosphorus, magnesium, and zinc requirements and toxicity as well as deficiency syndromes is included later in this chapter.

Other Additives

Many other additives are often included in the intravenous nutritional solution including 1000 or more units of heparin per liter, up to 25 g of albumin per liter, hydrochloric acid, cimetidine, and even occasionally antibiotics and steroids. As can be appreciated from the above discussion, intravenous nutritional solutions can be extremely complex. The chance of precipitate formation or adverse interactions is good and expertise in formulation and meticulous monitoring is critical for safe and effective nutritional support.

VASCULAR ACCESS, SOLUTION PREPARATION, AND ADMINISTRATION

Solutions formulated to provide calorie, nitrogen, electrolyte, trace element, and vitamin requirements by necessity are quite hypertonic, a quality that prohibits their administration through peripheral veins. Central access via the superior vena cava or inferior vena cava is therefore necessary for total nutritional support. In clinical practice, catheters are typically placed percutaneously into the superior vena cava by either the infraclavicular or supraclavicular approach to the subclavian vein, or, less commonly, via the external or internal jugular veins. Occasionally, when there is no access in the neck or shoulder due to skin lesions or draining infections, catheters are placed in an antecubital vein and advanced into the superior vena cava. If the superior vena cava is not available due to thrombosis, access can be achieved through a small anterior thoracotomy with placement of tubes directly into the right atrium through the right atrial appendage. In addition, catheters have been placed through the femoral system and they are advanced well into the inferior vena cava, although this carries the risk of venous thrombosis. More recently long-term access catheters have been utilized for nutritional support. These catheters are made of silastic and are anchored to the subcutaneous tissues by a Dacron cuff. They are placed percutaneously in the operating room via the subclavian vein or through a small cutdown over the internal or external jugular vein, advanced into the right atrium, and then tunneled subcutaneously to exit on the anterior chest wall. The long subcutaneous tract appears to reduce infectious complications. Newer catheters now

Table 44.2
Recommended Daily Allowances of Vitamins[a]

Method	Fat-Soluble Vitamins				Water-Soluble Vitamins							
	A (IU)	D (IU)	E (IU)	K (mg)	B$_1$ (mg)	B$_2$ (mg)	B$_3$ (mg)	B$_5$ (mg)	B$_6$ (mg)	B$_9$ (mg)	B$_{12}$ (mg)	C (mg)
Oral FAO/WHO	2500	100	12		0.9[b]/1.2	1.3/1.8		14.5/19.8		200	2.0	30
NRC	5000	400	15		1.2/1.5	1.4/1.8	5–10	14/20	2.0	400	3.0	45
Normal serum concentration per 100 ml	90–233	112–168	0.5–1.2		0.001–0.006		0.015–0.04	0.3–0.6	0.003–0.008	0.4–2.0	0.02–0.09	0.4–1.0
Intravenous	3300	200	10.0		3.0	3.6	15.0	40.0	4.0	400.0	5.0	100.0

[a]Modified from Grant JP: *Handbook of Total Parenteral Nutrition.* Philadelphia, WB Saunders, 1980, p 172.
[b]Top figure is daily allowance for females; bottom figure is for males.

Table 44.3
Trace Elements

Element	Excretion	RDA[a]	Body Stores	Measured Level
Iron	0.1 mg urine; 0.3–0.5 mg feces ± sweat/skin; Total = 0.5–1.0 mg/day	16–18 mg/day p.o.; 0.5–1.0 mg/day i.v.	3–5 g (50% Hgb, 35% bone marrow, 15% tissues and enzymes)	Serum: 45–160 µg/dl
Zinc	0.3–0.7 mg/d urine (8 mg/day stress); 17.1 mg/kg stool or ileostomy; 12.2 mg/kg UGI drainage	10–15 mg p.o.; 2.5–4.0 mg i.v.	1–2.3 g	Plasma: 80 µg/dl; Hair: 103 PPM
Copper	25 ± 13 µg/kg/day via vile	30 µg/kg/day p.o.; 20 µg/kg/day i.v.	75–150 mg (brain, liver, heart, spleen, kidney, blood)	Serum: 75–150 µg/dl
Manganese	Mainly via bile and pancreatic juice	0.7–22 mg/day p.o.; 2–10 µg/kg/day i.v.	12–20 mg (brain, kidney, pancreas, liver, bone)	Serum: 0.8 µg/dl
Selenium	?	? 120 µg/day i.v.	6–10 mg	Serum: 2–22 µg/dl
Iodine		1 µg/kg/day		Plasma: 3.6–6.0 µg/dl
Chromium	7–10 µg/d urine	70–80 µg/day p.o.; 0.14–0.2 µg/kg/day i.v.	6 mg (skin, muscle, fat, testes, bone, liver, spleen)	Serum: 0.3–0.72 µg/dl
Molybdenum	?	2.0 µg/kg/day p.o.	?	?

[a] RDA, recommended daily allowance.

have double or triple lumens, allowing general access while one lumen is reserved for nutritional support. On rare occasions a port of the Swan Ganz catheter or the central port of a dual lumen percutaneous subclavian vein dialysis catheter can be employed for feeding, but because of infectious complications these methods should be avoided unless absolutely necessary. Care of central venous catheters must be meticulous to avoid infectious complications. With appropriate care, catheter related infections should be less than 1%. Complications of catheter insertion can be significant but are generally preventable with proper knowledge of anatomy and care during insertion.

Solutions Used for Intravenous Support

Multiple protein sources are now available for intravenous infusion. Initially these sources were casein or fibrin hydrolysates. More recently, crystalline amino acid solutions have replaced the hydrolysate solutions and are available as 3.5–10% solutions. Protein and electrolyte content of these solutions vary widely, and each solution should be carefully evaluated prior to mixing a patient's formula. Although various solutions have slightly different amino acid compositions, there are no apparent clinical differences between products. Specialized amino acid solutions for renal failure and liver failure are available and branched-chain amino acid enriched solutions are available for use in critically ill patients.

Carbohydrate is provided as a 10% to 70% solution and is mixed in various ratios with the protein solutions. Patients with volume intolerance may have special formulas mixed with 70% dextrose and 10% amino acids to reduce free water.

Since 1973 fat emulsions have been available for intravenous use. They are particularly useful in meeting essential fatty acid requirements of patients during long-term intravenous nutrition and are useful as a caloric source as well, especially during acute stress and sepsis. Fat emulsions are available in 10% and 20% concentrations.

Multiple additives are available in combination or singly so that all electrolytes, trace elements, and minerals can be added with little danger of contamination and pyrogenicity. Solutions of multivitamins that contain both fat-soluble and water-soluble vitamins are also available. Vitamin K must be given orally or by intramuscular injection.

These solutions must be mixed in a specific order to avoid complexing and precipitation. Exposure to light may result in vitamin and amino acid deterioration. Interactions between vitamin C and heparin and the various trace elements, although rarely clinically important, are theoretically possible.

Writing Orders for Parenteral Nutrition

Patients requiring TPN should begin on approximately 2000 ml a day of a 25% dextrose solution with approximately 4% amino acids. This will provide approximately 500 g of carbohydrate, which is generally well tolerated during initiation of intravenous support, and 80 g of protein. In patients with volume restrictions, either the solutions should be concentrated, or the starting volume of the standard solution should be reduced. If glucose intolerance on 5% dextrose solutions or diabetes is present, insulin should be added to the initial order. If the blood glucose concentration is above 150 mg/dl, 10 U of insulin should be added per 250 g of carbohydrate. If the blood glucose concentration is greater than 200 mg/dl, 20–25 units of insulin should be added and if greater than 250 mg/dl, 30–50 units insulin per 250 g carbohydrate are called for. If after the first 24 hours, the patient is stable on the 2-liter infusion, the infusion rate should be advanced to the required caloric support, increasing by 1000 kcal/day. If glucose intolerance is observed even with the addition of insulin, lipid calories should be substituted for carbohydrate. When the feeding solution is discontinued, the amount infused should be reduced by 1000 kcal/day until the patient is receiving 2000 kcal in 24 hours. At this point the solution is converted overnight to 5% dextrose and then discontinued the following morning. Whenever the solution must be suddenly interrupted, it is recommended that a 5% dextrose solution with appropriate electrolytes be substituted via a peripheral vein to run at the same rate as the previous intravenous nutrition solution. At no time is 10% dextrose necessary. When converting to 5% dextrose by a peripheral vein, one must be careful be taken to assure adequate insulin coverage in those patients who are glucose intolerant.

Patient Monitoring

Patients in the critical care unit should have serum electrolytes, urea nitrogen, and glucose concentrations evaluated daily until stability is achieved. Serum calcium, phosphorus and magnesium concentrations should be initially monitored every other day and the prothrombin time and white blood count two to three times a week. After stability has been reached, electrolytes and minerals should be monitored twice a week for the next week and then, depending on the degree of stability, reduced to once a week. Patients are observed carefully for evidence of sepsis, which may be heralded by glucose intolerance 12–24 hours before obvious clinical sepsis. In addition, body weight is monitored carefully to avoid fluid overload with the expectation of no more than 0.5-kg weight gain per day in malnourished patients receiving intensive support. Finally, careful observation of the access catheter with routine dressing changes is necessary to avoid septic complications.

Other Techniques of Administration

New innovations in nutritional support are being evaluated in the critical care setting. The first of these is cyclic intravenous feeding, whereby for 12–16 hours a day patients receive intensive nutritional support and during the remaining 8–12 hours a day they are either on protein solutions alone or converted to a heparin lock (50, 116). Whether cyclic feeding is more advantageous from a metabolic viewpoint remains to be determined. Another method to consider in the critical care unit is modular feeding in which some nutrition substrates are given enterally and the rest are given parenterally through intravenous catheters. An example might be the administration of amino acids and fats through a peripheral vein with glucose via an enteric feeding tube. This is especially useful when the gastrointestinal tract is only partially usable and one wishes to avoid the risks of central venous cannulation.

CATHETER-RELATED COMPLICATIONS OF TPN

Subclavian catheter insertion has the potential for numerous complications and should be performed or directly supervised only by experienced physicians. Full knowledge of the subclavian vein anatomy and attention to minute details minimizes the occurrence of pneumothorax, arterial puncture, hemomediastinum, hemothorax, hydrothorax and hydromediastinum, and virtually eliminates brachial plexus injury, thoracic duct injury, air embolism, and catheter emboli. In large-series catheter insertion complications occur between 1% and 5% of the time, with 1% or less being major complications (13, 17, 30, 166).

The majority of pneumothoraces are small and nonprogressive and usually resolve over several days without treatment. However, some are large and progressive, requiring chest tube placement. If after tube placement an air leak persists for several days, it may be necessary to remove the catheter as it may be passing through lung and pleura which would cause a bronchopleural fistula. A pneumothorax is an especially serious problem in the patient receiving mechanical ventilation. The positive pressure ventilation can delay closure of a small leak, and if the pneumothorax is not recognized, the patient can develop a tension pneumothorax.

Arterial puncture is a risk associated with most approaches to the great veins. Usually puncture of an artery does not pose a serious problem if the needle is carefully removed as normal muscular contraction of the artery prevents significant leakage of blood. If the direction of the needle is altered during insertion or withdrawal, however, the artery and/or vein may be lacerated resulting in development of hemothorax or hemomediastinum with possible cardiac tamponade requiring emergent surgical decompression.

Air embolism is a completely avoidable and potentially lethal complication (24). Aspiration of air may occur during insertion of the catheter (84), during changing of the intravenous tubing (49), upon accidental separation of the intravenous tubing (142), or through the subcutaneous tract, which may fail to close after removal of the catheter (145). Treatment consists of placing the patient in a head-down, left lateral decubitus position (141). Needle aspiration of the right ventricle and even emergency thoracotomy may be necessary to remove the air in the pulmonary outflow tract (178).

Catheter shearing and embolization may occur if the catheter is unwisely manipulated in and out through a metal insertion needle. If the catheter is severed, it may embolize to the subclavian or inominant vein, right atrium, right ventricle, or pulmonary artery. In any case, it should be removed promptly by vascular radiology or by surgery to avoid thrombus formation, infection, cardiac arrhythmias, and possible perforation of the vessels or heart. Use of a smaller needle and guidewire in the Seldinger technique greatly reduces all of the above risks.

With the development of newer and more pliable catheter materials great vein perforation, leading to hemothorax and hemomediastinum or the perforation of the right atrium, is very infrequent.

Another difficulty related to placement of the TPN catheter is improper catheter tip location. The catheter should be a few centimeters superior to the right atrium in the superior vena cava. Improper location can lead to thrombophlebitis, atrial or ventricular perforation, and cardiac arrhythmias. Subclavian vein phlebitis and thrombosis can result in edema of the arm, face, and neck and can be a cryptic source of infection or pulmonary emboli (17, 46). Treatment consists of removal of the catheter, blood and catheter cultures, and initiation of intravenous heparin therapy. If infection is present, vigorous antibiotic therapy is warranted.

Sepsis is a serious complication of TPN. Patients who require TPN are already at high risk due to malnutrition, broad-spectrum antimicrobial therapy, use of corticosteroids, and concominant infection in the lungs, urine, and wounds. Most septic problems related to TPN can be eliminated by scrupulous attention to aseptic catheter placement, solution preparation, and administration (55, 166, 167). Primary catheter sepsis is defined as a septic episode in which no other source is found and the septic episode resolves upon catheter removal with culture-positive identification of the same microorganism on the catheter or in blood drawn through the catheter as is present in the peripheral blood (46). Management of patients who become febrile while receiving TPN begins with a detailed investigation for a possible etiology of the fever. An effort should be made to preserve the central catheter. If the etiology of the fever is still elusive, and there is a fever of 38.5°C often with shaking chills every 4–8 hours, leukocytosis with increased polymorphonucleocytes, and glucose intolerance, the catheter should be removed and blood, catheter tip, and feeding solution cultures obtained. If the clinical condition is not urgent and the diagnosis of catheter-related sepsis is not obvious, cultures can be obtained through the catheter and the administration of the TPN solution can be continued until the culture results are available (115). If the patient's fever is greater than 38.5°C with shaking chills while the medical staff is waiting for the culture results, peripheral infusion of 5% dextrose should be initiated and the central catheter removed and cultured.

METABAOLIC COMPLICATIONS OF TPN

Hyperglycemia

The normal adult in good health is able to metabolize 400–500 g carbohydrate/day and, if increased gradually over several days, upward to 1500 g/day. Attention must be paid to patients with stress, extremes of age, malnutrition, diabetes, and sepsis. Often these patients need nutrition the most, but are the least tolerant to glucose loading, often developing severe hyperglycemia and glucosuria. If 2 g glucose/100 ml urine is permitted to continue, a vigorous osmotic diuresis will ensue, leading to a syndrome of hyperglycemic, hyperosmolar, nonketotic acidosis with an associated mortality approaching 40–50% (32). Optimal therapy is obviously prevention, but survival is improved by early intervention, with rapid fluid replacement with 0.5 N saline (½ NS) + 20 mEq KCl at 250 ml/hour. Insulin should be added to the intravenous solution at 15–20 units/hour while carefully monitoring blood glucose and potassium concentrations. Correction of the acidosis with sodium bicarbonate should be gradual. The goal is to achieve a slow return to normal serum glucose therapy permitting equilibration between the blood and the cerebral spinal fluid, preventing cerebral edema.

Normal serum glucose concentrations during TPN should be less than 200 mg/dl with no more than 2+ or 1% glucosuria. Values greater than 200 mg/dl should be treated. Normal insulin supplementation was discussed earlier but if a patient is glucose tolerant and suddenly develops glucose intolerance, the following should be evaluated as a potential source of hyperglycemia and/or glucosuria:

1. MEDICATION CHANGE. Many medications interfere with the urinary sugar determination by standard Clinitest or Tes-Tape techniques (Table 44.4). There are some medications that effect glucose metabolism directly

Table 44.4
Drug Interference with Urine Glucose Determinations[a]

Drug	Effect on Copper Reduction (Clinitest)	Effect on Glucose Oxidase (Tes-Tape)	Dealing with Potential Interferences
Cephalosporins Keflin Keflex Kefzol, Ancef Kafocin Loridine	False positive (black-brown color)	No effect	Use glucose oxidase test
Vitamin C (in large doses)	False positive	False negative	Also may monitor blood glucose[a]
Aspirin and other salicylates (in very large doses)	False positive	False negative	Also may monitor blood glucose[a]
Aldomet (methyldopa) (in very large doses)	False positive	No effect	Use glucose oxidase test
Benemid (probenecid)	False positive	No effect	Use glucose oxidase test
Achromycin (tetracycline, injection only)	False positive	False negative	Also may monitor blood glucose[a]
Pyridium (phenazopyridine)	No effect	False positive and false negative	Use copper reduction method
Chloromycetin (chloramphenicol)	False positive (potentially)	No effect	If in doubt, use glucose oxidase test
Levodopa (in large doses)	False positive	False negative	Also may monitor blood glucose[a]

[a] *Note*: Potential interferences with glucose oxidase tests (Tes-Tape) can be eliminated by careful testing. While interfering substances will prevent color development in the part of the paper actually dipped into the urine sample, they will not prevent accurate development in a band across the very highest portion of the wetted tape. A true-negative test occurs when the band remains the same color as the rest of the tape, and a true-positive test occurs when the band changes to one of the colors shown on the color chart. (Reprinted with permission. From Grant JP: *Handbook of Total Parenteral Nutrition*. Philadelphia, WB Saunders, 1980.)

(corticosteroids, certain diuretics, phenytoin, and phenothiazines).

2. ERROR IN RATE OF FLUID ADMINISTRATION. A sudden increase in the infusion rate commonly leads to glucose intolerance.

3. IMPENDING SEPSIS. Glucosuria, hyperglycemia, and hyperkalemia may occur up to 12 hours before a temperature elevation or any other sign of sepsis.

4. INSULIN NEEDS. A change in insulin requirements with persistently elevated serum glucose may indicate the formation of antibodies to insulin or resistance of peripheral tissues to the effects of insulin possibly due to chromium deficiency (82). Some patients who tolerate low doses of glucose will, as doses are increased, exhibit evidence of a diabetic state and require insulin during TPN.

Hypoglycemia

Administration of a hypertonic dextrose solution to a nondiabetic patient is associated with a rapid rise in serum insulin, which reaches a steady state four to six times greater than basal within 6 hours (168). As the infusion continues, serum glucose and insulin concentrations gradually decrease. With interruption of the carbohydrate infusion, serum insulin falls to basal levels within 60 minutes and blood glucose decreases to below previous basal levels, but seldom to less than 60 mg/dl. In spite of a rapid decline in serum insulin, reactive hypoglycemia is occasionally observed with abrupt discontinuance of TPN (35). It may occur if the infusion is interrupted for as little as 15–30 minutes. Therefore, in patients receiving greater than 2000 kcal/day of TPN, the solution should be tapered by 1000 kcal/day to 2000 kcal, then changed to 5% dextrose at 100–125 ml/hour for 12–24 hours, at which time the catheter can safely be removed. If abrupt cessation of TPN is necessary, a peripheral infusion of 5% dextrose with appropriate electrolytes at the same rate as the TPN should be given for 12–24 hours.

Anabolic Electrolytes

POTASSIUM

Potassium is the most abundant intracellular cation. Ninety-eight percent of the total body potassium is within the intracellular fluid pool with an average intracellular concentration of 150 mEq/liter. Intravascular potassium is a mere 2% of total body potassium, 3.5–5.0 mEq/liter. Serum concentrations are, therefore, a poor indicator of total body potassium. The kidneys are the major route of potassium excretion, eliminating approximately 100 mEq/day in the normal healthy person. In certain situations, the kidneys can preserve potassium, but not as efficiently as it can preserve sodium. Potassium is essential to the function and operation of the cell, to the maintenance of the resting potential of the cell membrane by maintaining an extracellular/intracellular gradient, to various enzyme systems, to carbohydrate metabolism, and to protein metabolism (7, 23, 41).

Hypokalemia (Table 44.5) reflects a decrease in extracellular potassium, and is usually the result of insufficient administration or gastrointestinal or urinary losses. The lost potassium should be replaced with either the chloride, acetate, or phosphate salts at 10 mEq/hour to a maximum of 40 mEq/hour.

Hyperkalemia is usually the result of excessive exogenous administration or decreased urinary output. On rare occasions hyperkalemia is factitious, resulting from red cell lysis or forearm acidosis caused by improper blood-drawing techniques. Hyperkalemia is especially prominent in renal failure when the glomerular filtration rate is below 5 ml/min, but may also result from transfusion of aged blood, Addison's disease, tissue trauma, or

Table 44.5
Clinical Symptoms of Potassium Alterations

System	Hyperkalemia	Hypokalemia
Neuromuscular	Diarrhea, weakness, intestinal colic	Paralytic ileus, muscular weakness, possible paralysis
Cardiac	Ventricular arrhythmias, ECG changes: peaked T waves, prolonged PR interval, possible cardiac arrest	Atrial and ventricular premature contractions, myocardial fibrosis, ECG changes: flat T waves, U waves
Metabolic		Abnormal carbohydrate metabolism, negative nitrogen balance

potassium-sparing diuretics (triamterene or spironolactone). Treatment should be rapid and aggressive as hyperkalemia can lead to cardiac arrest. Specific treatment consists of glucose and insulin administration to increase intracellular transport of potassium; correction of metabolic acidosis with sodium bicarbonate transporting potassium, intracellularly; kaluretic diuretics; ion exchange resins; dialysis; and intravenous calcium which lowers the threshold away from the resting potential of the cell membrane (42).

PHOSPHORUS

The phosphate ion is an integral modulator of human metabolism. It participates in energy transfer through high energy phosphates (ATP), oxygen transport and release, leukocyte phagocytosis and microbial resistance (26, 61). Approximately 80% of the adult body's phosphorus is located in bones and teeth, while 9% is within skeletal muscle. Serum phosphorus is a small fraction of total body phosphorus (2.5–4.3 mg/100 ml) and is normally inversely related to serum calcium. Serum phosphate concentrations are regulated by the kidneys and excretion is directly related to phosphate ingestion, as well as serum parathormone level.

Hypophosphatemia may result from insufficient administration in the TPN fluid, alkalosis due to increased phosphorylation of carbohydrate (respiratory greater than metabolic), Gram-negative bacteremia, salicylate intoxication, impaired absorption (phosphate binding antacids—Mg^{2+}, A^{2+}), increased renal clearance (hyperparathyroidism, vitamin D deficiency, Fanconi syndrome, hypomagnesemia, hypokalemia), metabolic acidosis, and alcoholism. Phosphate deficiency may develop within the first 24 hours of TPN if inadequate or no supplemental phosphate is given (179, 190). Glucose administration stimulates insulin secretion, which facilitates transport of glucose and phosphate into the liver and skeletal muscle thus acutely lowering blood concentrations. In addition phosphorus is taken up rapidly in skeletal muscle upon initiation of nutritional support following starvation leading to hypophosphatemia. Renal losses and amino acid binding of phosphate are minimal.

Clinical symptoms of phosphate depletion usually appear when the inorganic phosphate concentration is less than 1.0 mg/100 ml. Symptoms and signs include weakness of the muscles of extremities, neck, mastication, and respiration. There may be paresthesias, absent deep tendon reflexes, anisocoria, hyperventilation, mental obtundity, and an abnormal EMG (179, 190). Bone pain may mimic ankylosing spondylitis. There is a depletion of ATP that conformationally affects RBC membranes leading to rigid spherocytes. Also seen are abnormal red blood cell and platelet survival times, shift of the oxyhemoglobin curve to the left, and impaired white blood cell chemotaxis and phagocytosis (80, 190).

Phosphate replacement can be accomplished by adding sodium or potassium phosphate to the TPN solution in excess of maintenance until normal serum inorganic phosphate concentrations are re-established. To avoid a rapid decrease in calcium and associated tetany, phosphate supplements should be accompanied with 0.2–0.3 mEq/liter calcium infusion.

Hyperphosphatemia is usually the result of renal failure. In this setting a large portion of the phosphate becomes nonultrafilterable and forms colloidal complexes with calcium. This usually occurs when the glomerular filtration rate is 20–25 ml/minute. These complexes may be responsible for the development of metastatic calcifications in soft tissues and organs. Other etiologies of hyperphosphatemia include neoplastic diseases treated with cytotoxic agents, oral phosphate, and phosphate-containing enemas. Hyperphosphatemia may lead to hypocalcemia with possible tetany. Effective treatment consists of the administration of phosphate binding antacids (aluminum hydroxide), which decreases the gastrointestinal absorption of phosphate.

MAGNESIUM

Magnesium is the second most abundant intracellular cation, exceeded only by potassium. The average adult body contains about 330 mEq magnesium per kilogram, of which 60% is bound to the bony skeleton. Most of the remaining magnesium is concentrated in the body cells, particularly the liver, muscle, and heart. Only about 1% of the body's magnesium is in serum (1.4–2.2 mEq/liter). In magnesium deprivation, the kidney can reduce losses to less than 1 mEq/day.

Magnesium has vital metabolic functions important in the activation of many metabolic enzyme systems (especially the ATPases) (197). Many cellular energy processes are catalyzed by magnesium (196). Magnesium is essential in protein synthesis as well as synthesis of nucleic acids (15). Magnesium is of special importance to the normal function of nervous tissue, skeletal muscle, and the heart (174).

Hypomagnesemia may be the result of inadequate intake, impaired absorption, or excessive losses. Inadequate intake can result from prolonged administration of magnesium-free TPN solutions or severe starvation. Magnesium depletion may be associated with various malabsorption syndromes, extensive small bowel resections, intestinal or biliary tract fistulas, prolonged vomiting or nasogastric suction, chronic alcoholism, pancreatitis, parathyroid disease, and diabetes, especially if large insulin doses are required. Renal losses of magnesium may be secondary to diuretic abuse with mercurials, ammonium chloride, and thiazides; the diuretic phase of acute renal failure; or various intrinsic renal diseases such as glomerulonephritis, pyelonephritis, and nephrosclerosis (3). Clinical manifestations are usually present when the serum concentration is less than 1.0 mEq/liter. Many signs and symptoms resemble hypocalcemia and differentiation is essential as tetany from hypocalcemia is only temporarily corrected by magnesium administration and vice versa. Most clinical signs of hypomagnesemia are related to increased neuromuscular irritability such as confusion, hyperactive deep tendon reflexes, convulsions, tetany, positive Chvostek's sign, tremor, clonus, nystagmus, muscle fasiculation, paresthesias, and weakness (177). Magnesium deficiency also affects the cardiovascular system as evidenced by depression of ST segments and inverted T waves in precordial leads and tachycardia. Finally, magnesium deficiency can result in severe potassium wasting in the urine. Treatment is by administration of up to 40 mEq of magnesium sulfate per day, the rate of administration depending on the clinical situation.

Hypermagnesemia is rare during TPN except in patients with renal failure, diabetic acidosis, aldosterone deficiency, hyperparathyroidism, and those who use magnesium-containing laxatives and enemas excessively (3, 46). The clinical spectrum of hypermagnesemia usually involves impairment of neuromuscular transmission as reflected by hypotension, nausea, vomiting, lethargy, drowsiness, hyporeflexia, weakness, respiratory depression, coma, and cardiac arrest. ECG changes reveal QT prolongations, a prolonged PR interval, and various degrees of atrioventricular block. Intravenous calcium can temporarily reverse the depressant effects of excess magnesium. Cardiac and pulmonary support may be necessary, but the best therapy is prevention. Dialysis can be used to lower the serum magnesium concentration.

TRACE ELEMENT DEFICIENCY

Trace element metabolism during nutritional support is a new and largely unexplored area. The term "trace element" refers to those elements present in such small quantities that their precise concentrations can not be measured accurately using conventional equipment. Usually the elements are present in concentrations less than 100 $\mu g/g$ (122). With the development of TPN and the refinement of highly purified constituents, various deficiency syndromes have been recognized (54). Trace element deficiencies develop during TPN for several reasons: There may be reduced intake, increased utilization, decreased plasma binding of the elements secondary to either a decrease in synthesis or an increase in loss of the plasma binding proteins, or there may be increased excretion of the trace elements through primary or secondary routes of elimination. Iron, zinc, copper, manganese, selinium, iodine, chromium, cobalt, and molybdenum are essential to human nutrition. Fluorine, vanadium, nickel, silicon, and tin are felt to be only possibly important during TPN. Administration of these elements must be individualized because toxic concentrations and manifestations have yet to be recognized. In patients with renal and hepatic dysfunction, appropriate adjustments in dosage must be made. Table 44.3 details the route of excretion, recommended daily supplementation, body stores, and measured levels of the nine essential trace elements (53). Often clinical symptoms may take months to become evident because of large body stores of the trace elements.

IRON

Iron is necessary for the production of hemoglobin and myoglobin as well as for the functioning of some essential metabolic enzymes (148). Deficiency is demonstrated by a hypochromic, microcytic anemia, low serum iron, and high total iron binding capacity. Its deficiency leads to increased susceptibility to helminth infections, depression of cellular immunity, and a decrease in bactericidal activity of leukocytes (20, 85, 201). To calculate replacement of a preexisting iron deficiency the following formula is useful:

$$\text{Iron (mg) needed} = 0.3 \text{ (wt in lb)} \times \frac{100\text{-Hgb} \times 100}{14.8}$$

ZINC

Zinc was first shown to be essential in 1934 (188). It is required for both RNA and DNA synthesis, as well as for the proper functioning of a number of zinc-dependent metabolic enzymes including aldolases, dehydrogenases, peptidases, and thymidine kinases (119). Much of our knowledge of zinc comes from the various manifestations of zinc deficiency such as growth retardation (57), impaired wound healing (153), alopecia (87, 88), depressed cellular immunity (150), acrodermatitis enteropathica-like skin lesions (58), anorexia with impairment of taste and smell, hypogonadism, diarrhea, and glucose intolerance (155). Patients prone to zinc deficiency include those on long-term corticosteroid therapy, those with bilateral adrenalectomies, major surgical, traumatized, and septic patients, and those with malabsorption syndromes, fistulous disease, and low dietary intake (40, 66, 198). Zinc toxicity results in fever, nausea, vomiting, and diarrhea.

COPPER

Copper deficiency in adults during TPN typically presents as a hematological abnormality usually consisting of anemia, leukopenia, and neutropenia (195). The precise mechanism for these changes is unclear, but it is known that in copper deficiency iron stores are not effectively utilized for heme formation. Zidar et al. (209) show an inappropriately low level of erythropoietin for the degree of anemia and demonstrate ineffective granulopoesis. In children, copper deficiency may lead to osteoporosis by an unknown mechanism (65). In addition, copper is important in the electron transport system (110), connective tissue integrity, and wound healing (92). Acute copper toxicity follows ingestion of greater than 15 mg of elemental copper and is associated with nausea, vomiting, intestinal cramps, diarrhea, intravascular hemolysis, and renal impairment.

MANGANESE

Mangnaese participates in the activation of many enzyme systems (136), such as chondroitin sulfate synthesis (105) and protein synthesis via stimulation of RNA, and DNA polymerase activity. Doisy et al. report a case of manganese deficiency manifested by weight loss, dermatitis, slow growth, change in hair color, alteration of protein synthesis, and hypocholesterolemia (34). Manganese is also possibly involved in glucose utilization. Toxicity of manganese is rare but it may damage the extrapyirmidal system causing symptoms resembling Parkinson's disease.

SELENIUM

In experimental animals, selenium deficiency can cause liver necrosis, pancreatic atrophy, and a form of muscular dystrophy (171). In the human, several case reports have been published describing severe muscle pain, thigh tenderness and cardiomyopthy (15a, 39a, 156a, 193, 198a). Most importantly, selenium is involved as a catalyst for the important enzyme glutathione peroxidase (183). This enzyme protects against oxidative stress and cellular damage by peroxides. Selenium can function as an antioxidant and probably important in drug metabolizing systems.

IODINE

Much has been written about iodine and its deficiency syndrome of thyroid goiter. Iodine is an integral part of the thyroid hormones thyroxine and triiodothyronine, and therefore is important in the regulation of body metabolism.

CHROMIUM

Chromium has only recently been recognized as an important element in carbohydrate metabolism through its close association with the glucose tolerance factor (GTF). Chromium through GTF, appears to exert its effect peripherally by potentiating the effect of insulin upon muscle and fat calls. Jeejeebhoy et al. (82) describe a case of chromium deficiency in a patient receiving home TPN for 3 years. Symptoms included weight loss, hyperglycemia, abnormal glucose tolerance, and a diabetic-like peripheral neuropathy.

COBALT

The only human requirement for cobalt is the amount necessary for the structure of vitamin B_{12}. Humans are unable to incorporate cobalt into the corrinoid ring of this vitamin, therefore the cobalt is absorbed in total with vitamin B_{12}. Deficiency of B_{12} is described later.

MOLYBDENUM

This metal is essential in xanthine oxidase (160). There are no documented deficiency syndromes in humans.

FLUROINE

Fluorine may play an important role in fertility, growth, and maintenance of a normal hematocrit (191). It also benefits maintenance of teeth and the skeleton.

NICKEL

In animals, deficiency has led to impairment of reproduction, hair loss, and hepatocyte dysfunction (134). There has been no documented deficiency in humans.

SILICON

Silicon appears to be involved in bone calcification, structure of cartilage matrix, and possibly mucopolysaccharide metabolism (19). No human deficiency syndrome is known.

VANADIUM

In animals, deficiency of this element reduces body growth, increases packed red blood cell values, increases plasma triglycerides, impairs reproduction, and impairs bony development (172). No human deficiency is documented.

TIN

Tin may contribute to the tertiary structure of proteins. No deficiency syndrome is documented.

VITAMIN DEFICIENCIES

Vitamins are essential components in the metabolism of carbohydrates, protein, and fat. It is only over the past 40–50 years that the symptoms of various vitamin deficiencies have been well delineated. Recommended daily allowances (Table 44.2) for each vitamin are established by the World Health Organization (146) and others (31, 132). Unfortunately, these values are based on oral not intravenous intake and changes in requirements with disease and injury are unknown. When work was first started in vitamin research it was convenient to divide them into two groups: fat-soluble and water-soluble.

Fat-Soluble Vitamins (A, D, E, K)

VITAMIN A

The activity of vitamin A is measured in international units (IU) where 1 IU is equal to 0.3 μg of crystalline vitamin A alcohol or 0.6 μg of β-carotene. The decreased biological activity of carotene is due to the less efficient absorption from the intestine and to a low efficiency in converting carotene to vitamin A (147). In the normal healthy person stores of vitamin A (600,000 IU) can support the body for 3 months to a year. However, infection, hypothermia and other stresses rapidly decrease the supply of vitamin A. Serum vitamin A levels are not a good reflection of total body stores (161). The functions of vitamin A include contributions to vision, growth, and reproduction. Deficiencies usually arise because of interference with absorption or storage, inadequate dietary intake, interference with conversion from carotene to vitamin A, and rapid loss of vitamin A from the body (161). Deficiencies of vitamin A are associated with nyetalopia, xerophthalmia, phyrnoderma, decreased resistance to infection, retardation of growth, depressed production of corticosteroids, and mild leukopenia with a decrease in polymorphonuclear leukocytes and an increase in juvenile forms. Prevention of vitamin A deficiency is possible by maintenance therapy. The recommended oral intake of vitamin A is 2500–5000 IU/day. Suggestions for intravenous infusion of vitamin A are slightly higher, 2500–8000 IU/day, due to binding to glass and plastic (132).

VITAMIN D

The activity of vitamin D is also measured in international units, where 1 mg vitamin D equals 40,000 IU. Vitamin D stores are maintained normally by both dietary intake and conversion of vitamin D from the action of ultraviolet light on the skin. It is transported to the liver, where it is hydroxylated to 25-(OH)D$_3$ and then converted by the renal mitochondria to the highly active form 1,25-(OH)$_2$D$_3$. In this form vitamin D regulates calcium and phosphorus homeostasis in conjunction with parathormone and thyrocalcitonin (139). Vitamin D increases the absorption of calcium and phosphate from the intestine and also regulates the rate of reabsorption of phosphates by the renal tubules. Deficiency of vitamin D leads to osteomalacia (rickets), decreased serum calcium and phosphorus, and elevated alkaline phosphatase levels. Tetany due to hypocalcemia may occur. Proposed maintenance therapy for vitamin D is 100–400 IU/day orally or 200–420 IU/day (132).

VITAMIN K

Vitamin K is synthesized by gut flora or acquired from food. Absorption requires the presence of bile salts and pancreatic juices (51). Vitamin K plays an essential role in synthesis of clotting factors (II, VII, IX, X) (184). Deficiency of vitamin K leads to a prolongation of the prothrombin time. There is no recommended daily intake, but 0.7–2.0 mg/day is suggested. While on TPN, Jeejeebhoy et al. (83) suggest 5 mg/week administered intramuscularly.

VITAMIN E

There is much speculation about the function of vitamin E in human nutrition. It may serve primarily as an antioxidant, thereby inhibiting the oxidation of unsaturated free fatty acids (173, 185). Deficiency states of vitamin E are well described and include anemia secondary to hemolysis (74), excessive creatinuria (135), deposition of a ceroid material in smooth muscle, lesions in skeletal muscles similar to muscular dystrophy (8), and increased platelet aggregation (102). The recommended daily oral allowance for vitamin E is 12–15 IU. Suggested intravenous support ranges from 2.1 to 60 IU/day. In our experience, 25–50 IU are needed during TPN. The requirements for vitamin E are increased by the presence of polyunsaturated fatty acids in the diet. Therefore, additional vitamin E should be given when fat is administered during TPN (162).

Water-Soluble Vitamins

The clinical syndromes of water-soluble vitamin deficiencies are often similar and therefore therapy is usually directed towards multiple replacement. The tissue stores of water soluable vitamins are small and deficiencies develop early with dietary restriction. Patients receiving TPN must be supplemented early with these vitamins. Excess water soluable vitamins are excreted in the urine, therefore toxic manifestations are rare.

THIAMINE-VITAMIN B$_1$

Thiamine functions as a coenzyme for the enzyme transketolase which is important in the phosphogluconate pathway. Thiamine is also believed to be a structural component of nervous system membranes (78). Nutritional deficiencies are common owing to its limited distribution in foods. Mild deficiency leads to peripheral neuropathy characterized by paresthesias, hyperesthesia, anesthesia, and weakness. Muscles become tender with atrophy and there may be foot and wrist drop. With more severe deficiency cardiomegaly may develop especially right sided, along with tachycardia, palpitations, dependent edema, and arterial-venous shunting (138).

Acute pernicious beriberi may occur if a patient becomes thiamine deficient during TPN and is associated with mortality rates up to 50%. High output cardiac failure may be severe. Prolonged thiamine deficiency can lead to Wernicke's encephalopathy (12).

Early recognition and adequate replacement of thiamine deficiency brings rapid recovery. Maintenance requirements for thiamine vary with caloric intake. Recommended doses are approximately 0.5 mg of thiamine/1000 kcal taken orally (169) or 3–21 mg/day during TPN, although intravenous requirements are still unknown.

RIBOFLAVIN-VITAMIN B$_2$

Riboflavin is a constituent of two coenzymes, riboflavin-5′-phosphate and flavin adenine dinucleotide. These coenzymes are important components of several oxidative enzyme systems involved in electron transport.

There are essentially no stores of riboflavin and deficiency symptoms develop rapidly with dietary restriction (187). Symptoms include inflammation of lips, fissures at the corners of the mouth, scaliness, greasiness, seborrheic dermatitis about nose and scrotum, and vascularization of the cornea. Riboflavin requirements are 1.3–1.7 mg/day orally or 3.6–7.5 mg/day intravenously (132).

PANTOTHENIC ACID-VITAMIN B$_3$

The only functional form of panthothenic acid is coenzyme A which takes part in all acylation reactions. There is no documented deficiency syndrome of pantothenic acid. There is no specified daily allowance, but recommended oral intake is 5–10 mg/day while the suggested intravenous dose is 10–29 mg/day (132).

NIACIN-VITAMIN B$_5$

Niacin plays an important role in body metabolism in the form of coenzymes NAD and NADP. These coenzymes participate in the intracellular respiratory mechanism of all cells by assisting in the stepwise transfer of hydrogen from glycolysis to the flavin mononucleotide. The reduced forms of the coenzymes also participate in many biosynthetic pathways such as fatty acid synthesis.

Clinical symptoms of niacin deficiency include weakness, lassitude, anorexia, dermatitis, inflammation of the mouth, and pellagra. Effective prevention of niacin deficiency is accomplished by providing 14.5–19.8 mg niacin/day orally or 40–140 mg/day intravenously (132).

PYRIDOXINE-VITAMIN B$_6$

Pyridoxine functions as a coenzyme for transaminases, decarboxylases, for the two enzyme systems involved in the metabolism of sulfur-containing amino acids, and phosphorylase. Pyridoxine also functions as a cofactor for hydroxylases, synthetases, and many other enzymes. Deficiency of vitamin B$_6$ is well described. Personality changes, irritability, depression, filiform hypertrophy of the lingual papilla, and stomatitis characterize the deficiency syndrome. There is also a strong tendency to develop genitourinary infections (200). Prolonged vitamin B$_6$ deficiency leads to sideroblastic anemia (202). Vitamin B$_6$ deficiency is accentuated by certain antagonists such as isoniazid, pencillamine, and cycloserine (91). The recommended oral intake pyridoxine is 2.0 mg/day for adult men and 1.5 mg/day for adult women. Intravenous doses of 4.0–6.3 mg are suggested (132).

BIOTIN-VITAMIN B$_7$

Biotin can be synthesized by the intestinal flora, therefore deficiency syndromes are rare (140). The main metabolic activity of biotin is in carboxylation reactions. Deficiencies of biotin lead to a fine-scale desquamation of skin. Adult requirements for biotin are not determined.

FOLIC ACID-VITAMIN B$_9$

Because serum folate concentrations are normally 5–16 ng/ml and body folate stores range from 5–10 mg, serum measurements do not accurately reflect tissue stores. Folate participates in the uptake and transfer of 1-carbon fragments. It is involved in a multitude of metabolic processes such as purine synthesis, pyrimidine nucleotide biosynthesis, and various 3-carbon amino acid conversions. Stores of folate can usually last 3–6 months upon complete dietary restriction (67), but in stressed patients, depletion may be more rapid (37). Deficiencies also result from inadequate absorption secondary to a host of diseases or competing drugs (199); deficiency of vitamin B$_{12}$, which participates in removal of a methyl group to form the active tetrahydrofolic acid; and because of increased requirements associated with pregnancy, malignancy, sepsis, and anemias.

Symptoms include megaloblastic anemia and possibly diarrhea. Recommended daily intake for folate is 200–400 μg/day orally and 0.4–1.0 mg/day intravenously (132).

CYANOCOBALAMIN-VITAMIN B$_{12}$

Vitamin B$_{12}$ absorption is extremely dependent upon two mechanisms: gastric acid and intestinal enzyme separation from food and the gastric intrinsic factor. The normal stores of vitamin B$_{12}$ are 1–10 mg with liver containing 50–90% of total (157). The normal serum concentration is 200–900 g/ml.

Vitamin B$_{12}$ has many metabolic functions, but primarily it acts as a transmethylating agent thereby functioning in biosynthesis of thiamine, methionine, and possibly choline. By an unknown mechanism, vitamin B$_{12}$ assists in movement of folate into cells. It is also involved in seven to eight enzyme reactions and therefore is important in normal fat, carbohydrate, and protein metabolism.

A deficiency of vitamin B$_{12}$ during short-term dietary restriction is rare because of large stores as well as an efficient enterohepatic circulation. When it does occur, it takes 3–6 years to become evident. Deficiencies are characterized by a megaloblastic anemia (pernicious anemia) (25), glossitis, impairment of myelinization of peripheral nerves, and platelet aggregation defects resulting in a prolonged bleeding time (107). Neurological symptoms develop insideously with peripheral paresthesias, decreased vibratory sense, ataxia, central scotomata, confusion, and possibly psychosis.

The recommended daily maintenance for vitamin B_{12} is 2–3 μg/day orally and 5–15 μg/day intravenously. Deficiency symptoms can usually be treated with a single injection of 100–1000 μg of vitamin B_{12} (132). (*Note:* Begin with no more than 100μg as larger doses may cause severe hypokalemia.)

ASCORBIC ACID-VITAMIN C

Vitamin C is active in forming collagen, transporting mitochondrial electrons, metabolizing tyrosine, converting folate to tetrahydrofolic acid, and metabolizing cholesterol. It prevents and cures scurvy, which is characterized by anemia, joint pain, mucous membrane hemorrhages, weakness, and emaciation. Less severe deficiency impairs wound healing, diminishes host immunity, and decreases tyrosine metabolism (46).

No specific daily requirements are known, but 30–45 mg/day orally is recommended while suggested intravenous supplementation is 100–500 mg/day (132). Body stores of vitamin C are minimal, and coupled with increased urinary losses with stress, a deficiency may develop rapidly during TPN if inadequate supplements are given (70). Vitamin C administration interferes with the anticoagulant effects of heparin; 2 mg ascorbic acid neutralizes 1 U of heparin (143).

OTHER COMPLICATIONS OF TPN

Elevated Liver Function Test

Many investigators note a high percentage of patients receiving parenteral nutrition develop elevations of serum bilirubin and hepatic enzymes (SGOT, SGPT, alkaline phosphatase, LDH) (44, 48, 50, 75, 114, 144, 205). Liver biopsies obtained at these times reveal periportal fatty changes with little evidence of inflammation or other abnormalities (75). There is much speculation as to the etiology of these liver changes, but attempted correlation with various parameters has been unsuccessful (48, 64, 149, 152, 176, 189). Changes are seen with equal frequency when casein or protein hydrolysates or crystalline amino acids are used

as protein sources. The liver enzyme elevations also do not correlate with the initiation of feeding preoperatively versus postoperatively, with the mean serum glucose level, or with the amount of exogenous insulin administered.

It has been proposed that early changes are secondary to toxic conversion products of the amino acid tryptophan in the presence of sodium bisulfite (48). Sheldon et al. (176) found evidence of progressive intrahepatic cholestases, bile duct proliferation, and bile plugs associated with serum hepatic enzyme changes, and felt that this was due to an imbalance in the caloric:nitrogen ratio. Langer et al. (103) theorized that the changes were secondary to lack of essential fatty acids, whereas others have reported these changes while patients received intravenous fat. Kaminski et al. (86) postulated that fatty infiltration was associated with a decreased ability to transport lipid away from the liver due to a deficiency of lipotropic factors and Hall et al. (56a) documented abnormalities in fat synthesis, fat oxidation, fat uptake, and fat mobilization by the liver. Others feel that changes are secondary to protein allergies (64, 149, 189). The precise etiology of these changes remains to be determined. Most investigators feel it is due to glucose overloading (50, 114, 162a).

Elevation of Blood Urea Nitrogen (BUN)

Almost all patients receiving parenteral nutrition demonstrate some elevations of BUN regardless of renal function. The elevation rarely exceeds normal limits in patients with normal renal function; if it does it usually plateaus at less than 80 mg/dl. Some of the elevation can be attributed to dehydration. However, in patients with compromised renal function (creatine clearance < 20 ml/minute) the BUN may progressively increase, thereby limiting the amount of nitrogen that can be infused. In patients with a creatinine clearance > 20 ml/minute, usually 9 g or more of nitrogen per day will be well tolerated. In more severe renal failure, special formulas may be required to reduce nitrogen support to 6–9 g or less per day (1a, 46).

Essential Fatty Acid Deficiency

There are three polyunsaturated fatty acids that cannot be synthesized by humans (linoleic, arachidonic, and linolenic); however, only linoleic acid is essential in the adult diet. Arachidonic acid can be synthesized when linoleic acid is present. The precise role and need for linolenic acid in the adult is undetermined. The average daily intake of fat in the human diet is approximately 100–180 g, approximately 12–125 g of which are essential fatty acids (EFA). The RDA for EFA is not established, but suggested intravenous supplementation ranges from 1% to 4% of the total caloric intake or 25–100 mg/kg/day of linoleic acid (18, 59, 72, 186).

EFA play a primary role in the structure and maintenance of cell membranes, prostaglandin synthesis, and various transport mechanisms (106). EFA deficiency leads to a decrease in the efficiency of calorie utilization, and possibly the dissociation of oxidative phosphorylation and the impairment of production of high-energy phosphate bonds. The clinical symptoms of EFA deficiency include diarrhea, dryness of skin, hair loss, impaired wound healing, and brittle and osteoporotic bones (18, 59, 72). Biochemical changes include decreased cholesterol levels thrombocytopenia, increased platelet aggregation, increased capillary permeability, anemia, increased RBC fragility, elevations of serum hepatic enzymes, and fatty infiltration of the liver (181, 186).

EFA deficiency can be documented by an elevated serum 5,8,11-eicosatrienoic: arachiodonic acid ratio that is normally less than 0.4 (72, 73). All symptoms can be reversed with the administration of linoleic acid. If the oral route is available, oils high in linoleic acid such as corn oil or safflower oil may be administered (5 ml twice or three times a day). Other available routes include topical administration of corn oil or safflower oil (15 ml three times a day) (156), or intravenous administration of 25–100 mg/kg/day of linoleic acid as a 10% or 20% fat emulsion (60). Biochemical signs of EFA deficiency may develop early over the first few days of fat-free TPN, whereas clinical symptoms may require several weeks to become obvious, in any case, fat administration should be started early in the course of TPN therapy.

Hypoalbuminemia

Albumin is a major synthetic product of the liver, and averages about 130–200 mg/kg/day, but may be as high as 860 mg/kg/day during maximum synthesis. Depressed serum albumin concentrations may result from decreased synthesis, increased degradation, or altered fluid status.

Depressed synthesis is associated with many conditions including malnutrition, cancer, acute stress, cirrhosis, hypothyroidism, and exposure to hepatic toxins. The main clinical condition associated with increased degradation is catabolism (36). Because of the redistribution of extravascular albumin into the plasma pool, serum concentrations of albumin decrease slowly and do not always reflect the total body pool. When the serum albumin concentration is 2.5 mg/100 ml, the total exchangeable albumin pool may be less than one-half its normal level.

Hypoalbuminemia has been associated with impairment of soft and bony tissue healing (43), decreased immune defense (104), depressed gastrointestinal motility (120), and impaired intestinal absorption of water and electrolytes (130). A major function of albumin is regulating the distribution of body water through its osmotic properties (76). We therefore try to reestablish normal total body albumin content rapidly in catabolic patients by adding up to 25 g albumin/liter TPN. The approximate amount of total body albumin deficit can be determined by the formula: grams albumin deficit $= (4.0 - \text{Alb})\text{BW(kg)}$. When albumin is given alone without adequate nutritional support, it is used as a calorie substrate but when given with adequate caloric support, its half-life approaches normal. In patients who have acute respiratory distress or possible damage to pulmonary capillary integrity, it may be wise not to administer albumin because it may leak into the perivascular pulmonary tissues (71). Use personal judgement in deciding whether to administer albumin during TPN.

Acid-Base Derangements

Acid-base balance is an extremely complex system involving multiple feedback mechanisms. An in-depth discussion is beyond the scope of this section.

Parenteral nutrition has the potential for either causing or magnifying acid-base disturbances. Most enzymatic and metabolic processes in the human are pH sensitive and the body strives to preserve acid-base homeostasis. Therefore frequent monitoring of the serum pH is made in critically ill patients receiving parenteral nutrition.

Metabolic acidosis can usually be attributed to either abnormal production of acid or to excessive loss of base. Diseases or processes leading to excess production of acid include diabetes mellitus, hyperthryoidism, high fat diets, hepatitis, anesthesia, sepsis, low cardiac output syndromes leading to lactic acidosis, and many others. Disease states which may lead to excess loss of bicarbonate include diarrhea, pancreatic, biliary, or small intestinal drainage, renal insufficiency and the administration of acidifying salts.

There are, however, two other potential causes which should be considered in patients receiving TPN:

1. Synthetic L-amino acids contain one-third to one-fifth the titratable acidity of the older protein hydrolysates, but they too can induce metabolic acidosis due to an increased amount of cationic amino acids compared to anionic amino acids (63).
2. Metabolic acidosis may result from excessive chloride administration (56, 158). An increased quantity of chloride ions are filtered at the renal glomerulus, thereby providing more chloride to be reabosrbed in the distal renal tubules with sodium. This increased sodium chloride reabsorption inversely effects hydrogen ion secretion into the tubules leading to a hyperchloremic metabolic acidosis.

Metabolic alkalosis may result from gastric suctioning, vomiting, diarrhea, diuretic intake, excessive administration of potassium-free solution, excessive ingestion of antacids, and hyperadrenocorticism. However, during parenteral nutrition, special attention should be paid to patients on prolonged nasogastric suctioning. In addition to the loss of hydrogen ions, the loss of chloride ions leads to less chloride filtration by the renal glomerulus and therefore greater amounts of H^+ ion secreted in the distal tubule in exchange for sodium.

Prevention of acid-base disturbances is the best treatment. To avoid difficulties of excess chloride infusion, the Na:Cl ratio is adjusted to 1:1 and additional anions are given as acetate, lactate, or phosphate. Nasogastric losses are replaced carefully with appropriate electrolyte solutions. If acid losses are extreme, it may be necessary to administer an H_2 blocker or even to infuse dilute hydrochloric acid intravenously. Hydrochloric acid up to 0.2 N is compatible with crystalline amino acid solutions or standard dextrose solutions and can be administered via central venous line. It is suggested that trace elements, vitamin, and other low-priority additives be removed when hydrochloric acid is added to prevent untoward reactions.

Lethargy

Patients will occasionally become weak, tired, lethargic, and even semicomatose upon initiation of TPN. The cause of this lethargy is unknown. One suggestion is that the change from starvation to full nutritional support may result in metabolic or hormonal changes that lead to sedation (108). An increase in serum tryptophan enhances its passage into the brain, which leads to serotonin production and lethargy. There is no specific therapy and symptoms usually diminish after 6–10 days. Exercise may be safely encouraged.

Alopecia

Excessive or complete loss of hair is common during TPN but is usually not due to the nutrition solution. The most common cause is an interruption of the normal hair cycle in response to a stressful event (trauma, sepsis, malnutrition). Hair undergoes three phases of growth. The anagen phase is the period of intense mitotic activity, formation of the hair root, and growth of the hair shaft. The catagen phase is a short period of transition when the hair follicle stops growing and regresses to a state similar to the embryologic follicle germ. The final resting stage, the telogen phase, is when the keratinized hair shaft and hair bulb are lying within the resting follicle. At some point the follicles are reactivated and the old hair is shed. Normally, 85% of hairs in the scalp are in the anagen phase while 15% are in the telogen phase. With stress, many hair follicles simultaneously enter the telogen phase (97). Shortly thereafter, the hair is shed and the follicles start over in the anagen phase. Hair loss is therefore a common but temporary event. Other causes of hair loss include severe protein depletion and zinc deficiency.

NUTRITIONAL SUPPORT IN SPECIAL CLINICAL SETTINGS

Renal Failure

Renal failure is a frequent complication in the critically ill patient. Metabolic requirements of these patients are no different than requirements of patients without renal failure (182). Any initial attempt to reduce metabolic support to avoid volume or protein tolerance is avoided. Rather, effective hemodialysis or peritoneal dialysis is established early to permit aggressive TPN. If dialysis is established, no reduction need be made in the routine supply of nutrients as dialysis will clear any excesses or waste by-products. Indeed, it must be recognized that there is a loss of nitrogen during dialysis that requires replacement. Hemodialysis results in loss of up to 9 g amino acids and 3–4 g peptides over 4 hours while in peritoneal dialysis up to 15 g of amino acids and 40 g of protein may be lost. Only in cases in which dialysis is contraindicated or not available should consideration be given to modification of nutritional support reducing both volume and protein content. In this setting, if intravenous protein support is reduced below 30–40 g a day (the minimum protein support providing adequate essential amino acids in currently available solutions) administration of essential amino acids as supplements or essential amino acids alone should be considered. Renal failure solutions containing only essential amino acids are commercially available. They are packaged in 200- to 250-ml volume and provide approximately 6 g of protein as essential amino acids plus histadine. These are mixed with 500 ml of 70% dextrose to provide calories. One or two bottles are administered daily until renal function recovers adequately or dialysis becomes available, permitting administration of more balanced solutions. The routine supplementation of vitamins, essential fatty acids, trace elements, and minerals must be emphasized during the feeding program whether specialized renal failure formulas or standard products are used. Morbidity and mortality of renal failure is in part due to the subsequent metabolic alteration and nutritional depletion that results when nutritional support is inadequate. Aggressive nutritional support coupled with adequate dialysis offers significantly improved care for these high-risk patients.

Hepatic Failure

Providing adequate nutritional support to patients with hepatic failure poses a major metabolic problem. These patients often manifest protein intolerance, which is characterized by increased serum ammonia concentrations and hepatic encephalopathy. Studies by Fischer et al. (38) suggest the onset of hepatic encephalopathy may be due to abnormal amino acid profiles due to the altered hepatic function. In particular, straight-chain and aromatic amino acids are increased in the blood and brain, whereas branched-chain amino acids are decreased. The resulting abnormal ratio between aromatic and branched-chain amino acids contributes to altered amino acid transport through the blood-brain barrier and an abnormal neurotransmitter profile (81). Experimentation in the animal as well as clinical trials in humans have demonstrated that products containing high concentrations of branched-chain amino acids and low concentrations of aromatic amino acids improve or prevent hepatic encephalopathy while permitting aggressive protein supplementation of up to 100–150 g per day (73a). Coupled with adequate caloric, vitamin, electrolyte, mineral, and trace element supplementation, anabolism can often be achieved even in the patient with significant hepatic failure. Recent studies, however, have not confirmed the earlier findings (19a, 122a, 197a). Current recommendations are to provide routine protein loading until or unless encephalopathy is present at which time use of branched-chain enriched products may be useful.

Respiratory Failure

Respiratory failure due to malnutrition is manifested in two ways. The first and most common is a decrease in respiratory skeletal and diaphragmatic muscle function with a subsequent decrease in ventilatory effort. In these cases, nutritional support must be aggressive and complete in hopes of regenerating skeletal and diaphragmatic muscle mass. Excessive carbohydrate administration in patients with respiratory failure leads to increased carbon dioxide production and perhaps respirator dependency (5). In these situations it is perhaps best to continue the administration of a nutrient solution until muscle mass is regenerated, and then either interrupt the feeding solution or convert to a more balanced carbohydrate-fat caloric substrate in order to reduce carbon dioxide production, allowing for ventilation weaning.

The second form of respiratory failure results from loss of chemoreceptor sensitivity as outlined earlier. Receptors sensitive to hypoxic states are impaired by combined protein-caloric depletion, whereas chemoreceptors sensitive to hypercarbia are impaired mainly by protein depletion. Sensitivity of both receptors is rapidly restored with nutritional support.

Frequently, critically ill patients also have chronic obstructive pulmonary disease. In selected cases, these patients can be weaned from respirators and gradually advanced to a significantly improved quality of life with instigation of aggressive intravenous nutritional support coupled with an active physical therapy program (73a).

Cardiac Failure

Cardiac dysfunction in the malnourished, critically ill patient can occur by two mechanisms (69). In the first, patients have intrinsic cardiac disease such as valvular or coronary artery disease, which leads to progressive cardiac failure and subsequent decreased nutritional intake and cardiac cachexia. Attempts at nutritional rehabilitation without correction of the intrinsic cardiac disease, and sometimes even after correction of their cardiac disease, can be catastrophic. The additional burden on the myocardium of regenerated body cell mass can lead to irreversible cardiac failure. Maintenance of body cell mass should be the priority rather than restoration of normal body cell mass. Only as myocardial function improves should one attempt to increase body mass.

Other patients present with malnutrition as a primary diagnosis with subsequent nutritional injury to the myocardium and cardiac failure. They demonstrate the same picture of cardiac cachexia but require nutritional support as specific therapy. Nutritional support is begun slowly and advanced gradually, allowing time for recovery of myocardial function. Patients should be observed carefully for tachycardia and congestion as they are quite prone to develop congestive heart failure. An exercise program is important during nutritional rehabilitation.

Cancer

The value of nutritional support of patients with malignant processes remains controversial (14). Although it does not improve survival, there is evidence of improved tolerance and response to therapy and improved quality of life. Cancer patients often demonstrate a marked increase in metabolic rate and altered metabolic pathways probably because of an effect of the cancer on the host. Failure to meet the increased metabolic demands results in rapid development of cachexia. Hospitalized patients who undergo intensive chemotherapy, radiotherapy, or surgical therapy should be nutritionally supported during their therapy to afford the best change of response. On the other hand, patients who have no further effective therapeutic intervention available and who are terminally ill should not have intravenous nutritional support initiated.

Burns

Data are now available supporting the use of intensive nutritional support in patients with extensive body burns (28). The increase in metabolic rate is well documented and complications resulting from rapid nutritional decay are extensively reported. Often nutritional support is administered solely via the gastrointestinal tract, but at times supplementation via the intravenous route is also required. As with volume supplementation in burn patients, formulas have been developed to calculate nitrogen and caloric requirements based on the degree and percent of body burn.

Spinal Cord Injury

Little is known of the metabolic requirements of the patient with spinal cord injury. Psychological stress is felt to increase basal metabolic rate, whereas neurological injury eliminates much muscular activity. Denervation of skeletal muscles results in mandatory wasting of skeletal muscle mass, rendering nitrogen balance studies of little value. Of some value is actual measurement of oxygen consumption and carbon dioxide production to determine the RME.

References

1. Abel RM, Fischer JE, Buckley ML, et al: Malnutrition in cardiac surgical patients. *Arch Surg* 111:45–50, 1976.
1a. Abel RM, Shik VE, Abbott WM, et al: Amino acid metabolism in acute renal failure: Influence of intravenous essential L-amino acid hyperalimentation therapy. *Ann Surg* 180:350–355, 1974.
2. Addis P, Poo LJ, Lew W: The quantities of proteins lost by the various organs and tissues of the body during a fast. *J Biol Chem* 115:111–116, 1936.
3. Alfrey AC: Disorders of magnesium metabolism. In Shrier RW: *Renal and Electrolyte Disorders* Boston, Little, Brown, 1976, pp 223–242.

4. Anderson GH, Patel DG, Jeejeebhoy KN: Design and evaluation by nitrogen balance and blood aminograms of an amino acid mixture for total parenteral nutrition of adults with gastrointestinal disease. *J Clin Invest* 53:904–912, 1974.

5. Askanazi J, Weissman C, Rosenbaum SH, et al: Nutrition and the respiratory system. *Crit Care Med* 10:163–172, 1982.

6. Askanazi J, Carpentier YA, Elwyn DH, et al: Influence of total parenteral nutrition on fuel utilization in injury and sepsis. *Ann Surg* 191:40–46, 1980.

7. Beal JM, Frost PM, Smith JL: The influence of caloric and potassium intake on nitrogen retention in man. *Ann Surg* 138:842–845, 1953.

8. Binder HJ, Hertin DC, Hurst V, et al: Tocopherol deficiency in man. *N Engl J Med* 273:1287–1297, 1965.

9. Bingham JG, Krischer JP, Shuster JJ et al: Effects of nutrition on length of stay and survival for burned patients. *Burns* 7:252–257, 1981.

10. Bistrian BR, Sherman M, Blackburn GL, et al: Cellular immunity in adult marasmus. *Arch Intern Med* 137:408–412, 1977.

11. Black PR, Brooks DC, Bessey PQ, et al: Mechanisms of insulin resistance following injury. *Ann Surg* 196:420–435, 1982.

11a. Blackburn GL, Moldawer LL, Usui S, et al: Branched chain amino acid administration and metabolism during starvation, injury and infection. *Surgery* 86:307–315, 1979.

12. Blennow G: Wernicke's encephalopathy following prolonged artificial nutrition. *Am J Dis Child* 129:1456, 1975.

13. Borja AR: Current status of infraclavicular subclavian vein catheterization. *Ann Thorac Surg* 13:615–624, 1972.

13a. Borum PR (ed): Role of carnitine supplementation in clinical nutrition. In *Clinical Aspects of Human Carnitine Deficiency*. Pergamon Press, NY, 1986.

14. Brennan MF: Total parenteral nutrition in the cancer patient. *N Engl J Med* 305:375–382, 1981.

15. Brenner S, Jacob F, Meselson M: An unstable intermediate carrying information from genes to ribosomes for protein synthesis. *Nature (Lond)* 190:576–581, 1961.

15a. Brown MR, Cohen HJ, Lyons JM, et al: Proximal muscle weakness and selenium deficiency associated with long term parenteral nutrition. *Am J Clin Nutr* 43:549–554, 1986.

16. Buchanan N, Davis MD, Eyberg C: Gentamycin pharmacokinetics in kwashiorkor. *Br J Clin Pharmacol* 8:451–453, 1979.

16a. Burke JF, Wolfe RR, Mullany CJ, et al: Glucose requirements following burn injury. *Ann Surg* 190:274–285, 1979.

17. Burni C, Krischak G: Techniques and complications of administration of total parenteral nutrition. In Manni C, Magalini SI, Scrascia E: *Total Parenteral Nutrition*. New York, American Elsevier, 1976, pp 306–315.

18. Caldwell MD, Jonsson HT, Othersen HB Jr: Essential fatty acid deficiency in an infant receiving prolonged parenteral alimentation. *J Pediatr* 81:894–898, 1972.

19. Carlisle EM: Silicon: an essential element for the chick. *Science* 178:619–521, 1972.

19a. Cerra FB: A multi-center trial of branched chain enriched amino acid infusion (FO80) in hepatic encephalopathy. *Hepatology* 2:699, 1982.

19b. Cerra FB, Mazuski JE, Chute E, et al: Branched chain metabolic support. A prospective, randomized, double-blind trial in surgical stress. *Ann Surg* 199:286–291, 1984.

20. Chandra RK: Reduced bactericidal capacity of polymorphs in iron deficiency. *Arch Dis Child* 48:864–866, 1973.

21. Clark I: Effect of cortisone upon protein synthesis. *J Biol Chem* 200:69–76, 1953.

22. Committee on Trauma, National Academy of Sciences-National Research Council: Postoperative wound, infections: the influence of ultraviolet irradiation of the operating room and of various other factors. *Ann Surg (Suppl)* 16:1–192, 1964.

23. Conn J: Hypertension, the potassium ion and impaired carbohydrate tolerance. *N Engl J Med* 273:1135–1142, 1965.

24. Coppa GF, Gouge TH, Hofstetter SR: Air embolism: a lethal but preventable complication of subclavian vein catheterization. *J Parent Enter Nutr* 5:116–168, 1981.

25. Cooper BA, Lowenstein L: Relative folate deficiency of erythrocytes in pernicious anemia and its correction with cyanocobalamin. *Blood* 24:502–521, 1964.

26. Craddock PR, Yawata Y, Van Santen L, et al: Acquired phagocyte dysfunction. A complication of the hypophosphatemia of parenteral hyperalimentation. *N Engl J Med* 290:1403–1407, 1974.

27. Cruse PJE, Foord R: A five-year prospective study of 23,649 surgical wounds. *Arch Surg* 107:206–210, 1973.

28. Curreri PW: Nutritional support of burn patients. *World J Surg* 2:215–221, 1978.

29. Cuthbertson DP: The disturbances of metabolism produced by bony and non-bony injury, with notes on certain abnormal conditions of bone. *Biochem J* 24:1224–1263, 1930.

30. Daly JM, Lawson M, Speir A: Intravenous access in chemotherapy patients. *Int Adv Surg Oncol* 4:59–82, 1981.

31. Dietary Allowances Committee and Food and Nutrition Board: *Recommended Dietary Allowances*, ed 8. Washington, DC, National Academy of Sciences, 1974.

32. Docomal M, Cantos JW: Hyperosmolar nonketotic coma complicating intravenous hyperalimentation. *Surg Gynecol Obstet* 136:729–732, 1973.

33. Doekel RC, Zwillich CW, Scoggin CH, et al: Clinical semi-starvation: depression of the hypoxic ventilatory response. *N Engl J Med* 295:358–361, 1976.

34. Doisy EA Jr: Micronutrient control on biosynthesis of clotting proteins and cholesterol. In Hemphill DD: *Proceedings of the University of Missouri's 6th Annual Conference on Trace Substances in Environmental Health*. Columbia, MO, University of Missouri Press, 1973, p 193.

35. Dudrick SJ, MacFaydyen BV Jr, Van Buren CT, et al: Parenteral hyperalimentation. Metabolic problems and solutions. *Ann Surg* 176:259–264, 1972.

36. Eckart J, Tempel G, Schreiber V, et al: The turnover of I-125-labeled serum albumin after surgery and injury. In Wilkinson AW: *Parenteral Nutrition*. Edinburgh, Churchill Livingstone, 1972, pp 288–298.

37. Eichner ER, Pierce HI, Hillman RS: Folate balance in dietary-induced megaloblastic anemia. *N Engl J Med* 284:933–938, 1971.

38. Fischer JE, Rosen HM, Ebeid AM, et al: The effect of normalization of plasma amino acids on hepatic encephalopathy in man. *Surgery* 80:77–91, 1976.

39. Fleck A: Metabolic response to injury. In Ledingham IM, Mackay G: *Jamieson and Kay's Textbook of Surgical Physiology*. New York, Churchill Livingstone, 1978.

39a. Fleming CR, Lie JT, McCall JT, et al: Selenium deficiency and fatal cardiomyopathy in a patient on home parenteral nutrition. *Gastroenterology* 83:689–693, 1982.

40. Flynn A, Strain WH, Pories WJ, et al: Zinc deficiency with altered adrenocortical function and its relation to delayed healing. *Lancet* 1:789–791, 1973.

41. Fourman PS: Experimental observations of the tetany of potassium deficiency. *Lancet* 2:575, 1954.

42. Gabow P: Disorders of potassium metabolism. In Schrier RW: *Renal and Electrolyte Disorders*. Boston, Little, Brown, 1976, pp 143–165.

43. Garrow JS: Protein nutrition and wound healing. *Proc Nutr Soc* 28:242–248, 1969.

44. Ghadimi H, Abaci F, Kumar S, et al: Biochemical aspects of intravenous alimentation. *Pediatrics* 48:955–965, 1971.
44a. Goodenough RD, Wolfe RR: Effect of total parenteral nutrition on free fatty acid metabolism in burned patients. *J Parent Enter Nutri* 8:357–360, 1984.
45. Gracey M, Suharjono S, Stone DE: Microbial contamination of the gut: another feature of malnutrition. *Am J Clin Nutr* 26:1170–1174, 1973.
46. Grant JP: *Handbook of Total Parenteral Nutrition.* Philadelphia, WB Saunders, 1980.
47. Grant JP: Clinical impact of protein malnutrition on organ mass and function. In Blackburn GL, Grant JP, Young VR: *Amino Acids Metabolism and Medical Applications.* Boston, John Wright PSG Inc., 1983, pp 347–358.
48. Grant JP, Cox CE, Kleinman LM: Serum hepatic enzyme and bilirubin elevations during parenteral nutrition. *Surg Gynecol Obstet* 145:573–580, 1977.
48a. Grant J, Snyder P: Use of L-glutamine in TPN. *J Surg Res* (in press).
49. Green HL, Nemir P Jr: Air embolism as a complication during parenteral alimentation. *Am J Surg* 121:614–616, 1971.
50. Greenlaw C: Liver enzyme elevations associated with total parenteral nutrition. *Drug Intell Clin Pharm* 14:702–709, 1980.
51. Gross L, Brotman M: Hypoprothrombinemia and hemorrhage associated with cholestyramine therapy. *Ann Intern Med* 72:95–96, 1970.
52. Groves AC, Griffiths J, Leung F, et al: Plasma catecholamines in patients with serious postoperative infection. *Ann Surg* 178:102–107, 1973.
53. Guidelines for Essential Trace Element Preparations for Parenteral Use: A statement by the Nutrition Advisory Group *J Paren Enter Nutr* 3:263–267, 1979.
54. Guidelines for Essential Trace Element Preparations for Parenteral use. AMA Department of Foods and Nutrition. *JAMA* 241:2051–2054, 1979.
55. Guidelines for Infectious Control in Hyperalimentation Therapy: National Nosocomial Infection Study Quarterly Report, May, 1972, p 22.
56. Guyton AC: *Textbook of Medical Physiology,* ed 4. Philadelphia, WB Saunders, 1971, p 437.
56a. Hall RI, Grant JP, Ross HL, et al: Pathogenesis of hepatic steatosis in the parenterally fed rat. *J Clin Invest* 74:1658–1668, 1984.
56b. Hallberg D: Studies on the elimination of exogenous lipids from the bloodstream. The effect of fasting and surgical trauma in man on the elimination rate of a fat emulsion injected intravenously. *Acta Physiol Scand* 65:151–163, 1965.
57. Hambidge RM, Hambidge C, Jacobs M, et al: Low levels of zinc in hair, anorexia, poor growth, and hypogeusia in children. *Pediatr Res* 6:868–874, 1972.
58. Hambidge KM, Neldnes KH, Walravens PA: Zinc and acrodermatitis, enteropathica. In Hambidge KM, Nichols BL (eds): *Zinc and Copper in Clinical Medicine.* New York, Spectrum Publications, 1978, pp 81–98.
59. Hansen AE, Haggard ME, Boeloche AN, et al: Essential fatty acids in infant nutrition. III. Clinical manifestations of linoleic acid deficiency. *J Nutr* 66:565–576, 1958.
60. Hansen LM, Hardie WR, Hidalgo J: Fat emulsion for intravenous administration: clinical experience with intralipid 10%. *Ann Surg* 184:80–88, 1976.
61. Harken AH, Woods M: The influence of oxyhemoglobin affinity on tissue oxygen consumption. *Ann Surg* 183:130–135, 1976.
62. Harris JA, Benedict FG: Biometric studies of basal metabolism in man. Carnegie Institution of Washington, Publication No. 279, 1919.
62a. Harvey KB, Moldawer LL, Bistrian BR, et al: Biological measures for the formation of a hospital prognostic index. *Am J Clin Nutr* 34:2013–2022, 1981.
63. Heird WC, Dell RB, Driscoll JM Jr, et al: Metabolic acidosis resulting from intravenous alimentation mixtures containing synthetic amino acids. *N Engl J Med* 287:943–948, 1972.
64. Heird WC, Driscoll JM, Schullinger JN, et al: Intravenous alimentation in pediatric patients. *J Pediatr* 80:351–372, 1972.
65. Heller RM, Kirchner SG, O'Neill JA Jr, et al: Skeletal changes of copper deficiency in infants receiving prolonged total parenteral nutrition. *J Pediatr* 92:947–948, 1978.
66. Henzel JH, DeWeese MS, Pories WJ: Significance of magnesium and zinc metabolism in the surgical patient. *Arch Surg* 95:991–999, 1967.
67. Herbert V: Experimental nutritional folate deficiency in men. *Trans Assoc Am Physicians* 75:307–320, 1962.
68. Heymsfield SB, Bethel RA, Ansley JD, et al: Cardiac abnormalities in cachectic patients before and during nutritional repletion. *Am Heart J* 95:584–594, 1978.
69. Heymsfield SB, Smith J, Redd S, et al: Nutritional support in cardiac failure. *Surg Clin North Am* 61:635–652, 1981.
70. Hodges RE, Hood J, Canham JE, et al: Clinical manifestations of ascorbic acid deficiency in man. *Am J Clin Nutr* 24:432–443, 1971.
71. Holcroft JW, Trunkey DD: Pulmonary extravasation of albumin during and after hemorrhagic shock in baboons. *J Surg Res* 18:91–97, 1975.
72. Holman RT: The ratio of trienoic-tetraenoic acids in tissue lipids as a measure of essential fatty acid requirement. *J Nutr* 70:405–410, 1960.
73. Holman RT: Essential fatty acid deficiency. *Prog Chem Fats Other Lipids* 9:329–331, 1971.
73a. Horst D, Graze N, Conn HO: A double-blind randomized comparison of dietary protein and an oral branched chain amino acid (BCAA) solution in cirrhotic patients with chronic portal-systemic encephalopathy. *Hepatology* 2:184, 1982.
74. Horwitt MK, Harvey CC, Duncan GD, et al: Symposium on the role of some of the newer vitamins in human metabolism and nutrition; effects of limited tocopherol intake in man with relationships to erythrocyte hemolysis and lipid oxidations. *Am J Clin Nutr* 4:408–419, 1956.
75. Host WR, Serlin O, Rush BF Jr: Hyperalimentation in cirrhotic patients. *Am J Surg* 123:57–62, 1971.
76. Howland WS, Schweizer O, Ragasa J, et al: Colloid oncotic pressure and levels of albumin and total protein during major surgical procedures. *Surg Gynecol Obstet* 143:592–596, 1976.
77. Hume DM: The neuro-endocrine response to injury: present status of the problem. *Ann Surg* 138:548–557, 1953.
78. Itokawa Y, Schultz RA, Cooper JR: Thiamine in nerve membranes. *Biochim Biophys Acta* 266:293–299, 1972.
79. Jackson CM: Effect of acute and chronic inanition upon the relative weights of the various organs and systems of adult albino rats. *Am J Anat* 18:75–116, 1915.
80. Jacob HS, Amsden T: Acute hemolytic anemia with rigid red cells in hypophosphatemia. *N Engl J Med* 285:1446–1450, 1971.
81. James JH, Jeppsson B, Ziparo V, et al: Hyperammonaemia, plasma amino acid imbalance, and blood-brain amino acid transport: A unified theory of portal-systemic encephalopathy. *Lancet* 2:772–775, 1979.
82. Jeejeebhoy KN, Chu RC, Marliss EB, et al: Chromium deficiency, glucose intolerance, and neuropathy reversed by chromium supplementation in a patient receiving long-term total parenteral nutrition. *Am J Clin Nutr* 30:531–538, 1977.
83. Jeejeebhoy KN, Langer B, Tsallas G, et al: Total parenteral nutrition at home: studies in patients surviving 4 months to 5 years. *Gastroenterology* 71:943–953, 1976.

84. Johnson CL, Lazarchick J, Lynn HI: Subclavian venipuncture: preventable complications; report of two cases. *Mayo Clin Proc* 45:712–719, 1970.

85. Joynson DHM, Walker DM, Jacobs A, et al: Defect of cell-mediataed immunity in patients with iron-deficiency anaemia. *Lancet* 2:1058–1059, 1972.

86. Kaminski DL, Adams A, Jellinek M: The effect of hyperalimentation on hepatic lipid content and lipogenic enzyme activity in rats and man. *Surgery* 88:93–100, 1980.

87. Kay RG, Tasman-Jones C, Pybus J, et al: A syndrome of acute zinc deficiency during total parenteral alimentation in man. *Ann Surg* 183:331–340, 1976.

88. Kay RG, Tasman-Jones C: Acute zinc deficiency in man during intravenous alimentation. *Aust NZ J Surg* 45:325–330, 1975.

88a. Kern KA, Bower RJ, Atamian S, et al: The effect of a new branched chain-enriched amino acid solution on postoperative catabolism. *Surgery* 92:780–785, 1982.

89. Keys A, Brozek J, Henschel A, et al: *The Biology of Human Starvation.* Minneapolis, University of Minnesota Press, 1950, pp 714–748.

90. Keys A, Brozek J, Henschel A, et al: *The Biology of Human Starvation.* Minneapolis, University of Minnesota Press, 1950, pp 601–606.

91. Kilsell ME: Vitamin B₆ in metabolism of the nervous system. *Ann NY Acad Sci* 166:1–364, 1969.

92. Kim CS, Hill CH: The interrelationship of dietary copper and amine oxidase in the formation of elastin. *Biochem Biophys Res Commun* 24:395–400, 1966.

93. Kinney JM, Long CL, Duke JH: Carbohydrate and nitrogen metabolism after injury. In Porter R, Knight J: *Injury Metabolism in Trauma.* London, J & A Churchill, 1970, p 103.

94. Kinney JM: The metabolic response to injury. In Richards JR, Kinney JM: *Nutritional Aspects of Care in the Critically Ill.* New York, Churchill Livingstone, 1977.

95. Kinney JM: Energy requirements of the surgical patient. In American College of Surgeons, Committee on Pre- and Postoperative Care: *Manual of Surgical Nutrition.* Philadelphia, WB Saunders, 1975, pp 233–234.

96. Klein PD, Johnson RM: Phosphorus metabolism in unsaturated fatty acid deficient rats. *J Biol Chem* 211:103–110, 1954.

97. Klingman AM: Pathologic dynamics of human hair loss. *Arch Dermatol* 83:175–198, 1961.

98. Krishnaswamy K, Naidu AN: Microsomal enzymes in malnutrition as determined by plasma half life of antipyrine. *Br Med J* 1:538–540, 1977.

99. Klahr S, Tipathy K, Garcia FT, et al: On the nature of the renal concentrating defect in malnutrition. *Am J Med* 43:84–95, 1967.

100. Klahr S, Tipathy K, Lotero H: Renal regulation of acid-base in malnourished man. *Am J Med* 48:325–331, 1970.

101. Krieger M: Ueber die Atrophie der menschlichen Organe bei Inanition. *Z Angew Anat Konstitutional* 7:87–134, 1921.

102. Lake AM, Stuart MJ, Oski FA: Vitamin E deficiency and enhanced platelet function. Reversal following E supplementation. *J Pediatr* 90:722–725, 1977.

103. Langer B, McHattie JD, Zohrab WJ, et al: Prolonged survival after complete bowel resection using intravenous alimentation at home. *J Surg Res* 15:226–233, 1973.

104. Law DK, Dudrick SJ, Abdou HI: Immunocompetence of patients with protein-calorie malnutrition: the side effects of nutritional repletion. *Ann Intern Med* 79:545–550, 1973.

104a. Lawson LJ: Parenteral nutrition in surgery. *Br J Surg* 52:795–800, 1965.

105. Leach RM Jr, Muenstes AM, Wien EM: Studies on the role of manganese in bone formation. II. Effect upon chondroitin sulfate syntheses in chick epiphyseal cartilage. *Arch Biochem Biophys* 133:22–28, 1969.

106. Lehninger AL: The enzymatic and morphologic organization of the mitochondria. *Pediatrics* 26:466–475, 1960.

107. Levin PH: A qualitative platelet defect in severe vitamin B₁₂ deficiency. Response, hyperresponse, and thrombosis after vitamin B₁₂ therapy. *Ann Intern Med* 78:533–539, 1973.

108. Levine R: Analysis of the actions of the hormonal antagonists of insulin. *Diabetes* 13:362–365, 1964.

109. Levine R, Haft DE: Carbohydrate homeostasis. *N Engl J Med* 283:175–183, 1970.

110. Linder MC, Munro HN: Iron and copper metabolism during development. *Enzyme* 15:111–138, 1973.

110a. Lindholm M, Rossner S: Rate of elimination of the Intralipid fat emulsion from the circulation in ICU patients. *Crit Care Med* 10:740–746, 1982.

111. Long CL, Schaffel N, Geiger JW, et al: Metabolic response to injury and illness: estimation of energy and protein needs from indirect calorimetry and nitrogen balance. *J Paren Enter Nutr* 3:452–456, 1979.

112. Long CL, Kinney JM, Gerger JW: Nonsuppressability of gluconeogenesis by glucose in septic patients. *Metabolism* 25:193–201, 1976.

113. Long JM III, Wilmore DW, Mason AD Jr, et al: Effect of carbohydrate and fat intake on nitrogen excretion during total parenteral feeding. *Ann Surg* 185:417–422, 1977.

113a. Lopes J, Russell D, Whitwell J, et al: Skeletal muscle function in malnutrition. *Am J Clin Nutr* 36:602–610, 1982.

114. Lowry SF, Brennan MF: Abnormal liver function during parenteral nutrition: relation to infusion excess. *J Surg Res* 26:300–307, 1979.

115. Macht SD: A technique for evaluating sepsis in TPN patients. *J Paren Enter Nutr* 1:92–99, 1977.

116. Maini B, Blackburn GL, Bistrian BR: Cyclic hyperalimentation: an optimal technique for preservation of visceral protein. *J Surg Res* 20:515–525, 1976.

116a. Maiz A, Yamazaki K, Sobrado J, et al: Protein metabolism during total parenteral nutrition in injured rats using medium-chain triglycerides. *Metabolism* 33:901–909, 1984.

117. Marco J, Calle C, Roman D, et al: Hyperglucagonism induced by glucocorticoid treatment in man. *N Engl J Med* 288:128–131, 1973.

118. Mayoral LG, Tripathy K, Bolanos O, et al: Intestinal, functional, and morphologic abnormalities in severely protein-malnourished adults. *Am J Clin Nutr* 25:1084–1091, 1972.

119. McClain CJ: Trace metal abnormalities in adults during hyperalimentation. *J Paren Enter Nutr* 5:424–429, 1981.

120. Mecray PM Jr, Barden RP, Ravdin IS: Nutritional edema: its effect on gastric emptying time before and after gastric operations. *Surgery* 1:53–64, 1927.

121. Meguid M, Brennan MF, Aoki TT, et al: Hormone-substrate interrelationships following trauma. *Arch Surg* 109:776–783, 1974.

122. Meurling S, Plantin LO: The concentrations of trace elements in blood from healthy newborn infants. *Acta Chir Scand* 147:481–485, 1981.

122a. Millikan WJ, Henderson JM, Warren WD, et al: Total parenteral nutrition with FO80 in cirrhotics with subclinical encephalopathy. *Ann Surg* 52:294–304, 1983.

123. Moore FD: *Metabolic Care of the Surgical Patient.* Philadelphia, WB Saunders, 1959, p 460.

124. Moore FD, Steenburg RW, Ball MR, et al: Studies in surgical endocrinology. I. The urinary excretion of 17-hydroxycorticoids, and associated metabolic changes in cases of soft tissue trauma of varying severity and in bone trauma. *Ann Surg* 141:145–174, 1955.

125. Moore FD, Megurd MM: Homeostasis and nutrition in the surgical patient: The metabolic and endocrine re-

sponse to injury. In Byrne JJ, Goldsmith HS: *General Surgery I.* Philadelphia, Harper & Row, 1982.

126. Moore FD: *Metabolic Care of the Surgical Patient.* Philadelphia, WB Saunders, 1959.

127. Moore FD, Ball MR: *The Metabolic Response to Surgery.* Springfield, IL, Charles C Thomas, 1952.

128. Moore FD: Homeostasis: bodily changes in trauma and surgery. In Sabiston DC: *Davis-Christopher Textbook of Surgery,* ed 11. Philadelphia, WB Saunders, 1977, pp 27–64.

129. Moran LR, Thurlow J, Custer P, et al: Nutritional assessment as a predictor of physical performance (abstr). *J Paren Enter Nutr* 3:514, 1980.

130. Moss G: Postoperative metabolism. The role of plasma albumin in the absorption of water and electrolytes. *Pacific Med Surg* 75:355–358, 1967.

131. Mullen JL: Consequences of malnutrition in the surgical patient. *Surg Clin North Am* 61:465–487, 1981.

132. Multivitamin Preparations for Parenteral Use: A statement by the Nutrition Advisory Group. *J Paren Enter Nutr* 3:258–262, 1979.

133. Munro HN: General aspects of the regulation of protein metabolism by diet and hormones. In Munro HN, Allison JB: *Mammalian Protein Metabolism.* New York, Academic Press, 1964, vol 1, pp 381–481.

133a. Nachbauer CA, James JH, Edwards LL, et al: Infusion of branched chain-enriched amino acid solutions in sepsis. *Am J Surg* 147:743–752, 1984.

134. Nielsen FH, Ollerich DA: Nickel: a new essential trace element. *Fed Proc* 33:1767–1772, 1974.

135. Nitowsky HM, Tildon JT, Levin S, et al: Studies of tocopherol deficiency in infants and children. VII. The effect of tocopherol on urinary, plasma, and muscle creatine. *Am J Clin Nutr* 10:368–378, 1962.

136. O'Dell BL, Campbell BJ: Trace elements: metabolism and metabolic function. In Florkin M, Stotz E: *Comprehensive Biochemistry.* New York, Elsevier North-Holland, 1971, p 223.

137. Oji N, Shreeve WW: Gluconeogenesis from 14-C and 3-H-labeled substrates in normal and cortisone-treated rats. *Endocrinology* 78:765–772, 1966.

138. Olson RE: Proceeding of a conference on beriberi. *Fed Proc* 17 (Suppl 2):24–27, 1958.

139. Omdahl JL, Deluca HF: Vitamin D. In Goodheart RS, Shils ME: *Modern Nutrition in Health and Disease,* ed 5. Philadelphia, Lea & Febiger, 1973, pp 158–165.

140. Oppel TW: Studies of biotin metabolism in man; excretion of biotin in human urine, relationship between biotin content of diet and its output in urine and feces; excretion of 2 biotin-like substances in urine. *Am J Med Sci* 204:856–875, 1942.

141. Oppenheimer MJ, Durant TM, Lynch P: Body position in relation to venous air embolism and the associated cardiovascular respiratory changes. *Am J Med Sci* 225:362–373, 1953.

142. Ordway CB: Air embolus via CVP catheter without positive pressure: presentation of case and review. *Ann Surg* 179:479–481, 1974.

143. Owen CA Jr, Tyce GM, Glock EV, et al: Heparin-ascorbic acid antagonism. *Mayo Clin Proc* 45:140–145, 1970.

144. Parsa MH, Habif DV, Ferrer JM, et al: Intravenous hyperalimentation: Indications, technique and complications. *Bull NY Acad Med* 48:920–942, 1972.

145. Paskin DL, Hoffman WS, Tuddenham WJ: A new complication of subclavian vein catheterization. *Ann Surg* 179:266–268, 1974.

146. Passmore R, Nicol BM, Rao MN, et al: Handbook of human nutritional requirements. *WHO Monogr Ser* 0(61):1–66, 1974.

147. Patel SM, Mehl JW, Denel HJ Jr: Studies on carotenoid metabolism; site of conversion of cryptoxanthen to vitamin A in the rat. *Arch Biochem Biophys* 30:103–109, 1951.

148. Peden JC: Present knowledge of iron and copper. *Nutr Rev* 25:321–324, 1967.

149. Peden VH, Witzelben CL, Skelton MA: Total parenteral nutrition. *J Pediatr* 78:180, 1971.

150. Pekarek RS, Sandstead HH, Jacob RA, et al: Abnormal cellular responses during acquired zinc deficiency. *Ann J Clin Nutr* 32:1466–1471, 1979.

151. Perley M, Kipnis DM: Effects of glucocorticoids on plasma insulin. *N Engl J Med* 274:1237–1241, 1966.

152. Popper H: Cholestasis. *Am Rev Med* 19:39–56, 1968.

153. Pories WJ, Strain WH: Zinc and wound healing. In Prasad AS: *Zinc Metabolism.* Springfield, IL, Charles C Thomas, 1966, p 378.

154. Porte D, Robertson RP: Control of insulin secretion by catecholamine, stress, and the sympathetic nervous system. *Fed Proc* 32:1792–1796, 1973.

155. Prasad AS, Miale A Jr, Farid Z, et al: Zinc metabolism in patients with the syndrome of iron deficiency anemia, hepatosplenomegaly, dwarfism, and hypogonadism. *J Lab Clin Med* 61:537–549, 1963.

156. Press M, Hartop PJ, Prottey C: Correction of essential fatty acid deficiency in man by the cutaneous application of sunflower seed oil. *Lancet* 1:597–599, 1974.

156a. Quercia RA, Korn S, O'Neill D, et al: Selenium deficiency and fatal cardiomyopathy in a patient receiving long-term home parenteral nutrition. *Clin Pharmacol* 3:531–535, 1984.

157. Rappazzo ME, Salmi HA, Hall CA: The content of vitamin B_{12} in adult and foetal tissue: a comparative study. *Br J Haematol* 18:425–433, 1970.

158. Rector FC JR: Acidification of the urine. In Orloff J, Berline RW, Geiger SR: *Handbook of Physiology.* Washington, DC, American Physiological Society, 1973, p 447.

159. Reinhardt GF, Myscofski JW, Wilkens DB, et al: Incidence and mortality of hypoalbuminemic patients in hospitalized veterans. *J Paren Enter Nutr* 4:357–359, 1980.

160. Richert DA, Westerfeld WW: Isolation and identification of the xanthene oxidase factor as molybdenum. *J Biol Chem* 203:915–923, 1953.

161. Roels OA, Lui NST: The vitamins. Vitamin A and carotene. In Goodheart RS, Shils ME: *Modern Nutrition in Health and Disease.* ed 5. Philadelphia, Lea & Febiger, 1973, pp 142–157.

162. Roels OA: Present knowledge of vitamin E. In *Present Knowledge in Nutrition,* ed 3. New York, Nutrition Foundation, 1967, pp 86–88.

162a. Ross LH, Griffeth L, Hall RI, et al: Elimination of hepatotoxicity of total parenteral nutrition using fat-carbohydrate mixture. *Surg Forum* 35:97–99, 1984.

163. Rothschild MA, Oratz M, Schreiber SS: Albumin synthesis. *N Engl J Med* 286:748–757, 816–821, 1972.

164. Rudman D, Millikan WJ, Richardson TJ, et al: Elemental balances during intravenous hyperalimentation of underweight adult subjects. *J Clin Invest* 55:94–104, 1975.

165. Rush BF Jr, Richardson JD, Griffen WO: Positive nitrogen balance immediately after abdominal operations. *Am J Surg* 119:70–76, 1970.

166. Ryan JA, Abel RM, Abbott WM, et al: Catheter complications in total parenteral nutrition. *N Engl J Med* 290:757–761, 1974.

167. Sanderson I, Deitel M: Intravenous hyperalimentation without sepsis. *Surg Gynecol Obstet* 136:572–585, 1973.

168. Sanderson I, Deitel M: Insulin response in patients receiving concentrated infusions of glucose and casein hydrolysate for complete parenteral nutrition. *Ann Surg* 179:387–394, 1974.

169. Sauberlich HE, Herman YF, Stevens CO: Thiamine requirements of the adult human. *Am J Clin Nutr* 23:671–672, 1970.

170. Schumner W: The metabolic effects of trauma. *Contemp Surg* 1:39–45, 1972.

171. Schwartz K: Essentiality and metabolic functions of selenium. In Burch RE, Sullivan JF: *The Medical Clinics of North America Symposium on Trace Metals.* Philadelphia, WB Saunders, 1976, pp 745–758.

172. Schwarz K, Milne DB: Growth effect of vanadium in the rat. *Science* 174:426–428, 1971.

173. Schwarz K: Role of vitamin E, selenium, and related factors in experimental nutritional liver diseases. *Fed Proc* 20:58–67, 1965.

174. Seelig MS, Heggtveit HA: Magnesium interrelationships in ischemic heart disease: a review. *Am J Clin Nutr* 27:59–79, 1974.

175. Selvaraj RJ, Bhat KS: Phagocytosis and leukocyte enzymes in protein-calorie malnutrition. *Biochem J* 127:255–259, 1972.

176. Sheldon GF, Peterson SR, Sanders R: Hepatic dysfunction during hyperalimentations. *Arch Surg* 113:504–508, 1978.

176a. Sherwin RS, Hendler RG, Felig P: Effect of ketone infusions on amino acid and nitrogen metabolism. *J Clin Invest* 55:1382–1390, 1975.

177. Shils ME: Experimental human magnesium depletion. *Medicine* 48:61–81, 1969.

178. Shires T, O'Banion J: Successful treatment of massive air embolism producing cardiac arrest. *JAMA* 167:1483–1484, 1958.

179. Silvis SE, Paragas PD Jr: Paresthesias, weakness, seizures, and hypophosphatemia in patients receiving hyperalimentation. *Gastroenterology* 62:513–520, 1972.

180. Skillman JJ, Lauler DP, Hickler RB, et al: Hemorrhage in normal man: effect on renin, cortisol, aldosterone, and urine composition. *Ann Surg* 166:865–885, 1967.

181. Soderhjelm L, Wiese HF, Holman RT: The role of polyunsaturated acids in human nutrition and metabolism. *Prog Chem Fats Other Lipids* 9:555–585, 1970.

182. Steffee WP: Nutritional support in renal failure. *Surg Clin North Am* 61:661–670, 1981.

183. Sunde RA, Hoekstra WG: Structure, synthesis and function of glutathione peroxidase. *Nutr Rev* 38:265–273, 1980.

184. Suttie JW: Mechanism of action of vitamin K: demonstration of a liver precursor of prothrombin. *Science* 179:192–194, 1973.

184a. Tao RC, Yoshimura NN: Carnitine metabolism and its application in parenteral nutrition. *J Parent Enter Nutr* 4:469–486, 1980.

185. Tappel AL: Free-radical lipid peroxidation damage and its inhibition by vitamin E and selenium. *Fed Proc* 20:58–67, 1965.

186. Tashiro T, Ogata H, Yokoyama H, et al: The effects of fat emulsion on essential fatty acid deficiency during intravenous hyperalimentation in pediatric patients. *J Pediatr Surg* 10:203–213, 1975.

187. Tillotson JA, Baker EM: An enzymatic measurement of the riboflavin status in man. *Am J Clin Nutr* 25:425–431, 1972.

188. Todd WR, Elvehjem CA, Hart EB: Zinc in the nutrition of the rat. *Am J Physiol* 107:146–156, 1934.

189. Touloukian RJ, Downing SE: Cholestasis associated with long term parenteral hyperalimentation. *Arch Surg* 106:56–62, 1973.

190. Travis SF, Sugerman JH, Ruberg RL, et al: Alterations of red cell glycolytic intermediates and oxygen transport as a consequence of hypophosphatemia in patients receiving intravenous hyperalimentation. *N Engl J Med* 285:763–768, 1971.

191. Underwood EJ: *Trace Elements in Human and Animal Nutrition,* ed 3. New York, Academic Press, 1971, p 369.

192. Unger RH, Orci L: Physiology and pathophysiology of glucagon. *Physiol Rev* 56:778–826, 1976.

193. Van Rij AM, McKenzie JM, Thomson CD, et al: Selenium supplementation in total parenteral nutrition. *J Paren Enter Nutr* 5:120–124, 1981.

194. Van Rij AM, Thomson CD, McKenzie JM, et al: Selenium deficiency in total parenteral nutrition. *Am J Clin Nutr* 32:2076–2085, 1979.

194a. Vary TC, Siegel JH, Nakatani T, et al: Regulation of glucose metabolism by altered pyruvate dehydrogenase activity. I. Potential site of insulin resistance in sepsis. *JPEN* 10:351–355, 1986.

195. Vilter RW, Bozian RC, Hess EV, et al: Manifestations of copper deficiency in a patient with systemic sclerosis on intravenous hyperalimentation. *N Engl J Med* 291:188–191, 1974.

196. Vitale JJ, Nakamura M, Hegsted DM: The effect of magnesium deficiency on oxidative phosphorylation. *J Biol Chem* 228:573–576, 1957.

197. Wacker WEC, Parisi AF: Magnesium metabolism. *N Engl J Med* 278:658–662, 712–717, 772–776, 1968.

197a. Wahren J, Jacques D, Desurmont P, et al: Is intravenous administration of branched chain amino acids effective in the treatment of hepatic encephalopathy? *Hepatology* 3:475–480, 1983.

198. Walker BE, Dawson JB, Kelleher J, et al: Plasma and urinary zinc in patients with malabsorption syndromes or hepatic cirrhosis. *Gut* 14:943–948, 1973.

198a. Watson RD, Cannon RA, Kurland GS, et al: Selenium responsive myositis during prolonged home total parenteral nutrition in cystic fibrosis. *J Paren Enter Nutr* 9:58–60, 1985.

199. Waxman S, Corcino JJ, Herbert V: Drugs, toxins, and dietary amino acids affecting vitamin B_{12} or folic acid absorption or utilization. *Am J Med* 48:599–608, 1970.

200. Wayne L, Well JJ, Friedman BI, et al: Vitamin B_6 in internal medicine. *Arch Intern Med* 101:143–155, 1958.

201. Weinberg ED: Iron and susceptibility to infectious disease. *Science* 184:952–956, 1974.

202. Weintraub LR, Conrad ME, Crosby WH: Iron-loading anemia. Treatment with repeated phlebotomies and pyridoxine. *N Engl J Med* 275:169–176, 1966.

203. Weissman C, Askanazi J, Rosenbaum SH: Amino acids and respiration (in press).

204. Welt IO, Stetten D Jr: Effect of cortisone upon rates of glucose production and oxidation in the rat. *J Biol Chem* 197:57–66, 1952.

205. Wigger JH: Hepatic changes in premature infants receiving intravenous alimentation (abstr). Toronto, Pediatric Pathology Club, 1971.

206. Wilmore DW: *The Metabolic Management of the Critically Ill.* New York, Plenum Press, 1977, p 197.

207. Wilmore DW, Moylan JA, Bristow BF, et al: Anabolic effects of human growth hormone and high caloric feedings following thermal injury. *Surg Gynecol Obstet* 138:875–884, 1974.

208. Wright PD, Johnson IDA: The effect of surgical operation on growth hormone levels in a plasma. *Surgery* 77:479–486, 1975.

209. Zidar BL, Shaddus RK, Zeigler Z, et al: Observations on the anemia and neutropenia of human copper deficiency. *Am J Hematol* 3:177–185, 1977.

45

Management of the Critically Ill Marrow Transplant Patient

Carl H. June, M.D.
Craig B. Thompson, M.D., Ph.D.
H. Joachim Deeg, M.D.

The management of the immunosuppressed patient is of increasing importance for intensivists. The average length of hospitalization for marrow transplantation is 4–6 weeks, and ~25% of patients will spend one month in an intensive care unit. Optimal care of the patient during marrow transplantation requires the skills of oncologists, infectious disease specialists, and often, input from intensivists is required, most commonly to assist in the management of renal and pulmonary complications. Marrow transplantation represents a curative attempt at the treatment of malignant diseases of hematopoietic and nonhematopoietic origin, to correct marrow failure of diverse causes, and to treat a variety of genetic disorders (Table 45.1). In this chapter, we will focus on (a) the drugs that are commonly given

during the course of marrow transplantation, and that are otherwise not commonly used in the ICU, (b) management of the immunosuppressed patient, and (c) acute complications such as graft-versus-host disease (GVHD) and hepatic venoocclusive disease (VOD) that are relatively specific to marrow transplantation. Various aspects of marrow transplantation have been reviewed in recent years (1, 14, 19, 33, 45, 49, 55, 80, 81, 83).

Bone marrow transplantation can be divided into three phases consisting of (a) the preparative regimen, (b) marrow aspiration and infusion, and (c) engraftment and subsequent events. Preparative regimens are required both for their immunosuppressive and their antineoplastic potential (90). In order for cells from a genetically different donor to survive

Table 45.1
Applications of Marrow Transplantation

Malignant Disorders	Acquired Nonmalignant Disorders	Inherited Disorders
Acute lymphoblastic leukemia	Aplastic anemia	Ataxia telangietasia
Acute nonlymphoblastic leukemia	Myelofibrosis	Blackfan-Diamond anemia
Chronic granulocytic leukemia	Paroxysmal nocturnal hemoglobinuria	Chediak-Higashi syndrome
Hairy cell leukemia	Pure red cell aplasia	Chronic granulomatous disease
Histiocytosis X		Chronic mucocutaneous candidiasis
Hodgkin's disease		Congenital agranulocytosis
Myelodysplastic syndrome		Congenital red cell aplasia
Myeloma		Fanconi's anemia
Neuroblastoma		Gaucher's disease
Non-Hodgkin's lymphoma		Infantile agranulocytosis
Selected "solid" tumors		Metachromatic leukodystrophy
		Mucopolysaccharidosis types I,II,VI
		Osteopetrosis
		Severe combined immunodeficiency
		Sickle cell anemia
		Thalassemia
		Wiskott-Aldrich syndrome

and replicate, the patient's immune system must be paralyzed or eradicated. To achieve this, immunosuppressive therapy ("conditioning") is given in preparation for the marrow infusion. For autologous (self) marrow transplantation, the regimen need only to be optimized for maximal tumor eradication since there is no immunological barrier to overcome. One advantage of chemotherapy in the setting of marrow transplantation is that "supralethal" doses can be given and the patient rescued by marrow infusion, thereby permitting dose escalation in settings in which marrow toxicity is normally the dose-limiting factor (21, 81). In addition, in allogeneic (non-self) transplantation, there is clinical and experimental evidence that the genetic nonidentity may also result in a graft-versus-tumor effect of immunocompetent donor cells (96). Such an effect could of course not be expected with syngeneic (identical twin) or autologous marrow.

The conditioning regimen must be chosen by an experienced clinician with attention to detail in order to avoid potentially lethal complications. For example, patients with Fanconi's anemia appear to be overly sensitive to the cytotoxic effects of cyclophosphamide and radiation, and therefore, require specially tailored conditioning protocols (30). In rare cases such as children with severe congenital immunodeficiency syndrome, a preparative regimen is not required and allogeneic engraftment can often be achieved simply by infusion of donor marrow since the patient's immune system is defective. Similarly, some patients with aplastic anemia who have identical twins may be cured simply by infusion of syngeneic marrow.

MODALITIES USED IN MARROW TRANSPLANTATION

Total-Body Irradiation

Conditioning regimens utilized for the treatment of malignant diseases classically have included total body irradiation (TBI) followed or preceded by chemotherapy. Radiation-induced marrow aplasia occurs after exposure to ~300–500 cGy (rad) TBI, and in a single exposure, ~1000 rad (10 Gy, 1 Gray unit = 100 rad) of TBI is the maximum tolerated dose that can be administered without causing lethal extramedullary damage. (Related information

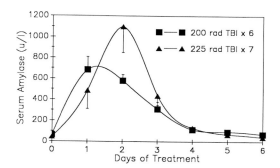

Figure 45.1. Effects of fractionated total-body irradiation (TBI) on serum amylase. Total serum amylase was measured on 30 patients treated with either 200 rad TBI daily for 6 days or 225 rad TBI daily for 7 days as preparation for marrow transplantation. Mean ± SEM is indicated.

may be found in Chapter 42). Because most tumor cells repair radiation-induced DNA damage poorly as compared with normal cells, fractionated doses of TBI permit the administration of higher cumulative doses (82). Severe mucositis, nausea, vomiting, diarrhea, and parotitis commonly develop during the several days following TBI (4, 12, 45, 69, 83). Some patients, particularly those who have been given chemotherapy that may sensitize ("radiation recall") to the effects of radiation, develop dermal erythema and desquamation after TBI. Pancreatitis develops occasionally after TBI. It is not commonly realized the TBI causes elevation of serum amylase levels in all patients following single-dose and fractionated TBI (Fig. 45.1), thus invalidating this commonly performed test in marrow graft recipients in the first week after TBI. The hyperamylasemia following TBI is self-limiting and involves parotid isoforms, so that patients with abdominal pain can still be evaluated for pancreatic disorders if isoenzyme fractionation is done.

Patients are treated with antiemetics to prevent emesis during TBI. Symptomatic relief from diarrhea has been reported with cholestyramine therapy (34). Allopurinol is given and the intravascular volume maintained during TBI in order to prevent tumor lysis syndrome. Approximately 80% of adults will develop reactivation of herpes simplex virus as a superinfection due to the immunosuppression that accompanies radiation-induced mucositis; these patients benefit from prophylactic administration of acyclovir (71). Late complications of TBI include growth retardation, cataracts, infertility, and malignancy (19, 77).

Cyclophosphamide

The most common chemotherapeutic agent employed for conditioning is cyclophosphamide in large doses (81). High-dose cyclophospamide causes nausea, vomiting, and alopecia in all patients. The dose-limiting toxicity, however, is cardiac. Cardiac failure affects equally patients with autologous and allogeneic grafts. Conditioning protocols for marrow transplantation commonly employ total doses of cyclophosphamide of 120–200 mg/kg given over 2–4 days, and at these doses, > 90% of patients develop decreased ECG voltage of the QRS complex, and the incidence of clinically significant cardiac toxicity may be as high as 15% (32). When heart failure develops, it usually occurs in the first week after therapy with cyclophosphamide and is encountered particularly with patients who had prior mediastinal radiation, concurrent TBI, or therapy with anthracylines (13). It has recently been reported that the addition of cytosine arabinoside to the preparative regimen also potentiates the cardiac toxicity of cyclophosphamide (87). Clinically, patients develop tachycardia, rapid weight gain, cardiomegaly with or without a pericardial effusion, a loss of voltage on surface ECG, and a decrease in ejection fracton (13). The syndrome is acute and often refractory to therapy. Most patients die within a week of onset of symptoms. It is therefore important to carefully evaluate the past medical history in order to avoid cardiac toxicity from cyclophosphamide. There is evidence that the development of cardiac toxicity correlates better with dose per body surface area than with weight, and that in the absence of TBI, the maximum tolerated dose of cyclophosphamide is 1.55 g/m^2/day for 4 days (32).

Other potential complications of high-dose cyclophosphamide therapy are also of importance. Plasma cholinesterase can be depleted and, as a consequence, the clearance of local anesthetics or neuromuscular blocking agents may be substantially prolonged (22, 103). Plasma cholinesterase levels should be measured, if possible, prior to any surgical procedure in a patient who has recently been prepared for marrow transplantation.

Hemorrhagic cystitis of varying severity occurs in ~30% of patients after high-dose cyclophosphamide. Therapy of cystitis is difficult as patients are thrombocytopenic, and in extreme cases, fulguration, bilateral nephrostomies, and even cystectomy may be required. Cystitis is mostly related to the cyclophosphamide metabolite acrolein. In order to minimize or prevent cystitis, a three-way Foley catheter should be inserted and the bladder continuously irrigated and drained. In addition, a brisk saline diuresis is initiated before administration of cyclophosphamide. Mesna (2-mercaptoethane sodium sulfonate), an investigational drug that acts as a sulfhydryl donor, has been shown to be effective in most instances in preventing cystitis (36). Mesna appears to have a role in patients who are particularly predisposed to hemorrhagic cystitis such as those with Fanconi's anemia (20, 30); however, it is not yet available commercially in this country.

In the differential diagnosis of hematuria, in addition to cyclophosphamide and the usual causes of hematuria, other disorders more specific to the marrow transplant patient should be considered. Reactivation of the BK type of human polyoma virus has recently been reported to be a common cause of hematuria in patients with allogeneic but not autologous marrow grafts (2). In addition, infection with other viruses such as adenovirus should be excluded. Hematuria that occurs in association with hypertension may be caused by radiation-induced nephritis (6). Finally, some patients develop the syndrome of inappropriate secretion of antidiuretic hormone or nephrogenic diabetes insipidus in association with high-dose cyclophosphamide treatment (26).

Treatment with cyclophosphamide alone (200 mg/kg) is sufficiently immunosuppressive to allow allogeneic engraftment, and is used without TBI as the conditioning regimen of choice for patients with aplastic anemia (61, 83). Similarly, in combination with busulfan, cyclophosphamide has been used successfully as a conditioning protocol for patients with acute nonlymphocytic leukemia (68). In attempts to increase tumor kill, other agents such as cytosine arabinoside, etoposide (VP-16), daunomycin, and BCNU have been added to preparative regimens, or substituted for cyclophosphamide. The addition of these drugs, particularly in combination, often causes a substantial increase in acute toxicity that is frequently manifest as hepatic VOD (see "Veno-occulsive Disease").

Cyclosporine

Cyclosporine is the first agent that has reversible immunosuppressive effects that are relatively specific for T lymphocytes (3, 62). It is approved by the Food and Drug Administration (FDA) to be used for prevention of solid-organ rejection. In patients given marrow transplantation, it is commonly used, non-FDA approved, to prevent or treat GVHD and to reduce the risk of marrow graft rejection. Cyclosporine is most effective when given with other agents such as glucocorticoids or methotrexate (see "Methotrexate"). The drug is usually administered intravenously beginning several days before marrow transplantation. The drug is water insoluble; when administered orally, it must be given with lipids such as olive oil or milk in order to promote absorption. There can be severe impairments of cyclosporine absorption after marrow transplantation due to chemoradiotherapy-induced enteritis and to intestinal GVHD (99). Patients commonly have trough serum or whole blood cyclosporine levels measured by radioimmunoassay (RIA) two or three times weekly during the first month after transplantation. The dose is adjusted to maintain serum levels at ~100 ng/ml in order to minimize nephrotoxicity, although there is little information currently available to support the concept of "therapeutic" levels. The drug has a large volume of distribution and is predominantly metabolized in the liver. It is subject to enterohepatic recirculation and only a small fraction is excreted by the kidneys (99). Plasma clearance is age related; children require higher doses on a milligram-per-kilogram basis than do adults.

A number of drug-drug interactions have been reported (15, 62). Ketoconazole, cimetidine, diltiazem, and oral contraceptives have been reported to increase the plasma concentration of cyclosporine. Rifampin, trimethoprim, phenobarbital, and phenytoin may reduce the concentration of cyclosporine.

The hallmark of cyclosporine toxicity is renal impairment that is first recognized by an asymptomatic increase in the serum creatinine concentration. This is usually associated with increased serum levels of cyclosporine. Renal toxicity is potentiated by aminoglycosides and amphotericin B, and therefore, dose reduction is often necessary when given concurrently with drugs such as aminoglycosides, vancomycin, or amphotericin B (15, 40). Severe hypomagnesemia due to renal magnesium wasting is common in patients treated with cyclosporine after marrow transplantation but not after renal transplantation (38). Cyclosporine causes arterial hypertension, especially in patients treated concomitantly with glucocorticoids (37, 44). In the treatment of cyclosporine-induced hypertension it is best to avoid diuretics and β-blockers that may precipitate or exacerbate renal impairment, to correct serum magnesium levels, and give calcium channel antagonists such as nifedipine. Hepatotoxicity has been ascribed to cyclosporine and is manifest by conjugated hyperbilirubinemia; in this setting, it must be distinguished from VOD and GVHD (62). Neurotoxicity consisting of tremor, seizures, and cerebellar symptoms has been reported and may in some cases be secondary to hypomagnesemia (84). Some patients experience paresthesia in palms and soles with intravenous infusion of cyclosporine that is likely due to cremophore, the vehicle used to dissolve cyclosporine.

Methotrexate

Methotrexate is commonly given to marrow transplant patients for the prevention of GVHD and for the treatment of leukemia involving the central nervous system. Until recently a standard regimen involved the use of methotrexate; 15 mg/m² on day 1 and 10 mg/m² on days 3, 6, 11; and then biweekly for the first 3 months after transplant for the prevention of GVHD (76, 83). For the prevention of CNS leukemia intrathecal methotrexate is often given 12 mg/m² for two doses before transplantation and approximately five doses biweekly beginning 1 month after transplantation. The use of methotrexate in the general oncology patient in such modest doses would ordinarily be expected to result in little toxicity. The marrow transplant patient is, however, subject to rapid deterioration in renal function, generally from the concurrent administration of nephrotoxic agents, or from the sudden accumulation of ascites from VOD. It is important therefore for the intensivist to realize that decreased renal function and third-space fluids have profound impact on the pharmacokinetics of methotrexate that may severely aggravate mucositis and impair or prevent hematopoietic recovery. Folinic acid is an antidote of methotrexate and may be used to prevent toxicity in cases of delayed renal excretion. Serum methotrexate levels should be obtained 24 hours after each dose, and if the level is $> 5 \times 10^{-8}$ M, therapy is started with folinic acid. Methotrexate levels should again be obtained at 48 hours and if the level remains elevated, folinic acid "rescue" continued. (Further details on the pharmacology of methotrexate can be found in Chapter 29.)

Antibody Therapy

Polyclonal immune serum globulin (ISG) or antilymphocyte immunoglobulin (ALG) antibodies or murine monoclonal antibodies are used with increasing frequency in marrow transplant patients (Table 45.2). ISG consists of purified human immunoglobulin preparations derived from multiple donors. ISG and CMV hyperimmune globulin, obtained from donors with high titers of antibodies to cytomegalovirus, are currently being tested in marrow transplant patients in order to prevent viral and bacterial infections. Both ISG and CMV hyperimmune globulin have been shown to prevent seroconversion and prevent intersitial pneumonitis in patients who are not infected with CMV before marrow transplantation (10, 98). However, the same effect can be achieved in CMV-seronegative transplant patients by giving CMV-negative blood products and by avoiding the use of CMV-positive marrow donors when possible (10). The role of ISG in the prevention of CMV pneumonia in seropositive patients is controversial. Complications from ISG are unusual, although patients can develop a positive Coombs test during therapy because ISG may contain red cell isoagglutinins (anti-A, anti-B and anti-A,B antibodies) (101).

ALG, usually prepared from horses or goats immunized with human lymphocytes or thymocytes, is used to treat acute GVHD. ALG is also used to treat patients with aplastic anemia who are not candidates for marrow transplantation. ALG, in contrast to ISG, is highly toxic. A test dose of 0.1 ml of ALG and normal horse serum (both diluted 1:1000 in normal saline) is given intradermally as two separate injections in order to test for an immediate hypersensitivity reaction; a positive reaction consists of any systemic symptoms or local erythema and/or wheal formation > 10 mm to both horse serum, and ALG is a contraindication for therapy due to the risk of anaphylaxis. Patients must be premedicated with antipyretics and corticosteriods as severe febrile reactions are common during antibody infusion. Other major complications of ALG include thrombocytopenia and the development of serum sickness. In addition, ALG often contains antibodies to human marrow progenitor cells and can result in graft failure. Lymphocytes in the peripheral blood are rare or undectectable during therapy with ALG, and therefore patients are severely immunosuppressed and prone to infection.

ALG often is effective for treatment of GVHD that has been refractory to other therapy. By nature of the production process, however, ALG batches may differ significantly with regard to efficacy and toxicity.

Murine monoclonal antibodies are increasingly used because of specificity and lack of lot-to-lot variability. OKT3 is the first murine monoclonal antibody that has been approved by the FDA for prevention of solid-organ-graft rejection, and it is used without FDA approval to prevent or treat acute GVHD (25, 47). OKT3 is directed against the CD3 T cell antigen, and like ALG, is a potent immunosuppressant because it clears T cells from the circulation and blocks their biological effects. An acute symptom complex consisting of chills and high-grade fever occurs in nearly all patients with the first dose. This reaction is probably caused by lymphokines that are released upon destruction of lymphocytes. In severe cases, hypotension and pulmonary edema occur. As with ALG, patients should be premedicated with antipyretics and corticosteroids prior to therapy with OKT3. Delayed toxicity from OKT3 can also be formidable. Patients often develop antibodies to the murine antibody that prevent further therapy. In addition, potent immunosuppression may result in the development of lymphomas. The lymphomas are usually of B-cell origin and appear to be due to Epstein-Barr virus reactivation. They are unusual in renal transplant recipients and may be more common in marrow transplant patients, particularly those given prolonged courses of therapy (47, 67). Serum sickness also occurs 2–3 weeks after therapy in some patients, although this is unusual in marrow transplant patients, perhaps because they are unable to mount a sufficient immune response.

MARROW ABLATION

The major difference between bone marrow transplation and cardiac and renal transplantation is that the conditioning protocol ablates rather than suppresses the host immune and hematopoetic systems. The intent of a successful marrow transplant is to reconstitute the hematoimmunopoetic system of the recipient with donor-derived hematopoetic and immu-

Table 45.2
Experimental Use of Immunoglobulins in Marrow Transplantation[a]

Antibody Preparation	Dose (mg/kg)	Indication	Comments	Reference
Polyclonal antibodies				
Hyperimmune CMV	0.1–0.15 g/kg i.v. every 1–3 weeks	Prevention of CMV infection	Appears more effective when combined with ganciclovir (DHPG)	10
Immune globulin	0.5–1.5 g/kg i.v. every 2–3 weeks	Chronic GVHD, prevention of CMV infection	May cause false-positive Coombs test	99
Antilymphocyte globulin	15 mg/kg i.v. q.o.d. for 7 doses	Acute GVHD, aplastic anemia	Premedicate with methylprednisolone 1 mg/kg i.v. and give diphenhydramine and acteominophen p.r.n. Chills, fever and thrombocytopenia are common, serum sickness, pulmonary edema and hypotension occur occasionally	60
Monoclonal antibodies				
CD3 (OKT3)	5 mg/day i.v. for 2 weeks	Acute GVHD	Premedicate for first dose with methylprednisolone and acetominophen; side effects similar to ATG	25
CD18 (anti-LFA-1)	0.1 mg/kg i.v. daily for 5 doses	Prevention of graft failure		28

[a]These agents are being tested experimentally and should only be used on an investigational basis. GVHD, graft-versus-host disease; CMV, cytomegalovirus; ATG, antithymocyte globulin.

nological precursors. The most serious complications that result from marrow ablation are bleeding and infection (Table 45.3) (23, 49, 86).

Bleeding Complications

Bleeding complications result primarily from the combination of thrombocytopenia and mucosal damage. Thrombocytopenia occurs as a necessary side effect of all conditioning regimens and develops within a week following initiation of therapy. Platelet transfusions are then necessary to support the patient's platelet count and prevent bleeding complications until the third or fourth week post-transplant platelet, when production usually becomes self-sustaining. Bleeding that occurs in the first several weeks post-transplant is usually from mucosal surfaces that have been damaged as a result of the conditioning regimen. Mucosal damage can be worsened in the early transplant period by multiple factors such as herpes simplex stomatitis, methotrexate therapy for the prevention of GVHD, and the onset of acute GVHD itself. Serious internal bleeding as a result of clotting factor deficiencies is not common in the setting of marrow transplantation, presumably because of the plasma present in the other blood products the patients receive,

the relatively long half-life of the clotting proteins, and extramedullary sources of factor production.

Several syndromes are now recognized that may cause a delayed risk of bleeding as a result of recurrent thrombocytopenia. As many as 37% of patients after transplantation will develop an isolated acquired thrombocytopenia that occurs more than a month after marrow infusion and subsequent to the initial recovery of the megakaryocytic lineage (27). In some patients this has been attributed to the suppressive effects of concomitant cytotoxic drug therapy. Trimethoprim/sulfamethoxazole has been implicated in several cases of transient drug-induced thrombocytopenia. Transient thrombocytopenia has also been associated with acute GVHD due to both marrow suppression and to decreased platelet survival. A more chronic and persistent form of thrombocytopenia can present in as many as a quarter of bone marrow transplant survivors that develop chronic GVHD, and is associated with a poor prognosis.

Topical agents such as thrombin, sucralfate, and silver nitrate are often used as therapy of mucosal bleeding. The mainstay of therapy for the treatment of bleeding complications of marrow transplantation, however, is the transfusion of platelets and red cells. In addition to the usual serology for hepatitis B and HIV,

Table 45.3
Major Post-transplant Periods and Their Associated Complications[a]

	Early (0–30 days)	Middle (30–100 days)	Late (>100 days)
Patient Condition	Patient usually hospitalized the entire period; central venous access required for support	Patient usually can be followed in a closely monitored outpatient setting	Patient usually independent of i.v. support and able to return to care by referring physician. If all goes well, a patient should be able to resume full activities, including work and school, by 1 yr.
Requirements	Complete transfusion support; hyperalimentation; vigorous hygiene and/or isolation; pain control; surveillance cultures and/or prophylactic antibiotics	Available transfusion and alimentary support (central venous access maintained); limited external contact; physiological support; frequent observation and monitoring; antibiotic prophylaxis for *P. carinii* and encapsulated organisms	Continued bacterial prophylaxis for 1 yr; regular visits with referring physician; periodic visits with marrow transplant unit
Major Complications	Bacterial infection; fungal infections; herpes simplex; stomatitis/cystitis; veno-occlusive disease of the liver	Acute GVHD; interstitial pneumonia; CMV infection	Chronic GVHD; relapse; bacterial infections with encapsulated organisms; varicella zoster; cataracts

[a] From Thompson CB, Thomas ED: Bone marrow transplantation. *Surg Clin North Am* 66:589–601, 1986.

etc., it is important that the products be evaluated for cytomegalovirus (see "Infections Complications"). Finally, a unique risk of transfusion therapy in marrow graft recipients is the possibility that red cells and platelets will contain sufficient "passenger" lymphocytes to cause GVHD (95). To avoid this complication, all blood products which transplant patients receive for at least the first year after marrow transplantation should be irradiated (2000 rad) to prevent proliferation of the transfused immune cells.

There is frequently ABO incompatibility of donor and recipient in allogeneic marrow grafts because of the independent inheritance of the ABO and HLA regions. This is managed by either removing the red blood cells from the bone marrow to be infused or using procedures to deplete the recipient of isoagglutinins (5, 8). Both procedures are effective in preventing transfusion reactions at the time of bone marrow infusion. If required, isoagglutinins in the donor's marrow can be removed by separating cells from the plasma. Conversion to the donor's ABO blood group can usually be expected to occur within 2–3 months following marrow engraftment. In cases of ABO incompatibility with the marrow donor, the patient is usually supported with recipient type or group O blood products, and units are screened and selected to prevent transfusion of units containing high titer anti-AB antibodies. Blood products can also be concentrated to minimize plasma content. Once a significant proportion of circulating red blood cells is of donor type, a switch in red cell transfusion can be made to the donor's blood group. In addition, the presence of circulating blood cells of donor type can be used as evidence of successful allogeneic marrow engraftment.

Infectious Complications

In the early post-transplant period, the principal infectious complications are associated with granulocytopenia (23, 49). Following ablation and reinfusion of marrow, granulocyte counts are less than 0.1×10^9/liter for ~2 weeks. The granulocyte count does not usually exceed 1×10^9/liter until the third or fourth week after transplant. A rise in the serum transcobalamin II level procedes the rise in the peripheral granulocyte count and therefore may serve as an early marker of marrow regeneration (53). The use of cyclosporine rather than methotrexate for GVHD prophylaxis has short-

ened this period of severe neutropenia. The disruption of mucosal immunity as a result of the toxic effects of the conditioning regimen on the gastrointestinal mucosa contributes to the risk of infection. Long-term indwelling central venous catheters, used in virtually all patients, also provide a portal for infection (59). This early period of neutropenia is usually characterized by bacterial infections predominantly of a bacteremic nature and occasional fungal infections. The hallmark of bacteremia in this early neutropenic period is fever, and with the initial manifestation of a fever patients are treated with broad spectrum antibiotics that confer converage consistent with the epidemiological experience of the transplant center. Therapy is maintained until appropriate culture information has been obtained and a suitable antibiotic choice can be made, or until neutropenia resolves. Fever unresponsive to therapy with broad-spectrum antibiotics after 72 hours and the absence of microbiological diagnosis often warrants the addition of systemic antifungal therapy. The most common viral infection in the early post-transplant period is herpes simplex (HSV). Oropharyngeal herpes simplex infection often causes severe local disease that predisposes to secondary bacterial infections and may spread to involve both the esophagus and the lungs. The use of acyclovir for both treatment and prophylaxis of HSV infections has substantially reduced this complication of the early post-transplant period (71).

Following the recovery of neutropenia as a result of successful marrow engraftment, the spectrum of organisms that induces infectious complications in marrow transplant recipients shifts. Bacterial infections with enteric pathogens remain common in the intermediate time period, however, infections resulting from encapsulated bacterial organisms and *Pneumocystis carinii*, which were previously seen in high frequency during this time period, are now seen rarely because of the instigation of trimethoprim/sulfamethoxazole prophylaxis. A variety of fungal infections can occur in this time period. While infection with *Candida* and *Aspergillus* species are most common, a number of rare fungal infections caused by organisms usually considered "nonpathogenic" have been reported.

The most serious of the infections during this intermediate time period are the viral infections. Reactivation or primary infection with cytomegalovirus (CMV) is the most severe of the infections, with CMV pneumonia occurring in approximately 15% of all patients undergoing allogeneic marrow transplantation and having an approximate 85% fatality rate. Other viruses that occur frequently in this time period are adenovirus and Epstein-Barr virus (EBV). Fatal lymphoproliferative diseases associated with EBV infection have occurred, predominantly in patients treated with either antithymocyte globulin or anti-T-cell monoclonal antibodies for the treatment of acute GVHD (47, 70). Some of the lymphomas appear to respond to therapy with acylcovir and discontinuation of immunosuppressive therapy.

The final period of infectious complications from marrow transplantation begins 3–4 months after transplantation at a time when the marrow graft is fully established and mucosal injury has been repaired. Bacterial infections at this time are usually associated with the development of chronic GVHD and include frequent sinopulmonary infections thought to be related to IgA deficiency and sicca syndromes. In addition, the presence of functional hyposplenia or asplenia that occurs in most patients in combination with a naive immune system predisposes to spontaneous bacteremias associated with encapsulated organisms. Most patients receive trimethoprim/sulfamethoxazole, daily oral penicillin, or infusions of immune serum globulins as prophylaxis. The major viral syndrome associated with this time period is the recurrence of varicella-zoster, which occurs in approximately one-third of all patients and in half of patients with chronic GVHD. Virtually all of these infections are due to reactivation of latent virus, although the clinical syndrome may resemble that of primary varicella infection. It is important for the physician caring for these patients to remember that it takes at least a year for the immune system to fully develop after successful transplantation, and that live viral vaccines are contraindicated. The tempo of immune recovery is delayed, however, in patients who develop chronic GVHD. Vaccinations involving killed organisms are unlikely to be effective.

ACUTE GRAFT-VERSUS-HOST DISEASE

Background and Epidemiology

For graft-versus-host diseases (GVHD) to occur, three conditions must be met (7): (a) Immunocompetent cells, capable of replication must be transferred from one individual to another. (b) There must be a histoincompatibility between the two individuals. (c) The recipient must be unable to reject and destroy the transferred cells. All those requirements are met with allogeneic marrow transplantation, as well as in some instances of blood (leukocyte) transfusions to patients who receive chemotherapy or fetuses who receive accidental intrauterine maternofetal transfusions or therapeutic exchange transfusions (95). Unexpectedly a GVHD-like syndrome has also been observed occasionally with syngeneic transplants or autologous marrow reinfusion (35).

GVHD is more frequent and often more severe in patients who are given an HLA-nonidentical ("mismatched") transplant. For unclear reasons the incidence of GVHD increases with age. It is conjectural whether the probability of GVHD is influenced by the patient's original diagnosis or whether GVHD is more frequent in male patients given a graft from a female donor (18).

GVHD can occur in an acute form, usually within 2–8 weeks (31) or in a chronic form which generally develops within 3 months to 1 year of transplantation (79). Often acute GVHD will progress into the chronic form. The present discussion will be limited to acute GVHD.

Pathophysiology

Donor T lymphocytes react to recipient histocompatibility antigens, proliferate, and attack recipient tissues, leading to tissue damage and the clinical syndrome of GVHD. The immunological attack, usually associated with organ dysfunction, subsides as donor T cells begin to accept the new environment as "self". The onset of GVHD is associated with the presence of nonspecific suppressor cells that are replaced by specific (host-directed) suppressor cells as tolerance develops and GVHD resolves. GVHD and nonspecific suppression are associated with profound immunoincompetence, while patients regain immunocompetence with the emergence of specific suppressor T cells (88, 89). Damage suffered by target organs may require prolonged periods of time for complete healing.

It is thought that acute GVHD can be aggravated and propagated by cross-reactivity of donor T cells with microorganisms contaminating skin and gastrointestinal tract (91). There is experimental and clinical evidence that the treatment of patients in laminar airflow isolation rooms and attempts at decontamination of skin and intestinal tract decreases the incidence and severity of acute GVHD (75). Exposure to ultraviolet light with sunburn may initiate or cause chronic GVHD to flare.

Clinical Spectrum of the Disease

The three major target organs are the skin, liver, and intestinal tract. Clinical onset is often marked by pruritus and a maculopapular rash that characteristically involves palms and soles but may spread over the entire body. The median time to onset of the rash is ~19 days after marrow infusion. The rash can progress to bullae and burn-like blister formation. Breakdown of the skin may result in considerable fluid, electrolyte, and protein loss and further increase the risk of infections. In some patients, in particular after HLA incompatible transplants or if no GVHD prophylaxis is given, GVHD can present within a few days of transplantation in a hyperacute form (78). These patients have high fever, hyperemia of skin and internal organs, diffuse edema, and may appear quite toxic. Presumably, there is endothelial damage and capillary leak associated with this syndrome (58). With hepatic GVHD the only symptom may be right-upper-quadrant pain. Often there is a striking rise of serum bilirubin (indirect and direct) associated with elevated serum alkaline phosphatase, aspartate

aminotransferase, and γ-glutamyltranspeptidase. Liver dysfunction can progress relentlessly and lead to hepatic encephalopathy and, in rare instances, death due to hepatic failure.

The first intestinal manifestation is usually diarrhea; however, patients may present with nausea and vomiting, often associated with abdominal pain and distension. In severe cases paralytic ileus may develop. Lesions in the gastrointestinal tract range from single-cell necrosis of mucosal epithelial cells and crypt abscesses to diffuse mucosal denudation (66). The mucosal damage may be so profound that drugs normally considered nonabsorbable, such as vancomycin and oral aminoglycosides, may achieve potentially nephrotoxic serum concentrations (63). The stool often is of greenish color. The fluid and electrolyte loss may be severe with stool volumes up to several liters per day (45).

A grading scheme for severity of GVHD is given in Table 45.4 (18, 31, 83). The grading system is based upon the degree of individual organ dysfunction of the skin, liver, and intestinal tract, and on overall performance status so that a clinical grade II would be assigned to a patient with 1^+ to 3^+ skin rash, 1^+ gut or 1^+ liver involvement (or both), and a mild decrease in performance status. In cases where the severity of one organ-related symptom differs widely from that in another, the overall clinical grade assigned is that of the most severely affected organ. For example, a patient with a serum bilirubin concentration of 20 mg/dl, severe intestinal cramping and 1^+ skin

Table 45.4
Clinical Grading of Acute GVHD

Organ	Extent of Involvement		Severity	I	II	III	IV
	Grading by Organ System				Overall Clinical Grade		
Skin	Rash (% of body surface)	<25	1+	x	x		
		25–50	2+	x	x	x	x
		>50	3+		x	x	x
	Desquamation		4+				x
Liver	Bilirubin (mg%)	2–3	1+		x		
		3–6	2+			x	x
		6–15	3+			x	x
		>15	4+				x
Intestine	Diarrhea (ml/day)	>500	1+		x		
		>1000	2+			x	x
		>1500	3+			x	x
	Pain/Ileus		4+			x	x
	Impairment of Performance		1+		x		
			2+			x	
			3+				x

involvement (rash limited to the palms and soles) would be assigned an overall clinical grade IV. The incidence of moderate to severe (grades II to IV) GVHD in patients given HLA-matched marrow varies from ~30–50%. Grade I acute GVHD is often self-limited and may not require any specific therapy. In contrast, mortality with grade IV acute GVHD is ~90%.

Differential Diagnosis

The fully developed picture of acute GVHD with typical involvement of skin, intestinal tract, and liver is clinically quite specific. However, all these organs can be affected by other diseases, and when only a single organ is involved the diagnosis is more difficult. A tissue biopsy with characteristic histology often (but not always) will be helpful. Histologically, the skin alterations due to radiochemotherapy cannot be differentiated reliably from GVHD until about 2½ weeks post-transplant. Viral exanthems and drug reactions can resemble GVHD. The typical involvement of palms and soles is often helpful. Hepatic dysfunction after transplantation can have numerous causes. It may be related to chemoradiotherapy given in preparation for transplantation and must be differentiated from VOD, which usually develops within 1–3 weeks of transplant or from cyclosporine-induced hyperbilirubinemia (45). In patients conditioned with high-dose cyclophosphamide there may be a transient rise of serum bilirubin and lactate dehydrogenase (but not other enzymes) due to hemolysis. It may be difficult or impossible to differentiate non-A, non-B hepatitis from hepatic GVHD. Hepatic biopsy—if not contraindicated by thrombocytopenia or ascites—may be helpful.

The intestinal tract can be severely affected by chemoradiotherapy, resulting in nausea, vomiting, and profuse diarrhea, often lasting through the first week post-transplant. If diarrhea persists longer than 1 week an infectious cause or GVHD must be considered. Pathogens such as adenovirus, coxsackievirus, and rotavirus that often cause mild diarrhea can cause severe infection in marrow graft recipients (100). GVHD may be a diagnosis of exclusion unless a rectal or endoscopic gastric/duodenal biopsy reveals characteristic changes of GVHD (65). Biopsy is not useful in the diagnosis of GVHD in the first 3 weeks after transplantation as histologic abnormalities due to the conditioning therapy may be confused with GVHD; in the absence of GVHD, intestinal histology be-

comes normal by day 21 after transplantation (45).

Prevention

The classic approach to GVHD prevention has been the administration of immunosuppressive drugs to the patient following infusion of bone marrow. Several agents used in a standard fashion or on an experimental basis are listed in Table 45.5.

The use of methotrexate was described previously. Alternatively, cyclophosphamide has been given at 7.5 mg/m² on days 1, 3, 5, 9 and then weekly (67). With this approach the incidence of acute GVHD has ranged from 40 to 70%. Although the usefulness of both methotrexate and cyclophosphamide for GVHD prevention has at times been questioned (43), it is now generally accepted that omission of GVHD prophylaxis results in a very high incidence of GVHD and transplant related mortality (78). Both drugs are myelosuppressive, which may delay hemopoietic recovery, and both can prolong or aggravate mucositis.

More recently, cyclosporine, a new drug apparently lacking marrow toxicity, has been used widely for GVHD prophylaxis (3, 62). Initially only a poorly tolerated intramuscular preparation and an oral preparation with a bioavailability of approximately 27% were used. Subsequently an intravenous preparation became available. Several randomized studies compared cyclosporine (3–5 mg/kg/day intravenously or 10–12.5 mg/kg/day orally) with either methotrexate or cyclophosphamide and failed to show significant differences in the incidence of GVHD (reviewed in 17, 62).

Table 45.5
Drugs for Prevention and Treatment of Graft-versus-Host Disease

Methotrexate
Azathioprine
6-Mercaptopurine
2-Deoxycoformicin
Cyclophosphamide
Procarbazine
Cytosine arabinoside
Chlorambucil
L-Asparaginase
Glucocorticoids
Cyclosporine
Antithymocyte globulin (ATG)
Monoclonal antibodies
4-Hydroperoxycyclophosphamide
Thalidomide

Next, several agents were combined in an attempt to improve results. A combination of methotrexate, prednisone, and antithymocyte globulin significantly reduced the incidence of GVHD to 21% as compared with 48% in a control group given methotrexate only (60). With a regimen of methotrexate on days 1, 3, 6, and 11 combined with daily cyclosporine starting the day before marrow infusion the incidence of acute GVHD in two trials was 33% and 18% respectively compared with 54% and 53% in the control arms given single-agent cyclosporine or methotrexate respectively (73, 74). Similar results are achieved with combinations of cyclosporine and methylprednisolone (29).

Other agents listed in Table 45.5 have so far only been used experimentally. For example, thalidomide, initially used as a sedative, was found to be effective in the treatment of hypersensitivity reactions that occur during the treatment of leprosy. The immunosuppressive effects of thalidomide were tested in rats given marrow transplants and found to be effective in the therapy of GVHD (92). A more recent approach to GVHD has been the elimination of T lymphocytes in vitro from the donor marrow (9). A major benefit of this technique is that the profound immunosuppression associated with drug administration that renders patients highly susceptible to infections, by viral, bacterial, fungal, and protozoan organisms could be avoided. Of concern, however, is the observation that this approach may result in an increased graft failure rate (in some reports 30–40%) not only with HLA-incompatible but even with HLA-identical transplants (9, 57). A second concern is that an increased recurrence rate of leukemia was reported for both chronic myelocytic leukemia and acute leukemias, which were presumably due to the loss of graft-versus-leukemic effect.

Treatment

The development of acute GVHD, unless it is mild and self-limited, always presents a dilemma. GVHD by itself is immunosuppressive, the patient is usually receiving immunosuppressive drugs for GVHD prophylaxis, and finally, virtually all known therapeutic options for GVHD again involve immunosuppressive drugs (17). All this sets the stage for overwhelming infectious complications and interstitial pneumonitis (51). Although there is no clear indication that the response to treatment is more likely with early institution

of therapy, it is likely that progression of GVHD will cause more tissue damage and increase the probability of infection. It is generally agreed that acute GVHD of grades II–IV requires treatment. Glucocorticoids, ATG, cyclosporine, and monoclonal antibodies are being used widely. With individual drugs, generally either glucocorticoids or ATG, responses are achieved in 30% of patients. With combinations of drugs such as cyclosporine plus ATG as many as 60% of patients have responded. The usual dose of methylprednisolone is 2 mg/kg/day in divided doses given for 1–2 weeks and then gradually tapered. ATG is given at doses of 10–15 mg of IgG/kg for six to eight doses over 2 weeks.

ORGAN FAILURE SYNDROMES

Pulmonary Complications

Approximately half of patients develop respiratory complications after marrow transplantation and pneumonia is the major cause of mortality in the first 100 days following transplantation (33, 42, 49). The differential diagnosis of new-onset pulmonary symptoms varies with respect to time from transplantation. In the first 2 weeks after transplantation there are two conditions to consider in addition to the myriad of disorders that result in pulmonary infiltrates in the immunocompromised host (97). Patients may develop a generalized "capillary leak" syndrome due to what has been termed "hyperacute GVHD" (58, 78). This generally occurs in the setting of HLA-nonidentical transplantation. One must exclude acute congestive heart failure due to cardiac necrosis consequent to the conditioning regimen (13). Fat embolism may rarely occur in the first several days after transplantation if the marrow infusion was inadequately filtered (56, 72). Unlike the case of the multiple-trauma victim, this syndrome may be difficult to recognize because of the nonspecificity of petecchiae in a thrombocytopenic patient.

In the intermediate period (30–100 days) after transplantation, nonbacterial interstitial pneumonia is the major complication (Table 45.3) (42, 49, 50). Viral pneumonia due to cytomegalovirus occurs in ~25% of patients and has a mortality rate approaching 100% in those patients who require tracheal intubation and mechanical ventilation. Severe pneumonia due to CMV rarely occurs in non-marrow-transplant patients, and in fact, occurs almost exclusively in patients after allogeneic grafts and rarely after syngeneic (identical twin) or autologous grafts. Acute GVHD is a major risk factor for the development of CMV pneumonia (51, 52), presumably due to the immunusuppression cause by GVHD, or from the immunosuppressive treatment given for GVHD. The clinical presentation varies from a prolonged fever followed by the development of a nonproductive cough to a fulminant case of acute respiratory distress syndrome that is fatal within 24 hours of clinical onset. Effective therapy for established CMV pneumonia has not been available until recently. New drugs that are relatively specific for CMV such as ganciclovir (dihydroxypropoxymethyl guanine, DHPG) may prove useful (24), particularly when combined with ISG; a preliminary report indicates that mortality of CMV pneumonia may be decreased to < 50% (11). Fortunately, there is an established role for the prophylaxis of CMV infection after marrow grafting. CMV pneumonia may result from a primary infection acquired during the peritransplant period or from reactivation of latent infection. Approximately 30% of patients are seronegative prior to transplantation, and they may be prevented from acquiring the infection by the use of blood products derived exclusively from CMV seronegative donors (10). Finally, if available, a seronegative marrow donor should be used for seronegative recipients.

The other major cause of nonbacterial pneumonia during the intermediate period after transplantation is termed "idiopathic" pneumonia and is presumably caused by damage from radiation and chemotherapy (39, 41, 42, 50, 102). The presentation may be identical to CMV pneumonia, and in order to obtain a diagnosis, an open lung biopsy is often required in order to exclude infectious etiologies, recurrent neoplasm, etc. The prognosis of "idiopathic" pneumonia is better than for CMV pneumonia as up to 50% of patients will recover. There is no established therapy other than supportive measures and the withdrawal of potentially harmful antimicrobial agents such as amphotericin B. Corticosteroids are often given although they have never been shown to be helpful.

P. carinii pneumonia was formerly a frequent pathogen in marrow graft recipients although presently, it rarely occurs due to the routine prophylactic administration of trimethoprim/sulfamethoxazole. All patients should be evaluated for latent mycobacterial infections prior to transplantation; antituber-

culous prophylaxis is indicated in patients with evidence of past infection (54). Pulmonary thromboembolism is rarely documented in patients following marrow transplant, suggesting that they do not become "hypercoaguable" in the presence of prolonged hospitalization.

Gastrointestinal and Hepatic Complications

The most pervasive gastrointestinal problems associated with marrow transplantation are the result of the intensive chemotherapy and radiation required for marrow conditioning (45). The combined modality therapy required for successful bone marrow ablation frequently leads to extensive necrosis of the intestinal crypts. This damage results in diffuse mucositis, anorexia, crampy abdominal pain, and watery diarrhea (12, 45, 69). As a rule, the intestinal damage consequent to the conditioning protocol is entirely reversible, unlike the liver injury that may occur (see below). Most patients receiving allogeneic marrow transplantation require complete parenteral alimentation during the 3–4 weeks required for resolution of this intestinal damage. Because of the protein loss it is difficult to prevent the patients from developing a negative nitrogen balance, even with aggressive nutritional support. Complications of prolonged hyperalimentation include abnormal liver function tests, gallbladder atony, and sludge formation in the biliary tract (48, 94). Severe gastrointestinal bleeding is rarely seen during this time period, although gastrointestinal fluid losses need to be monitored and replaced appropriately.

Patients with chronic GVHD usually have hepatic and esophageal involvement (45). Intestinal fibrosis resembling that caused by scleroderma may result in dysphagia, retrosternal pain, and aspiration associated with esophageal dysfunction. Webs and strictures of the distal esophagus are also frequently seen and may require bougienage. Chronic liver disease occurs in almost 90% of patients with chronic GVHD. Because of the high incidence of infectious complications in patients with chronic GVHD, vigilance must be maintained to exclude infectious etiologies for deteriorating liver function. Among the agents to be excluded are chronic viral infections with non-A, non-B hepatitis, cytomegalovirus, and hepatitis B virus or infiltrative bacterial liver disease with agents such as tuberculosis. In addition, hepatotoxic reactions can occur, most frequently from trimethoprim/sulfamethoxazole, and cholestasis has been associated with the use of cyclosporine and azathioprine for the treatment of chronic GVHD. The possibility of extrahepatic biliary obstruction due to cholelithiasis must always be considered as a potential underlying etiology of worsening liver disease. Although some patients with chronic GVHD may have hyperbilirubinemia for years, hepatic failure, portal hypertention and cirrhosis are unusual complications of this disease.

Veno-occlusive Disease

Veno-occlusive disease of the liver (VOD) occurs in up to 20% of patients after transplantation and is becoming more common due to the use of more aggressive conditioning protocols, and to the fact that patients have been more intensively pretreated prior to transplantation (45, 46, 64). The signs of VOD usually develop during the first 2 weeks after marrow transplantation. Most patients first develop a gradual weight gain with jaundice appearing at 1 week. These signs are followed by the development of abdominal pain, hepatomegaly, ascites, and even encephalopathy within 6–10 days. Weight gain is due to prerenal oliguria, suggesting that postsinusoidal obstruction activates renal salt retention prior to the onset of ascites. Jaundice is a virtual sine qua non of the syndrome, with the serum bilirubin reaching a maximum usually between 2 and 3 weeks after transplant. Abdominal pain can be a prominent symptom, and encephalopathy will develop in as many as half of the patients. VOD is characterized histologically by a centrolobular hemorrhage. The terminal hepatic venules and sublobular veins may be damaged and activation of clotting factors within the venules may be responsible for the early manifestations of VOD.

The clinical course of patients with VOD ranges from cases of fulminant hepatic failure leading to death within 1–2 weeks after transplant to a mild transient illness with complete recovery by week 3. To date, no intervention appears likely to alter the course of this disease, and therapy is directed at maintaining intravascular volume and renal perfusion while simultaneously attempting to minimize extravascular fluid accumulation (45, 46). Sodium intake should be restricted and the judicious use of spironolactone or triamterene can help

achieve a negative sodium balance. Encephalopathy should be treated with protein restriction and lactulose. Drugs that are metabolized in the liver should be monitored carefully during periods in which ongoing liver disease is present. Drugs associated with renal toxicity should also be reduced and monitored closely because of renal hypoperfusion. Drugs that distribute into third-space fluids usually have to be reduced or withheld if ascites develops. While other forms of VOD are thought to be responsive to anticoagulant therapy, this approach is relatively contraindicated in marrow graft recipients during this time period of marrow transplantation.

The diagnosis of VOD must be made on a clinical basis as liver biopsy is usually contraindicated due to thrombocytopenia and ascites. Patients that exhibit any two of the three major criteria of VOD (jaundice, hepatomegaly or hepatic pain, ascites or unexplained weight gain) within 30 days of transplantation have an ~85% probability of having VOD (46). The major differential diagnoses that require consideration are acute GVHD of the liver, post-transfusion hepatitis, and the Budd-Chiari syndrome (64). Liver involvement in acute GVHD usually manifests as cholestatic jaundice without evidence of significant hepatocellular damage or portal hypertension and occurs 3 weeks or later after transplantation, whereas VOD occurs in the first 3 weeks of transplantation. The patient with acute GVHD develops mild hepatomegaly with an increased serum alkaline phosphatase concentration and hyperbilirubinemia, and elevations of transaminase levels are not usually pronounced. Imaging techniques such as computed tomography and magnetic resonance imaging (MRI) usually reveal sparing of the caudate lobe of the liver in patients with the Budd-Chiari syndrome, while patients with VOD have total hepatic involvement. Pericentral hepatocyte necrosis is a pathologically distinct lesion from VOD that produces a clinical syndrome that is similar to VOD (45).

Neurological Complications

The most common CNS side effect reported in association with bone marrow transplantation is metabolic encephalopathy as a result of failure of other organ systems. Metabolic encephalopathy is treated primarily by therapy for the underlying condition such as hemodialysis for acute renal failure. The second most common CNS complications are adverse effects from various drugs. As with other patients in the ICU, corticosteroids have been associated with psychosis reactions. Parenteral acyclovir therapy has been reported to induce tremors and transient hemiparesis (93). Cyclosporine has been associated with seizure disorders, cerebellar ataxia, tremors, and depression, all which appear to be corrected by magnesium therapy (84). Infectious CNS complications are also reported in marrow transplant patients and fatal CNS infections have been reported involving *Aspergillosis*, herpes simplex virus types I and II, *Listeria monocytogenes*, and toxoplasmosis. Despite the frequency of bacteremia in the post-transplant period, however, surprisingly few episodes of bacterial meningitis/encephalitis are seen. This suggests that, contrary to some reports, the blood-brain barrier is remarkably resistant to the conditioning protocols used for allogeneic marrow transplantation.

The most devastating neurological complication of marrow transplantation is the development of idiopathic leukoencephalopathy. Patients develop a progressive syndrome consisting of lethargy, slurred speech, ataxia, seizures, confusion, spasticity, and decerebrate posturing. Pathological findings are those of degeneration of the white matter with a multifocal pattern of noninflammatory necrosis. Onset is usually insidious, beginning 3–6 months following marrow transplantation and is nearly always fatal. Leukoencephalopathy has not been reported in patients transplanted for nonmaligant disorders, suggesting that the prior cytotoxic therapy may predispose to the development of leukoencephalopathy. In addition, almost all of these patients have been treated with post-transplant intrathecal methotrexate to prevent CNS recurrences of hematological malignancy. A recent report suggests that the incidence of leukoencephalopathy is associated not only with the preparative regimen but also with a history of pretransplant CNS therapy and the extent of post-transplant CNS therapy (85). In patients with a history of previous CNS therapy who received post-transplant intrathecal methotrexate as prophylaxis to prevent recurrent CNS disease, the incidence of leukoencephalopathy may be as high as 15%. At the onset of symptoms consistent with leukoencephalopathy other reversible etiologies should be excluded. For example, hypomagnesemia is common in patients that are treated with cyclosporine and may result in seizures, Parkinsonian symptoms, and cerebellar signs similar to leukoen-

cephalopathy (84). Similarly, the syndrome of D-lactic acidosis found in patients with severe intestinal malabsorption that may occur with chronic GVHD can cause slurred speech and cerebellar symptoms that resolve after treatment with antimicrobials and correction of metabolic acidosis (16). Finally, progrssive multifocal leukoencephalopathy, caused by infection with JC virus, must be distinguished by brain biopsy, from idiopathic leukoencephalopathy.

Acknowledgments

The opinions and assertions expressed herein are those of the authors and are not to be construed as official or reflecting the views of the Navy Department.
This work was supported in part by Naval Medical Research Development Command, Research Task M0095.001.0045.

References

1. Appelbaum FR, Buckner CD: Overview of the clinical relevance of autologous bone marrow transplantation. *Clin Haematol* 15:1–18, 1986.
2. Arthur RR, Shah KV, Baust SJ, Santos GW, Saral R: Association of BK viruria with hemorrhagic cystitis in recipients of bone marrow transplants. *N Engl J Med* 315:230–234, 1986.
3. Atkinson K: Cyclosporin in bone marrow transplantation. *Bone Marrow Transpl* 1:265–270, 1987.
4. Barrett AP: Oral complications of bone marrow transplantation. *Aust NZ J Med* 16:239–240, 1986.
5. Bensinger WI, Baker DA, Buckner CD, Clift RA, Thomas ED: Immunoadsorption for removal of A and B blood-group antibodies. *N Engl J Med* 304:160–162, 1981.
6. Bergstein J, Andreoli SP, Provisor AJ, Yum M: Radiation nephritis following total-body irradiation and cyclophosphamide in preparation for bone marrow transplantation. *Transplantation* 41:63–66, 1986.
7. Billingham RE: The biology of graft-versus-host reactions. In *Harvey Lectures 1966–67*. New York, Academic Press, vol 62, pp 21–78.
8. Blacklock HA, Gilmore MJ, Prentice HG, Hazlehurst GR, Evans JP, Ma DD, Knight CB, Hoffbrand AV: ABO-incompatible bone-marrow transplantation: removal of red blood cells from donor marrow avoiding recipient antibody depletion. *Lancet* 2:1061–1064, 1982.
9. Blazar BR, Filipovich AH, Kersey JH, et al: T-cell depletion of donor marrow allografts: effects on graft-versus-host disease and engraftment. In Gale RP, Champlin R (eds): *Progress in Bone Marrow Transplantation*. New York Alan R. Liss 1987, pp 381–397.
10. Bowden RA, Sayers M, Flournoy N, Newton B, Banaji M, Thomas ED, Meyers JD: Cytomeglovirus immune globulin and seronegative blood products to prevent primary cytomegalovirus infection after marrow transplantation. *N Engl J Med* 314:1006–1010, 1986.
11. Bratanow NC, Ash RC, Turner PA, Smith R, Chitamber C, Hansen R, Casper J: Successful treatment of serious cytomegalovirus disease with (1,3-dihydroxy-2-propoxymethyl) guanine in bone marrow transplant (BMT) patients. *Blood* 70 (Suppl 1):302a, 1987.
12. Carl W, Higby DJ: Oral manifestations of bone marrow transplantation. *Am J Clin Oncol* 8:81–87, 1985.
13. Cazin B, Gorin NC, Laporte JP, Gallet B, Douay J, Lopez

M, Najman A, Duhamel G: Cardiac complications after bone marrow transplantation. A report on a series of 63 consecutive transplantations. *Cancer* 57:2061–2069, 1986.

14. Champlin R, Gale RP: Bone marrow transplantation for acute leukemia: recent advances and comparison with alternative therapies. *Semin Hematol* 24:55–67, 1987.

15. Cockburn I: Cyclosporine A: a clinical evaluation of drug interactions. *Transplant Proc* 18:50–55, 1986.

16. Cross SA, Callaway CW: D-Lactic acidosis and selected cerebellar ataxias. *Mayo Clin Proc* 59:202–205, 1984.

17. Deeg HJ, Doney K, Sullivan KM, et al: Prevention and treatment of graft-versus-host disease (GVHD) with drugs. In Gale RP, Champlin R (eds): *Progress in Bone Marrow Transplantation.* New York, Alan R. Liss, 1987, pp 265–276.

18. Deeg HJ, Storb R: Graft-versus-host disease: pathophysiological and clinical aspects. *Ann Rev Med* 35:11–24, 1984.

19. Deeg HJ, Storb R, Thomas ED: Bone marrow transplantation: a review of delayed complications. *Br J Haematol* 57:185–208, 1984.

20. Deeg HJ, Storb R, Thomas ED, Appelbaum F, Buckner CD, Clift RA, Doney K, Johnson L, Sanders JE, Stewart P, Sullivan KM, Witherspoon RP: Fanconi's anemia treated by allogeneic marrow transplantation. *Blood* 61:954–959, 1983.

21. Dicke KA, Spitzer G: Evaluation of the use of high-dose cytoreduction with autologous marrow rescue in various malignancies. *Transplantation* 41:4–20, 1986.

22. Dillman JB: Safe use of succinylcholine during repeated anesthetics in a patient treated with cyclophosphamide. *Anesth Analg* 66:351–353, 1987.

23. Engelhard D, Marks MI, Good RA: Infections in bone marrow transplant recipients. *J Pediatr* 108:335–346, 1986.

24. Erice A, Jordan MC, Chace BA, Fletcher C, Chinnock BJ, Balfour HH Jr: Ganciclovir treatment of cytomegalovirus disease in transplant recipients and other immunocompromised hosts. *JAMA* 257:3082–3087, 1987.

25. Filipovich AH, Krawczak CL, Kersey JH, McGlave P, Ramsay NK, Goldman A, Goldstein G: Graft-versus-host disease prophylaxis with anti-T-cell monoclonal antibody OKT3, prednisone and methotrexate in allogeneic bone-marrow transplantation. *Br J Haematol* 60:143–152, 1985.

26. Finn G, Denning D: Transient nephrogenic diabetes insipidus following high-dose cyclophosphamide chemotherapy and autologous bone marrow transplantation. *Cancer Treat Rep* 71:220–221, 1987.

27. First LR, Smith BR, Lipton J, Nathan DG, Parkman R, Rappeport JM: Isolated thrombocytopenia after allogeneic bone marrow transplantation: existence of transient and chronic thrombocytopenic syndromes. *Blood* 65:368–374, 1985.

28. Fischer A, Griscelli C, Blanche S, Le Deist F, Veber F, Lopez M, Delaage M, Olive D, Mawas C, Janossy G: Prevention of graft failure by an anti-HLFA-1 monoclonal antibody in HLA-mismatched bone-marrow transplantation. *Lancet* 2:1058–1061, 1986.

29. Forman SJ, Blume KG, Krance RA, et al: A prospective randomized study of acute graft-v-host disease in 107 patients with leukemia: Methotrexate/prednisone v cyclosporine A/prednisone. *Transplant Proc* 19:2605–2607, 1987.

30. Gluckman E, Devergie A, Dutreix J: Radiosensitivity in Fanconi anaemia: application to the conditioning regimen for bone marrow transplantation. *Br J Haematol* 54:431–440, 1983.

31. Glucksberg H, Storb R, Fefer A, et al: Clinical manifestations of graft-versus-host disease in human recipients of marrow from HL-A- matched sibling donors. *Transplantation* 18:295–304, 1974.

32. Goldberg MA, Antin JH, Guinan EC, Rappeport JM: Cyclophosphamide cardiotoxicity: an analysis of dosing as a risk factor. *Blood* 68:1114–1118, 1986.

33. Hamilton PJ, Pearson AD: Bone marrow transplantation and the lung. *Thorax* 41:497–502, 1986.

34. Heusinkveld RS, Manning MR, Aristizabal SA: Control of radiation-induced diarrhea with cholestyramine. *Int J Radiat Oncol Biol Phys* 4:687–690, 1978.

35. Hood AF, Vogelsang GB, Black LP, Farmer ER, Santos GW: Acute graft-versus-host disease. Development following autologous and syngeneic bone marrow transplantation. *Arch Dermatol* 123:745–750, 1987.

36. Hows JM, Mehta A, Ward L, Woods K, Perez R, Gordon MY, Gordon-Smith EC: Comparison of mesna with forced diuresis to prevent cyclophosphamide induced haemorrhagic cystitis in marrow transplantation: a prospective randomised study. *Br J Cancer* 50:753–756, 1984.

37. June GH, Thompson CB, Kennedy MS, Loughran TP, Deeg HJ: Correlation of hypomagnesemia with the onset of cyclosporine-associated hypertension in marrow transplant patients. *Transplantation* 41:47–51, 1986.

38. June CH, Thompson CB, Kennedy MS, Nims J, Thomas ED: Profound hypomagnesemia and renal magnesium wasting associated with the use of cyclosporine for marrow transplantation. *Transplantation* 39:620–624, 1985.

39. Keane TJ, Van Dyk J, Rider WD: Idiopathic interstitial pneumonia following bone marrow transplantation: the relationship with total body irradiation. *Int J Radiat Oncol Biol Phys* 7:1365–1370, 1981.

40. Kennedy MS, Deeg HJ, Siegel M, Crowley JJ, Storb R, Thomas ED: Acute renal toxicity with combined use of amphotericin B and cyclosporine after marrow transplantation. *Transplantation* 35:211–215, 1983.

41. Kim TH, Rybka WB, Lehnert S, Podgorsak EB, Freeman CR: Interstitial pneumonitis following total body irradiation for bone marrow transplantation using two different dose rates. *Int J Radiat Oncol Biol Phys* 11:1285–2491, 1985.

42. Krowka MJ, Rosenow EC, Hoagland HC: Pulmonary complications of bone marrow transplantation. *Chest* 87:237–246, 1985.

43. Lazarus HM, Coccia PF, Herzig RH, et al: Incidence of acute graft-versus-disease with and without methotrexate prophylaxis in allogeneic bone marrow transplant patients. *Blood* 64:215–220, 1984.

44. Loughran TP Jr, Deeg HJ, Dahlberg S, Kennedy MS, Storb R, Thomas ED: Incidence of hypertension after marrow transplantation among 112 patients randomized to either cyclosporine or methotrexate as graft-versus-host disease prophylaxis. *Br J Haematol* 59:547–553, 1985.

45. McDonald GB, Shulman HM, Sullivan KM, Spencer GD: Intestinal and hepatic complications of human bone marrow transplantation. Part I and part II. *Gastroenterology* 90:460–477, 770–84, 1986.

46. McDonald GB, Sharma P, Mathews DE, Shulman HM, Thomas ED: The clinical course of 53 patients with venocclusive disease of the liver after marrow transplantation. *Transplantation* 39:603–608, 1985.

47. Martin PJ, Shulman HM, Schubach WH, Hansen JA, Fefer A, Miller G, Thomas ED: Fatal Epstein-Barr-virus-associated proliferation of donor B cells after treatment of acute graft-versus-host disease with a murine anti-T-cell antibody. *Ann Intern Med* 101:310–315, 1984.

48. Messing B, Bories C, Kunstlinger F, Bernier J-J: Does total parenteral nutrition induce gallbladder sludge formation and lithiasis? *Gastroenterology* 84:1012–1019, 1983.

49. Meyers JD: Infection in bone marrow transplant recipients. *Am J Med* 81:27–38, 1986.

50. Meyers JD, Flournoy N, Thomas ED: Nonbacterial pneumonia after allogeneic marrow transplantation: a

review of ten years' experience. *Rev Infect Dis* 4:1119–1132, 1982.

51. Meyers JD, Flournoy N, Thomas ED: Risk factors for cytomegalovirus infection after human marrow transplantation. *J Infect Diseases* 153:478–489, 1986.

52. Miller W, Flynn P, McCullough J, Balfour HHJr, Goldman A, Haake R, McGlave P, Ramsay N, Kersey J: Cytomegalovirus infection after bone marrow transplantation: an association with acute graft-v-host disease. *Blood* 67:1162–1167, 1986.

53. Naparstek E, Rachmilewitz B, Rachmilewitz M, Fuks Z, Slavin S: Serum transcobalamin levels as an early indicator of bone marrow engraftment following transplantation. *Br J Haematol* 55:229–234, 1983.

54. Navari RM, Sullivan KM, Springmeyer SC, Siegel MS, Meyers JD, Buckner CD, Sanders JE, Stewart PS, Clift RA, Fefer A, et al: Mycobacterial infections in marrow transplant patients. *Transplantation* 36:509–513, 1983.

55. O'Reilly RJ: Allogeneic bone marrow transplantation: current status and future directions. *Blood* 62:941–964, 1983.

56. Paradinas FJ, Sloane JP, Depledge MH, Morgenstern GR, Monaghan P, Roberts JD, Corrin B: Pulmonary fat embolization after bone marrow transplantation (letter) *Lancet* 26:1:715–716, 1983.

57. Patterson J, Prentice HG, Brenner MK, Gilmore M, Janossy G, Ivory K, Skeggs D, Morgan H, Lord J, Blacklock HA, et al: Graft rejection following HLA matched T-lymphocyte depleted bone marrow transplantation. *Br J Haematol* 63:221–230, 1986.

58. Powles RL, Morgenstern GR, Kay HEM et al: Mismatched family donors for bone-marrow transplantation as treatment for acute leukaemia. *Lancet* I:612–614, 1983.

59. Press OW, Ramsey PG, Larson EB, Fefer A, Hickman RO: Hickman catheter infections in patients with malignancies. *Medicine (Baltimore)* 63:189–200, 1984.

60. Ramsay NK, Kersey JH, Robison LL, et al: A randomized study of the prevention of acute graft-versus-host disease. *N Engl J Med* 306:392–397, 1982.

61. Ramsay NK, Kim TH, McGlave P, Goldman A, Nesbit ME Jr, Krivit W, Woods WG, Kersey JH: Total lymphoid irradiation and cyclophosphamide conditioning prior to bone marrow transplantation for patients with severe aplastic anemia. *Blood* 62:622–626, 1983.

62. Ringden O: Cyclosporine in allogeneic bone marrow transplantation. *Transplantation* 42:445–452, 1986.

63. Rohrbaugh TM, Anolik R, August CS, Serota FT, Koch PA: Absorption of oral aminoglycosides following bone marrow transplantation. *Cancer* 53:1502–1506, 1984.

64. Rollins BJ: Hepatic veno-occulsive disease. *Am J Med* 81:297–306, 1986.

65. Sale GE, McDonald GB, Shulman HM, Thomas ED: Gastrointestinal graft-versus-host disease in man. A clinicopathologic study of the rectal biopsy. *Am J Surg Pathol* 3:291–299, 1979.

66. Sale GE, Shulman HM: *The Pathology of Bone Marrow Transplantation.* New York, Masson 1984.

67. Santos GW, Hess AD, Vogelsang GB: Graft-versus-host reactions and disease. *Immunol Rev* 88:169–192, 1985.

68. Santos GW, Tutschka PJ, Brookmeyer R, Saral R, Beschorner WE, Bias WB, Braine HG, Burns WH, Elfenbein GJ, Kaizer H, et al: Marrow transplantation for acute nonlymphocytic leukemia after treatment with busulfan and cyclophosphamide. *N Engl J Med* 309:1347–1353, 1983.

69. Seto BG, Kim M, Wolinsky L, Mito RS, Champlin R: Oral mucositis in patients undergoing bone marrow transplantation. *Oral Surg Oral Med Oral Pathol* 60:493–497, 1985.

70. Shapiro RS, Pietryga D, Blazar BR, et al: B cell lymphoproliferative disorders following bone marrow transplantation. In Gale RP, Champlin R (eds): *Pro-gress in Bone Marrow Transplantation.* New York, Alan R. Liss, 1987, pp 647–657.

71. Shepp DH, Dandliker PS, Flournoy N, Meyers JD: Sequential intravenous and twice-daily oral acyclovir for extended prophylaxis of herpes simplex virus infection in marrow transplant patients. *Transplantation* 43:654–658, 1987.

72. Springmeyer SC, Silvestri RC, Flournoy N, Kosanke CW, Peterson DL, Huseby JS, Hudson LD, Storb R, Thomas ED: Pulmonary function of marrow transplant patients. I. Effects of marrow infusion, acute graft-versus-host disease, and interstitial pneumonitis. *Exp Hematol* 12:805–810, 1984.

73. Storb R, Deeg HJ, Whitehead J, et al: Methotrexate and cyclosporine compared with cyclosporine alone for prophylaxis of acute graft-versus-host disease after marrow transplantation for leukemia. *N Engl J Med* 314:729–735, 1986.

74. Storb R, Deeg HJ, Whitehead J, et al: Marrow transplantation for leukemia and aplastic anemia: two controlled trials of a combination of methotrexate and cyclosporine v cyclosporine alone or methotrexate alone for prophylaxis of acute-graft-v-host disease. *Transplantation Proc* 19:2608–2613, 1987.

75. Storb R, Prentice RL, Buckner CD, et al: Graft-versus-host disease and survival in patients with aplastic anemia treated by marrow grafts from HLA-identical siblings. Beneficial effect of a protective environment. *N Engl J Med* 308:302–307, 1983.

76. Storb R, Thomas ED: Graft-versus-host disease in dog and man: the Seattle experience. *Immunol Rev* 88:215–238, 1985.

77. Sullivan KM, Deeg HJ, Sanders JE, Shulman HM, Witherspoon RP, Doney K, Appelbaum FR, Schubert MM, Stewart P, Springmeyer S, et al: Late complications after marrow transplantation. *Semin Hematol* 21:53–63, 1984.

78. Sullivan KM, Deeg HJ, Sanders J, et al: Hyperacute graft-v-host disease in patients not given immunosuppression after allogeneic marrow transplantation. *Blood* 67:1172–1175, 1986.

79. Sullivan KM, Shulman HM, Storb R, et al: Chronic graft-versus-host disease in 52 patients: adverse natural course and successful treatment with combination immunosuppression. *Blood* 57:267–276, 1981.

80. Thomas ED: Karnofsky Memorial Lecture. Marrow transplantation for malignant diseases. *J Clin Oncol* 1:517–531, 1983.

81. Thomas ED: High-dose therapy and bone marrow transplantation. *Semin Oncol* 12(4 Suppl 6):15–20, 1985.

82. Thomas ED, Clift RA, Hersman J, Sanders JE, Stewart P, Buckner CD, Fefer A, McGuffin R, Smith JW, Storb R: Marrow transplantation for acute nonlymphoblastic leukemia in first remission using fractionated or single-dose irradiation. *Int J Radiat Oncol Biol Phys* 8:817–821, 1982.

83. Thomas ED, Storb R, Clift RA, Fefer A, Johnson FL, Neiman PE, Lerner KG, Glucksberg H, Buckner CD: Bone-marrow transplantation (in two parts). *N Engl J Med* 292:832–843, 895–902, 1975.

84. Thompson CB, June CH, Sullivan KM, Thomas ED: Association between cyclosporine neurotoxicity and hypomagnesaemia. *Lancet* 2:1116–1120, 1984.

85. Thompson CB, Sanders JE, Flournoy N, Buckner CD, Thomas ED: The risks of central nervous system relapse and leukoencephalopathy in patients receiving marrow transplants for acute leukemia. *Blood* 67:195–199, 1986.

86. Thompson CB, Thomas ED: Bone marrow transplantation. *Surg Clin North Am* 66:589–601, 1986.

87. Trigg ME, Finlay JL, Bozdech M, Gilbert E: Fatal cardiac toxicity in bone marrow transplant patients receiving cytosine arabinoside, cyclophosphamide, and total body irradiation. *Cancer* 1;59:38–42, 1987.

88. Tsoi MS: Immunological mechanisms of graft-versus-host disease in man. *Transplantation* 33:459–463, 1982.

89. Tutschka PJ, Hess AD, Beschorner WE, Santos GW: Suppressor cells in transplantation tolerance. I. Suppressor cells in the mechanisms of tolerance in radiation chimeras. *Transplantation* 32:203–209, 1981.

90. van Bekkum DW: Conditioning regimens for marrow grafting. *Semin Hematol* 21:81–90, 1984.

91. van Bekkum DW, Roodenburg J, Heidt PJ, van der Waaij D: Mitigation of secondary disease of allogeneic mouse radiation chimeras by modification of the intestinal microflora. *J Natl Cancer Inst* 52:401–404, 1974.

92. Vogelsang GB, Hess AD, Gordon G, Santos GW: Treatment and prevention of acute graft-versus-host disease with thalidomide in a rat model. *Transplantation* 41:644–647, 1986.

93. Wade JC, Meyers JD: Neurologic symptoms associated with parenteral acyclovir treatment after marrow transplantation. *Ann Intern Med* 98:921–925, 1983.

94. Wagman LD, Burt ME, Brennan MF: The impact of total parenteral nutrition on liver function tests in patients with cancer. *Cancer* 49:1249–1257, 1982.

95. Weiden P: Graft-v-host disease following blood transfusions. *Arch Intern Med* 144:1557–1558, 1984.

96. Weiden PL, Sullivan KM, Flournoy N, Storb R, Thomas ED: Antileukemic effect of chronic graft-versus-host disease: contribution to improved survival after allo-geneic marrow transplantation. *N Engl J Med* 304:1529–1533, 1981.

97. Wilson WR, Cockerill FR, Rosenow EC: Pulmonary disease in the immunocompromised host. *Mayo Clin Proc* 60:610–631, 1985.

98. Winston DJ, Ho WG, Lin CH, Bartoni K, Budinger MD, Gale RP, Champlin RE: Intravenous immune globulin for prevention of cytomegalovirus infection and interstitial pneumonia after bone marrow transplantation. *Ann Intern Med* 106:12–18, 1987.

99. Yee GC, Lennon TP, Gmur DG, Carlin J, Schaffer RL, Kennedy MS, Deeg HJ: Clinical pharmacology of cyclosporine in patients undergoing bone marrow transplantation. *Transplant Proc* 18(6 Suppl 5):153–159, 1986.

100. Yolken RH, Bishop CA, Townsend TR, Bolyard EA, Bartlett J, Santos GW, Saral R: Infectious gastroenteritis in bone-marrow-transplant recipients. *N Engl J Med* 306:1010–1012, 1982.

101. Whitsett CF, Pierce JA, Daffin LE: Positive direct antiglobulin tests associated with intravenous gamma globulin use in bone marrow transplant recipients. *Transplantation* 41:663–664, 1986.

102. Wingard JR, Santos GW: Saral R. Late-onset interstitial pneumonia following allogeneic bone marrow transplantation. *Transplantation* 39:21–23, 1985.

103. Zsigmond E, Robins G: The effect of a series of anticancer drugs on plasma cholinesterase activity. *Can Anaesth Soc J* 19:75–82, 1972.

46

Computer-Controlled Vasoactive Drug Therapy

L. C. Sheppard, Ph.D.
T. C. Jannett, Ph.D.

Hypertension following intracardiac operations may be the result of pain, hypothermia, reflex vasoconstriction following cardipulmonary bypass, activation of the renin-angiotensin system, ventilatory difficulties, and recovery from anesthesia. Complications of postoperative hypertension include myocardial ischemia, myocardial infarction, rupture of suture lines, increased bleeding, cerebrovascular accident, and arrhythmia. The fast-acting vasodilator sodium nitroprusside (SNP) is the most frequently used hypotensive agent in postoperative patients. With SNP infusion, the reduction of peripheral vascular resistance, and the resulting reduction in the arterial pressure, has a rapid onset and quickly subsides when the infusion is stopped. Control of arterial pressure with this drug requires frequent adjustment of the infusion rate based on measurement of systolic or mean arterial pressure (MAP). An intra-arterial cannula, pressure transducer, and preamplifier system is necessary for reliable pressure measurement. The MAP signal is obtained by low-pass filtering of the arterial pressure signal, thus attenuating the signal variation during the cardiac cycle and recovering the mean, or average, arterial pressure value.

Manual regulation of MAP with hypotensive agents is difficult and time consuming. The drug infusion rate must be frequently adjusted because of spontaneous pressure variations and the changing condition of the patient. Difficulties in control are also encountered because the response of blood pressure to infusion rate changes is delayed, may change with time, and varies among patients. Inadequate adjustments of the SNP infusion rate by clinical personnel often cause poor pressure regulation. In patients where pressure regulation is difficult, the nurse must monitor the MAP constantly, and make frequent changes in the infusion rate

to avoid pressure fluctuations that could be catastrophic. In such situations, the nurse is not free to undertake other tasks, and the quality of blood pressure control may suffer because of the distraction of the nurse in an emergency, or because of the nurse's inexperience.

An automated system for infusing vasodilating agents in postoperative patients is used in the Cardiac Surgical Intensive Care Unit (CICU) of University Hospital at The University of Alabama at Birmingham (8). Automated control of MAP has the following advantages:

1. The benefits of feedback control are provided. These benefits include the control of the blood pressure response to changes in the setpoint, reduction of the effect of spontaneous pressure variations, and reduction of the sensitivity of the system to variations in the patient response to the drug.
2. Infusion rate adjustments are based on pressure measurements made at a higher frequency than is possible with manual control.
3. A rigid set of rules is applied to calculate the infusion rate adjustments.

AUTOMATED BLOOD PRESSURE CONTROL SYSTEM

Development of the automated blood pressure control system was based on investigation of the dynamics of physiological responses of hypertensive patients to SNP. In computer simulations, representative patient responses were used for evaluation of the control algorithm, which determines the change in SNP infusion rate. The control algorithm was tuned further in clinical trials.

Dynamic Response Investigations

Control of a physiological variable with a pharmacological agent in the clinical environment requires knowledge of the dynamics of the response produced by drug infusion. The dynamic response characteristics of a linear system are described by its impulse response. The impulse response can be identified by observing the system output response to the application of an appropriate excitation signal, such as pure white noise. The impulse response is similar to the response of a biological system to the bolus injection of a pharmacological agent. Overdriving the system with a large input may produce an output that contains undesirable nonlinear components. It is theoretically feasible to obtain an impulse response with a cross-correlation technique since the cross-correlation function of a white random input signal with the output signal is directly proportional to the impulse response. The advantage of the cross-correlation method is that the system response can be evaluated in the linear range near the operating state without introducing an unacceptably large disturbance.

The cross-correlation method was used to determine the dynamic response of cardiovascular system variables to vasodilating agents. Pseudo-random-binary sequences (PRBS) were used to vary the SNP infusion rate to provide an appropriate input signal for system excitation. This class of periodic signals meets the randomness criteria over the sequence length and is easy to generate by computer programming. Also, conversion of the PRBS to the appropriate system input variable is easily achieved since there are only two states (off and on).

The dynamic responses of heart rate, MAP, and mean left atrial pressure (LAP) to the infusion of SNP through the right atrium (Fig. 46.1) were investigated. Signals were each digitized at one sample per second and recorded. For analysis, the system was considered to have a single input (SNP infusion rate) and multiple outputs. The input signal was cross-correlated with each output to determine the impulse response of each output variable to the drug infusion rate. Subjects were selected from postoperative patients who exhibited MAP above 100 mm Hg following an open intracardiac operation. MAP was recorded from a radial artery cannula; LAP was recorded from an intracardiac cannula. Heart rate was determined from recording of the electrocardiogram (ECG).

Impulse responses were serially reproducible for a given patient and exhibited common features among patients. The duration of the impulse responses ranged from 2.0 to 3.5 minutes. The MAP response to drug infusion is delayed by a period that corresponds to one circulation time (20–45 seconds), reaches a minimum at 1.2–1.9 minutes, and rises as the drug effect dissipates.

Controller Design and Simulation

For controller evaluation, representative impulse responses were selected to model the patient MAP response to SNP infusion in com-

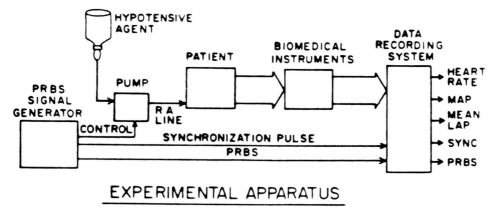

Figure 46.1. Equipment arrangement for programming the infusion of the agent and recording of the physiological response. (Reprinted with permission from Sheppard LC: Computer control of the infusion of vasoactive drugs. *Ann Biomed Eng* 8:431, 1980. Copyright 1980, Pergamon Press, Ltd.)

puter simulations. The impulse response was considered to be a simple exponential for simulation of patient responses. A computer programmed version of a proportional-integral-derivative (PID) controller was selected because the impulse responses were not complicated. The control algorithm was initially adjusted in simulations to provide a simulated patient response with minimal overshoot and acceptable settling time in the reduction of MAP from 120 to a set point of 100 mm Hg. In the control algorithm an error signal (e) was calculated as the difference between the simulated MAP (P) and the setpoint (desired pressure, $P_D = 100$ mm Hg). The error signal was used to calculate the infusion rate required to reduce the error by increasing, holding constant, or decreasing the drug infusion rate in the simulations.

Further tuning of the algorithm was required in the CICU to achieve good controller performance. The following equations and coefficients gave the best clinical performance for the computerized controller:

$$e = P_D - P$$
$$A = (0.4512)e + (0.4512)(e - e')$$
$$\Delta I = KA$$
$$I = I' + \Delta I$$

where P_D is the desired pressure; P is the mean arterial pressure; e is the current error, $P_D - P$; e' is the previous error, 1 minute earlier; A is the calculated pressure change required; I is new infusion rate; I' is the present rate, initiated 1 minute earlier; ΔI is the incremental infusion rate; and K is the controller gain. P_D,

P, e, e', and A are measured in millimeters of mercury; I, I', and ΔI are measured in milliliters per hour; and K is measured in milliliters per hour per millimeter of mercury.

The measured MAP is digitally filtered by taking a six-point average of samples acquired at 1-second intervals to reduce disturbances produced by respiration. In the control algorithm, an incremental infusion rate change is calculated from proportional and derivative error terms where the first difference of the error signal approximates its derivative. The proportional component in the control algorithm is needed to increase the infusion rate in proportion to the degree of MAP elevation above the set point. Derivative control assists in reducing overshoot by taking into account the rate at which MAP is approaching the target value. This incremental action is multiplied by the overall controller gain and is then integrated to determine the infusion rate.

To minimize pharmacological intervention, we have applied rules that bias the algorithm to minimize the infusion rate and the total amount of drug infused. Intentional nonlinearities are introduced into the calculation of the incremental infusion rate change using a decision table (Table 46.1). These rules were developed to improve the transient response of the PID controller and for patient safety.

The incremental infusion rate per unit of pressure correction (K, in milliliters per hour per millimeter of mercury) depends on the measured MAP (P). This gain scheduling (rules 1–4) reduces overshoot, improves the speed of response, and biases the controller to turn off

Table 46.1
Decision Table for Controller Gain and Infusion Rate Increment

Criteria	Rules						
	1	2	3	4	5	6	7
$P > P_D + 5$	+					+	
$P \leq P_D + 5$		+					
$P > P_D$		+		+			
$P \leq P_D$			+				
$P \geq P_D - 5$			+				
$P < P_D - 5$				+			+
$\Delta I > 7$					+		
$\Delta I > 0$							+
Action							
1 $K = -1$	1						
2 $K = -0.5$		2					
3 $K = -1$			3				
4 $K = -2$				4			
5 $\Delta I = 7$					5		
6 $\Delta I = \Delta I - 2$						6	
7 $\Delta I = 0$							7

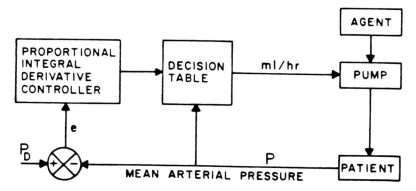

Figure 46.2. Schematic diagram of the control loop. (Reprinted with permission from Sheppard LC: Computer control of the infusion of vasoactive drugs. *Ann Biomed Eng* 8:431, 1980. Copyright 1980, Pergamon Press, Ltd.)

the infusion if pressure is persistently below the set point. Infusion rate increases are limited to +7 ml/hour (rule 5), but infusion rate decreases are not constrained. To reduce overshoot, the increment is reduced (−2 ml/hour) if the MAP is above the set point by 5 mm Hg more than (rule 6) during the transient control phase. If MAP is more than 5 mm Hg below the set point, infusion is not allowed to increase (rule 7). Also, the infusion rate is limited to prevent negative infusion rates and to avoid exceeding the maximum recommended dose rate (10 μg/kg/minute). All rules are evaluated each minute.

IMED Corporation, San Diego, California, developed a pump (IMED 929) that is digitally controlled by our computer system (Hewlett-Packard 21MX). The eight infusion pumps in our unit accept numerically coded information (RS-232, serial, asynchronous, ASCII) that specifies infusion rates from 0–399 ml/hour in 1 ml/hour increments. The infusion rates for each patient are calculated at 1-minute intervals using the control algorithm. The incremental infusion rate adjustment is summed with the previous rate to calculate a new infusion rate that is transmitted to each pump in turn. A schematic diagram of the control loop is shown in Figure 46.2.

Discussion

The automated blood pressure control system is used in the CICU to treat patients with high arterial blood pressure or high afterload (which impairs the pumping ability of the heart). Automated control may be started when the patient is moved to the intensive care unit if SNP infusion is begun in the operating room.

MAP above 100–110 mm Hg is usually treated, and the pressure is usually maintained at a level between 75 and 110 mm Hg. Automated control of MAP exhibits approximately half the variation observed during manual control; MAP measurements are more tightly distributed about the mean (Fig. 46.3).

The incidence of transient MAP variations caused by patient care procedures is minimized by affixing a label to the pressure transducer mount at the bedside to inform clinical personnel that the patient is on "computer nipride". Also, a label is placed on the patient's arm adjacent to the stopcock attached to the radial artery cannula. Clinical personnel temporarily interrupt automatic control when arterial blood samples are withdrawn for cardiac output measurements and blood gases. The computer system is directed to maintain a constant rate of SNP infusion during any event likely to disturb the MAP measurement. Since short-lived transients induced by patient care procedures or by patient movement may sometimes bring about higher or lower infusion rates than are necessary, the stability of blood pressure regulation must be observed by the bedside nurse or physician to ensure the selection of an appropriate constant infusion rate.

The use of computer-controlled drug infusion requires implementation of highly structured, complete, and explicit operating procedures that are rigidly enforced. Strict adherence to these rules is necessary to avoid operator error and to prevent negligent use of devices and systems. Training and experience are required to avoid erratic performance and to prevent system malfunctions. Clinical personnel must monitor system performance to detect malfunctions and to take corrective ac-

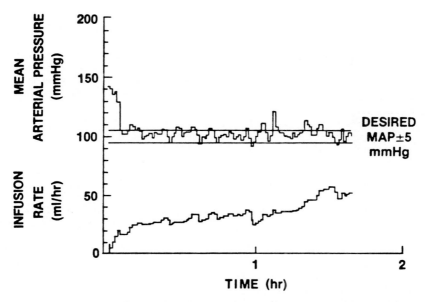

Figure 46.3 Regulation of MAP with automatic control of SNP infusion. (Reprinted with permission. From Sheppard LC: Computer control of the infusion of vasoactive drugs. *Ann Biomed Eng* 8:431, 1980. Copyright 1980, Pergamon Press, Ltd.)

tions. Safeguards are employed to minimize the severity of operator errors.

The infusion pumps are equipped with air embolism detectors and empty reservoir alarms that signal malfunctions to personnel and to the computer. Two steps are required for the nurse to modify the desired pressure (P_D). First, the new value is entered by means of a bedside computer terminal. The newly entered value must then be verified by the entry of a code before the current set point is replaced. Extremely high or low pressure measurements are identified as invalid; the infusion rate is not adjusted during that minute. The computer stops the infusion of SNP if two very low pressure measurements occur in succession.

The system can be used to control the MAP of six patients simultaneously, but the requirement seldom exceeds three patients during a 24-hour period. Typically, two or three patients are hypertensive upon arrival in the CICU or become so during the early hours following operation. The infusion of a hypotensive agent is discontinued after 12–24 hours of treatment in most patients.

Factors That May Affect Controller Performance

Controller performance is influenced by several factors (Table 46.2). Time is required for

the circulation to carry the agent from the infusion site to the vascular receptors, which may be located an appreciable distance away. We use a right atrial cannula for SNP infusion; if infusion is more peripheral, controller performance may be degraded by the additional transport delay.

Fluctuations in MAP measurements that are not attributable to drug infusion have been observed. Variations in the background pressure may be the result of spontaneous fluctuations in sympathetic nervous system activity. During routine patient care, a number of maneuvers introduce short-lived variations in the MAP. Many of these variations are directly attributable to activities such as suctioning of the endotracheal tube, bathing, chest film plate placement and withdrawal, flushing the arterial line, administration of pain medication, extubation, and the ventilatory cycle. Nausea, restlessness, shivering, pain, and anxiety are other factors that may introduce more pro-

Table 46.2
Factors That May Affect Controller Performance

Infusion Site
Background Variation
Variable Sensitivity to SNP
Reflex Responses
Blood Volume
Arrhythmias

longed pressure changes. The conservative rules and limits applied to the control action tend to reduce the impact of MAP variations.

Sensitivity to SNP may vary over a 30 to 1 range among patients; the sensitivity of an individual patient may also change with time. Since SNP is photosensitive, it may appear that the patient is becoming less responsive to SNP as the drug deteriorates over a few hours. Lowering the blood pressure may trigger reflex responses that cause changes in the background pressure; slow drifts and pressure oscillations exhibiting periods from 1 to 8 minutes have been observed (10). The reflex response model has assisted in interpreting certain clinically observed responses. Lowering the blood pressure may trigger reflex responses with relatively long time constants such as increased renal secretion of renin. For example, the requirement for a gradually increasing infusion rate for maintenance of a desired arterial pressure, which was previously not understood, is now attributed to this reflex response. Also, the patient's endogenous neurohumoral control system, which may be severely disturbed following open-heart surgery, causes pressure fluctuations and oscillations. Other reflex responses appear to be of neurohumoral origin (endogenous epinephrine and norepinephrine).

The main effect of SNP is the reduction of arteriolar resistance through the relaxation of vascular smooth muscle. However, venous capacitance is also increased. If this results in a sufficient pooling of blood, venous return and cardiac output may be reduced as ventricular filling pressure is lowered (Frank-Starling Mechanism).

Cardiac arrhythmias, particularly atrial flutter and tachycardia, may cause disturbances in the MAP that degrade the performance of both manual and automatic control.

RESEARCH

Clinical experiences with the controller indicate that system performance needs improvement for patients who are relatively sensitive or insensitive to SNP and for patients whose blood pressure exhibits large fluctuations. To facilitate the design of an improved control algorithm, Slate formulated a mathematical model to represent the essential aspects of the MAP and its response to the infusion of SNP (9). The design of an adaptive controller that provides robust performance has been the topic of significant research. With adaptive control, the control algorithm adapts to individual patients to provide improved performance.

Modeling

Slate used physiological and pharmacological concepts in structuring model input-output relationships from patient data (9). The

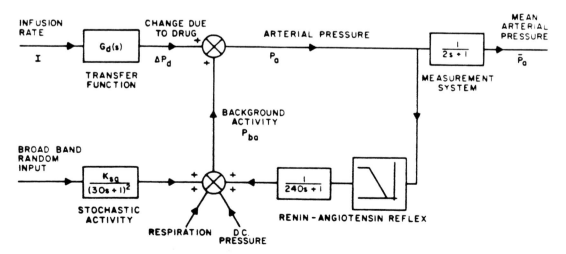

Figure 46.4. Model of MAP and its response to SNP infusion. (Reprinted with permission. From Sheppard LC: Computer control of the infusion of vasoactive drugs. *Ann Biomed Eng* 8:431, 1980. Copyright 1980, Pergamon Press, Ltd.)

MAP is considered to be the sum of a background pressure (P_{ba}) and a change in the pressure due to drug infusion ($\triangle P_d$), which is related to the drug infusion rate (I) by a linear transfer function ($G_d(s)$) (Fig. 46.4). The transfer function was derived from impulse response data obtained using cross-correlation analysis in Sheppard's dynamic response investigations (8). A first-order transfer function provides an adequate and parsimonious representation of the human MAP response to SNP infusion:

$$G_d(s) = \frac{\triangle P_d(s)}{I(s)} = \frac{Ke^{-T_i s}(1 + \alpha e^{-T_c s})}{(1 + \tau s)}$$

The gain K represents the patient's sensitivity to the drug (in millimeters of mercury per milliliter per hour) while α is the recirculating fraction ($\alpha = 0.4$). The lag with time constant $\tau = 50$ s represents the uptake, distribution and metabolism of the drug. The time delays represent the delay in response caused by transport of the drug from the infusion site ($T_i = 30$ seconds) and the recirculation time ($T_c = 45$ seconds).

The background pressure consists of a constant term, a low-amplitude sinusoid that represents activity caused by respiration or ventilation, stochastic activity, and a component representing the neurohumoral reflex response to a reduction in pressure. Other disturbances, including those associated with changes in the condition of the patient or procedures related to patient care, can be approximately modeled as step, ramp, or pulse changes in the background activity. The stochastic activity is modeled as the output of a second-order filter with a corner frequency corresponding to a period of 30 seconds and a broadband random noise input. The renin-angiotensin reflex response is modeled as a one-sided dead zone with saturation followed by a first-order lag. The effect of this model of renin-angiotensin reflex response is to increase the background pressure level when the MAP drops below a threshold value.

Adaptive Blood Pressure Control

Adaptation of the control algorithm allows variations in the patient sensitivity to SNP to be accommodated. Slate used the model (Fig. 46.4) to design a controller in which an adaptive mechanism adjusts controller parameters based on the estimated sensitivity of a patient to the drug. Adaptation is performed during an initial 15-minute control period. Controller parameters are fixed after the adaptation period, which may be repeated if necessary. Improved performance of this adaptive controller was demonstrated in simulations, dog experiments, and clinical trials.

Other adaptive control methods have been investigated (2, 4, 5, 11). If parameter values in an appropriate model of the patient are known, the control algorithm can be designed to optimize a performance index in which factors such as the control performance (pressure variance) and the cost of control (variance of the drug infusion rate) are weighed (1, 6). Such controllers are usually used in conjunction with on-line parameter estimation to form adaptive control algorithms because the performance index is optimized only if accurate model parameter values are used to calculate the optimal control.

Although many adaptive blood pressure control systems have been tested in the laboratory, there have been few clinical applications. For the design of a clinically useful system, patient care practices and other aspects of the clinical environment must be considered. Stable operation of the adaptive controller must be assured by the use of supervisory algorithms (9, 11).

OTHER CLINICAL EXPERIENCE

A computerized bedside system for automated delivery of SNP has been developed and clinically tested at the Mount Sinai Medical Center in New York City (2). The control algorithm is based on the work of Sheppard (8) and Slate (9). The system was used to investigate the hypothesis that automated control of SNP infusion is superior to manual control. In a group of 37 patients managed with manual control, the measured MAP was within 5 mm Hg of the desired MAP only 52% of the time; in a group of 49 patients managed by computer control, the measured MAP was within the prescribed range 94% of the time.

The use of automated SNP infusion for blood pressure control in medical emergencies has also been investigated (3). The algorithm for blood pressure control reflects a series of decision pathways that is based on clinical experience. Potentially dangerous blood pressure levels are reduced in a stepwise and predictable fashion, and long-term regulation is achieved.

CONCLUSION

The rapid and powerful action of SNP makes frequent monitoring of MAP followed by appropriate adjustment of the infusion rate necessary for MAP regulation. Because of many other nursing duties, there may not be sufficient time available for achieving good control manually (7). Automated blood pressure control has been used at The University of Alabama at Birmingham to provide minute-by-minute monitoring and control of MAP in several thousand patients for more than 10 years. The automated controller performs satisfactorily over a wide range of conditions and is operated by personnel without knowledge of control theory. The success of the system is attributed to the fact that it was designed to reduce the workload in the clinical environment.

References

1. Arnsparger JM, McInnis BC, Glover JR, et al: Adaptive control of blood pressure. *IEEE Trans Biomed Eng* 30:168, 1983.
2. de Asla RA, Benis AM, Jurado RA, et al: Management of postcardiotomy hypertension by microcomputer-controlled administration of sodium nitroprusside. *J Thorac Cardiovasc Surg.* 89:115, 1985.
3. Hammond JJ, Kirkendall WM, Calfee RV: Hypertensive crisis management by computer controlled infusion of sodium nitroprusside: a model for the closed loop administration of short acting vasoactive agents. *Comput Biomed Res* 12:97, 1979.
4. He WG, Kaufman H, Roy R: Multiple model adaptive control procedure for blood pressure control. *IEEE Trans Biomed Eng* BME-33:10, 1986.
5. Kaufman H, Roy R, Xu X: Model reference adaptive control of drug infusion rate. *Automatica* 20:205, 1984.
6. Meline LJ, Westenskow DR, Pace NL, et al: Computer-controlled regulation of sodium nitroprusside infusion. *Anesth Analg* 64:38, 1985.
7. Mitchell RM: The need for closed-loop therapy. *Crit Care Med* 10:831, 1982.
8. Sheppard LC: Computer control of the infusion of vasoactive drugs. *Ann Biomed Eng* 8:431, 1980.
9. Slate JB: Model-based design of a controller for infusing sodium nitroprusside during postsurgical hypertension. Ph.D. thesis, University of Wisconsin, Madison, 1980.
10. Slate JB, Sheppard LC: Automatic control of blood pressure by drug infusion. *IEE Proc* 129:639, 1982.
11. Stern KS, Chizeck HJ, Walker, BK, et al: The self-tuning controller: comparison with human performance in the control of arterial pressure. *Ann Biomed Eng* 813:341, 1985

47

Special Pediatric Problems

Curt M. Steinhart, M.D.
Albert W. Pruitt, M.D.

Certain clinical problems are encountered with much greater frequency in the pediatric intensive care unit (PICU) than in the adult ICU and vice versa. Specific aspects of drug absorption, distribution, metabolism and action in pediatric patients are presented in Chapter 7. Application of these principles during bedside management presents a special challenge to the critical care specialist. This chapter contains some pharmacological and toxicological considerations unique to pediatric critical care. Discussions regarding the use of intravenous isoproterenol for status asthmaticus, ribavirin for respiratory syncytial virus, racemic epinephrine for croup, and prostaglandin E_1 for congenital heart diseases are presented. Pediatric approaches to status epilepticus and supraventricular tachycardia as well as sedation and neuromuscular paralysis are addressed in a framework for care in the PICU. In addition, three toxicological problems (clonidine overdose, iron intoxication, organophosphate poisoning) are discussed both because of their relative frequency of occurrence and their unique pharmacotherapy.

INTRAVENOUS ISOPROTERENOL FOR STATUS ASTHMATICUS

Although most children with status asthmaticus respond adequately to some combination of inhaled β-agonists, intravenous aminophylline, parenteral epinephrine, and corticosteroid administration, a small percentage develop respiratory failure and require admission to a pediatric ICU. Unlike most other lower airway causes of respiratory failure, status asthmaticus in children often is treated successfully without the need for endotracheal intubation and mechanical ventilation (55, 69, 91, 120, 121). Isoproterenol by continuous intravenous infusion is utilized both in children

and adults in an effort to avoid intubation (55, 65, 91). Because of concerns about isoproterenol-induced tachycardia (65, 69, 91), myocardial oxygen supply and demand (67, 70), and a previous report of myonecrosis (70) this therapy is employed more frequently for children and adolescents (55, 69, 91, 120, 121) than for adults (65). In pediatric patients with severe hypercarbia (arterial $PCO_2 \geq 55$ torr) and/or hypoxemia (arterial $PO_2 \leq 60$ torr on 60% FIO_2), continuously infused isoproterenol reverses respiratory failure without the need for mechanical ventilation in up to 85% of cases (55, 91, 121).

For administration, isoproterenol hydrochloride is diluted in 5% dextrose or dextrose 5% in 0.2 normal saline (D_5.2NS). The number of milligrams of isoproterenol to be diluted to 100 ml is equal to the child's weight in kilograms multiplied by 0.15. When one uses a microdrip infusion pump, an initial rate of 2.0 ml/hour gives 0.05 μg/kg/minute. Incremental increases in rate of infusion of 1.0 ml/hour increases the amount infused by 0.025 μg/kg/minute. This dilution and adjustment of infusion rate allows for very careful titration to the desired effect. The use of infused isoproterenol requires monitoring of the ECG, heart rate, and respiratory rate. An indwelling arterial catheter is required for continuous blood pressure measurement and also allows for frequent arterial blood gas determinations. Fluid intake and output should also be carefully monitored. The isoproterenol infusion rate is increased every 15–20 minutes until (a) the $PaCO_2$ is ≤45 torr, (b) the heart rate becomes excessive (≥200 beats/minute for infants and small children; ≥180 for older children and adolescents), or (c) other evidence of toxicity (usually an arrhythmia) is noted. Dose requirements are usually in a range from 0.20 to 0.50 μg/kg/minute (55, 91, 121), but infusion rates greater than 1.0 μg/kg/minute have been successfully administered without untoward occurrences (121).

Because isoproterenol has a very short plasma half-life (61), a continuous infusion is necessary to maintain effective plasma drug levels. On the other hand, dose-related toxic effects are readily controlled. Tachycardia is the most common side effect. Concomitant use of aminophylline and the presence of relative dehydration, respiratory distress, and anxiety may compound the increased chronotropy inherent with isoproterenol. Isoproterenol-induced increases in heart rate of 10–20 beats/minute should be anticipated; however, in some cases relief of respiratory distress and anxiety after initiating isoproterenol infusion causes the heart rate to decrease. Aminophylline administration, usually as a continuous infusion, should be continued during isoproterenol therapy. Theophylline clearance increases when administered with isoproterenol (52). Therefore in isoproterenol treated patients, adjustments in aminophylline infusion rates should be based on frequent serum theophylline determinations. Caution is required when using β-agonists with aminophylline based upon evidence for increased myocardial toxicity with this combination (72). It is prudent to achieve low therapeutic serum theophylline levels (10–15 μg/ml) when using isoproterenol.

Reports of both myocardial ischemia (123) and myonecrosis (70) indicate potentially dangerous cardiovascular consequences from isoproterenol infusion. As a nonselective β-adrenergic receptor agonist with marked inotropic and chronotropic activity, isoproterenol increases myocardial oxygen consumption that, in the presence of hypoxemia, may potentiate myocardial cell injury. Continuous ECG recording and frequent careful bedside evaluation should provide detection of overt toxicity in most instances. A daily 12-lead ECG and determination of myocardial creatine kinase (CPK-MB) are advocated by some authors to assist in this assessment (69, 121).

Because isoproterenol-induced pulmonary arteriolar dilatation may occur before bronchial dilatation, intrapulmonary shunting may increase. The resultant worsening of hypoxemia can be extremely troublesome, but is usually transient. Frequent assessment of the arterial PO_2 in the first several hours after initiating isoproterenol therapy aided by continuous pulse oximetry and coupled with additional supplemental oxygen via face mask provides ample monitoring and therapy for this circumstance.

When an effective isoproterenol infusion rate is achieved, that rate should be continued for 24 hours unless complications occur. Subsequently, the infusion rate is slowly reduced over 24–48 hours with careful, repeated evaluation of clinical status and arterial blood gases.

Should respiratory failure persist or worsen despite the isoproterenol infusion, the infusion is continued during mechanical ventilation in a persistent effort to control bronchospasm. This approach may allow for a shorter ventilator time and improve chances for successful extubation.

STATUS EPILEPTICUS IN CHILDREN

Status epilepticus may be defined as seizures that last more than 30 minutes or recur so frequently during a given period as to be nearly continuous. Prolonged seizures in children may result from infection, drug ingestion, trauma, tumors, hypoxia, cerebral ischemia, metabolic derangements, fever, and from uncertain (idiopathic) causes. A variety of effective anticonvulsant medications are presently available; however, a single method of treatment for status epilepticus is appropriate. Moreover, dosage and drug-drug interactions warrant careful attention.

Seizures from metabolic causes (e.g., from hypoglycemia, hypocalcemia, or hyponatremia) are usually resistant to anticonvulsants and require correction of the metabolic abnormality. Proper diagnosis by blood chemistry analysis is essential in order to suitably manage such seizures.

For status epilepticus due to causes other than metabolic derangements, diazepam (0.1–0.2 mg/kg, slow intravenous push) has become the mainstay for acute convulsive states in both children and adults (10, 21, 42, 98, 104, 113). Readily available in nearly all emergency rooms and intensive care units, its rapid onset of action (often less than 1 minute) makes it a nearly ideal and effective agent. Diazepam, however, has several properties that necessitate cautious use in pediatric patients. It has a relatively short anticonvulsant duration of action (20–30 minutes), but may have a more prolonged effect on respiratory activity (101). For these reasons, repeated administration is often necessary to maintain seizure control but may result in cumulative respiratory depressant effects.

A common approach is to stop the acute convulsions with diazepam and then initiate treatment with a longer acting preparation. Phenobarbital administration following diazepam therapy results in such potent respiratory depression that their concomitant use is not advised. Initial anticonvulsant therapy with phenobarbital alone can be given more safely than when used after diazepam (98, 113, 124). Children who are not receiving chronic therapy should receive an initial intravenous dose of phenobarbital of 10 mg/kg over 1–2 minutes. Seizures may take 5 minutes or longer to abate, therefore careful observation of the airway and the cardiovascular system are needed while convulsions persist. Subsequently, phenobarbital doses of 5 mg/kg (maximum 20–30 mg/kg) are given every 5–15 minutes until the seizures cease. The decision to administer further therapy should be governed by serum phenobarbital levels.

The use of phenobarbital therapy after diazepam should be undertaken only when facilities and personnel can rapidly provide endotracheal intubation and subsequent ventilatory support. Numerous cases of respiratory arrest following combination therapy with diazepam and phenobarbital have been observed. Conversely, if the airway has been secured via endotracheal intubation, the early use of diazepam to halt the convulsions and subsequent use of phenobarbital for maintenance therapy is appropriate.

Phenytoin is an excellent agent for use in status epilepticus (98, 104, 119). In combination with diazepam, it provides long-acting anticonvulsant activity without the respiratory depressant synergism seen with phenobarbital. It may also be used as the initial agent. A first phenytoin dose of 10 mg/kg (maximum 500 mg) is slowly (over 10 minutes) given intravenously. Subsequent doses of 5 mg/kg to a total of 20–25 mg/kg result in therapeutic serum levels of 10–25 μg/ml. If the initial dose stops the seizures, the remainder of the total dose should be given over 12–18 hours in order to reach therapeutic levels needed for chronic therapy.

To avoid potential phenytoin toxicity and to avert respiratory depression created when using phenobarbital (with or without diazepam), some clinicians use lorazepam for status epilepticus in children (71). Lorazepam has a relatively rapid onset (usually less than 3 minutes), a longer duration of action (2–4 hours) than that of diazepam, and minimal respiratory depressant activity (25). An initial lorazepam dose of 0.05–0.10 mg/kg slow intravenous push is usually effective, but subsequent

similar doses every 15 minutes may be necessary in more refractory states. A maximum of three doses has been recommended. Anticonvulsant activity lasted more than 3 hours in 83% and greater than 24 hours in 50% of the children in one study (71), with no adverse systemic or local effects. Maintenance therapy with phenobarbital or phenytoin following lorazepam administration appears to be safe (71).

Paraldehyde remains a useful anticonvulsant for status epilepticus (10, 98, 124). Its primary drawback is difficulty with administration. Although effective orally and per rectum, we prefer the intravenous route of administration. A 5% or 10% solution prepared in a glass bottle or syringe should be attached to the intravenous catheter using a minimum amount of intravenous tubing since paraldehyde may slowly react with some intravenous tubing. A large peripheral or central vein is preferred to avoid local phlebitis. A dose of 0.15 mg/kg (1.5 ml/kg of 10% solution) is suggested per hour (98), but optimal therapy requires careful, bedside titration. Paraldehyde is partially eliminated through the lungs, and pulmonary edema is associated with excessive doses. Arterial blood gas measurements and chest roentgenograms are strongly suggested. Paraldehyde is primarily eliminated by hepatic metabolism. Cautious use of paraldehyde in patients with liver disease is advised. Solutions containing paraldehyde should be shielded from light to prevent oxidation to acetic acid.

For cases refractory to a combination of agents, diazepam by continuous infusion is usually effective, but is used only after endotracheal intubation. Diazepam should be diluted in normal saline and administered through a large peripheral or central vein at a rate of 0.2 mg/kg/hour and titrated to achieve total seizure control. Cardiovascular depression may be noted with diazepam infusion and inotropic support may be required.

RIBAVIRIN FOR RESPIRATORY SYNCYTIAL VIRUS INFECTIONS

Respiratory syncytial virus (RSV) is a common respiratory pathogen in infants and young children and may be particularly troublesome in infants with underlying pulmonary or cardiovascular disease. This RNA virus causes epidemic bronchiolitis and pneumonia during yearly outbreaks (45, 50, 90). Following infection, immunity is only for a short term and no effective immunization is presently available (48, 53).

Ribavirin (1-β-D-ribofuranosyl -1, 2, 4-triazole-3-carboxamide), a synthetic nucleoside analog, possesses activity against several different viruses apparently through RNA synthesis inhibition (107). It may also act by interfering with the expression of viral messenger RNA without becoming incorporated into host cell RNA or DNA. The drug was approved in 1985 by the Food and Drug Administration (FDA) in aerosol form only for respiratory infections caused by RSV. It has been safely administered to both previously well infants (50, 110) and in those with underlying cardiopulmonary disorders (49, 109) such as bronchopulmonary dysplasia and congenital heart diseases. A rapid diagnostic test utilizing fluorescent antibodies makes it possible to select patients for treatment.

Ribavirin is administered using a Collison generator to create an aerosol with a mass median diameter of 1.3–1.4 μm. The 6-g vial is diluted in 300 ml of sterile water and placed in a reservoir that then has a concentration of 20 mg/ml. The generator flow is adjusted to 12–14 liters/minute and delivered into an oxygen hood. No exact administered dosage has been determined as this dose depends upon the patient's minute ventilation, but delivery over 18–21 hours/day has been recommended (48, 50).

Respiratory failure, endotracheal intubation, and mechanical ventilation do not preclude ribavirin usage despite FDA-required product labeling, which states therapy during mechanical ventilation is contraindicated. That warning is related to the hygroscopic nature of the drug that, when aerosolized, may deposit onto ventilator circuit tubing and the endotracheal tube. With careful monitoring and strong technical support from respiratory therapists, complications from ribavirin during mechanical ventilation can be reduced and even eliminated. It is crucial that aerosol flow from the Collison generator be connected to the inspiratory limb of the ventilator circuit as near to the endotracheal tube as is feasible. Ventilator gas flow should be well humidified and warmed to 32–34°C. Filters on the expiratory limb of the ventilator circuit must be changed frequently (every 1–2 hours) to avoid residue accumulation that can result in inadvertent positive end-expiratory pressure (PEEP). Both the aerosol generator flow rate and the ventilator gas flow rate must be adjusted at frequent intervals so that most of the 300 ml of ribavirin solution is delivered from the reservoir during an 18–24 hour period. Close monitoring of peak inspiratory pressure and PEEP is essential, and continuous pulse oximetry or frequent measurement of arterial blood gases is important when ribavirin is administered to patients requiring mechanical ventilation to ensure adequate ventilation and oxygenation.

Toxicity studies have revealed no consistent patterns (50, 110). Minor variations in hematological values and serum chemistries have been transient and trivial. No long-term untoward effects have yet been found. Treatment usually lasts 3–5 days but long-term therapy has been undertaken in an infant with an immunodeficiency (82).

Recommendations regarding indications for treatment are still evolving; however, recent recommendations (1) for ribavirin therapy include infants at high risk for severe or complicated RSV infection and infants already severely ill because of RSV lower respiratory tract disease. RSV often causes only mild upper respiratory tract symptoms, but lower respiratory tract disease may require hospital admission. During epidemics, it has been recommended that all hospitalized infants with a clinical presentation strongly suggesting RSV infection should receive ribavirin prior to laboratory confirmation (48, 51). Where diagnostic studies for RSV can be done without delays, it may be prudent to hold treatment pending laboratory diagnosis. In those patients with underlying cardiac or pulmonary disease, therapy should be begun even without diagnostic certainty.

SUPRAVENTRICULAR TACHYCARDIA IN CHILDREN

Supraventricular tachycardia (SVT) in infants and children can occur as a single episode or as a chronic condition (8, 40, 44, 76). It may result from drug ingestion (22) or infection (41) as well as from an abnormal cardiac conduction pathway, both in the presence and absence of congenital heart disease (8, 40, 44, 76, 118). Although often presenting with nonspecific symptoms (poor weight gain, poor appetite), SVT may also present as an acute, life-threatening emergency requiring admission to the pediatric ICU (28, 76, 103). Whereas verapamil has become the treatment of choice for SVT in adults (54, 99), controversy continues as to the proper management of SVT in pediatric patients (8, 28, 39, 92, 94, 103, 118). Careful consideration of patient age, hemodynamic status, and underying cardiac disorder is required for optimal results.

The primary consideration at the time of initial evaluation should be the hemodynamic and respiratory status of the patient. If significant respiratory distress is present, endotracheal intubation should be considered as an initial step. In the presence of hypotension, poor perfusion, or other evidence of a decreased cardiac output, continuous ECG and blood pressure monitoring are required. Immediate DC cardioversion, at 0.2–0.5 watt-seconds per kilogram, should be tried and repeated if necessary. Cardioversion does not preclude early attempts at vagal stimulation (carotid massage, gag reflex, Valsalva maneuver), but repeated efforts to induce vagal slowing in the hemodynamically compromised patient are discouraged.

Intravenous digoxin must be readily available. Should DC cardioversion be successful, a total digitalizing dose of 20–40 μg/kg is used, with one-fourth to one-half given as the first dose over 1–2 minutes; the remainder is prescribed as two or three equal doses 6–8 hours apart. If DC cardioversion is unsuccessful, the loading dose of digoxin is administered in the same manner as with successful cardioversion. A rapid conversion with digoxin after failed DC cardioversion is unlikely, but may be a safer approach than immediate use of other antiarrhythmic agents.

Diving reflex stimulation via ice water immersion (less than 5 seconds) or application for 15–30 seconds to the face (e.g., an ice-water-filled bag over the patient's face) are both rapid and safe but only occasionally successful. An α-adrenergic agonist such as phenylephrine hydrochloride via intravenous infusion (0.5–5.0 μg/kg/minute) may be utilized to induce reflex slowing of heart rate and to correct hypotension through vasoconstriction, but often does so at the expense of worsened tissue perfusion.

When hemodynamic decompensation and SVT persist, "overdrive" pacing through the transvenous approach is recommended. The pacemaker rate is gradually increased until capture of the rate occurs. Once captured, the rate can then be reduced to achieve ventricular slowing; if SVT resumes upon a reduction of pacemaker rate, the pacemaker rate can be increased in an effort to obtain a 2:1 block with a reduced ventricular rate.

When hemodynamically stable, verapamil hydrochloride in small doses successfully converts up to 93% of pediatric patients with acute SVT (103). Continuous ECG and blood pressure monitoring are required during verapamil administration (0.1 mg/kg) infused intravenously over 30–60 seconds. When successful, the rhythm often reverts to normal sinus or sinus tachycardia within 1–3 minutes. If needed, verapamil may be repeated at 15-minute intervals for a total of three doses (0.3 mg/kg total dose). Calcium chloride (10%) at 10 mg/kg must be available and administered if sudden hypotension or asystole occur as a result of the verapamil infusion. Atropine sulfate (0.01 mg/kg, minimum 0.1 mg) may be useful if problematic bradycardia develops. However, should SVT return, the rate may be more rapid than previously noted. Since verapamil may cause peripheral vasodilation, volume expansion with normal saline or lactated Ringer's solution (10 ml/kg) may be required. Depressed inotropic activity caused by verapamil can be counteracted by dopamine or epinephrine infusion, but recurrence of SVT with these catecholamines is common.

Verapamil should be avoided in pediatric patients with hypotension, low cardiac output, unstable second-degree atrioventricular block and third-degree atrioventricular block, as well as those in the tachycardic phase of the sick sinus syndrome (28, 93). Its use in patients who have received β-blockers (93) and in newborn infants (28) may be particularly dangerous.

In certain instances, the electrophysiology of the child's SVT may be known from a previous electrophysiological study. In SVT due to re-entry (atrioventricular re-entry or accessory pathway), verapamil is likely to be very effective. It is generally ineffective in SVT because of ectopic tachycardias (atrial or junctional) and may lead to further deterioration (93, 94).

In conclusion, the relative safety of digoxin and its frequent use as an agent for chronic SVT make it a good agent for all forms of SVT in all pediatric age groups. Concerns about DC cardioversion in patients receiving digoxin are warranted. We therefore choose to use DC cardioversion as the initial treatment when SVT presents with hypotension or poor cardiac output and then administer digoxin to the patient after a slower rate is achieved. We prefer verapamil only in the older child or adolescent in whom hypotension is not present.

RACEMIC EPINEPHRINE FOR RESPIRATORY DISTRESS

Acute upper airway problems are a frequent cause for admissions to pediatric ICUs. Croup syndromes (viral laryngotracheobronchitis, spasmodic croup) and postextubation subglottic edema present as stridor, which may portend significant respiratory distress and eventual respiratory failure. These maladies affect pediatric patients far more frequently than adults because of anatomic airway differences, particularly in the subglottic area where the narrowest portion is at the level of the cricoid cartilage.

As treatment for respiratory distress, racemic ephinephrine, a mixture of the optically active epinephrine isomers (L-epinephrine and D-epinephrine) can be diluted in 0.9% normal saline and then delivered as a nebulized aerosol (32, 38, 62, 79). In this form, it is a rapidly acting, effective means of controlling acute subglottic swelling and perhaps avoiding the need for endotracheal intubation or tracheostomy (95, 106, 115). Supplied as a 2.5% solution, 0.25–0.50 ml of the drug should be diluted in 3.0–4.0 ml of normal saline, aerosolized by jet nebulizer, and given by either face mask or simply by holding the mist close to the patient's face. This localized delivery to the upper airway avoids many of the side effects from parenterally administered epinephrine, such as systemic vasoconstriction. Tachycardia is not uncommon, but excessively high heart rates and ectopy are infrequent (32, 106, 111, 115).

Racemic epinephrine has a duration of action of 30–120 minutes. Therefore, to discharge the patient from the emergency room after treatment with this medicine is contraindicated without a long observation period (at least 6 hours). Whether rebound swelling in excess of that already present occurs after therapy is uncertain (79, 111, 115), but there is little disagreement that despite epinephrine's palliative, temporizing effect, the natural history of viral croup is not altered (111, 115). We feel that any child whose airway abnormality is severe enough to require racemic epinephrine should be hospitalized. A false sense of security following a simple treatment and an early discharge home can lead to catastrophic results.

Treatment with racemic epinephrine should be construed as a palliative effort to avoid endotracheal intubation or tracheostomy. The croup score (24) is extremely useful for initial and repeated evaluation for those with subglottic swelling. A score of 5 or more should necessitate admission to a unit where direct observation is possible. Scores of 7 or 8 imply respiratory difficulty that often responds to racemic epinephrine treatment and continued use of other therapies such as cool mist and mild sedation. When the croup score is 9 or 10, impending or actual respiratory failure exists. Rapid improvement with racemic epinephrine may still be possible, but preparation for emergency intubation and/or tracheostomy in the operating room should be made with an anesthesiologist and otolaryngologist in attendance. If a patient requires racemic epinephrine nearly continuously (more than every 30 minutes), it is prudent to establish an airway via intubation or tracheostomy and to avoid the risk of respiratory fatigue, sudden obstruction, hypoxemia, or hypercarbia.

PROSTAGLANDIN E_1 FOR DUCTAL PATENCY

Although an understanding of prostaglandin biosynthesis and pharmacology have provided potential therapeutic modalities for sepsis and cerebral ischemia (9, 36, 105, 116), nowhere has the ability to manipulate prostaglandin-mediated events been more profound than with therapies aimed at constricting or dilating the ductus arteriosus early in life. The premature infant may sustain prolonged cardiorespiratory failure secondary to a patent ductus arteriosus (20, 64, 74) that may respond to nonsurgical closure using the prostaglandin synthetase inhibitor indomethacin (58, 80). To the contrary, maintaining ductal patency in certain forms of cyanotic and acyanotic congenital heart disease may provide preoperative stabilization (35, 46, 57).

Since Coceani and Olley (12) showed that prostaglandins E_1 and E_2 relaxed the isolated ductus arteriosus of fetal lambs, many large clinical trials have provided ample support for the use of prostaglandin E_1 in the presence of cyanotic or acyanotic lesions in which ductal patency is required for adequate pulmonary or systemic flow (14, 35, 46, 57, 75). Infants with pulmonary atresia, hypoplastic right ventricle, and severe pulmonic stenosis may sustain a large increase in arterial PO_2 following prostaglandin E_1 initiation. Other forms of cyanotic congenital heart disease including transposition of the great vessels, tricuspid atresia, truncus arteriosus and total anomalous pulmonary venous return may also benefit from prostaglandin E_1 infusion to improve arteriovenous mixing. Since severe cyanosis with resultant acidemia and cardiovascular collapse may occur prior to diagnosis, most pediatric heart centers advocate prostaglandin E_1 therapy for all critically ill neonates in whom cyanotic congenital heart disease is strongly suspected.

Infants with systemic cardiovascular collapse due to aortic arch anomalies (interrupted aortic arch, juxtaductal aortic coarctation) may develop severe acidemia and renal failure during spontaneous ductal closure. Many such infants show marked improvement in lower body perfusion, urine output, and arterial pH when prostaglandin E_1 is used to obtain ductal patency (35, 57). As with cyanotic lesions, prostaglandin E_1 should be instituted in all critically ill infants suspected to have aortic arch anomalies even before exact diagnosis is established.

Prostaglandin E_1 therapy can be administered via a peripheral venous, central venous, or umbilical arterial site. The intravenous route is preferred since cutaneous vasodilation is more pronounced with intra-arterial infusion (75). The amount of prostaglandin E_1 in milligrams to be diluted in 100 ml 5% dextrose water is the product of the body weight in kilograms times 0.3. An initial dose of 0.05 μg/kg/minute is achieved with an infusion rate of 1.0 ml/hour. Clinical efficacy is usually achieved at doses ranging from 0.05 to 0.20 μg/kg/minute; however, both lower and higher doses have been utilized (35, 57). The infusion should be continued until surgical palliation or correction is performed, or until further assessment shows no need to maintain ductal patency.

Side effects from prostaglandin E_1 infusion merit considerable attention. Apnea and/or hypoventilation, presumably attributed to CNS effects, are extremely common. Provision should be made for immediate airway management, including endotracheal intubation for all infants receiving prostaglandin E_1. Intubation should be performed prior to transport of an infant to another center. Because there is concern about susceptibility to infection, concurrent antibiotic therapy is usually warranted. Cardiovascular effects secondary to vasodilation should be anticipated and volume replacement and inotropic agents (usually dopamine) are often necessary to avoid systemic

hypotension. Fever, even in the absence of sepsis, is not unusual while seizures, jitteriness, hypoglycemia, hypocalcemia, diarrhea, renal failure, and clotting abnormalities have been reported (14, 75). Despite these associated risks, prostaglandin E_1 is often life sustaining in critically ill infants with congenital heart disease prior to surgical correction or palliation.

SEDATION IN THE PEDIATRIC ICU

Numerous pharmacological agents are used routinely in the pediatric ICU to relieve pain, prevent anxiety, facilitate endotracheal intubation, and provide muscle relaxation for those requiring mechanical ventilation. The following commentary is a review of these drugs as utilized in the pediatric ICU.

Morphine sulfate is one of the more commonly used analgesics in the pediatric ICU. Its uses include (a) relief of postoperative pain, (b) sedation for infants and children who require neuromuscular blockade, (c) afterload reduction in patients with congestive cardiac states or low cardiac output, and (d) sleep in anxious patients. Morphine's popularity is based upon its easy dosing, fairly predictable responses, duration of action, and the ability to reverse its action with the opiate antagonist, naloxone.

To provide sedation for those patients requiring neuromuscular blockade, an intravenous morphine dose of 0.1 mg/kg given over 1–5 minutes appears to be effective. Common practice is to repeat the dose every 2–6 hours based on evidence that desired effects have dissipated (return of tachycardia, hypertension, decreased perfusion, movement). Precautions should be taken in patients with altered cardiovascular performance as a slight, transient reduction in blood pressure, presumably due to decreased peripheral vascular resistance, is quite common (unpublished observation) and/or via relaxation of venous tone resulting in decreased preload. Dosing for postoperative analgesia, afterload reduction, and sleep induction more commonly requires individual titration, but intravenous doses of 0.05–0.10 mg/kg are commonly employed. We prefer to avoid intramuscular administration as this is painful and offers no advantage to the ICU patient, who must always have an intravenous line in place.

Infants and children seem to develop dependency or addiction only rarely when morphine is used in the pediatric ICU setting. Other than cardiovascular changes, the primary concern with prolonged use is reduced gastrointestinal motility. Morphine may impair the ability to enterally feed these patients. Metoclopramide may alleviate gastric atony, but seems ineffective in improving lower gastrointestinal immotility (unpublished observation). Despite its potential problems, morphine remains in frequent use in most pediatric ICUs. Morphine has been given by continuous intravenous infusion in both infants (66) and children (77). Dosages of $10-30$ μg/kg/hour seem to provide effective analgesia and may reduce the hemodynamic variations seen with intermittent bolus infusions. Neonates developed higher serum morphine levels than older children, and doses not exceeding 15 μg/kg/hour have been recommended for infants (66).

Some pediatric intensivists prefer the potent synthetic opioid fentanyl over morphine because of fentanyl's lack of histamine release and minimal cardiovascular effects (108). Fentanyl is approximately 500 times more potent than morphine because of its greater lipid solubility (78). Although its duration of action may be only $30-90$ minutes following a single dose, far longer activity may be seen after higher doses or following repeated usage.

Chloral hydrate provides mild sedation without analgesia. Its advantages are a lack of cardiovascular effects and minimal, or no, respiratory depression. Given as an oral or rectal dose of $20-50$ mg/kg, chloral hydrate generally induces sleep in $20-30$ minutes. It is not available in parenteral form and provides no pain relief, which are its two major disadvantages. Despite these shortcomings, it remains a valuable adjunct for sedation.

The benzodiazepines, diazepam and lorazepam, both provide effective sedation and amnesia. Diazepam in doses of 0.1 to 0.2 mg/kg given slowly via the intravenous route, provides amnesia up to 3 hours (34) with a rapid onset of action. These properties make it an ideal agent for use during endotracheal intubation in children and adolescents and for other uncomfortable procedures such as DC cardioversion and fiberoptic bronchoscopy. We frequently employ diazepam alternately with morphine for patients requiring neuromuscular paralysis. In this setting, diazepam adds amnesia to the analgesic and muscle relaxation provided by morphine and pancuronium respectively. Diazepam cannot be administered with dextrose-containing solutions and may cause hypotension if infused too rapidly. For the latter reason, lorazepam at an intravenous dose of $0.5-0.10$ mg/kg may be preferred to diazepam for inducing amnesia with less potent cardiovascular effects (25).

A variety of neuromuscular blocking agents are available to assist with endotracheal intubation or for more prolonged use during mechanical ventilation or both. Succinylcholine chloride, a depolarizing neuromuscular blocker, is usually the drug of choice for endotracheal intubation particularly in young children and infants. Adequate muscle relaxation for intubation occurs within $10-20$ seconds after a dose of $1.0-2.0$ mg/kg given as an intravenous bolus and usually lasts $3-5$ minutes. The higher dose (2 mg/kg) is primarily recommended for infants and young children who have a relatively greater blood volume and extracellular fluid volume than older children on a weight basis, as succinylcholine is rapidly distributed to the extracellular spaces (16, 17, 88). Elimination of the drug is rapid because of hydrolysis by plasma (pseudo-) cholinesterase. Succinylcholine activity is potentiated by decreased or abnormal plasma cholinesterase, alkalosis, increased extracellular potassium (hyperkalemia), decreased temperature, quinidine, concomitant magnesium sulfate administration, liver disease, and certain antibiotics (aminoglycosides, polymixins, tetracyclines) (88). Antagonism and/or a shortened duration of action may occur with hypokalemia, acidosis, decreased cardiac output or increased skeletal muscle blood flow (88).

Succinylcholine frequently induces vagal stimulation, which may be further augmented during laryngoscopy, resulting in clinically significant bradycardia. It should always be administered with, or preferably after intravenous atropine (0.01 mg/kg, minimum 0.10 mg). Older children and adolescents should be given an "obtundation dose" of thiopental ($2-4$ mg/kg) or ketamine ($1-2$ mg/kg) or, as we prefer diazepam ($0.2-0.4$ mg/kg) prior to succinylcholine administration.

The major drawbacks of succinylcholine are a very short duration of action, induction of muscle fasciculations particularly in older children and its contraindication in patients with burns, massive muscle trauma, and certain motor neurological defects (88) as well as those at risk for the malignant hyperthermia syndrome (determined by history, familial predisposition, or provocative muscle testing). Succinylcholine also causes increased intracranial, intragastric, and intraocular pressures. "Crash induction" techniques with the use of thiopental coupled with cricoid pressure and then atropine-succinylcholine block increase in intracranial pressure and also lessen the hazards of aspiration.

The nondepolarizing neuromuscular blockers most commonly used are d-tubocurarine chloride and pancuronium bromide, but vecuronium bromide, metocurine iodide, and atracurium besylate are also available. Equipotent doses for these agents have been established for both infants and children (Table 47.1). Advantages and disadvantages for each of these agents are also noted in the table, with a few requiring specific commentary.

Histamine release by d-tubocurarine can potentially aggravate bronchospasm in those with asthma or other allergic disorders. However, in newborn infants histamine appears to be a bronchodilator and vasodilator (73). This fact makes histamine release potentially helpful in early postnatal circulatory derangements caused by high pulmonary vascular resistance (persistent pulmonary hypertension syndrome), wherein pulmonary vasodilation via histamine release would be advantageous.

Pancuronium has great appeal because of its longer duration of action. This characteristic makes dosing less frequent, a major advantage to nursing personnel who must administer these agents often around the clock for several days and/or weeks. This advantage is somewhat offset by its often profound cardiovascular effects, particularly tachycardia and hypertension. These responses may be particularly troublesome in patients with cardiovascular compromise or in those in whom other pharmacological agents may already have created or may further enhance tachyarrhythmias (methylxanthines, β-agonists, catecholamines).

For the reasons just mentioned, we prefer to use vecuronium as the agent of choice whenever pancuronium has created or may potentially elicit an untoward response. Vecuronium has almost no cardiovascular side effects and although not as "long acting" as pancuronium, its duration of action is acceptable in most circumstances.

Atracurium is cleared by rapid, nonenzymatic degradation (Hofmann elimination) (6), a potential advantage over other agents that may require renal or hepatic removal. Since many PICU patients have altered renal and hepatic function, atracurium may be more predictable in certain patients. To our knowledge, however, its use is relatively uncommon.

Ketamine hydrochloride, a so-called dissociative anesthetic, has been used for pediatric patients during dental (13) and other minor surgical procedures (11). As such, its use for minor surgical procedures in the pediatric ICU seems reasonable. Intravenous doses of 0.5–2.0 mg/kg have been utilized (117). Ketamine creates cardiovascular stimulation, primarily through CNS mechanisms, which offers a potential advantage over morphine and other depressant agents. Paradoxically, ketamine is a direct myocardial depressant (102), which may explain the sudden, unexpected hypotension reported in critically ill patients (114). Well-described, unpleasant psychic disturbances during emergence from ketamine may make its use less preferable than other agents, and unpleasant dreams even weeks following its use have been reported (84). In the unfamiliar pediatric ICU environment, further psychiatric stresses should be eliminated; thus, we have chosen to avoid ketamine use except when other agents are more contraindicated.

Table 47.1
Equipotent Doses of Nondepolarizing Neuromuscular Blockers

	Usual Dose (mg/kg)	Onset of Action (min)	Duration of Action (min)	Metabolism/ Clearance	Comments
Pancuronium	0.08–0.12	2–4	65	40% unchanged (urine) 87% bound	Somewhat longer action; tachycardia frequent
Vecuronium	0.06–0.10	2–3	35–55	35% unchanged (urine) 25–50% bile 60–80% bound	Few cardiovascular changes; shorter duration of action
Atracurium	0.4–0.5	2–2½	40–60	Hofmann elimination and ester hydrolysis	Predictable duration in renal and hepatic failure
d-Tubocurarine	0.3–0.6	2–4	50	45% unchanged (urine)	Released histamine may be beneficial in neonates
Metocurine	0.2–0.4	1½–2	40–60	50% unchanged (urine) 35% bound	Somewhat shorter onset of action

CLONIDINE OVERDOSE

Clonidine hydrochloride is a frequently prescribed oral antihypertensive agent. Because of its popularity, it is a relatively frequent cause of drug overdose in children admitted to intensive care units. The drug achieves its antihypertensive effect through central sympathetic mechanisms that reduce peripheral vascular tone and heart rate. Conversely, the drug may act on peripheral receptors to transiently increase vascular tone. These dual, somewhat competitive, actions can create a variety of clinical manifestations when ingested by small children or when overdose occurs in adolescents. Symptoms of overdose include drowsiness, impaired sensorium, respiratory depression, apnea, bradycardia, miosis, hypertension, and hypothermia as probable consequences of the central action. Hypertension, due to peripheral α-adrenergic agonist effect, has also been reported (2, 15, 60). The balance between central sympathetic inhibition and peripheral α-adrenergic stimulation determines which effects predominate.

In infants and young children who ingest clonidine by accident, central sympathetic depression often predominates. Drowsiness often ensues within 1 hour of ingestion of a very small amount and may progress to obtundation, coma, and apnea. Cardiovascular effects range from mild bradycardia with a normal or minimally decreased blood pressure to overt hypotension (4, 83). Adolescents who have ingested an overdose of clonidine may manifest hypertension along with respiratory depression and depressed level of consciousness.

Initial treatment must include attention to the airway and adequacy of ventilation. Endotracheal intubation has been required especially in young children because of marked slowing of respiration (4). Cardiovascular support may be necessary to correct either hypotension or bradycardia, and less often for hypertension. Atropine sulfate (0.01 mg/kg, minimum 0.1 mg) is generally effective for bradycardia and may improve blood pressure in the heart rate–dependent cardiovascular system of the infant. Although the α-adrenergic blocker tolazoline has been recommended in both hypotensive and hypertensive states, patients respond unpredictably (100, 122). Volume expansion with 10 ml/kg of 0.9% normal saline or lactated Ringer's solution, often accompanied by dopamine (5–10 μg/kg/minute) or epinephrine (0.1 to 0.3 μg/kg/minute)

by continuous infusion, reverses both the bradycardia and hypotension. The short half-life of dopamine and epinephrine permits rapid discontinuation as the clonidine effects subside. The infrequent hypertensive state induced by clonidine may be better treated with tolazoline (100, 122). An initial dose of 1.0 mg/kg (followed by a continuous infusion of 1.0–2.0 mg/kg/hour when necessary) may be effective, but alternative therapy with a more predictable peripheral vasodilator such as sodium nitroprusside (0.5–5.0 μg/kg/minute) should also be considered.

Such supportive and specific treatment is in addition to routine measures for acute ingestions, which include emetics, activated charcoal, and cathartics. Clonidine is cleared mostly in the urine (15), while poorly defined extrarenal clearance mechanisms also exist with an overall plasma half-life of approximately 12 hours. Although forced diuresis with loop and/or osmotic diuretics has been advocated, most authors feel such is not necessary and may even worsen hypotension (89). As expected from its half-life, most symptoms of clonidine ingestion resolve within 12–24 hours.

The opiate antagonist naloxone has been debated as a specific agent for management of clonidine intoxication. Such use has some pharmacological justification in that naloxone reverses clonidine's hypotensive effects in spontaneously hypertensive rats (30) and is efficacious in models of respiratory and cardiovascular depression (18, 29, 47, 56, 59, 68, 97). Nevertheless Banner et al. (4) reported that five children, aged 17 months to 2 years, had no detectable response to intravenous naloxone (0.03–0.05 mg/kg). Its efficacy therefore appears to remain anecdotal and unsubstantiated.

IRON INTOXICATION

The ingestion of iron-containing compounds, particularly by young children, remains a frequent cause for pediatric ICU admission (47, 56, 68, 97). These products are widely available, and their use during pregnancy, when mothers may be less able to adequately supervise the younger children in the household, as well as an underappreciation by the general public regarding the danger associated with iron ingestion, creates a scenario for accidental iron intoxication.

The clinical effects from acute iron ingestion are well described (5, 23). The characteristic stages are (a) gastrointestinal, (b) relative stability, (c) shock, (d) hepatic necrosis, and (e) gastrointestinal scarring. Clearly, not all patients manifest each stage, but the more severe cases may likely do so. The initial gastrointestinal stage begins shortly after the iron-containing product has been ingested. Symptoms usually include vomiting and abdominal pain, but may also include diarrhea and/or gastrointestinal hemorrhage. A quiescent stage of relative stability may ensue between 4 and 48 hours after ingestion, but in severe cases this "eye of the hurricane" period may only be a failure to recognize the subtle signs of impending cardiovascular collapse. The third stage is characterized by circulatory derangements attributed to both the direct and indirect effects of iron. A reduction in the circulating plasma volume may be due to vomiting, diarrhea, hemorrhage, or "third spacing" of fluid into the irritated gastrointestinal tract. Metabolic acidosis results from conversion of ferrous to ferric ions (96), from inhibitory effects of iron on cellular oxidative metabolism (96), and from a hypoperfusion–low cardiac output state. Coagulation may become impaired with further bleeding and continued cardiovascular deterioration. Hepatic necrosis may develop even if circulatory impairment is corrected. The liver appears to be a target organ for the direct toxic effects of iron. The hepatic toxicity stage fortunately occurs only rarely. The acute, corrosive injury to bowel usually heals within several weeks; however, such healing may leave stenotic areas in both the gastric outlet and the proximal small bowel that later may present as acute gastrointestinal obstruction (31, 37).

Despite the availability of deferoxamine mesylate as an effective chelating agent, some controversy persists as to the actual procedures for treating acute iron intoxication. Certain recommendations can be reasonably made. Emesis should be induced unless the sensorium precludes it. Mechanical lavage to remove iron in the neurologically depressed patient is always indicated. Some have proposed using sodium bicarbonate (26) or sodium phosphate (3) as the lavage fluid, based on the relatively water insoluble complexes these agents form with iron (19). Because of the risk of excessive phosphate absorption (43), approximately 100 ml of a 5% sodium bicarbonate solution in water is preferable, and should be left in the stomach after lavage to produce poorly soluble ferrous carbonate (7). Activated charcoal is of little value in inhibiting absorption, but a cathartic should be used to assist in intestinal emptying. Although deferoxamine has been administered by the enteral route, absorption of the iron-deferoxamine complex may occur from the gastrointestinal tract (5). Thus, we feel its safety has not been adequately demonstrated (5).

The serum iron concentration should be determined. Patients with levels greater than 300 µg/dl usually require parenteral deferoxamine therapy. Unless there is evidence of poor tissue perfusion, deferoxamine (40 mg/kg) should be given intramuscularly. In the presence of hypotension, a secure intravenous line is required for blood volume expansion and intravenous deferoxamine administration is indicated. A continuous infusion at 15 mg/kg/hour is generally safe, but continuous ECG and frequent blood pressure measurements are necessary. Hypotension is generally reversible with further volume expansion although catecholamine (dopamine or epinephrine) infusion may occasionally be required.

The iron-deferoxamine complex may produce a pink color in the urine. When present, the color serves as a simple method to assess excretion of the complex. A simple qualitative test has been proposed as a screen for iron ingestion (81) when the intoxicant is unknown. Monitoring urine color as well as serial serum iron determinations indicate when chelation therapy may be discontinued.

More invasive treatments aimed at removing iron have been advocated, including surgical gastrotomy (33), hemodialysis (23), and total body exchange transfusion (86). Although each of these has been helpful in specific, unusual cases, their routine use is generally not advised. Further supportive care requirements should be based on the severity of the ingestion and the clinical response to initial therapy.

ORGANOPHOSPHATE POISONING

Children exposed to organophosphate insecticides through inhalation, ingestion, or skin absorption may represent a serious medical emergency. Other insecticides may also cause severe toxic reactions and may occasionally prove fatal, but the relative availability of organophosphates in both household and agricultural pesticides warrant their specific mention here.

Organophosphate compounds bind irreversibly to the two cholinesterases found in humans. Acetylcholinesterase (true cholinesterase) is found primarily in neurons, at the neuromuscular junction, and in red blood cells; whereas pseudocholinesterase (serum cholinesterase) is found in serum, liver, and other organs. These enzymes are responsible for terminating the effects of acetylcholine, a central and peripheral neurotransmitter responsible for central respiratory and cardiovascular control and peripheral nicotinic and muscarinic receptor activity. Failure to deactivate acetylcholine at the neuroeffector junction occurs when organophosphates bind to the cholinesterase enzymes and create the symptoms that can be classified as nicotinic (muscle fasciculations, cramps, incoordination, weakness, paralysis), muscarinic (miosis, sweating, salivation, lacrimation, bronchospasm, bronchorrhea, bradycardia, hypertension, nausea, vomiting, diarrhea), and central (apathy, obtundation, coma, convulsions).

Highly toxic organophosphates include tetraethylpyrophosphate (TEPP), methyl parathion, ethyl parathion, and bomyl (27, 85). Moderately toxic agents such as fenthion, diazinon, dichlorvos, and malathion (27, 85) are more commonly used in household products than for agricultural use. In addition, most household products are provided in diluted formulations. Petroleum distillates may be used as the organic solvent for certain organophosphates and further complicate therapy.

Initial therapy should be promptly administered. For preparations not containing petroleum distillates, emesis should be induced. Gastric lavage, if indicated, should be performed in the usual manner. Skin cleaning with copious amounts of soap and water is required to remove the compounds from the skin. Health professionals must be careful to wear rubber gloves and other protective garments to prevent contamination by the toxin and subsequent absorption. Atropine antagonizes the central and muscarinic effects, but does not reverse the nicotinic receptor–mediated muscle weakness. Dosing should be directed toward atropinization, which may require large and frequent intravenous infusions. Younger children are treated with an initial dose of 0.05 mg/kg followed by a maintenance dose of 0.02–0.05 mg/kg every 10–30 minutes until cholinergic signs are reversed. Older children (12 years of age and older) may be given 1.0–2.0 mg initially and then every 15–30 minutes until complete reversal of cholin-

ergic signs. Careful, repeated assessment of airway adequacy and respiratory muscle strength is required even in the fully atropinized patient. The presence of a dry mouth; warm, flushed skin; dilated pupils; and increased heart rate indicate adequate atropinization. Atropine therapy should be continued for at least 24 hours in moderate and severe cases to allow time for the organophosphate compound to be eliminated. Atropine toxicity manifest by fever, muscle fasciculations, and delirium requires halting further atropine administration. If cholinergic signs return during withdrawal of atropine therapy, it should be reinstituted.

The cholinesterase reactivating oximes PAM (2-PAM, pralidoxime iodide) or protopam (pralidoxime chloride) counteract the nicotinic and muscarinic effects but not the central effects incurred with organophosphate intoxication. Atropine therapy must continue concurrently with either of these agents. There does not appear to be any particular advantage of one agent over the other. An intravenous infusion of 25–50 mg/kg prepared in 5% dextrose and 0.45% normal saline (D_5.45NS) should be administered over 10–30 minutes. A dose of 0.5–1.0 g may be given to larger children or adolescents. Nausea, headache, dizziness, diplopia, respiratory depression, and hypertension are side effects of pralidoxime. The initial infusion should be followed by a second infusion using the same dose 1–2 hours later and then again after around 12 hours if cholinergic signs recur. Treatment for more than 24 hours is generally not required except with fenthion exposure, which undergoes very slow elimination (85). Although measurements of acetylcholinesterase and pseudocholinesterase are helpful in determining the response to pralidoxime and assessing the severity of organophosphate exposure, these tests often are not readily available and delay in providing pralidoxime therapy must be avoided. We make this recommendation because the enzyme-organophosphate complexes become more resistant to the reactivating effects of pralidoxime as time passes (112).

Morphine, methylxanthines, and loop diuretics are specifically contraindicated in organophosphate poisoning (85). Supportive care, including endotracheal intubation and mechanical ventilation, is based upon the severity of exposure, physical findings, arterial blood gases and other laboratory assessments (27, 63, 85, 87).

References

1. American Academy of Pediatrics Committee on Infectious Diseases: Ribavirin therapy of respiratory syncytial virus. *Pediatrics* 79:475, 1987.
2. Anderson RJ, Hart GR, Crumpler CP, et al: Clonidine overdose: report of six cases and review of the literature. *Ann Emerg Med* 10:107, 1981.
3. Arron: Iron. In Rumack BH (ed): *Poisindex.* Englewood, CO, Micromedex, 1980.
4. Banner W, Lund ME, Clawson L: Failure of naloxone to reverse clonidine toxic effect. *Am J Dis Child* 137:1170, 1983.
5. Banner W, Tong TG: Iron poisoning. *Pediatr Clin North Am* 33:393, 1986.
6. Basta, SJ, Ali HH, Savarese JJ, et al: Clinical pharmacology of atracurium besylate (BW 33A). *Anesth Analg* 61:723, 1982.
7. Benjamin, BI, Cortell S, Conrad, ME: Bicarbonate-induced iron complexes and iron absorption: one effect of pancreatic secretions. *Gastroenterology* 53:389, 1967.
8. Benson DW Jr, Dunningan A, Benditt DG, et al: Prediction of digoxin treatment failure in infants with supraventricular tachycardia: role of transesophageal pacing. *Pediatrics* 75:228, 1985.
9. Butler RR, Wise WC, Haluska PV, et al: Thromboxane and prostacyclin production during septic shock. *Adv Shock Res* 7:133, 1982.
10. Camfield PR: Treatment of status epilepticus in children. *Can Med Assoc J* 128:671, 1983.
11. Carrel R: Ketamine: a general anesthetic for unmanageable ambulatory patients. *ASDC J Dent Child* 40:288, 1973.
12. Coceani F, Olley PM: The response of the ductus arteriosus to prostaglandins. *Can J Physiol Pharmacol* 51:220, 1973.
13. Cohenhour K, Gamble JW, Metzgar MT, et al: A composite general anesthesia for pediatric outpatients. *J Oral Surg* 36:594, 1978.
14. Cole RB, Alman S, Aziz KU, et al: Prolonged prostaglandin E1 infusion: histologic effects on the patent ductus arteriosus. *Pediatrics* 67:816, 1981.
15. Conner CS, Watanabe AS: Clonidine overdose: a review. *Am J Hosp Pharm* 36:906, 1979.
16. Cook DR: Muscle relaxants in infants and children. *Anesth Analg* 60:335, 1981.
17. Cook, DR, Fischer CG: Neuromuscular blocking effects of succinylcholine in infants and children. *Anesthesiology* 42:662, 1975.
18. Curtis MT, Lefer AM: Protective actions of naloxone in hemorrhagic shock. *Am J Physiol* 239:H416, 1980.
19. Czajka PA, Konrad JD, Duffy JP: Iron poisoning: an in vitro comparison of bicarbonate and phosphate lavage solutions. *J Pediatr* 98:491, 1981.
20. Danielowicz D, Rudolph AM, Hoffman JIE: Delayed closure of the ductus arteriosus in premature infants. *Pediatrics* 37:74, 1966.
21. Delgado-Escueta AV, Wasterlain C, Treiman DM, et al: Management of status epilepticus. *N Engl J Med* 306:1337, 1982.
22. Dobmeyer DJ, Stine RA, Leier CV, et al: The arrhythmogenic effects of caffeine in human beings. *N Engl J Med* 308:814, 1983.
23. Doolin EJ, Drueck C: Fatal iron intoxication in an adult. *J Trauma* 20:518, 1980.
24. Downes JJ, Raphaely R: Pediatric intensive care. *Anesthesiology* 43:242, 1975.
25. Dundee, JW, McGowan WAW, Lilburn JK, et al: Comparison of the actions of diazepam and lorazepam. *Br J Anaesth* 51:439, 1979.
26. Einhorn AH: Iron poisoning. In Rudolph AM (ed): *Pediatrics,* ed 16. New York, Appleton-Century-Crofts, 1977, pp 790–793.
27. Einhorn, AH: Organophosphate insecticide poisoning. In Rudolph AM (ed): *Pediatrics,* ed 16. New York, Appleton-Century-Crofts, 1977, pp 793–795.
28. Epstein ML, Kiel EA, Victorica BE: Cardiac decompensation following verapamil therapy in infants with supraventricular tachycardia. *Pediatrics* 75:737, 1985.
29. Faden AL, Holaday JW: Opiate antagonists: a role in the treatment of hypovolemic shock. *Science* 205:317, 1979.
30. Farsong C, Kunas G: Naloxone reverses the antihypertensive effect of clonidine. *Br J Pharmacol* 67:161, 1979.
31. Filpi RG, Majd M, LoPresti JM: Reversible gastric stricture following iron ingestion. *South Med J* 66:845, 1973.
32. Fogel JM, Berg IJ, Gerber MA, et al: Racemic epinephrine in the treatment of croup: nebulization alone versus nebulization with intermittent positive pressure breathing. *J Pediatr* 101:1028, 1982.
33. Foxford R, Goldfrank L: Gastrotomy—a surgical approach to iron overdose. *Ann Emerg Med* 14:1223, 1985.
34. Fragen RJ, Caldwell N: Lorazepam premedication-lack of recall and relief of anxiety. *Anesth Analg* 55:792, 1976.
35. Freed MD, Heymann MA, Lewis AB, et al: Prostaglandin E1 in infants with ductus arteriosus-dependent congenital heart disease. *Circulation* 64:988, 1981.
36. Fukumori T, Tani E, Maeda Y, et al: Effects of selective inhibitor of thromboxane A_2 synthetase on experimental cerebral vasospasm. *Stroke* 15:306, 1984.
37. Gandhi RK, Robarts FH: Hour-glass stricture of the stomach and pyloric stenosis due to ferrous sulfate poisoning. *Br J Surg* 49:613, 1962.
38. Gardner HG, Powell KR, Roden VJ, et al: The evaluation of racemic epinephrine in the treatment of infectious croup. *Pediatrics* 52:52, 1973.
39. Garson A: Medicolegal problems in the management of cardiac arrhythmias in children. *Pediatrics* 79:84, 1987.
40. Garson A, Gillette PC: Electrophysiologic studies of supraventricular tachycardia in children. I. Clinical-electrophysiologic correlations. *Am Heart J* 102:223, 1981.
41. Garson A, Gillette PC, McNamara DG: Supraventricular tachycardia in children: clinical features, response to treatment and long-term follow-up in 217 patients. *J Pediatr* 98:875, 1981.
42. Gastaut H, Naquet R, Poire R, et al: Treatment of status epilepticus with diazepam (Valium). *Epilepsia* 6:167, 1965.
43. Geffner ME, Opas LM: Phosphate poisoning complicating treatment for iron ingestion. *Am J Dis Child* 134:509, 1980.
44. Gillette PC, Garson A, Kugler JD: Wolff-Parkinson-White syndrome in children: electrophysiologic and pharmacologic characteristics. *Circulation* 60:1487, 1979.
45. Glezen WP, Denny FW: Epidemiology of acute lower respiratory disease in children. *N Engl J Med* 288:498, 1973.
46. Graham TP, Atwood GF, Boucek RJ: Pharmacologic dilatation of the ductus arteriosus with prostaglandin E1 in infants with congenital heart disease. *South Med J* 71:1238, 1978.
47. Greenblatt DJ, Allen MD, Koch-Weser J: Accidental iron poisoning in childhood. *Clin Pediatr* 15:835, 1976.
48. Hall CB, McBride JT: Vapors viruses, and views—ribavirin and respiratory syncytial virus (editorial). *Am J Dis Child* 140:331, 1986.
49. Hall CB, McBride JT, Gala CL: Ribavirin therapy of respiratory syncytial virus in infants with cardiopulmonary disease. *Pediatr Res* 19:295A, 1985.
50. Hall CB, McBride JT, Walsh EE, et al: Aerosolized ribavirin treatment of infants with respiratory syncy-

tial viral infection—a randomized double-blind study. *N Engl J Med* 308:1443, 1983.

51. Hall CB: Ribavirin: beginning the blitz on respiratory viruses? *Pediatr Infect Dis* 4:668, 1985.

52. Hemstreet MP, Miles MV, Rutland RO: Effect of intravenous isoproterenol on theophylline kinetics. *J Allergy Clin Immunol* 69:360, 1982.

53. Henderson FW, Collier AM, Clyde WA, et al: Respiratory syncytial virus infections, reinfection, and immunity: a prospective, longitudinal study in young children. *N Engl J Med* 300:530, 1979.

54. Heng MK, Singh BN, Roch AHG, et al: Effects of intravenous verapramil on cardiac arrhythmias and on the electrocardiogram. *Am Heart J* 90:487, 1975.

55. Herman JJ, Noah ZL, Moody RR: Use of intravenous isoproterenol for status asthmaticus in children. *Crit Care Med* 11:716, 1983.

56. Herretig FM, Karl SR, Weintraub WH: Severe iron poisoning treated with enteral and intravenous deferoxamine. *Ann Emerg Med* 12:306, 1983.

57. Heymann MA, Berman W, Rudolph AM, et al: Dilatation of the ductus arteriosus by Prostaglandin E1 in aortic arch abnormalities. *Circulation* 59:169, 1979.

58. Heymann MA, Rudolph AM, Silverman NH: Closure of the ductus arteriosus in premature infants by inhibition of prostaglandin synthesis. *N Engl J Med* 295:530, 1976.

59. Holaday JW, Faden AL: Naloxone acts at central opiate receptors to reverse hypotension, hypothermia and hypoventilation in spinal shock. *Brain Res* 189:295, 1980.

60. Hunyor SN, Bradstock K, Somerville PJ, et al: Clonidine overdose. *Br Med J* 4:23, 1975.

61. Kadar D, Tang HY, Conn AW: Isoproterenol metabolism in children after intravenous administration. *Clin Pharmacol Ther* 16:789, 1974.

62. Kepes ER, Martinez LR, Andrews IC, et al: Racemic epinephrine in postintubation laryngeal edema. *NY State Med J* 7:583, 1972.

63. Kiss Z, Fazekas T: Arrhythmias in organophosphate poisonings. *Acta Cardiol* 34:323, 1979.

64. Kitterman JA, Edmunds LH, Gregory GA: Patent ductus arteriosus in premature infants: incidence, relation of pulmonary disease and management. *N Engl J Med* 287:473, 1972.

65. Klaustermeyer WB, DiBernardo RL, Hale FC: Intravenous isoproterenol: Rationale for bronchial asthma. *J Allergy Immunol* 55:325, 1975.

66. Koren G, Butt W, Chinyanga H, et al: Post-operative morphine infusion in newborn infants: Assessment of disposition characteristics and safety. *J Pediatr* 107:963, 1985.

67. Krasnon N, Rolett EL, Yurchak D, et al: Isoproterenol and cardiovascular performance. *Am J Med* 37:514, 1964.

68. Krenzelok EP, Hoff JV: Accidental childhood iron poisoning: a problem of marketing and labeling. *Pediatrics* 63:591, 1979.

69. Kurland G, Leong AB: The management of status asthmaticus in infants and children. *Clin Rev Allergy* 3:37, 1985.

70. Kurland G, Williams J, Lewiston NJ: Fatal myocardial toxicity during continuous infusion intravenous isoproterenol therapy of asthma. *J Allergy Clin Immunol* 63:407, 1979.

71. Lacey DJ, Singer WC, Horwitz SJ, et al: Lorazepam therapy of status epilepticus in children and adolescents. *J Pediatr* 108:771, 1986.

72. Lehr D, Guideri G: More on combined beta-agonists and methylxanthines in asthma. *N Engl J Med* 30:1581, 1983.

73. Levin DL, Heymann MA, Kitterman JA, et al: Persistent pulmonary hypertension of the newborn infant. *J Pediatr* 89:626, 1976.

74. Levin DL, Stanger P, Kitterman JA, et al: Congenital heart disease in low-birth-weight infants. *Circulation* 52:500, 1975.

75. Lewis AB, Freed MD, Heymann MA, et al: Side effects of therapy with prostaglandin E₁ in infants with critical congenital heart disease. *Circulation* 64:893, 1981.

76. Linde LM, Turner SW, Awa S: Present status and treatment of paroxysmal supraventricular tachycardia. *Pediatrics* 50:127, 1972.

77. Lynn AM, Opheim KE, Tyler DC: Morphine infusion after pediatric cardiac surgery. *Crit Care Med* 12:863, 1984.

78. Mather LE, Phillips GD: Opioids and Adjuvants: Principles of use. In Cousins MJ, Phillips GD (eds): *Acute Pain Management*. New York, Churchill Livingston, 1986, pp 77–103.

79. McBride JT: Stridor in childhood. *J Fam Pract* 19:782, 1984.

80. McCarthy JS, Zies LG, Gelband H: Age-dependent closure of the patent ductus arteriosus by indomethacin. *Pediatrics* 62:706, 1978.

81. McGuigan MA, Lovejoy FH, Marino SK, et al: Qualitative deferoxamine color test for iron ingestion. *J Pediatr* 94:940, 1979.

82. McIntosh K, Kurachek SC, Cairns LM, et al: Treatment of respiratory viral infection in an immunodeficient infant with ribavirin aerosol. *Am J Dis Child* 138:305, 1984.

83. Mendoza JE, Medalie M: Clonidine poisoning with marked hypotension in a 2½ year-old child. *Clin Pediatr* 18:123, 1979.

84. Meyers EF, Charles P: Prolonged adverse reactions to ketamine in children. *Anesthesiology* 49:39, 1978.

85. Mortensen ML: Management of acute childhood poisonings caused by selected insecticides and herbicides. *Pediatr Clin North Am* 33:421, 1986.

86. Movassaghi N, Purugganan MD, Leikin S: Comparison of exchange transfusion and deferoxamine in the treatment of acute iron poisoning. *J Pediatr* 75:604, 1969.

87. Namba T, Nolte CT, Jackson J, et al: Poisoning due to organophosphate insecticides. *Am J Med* 50:475, 1971.

88. Nugent SK, Laravuso R, Rogers MC: Pharmacology and use of muscle relaxants in infants and children. *J Pediatr* 94:481, 1979.

89. Pai GA, Lipsitz DJ: Clonidine poisoning. *Pediatrics* 58:749, 1976.

90. Parrott RH, Kim HW, Brandt CD, et al: Respiratory syncytial virus in infants and children. *Prev Med* 3:473, 1974.

91. Parry WH, Martorano F, Cotton EK: Management of life-threatening asthma with intravenous isoproterenol infusions. *Am J Dis Child* 130:39, 1976.

92. Pickoff AS, Zies L, Ferrer PL, et al: High-dose propranolol therapy in the management of supraventricular tachycardia. *J Pediatr* 94:144, 1979.

93. Porter CJ, Garson A, Gillette PC: Verapamil: an effective calcium blocking agent for pediatric patients. *Pediatrics* 71:748, 1983.

94. Porter CJ, Gillette PC, Garson A, et al: Effects of verapamil on supraventricular tachycardia in children. *Am J Cardiol* 48:487, 1981.

95. Postma DS, Jones RO, Pillsbury HC: Severe hospitalized croup: treatment trends and prognosis. *Laryngoscope* 94:1170, 1984.

96. Reissman KR, Coleman TJ: Acute intestinal iron intoxication. II. Metabolic, respiratory and circulatory effects of absorbed iron salts. *Blood* 10:46, 1955.

97. Reynolds LG, Kelin M: Iron poisoning—a preventable hazard of childhood. *S Afr Med J* 67:680, 1985.

98. Rothner AD, Erenberg G: Status epilepticus. *Pediatr Clin North Am* 27:593, 1980.

99. Schamroth L, Krikler DM, Garret C: Immediate effects of intravenous verapamil in cardiac arrhythmias. *Br Med J* 1:660, 1972.

100. Schieber RA, Kaufman ND: Use of tolazoline in massive clonidine poisoning. *Am J Dis Child* 135:77, 1981.

101. Schmidt D: Benzodiazepines—diazepam. In Woodbury DM, Penry JK, Pippenger CE (eds): *Antiepileptic Drugs.* New York, Raven Press, 1982, pp 711–735.

102. Schwartz DA, Horwitz LD: Effects of Ketamine on left ventricular performance. *J Pharmacol Exp Ther* 194:410, 1975.

103. Shahar E, Barzilay Z, Frand M: Verapamil in the treatment of paroxysmal supraventricular tachycardia in infants and children. *J Pediatr* 98:323, 1981.

104. Shaywitz BA: Management of acute neurologic syndromes in infants and children. *Yale J Biol Med* 57:83, 1984.

105. Short BL, Gardiner WM, Walker R, et al: Indomethacin improves survival in gram negative sepsis. *Adv Shock Res* 6:27, 1981.

106. Singer OP, Wilson WJ: Laryngotracheobronchitis: 2 years' experience with racemic epinephrine. *Can Med Assoc J* 115:132, 1976.

107. Smith RA: Background and mechanisms of action of ribavirin. In Smith RA, Knight V, Smith JAD, (eds): *Clinical Application of Ribavirin.* Orlando, Academic Press, 1984, p 1.

108. Sonntag H, Larsen R, Hilfiker D, et al: Myocardial blood flow and oxygen consumption during high dose fentanyl anesthesia in patients with coronary artery disease. *Anesthesiology* 56:417, 1982.

109. Spinelli M, Ciardullo-Geraci K, Palumbo PE, et al: Efficacy of ribavirin for treating respiratory syncytial virus (RSV) pneumonia in high-risk infants. *Pediatr Res* 19:304A, 1985.

110. Taber LH, Knight V, Gilbert BE, et al: Ribavirin aerosol treatment of bronchiolitis associated with respiratory syncytial virus infection in infants. *Pediatrics* 72:613, 1983.

111. Taussig LM, Castro O, Beaudry PH, et al: Treatment of laryngotracheobronchitis (croup). *Am J Dis Child* 129:790, 1975.

112. Taylor P: Anticholinesterase agents. In Gilman AG, Goodman LS, Gilman A (eds): *The Pharmacologic Basis of Therapeutics,* ed 6. New York, Macmillan Publishing Company, 1980, pp 100–119.

113. Trauner DA: Acute management of seizures. In James HE, Anas NG, Perkin RM (eds): *Brain Insults in Infants and Children.* Orlando, FL, Grune & Stratton, 1985, pp 213–218.

114. Waxman K, Shoemaker WC, Lippmann M: Cardiovascular effects of anesthetic induction with ketamine. *Anesth Analg* 59:355, 1980.

115. Westley CR, Cotton EK, Brooks JG: Nebulized racemic epinephrine by IPPB for the treatment of croup. *Am J Dis Child* 132:484, 1978.

116. White BC, Wiegenstein JG, Winegar CD: Brain ischemic anoxia—mechanisms of injury. *JAMA* 251:1586, 1984.

117. White PF, Way WL, Trevor AJ: Ketamine—its pharmacology and therapeutic uses. *Anesthesiology* 56:119, 1982.

118. Whitman V, Friedman Z, Berman W Jr, et al: Supraventricular tachycardia in newborn infants: an approach to therapy. *J Pediatr* 91:304, 1977.

119. Wilder BJ, Ramsay RE, Wilmore, LJ, et al: Efficacy of intravenous phenytoin in the treatment of status epilepticus: kinetics of central nervous system penetration. *Ann Neurol* 6:515, 1977.

120. Wood DW, Downes J: Intravenous isoproterenol in the treatment of respiratory failure in childhood status asthmaticus. *Ann Allergy* 31:607, 1973.

121. Wood DW, Downes JJ, Scheinkopf H, et al: Intravenous isoproterenol in the management of respiratory failure in childhood status asthmaticus. *J Allergy Clin Immunol* 50:75, 1972.

122. Yagupsky P, Gorodischer R: Massive clonidine ingestion with hypertension in a 9-month-old infant. *Pediatrics* 72:500, 1983.

123. Yossef A, Laks MM, Beall G: An electrocardiographic pattern of acute myocardial infarction associated with excessive use of aerosolized isoproterenol. *Chest* 68:107, 1975.

124. Zimmerman SS, Fish I: Status epilepticus. In Zimmerman SS, Gildea JH (eds): *Critical Care Pediatrics.* Philadelphia, WB Saunders Company, 1985, pp 397–400.

48

Calcium and Calcium Antagonists in Shock and Ischemia[a]

Diana S. Malcolm, Ph.D.
John W. Holaday, Ph.D.
Bart Chernow, M.D., F.A.C.P.
Gary P. Zaloga, M.D., F.A.C.P.

One of the primary characteristics of the shock syndrome in humans is a profound alteration of the physiological regulation of the circulation, resulting in inadequate tissue oxygenation, anaerobic metabolism, organ failure, and death. Prolonged hemorrhage, cardiac failure, trauma, and sepsis are a few of the many recognized causes of shock. Septic shock develops in approximately 25% of the estimated 330,000 Gram-negative bacteremias that occur in the United States each year (45). Sepsis and septic shock may result from many causes, such as wound contamination in a traumatized patient, postoperative surgical complications, dissemination of a localized infection, and invasion of microorganisms through or around invasive instruments. Often, sepsis is further complicated by immune suppression, as often occurs during critical illnesses. Gram-negative sepsis is associated with an overall 50% mortality, even when treated under optimal situations (55). When further complicated by renal or respiratory failure, the mortality rate approaches 90–100% (18). Most of these patients die from progressive multiorgan failure, which is thought to be due to the release of toxic substances from the infecting organisms (e.g., endotoxin), the release of secondary endogenous mediators, and altered metabolic status, resulting in progressive tissue ischemia.

Current clinical management of circulatory shock involves aggressive ventilatory support, fluid resuscitation, and pharmacotherapy directed at maintaining blood pressure and cardiac output. Despite these medical interventions and the availability of new and effective antibiotics, the mortality rate for septic shock has remained virtually unchanged (35). It is clear that new pharmacological strategies, based on a better knowledge and understanding of the pathophysiological mechanisms involved in shock, are necessary for more effective treatment. The purpose of this chapter is to review the pertinent basic and clinical research findings suggesting that calcium (Ca) plays an important role in the pathophysiology of ischemia and shock. Although septic shock will be emphasized, the role of Ca in other forms of circulatory shock will also be addressed.

ROLE OF CALCIUM IN THE PATHOPHYSIOLOGY OF SHOCK

Calcium plays a critical role as a modulator and initiator of many essential cellular functions during physiological or pathophysiological conditions. Chief among these are muscle contraction, electrical activation of various excitable cells, neurotransmitter release, platelet aggregation, chemotaxis, enzyme activity, and endocrine and exocrine secretion. Cellular responses to drugs, hormones, neurotransmitters, and other biological messengers include the activation of specific receptors that in turn alter Ca channels or couple to second messenger systems such as cyclic AMP and phosphatidylinositol. These major intracellular second messengers further modify biochemical events within the cell, in part through alteration of

[a] The opinions or assertions contained herein are the private views of the authors and should not be construed as official or as necessarily reflecting the views of the Uniformed Services University of the Health Sciences, U.S. Army Medical Research Development and Command, or the Department of Defense. There is no objection to its presentation and/or publication.

intracellular Ca availability. Recently, much attention has focused on the role of Ca in mediating or propagating the ischemic cell injury that occurs during shock. In order to better understand the possible mechanisms by which Ca may alter cellular function, it may be helpful to review the major steps involved in the regulation of cellular Ca homeostasis.

The vast majority of Ca in the circulation is bound to proteins such as albumin. However, it is the free (ionized) Ca^{2+}, in equilibrium with the bound Ca, that provides the biologically functional Ca pool. In unstimulated cardiac and smooth muscle cells, free cytosolic Ca^{2+} concentrations range between 0.05 and 0.5 μmol, whereas Ca^{2+} concentrations in the extracellular milieu are approximately 1–5 μmol. Thus, the concentration gradient for free Ca^{2+} across the cell membrane is approximately 1 to 10,000 (intracellular to extracellular). The maintenance of this gradient is essential for cell viability since excessive elevations in intracellular Ca can be destructive to the cell. The Ca gradient across the cell is maintained primarily by (a) the cell membrane which is relatively impermeable to Ca, (b) Ca pumps within the membrane (Ca-ATPase, Ca-sodium exchange), and (c) cellular organelles [sarco(endo)plasmic reticulum and mitochondria] that remove Ca from the cytosol. Many of these processes require a constant supply of energy.

In shock or other ischemic disorders, Ca homeostasis is disrupted, usually resulting in an abnormal accumulation of Ca within the cell (44, 56, 58, 67). This accumulation of cytosolic Ca can be a consequence of either an increase in cell membrane Ca permeability and/or a decrease in activity of the cellular pumps or cellular organelles that sequester or remove Ca from the cell (e.g., as a result of ATP depletion). In septic shock, infecting agents may act directly on these Ca systems or indirectly, such as through the release of bacterial endotoxins, to increase intracellular Ca levels.

An uncontrolled rise in cystolic Ca can disrupt a number of intracellular processes (16) which include excitation-contraction coupling, endocytosis and exocytosis, and enzyme activation. These processes may further exacerbate the hemodynamic and metabolic insufficiencies underlying the shock syndrome. For example, Ca-induced smooth muscle contraction in blood vessels (vasoconstriction) may produce or worsen ischemia by decreasing nutrient blood flow to tissues and cells. Among the intracellular mechanisms that may be in-

volved, phospholipase activation (by Ca) can produce membrane damage and liberate free fatty acids (89). Furthermore, free fatty acid elevations can stimulate the production of free radicals and increase the production of platelet activating factor and eicosanoids, including thromboxanes, prostacyclins, and leukotrienes (89). Some of these toxic products may cause additional cellular damage and a further disruption of Ca homeostasis. Elevations in cytosolic Ca may also activate proteases, nucleases, and Ca-dependent ATPases and uncouple oxidative phosphorylation (12, 47, 83). Thus, although Ca is essential for cellular function, excessive increases in intracellular Ca may also damage the cell.

It is unclear whether the alterations in Ca fluxes leading to intracellular Ca overload are a cause for the cellular metabolic derangements observed in shock or whether these changes are a result of other pathophysiological processes occuring in shock. In either case, the administration of agents that can block Ca entry into cells or block Ca action during shock may help prevent cellular injury and maintain organ function. In addition, the use of Ca antagonists may help to elucidate some of the underlying mechanisms involved in shock pathophysiology and offer new insights into potentially more effective strategies for treating shock.

RATIONALE FOR USING CALCIUM ANTAGONISTS IN SHOCK THERAPY

Figure 48.1 illustrates a proposed scheme of the pathophysiological events occurring during sepsis that ultimately lead to the irreversible stages of septic shock (multiorgan failure). A similar scheme of events may occur during other forms of circulatory shock or ischemic disorders. Although it is unknown whether ischemia is a primary (or causative) effect or a secondary consequence of shock, it is known that prolonged ischemia leads to hemodynamic and metabolic derangements that are detrimental to the cell. These derangements include decreased tissue oxygenation, decreased ATP levels, and accumulation of cellular metabolic products resulting in metabolic acidosis. As reviewed above, an increase in cell membrane permeability, whether due to the release of biochemical mediators (e.g., free radicals, eicosanoids), depletion of energy stores, or a direct result of endotoxemia, can result in an influx of Ca into the cell, resulting

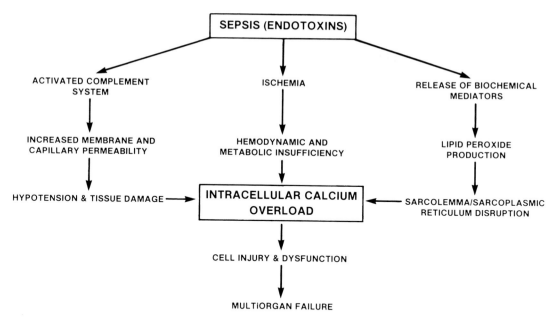

Figure 48.1. A proposed scheme of the pathophysiologic events occurring during sepsis and leading to multiorgan failure (see text).

in an intracellular Ca overload. Elevated cytosolic Ca activates a host of intracellular processes that, if left unchecked, can lead to cellular destruction and eventual organ dysfunction and death. Thus, intracellular Ca accumulation or overload can be thought of as a common pathway for ischemic injury in shock.

Based on the hypothesis that intracellular Ca overload is a mediator for cellular dysfunction in shock, it would be reasonable to assume that Ca antagonists may prevent Ca accumulation within the cell and thus preserve cell/organ function and ultimately improve outcome. Indeed, several lines of evidence support the potential use of Ca blockers in the treatment of shock and other ischemic diseases.

A variety of pharmacological agents are currently available that may be useful in preventing intracellular Ca overload during shock. As a group, these drugs may be classified as Ca "antagonists". A Ca antagonist may be loosely defined as a drug that alters the cellular action of Ca by inhibiting its entry and/or release or by interfering with one of its intracellular actions. Specifically, Ca antagonists may be divided into at least three catagories: (a) Ca chelators (e.g., EGTA), which lower circulating extracellular Ca levels and thus decrease Ca availability for entry into cells; (b) Ca channel blockers (e.g., verapamil, nifedipine, dilti-

azem), which block Ca entry into cells by interacting with Ca specific channels (18); and (c) intracellular Ca antagonists, which either inhibit sarcoplasmic reticular release of Ca (e.g., dantrolene) or inhibit intracellular Ca action (e.g., calmodulin antagonists). It is not the objective of this chapter to provide a comprehensive review of Ca antagonists and their mechanisms of action (31). Instead, we will focus on the use of Ca channel blockers in the treatment of shock and ischemic disorders.

EFFECTS OF CALCIUM ANTAGONISTS IN ISCHEMIC DISORDERS

Ca antagonists have been used extensively (and successfully) in the treatment of cardiac arrhythmias, myocardial ischemic syndromes, and systemic hypertension (see "Clinical Perspectives"). In particular, extensive laboratory and clinical evidence has accumulated to suggest that Ca antagonists may be useful in the treatment of myocardial infarction (81). In the ischemic heart, the Ca antagonists verapamil and nifedipine have been shown to preserve high-energy phosphate compounds (ATP), improve cardiac function, improve myocardial perfusion, preserve normal metabolic activity, reduce infarct size, decrease oxygen demand, prevent intracellular Ca accumulation, and improve survival (40, 57, 65, 69, 70, 85). In contrast, agents that increase Ca entry into the cell or elevate extracellular Ca levels during ischemia have been shown to result in elevated myocardial muscle resting tensions and to exacerbate myocardial injury (56). Together, these findings support the hypothesis that elevated intracellular Ca levels contribute to myocardial cell necrosis during low perfusion states.

There is also evidence that Ca may be responsible for producing vasospasm and cellular dysfunction following cerebral ischemia. Although evidence to the contrary exists (26), Ca channel antagonists have been shown to improve cerebral tissue oxygenation, reduce cerebral vasospasm, and improve neurological recovery and survival in cats and rats following cerebral embolization (90, 91). Others have shown that Ca channel antagonists also improve cerebral perfusion and neurological recovery following cardiac arrest (42, 88, 93).

Similar evidence is accumulating to suggest that Ca is a pathogenic mediator of cellular

injury during ischemia in the kidney, liver, and skeletal muscle. In the kidney, verapamil treatment preserves inulin clearance and renal blood flow, protects against tubular necrosis, and prevents intracellular Ca accumulation following norepinephrine infusion (11, 49) and renal artery occlusion (84). Incubation of hepatocytes with Ca-free solutions has been shown to protect the cells against death due to anoxia and hepatotoxins (67). Other studies show that elevated intracellular Ca levels can cause major ultrastructural damage to mitochondria and myofilaments within skeletal muscle (24, 64).

SPECIFIC EFFECTS OF CALCIUM ANTAGONISTS IN EXPERIMENTAL MODELS OF SHOCK

Endotoxic and Septic Shock

As reviewed in the preceding section, Gram-negative bacteria are the most common cause

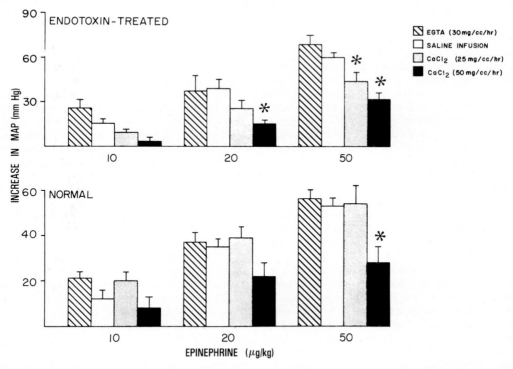

Figure 48.2. Effects of hypocalcemia and hypercalcemia on epinephrine-induced increases in mean arterial pressure (MAP) in normal and endotoxin-treated rats. Rats ($n = 8$) were rendered hypocalcemic (with EGTA infusion) or hypercalcemic (with $CaCl_2$ infusion) and then subjected to bolus injection of *Escherichia coli* endotoxin (5 mg/kg, i.v.) or saline (normal group). Control rats were infused with saline (1 ml/hr, i.v.). Sixty minutes postendotoxin or saline, rats were injected with incremental bolus doses of epinephrine (10, 20, 50 μg/kg, i.v.) approximately 15 minutes apart. $CaCl_2$ infusions (50 mg/cc/hr) blunted epinephrine's pressor effects in normal and endotoxemic rats. EGTA infusions did not alter epinephrine's pressor effects. ($^* = P < 0.05$)

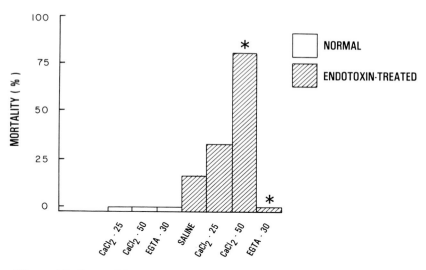

Figure 48.3. Effects of CaCl$_2$ and EGTA infusions on endotoxin mortality. Rats ($n = 8$) were infused with saline, CaCl$_2$, or EGTA and 30 minutes later injected with either saline (normals) or endotoxin (5 mg/kg, i.v.). Animals were infused a total of 2 hours. Mortality was determined 24 hours postendotoxin injection. CaCl$_2$ infusions (50 mg/cc/hr) significantly increased endotoxin mortality, whereas EGTA infusions (30 mg/cc/hr) significantly decreased endotoxin mortality. (* = $P < 0.05$)

of sepsis and septic shock, and bacterial lipopolysaccharides (endotoxins) are considered to be primary factors in the development of the shock state (51). Like other shock syndromes, endotoxic shock is characterized by decreased organ perfusion leading to a decrease in cellular oxygen supply and nutrient delivery, with eventual cellular injury and death. Intracellular Ca overload has been postulated to be a common pathway for cellular injury and death in experimental endotoxic shock. Supporting this hypothesis are the findings that Ca channel antagonists improve cardiovascular function and survival in dogs (4) and rats (46) following endotoxin injections. In direct septic shock models, Bosson and colleagues (6) demonstrated that Ca antagonists decreased mortality in mice given live *Escherichia coli* infusions. These investigators also showed that Ca blockers improved cardiac output, arterial pressure and diminished intestinal damage in cats treated with live *E. coli* (5). Despite these studies, it remains unknown whether the beneficial effects of Ca antagonists such as verapamil, diltiazem, and nifedipine are a result of their blockade of Ca channels.

Although intracellular Ca has been reported to accumulate in cellular organelles following endotoxin administration (43, 66), the effects of bacterial endotoxins on intracellular Ca regulation also remain to be firmly defined. A depression in Ca^{2+} uptake by mitochondria

(52, 73) or the sarcoplasmic reticulum (72) may result in elevated free cytoplasmic Ca^{2+} levels, although contrary evidence also exists demonstrating no change in cellular or mitochondrial Ca uptake in animals treated with endotoxin or rendered septicemic by cecal ligation with puncture (74). Soulsby et al. (73) report a decrease in Ca ATPase activity in vascular sarcoplasmic reticulum of endotoxemic dogs. Nonetheless, endotoxin has been shown in vitro to impair sarcoplasmic reticular and mitochondrial Ca uptake in canine myocardial tissues (38) and bovine vascular tissues (71), both of which may lead to the accumulation of cytosolic Ca. Clearly, more definitive studies are needed to determine whether intracellular Ca overload does indeed occur in shock states; what tissues, cells, and organelles are affected by Ca overload; and whether Ca antagonists can prevent or reverse this cellular accumulation of Ca and thus improve outcome.

In addition to studies using Ca antagonists, other reports suggest a significant role for Ca in the pathophysiology of shock. We were among the first to show that Ca chloride (CaCl$_2$) infusions (producing hypercalcemia) are detrimental in shock (92). CaCl$_2$ (50 mg/cc/hour, intravenously) infusions elevated ionized circulating Ca levels by 100% and not only blunted epinephrine's pressor effects (Fig. 48.2), but also significantly increased mortality in endotoxemic rats (Fig. 48.3). In contrast, lower-

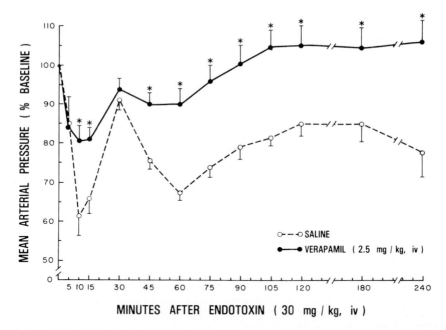

Figure 48.4. Effects of verapamil pretreatment on hemodynamic responses during endotoxic shock in rats. Verapamil pretreatment (2.5 mg/kg, i.v., 15 minutes) significantly (* = $P < 0.05$) improved mean arterial pressure throughout the 4 hours postendotoxin (30 mg/kg, i.v.) except at the 30-minute time point.

ing circulating Ca levels by the intravenous administration of a chelator (EGTA) improved survival in endotoxic shock (Fig. 48.3) and did not impair epinephrine's pressor actions (Fig. 48.2) (Zaloga GP, Malcolm D, Willey S et al., unpublished data). Interestingly, we observed that verapamil injection (2.5 mg/kg intravenously) also produced a decrease in circulating ionized Ca^{2+} levels (48). Confirming the results of others (4), we were able to demonstrate that verapamil improved mean arterial pressure (Fig. 48.4) and increased 24-hour survival from 50% to 90% (48). Together, these findings suggest that lowering circulating Ca levels (with EGTA) or blocking its entry into cells (with verapamil) may protect cells from Ca overload and thus improve the shock state. Obviously, in a syndrome as complex as shock and with a class of drugs with several different modes of action, more studies are needed in order to determine the precise mechanism(s) involved in the protective effects of Ca antagonists in shock.

Hemorrhagic Shock

During the course of hemorrhagic shock, there is a significant degree of ischemic injury to many organs, including the heart, kidney, brain, and liver. Since Ca antagonists have been shown to decrease ischemic damage and improve function in these organs, they should theoretically be of benefit in the treatment of hemorrhagic shock. Indeed, it has been shown by Hackel et al. (32) that verapamil infusions in hemorrhaged dogs partially or completely prevented the development of ventricular subendocardial hemorrhage and necrosis and resulted in less intestinal mucosal hemorrhage. In these studies, verapamil-treated animals also had a significantly higher survival rate. Others have confirmed and extended these findings to demonstrate that verapamil treatment significantly improves mean arterial pressure and coronary blood flow, improves cardiac index, and decreases heart rate and total peripheral resistance during the course of hemorrhagic shock (33, 40, 41).

Not only has cardiovascular function and myocardial histology been shown to be improved by verapamil, but subcellular function has also been documented to be protected by verapamil during the course of shock. Hess and Greenfield (39) have demonstrated a significant depression of Ca uptake by the sarcoplasmic reticulum and an uncoupling of Ca transport from ATP hydrolysis in the myocardium during hemorrhagic shock. In verapamil-treated animals, Ca uptake by the sarcoplasmic reticulum was not suppressed, and excitation-contraction remained tightly coupled. Although intracellular Ca levels were not measured in these studies, the observation that sarcoplasmic reticular Ca uptake was depressed suggests that intracellular Ca levels were consequently elevated above normal in the untreated shocked animals. This would support the hypothesis that (a) intracellular Ca overload occurs during hemorrhagic shock and (b) that a defect in the sarcoplasmic reticulum may be a potential site or cause for the Ca overload. Thus, verapamil's beneficial effects in shock and ischemia may be due to a stabilization of the sarcoplasmic reticulum with a subsequent decrease in intracellular Ca overload, resulting in improvement of myocardial function and overall survival (39).

In addition to the potential effects of verapamil in stabilizing the sarcoplasmic reticulum, other mechanism(s) by which Ca antagonists improve outcome in hemorrhagic shock may be involved. Some have suggested that the beneficial effects of verapamil are not mediated by calcium channel blockade per se, but rather by unknown metabolic effects that preserve ATP (7). In addition, verapamil's ability to mitigate myocardial and intestinal mucosal injury cannot be overlooked as a possible contributor to the overall increase in survival observed in verapamil-treated animals. The prominent effects of verapamil and other Ca antagonists on peripheral vascular smooth muscle may also play a significant role in improving shock outcome. Ca channel antagonists have a well-documented effect on Ca influx in vascular smooth muscle and are capable of directly producing peripheral and coronary artery vasodilation, reducing left ventricular afterload and improving cardiac output. Others have shown that verapamil inhibits the development of portal hypertension and lowers circulating renin levels (suggesting improved renal perfusion) during the course of hemorrhagic shock (87).

CLINICAL PERSPECTIVES

Calcium Administration

As reviewed in the preceding section, Ca is essential for normal cellular function, yet calcium may also be responsible for cellular injury during ischemia and shock. In this section, we review the clinical uses of calcium and calcium channel antagonists and make recommendations for their appropriate applications.

Calcium administration is known to prevent arrhythmias, to augment the action of Ca-dependent drugs (e.g., digitalis, norepinephrine, glucagon, milrinone), and to improve the signs and symptoms of hypocalcemia in hypocalcemic patients (see Chapter 32). As reviewed previously, Ca is also essential for excitation-contraction coupling in cardiac muscle. Hypocalcemia produces a depression of ventricular function that can be reversed by Ca administration, resulting in improved contractility and cardiac output (20, 22, 23).

Among the other therapeutic uses, Ca has been shown to reverse the cardiotoxic effects of hyperkalemia, hypermagnesemia, calcium channel antagonist overdose, and β-adrenergic antagonist overdose (54, 68, 95). Since these clinical conditions and drugs collectively decrease Ca entry into the myocardium, Ca administration in such situations elevates intracellular calcium concentrations and thus improves contractility. Calcium has also been used to reverse myocardial depression resulting from halothane (61) and nitrous oxide (62) anesthetics, both of which also decrease Ca entry into the heart. In addition, Ca effectively minimizes the hypotension that occurs when verapamil is used in the treatment of supraventricular tachycardias (34).

Patients with longstanding cardiomyopathy develop α- and β-adrenergic receptor downregulation as a result of chronic sympathetic stimulation (9). Under these circumstances, Ca may be an effective inotropic agent (25, 30), even when catecholamines fail to work. Ca has also been used successfully to maintain cardiovascular function in patients awaiting heart transplantation (9, 30) and to maintain cardiac output in patients with nonischemic cardiomyopathies (12).

The list of Ca's therapeutic effects in clinical settings continues to grow. For example, Ca is effective in improving cardiovascular function following cardiopulmonary bypass surgery (3, 14, 20). In these patients, Ca improves cardiac contractility, augments cardiac output, increases systemic vascular resistance, and improves blood pressure. Because of these effects, most centers performing cardiopulmonary bypass surgery add calcium chloride to their pump-priming solutions (14). Similarly, in patients with impaired ventricular function and hypotension undergoing hemodialysis because

Table 48.1
Clinical Uses of Calcium

Beneficial	Possibly Harmful	Harmful
Hypocalcemia	Normocalcemia	Cardiac Arrest?
Hyperkalemia		Sepsis
Hypermagnesemia		Ischemia
Calcium blocker overdose		
β-Blocker overdose		
Nonischemic cardiomyopathy		
After cardiopulmonary bypass		
Rapid blood transfusion		
Rapid albumin infusion		
Halothane, nitrous oxide		
Before heart transplant		
Dialysis		

of renal failure, increasing the Ca concentration in the dialysis bath can improve cardiac contractility and help maintain arterial pressure (36, 50). It has been shown that this effect is not a result of the removal of uremic toxins or correction of acidosis (36) but relates directly to the increase in circulating ionized Ca levels (50).

There are important caveats regarding the administration of Ca. First, the hemodynamic effects of Ca depend upon the endogenous Ca levels at the time of treatment. Thus, although vascular tone increases as Ca is raised from hypocalcemic to hypercalcemic levels (22, 23, 68), the elevation of circulating Ca levels above normal does not further augment cardiac output because increased contractility is offset by the increased afterload produced by Ca (13, 22, 23, 68). For these reasons, Ca infusions into hypocalcemic subjects are predominantly associated with an increase in ventricular function, cardiac output and tissue perfusion (15). On the other hand, Ca infusions initiated in normocalcemic subjects primarily result in an increase in systemic vascular resistance and decreased tissue perfusion (Table 48.1). As a second caveat, one must be cautious when using Ca to maintain cardiac function in patients with ischemic heart disease. In this situation, Ca may increase oxygen consumption in already ischemic tissues, cause vasospasm, and augment ischemic cellular injury and death (Table 48.1) (28, 37).

As mentioned previously, there are many clinical conditions that merit the judicious administration of Ca. When Ca administration is indicated, it should be given as an initial bolus followed by a constant infusion since the cardiovascular effects of a Ca bolus (10–15 mg/kg over 5 minutes) are transient (lasting 10–20 minutes) and frequently associated with a rebound reduction in inotropic activity (60, 68).

The inappropriate administration of Ca can be harmful in the treatment of cardiac arrest, shock, and ischemic disorders. Laboratory studies have shown that Ca increases cellular damage in the brain and heart during anoxia and therefore reduces the chances for successful resuscitation (80). Thus, the high levels of circulating Ca induced by Ca administration are believed to be detrimental, except in situations where Ca may be indicated for the treatment of hypocalcemia, hyperkalemia, hypermagnesemia, or calcium blocker toxicity (75). Ca administration was originally advocated for the treatment of cardiac arrest based on preliminary animal studies and anecdotal reports in humans (80). However, as of yet, clinical studies (both retrospective and prospective double-blind studies) have failed to find any benefit from Ca in the treatment of cardiac arrest associated with ventricular fibrillation, asystole, or electromechanical dissociation (78–80). Recent laboratory findings also suggest that Ca may be detrimental in patients with septic and hemorrhagic shock (see "Specific Effects of Calcium Antagonists in Experimental Models of Shock"). For the many reasons outlined above, Ca administration has been removed from the "Standards and Guidelines for Cardiopulmonary Resuscitation" (75).

Since citrated blood and albumin solutions used in shock resuscitation can produce a hypocalcemic state (by chelating Ca) and thus compromise cardiovascular function (10, 27, 94), Ca administration in these instances would be expected to reverse the hypocalcemia and to improve cardiac contractility and blood pressure. In this clinical situation, measure-

Table 48.2
Actions of Calcium Antagonists on Various Tissues

	Vascular Muscle (Hypotension)	Cardiac Muscle (LV Dysfunction)	Inhibition of Conduction (AV Block)
Verapamil[a−c]	+ +	+ +	+ + +
Nifedipine[a,c]	+ + +	+	
Diltiazem[a]	+	+ +	+

[a] Use for myocardial ischemia.
[b] Use for supraventricular arrhythmias.
[c] Use for hypertension.

ment of free Ca^{2+} levels would be useful in determining whether Ca administration is warranted.

Calcium Antagonist Administration

Ca channel antagonists inhibit the cellular entry of Ca through specific membrane channels and thus prevent a number of Ca-dependent processes, including excitation-contraction coupling in both cardiac and smooth muscle. In addition, Ca antagonists block the entry of Ca into the cells of the sinoatrial and atrioventricular conduction system. Verapamil, nifedipine, and diltiazem are the calcium-channel antagonists approved for human use in the United States. As shown in Table 48.2, these three Ca antagonists differ in their effects and sites of action on target tissues (8, 77), and these differences should be important considerations in choosing Ca antagonists for clinical usage.

Extensive clinical evidence has demonstrated the utility of Ca channel antagonists in the treatment of myocardial ischemia and angina (Table 48.3) (2, 8, 77). These drugs improve myocardial oxygen supply by: 1) increasing coronary blood flow, 2) decreasing myocardial oxygen demand and 3) decreasing peripheral vascular resistance, cardiac contractility, and heart rate (8, 77). Some evidence also suggests that these agents may be of benefit in reducing the size of myocardial infarcts, and in preserving myocardial tissue during open heart surgery and following cardiac arrest (2, 8, 17, 77, 86). However, it must also be remembered that these drugs have the potential of increasing ischemia by reducing blood pressure and coronary perfusion through their vasodilatory actions (e.g., hypotension).

Calcium channel blockers are useful in the treatment of supraventricular cardiac arrhythmias (8). Verapamil, the most potent of the approved drugs, prolongs atrioventricular nodal refractoriness. Verapamil is also useful in slowing ventricular response during supraventricular tachycardias (e.g., paroxysmal supraventricular tachycardia, atrial flutter, atrial fibrillation) and in converting supraventricular arrhythmias to a sinus rhythm. Supraventricular arrhythmias associated with atrial disease, mitral valve prolapse, and digitalis intoxication also respond well to verapamil treatment (8). Despite these therapeutic indications, Ca antagonists are of little value in treating ventricular arrhythmias, except when they result from vasospasm or hypercalcemia (96), and their hypotensive actions may even be harmful under these circumstances.

Table 48.3
Use of Calcium Channel Blockers

Beneficial	Possibly Beneficial	Harmful
Cardiac ischemia	Cerebral ischemia	Ventricular arrhythmias
Supraventricular arrhythmias	After cardiac arrest	Hypotension
Hypertension	After myocardial infarction	
Vasospasm	Cardiac bypass	
Hypercalcemia	Sepsis	
Hypertrophic cardiomyopathy	Hemorrhage	
Heart failure	Seizures	
Pulmonary hypertension		

Since Ca antagonists reduce calcium entry into smooth muscle and cause vasodilation, these drugs are useful in treating hypertension and hypertensive crisis (2, 77). A few scattered reports, as well as our clinical experiences, suggest that Ca antagonists may be useful in reducing pulmonary vascular resistance and improving cardiac output in patients with pulmonary hypertension (2, 59). The systemic vasodilatory actions of these drugs (especially nifedipine) make them particularly useful as afterload reducing agents in patients with left ventricular failure (8). Nifedipine is effective when administered sublingually or orally in the treatment of pulmonary edema associated with hypertension, aortic or mitral regurgitation, and in patients with congestive cardiomyopathy (2, 59, 63). Verapamil and nifedipine also improve cardiac relaxation in patients with hypertrophic cardiomyopathy (8, 77). In addition, nifedipine has been used for the treatment of vasospasm in patients with Raynaud's phenomenon, achalasia, migraine, and subarachnoid hemorrhage (1, 2). Whether Ca antagonists are superior to other vasodilators in the treatment of these disorders is not yet clear. Nonetheless, their capacity to dilate coronary arteries, to reduce myocardial oxygen requirements, to prevent ischemic damage, and to decrease vasospasms make them particularly attractive agents in several clinical situations.

Additionally, Ca antagonists may be of benefit in the treatment of ischemic disorders within the CNS (29, 76, 82, 90). These agents increase cerebral blood flow after experimentally induced CNS ischemic (anoxic) arrest, and several reports contend that cerebral deficits and survival following acute stroke and cardiac arrest may be improved by Ca antagonist administration (29, 76, 82, 90). Current research also suggests that calcium flux into the neuron may be a critical factor in the genesis of seizures since nimodipine has been shown in rabbits to prevent seizures resulting from ischemia or convulsant administration (53). Clinical trials evaluating the use of Ca antagonists in cerebral ischemia and seizure disorders are currently underway.

Although Ca antagonists have been of benefit in a variety of experimental models of circulatory shock (e.g., endotoxic, septic, and hemorrhagic shock), these data are preliminary and further animal studies are needed before these agents can be recommended for the clinical treatment of shock.

SUMMARY

Calcium is essential for normal cellular metabolic function. However, hypercalcemia is toxic, resulting in adverse hemodynamic changes, a disruption of cellular membranes, free radical generation, depletion of energy stores and activation of destructive enzyme systems. These harmful effects of Ca are most remarkable during low perfusion states typically seen during shock, and the use of Ca is contraindicated in these circumstances. Based upon the basic and clinical evidence reviewed in this chapter, we have made a variety of recommendations for the judicious clinical use of Ca. The effects of administered Ca depend upon whether the patient is hypocalcemic or normocalcemic, as measured by free Ca^{2+} concentrations. However, Ca administration is specifically contraindicated in patients with known ischemic disorders or shock. Conversely, several clinical situations in which excessive intracellular Ca is etiologically involved may be successfully treated with calcium antagonists, including ischemic disorders and circulatory shock. In these patients, future research may indicate that the use of Ca antagonists may be beneficial.

References

1. Allen GS, Ahn HS, Preziosi TJ, et al: Cerebral arterial spasm—a controlled trial of nimodipine in patients with subarachnoid hemorrhage. N Engl J Med 308:619–624, 1983.
2. Anonymous: Nifedipine in myocardial ischemia, systemic hypertension, and other cardiovascular disorders. Ann Intern Med 105:714–729, 1986.
3. Auffant RA, Downe JB, Amick R: Ionized calcium concentration and cardiovascular function after cardiopulmonary bypass. Arch Surg 116:1072–1076, 1981.
4. Bosson S, Kuenzig M, Schwartz SI: Verapamil improves cardiac function and increases survival in canine E. coli endotoxin shock. Circ Shock 16:307–316, 1985.
5. Bosson S, Haglund U: Effects of nifedipine in feline septic shock. Circ Shock 19:125, 1986.
6. Bosson S, Kuenzig M, Schwartz SI: Increased survival with calcium antagonists in antibiotic-treated bacteremia. Circ Shock 19:69–74, 1986.
7. Bourdillon PD, Poole-Wilson PA: The effects of verapamil, quiescence, and cardioplegia on calcium exchange and mechanical function in ischemic rabbit myocardium. Circ Res 50:360–368, 1982.
8. Braunwald E: Mechanism of action of calcium-channel blocking agents. N Engl J Med 307:1618–1626, 1982.
9. Bristow MR, Ginsburg R, Minobe W, et al: Decreased catecholamine sensitivity and beta-adrenergic receptor density in failing human hearts. N Engl J Med 307:205–211, 1982.
10. Bunker JP, Bendixen HH, Murphy AJ: Hemodynamic effects of intravenously administered sodium citrate. N Engl J Med 266:372–382, 1962.

11. Burke TJ, Arnold PE, Gordon JA, et al: Protective effect of intrarenal calcium membrane blockers before or after renal ischemia. *J Clin Invest* 74:1830–1841, 1984.
12. Carafoli E, Crampton M: Calcium ions and mitochondria. *Symp Soc Exp Biol* 30:89–115, 1976.
13. Carlon GC, Howland WS, Kahn RC, et al: Calcium chloride administration in normocalcemic critically ill patients. *Crit Care Med* 8:209–212, 1980.
14. Catinella FP, Cunningham JN, Strauss ED, et al: Variations in total and ionized calcium during cardiac surgery. *J Cardiovasc Surg* 24:593–602, 1983.
15. Chamdy B, Bell PD, Navar LG: Renal hemodynamic and autoregulatory responses to acute hypercalcemia. *Am J Physiol* 232:F490–F496, 1977.
16. Cheung JY, Bonventre JV, Malis CP, et al: Calcium and ischemic injury. *N Engl J Med* 314:1670–1676, 1986.
17. Clark RE, Christlieb IY, Henry PD, et al: A myocardial protective agent. *Am J Cardiol* 44:825, 1979.
18. Cohen CJ, Janis RA, Taylor DG, et al: Where do calcium antagonists act? In Opie LH (ed): *Calcium Antagonist and Cardiovascular Disease*. New York, Raven Press, 1984, pp 271–282.
19. Colson JJ: The pathology of sepsis, septic shock and multiple organ failure. In Sibbald WJ, Sprung CL (eds): *Prospectives on Sepsis and Septic Shock*. Fullerton CA, Society of Critical Care Medicine, 1986, pp 27–59.
20. Connor TB, Rosen BL, Blaustein MP, et al: Hypocalcemia precipitating congestive heart failure. *N Engl J Med* 307:869–872, 1982.
21. d'Hollander A, Primo G, Hennart D, et al: Compared efficacy of dobutamine and dopamine in association with calcium chloride on termination of cardiopulmonary bypass. *J Thorac Cardiovasc Surg* 83:264–271, 1982.
22. Drop LJ, Geffin GA, O'Keefe DD, et al: Left ventricular performance during sustained hypo- and hypercalcemia. *Surg Forum* 29:259–261, 1978.
23. Drop LJ, Scheidigger D: Plasma ionized calcium concentration: important determinant of the hemodynamic response to calcium infusion. *J Thoracic Cardiovasc Surg* 79:425–432, 1980.
24. Duncan CJ, Smith JL: The effect of the ionophore A23187 on the ultrastructure and electrophysiological properties of frog skeletal muscle. *Cell Tissue Res* 173:193–209, 1976.
25. Eriksen C, Sorensen MB, Bille-Brahe NE, et al: Hemodynamic effects of calcium chloride administered intravenously to patients with and without cardiac disease during neuroleptic anesthesia. *Acta Anesthesiol Scand* 27:13–17, 1983.
26. Faden AI, Jacobs TP, Smith T: Evaluation of the calcium channel antagonist nimodipine in experimental spinal cord ischemia. *J Neurosurg* 60:796–799, 1984.
27. Gain EA: The problem of cardiac collapse associated with the massive transfusion of citrated blood. *Can Anesth Soc J* 9:207–219, 1962.
28. Gefin GA, Drop LJ, O'Keefe DD, et al: Global and regional function in the regionally ischemic left ventricle related to plasma ionized calcium. *Cardiovasc Res* 17:415–426, 1983.
29. Gelmers HJ: Calcium-channel blockers: effects on cerebral blood flow and potential uses in acute stroke. *Am J Cardiol* 55(Suppl):144B–148B, 1985.
30. Ginsburg R, Esserman LJ, Bristow MR, et al: Myocardial performance and extracellular ionized calcium in a severely failing heart. *Ann Intern Med* 98:603–606, 1983.
31. Godfraind T, Miller R, Wibo M: Calcium antagonism and calcium entry blockade. *Pharmacol Rev* 38:321–416, 1986.
32. Hackel DB, Mikat EM, Whalen G, et al: Treatment of hemorrhagic shock in dogs with verapamil. *Lab Invest* 41:356–359, 1979.
33. Hackel DB, Mikat EM, Whalen G: Effects of verapamil

on heart and circulation in hemorrhagic shock in dogs. *Am J Physiol* 241:H12–H17, 1981.
34. Haft JI, Halbab, MA: Treatment of atrial arrhythmias—effectiveness of verapamil when preceded by calcium infusion. *Arch Intern Med* 146:1085–1089, 1986.
35. Hale DJ, Robinson JA, Loeb HS, et al: Pathophysiology of endotoxin shock in man. In Proctor RA: *Handbook of Endotoxin, vol 4, Clinical Aspects of Endotoxin Shock*. Amsterdam, Elsevier Sciece Publishers, 1986, pp 1–15.
36. Henrich WL, Hunt JM, Nixon JV, et al: Increased ionized calcium and left ventricular contractility during hemodialysis. *N Engl J Med* 310:19–23, 1984.
37. Henry PD, Schuchleib R, David J, et al: Myocardial contracture and accumulation of mitochondrial calcium in ischemic rabbit heart. *Am J Physiol* 233:H677–H684, 1977.
38. Hess ML, Briggs FN: The effect of Gram-negative endotoxin on the calcium uptake activity of sarcoplasmic reticulum isolated from canine myocardium. *Biochem Biophys Res Commun* 45:917–924, 1971.
39. Hess ML, Greenfield LJ: Calcium entry blockers: potential applications in shock. *Adv Shock Res* 10:15–25, 1983.
40. Hess ML, Mahany TM, Greenfield LJ: Calcium channel blockers in shock. In Lefer AM, Schumer W: *Molecular and Cellular Aspects of Shock and Trauma*. New York, Alan R Liss, 1983, pp 271–282.
41. Hess ML, Warner MF, Smith JM, et al: Improved myocardial hemodynamic and cellular function with calcium channel blockade (verapamil) during canine hemorrhagic shock. *Circ Shock* 10:119–130, 1983.
42. Hoffmuster F, Kazda S, Krause HP: Influence of nimodipine on the postischemic changes of brain function. *Acta Neurol Scand* 60(Suppl 72):58, 1979.
43. Hulsmann WC, Lamers JMJ, Stam H, Breenan WAP: Calcium overload in endotoxemia. *Life Sci* 29:1009–1014, 1981.
44. Katz AM, Reuter H: Cellular calcium and cardiac cell death. *Am J Cardiol* 44:188–190, 1979.
45. Kreger BE, Craven DE, McCabe WR: Gram-negative bactermia—re-evaluation of clinical features and treatment of 612 patients. *Am J Med* 68:344, 1980.
46. Lee HC, Lum BKB: Protective action of calcium entry blockers in endotoxin shock. *Circ Shock* 18:193–203, 1986.
47. Lehninger AL: Mitochondria and calcium transport. *Biochem J* 119:129–138, 1970.
48. Malcolm D, Zaloga G, Chernow B, et al: Calcium involvement in endotoxic shock: verapamil improves hemodynamics and survival in rats. *Circ Shock* 18:346, 1986.
49. Malis DC, Cheung JY, Leaf A, et al: Effects of verapamil in models of ischemic acute renal failure in the rat. *Am J Physiol* 245:F735–F742, 1983.
50. Maynard JC, Cruz C, Kleerekoper M, et al.: Blood pressure response to changes in serum ionized calcium during hemodialysis. *Ann Intern Med* 104:358–361, 1986.
51. McCabe WR: Gram-negative bacteremia. *Adv Intern Med* 19:135–158, 1974.
52. Mela L, Bacalzo LV, Miller LD: Defective oxidative metabolism of rat liver mitochondria in hemorrhagic and endotoxic shock. *Am J Physiol* 220:571–577, 1971.
53. Meyer FB, Anderson RE, Sundt TM, et al: Selective central nervous system calcium channel blockers—a new clan of anticonvulsant agents. *Mayo Clin Proc* 61:239–247, 1986.
54. Morris DL, Goldschlager N: Calcium infusions for reversal of adverse effects of intravenous verapamil. *JAMA* 249:3212–3213, 1983.
55. National Center of Health Statistics: Advance report, final mortality statistics. In *Monthly Vital Statistics Report* 33(3):(Suppl):DHHS (PHS)84–1120, 1981.

56. Nayler WG, Poole-Wilson PA, Williams A: Hypoxia and calcium. *J Molec Cell Cardiol* 11f:683–706, 1979.

57. Nayler WG, Ferrari R, Williams A: Protective effect of pretreatment with verapamil, nifedipine, and propanolol on mitochondrial function in the ischemic and reperfused myocardium. *Am J Cardiol* 46:242–248, 1980.

58. Okuno F, Orrego H, Israel Y: Calcium requirements for anoxic liver injury. *Res Commun Chem Pathol Pharmacol* 39:437–444, 1983.

59. Olivari MT, Levine TB, Weir EK, et al: Hemodynamic effects of nifedipine at rest and during exercise in primary pulmonary hypertension. *Chest* 86:14–19, 1984.

60. Porter DL, Ledgewood AM, Lucas CE, et al.: Effect of calcium infusion on heart function. *Am Surgeon* 49:369–372, 1983.

61. Price HL: Calcium reverses myocardial depression caused by halothane: site of action. *Anesthesiology* 41:576–579, 1974.

62. Price HL: Myocardial depression by nitrous oxide and its reversal by Ca^{++}. *Anesthesiology* 44:211–215, 1976.

63. Proceedings of a Symposium on Calcium Channel Blockers: A new dimension in antihypertensive therapy. *Am J Med* 77(2B):1–45, 1984.

64. Publicover SJ, Duncan CJ, Smith JL: The use of A23187 to demonstrate the role of intracellular calcium in causing ultrastructural damage in mammalian muscle. *J Neuropathol Exp Neurol* 37:544–557, 1978.

65. Reimer KA, Lowe JE, Jennings RB: Effect of the calcium antagonist verapamil on necrosis following temporary coronary artery occlusion in dogs. *Circulation* 55:581–587, 1977.

66. Sakaguchi S, Abe H, Sakaguchi O: Calcium behavior in endotoxin poisoned mice: especially calcium accumulation in mitochondria. *Microbiol Immunol* 28:517–527, 1984.

67. Schanne FAX, Kane AB, Young EE, et al: Calcium dependent toxic cell death: a final common pathway. *Science* 206:700–702, 1979.

68. Scheidigger D, Drop LJ: Calcium ion concentration and beta-adrenergic activity. *J Thorac Cardiovasc Surg* 80:441–446, 1980.

69. Sherman LG, Liang CS, Boden WE, et al: The effect of verapamil on mechanical performance of acutely ischemic and reperfused myocardium in the conscious dog. *Circ Res* 48:224–232, 1981.

70. Smith HJ, Singh BN, Nisbet HD, et al: Effects of verapamil on infarct size following experimental coronary occlusion. *Cardiovasc Res* 9:569, 1975.

71. Soulsby ME, Ford GD, Davis JA, et al: The effect of Gram-negative endotoxin on calcium accumulation by subcellular fractions of vascular smooth muscle. *Circ Shock* 3:325–335, 1976.

72. Soulsby ME, Bruni FD, Looney TJ, et al: Influence of endotoxin on myocardial calcium transport and the effect of augmented venous return. *Circ Shock* 5:23–34, 1978.

73. Soulsby ME, Bennet Cl, Hess ML: Canine arterial calcium transport during endotoxic shock. *Circ Shock* 7:139–148, 1980.

74. Spitzer JA, Deaciuc IV: Effect of endotoxins and sepsis on intracellular calcium homeostasis in rat liver: mitochondrial and microsomal calcium uptake. *Circ Shock* 18:81–93, 1986.

75. Standards and guidelines of cardiopulmonary resuscitation (CPR) and emergency cardiac care (ECC). *JAMA* 255:2905–2984, 1986.

76. Steen PA, Newberg LA, Milde JH, et al: Nimodipine improves cerebral blood flow and neurologic recovery after complete ischemia in the dog. *J Cereb Blood Flow Metab* 3:38–43, 1983.

77. Stone PH, Ontman EM, Muller JE, et al: Calcium channel blocking agents in the treatment of cardiovascular disorders. Part II: Hemodynamic effects and clinical applications. *Ann Intern Med* 93:886–904, 1980.

78. Stueren HA, Thompson BM, Aprahamian C, et al: Use of calcium in prehospital cardiac arrest. *Ann Emerg Med* 12:136, 1983.

79. Stureren HA, Thompson BM, Aprahamian C, et al: Calcium chloride: reassessment of use in asystole. *Ann Emerg Med* 9:820, 1984.

80. Thompson BM, Steuven HS, Tonsfeldt DJ, et al: Calcium: limited indications, some danger. *Circulation* 74(Suppl IV):90–93, 1986.

81. Urthaler F: Review: role of calcium channel blockers in clinical medicine. *Am J Med Sci* 29:217–230, 1986.

82. Vaagenes P, Cantadore R, Safar P, et al: Effect of lidoflazine on neurologic outcome after cardiac arrest in dogs. *Anesthesiology* 59:100, 1983.

83. Villabobo A, Lehninger Al: Inhibition of oxidative phosphorylation in ascites tumor mitochondria and cells by intramitochondrial calcium. *J Biol Chem* 255:2457–2464, 1980.

84. Wait RB, White G, Davis JH: Beneficial effects of verapamil on postischemic renal failure. *Surgery* 94:276–282, 1983.

85. Watts JA, Koch CD, Lanoue KF: Effects of calcium antagonism on energy metabolism: calcium and heart failure after ischemia. *Am J Physiol* 238:H909–H916, 1980.

86. Weaver WD: Calcium-channel blockers and advanced cardiac life support. *Circulation* 74(Suppl IV):94–97, 1986.

87. Whalen GF, Hackel DB, Mikat E: Prevention of portal hypertension and small bowel hemorrhage in dogs treated with verapamil during hemorrhagic shock. *Circ Shock* 70:399–404, 1980.

88. White BC, Gadzinski DS, Hoehmer PJ, et al: Correction of canine cerebral cortical blood flow and vascular resistance after cardiac arrest using flunarizine, a calcium antagonist. *Ann Emerg Med* 11:118, 1982.

89. White BC, Winegar CD, Wilson RF, et al: Possible role of calcium blockers in cerebral resuscitation: a review of the literature and synthesis for future studies. *Crit Care Med* 11:202–207, 1983.

90. White BC, Winegar DC, Wilson RF, et al: Calcium blockers in cerebral resuscitation. *J Trauma* 23:788–793, 1983.

91. Wiernsperger N, Gypax, P, Hofmann A: Calcium antagonist PY 108-068: demonstration of its efficacy in various types of experimental brain ischemia. *Stroke* 15:679–685, 1984.

92. Willey S, Zaloga G, Malcolm D, et al: Calcium inhibits epinephrine's hypertensive effects and increases mortality in normal and endotoxic rats. *Clin Res* 34:868A, 1986.

93. Winegar CD, Henderson O, White BC, et al: Early amelioration of neurologic deficit by lidoflazine after fifteen minutes of cardiopulmonary arrest in dogs. *Ann Neurol Med* 12:471–477, 1983.

94. Zaloga GP, Chernow B: Hypocalcemia in critical illness. *JAMA* 256:1924–1929, 1986.

95. Zaloga GP, Chernow B: Life-threatening electrolyte and metabolic abnormalities. In Parrillo JE: *Current Therapy in Critical Care Medicine*. Toronto, BC Decker, 1987, pp 245–257.

96. Zaloga GP, Malcolm DS, Holaday JW, et al: Verapamil reverses calcium cardiotoxicity. *Ann Emerg Med* 16:637–639, 1987.

Index

Index

A

Abnormalities
  metabolic, and constipation, 335
ABO (see also blood), 256
  compatibility, 265
Absorption, drug, 3, 7–10
  and lag time for, 8
  extent of bioavailability of, 8–10
  drug interactions with, 24
  pediatric, differences, 141–143
Acanthosis nigricans
  and insulin resistance, 639
ACE (see angiotensin-converting enzyme)
Acebutolol, 413 (see beta blockers)
  dosage of, 413
  half-life of, 413
  in antihypertensive therapies, 413
  in hypertension, 365, 368, 369, 370
  in renal failure, 61
  pharmacokinetics of, 413
  receptor selectivity of, 413
Acellular oxygen carriers (see red cell substitutes)
Acetaminophen, 267 (see acetaminophen overdose), 749
  alterations of, in liver failure, 99
  alterations of, in renal failure, 99
  and transfusions, 267
  and warfarin, 529
  characterization of, in liver elimination, 92
  half-life of, in renal failure, 57, 59
  hepatic damage, cause of, 96
  interaction with cimetidine, 33
  interaction with oral contraceptives, 29
  metabolism of, 59

pediatric, adverse effect of, 133
pediatric, rectal administration, 141
pharmacokinetics of, 99
psychiatric side effect of, 493
ranitidine, interaction with, 329
metoclopramide, interaction with, 333
Acetaminophen overdose, 33, 59, 749–751
  acetylcysteine for, 749
  activated charcoal for, 748
  clinical manifestations of, 749
  frequency of, 749
  metabolism of, 749
  therapeutic nomogram for, 750
  treatment of, 59, 749
Acetate
  compatibility with other intravenous medications, 160
Acetazolamide, 126, 303, 815 (see diuretics)
  and hyperphosphatemia, 633
  and thrombocytopenia, 518
  dosage, 815
  for metabolic alkalosis, 815
  in renal failure, 62, 303
  intracranial hypertension and, 212
  kidney secretion of, 34
  side effects, 304
Acetoacetate
  and renal phosphate handling, 627
  norepinephrine, effect on, 590
Acetohexamide, 654
  dose, 654
  in renal failure, 63
Acetylators
  fast/slow, 92
Acetylcholine, 248
  receptors, in respiratory system, 436
Acetylcholinesterase, 124
  pediatric, organophosphate, 885

Acetylcysteine (see N-acetylcysteine)
N-Acetylcysteine, 134
  cyclophosphamide, combination, 538
  for acetaminophen overdose, 59
  treatment, 134
Acetylsalicylic acid (see also aspirin and salicylates)
  hepatic damage from, 96
  effect on insulin, 637
N-Acetyltransferase
  activity, pediatric, 145
Achalasia, 665
  and glucagon, 665
Achlorhydria
  in hypocalcemia, 613
Acid-base disorders, 803, 839
Acidemia
  and hypophosphatemia, 628, 630
Acidification of urine
  for amphetamine overdose, 749
  for fenfluramine overdose, 749
  for phencyclidine overdose, 749
  for quinidine overdose, 749
  for quinine overdose, 749
  use of ammonium chloride for, 749
Acidosis, 113 (see metabolic acidosis)
  and hyperphosphatemia, 632
  and hypophosphatemia, 628
  and hyperkalemia, 810
  and pulmonary failure, 113, 116
  effect on calcium, 603
  from iron overload, 768
  from isopropanol overdose, 760
  from phenformin, 49
  from nitroprusside, 73
  from salicylate poisioning, 751
  from theophylline poisoning, 756
  in status epilepticus, 471